✦ PRIORITY CONCEPT EXEMPLARS

ACID-BASE BALANCE

Acidosis, 190

CELLULAR REGULATION

Breast Cancer, 1440
Cirrhosis, 1169
Colorectal Cancer, 1126
Head and Neck Cancer, 547
Hypothyroidism, 1270
Osteoporosis, 1015
Prostate Cancer, 1481

CLOTTING

Venous Thromboembolism, 742

COGNITION

Alzheimer's Disease, 857
Traumatic Brain Injury, 940

COMFORT

End of Life, 104
Pain, 45

ELIMINATION

Benign Prostatic Hyperplasia, 1474
Chronic Kidney Disease, 1398
Intestinal Obstruction, 1121
Pyelonephritis, 1372
Ulcerative Colitis, 1150
Urinary Incontinence, 1343

FLUID AND ELECTROLYTE BALANCE

Dehydration, 167
Hypercortisolism (Cushing's Disease), 1255

GAS EXCHANGE

Chronic Obstructive Pulmonary Disease, 572
Pneumonia, 598
Pulmonary Embolism, 616
Tracheostomy, 537

GLUCOSE REGULATION

Diabetes Mellitus, 1280

IMMUNITY

Acute Pancreatitis, 1197
Angioedema, 361
Guillain-Barré Syndrome, 912
Hepatitis, 1180
HIV Infection and AIDS, 337
Infection, 413
Leukemia, 817
Multiple Sclerosis, 888
Peptic Ulcer Disease (PUD), 1107
Peritonitis, 1144
Pulmonary Tuberculosis, 605
Rheumatoid Arthritis, 318
Sepsis and Septic Shock, 760

MOBILITY

Fractures, 1032
Osteoarthritis, 305
Parkinson Disease, 868
Spinal Cord Injury, 894

NUTRITION

Cholecystitis, 1191
Esophageal Tumors, 1095
Gastroesophageal Reflux Disease (GERD), 1087
Malnutrition, 1215
Obesity, 1225

PERFUSION

Acute Coronary Syndrome, 769
Amputations, 1050
Atrial Fibrillation, 678
Heart Failure, 691
Hypertension, 720
Hypovolemic Shock, 754
Sickle Cell Disease, 808
Stroke (Brain Attack), 928

SENSORY PERCEPTION

Cataract, 968
Glaucoma, 972
Hearing Loss, 996
Otitis Media, 991

SEXUALITY

Pelvic Inflammatory Disease, 1514
Uterine Leiomyoma, 1459

TISSUE INTEGRITY

Pressure Injuries, 447
Stomatitis, 1076

PRIORITY CONCEPT EXEMPLARS

ACID-BASE BALANCE
Acidosis, 190

CELLULAR REGULATION
Breast Cancer, 1240
Cirrhosis, 1159
Colorectal Cancer, 1126
Head and Neck Cancer, 512
Thrombocytopenia, 1270
Care-priorities, 1073
Prostate Cancer, 1441

CLOTTING
Venous Thromboembolism, 746

COGNITION
Alzheimer's Disease, 857
Traumatic Brain Injury, 940

COMFORT
End of Life, 104
Pain, 43

ELIMINATION
Benign Prostatic Hyperplasia, 1424
Chronic Kidney Disease, 1368
Intestinal Obstruction, 1131
Pyelonephritis, 1392
Ulcerative Colitis, 1147
Urinary Incontinence, 1442

FLUID AND ELECTROLYTE BALANCE
Dehydration, 165
Hypovolemia (Volume Deficit), 1236

GAS EXCHANGE
Chronic Obstructive Pulmonary Disease, 622
Pneumonia, 594
Pulmonary Embolism, 616
Tracheostomy, 537

GLUCOSE REGULATION
Diabetes Mellitus, 1296

IMMUNITY
Acute Pancreatitis, 1197
Appendicitis, 36
Guillain-Barre Syndrome, 912
Hepatitis, 1180
HIV Infection and AIDS, 37
Infection, 415
Leukemia, 817
Multiple Sclerosis, 888
Peptic Ulcer Disease (PUD), 1107
Peritonitis, 1134
Pulmonary Tuberculosis, 603
Rheumatoid Arthritis, 318
Sepsis and Septic Shock, 7

MOBILITY
Fractures, 1053
Osteoarthritis, 305
Parkinson Disease, 868
Spinal Cord Injury, 901

NUTRITION
Dehydration, 1191
Esophageal Tumors, 1095
Gastroesophageal Reflux Disease (GERD), 1089
Malnutrition, 1256
Obesity, 1272

PERFUSION
Acute Coronary Syndrome, 760
Amputations, 1026
Atrial Fibrillation, 675
Heart Failure, 691
Hypertension, 720
Hypovolemic Shock, 751
Sickle Cell Disease, 804
Stroke (Brain Attack), 934

SENSORY PERCEPTION
Cataract, 968
Glaucoma, 972
Hearing Loss, 996
Otitis Media, 991

SEXUALITY
Pelvic Inflammatory Disease, 1514
Uterine Leiomyoma, 1489

TISSUE INTEGRITY
Pressure Injuries, 447
Skin Infection, 1570

9th EDITION

Medical-Surgical Nursing

CONCEPTS FOR INTERPROFESSIONAL COLLABORATIVE CARE

Donna D. Ignatavicius, MS, RN, CNE, ANEF
Speaker and Curriculum Consultant for Academic Nursing
 Programs;
Founder, Boot Camp for Nurse Educators;
President, DI Associates, Inc.
Littleton, Colorado

M. Linda Workman, PhD, RN, FAAN
Author and Consultant
Cincinnati, Ohio

Cherie R. Rebar, PhD, MBA, RN, COI
Professor of Nursing
Wittenberg University
Springfield, Ohio

Section Editor:
Nicole M. Heimgartner, MSN, RN, COI
Former Associate Professor of Nursing
Kettering College;
Subject Matter Expert, Author, and Consultant
Louisville, Kentucky

ELSEVIER

ELSEVIER

3251 Riverport Lane
St. Louis, Missouri 63043

MEDICAL-SURGICAL NURSING:
CONCEPTS FOR INTERPROFESSIONAL
COLLABORATIVE CARE, NINTH EDITION

ISBN (single volume): 978-0-323-44419-4
ISBN (2-volume set): 978-0-323-46158-0

Copyright © 2018 by Elsevier Inc. All rights reserved.

No part of this publication may be reproduced or transmitted in any form or by any means, electronic or mechanical, including photocopying, recording, or any information storage and retrieval system, without permission in writing from the publisher. Details on how to seek permission, further information about the Publisher's permissions policies and our arrangements with organizations such as the Copyright Clearance Center and the Copyright Licensing Agency, can be found at our website: www.elsevier.com/permissions.

This book and the individual contributions contained in it are protected under copyright by the Publisher (other than as may be noted herein).

Notices

Practitioners and researchers must always rely on their own experience and knowledge in evaluating and using any information, methods, compounds or experiments described herein. Because of rapid advances in the medical sciences, in particular, independent verification of diagnoses and drug dosages should be made. To the fullest extent of the law, no responsibility is assumed by Elsevier, authors, editors or contributors for any injury and/or damage to persons or property as a matter of products liability, negligence or otherwise, or from any use or operation of any methods, products, instructions, or ideas contained in the material herein.

Previous editions copyrighted 2016, 2013, 2010, 2006, 2002, 1999, 1995, 1991

International Standard Book Number (single volume): 978-0-323-44419-4
International Standard Book Number (2-volume set): 978-0-323-46158-0

Executive Content Strategist: Lee Henderson
Senior Content Development Manager: Laurie Gower
Senior Content Development Specialist: Laura Goodrich
Publishing Services Manager: Jeff Patterson
Senior Project Manager: Jodi M. Willard
Design Direction: Brian Salisbury

Printed in Canada

Last digit is the print number: 9   8   7   6   5   4

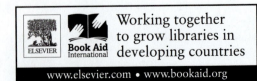

CONSULTANTS AND CONTRIBUTORS

CONSULTANTS

Deanne A. Blach, MSN, RN
President
DB Productions of NW AR, Inc.
Green Forest, Arkansas

Richard Lintner, RT (R), (CV), (MR), (CT)
Program Director, School of Interventional
  Radiology
The University of Kansas Health System
Kansas City, Kansas

CONTRIBUTORS

**Jeanette Spain Adams, PhD, RN, CRNI,
  ACNS, BC**
Consultant
University of Phoenix
Coconut Grove, Florida

Meg Blair, PhD, MSN, RN, CEN
Professor
Nursing Division
Nebraska Methodist College
Omaha, Nebraska

Andrea A. Borchers, PhD, RN
Assistant Professor
Northern Arizona University
Flagstaff, Arizona

Samuel A. Borchers, OD
Optometrist
Vision Clinic
Northern Arizona VA Healthcare System
Prescott, Arizona

Katherine L. Byar, MSN, APN, BC, BMTCN®
Nurse Practitioner
Nebraska Medicine
Omaha, Nebraska

**Michelle Camicia, PhD(c), MSN, CRRN,
  CCM, FAHA**
Director of Operations
Kaiser Foundation Rehabilitation Center
Kaiser Permanente
Vallejo, California;
PhD Candidate
The Betty Irene Moore School of Nursing
University of California, Davis
Davis, California

Lara Carver, PhD, RN, CNE
Professor
Department of Nursing
National University
Las Vegas, Nevada

Tammy Coffee, MSN, RN, ACNP
Nurse
MetroHealth Medical Center
Cleveland, Ohio

Keelin Cromar, MSN, RN
Adjunct Faculty
Mississippi Gulf Coast Community College
Perkinston, Mississippi

Janice Cuzzell, MSN, RN, CWS
Corstrata, Inc.
Savannah, Georgia

Cynthia Danko, DNP, RN
Instructor
Frances Payne Bolton School of Nursing
Case Western Reserve University
Cleveland, Ohio

**Laura M. Dechant, DNP, APRN, CCRN,
  CCNS**
Adjunct Clinical Instructor
School of Nursing
Widener University
Chester, Pennsylvania;
Clinical Nurse Specialist
Heart, Vascular and Interventional Services
Christiana Care Health System
Newark, Delaware

Stephanie M. Fox, PsyD
Clinical Psychologist
Littleton, Colorado

**Roberta Goff, MSN-Ed, RN-BC, ACNS-BC,
  ONC**
Senior Clinical Analyst
Information Systems
Munson Medical Center
Traverse City, Michigan

Saundra Hendricks, FNP, BC-ADM
Nurse Practitioner
Houston Methodist Hospital
Houston, Texas

Amy Jauch, MSN, RN
Clinical Instructor of Practice
College of Nursing
The Ohio State University
Columbus, Ohio

Gail B. Johnson, MSN, RN, AOCN, CNS
CNS, Midlevel Provider
Division of Surgical Oncology
UC/UCP—University of Cincinnati/
  University of Cincinnati Physicians, Inc.
UCMC—Barrett Cancer Center
Cincinnati, Ohio

Mary K. Kazanowski, PhD, APRN, ACHPN
Palliative Care Nurse Practitioner
Elliot Hospital;
VNA Hospice of Manchester and Southern
  New Hampshire
Manchester, New Hampshire

Harriet Kumar, MSN, ANP-BC
Nurse Practitioner
Division of Hematology/Oncology and Bone
  Marrow Transplantation
University of Cincinnati College of Medicine
Cincinnati, Ohio

**Linda Laskowski-Jones, MS, APRN,
  ACNS-BC, CEN, FAWM, FAAN**
Vice President Emergency & Trauma
  Services
Christiana Care Health System
Wilmington, Delaware

Kristin Oneail, MSN, RN
OK! Nurse Consultants
Walbridge, Ohio

Rebecca M. Patton, DNP, RN, CNOR, FAAN
Atkinson Scholar in Perioperative Nursing
Frances Payne Bolton School of Nursing
Case Western Reserve University
Cleveland, Ohio

Julie Ponto, PhD, APRN, CNS, AGCNS-BC, AOCNS®
Professor, Graduate Programs in Nursing
Winona State University—Rochester
Rochester, Minnesota

Jennifer Powers, MSN, RN, FNP-BC
Adjunct Faculty
Department of Nursing
National University
Henderson, Nevada

Harry Rees III, MSN, ACNP-BC
Acute Care Nurse Practitioner
Surgical Intensive Care
Ohio State University Wexner Medical
   Center
Columbus, Ohio

James G. Sampson, DNP, NP-C
Adjunct Assistant Professor
College of Nursing
University of Colorado
Aurora, Colorado;
Clinical Supervisor, Adult Nurse Practitioner
Department of Internal Medicine
Denver Health Medical Center
Denver, Colorado

Melanie H. Simpson, PhD, RN-BC, OCN, CHPN, CPE
Pain Team Coordinator
Department of Nursing
The University of Kansas Health System
Kansas City, Kansas

Tracy Taylor, MSN, RN
Clinical Instructor of Practice
College of Nursing
The Ohio State University
Columbus, Ohio

Karen L. Toulson, MSN, MBA, RN, CEN, NE-BC
Director, Emergency Department Clinical
   Operations
Christiana Care Health System
Newark, Delaware

Kathy Vanderbeck, ARNP, OCNS-C®, CNRN
Joint Center Program Coordinator
Baptist Health
Jacksonville, Florida

Constance G. Visovsky, PhD, RN, ACNP-BC
Associate Dean, Faculty Affairs &
   Partnerships
Director of Diversity
Associate Professor, School of Nursing
University of South Florida
Tampa, Florida

Laura M. Willis, DNP, APRN, FNP-C
Family Nurse Practitioner
Urbana Family Medicine and Pediatrics
Urbana, Ohio

Chris Winkelman, PhD, RN, CNS, CCRN, ACNP, FAANP, FCCM
Associate Professor
Frances Payne Bolton School of Nursing
Case Western Reserve Univesrity;
Clinical Support
Trauma/Critical Care Nursing
MetroHealth Medical Center
Cleveland, Ohio

CONTRIBUTORS TO TEACHING/LEARNING RESOURCES

PowerPoint Slides

Nicole M. Heimgartner, MSN, RN, COI
Former Associate Professor of Nursing
Kettering College;
Subject Matter Expert, Author, and Consultant
Louisville, Kentucky

Cherie R. Rebar, PhD, MBA, RN, COI
Professor of Nursing
Wittenberg University
Springfield, Ohio

TEACH for Nurses Lesson Plans

Carolyn Gersch, PhD, MSN, RN, CNE
Director of Nursing Education
Ohio Institute of Allied Health
Dayton, Ohio

Nicole M. Heimgartner, MSN, RN, COI
Former Associate Professor of Nursing
Kettering College;
Subject Matter Expert, Author, and Consultant
Louisville, Kentucky

Cherie R. Rebar, PhD, MBA, RN, COI
Professor of Nursing
Wittenberg University
Springfield, Ohio

Test Bank

Meg Blair, PhD, MSN, RN, CEN
Professor
Nursing Division
Nebraska Methodist College
Omaha, Nebraska

Tami Kathleen Little, RN, DNP, CNE
Dean of Nursing
Brookline College
Albuquerque, New Mexico

Marla Kniewel, EdD, MSN, RN
Associate Professor
Nursing Division
Nebraska Methodist College
Omaha, Nebraska

Case Studies

Candice Kumagai, MSN, RN
Former Clinical Instructor
University of Texas at Austin
Austin, Texas

Linda A. LaCharity, PhD, MN, BSN, RN
Adjunct Faculty
Former Accelerated Program Director and
   Assistant Professor
College of Nursing
University of Cincinnati
Cincinnati, Ohio

Concept Maps

Deanne A. Blach, MSN, RN
President, Nursing Education
DB Productions of NW AR, Inc.
Green Forest, Arkansas

Key Points

Deanne A. Blach, MSN, RN
President, Nursing Education
DB Productions of NW AR, Inc.
Green Forest, Arkansas

Review Questions for the NCLEX Examination

Lisa A. Hollett, MA, BSN, RN, MICN,
Certified Forensic Nurse
Stroke Coordinator
Hillcrest Medical Center
Tulsa, Oklahoma

Andrea R. Mann, MSN, RN, CNE
Interim Dean, Third Level Chair
Aria Health School of Nursing
Trevose, Pennsylvania

Molly McClelland, PhD, MSN, BSN,
ACNS-BC, CMSRN
Associate Professor
College of Health Professions
University of Detroit Mercy
Detroit, Michigan

Tara McMillan-Queen, MSN, BSN, AA,
ANP, GNP
Faculty II, NP
Mercy School of Nursing
Charlotte, North Carolina

Heidi Monroe, MSN
Assistant Professor
Nursing
Bellin College
Green Bay, Wisconsin

Denise Robinson, MS, RN, CNE
Assistant Professor of Nursing
Monroe County Community College
Monroe, Michigan

Kathryn Schartz, MSN, RN, PPCPNP-BC
Assistant Professor of Nursing
School of Nursing
Baker University
Topeka, Kansas

Bethany Sykes, EdD, MSN, BSN, RN, CEN
Emergency Department
St. Luke's Hospital;
CCRN
Critical Care Unit
St. Luke's Hospital
New Bedford, Massachusetts;
Adjunct Faculty
Department of Nursing
Salve Regina University
Newport, Rhode Island;
RN Refresher Course Coordinator
College of Nursing
University of Massachusetts
North Dartmouth, Massachusetts

REVIEWERS

Ramona Bartlow, DNP, MSN, RN
Assistant Professor, Course/Clinical
  Coordinator
Northwestern Oklahoma State University
College of Nursing
Enid, Oklahoma

**Marylee Bressie, DNP, RN, CCNS, CCRN-K,
  CEN**
Core Faculty/MSN Specialization Lead for
  Leadership & Administration
Capella University
School of Nursing & Health Sciences
Department of Nursing
Minneapolis, Minnesota

Ashley Leak Bryant, PhD, RN-BC, OCN
Assistant Professor
The University of North Carolina at Chapel
  Hill
School of Nursing
Chapel Hill, North Carolina

**Margaret-Ann Carno, PhD, MBA, MJ,
  CPNP, ABSM, FAAN**
Professor of Clinical Nursing and Pediatrics
University of Rochester
School of Nursing
Rochester, New York

Mary Cox
Professor
Clemson University
Clemson, South Carolina

**Diane Daddario, ANP-C, ACNS-BC,
  RN-BC, CMSRN**
Hospitalist CRNP in Behavioral Health Unit
Holy Spirit Hospital—A Geisinger Affiliate
Camp Hill, Pennsylvania;
Adjunct Nursing Faculty
Pennsylvania State University
University Park, Pennsylvania

Shirlee Proctor Davidson, MSN, RN
Independent Practitioner and Consultant,
Psychiatric Mental Health Nursing Clinical
  Specialist
Liaison Consultation and Education
Santa Fe, New Mexico

**Laura M. Dechant, APRN, MSN, CCRN,
  CCNS**
Clinical Nurse Specialist
Heart, Vascular and Interventional Services
Christiana Care Health System
Newark, Delaware

**Julie Eggert, NP, PhD, GNP-BC, AGN-BC,
  AOCN, FAAN**
Genetic Risk Consultant
Cancer Risk Screening Program
Bon Secours Hematology & Oncology
Greenville, South Carolina

Selena A. Gilles, DNP, ANP-BC, CCRN
Clinical Assistant Professor
New York University
New York, New York;
Nurse Practitioner
Garden State Pain Management
Clifton, New Jersey

Ruth Gladen, MS, RN
Associate Professor
North Dakota State College of Science
Nursing Department
Wahpeton, North Dakota

Cathy Glennon, RN, MHS, OCN, NE-BC
Director, Brandmeyer Resource Center
University of Kansas Hospital
Cancer Center
Kansas City, Kansas

**Roberta L. Goff, MSN, Ed, RN-BC,
  ACNS-BC, ONC**
Clinical Nurse Specialist
Orthopedics
Munson Medical Center
Traverse City, Michigan

Kathleen Griffith, MSN, RN
Full-Time Lecturer
California State University, Fullerton
School of Nursing
Fullerton, California

Linda Johanson, RN, MS, EdD, CNE
Associate Professor
Appalachian State University
Nursing Department, College of Health
  Sciences
Boone, North Carolina

Janie Lynn Jones, MSN, RN, CNE
Assistant Professor
University of Arkansas at Little Rock
Department of Nursing
Little Rock, Arkansas

**Deanna Jung, DNP, APRN, AGACNP-BC,
  ACCNS-AG**
Assistant Professor
California State University, Fullerton;
Bayside Medical Center
School of Nursing
Fullerton, California

**Marylyn Kajs-Wyllie, MSN, RN, CNS,
  CNRN, CCRN-K, SCRN**
Clinical Associate Professor
Texas State University
St. David's School of Nursing
Round Rock, Texas

Tamara M. Kear, PhD, RN, CNS, CNN
Assistant Professor of Nursing
Villanova University
College of Nursing
Villanova, Pennsylvania

Cheryl Kent, DNP, MS, RN, CNE
Assistant Professor of Nursing
Northwestern Oklahoma State University
Division of Nursing
Enid, Oklahoma

Kari Ksar, RN, MS, CPNP
Pediatric Nurse Practitioner
Lucile Packard Children's Hospital
Pediatric Gastroenterology, Hepatology and
  Nutrition
Palo Alto, California

**Martha E. Langhorne, MSN, RN, FNP,
  AOCN**
Nurse Practitioner
Binghamton Gastroenterology
Binghamton, New York

Shawn M. Mason, MEd, BSN, RN
Nursing Faculty
Kwantlen Polytechnic University, Langley
  Campus
Faculty of Health
Surrey, British Columbia, Canada

Maureen McDonald, MS, RN
Professor, Department Chair
Massasoit Community College
Brockton, Massachusetts

Predrag Miskin, DHSc, RN, PHN, CMSRN
Instructor
De Anza College
Department of Nursing
Cupertino, California

Jason Mott, PhD, RN, CNE
Assistant Professor
Bellin College
Green Bay, Wisconsin

Sandie Nadelson, RN, MSN, MSEd, PhD, CNE
Professor
Colorado Mesa University
Health Sciences
Grand Junction, Colorado

Casey L. Norris, MSN, RN, PCNS-BC
Assistant Clinical Professor
The University of Alabama in Huntsville
College of Nursing
Huntsville, Alabama

Rebecca Otten, EdD, RN
Associate Professor, Nursing
California State University, Fullerton
School of Nursing
Fullerton, California

Kaye Paladino, MSN, RN
Nursing Faculty
Baker College
School of Nursing
Cadillac, Michigan

Nancymarie Phillips, RN, PhD, RNFA, CNOR
Professor, Director
Lakeland Community College
Department of Perioperative Education
Kirtland, Ohio

Kimberly Priode, PhD, RN, CNE, CCRN
Assistant Professor
Appalachian State University
Department of Nursing
Boone, North Carolina

Mark Stevens, MSN, RN, CNS, CEN, CPEN
Clinical Nurse Specialist
Stanford Health Care
Stanford, California

Linda Turchin, MSN, RN, CNE
Associate Professor
Fairmont State University
College of Nursing and Allied Health
Fairmont, West Virginia

Tiffany W. Varner, MSN, RN
Director, School of Nursing
Southern University at Shreveport
School of Nursing
Shreveport, Louisiana

Wendy H. Vogel, MSN, FNP, AOCNP
Oncology Nurse Practitioner
Wellmont Cancer Institute
Kingsport, Tennessee

Tena Wheeler, PhD, MSN, RN, CNE
ASN Program Director
Ozarks Technical Community College
Allied Health Associate of Science in Nursing
Springfield, Missouri

ANCILLARY REVIEWERS

Donald Laurino, MSN, CCRN, CMSRN, PHN, RN-BC
Adjunct Professor
West Coast University
Anaheim, California

Bethany Sykes, EdD, MSN, BSN, RN, CEN
Emergency Department
St. Luke's Hospital;
CCRN
Critical Care Unit
St. Luke's Hospital
New Bedford, Massachusetts;
Adjunct Faculty
Department of Nursing
Salve Regina University
Newport, Rhode Island;
RN Refresher Course Coordinator
College of Nursing
University of Massachusetts
North Dartmouth, Massachusetts

Jane Tyerman, PhD, MScN, BScN, RN, BA
Faculty
Trent/Fleming School of Nursing
Ontario, Canada

PREFACE

The first edition of this textbook, entitled *Medical-Surgical Nursing: A Nursing Process Approach,* was a groundbreaking work in many ways. The following eight editions built on that achievement and further solidified the book's position as a major trendsetter for the practice of adult health nursing. Now, in its ninth edition, "Iggy" charts the cutting-edge approach for the future of adult nursing practice—an approach reflected in its current title: *Medical-Surgical Nursing: Concepts for Interprofessional Collaborative Care.* The focus of this new edition continues to help students learn how to provide safe, quality nursing care that is patient-centered, evidence-based, and interprofessionally collaborative. In addition to print formats as single- and two-volume texts, this edition is now available in a variety of electronic formats.

The subtitle for this ninth edition was carefully chosen to emphasize the interprofessional nature of today's care, in which the nurse serves as a central role in collaboration with the patient, family, and members of the interprofessional health care team in acute care, community-based, and home settings. This approach reflects the National Academy of Medicine, The Joint Commission, the Quality and Safety Education for Nurses (QSEN) Institute, and the 2010 *Future of Nursing* report that unanimously have called for all health professionals to coordinate and deliver safe, evidence-based, patient-centered care as a collaborative team.

KEY THEMES FOR THE 9TH EDITION

The key themes for this edition strengthen this text's conceptual focus on safety, quality care, patient-centeredness, and clinical judgment to best prepare the student for interprofessional practice in medical-surgical health settings. Each theme is outlined and described below.

- **Enhanced Focus on Professional Nursing and Health Concepts.** This edition uniquely balances a focus on concepts, and a conceptual approach to teaching and learning, with important underpinnings of content. Prelicensure programs that embrace concept-based nursing curriculum, system-focused curriculum, or a hybrid approach will find this edition easy to use. To help students connect previously learned concepts with new information in the text, Chapters 1 and 2 addresses the main concepts used in this edition, giving a working definition upon which the students will reflect and build as they learn new material. These unique features build on basic concepts learned in nursing fundamentals courses, such as gas exchange and safety, to help students make connections between foundational concepts and interprofessional patient care for medical-surgical conditions. For continuity and reinforcement, a list of specific Priority and Interrelated Nursing Concepts is highlighted at the beginning of each chapter. This placement is specifically designed to help students better understand the priority and associated needs that the nurse will address when providing safe, evidence-based, patient-centered care for individuals with selected health problems. When these concepts are discussed in the body of each chapter, they are presented in small capital letters (e.g.,

IMMUNITY) to help students relate and apply essential concepts to provide more focused nursing care.

- **Emphasis on Key Exemplars.** For each priority concept listed in selected chapters, the authors have identified key exemplars. The nursing and interprofesional collaborative care for patients experiencing these exemplar diseases and illnesses is discussed through the lens of the priority and interrelated concepts. In addition, patient problems are presented as a collaborative problem list rather than merely presenting nursing diagnoses.

- **Prioritized Focus on the Core Body of Knowledge and QSEN Competencies.** This edition not only continues to emphasize need-to-know content for the RN level of practice but also includes a continuing emphasis on Quality and Safety Education for Nurses (QSEN) Institute core competencies. Clinical practice settings emphasize the critical need for safe practices and quality improvement to provide interprofessional patient-centered care that is evidence-based. Many hospitals and other health care agencies have formally adopted these QSEN competencies as core values and goals for patient care, and many nursing programs have used these same competencies to build prelicensure nursing curriculum. To help prepare students for the work environment as new graduates, as well as to highlight the foundational underpinning of safety and quality into all nursing actions, this edition prioritizes a focus on these competencies.

- **Emphasis on Patient Safety.** Patient safety is emphasized throughout this edition, not only in the narrative but also in **Nursing Safety Priority boxes** that enable students to immediately identify the most important care needed for patients with specific health problems. These highlighted features are further classified as an Action Alert, Drug Alert, or Critical Rescue. We also continue to include our leading-edge Best Practice for Patient Safety & Quality Care charts to emphasize the most important nursing care. **Highlighted yellow text** also demonstrates the application of The Joint Commission's National Patient Safety Goals initiatives (http://www.jointcommission.org/standards_information/npsgs.aspx) and Core Measures content into everyday nursing practice. The Joint Commission's National Patient Safety Goals initiatives are also set in **boldface type** for further emphasis.

- **Focus on Patient-Centered Care.** Patient-centered care is enhanced in the ninth edition in several ways. The ninth edition continues to use the term "patient" instead of "client" throughout. Although the use of these terms remains a subject of discussion among nursing educators and health care organizations, we have not defined the patient as a dependent person. Rather, the patient can be an individual, a family, or a group—all of whom have rights that are respected in a mutually trusting nurse-patient relationship. Most health care agencies and professional organizations use "patient" in their practice and publications, and most professional nursing organizations support the term.

- **Focus on Gender Considerations.** To increase our emphasis on patient-centered care, **Gender Health Considerations** focus on important gender-associated information that impacts nursing care. Differences in patient values, preferences, and beliefs are addressed in **Chapter 73, Care of Transgender Patients**. Along with other individuals in the LGBTQ population, the health needs of transgender patients have gained national attention through their inclusion in *Healthy People 2020* and The Joint Commission's standards. This chapter, first introduced in the eighth edition, continues to provide tools to help prepare students and faculty to provide safe, evidence-based, patient-centered care for transgender patients who are considering or who have undergone the gender transition process.

- **Emphasis on Evidence-Based Practice.** The ninth edition focuses again on the importance of *using best current evidence in nursing practice* and how to locate and use this evidence to improve patient care. **Evidence-Based Practice boxes** offer a solid foundation in this essential component of nursing practice. Each box summarizes a useful research article and explains the implications of its findings for practice and further research, as well as a rating of the level of evidence based on a well-respected scale.

- **Focus on Quality Improvement.** The QSEN Institute emphasizes, and clinical practice agencies require, that all nurses have *quality improvement* knowledge, skills, and attitudes. To help prepare students for that role, this edition includes unique **Quality Improvement boxes.** Each box summarizes a quality improvement project published in the literature and discusses the implications of the project's success in improving nursing care. The inclusion of these boxes disseminates information and research and helps students understand that quality improvement begins at the bedside as the nurse identifies potential evidence-based solutions to practice problems.

- **Emphasis on Clinical Judgment.** Stressing the importance of clinical judgment skills via prioritization and delegation helps to best prepare students for practice and the NCLEX® Examination. As in the eighth edition, the ninth edition emphasizes the importance of nursing clinical judgment to make timely and appropriate decisions and prioritize care. To help achieve that focus, all-new case-based **Clinical Judgment Challenges** based primarily on QSEN core competencies are integrated throughout the text. Selected Clinical Judgment Challenges highlight ethical dilemmas, as well as delegation and supervision issues. These exercises provide clinical situations in which students can use evolving nursing clinical judgment to help prepare them for the fast-paced world of medical-surgical nursing. Suggested answer guidelines for these Clinical Judgment Challenges are provided on the companion Evolve website (http://evolve.elsevier.com/Iggy/).

  Dr. Christine Tanner's clinical judgment framework (Tanner, 2006) is integrated more deeply in this edition to help students apply selected concepts in the Disorders chapters. The components of this model match Tanner's terminology to each nursing process heading, thereby helping students use nursing judgment to provide safe, quality care by:
  - Assessment: Noticing
  - Analysis: Interpreting
  - Planning: Implementation and Responding
  - Evaluation: Reflecting

- **Emphasis on Preparation for the NCLEX® Examination.** An enhanced emphasis on the NCLEX Examination and consistency with the 2016 NCLEX-RN® test plan has been refined in this edition. The ninth edition emphasizes "readiness"—readiness for the NCLEX Examination, readiness for disaster and mass casualty events, readiness for safe drug administration, and readiness for the continually evolving world of genetics and genomics. An increased number of new **NCLEX Examination Challenges** are interspersed throughout the text to allow students the opportunity to practice test-taking and decision making. Answers to these Challenges are provided in the back of the book, and their rationales are provided on the Evolve website (http://evolve.elsevier.com/Iggy). In a world that needs more nurses than ever before, it is more critical than ever that students be ready to pass the licensure examination on the first try. To help students and faculty achieve that outcome, **Learning Outcomes** at the beginning of each chapter continue to be consistent with the competencies outlined in the detailed 2016 NCLEX-RN® Test Plan. The ninth edition continues to include an innovative end-of-chapter feature called **Get Ready for the NCLEX® Examination!** This unique and effective learning aid consists of a list of **Key Points** *organized by Client Needs Category* as found in the NCLEX-RN Test Plan. Relevant QSEN and Nurse of the Future competency categories are identified for selected Key Points.

- **New Focus on Care Coordination and Transition Management.** This edition includes a priority focus on continuity of care via a Care Coordination and Transition Management section in each Disorders chapter. Literature continues to emphasize the importance of care coordination and transition management between acute care and community-based care (Lattavo, 2014). To help students prepare for this role, the ninth edition of our text provides coverage focusing on Home Care Management, Self-Management Education, and Health Care Resources.

CLINICAL CURRENCY AND ACCURACY

To ensure currency and accuracy, we listened to students and faculty who have used the previous editions, focusing on their impressions of and experiences with the book. A thorough literature search of current best evidence regarding nursing education and clinical practice helped us validate best practices and national health care trends to shape the focus of the ninth edition.

In-depth reviews of every chapter were commissioned and conducted by a dedicated panel of instructors and clinicians across the United States and Canada. A well-respected interventional radiologist ensured the accuracy of diagnostic testing procedures and associated patient care. The input from these experts guided us in revising chapters into their final format.

The results of these efforts are reflected in the ninth edition's:
- Strong, consistent focus on NCLEX-RN® Examination preparation, clinical judgment, safe patient-centered interprofessional care, pathophysiology, drug therapy, quality improvement, evidence-based clinical practice, and care coordination and transition management
- Foundation of relevant research and best practice guidelines
- Emphasis on critical "need to know" information that entry-level nurses must master to provide safe patient care

With the amount of information that continues to evolve in health care practice and education, it is easy for a book to become larger with each new edition. The reality is that today's nursing students have a limited time to absorb and begin to apply essential information to provide safe medical-surgical nursing care. Materials in this edition were carefully scrutinized to determine what the essential information was that students will actively *use* when providing safe, patient-centered, inter-professional, quality nursing care for adults.

OUTSTANDING READABILITY

Today's students must maximize their study time to read information and quickly understand it. The average reading level of today's learner is 10th to 11th grade. To achieve this level of readability without reducing the quality or depth of material that students need to know, this text uses a direct-address style (where appropriate) that speaks directly to the reader, and sentences are as short as possible without sacrificing essential content. The new edition has improved consistency of difficulty level from chapter to chapter. The result of our efforts is a medical-surgical text of consistently outstanding readability in which content is clear, focused, and accessible.

EASE OF ACCESS

To make this text as easy to use as possible, we have maintained our approach of having smaller chapters of more uniform length. Consistent with our focus on "need to know" material, we chose exemplars to illustrate concepts of care versus detailing every health disorder. The focused ninth edition contains 74 chapters.

The overall presentation of the ninth edition has been updated, including more current, high-quality photographs for realism, as well as design changes to improve accessibility of material. The design of the ninth edition includes appropriate placement of display elements (e.g., figures, tables, and charts) for a chapter flow that enhances text reading without splintering content or confusing the reader. Additional ease-of-access features for this edition include tabbed markings for the answer key, glossary, and index for quick reference. To increase the smoothness of flow and reader concentration, side-turned tables and charts or tables and charts that span multiple pages are infrequently used. Drug tables have been reformatted for consistency and ease of use.

We have maintained the unit structure of previous editions, with vital body systems (cardiovascular, respiratory, and neurologic) appearing earlier in the book. In these three units we continue to provide complex care content in separate chapters that discuss managing critically ill patients with coronary artery disease, respiratory health problems, and neurologic health problems.

To break up long blocks of text and highlight key information, we continue to include streamlined yet eye-catching headings, bulleted lists, tables, charts, and in-text highlights. Key terms are in boldface color type and are defined in the text to foster the learning of need-to-know vocabulary. A glossary is located in the back of the book. Current bibliographic resources at the end of each chapter include research articles, nationally accepted clinical guidelines, and other sources of evidence when available for each chapter. Classic sources from before 2011 are noted with an asterisk (*).

A PATIENT-CENTERED, INTERPROFESSIONAL COLLABORATIVE CARE APPROACH

As in previous editions, we maintain in this edition a collaborative, interprofessional care approach to patient care. In the real world of health care, nurses, patients, and all other providers who are part of the interprofessional team *share* responsibility for the management of patient problems. Thus we present information in a collaborative framework with an increased emphasis on the interprofessional nature of care. In this framework we make no *artificial* distinctions between medical treatment and nursing care. Instead, under each Interprofessional Collaborative Care heading we discuss how the nurse coordinates care and transition management while interacting with members of the interprofessional team.

This edition includes newly redesigned patient-centered Concept Maps that underscore the interprofessional care approach. Each Concept Map contains a case scenario. It then shows how a selected complex health problem is addressed. Each Concept Map spells out the steps of the nursing process and related concepts to illustrate the relationships among disease processes, priority patient problems, collaborative management, and more.

Although our approach has a focus on interprofessional care, the text is first and foremost a *nursing* text. We therefore use a nursing process approach as a tool to organize discussions of patient health problems and their management. Discussions of *major* health problems follow a full nursing process format using this structure:

[Health problem]
Pathophysiology
    Etiology (and Genetic Risk when appropriate)
    Incidence and Prevalence
Health Promotion and Maintenance (when appropriate)
Interprofessional Collaborative Care
    Assessment: Noticing
    Analysis: Interpreting
    Planning and Implementation: Responding
        [Collaborative Intervention Statement (based on priority patient problems)]
        Planning: Expected Outcomes
        Interventions
    Care Coordination and Transition Management
        Home Care Management
        Self-Management Education
        Health Care Resources
    Evaluation: Reflecting

The Analysis sections list the priority patient problems associated with major health problems and disorders. The ninth edition identifies priority collaborative patient problems or needs as the basis for the interprofessional plan of care. These collaborative patient problems pair more clearly with the title's focus than the previous use of NANDA-I language, which addresses primarily nursing-oriented patient problems. With its concentration on collaborative patient problems or needs, the ninth edition aligns with the language of clinical practice.

Discussions of less common or less complex disorders follow a similar, yet abbreviated, format: a discussion of the problem itself (including pertinent information on pathophysiology) followed by a section on interprofessional collaborative care of patients with the disorder. To demonstrate our commitment to providing the content foundational to nursing education, and consistent with the recommendations of Benner and colleagues through the Carnegie Foundation for the Future of Nursing Education, we highlight essential pathophysiologic concepts that are key to understanding the basis for collaborative management.

Integral to the interprofessional care approach is a narrative of who on the health care team is involved in the care of the patient. When a responsibility is primarily the nurse's, the text says so. When a decision must be made jointly by various members of the team (e.g., by the patient, nurse, health care provider, and physical therapist), this is clearly stated. When health care practitioners in different care settings are involved in the patient's care, this is stated.

ORGANIZATION

The 74 chapters of *Medical-Surgical Nursing: Concepts for Interprofessional Collaborative Care* are grouped into 16 units. Unit 1, Foundations for Medical-Surgical Nursing, provides fundamental information for the health care concepts incorporated throughout the text. Unit 2 consists of three chapters on concepts of emergency and trauma care and disaster preparedness.

Unit 3 consists of three chapters on the management of patients with fluid, electrolyte, and acid-base imbalances. Chapters 11 and 12 review key assessments associated with fluid and electrolyte balance, acid-base balance, and related patient care in a clear, concise discussion. The chapter on infusion therapy (Chapter 13) is supplemented with an online Fluids & Electrolytes Tutorial on the companion Evolve website.

Unit 4 presents the perioperative nursing content that medical-surgical nurses need to know. This content provides a solid foundation to help the student better understand the interprofessional care required for the surgical patient regardless of setting. Emphasis is placed on continuous assessment during the perioperative period to prevent complications and improve outcomes as we continue to see an increase in ambulatory care.

Unit 5 provides core content on health problems related to immunity. This material includes information on inflammation and the immune response, altered cell growth and cancer development, and interventions for patients with connective tissue disease, HIV infection, and other immunologic disorders, cancers, and infections.

The remaining 11 units cover medical-surgical content by body system. Each of these units begins with an Assessment chapter and continues with one or more Nursing Care chapters for patients with selected health problems, highlighted via exemplars, in that body system. This framework is familiar to students who learn the body systems in preclinical foundational science courses such as anatomy and physiology.

MULTINATIONAL, MULTICULTURAL, MULTIGENERATIONAL FOCUS

To reflect the increasing diversity of our society, *Medical-Surgical Nursing: Concepts for Interprofessional Collaborative Care* takes a multinational, multicultural, and multigenerational focus. Addressing the needs of both U.S. and Canadian readers, we have included examples of trade names of drugs available in the United States and in Canada. Drugs that are available only in Canada are designated with the Canadian maple leaf symbol(🍁). When appropriate, we identify specific Canadian health care resources, including their websites. In many areas, Canadian health statistics are combined with those of the United States to provide an accurate "North American" picture.

To help nurses provide quality care for patients whose preferences, beliefs, and values may differ from their own, numerous **Cultural/Spiritual Considerations** and **Gender Health Considerations boxes** highlight important aspects of culturally competent care. Chapter 73 is dedicated to the special health care needs of transgender patients.

Increases in life expectancy and aging of the baby-boom generation contribute to a steadily increasing older adult population. To help nurses care for this population, the ninth edition continues to provide thorough coverage of the care of older adults. Chapter 3 offers content on the role of the nurse and interprofessional team in promoting health for older adults, with coverage of common health problems that older adults may experience, such as falls and inadequate nutrition. The text includes many **Nursing Focus on the Older Adult** charts. Laboratory values and drug considerations for older patients are also included throughout the book. Charts specifying normal physiologic changes to expect in the older population are found in each Assessment chapter, and **Considerations for Older Adults boxes** emphasize key points for the student to consider when caring for these patients. A new feature for the ninth edition is **Veterans' Health Considerations**. An increasing number of veterans of wars have multiple physical and mental health problems and require special attention in today's health care environment.

ADDITIONAL LEARNING AIDS

The ninth edition continues to include a rich array of learning aids geared toward adult learners that help students quickly identify and understand key information while serving as study aids.

- Written in "patient-friendly" language, **Patient and Family Education: Preparing for Self-Management charts** provide teaching information that nurses must know to safely transition patients and their families back to the community environment of care.
- **Laboratory Profile charts** summarize important laboratory test information commonly used to evaluate health status. Information typically includes the normal ranges of laboratory values (including differences for older adults, when appropriate) and the significance of abnormal findings.
- The streamlined **Common Examples of Drug Therapy charts** summarize important information about commonly used drugs. Charts include U.S. and Canadian trade names for typically used drugs along with nursing implications and rationales (rationales are indicated by italic type).
- **Key Features charts** highlight the clinical signs and symptoms of important health problems based on pathophysiologic concepts.
- **Evidence-Based Practice boxes**, provided in many chapters, give synopses of recent nursing research articles and other scientific articles applicable to nursing. Each box provides a summary of the research, its level of evidence (LOE), and a brief commentary with implications for nursing practice and future research. This feature helps students identify strengths and weaknesses of evidence while seeing how research guides nursing practice.

- **Quality Improvement boxes** offer anecdotes of recent nursing articles that focus on this important QSEN competency and how nurses at the bedside have an active hand in shaping best practice. Similar to the Evidence-Based Practice boxes, these features provide a brief summary of the research with commentary on the implications for practice.
- As in the previous editions, **Home Care Assessment charts** serve as a convenient summary of essential assessment points for patients who need follow-up home health nursing care.
- Subtypes of **Clinical Judgment Challenges** (CJCs) emphasize the six QSEN core competencies: Patient-Centered Care, Teamwork and Collaboration, Evidence-Based Practice, Quality Improvement, Safety, and Informatics.

AN INTEGRATED MULTIMEDIA RESOURCE BASED ON PROVEN STRATEGIES FOR STUDENT ENGAGEMENT AND LEARNING

Medical-Surgical Nursing: Concepts for Interprofessional Collaborative Care, 9th edition, is the centerpiece of a comprehensive package of electronic and print learning resources that break new ground in the application of proven strategies for student engagement, learning, and evidence-based educational practice. This integrated multimedia resource actively engages the student in problem solving and practicing clinical decision-making skills.

Resources for Instructors

For the convenience of faculty, all Instructor Resources are available on a streamlined, secure instructor area of the Evolve website (http://evolve.elsevier.com/Iggy/). Included among these Instructor Resources are the *TEACH for Nurses* Lesson Plans. These Lesson Plans focus on the most important content from each chapter and provide innovative strategies for student engagement and learning. This ninth edition *TEACH for Nurses* product incorporates numerous interprofessional activities that give students an opportunity to practice as an integral part of the health care team. Lesson Plans are provided for each chapter and are categorized into several parts:

    Learning Outcomes
    Teaching Focus
    Key Terms
    Nursing Curriculum Standards
        QSEN
        Concepts
        BSN Essentials
    Student Chapter Resources
    Instructor Chapter Resources
    Teaching Strategies

Additional Instructor Resources provided on the Evolve website include:

- A completely revised, updated, high-quality **Test Bank** consisting of more than 1750 items, both traditional multiple-choice and NCLEX-RN® "alternate-item" types. Each question is coded for correct answer, rationale, cognitive level, NCLEX Integrated Process, NCLEX Client Needs Category, and new key words to facilitate question searches. Page references are provided for Remembering (Knowledge)-level and Understanding (Comprehension)-level questions. (Questions at the Applying [Application] and above cognitive level require the student to draw on understanding of multiple or broader concepts not limited to a single textbook page, so page cross references are not provided for these higher-level critical thinking questions.) The Test Bank is provided in the Evolve Assessment Manager and in ExamView and ParTest formats.
- An electronic **Image Collection** containing all images from the book (approximately 550 images), delivered in a format that makes incorporation into lectures, presentations, and online courses easier than ever.
- **PowerPoint Presentations**—a completely revised collection of more than 2000 slides corresponding to each chapter in the text and highlighting key materials with integrated images and Unfolding Case Studies. Audience Response System Questions (three discussion-oriented questions per chapter for use with iClicker and other audience response systems) are included in these slide presentations. Answers and rationales to the Audience Response System Questions and Unfolding Case Studies are found in the "Notes" section of each slide.

Also available for adoption and separate purchase:

- Corresponding chapter-by-chapter to the textbook, *Elsevier Adaptive Quizzing (EAQ)* integrates seamlessly into your course to help students of all skill levels focus their study time and effectively prepare for class, course exams, and the NCLEX® certification exam. *EAQ* is comprised of a bank of high-quality practice questions that allows students to advance at their own pace—based on their performance—through multiple mastery levels for each chapter. A comprehensive dashboard allows students to view their progress and stay motivated. The educator dashboard, grade book, and reporting capabilities enable faculty to monitor the activity of individual students, assess overall class performance, and identify areas of strength and weakness, ultimately helping to achieve improved learning outcomes.
- *Simulation Learning System (SLS) for Medical-Surgical Nursing* is an online toolkit designed to help you effectively incorporate simulation into your nursing curriculum, with scenarios that promote and enhance the clinical decision-making skills of students at all levels. It offers detailed instructions for preparation and implementation of the simulation experience, debriefing questions that encourage critical thinking, and learning resources to reinforce student comprehension. Modularized simulation scenarios correspond to Elsevier's leading medical-surgical nursing texts, reinforcing students' classroom knowledge base, synthesizing lecture and clinicals, and offering the remediation content that is critical to debriefing.

Resources for Students

Resources for students include a revised, updated, and retitled Study Guide, a Clinical Companion, Elsevier Adaptive Learning (EAL), Virtual Clinical Excursions (VCE), and Evolve Learning Resources.

The *Study Guide* has been completely revised and updated and features a fresh emphasis on clinical decision making, priorities of delegation, management of care, and pharmacology.

The pocket-sized *Clinical Companion* is a handy clinical resource that retains its easy-to-use alphabetical organization and streamlined format. It includes "Critical Rescue," "Drug Alert," and "Action Alert" highlights throughout based on the Nursing Safety Priority features in the textbook. National Patient Safety Goals highlights have been expanded as a QSEN feature, focusing on one of six QSEN core competencies while still underscoring the importance of observing vital patient safety standards. This "pocket-sized Iggy" has been tailored to the special needs of students preparing for clinicals and clinical practice.

Corresponding chapter-by-chapter to the textbook, *Elsevier Adaptive Learning (EAL)* combines the power of brain science with sophisticated, patented Cerego algorithms to help students to learn faster and remember longer. It's fun, it's engaging, and it constantly tracks and adapts to student performance to deliver content precisely when it's needed to ensure core information is transformed into lasting knowledge.

Virtual Clinical Excursions, featuring an updated and easy-to-navigate "virtual" clinical setting, is once again available for the eighth edition. This unique learning tool guides students through a virtual clinical environment and helps them "learn by doing" in the safety of a "virtual" hospital.

Also available for students is a dynamic collection of Evolve Student Resources, available at http://evolve.elsevier.com/Iggy/. The Evolve Student Resources include the following:

- Review Questions for the NCLEX® Examination
- Answer Guidelines for NCLEX® Examination and Clinical Judgment Challenges

- Interactive Case Studies
- Concept Maps (digital versions of the 12 Concept Maps from the text)
- Concept Map Creator (a handy tool for creating customized Concept Maps)
- Fluid & Electrolyte Tutorial (a complete self-paced tutorial on this perennially difficult content)
- Key Points (downloadable expanded chapter reviews for each chapter)
- Audio Glossary
- Audio Clips and Video Clips
- Content Updates

In summary, *Medical-Surgical Nursing: Concepts for Interprofessional Collaborative Care,* 9th edition, together with its fully integrated multimedia ancillary package, provides the tools you will need to equip nursing students to meet the opportunities and challenges of nursing practice both now and in an evolving health care environment. The only elements that remain to be added to this package are those that you uniquely provide—your passion, your commitment, your innovation, *your nursing expertise.*

Donna D. Ignatavicius
M. Linda Workman
Cherie R. Rebar

To all the nursing educators who are passionate about teaching, and to all the nursing students who are passionate about learning.
To my husband, Charles, who has endured countless hours of loneliness while I've worked on this project, and to Stephanie, my daughter, who has educated me about the special needs of the LGBTQ community. Thank you!

DONNA

To students everywhere.
To John, still my one.

LINDA

To Michael…you are my everything.
To Gillian…all I do is for you, my beautiful girl.
To Mom and Dad…thank you for roots and wings.
To Donna and Linda…thank you for believing in me!
To our Elsevier team….thank you for your dedication!
To Carolyn, Laura, Nicole, Tracy, and Tracie…my kindred spirits.
To all who study, teach, and practice nursing….you are my heroes.

CHERIE

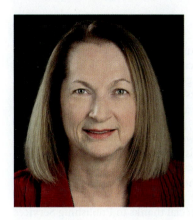

Donna D. Ignatavicius received her diploma in nursing from the Peninsula General School of Nursing in Salisbury, Maryland. After working as a charge nurse in medical-surgical nursing, she became an instructor in staff development at the University of Maryland Medical Center. She then received her BSN from the University of Maryland School of Nursing. For 5 years she taught in several schools of nursing while working toward her MS in Nursing, which she received in 1981. Donna then taught in the BSN program at the University of Maryland, after which she continued to pursue her interest in gerontology and accepted the position of Director of Nursing of a major skilled-nursing facility in her home state of Maryland. Since that time, she has served as an instructor in several associate degree nursing programs. Through her consulting activities, faculty development workshops, and international nursing education conferences (such as Boot Camp for Nurse Educators®),Donna is nationally recognized as an expert in nursing education. She is currently the President of DI Associates, Inc. (http://www.diassociates.com/), a company dedicated to improving health care through education and consultation for faculty. In recognition of her contributions to the field, she was inducted as a charter Fellow of the prestigious Academy of Nursing Education in 2007 and received her Certified Nurse Educator credential in 2016.

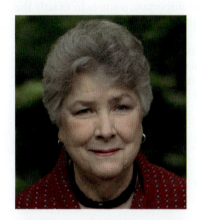

M. Linda Workman, a native of Canada, received her BSN from the University of Cincinnati College of Nursing and Health. After serving in the U.S. Army Nurse Corps and working as an Assistant Head Nurse and Head Nurse in civilian hospitals, Linda earned her MSN from the University of Cincinnati College of Nursing and a PhD in Developmental Biology from the University of Cincinnati College of Arts and Sciences. Linda's 30-plus years of academic experience include teaching at the diploma, associate degree, baccalaureate, master's, and doctoral levels. Her areas of teaching expertise include medical-surgical nursing, physiology, pathophysiology, genetics, oncology, and immunology. Linda has been recognized nationally for her teaching expertise and was inducted as a Fellow into the American Academy of Nursing in 1992. She received Excellence in Teaching awards at the University of Cincinnati and at Case Western Reserve University. She is a former American Cancer Society Professor of Oncology Nursing and held an endowed chair in oncology for 5 years. She has authored several additional textbooks and serves a consultant for major universities.

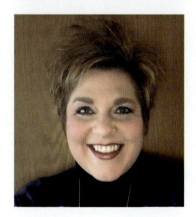

Cherie R. Rebar earned her first degree in education from Morehead State University in Morehead, Kentucky. She returned to school shortly thereafter to earn an Associate of Science degree in Nursing from Kettering College. Cherie's years of clinical practice includes medical-surgical, acute care, ear/nose/throat surgery and allergy, community, and psychiatric-mental health nursing. After earning her MSN and MBA from the University of Phoenix, Cherie combined her love of nursing and education and began teaching Associate and Baccalaureate Completion nursing students at Kettering College while pursuing her Family Nurse Practitioner post-Masters certificate from the University of Massachusetts Boston. Over a decade, Cherie served in numerous leadership positions at Kettering College, including Chair of AS, BSN Completion, and BSN Prelicensure Nursing Programs, as well as Director of the Division of Nursing. She currently is a Professor of Nursing at Wittenberg University, an Affiliate Faculty Member at Indiana Wesleyan University, a Psychiatric–Mental Health Nurse Practitioner Intern through the University of Cincinnati College of Nursing, and a frequent presenter at national nursing conferences. Cherie serves as a consultant with nursing programs and faculty, contributes regularly to professional publications, and holds student success at the heart of all she does.

ACKNOWLEDGMENTS

Publishing a textbook and ancillary package of this magnitude would not be possible without the combined efforts of many people. With that in mind, we would like to extend our deepest gratitude to many people who were such an integral part of this journey.

For the ninth edition, we welcomed section editor Nicole M. Heimgartner to assist in our revision process. Nicole has worked with our team in contributor and ancillary roles over the past editions. Within this edition, she updated and reviewed selected chapters of the text to provide her expertise.

Our contributing authors once again provided excellent manuscripts to underscore the clinical relevancy of this publication. We give special gratitude to Deanne Blach, who revised our Concept Maps, and to Dr. Richard Lintner, who provided expertise in interventional radiologic procedures and associated care. Our reviewers—expert clinicians and instructors from around the United States and Canada—provided invaluable suggestions and encouragement throughout the development of book.

The staff of Elsevier has, as always, provided us with meaningful guidance and support throughout every step of the planning, writing, revision, and production of the ninth edition. Executive Content Strategist Lee Henderson worked closely with us from the early stages of this edition to help us hone and focus our revision plan while coordinating the project from start to finish. Senior Content Development Specialist Laura Goodrich then worked with us to bring the logistics of the ninth edition from vision to publication. Laura also held the reins of our complex ancillary package and worked with a gifted group of writers and content experts to provide an outstanding library of resources to complement and enhance the text.

Senior Project Manager Jodi Willard was, as always, an absolute joy with whom to work. If the mark of a good editor is that his or her work is invisible to the reader, then Jodi is the consummate editor. Her unwavering attention to detail, flexibility, and conscientiousness helped to make the ninth edition consistently readable, while making the production process incredibly smooth. Also, a special thanks to Publishing Services Manager Jeff Patterson.

Designer Brian Salisbury is responsible for the beautiful cover and the new interior design of the ninth edition. Brian's work on this edition has cast important features in exactly the right light, contributing to the readability and colorful beauty of this edition.

Our acknowledgments would not be complete without recognizing our dedicated team of Educational Solutions Consultants and other key members of the Sales and Marketing staff who helped to put this book into your hands.

Donna D. Ignatavicius
M. Linda Workman
Cherie R. Rebar

CONTENTS

UNIT I Foundations for Medical-Surgical Nursing

1 Overview of Professional Nursing Concepts for Medical-Surgical Nursing, 1
Donna D. Ignatavicius
    Quality and Safety Education for Nurses Core Competencies, 2
    Patient-Centered Care, 2
    Safety, 3
    Teamwork and Interprofessional Collaboration, 5
    Evidence-Based Practice, 6
    Quality Improvement, 7
    Informatics and Technology, 7
    Clinical Judgment, 8
    Ethics, 8
    Health Care Organizations, 9
    Health Care Disparities, 10

2 Overview of Health Concepts for Medical-Surgical Nursing, 13
Donna D. Ignatavicius and Kristin Oneail
    Acid-Base Balance, 13
    Cellular Regulation, 14
    Clotting, 15
    Cognition, 16
    Comfort, 17
    Elimination, 18
    Fluid and Electrolyte Balance, 19
    Glucose Regulation, 20
    Gas Exchange, 20
    Immunity, 21
    Mobility, 23
    Nutrition, 24
    Perfusion, 25
    Sensory Perception, 26
    Sexuality, 27
    Tissue Integrity, 27

3 Common Health Problems of Older Adults, 29
Donna D. Ignatavicius
    Overview, 30
    Health Issues for Older Adults in Community-Based Settings, 30
    Decreased Nutrition and Hydration, 30
    Decreased Mobility, 31
    Stress, Loss, and Coping, 32
    Accidents, 33
    Drug Use and Misuse, 34
    Inadequate Cognition, 35
    Substance Use, 38
    Elder Neglect and Abuse, 39
    Health Issues for Older Adults in Hospitals and Long-Term Care Settings, 39
    Problems of Sleep, Nutrition, and Continence, 40
    Confusion, Falls, and Skin Breakdown, 40

    Care Coordination and Transition Management, 42

4 Assessment and Care of Patients With Pain, 45
Melanie H. Simpson and Donna D. Ignatavicius
    ***Pain,** 45
    Scope of the Problem, 45
    Definitions of Pain, 46
    Categorization of Pain by Duration, 46
    Categorization of Pain by Underlying Mechanisms, 47
    Interprofessional Collaborative Care, 48

5 Principles of Genetics and Genomics for Medical-Surgical Nursing, 71
M. Linda Workman
    Genetic Biology Review, 72
    DNA, 72
    Gene Structure and Function, 74
    Gene Expression, 76
    Protein Synthesis, 76
    Mutations and Variations, 76
    Microbiome, 77
    Patterns of Inheritance, 77
    Pedigree, 77
    Autosomal Dominant Pattern of Inheritance, 78
    Autosomal Recessive Pattern of Inheritance, 79
    Sex-Linked Recessive Pattern of Inheritance, 79
    Complex Inheritance and Familial Clustering, 80
    Genetic Testing, 80
    Purpose of Genetic Testing, 80
    Benefits and Risks of Genetic Testing, 80
    Genetic Counseling, 81
    Ethical Issues, 81
    The Role of the Medical-Surgical Nurse in Genetic Counseling, 82
    Communication, 82
    Privacy and Confidentiality, 83
    Information Accuracy, 83
    Patient Advocacy and Support, 83

6 Rehabilitation Concepts for Chronic and Disabling Health Problems, 86
Michelle Camicia and Donna D. Ignatavicius
    Overview, 87
    Chronic and Disabling Health Conditions, 87
    Rehabilitation Settings, 87
    The Rehabilitation Interprofessional Team, 88

7 End-of-Life Care Concepts, 103
Mary K. Kazanowski
    Overview of Death, Dying, and End of Life, 103
    Pathophysiology of Dying, 104
    ***End of Life,** 104
    Hospice and Palliative Care, 106
    Postmortem Care, 114
    Ethics and Dying, 114

Asterisk (*) denotes a Concept Exemplar.

UNIT II Principles of Emergency Care and Disaster Preparedness

8 Principles of Emergency and Trauma Nursing, 117
Linda Laskowski-Jones and Karen L. Toulson
The Emergency Department Environment of Care, 118
Demographic Data and Vulnerable Populations, 118
Special Nursing Teams—Members of the Interprofessional Team, 118
Interprofessional Team Collaboration, 119
Staff and Patient Safety Considerations, 120
Staff Safety, 120
Patient Safety, 121
Scope of Emergency Nursing Practice, 122
Core Competencies, 122
Training and Certification, 123
Emergency Nursing Principles, 123
Triage, 123
Disposition, 124
The Impact of Homelessness, 127
Trauma Nursing Principles, 127
Trauma Centers and Trauma Systems, 127
Mechanism of Injury, 128
Primary Survey and Resuscitation Interventions, 129
The Secondary Survey and Resuscitation Interventions, 130
Disposition, 130

9 Care of Patients With Common Environmental Emergencies, 133
Linda Laskowski-Jones
Heat-Related Illnesses, 133
Heat Exhaustion, 133
Heat Stroke, 134
Snakebites and Arthropod Bites and Stings, 135
Lightning Injuries, 141
Cold-Related Injuries, 142
Hypothermia, 142
Frostbite, 144
Altitude-Related Illnesses, 145
Drowning, 147

10 Principles of Emergency and Disaster Preparedness, 149
Linda Laskowski-Jones
Types of Disasters, 149
Impact of External Disasters, 150
Emergency Preparedness and Response, 151
Mass Casualty Triage, 151
Notification and Activation of Emergency Preparedness/Management Plans, 153
Hospital Emergency Preparedness: Personnel Roles and Responsibilities, 153
Event Resolution and Debriefing, 156
Critical Incident Stress Debriefing, 156
Administrative Review, 157
Role of Nursing in Community Emergency Preparedness and Response, 157
Psychosocial Response of Survivors to Mass Casualty Events, 157

UNIT III Interprofessional Collaboration for Patients With Problems of Fluid, Electrolyte, and Acid-Base Balance

11 Assessment and Care of Patients With Problems of Fluid and Electrolyte Balance, 160
M. Linda Workman
Anatomy and Physiology Review, 160
Filtration, 161
Diffusion, 162
Osmosis, 163
Fluid Balance, 164
Body Fluids, 164
Hormonal Regulation of Fluid Balance, 165
Significance of Fluid Balance, 166
Disturbances of Fluid and Electrolyte Balance, 167
*Dehydration, 167
Fluid Overload, 171
Electrolyte Balance and Imbalances, 172
Sodium, 173
Potassium, 175
Calcium, 179
Magnesium, 181

12 Assessment and Care of Patients With Problems of Acid-Base Balance, 185
M. Linda Workman
Maintaining Acid-Base Balance, 185
Acid-Base Chemistry, 186
Body Fluid Chemistry, 187
Acid-Base Regulatory Actions and Mechanisms, 188
Acid-Base Imbalances, 190
*Acidosis, 190
Alkalosis, 195

13 Concepts of Infusion Therapy, 199
Jeanette Spain Adams
Overview, 199
Types of Infusion Therapy Fluids, 200
Prescribing Infusion Therapy, 201
Vascular Access Devices, 201
Peripheral Intravenous Therapy, 202
Short Peripheral Catheters, 202
Midline Catheters, 204
Central Intravenous Therapy, 205
Peripherally Inserted Central Catheters, 205
Nontunneled Percutaneous Central Venous Catheters, 206
Tunneled Central Venous Catheters, 207
Implanted Ports, 207
Hemodialysis Catheters, 208
Infusion Systems, 208
Containers, 208
Administration Sets, 209
Rate-Controlling Infusion Devices, 211
Nursing Care for Patients Receiving Intravenous Therapy, 211
Educating the Patient, 211
Performing the Nursing Assessment, 212
Securing and Dressing the Catheter, 212
Changing Administration Sets and Needleless Connectors, 214

Controlling Infusion Pressure, 214
Flushing the Catheter, 214
Obtaining Blood Samples from Central Venous Catheters, 215
Removing the Vascular Access Device, 215
Documenting Intravenous Therapy, 216
Complications of Intravenous Therapy, 216
Catheter-Related Bloodstream Infection, 216
Other Complications of Intravenous Therapy, 216
Intravenous Therapy and Care of the Older Adult, 216
Skin Care, 216
Vein and Catheter Selection, 222
Cardiac and Renal Changes, 222
Subcutaneous Infusion Therapy, 223
Intraosseous Infusion Therapy, 223
Intra-Arterial Infusion Therapy, 224
Intraperitoneal Infusion Therapy, 225
Intraspinal Infusion Therapy, 225

UNIT IV Interprofessional Collaboration for Perioperative Patients

14 Care of Preoperative Patients, 228
Cynthia L. Danko and Rebecca M. Patton
Overview, 229
Categories and Purposes of Surgery, 229
Surgical Settings, 229
15 Care of Intraoperative Patients, 251
Cynthia L. Danko and Rebecca M. Patton
Overview, 251
Members of the Surgical Team, 252
The Surgical Suite—Patient and Team Safety, 252
Anesthesia, 256
16 Care of Postoperative Patients, 270
Rebecca M. Patton and Cynthia Danko
Overview, 270

UNIT V Interprofessional Collaboration for Patients With Problems of Immunity

17 Principles of Inflammation and Immunity, 289
M. Linda Workman
Overview, 289
Self Versus Non-Self, 289
Organization of the Immune System, 290
General Immunity: Inflammation, 291
Infection, 292
Cell Types Involved in Inflammation, 292
Phagocytosis, 294
Sequence of Inflammation, 294
Specific Immunity, 295
Antibody-Mediated Immunity, 295
Cell-Mediated Immunity, 299
Age-Related Changes in Immunity, 300
Transplant Rejection, 300
Hyperacute Rejection, 301
Acute Rejection, 301
Chronic Rejection, 301
Management of Transplant Rejection, 301

18 Care of Patients With Arthritis and Other Connective Tissue Diseases, 304
Roberta Goff and Kathy Vanderbeck
*Osteoarthritis, 305
*Rheumatoid Arthritis, 318
Lupus Erythematosus, 326
Systemic Sclerosis, 329
Gout, 330
Lyme Disease, 332
Disease-Associated Arthritis, 332
Fibromyalgia Syndrome, 333
19 Care of Patients With Problems of HIV Disease, 337
James G. Sampson and M. Linda Workman
*HIV Infection and AIDS, 337
20 Care of Patients With Hypersensitivity (Allergy) and Autoimmunity, 360
M. Linda Workman
HYPERSENSITIVITIES/ALLERGIES, 360
Type I: Rapid Hypersensitivity Reactions, 360
*Angioedema, 361
Allergic Rhinosinusitis, 365
Type II: Cytotoxic Reactions, 366
Type III: Immune Complex Reactions, 366
Type IV: Delayed Hypersensitivity Reactions, 367
AUTOIMMUNITY, 367
21 Principles of Cancer Development, 372
M. Linda Workman
Pathophysiology, 372
Biology of Normal Cells, 372
Biology of Abnormal Cells, 373
Cancer Development, 375
Carcinogenesis/Oncogenesis, 375
Cancer Classification, 375
Cancer Grading, Ploidy, and Staging, 376
Cancer Etiology and Genetic Risk, 377
Cancer Prevention, 381
Primary Prevention, 381
Secondary Prevention, 382
22 Care of Patients With Cancer, 384
Constance G. Visovsky and Julie Ponto
Impact of Cancer on Physical Function, 384
Impaired Immunity and Clotting, 385
Altered GI Function, 385
Altered Peripheral Nerve Function, 385
Motor and Sensory Deficits, 385
Cancer Pain, 385
Altered Respiratory and Cardiac Function, 386
Cancer Management, 386
Surgery, 386
Radiation Therapy, 387
Cytotoxic Systemic Therapy, 390
Oncologic Emergencies, 407
Sepsis and Disseminated Intravascular Coagulation, 407
Syndrome of Inappropriate Antidiuretic Hormone, 407
Spinal Cord Compression, 408
Hypercalcemia, 408
Superior Vena Cava Syndrome, 408
Tumor Lysis Syndrome, 409

23 Care of Patients With Infection, 413
Donna D. Ignatavicius
   *Infection, 413
      Transmission of Infectious Agents, 414
      Physiologic Defenses for Infection, 416
      Health Promotion and Maintenance, 417
      Infection Control in Health Care Settings, 417
      *Methods of Infection Control and
         Prevention, 417*
   **Multidrug-Resistant Organism Infections and
      Colonizations, 421**
      *Methicillin-Resistant Staphylococcus aureus
         (MRSA), 422*
      Vancomycin-Resistant Enterococcus (VRE), 422
      *Carbapenem-Resistant Enterobacteriaceae
         (CRE), 422*
   **Occupational and Environmental Exposure to
      Sources of Infection, 423**
   **Problems Resulting From Inadequate Antimicrobial
      Therapy, 423**
   **Critical Issues: Emerging Infections and Global
      Bioterrorism, 427**

**UNIT VI Interprofessional Collaboration for
         Patients With Problems of the Skin,
         Hair, and Nails**

24 Assessment of the Skin, Hair, and Nails, 431
Janice Cuzzell
   Anatomy and Physiology Review, 431
      Structure of the Skin, 431
      Structure of the Skin Appendages, 432
      Functions of the Skin, 433
      Skin Changes Associated With Aging, 433
   Assessment: Noticing and Interpreting, 433
      Patient History, 433
      Nutrition Status, 436
      Family History and Genetic Risk, 436
      Current Health Problems, 436
      Skin Assessment, 436
      Hair Assessment, 441
      Nail Assessment, 441
      *Skin Assessment Techniques for Patients With Darker
         Skin, 443*
      Psychosocial Assessment, 444
      Diagnostic Assessment, 444

25 Care of Patients With Skin Problems, 447
Janice Cuzzell
   *Pressure Injuries, 447
   Minor Skin Irritations, 461
      Pruritis, 461
      Urticaria, 462
   Common Inflammations, 462
   Psoriasis, 463
   Skin Infections, 466
   Parasitic Disorders, 470
      Pediculosis, 470
      Scabies, 470
      Bedbugs, 471
   Trauma, 471
   Skin Cancer, 474

   Other Skin Disorders, 478
      *Toxic Epidermal Necrolysis and Stevens-Johnson
         Syndrome, 478*

26 Care of Patients With Burns, 481
Tammy Coffee
   Introduction to Burn Injury, 481
   Health Promotion and Maintenance, 488
   Resuscitation Phase of Burn Injury, 489
   Acute Phase of Burn Injury, 497
   Rehabilitative Phase of Burn Injury, 504

**UNIT VII Interprofessional Collaboration for
          Patients With Problems of the
          Respiratory System**

27 Assessment of the Respiratory System, 508
Harry Rees
   Anatomy and Physiology Review, 508
      Upper Respiratory Tract, 509
      Lower Respiratory Tract, 510
      *Oxygen Delivery and the Oxygen-Hemoglobin
         Dissociation Curve, 512*
      Respiratory Changes Associated With Aging, 512
      Health Promotion and Maintenance, 512
   Assessment: Noticing and Interpreting, 515
      Patient History, 515
      Physical Assessment, 517
      Psychosocial Assessment, 521
      Diagnostic Assessment, 521

**28 Care of Patients Requiring Oxygen Therapy or
    Tracheostomy,** 529
Harry Rees
   Oxygen Therapy, 529
   *Tracheostomy, 537

**29 Care of Patients With Noninfectious Upper Respiratory
    Problems,** 547
M. Linda Workman
   *Head and Neck Cancer, 547
   Cancer of the Nose and Sinuses, 556
   Fractures of the Nose, 556
   Epistaxis, 557
   Facial Trauma, 558
   Obstructive Sleep Apnea, 559
   Laryngeal Trauma, 559
   Upper Airway Obstruction, 560

**30 Care of Patients With Noninfectious Lower Respiratory
    Problems,** 563
M. Linda Workman
   Asthma, 563
   *Chronic Obstructive Pulmonary Disease, 572
   Cystic Fibrosis, 581
   Pulmonary Arterial Hypertension, 584
   Idiopathic Pulmonary Fibrosis, 585
   Lung Cancer, 586

**31 Care of Patients With Infectious Respiratory
    Problems,** 596
Meg Blair
   Seasonal Influenza, 596
   Pandemic Influenza, 597
   **Middle East Respiratory Syndrome
      (MERS), 598**

*Pneumonia, 598
*Pulmonary Tuberculosis, 605
Rhinosinusitis, 610
Peritonsillar Abscess, 611
Inhalation Anthrax, 611
Pertussis, 613
Coccidioidomycosis, 613

32 Care of Critically Ill Patients With Respiratory Problems, 616
Harry Rees
*Pulmonary Embolism, 616
Acute Respiratory Failure, 624
Acute Respiratory Distress Syndrome, 626
The Patient Requiring Intubation and
    Ventilation, 628
Chest Trauma, 636
    Pulmonary Contusion, 636
    Rib Fracture, 636
    Flail Chest, 637
    Pneumothorax and Hemothorax, 637

UNIT VIII Interprofessional Collaboration for Patients With Problems of the Cardiovascular System

33 Assessment of the Cardiovascular System, 641
Laura M. Dechant
Anatomy and Physiology Review, 642
    Heart, 642
    Vascular System, 645
    Cardiovascular Changes Associated With Aging, 646
Assessment: Noticing and
    Interpreting, 646
    Patient History, 646
    Physical Assessment, 651
    Psychosocial Assessment, 655
    Diagnostic Assessment, 655

34 Care of Patients With Dysrhythmias, 664
Laura M. Dechant and Nicole M. Heimgartner
Review of Cardiac Conduction System, 664
Electrocardiography, 665
    Lead Systems, 666
    Continuous Electrocardiographic
        Monitoring, 667
    Electrocardiographic Complexes, Segments, and
        Intervals, 667
    Electrocardiographic Rhythm Analysis, 670
Overview of Normal Cardiac Rhythms, 671
Common Dysrhythmias, 671
Sinus Dysrhythmias, 672
    Sinus Tachycardia, 673
    Sinus Bradycardia, 674
Atrial Dysrhythmias, 675
    Premature Atrial Complex, 676
    Supraventricular Tachycardia, 676
*Atrial Fibrillation, 678
Ventricular Dysrhythmias, 683
    Premature Ventricular Complex, 683
    Ventricular Tachycardia, 684
    Ventricular Fibrillation, 684
    Ventricular Asystole, 686

35 Care of Patients With Cardiac Problems, 691
Laura M. Dechant
*Heart Failure, 691
Valvular Heart Disease, 705
Inflammations and Infections, 711
    Infective Endocarditis, 711
    Pericarditis, 712
    Rheumatic Carditis, 714
    Cardiomyopathy, 714

36 Care of Patients With Vascular Problems, 720
Nicole M. Heimgartner
*Hypertension, 720
Arteriosclerosis and Atherosclerosis, 728
Peripheral Arterial Disease, 731
Acute Peripheral Arterial Occlusion, 737
Aneurysms of the Central Arteries, 738
Aneurysms of the Peripheral Arteries, 740
Aortic Dissection, 740
Other Arterial Health Problems, 741
Peripheral Venous Disease, 741
*Venous Thromboembolism, 742
Venous Insufficiency, 746
Varicose Veins, 748

37 Care of Patients With Shock, 751
Nicole M. Heimgartner
Overview, 751
    Review of Gas Exchange and Tissue
        Perfusion, 752
    Types of Shock, 752
*Hypovolemic Shock, 754
*Sepsis and Septic Shock, 760

38 Care of Patients With Acute Coronary Syndromes, 768
Laura M. Dechant
Chronic Stable Angina Pectoris, 768
*Acute Coronary Syndrome, 769

UNIT IX Interprofessional Collaboration for Patients With Problems of the Hematologic System

39 Assessment of the Hematologic System, 795
M. Linda Workman
Anatomy and Physiology Review, 795
    Bone Marrow, 795
    Blood Components, 796
    Accessory Organs of Blood
        Formation, 797
    Hemostasis and Blood Clotting, 798
    Anti-Clotting Forces, 799
    Hematologic Changes Associated
        With Aging, 800
Assessment: Noticing and
    Interpreting, 800
    Patient History, 800
    Nutrition Status, 802
    Family History and Genetic Risk, 802
    Current Health Problems, 802
    Physical Assessment, 802
    Psychosocial Assessment, 803
    Diagnostic Assessment, 803

40 Care of Patients With Hematologic Problems, 808
Katherine L. Byar
  *Sickle Cell Disease, 808
  Anemia, 813
  Polycythemia Vera, 816
  Hereditary Hemochromatosis, 817
  Myelodysplastic Syndromes, 817
  *Leukemia, 817
  Malignant Lymphomas, 828
  Multiple Myeloma, 829
  Autoimmune Thrombocytopenic
    Purpura, 830
  Thrombotic Thrombocytopenic Purpura, 831
  Hemophilia, 831
  Heparin-Induced Thrombocytopenia, 832
  Transfusion Therapy, 832
    Pretransfusion Responsibilities, 832
    Transfusion Responsibilities, 833
    Types of Transfusions, 834
    Acute Transfusion Reactions, 835
    Autologous Blood Transfusions, 836

**UNIT X Interprofessional Collaboration
for Patients With Problems of
the Nervous System**

41 Assessment of the Nervous System, 839
Donna D. Ignatavicius
  Anatomy and Physiology Review, 839
    *Nervous System Cells: Structure and
      Function, 839*
    *Central Nervous System: Structure and
      Function, 840*
    *Peripheral Nervous System: Structure and
      Function, 842*
    *Autonomic Nervous System: Structure and
      Function, 842*
    Neurologic Changes Associated With Aging, 844
    Health Promotion and Maintenance, 845
  Assessment: Noticing and Interpreting, 846
    Patient History, 846
    Physical Assessment, 846
    Psychosocial Assessment, 850
    Diagnostic Assessment, 851

**42 Care of Patients With Problems of the Central Nervous
System: The Brain,** 857
Donna D. Ignatavicius
  *Alzheimer's Disease, 857
  *Parkinson Disease, 868
  Migraine Headache, 873
  Seizures and Epilepsy, 876
  Meningitis, 880
  Encephalitis, 883

**43 Care of Patients With Problems of the Central Nervous
System: The Spinal Cord,** 887
Laura M. Willis and Donna D. Ignatavicius
  *Multiple Sclerosis, 888
  *Spinal Cord Injury, 894
  Back Pain, 903
    Low Back Pain (Lumbosacral Back Pain), 903
    Cervical Neck Pain, 909

**44 Care of Patients With Problems of the Peripheral
Nervous System,** 912
Donna D. Ignatavicius
  *Guillain-Barré Syndrome, 912
  Myasthenia Gravis, 917
  Restless Legs Syndrome, 922
  Trigeminal Neuralgia, 923
  Facial Paralysis, 924

**45 Care of Critically Ill Patients With Neurologic
Problems,** 927
Laura M. Willis
  Transient Ischemic Attack, 927
  *Stroke (Brain Attack), 928
  *Traumatic Brain Injury, 940
  Brain Tumors, 950

**UNIT XI Interprofessional Collaboration
for Patients With Problems of
the Sensory System**

46 Assessment of the Eye and Vision, 957
Samuel A. Borchers and Andrea A. Borchers
  Anatomy and Physiology Review, 957
    Structure, 957
    Function, 960
    Eye Changes Associated With Aging, 961
    Health Promotion and Maintenance, 961
  Assessment: Noticing and Interpreting, 962
    Patient History, 962
    Physical Assessment, 963
    Psychosocial Assessment, 964
    Diagnostic Assessment, 965

47 Care of Patients With Eye and Vision Problems, 968
Samuel A. Borchers and Andrea A. Borchers
  *Cataract, 968
  *Glaucoma, 972
  Corneal Disorders, 977
    Corneal Abrasion, Ulceration, and Infection, 977
    Keratoconus and Corneal Opacities, 977
  Retinal Disorders, 979
    Macular Degeneration, 979
    Retinal Holes, Tears, and Detachments, 979
    Retinitis Pigmentosa, 980
  Refractive Errors, 980
  Trauma, 981
    Foreign Bodies, 981
    Lacerations, 981
    Penetrating Injuries, 982

**48 Assessment and Care of Patients With Ear and Hearing
Problems,** 984
Samuel A. Borchers and Andrea A. Borchers
  Anatomy and Physiology Review, 984
    Structure, 984
    Function, 986
  Assessment: Noticing and Interpreting, 986
    Patient History, 986
    Physical Assessment, 988
    General Hearing Assessment, 989
    Psychosocial Assessment, 990
    Diagnostic Assessment, 990
  *Otitis Media, 991

External Otitis, 993
Cerumen or Foreign Bodies, 994
Mastoiditis, 995
Trauma, 995
Tinnitus, 995
Ménière's Disease, 995
Acoustic Neuroma, 996
*Hearing Loss, 996

UNIT XII Interprofessional Collaboration for Patients With Problems of the Musculoskeletal System

49 Assessment of the Musculoskeletal System, 1004
Donna D. Ignatavicius
   Anatomy and Physiology Review, 1005
      Skeletal System, 1005
      Muscular System, 1007
      Musculoskeletal Changes Associated With Aging, 1007
      Health Promotion and Maintenance, 1007
   Assessment: Noticing and Interpreting, 1008
      Patient History, 1008
      Assessment of the Skeletal System, 1009
      Assessment of the Muscular System, 1011
      Psychosocial Assessment, 1011
      Diagnostic Assessment, 1011

50 Care of Patients With Musculoskeletal Problems, 1015
Donna D. Ignatavicius
   *Osteoporosis, 1015
   Osteomyelitis, 1022
   Bone Tumors, 1024
   Disorders of the Hand, 1028
   Disorders of the Foot, 1028
      Common Foot Deformities, 1028
      Plantar Fasciitis, 1029
      Other Problems of the Foot, 1029

51 Care of Patients With Musculoskeletal Trauma, 1031
Roberta Goff and Donna D. Ignatavicius
   *Fractures, 1032
   Selected Fractures of Specific Sites, 1046
      Upper-Extremity Fractures, 1046
      Lower-Extremity Fractures, 1047
      Fractures of the Chest and Pelvis, 1049
      Compression Fractures of the Spine, 1050
   *Amputations, 1050
   Knee Injuries, 1056
   Carpal Tunnel Syndrome, 1057
   Rotator Cuff Injuries, 1059

UNIT XIII Interprofessional Collaboration for Patients With Problems of the Gastrointestinal System

52 Assessment of the Gastrointestinal System, 1061
Amy Jauch
   Anatomy and Physiology Review, 1061
      Structure, 1061
      Function, 1062
      Gastrointestinal Changes Associated With Aging, 1064

Assessment: Noticing and Interpreting, 1065
   Patient History, 1065
   Physical Assessment, 1066
   Psychosocial Assessment, 1068
   Diagnostic Assessment, 1068

53 Care of Patients With Oral Cavity Problems, 1075
Tracy Taylor
   *Stomatitis, 1076
   Oral Cavity Disorders, 1078
      Oral Tumors: Premalignant Lesions, 1078
      Oral Cancer, 1079
   Disorders of the Salivary Glands, 1084
      Acute Sialadenitis, 1084
      Post-Irradiation Sialadenitis, 1085

54 Care of Patients With Esophageal Problems, 1087
Tracy Taylor
   *Gastroesophageal Reflux Disease (GERD), 1087
   Hiatal Hernias, 1092
   *Esophageal Tumors, 1095
   Esophageal Diverticula, 1101
   Esophageal Trauma, 1101

55 Care of Patients With Stomach Disorders, 1103
Lara Carver
   Gastritis, 1103
   *Peptic Ulcer Disease (PUD), 1107
   Gastric Cancer, 1115

56 Care of Patients With Noninflammatory Intestinal Disorders, 1121
Keelin Cromar
   *Intestinal Obstruction, 1121
   Polyps, 1126
   *Colorectal Cancer, 1126
   Irritable Bowel Syndrome, 1135
   Herniation, 1137
   Hemorrhoids, 1139
   Malabsorption Syndrome, 1141

57 Care of Patients With Inflammatory Intestinal Disorders, 1144
Keelin Cromar
   Acute Inflammatory Bowel Disorders, 1144
      Peritonitis, 1144
      Appendicitis, 1147
      Gastroenteritis, 1148
   Chronic Inflammatory Bowel Disease, 1150
      Ulcerative Colitis, 1150
      Crohn's Disease, 1157
      Diverticular Disease, 1162
      Celiac Disease, 1164
   Anal Disorders, 1164
      Anorectal Abscess, 1164
      Anal Fissure, 1165
      Anal Fistula, 1165
   Parasitic Infection, 1165

58 Care of Patients With Liver Problems, 1169
Lara Carver and Jennifer Powers
   *Cirrhosis, 1169
   *Hepatitis, 1180
   Fatty Liver (Steatosis), 1185
   Liver Trauma, 1186
   Cancer of the Liver, 1186
   Liver Transplantation, 1187

59 Care of Patients With Problems of the Biliary System and Pancreas, 1191
    Lara Carver and Jennifer Powers
        *Cholecystitis, 1191
        *Acute Pancreatitis, 1197
        Chronic Pancreatitis, 1202
        Pancreatic Abscess, 1205
        Pancreatic Pseudocyst, 1205
        Pancreatic Cancer, 1205

60 Care of Patients With Malnutrition: Undernutrition and Obesity, 1211
    Laura M. Willis and Cherie Rebar
        Nutrition Standards for Health Promotion and Maintenance, 1211
        Nutrition Assessment, 1212
            Initial Nutrition Screening, 1212
            Anthropometric Measurements, 1213
        *Malnutrition, 1215
        *Obesity, 1225

UNIT XIV Interprofessional Collaboration for Patients With Problems of the Endocrine System

61 Assessment of the Endocrine System, 1234
    M. Linda Workman
        Anatomy and Physiology Review, 1235
            Hypothalamus and Pituitary Glands, 1236
            Gonads, 1237
            Adrenal Glands, 1237
            Thyroid Gland, 1238
            Parathyroid Glands, 1239
            Pancreas, 1239
            Endocrine Changes Associated With Aging, 1240
        Assessment: Noticing and Interpreting, 1240
            Patient History, 1240
            Physical Assessment, 1241
            Psychosocial Assessment, 1242
            Diagnostic Assessment, 1242

62 Care of Patients With Pituitary and Adrenal Gland Problems, 1245
    M. Linda Workman
        Disorders of the Anterior Pituitary Gland, 1245
            Hypopituitarism, 1245
            Hyperpituitarism, 1247
        Disorders of the Posterior Pituitary Gland, 1250
            Diabetes Insipidus, 1250
            Syndrome of Inappropriate Antidiuretic Hormone, 1251
        Disorders of the Adrenal Gland, 1253
            Adrenal Gland Hypofunction, 1253
            *Hypercortisolism (Cushing's Disease), 1255
            Hyperaldosteronism, 1260
            Pheochromocytoma, 1261

63 Care of Patients With Problems of the Thyroid and Parathyroid Glands, 1264
    M. Linda Workman
        Thyroid Disorders, 1264
            Hyperthyroidism, 1264
            *Hypothyroidism, 1270
            Thyroiditis, 1275
            Thyroid Cancer, 1275

        Parathyroid Disorders, 1275
            Hyperparathyroidism, 1275
            Hypoparathyroidism, 1277

64 Care of Patients With Diabetes Mellitus, 1280
    Saundra Hendricks
        *Diabetes Mellitus, 1280

UNIT XV Interprofessional Collaboration for Patients With Problems of the Renal/Urinary System

65 Assessment of the Renal/Urinary System, 1321
    Chris Winkelman
        Anatomy and Physiology Review, 1322
            Kidneys, 1322
            Ureters, 1327
            Urinary Bladder, 1327
            Urethra, 1327
            Kidney and Urinary Changes Associated With Aging, 1328
        Assessment: Noticing and Interpreting, 1329
            Patient History, 1329
            Physical Assessment, 1330
            Psychosocial Assessment, 1331
            Diagnostic Assessment, 1331

66 Care of Patients With Urinary Problems, 1343
    Chris Winkelman
        *Urinary Incontinence, 1343
        Cystitis, 1354
        Urethritis, 1359
        Urolithiasis, 1361
        Urothelial Cancer, 1366
        Bladder Trauma, 1369

67 Care of Patients With Kidney Disorders, 1372
    Chris Winkelman
        *Pyelonephritis, 1372
        Acute Glomerulonephritis, 1376
        Chronic Glomerulonephritis, 1378
        Nephrotic Syndrome, 1378
        Nephrosclerosis, 1379
        Polycystic Kidney Disease, 1379
        Hydronephrosis and Hydroureter, 1382
        Renovascular Disease, 1384
        Diabetic Nephropathy, 1384
        Renal Cell Carcinoma, 1385
        Kidney Trauma, 1387

68 Care of Patients With Acute Kidney Injury and Chronic Kidney Disease, 1390
    Chris Winkelman
        Acute Kidney Injury, 1391
        *Chronic Kidney Disease, 1398

UNIT XVI Interprofessional Collaboration for Patients With Problems of the Reproductive System

69 Assessment of the Reproductive System, 1428
    Donna D. Ignatavicius
        Anatomy and Physiology Review, 1428
            Structure and Function of the Female Reproductive System, 1428

Structure and Function of the Male Reproductive System, 1430
Reproductive Changes Associated With Aging, 1431
Health Promotion and Maintenance, 1431
Assessment: Noticing and Interpreting, 1431
Patient History, 1431
Physical Assessment, 1433
Psychosocial Assessment, 1433
Diagnostic Assessment, 1433

70 Care of Patients With Breast Disorders, 1440
Gail B. Johnson and Harriet Kumar
*Breast Cancer, 1440
Benign Breast Disorders, 1455
Fibroadenoma, 1455
Fibrocystic Breast Condition, 1455
Issues of Large-Breasted Women, 1456
Issues of Small-Breasted Women, 1456

71 Care of Patients With Gynecologic Problems, 1459
Donna D. Ignatavicius
*Uterine Leiomyoma, 1459
Pelvic Organ Prolapse, 1464
Endometrial (Uterine) Cancer, 1465
Ovarian Cancer, 1467
Cervical Cancer, 1469
Vulvovaginitis, 1470
Toxic Shock Syndrome, 1471

72 Care of Patients With Male Reproductive Problems, 1473
Donna D. Ignatavicius
*Benign Prostatic Hyperplasia, 1474
*Prostate Cancer, 1481
Testicular Cancer, 1486
Erectile Dysfunction, 1489

73 Care of Transgender Patients, 1492
Donna D. Ignatavicius and Stephanie M. Fox
Patient-Centered Terminology, 1493
Transgender Health Issues, 1494
Stress and Transgender Health, 1494
The Need to Improve Transgender Health Care, 1494

74 Care of Patients With Sexually Transmitted Infections, 1504
Donna D. Ignatavicius
Overview, 1504
Health Promotion and Maintenance, 1505
Genital Herpes, 1506
Syphilis, 1508
Condylomata Acuminata (Genital Warts), 1510
Chlamydia Infection, 1511
Gonorrhea, 1512
*Pelvic Inflammatory Disease, 1514

Glossary, G-1
NCLEX® Examination Challenges Answer Key, AK-1

GUIDE TO SPECIAL FEATURES

BEST PRACTICE FOR PATIENT SAFETY AND QUALITY CARE

Acute Adrenal Insufficiency, 1253

AIDS, Infection Control for Home Care, 357

Alteplase, Nursing Interventions During and After Administration, 936

Altitude-Related Illnesses, 146

Alzheimer's Disease, Promoting Communication, 863

Anaphylaxis, 365

Anesthesia, Spinal and Epidural, Recognizing Serious Complications, 275

Anticoagulant Therapy, 744

Anticoagulant, Fibrinolytic, or Antiplatelet Therapy and Prevention of Injury, 623

Arteriovenous Fistula or Arteriovenous Graft, 1415

Artificial Airway Suctioning, 541

Aspiration Prevention During Swallowing, 543

Autologous Blood Salvage and Transfusion, Intraoperative, 264

Autonomic Dysreflexia: Immediate Interventions, 898

Benzodiazepine Overdose, 281

Breast Mass Assessment, 1445

Breast Reconstruction, Postoperative Care, 1451

Breast Self-Examination, 1444

Burn Patient and Fluid Resuscitation, 495

Burns, Emergency Management, 489

Cancer Pain Management with Intrathecal Pump, 62

Carpal Tunnel Syndrome Prevention, 1058

Catheter-Associated Urinary Tract Infections (CAUTI), 1356

Cervical Diskectomy and Fusion, 910

Chest Discomfort, 775

Chest Tube Drainage System Management, 592

Chronic Diarrhea, Special Skin Care, 1142

Cognition Assessment, 847

Colonoscopy, 1073

Colorectal Cancer Screening Recommendations, 1128

Communicating With Patients Unable To Speak, 550

Continuous Passive Motion (CPM) Machine, 316

Contractures, Positioning to Prevent, 503

Dark Skin, Assessing Changes, 444

Death Pronouncement, 114

Dehydration, 169

Diagnostic Testing, Precautions for Use of Iodine-Based or Gadolinium Contrast, 852

Diarrhea, 19

Driver Safety Improvement in Older Adults, 34

Dysrhythmias, 672

Ear Irrigation, 994

Eardrops Instillation, 993

Emergency Department and Patient and Staff Safety, 120

Endocrine Testing, 1243

Energy Conservation, 826

Esophageal Surgery and Nasogastric Tube, 1100

Extremity Fracture, 1038

Eyedrops Instillation, 966

Fall Prevention in Older Adults, 41

Feeding Tube Maintenance, 1222

Fires in Health Care Facility, 150

Fluid Volume Management, 1405

Fundoplication Procedures and Postoperative Complications, 1094

Gait Training, 95

Gastrointestinal Health History, 1065

Genetic Testing and Counseling, 82

Genital Herpes, Self-Management, 1507

Gynecologic Cancer, Brachytherapy and Health Teaching, 1466

Hand Hygiene, 418

Hearing Impairment and Communication, 998

Heart Transplant, Signs and Symptoms of Rejection, 716

Heat Stroke, 135

Hemodialysis, 1416

HIV, Recommendations for Preventing Transmission by Health Care Workers, 345

Hypertensive Urgency or Crisis, 727

Hypokalemia, 177

Hypophysectomy, 1249

Hypovolemic Shock, 759

Immunity, Reduced, Care of Hospitalized Patients, 351

Infection, Nursing Interventions for the Patient at Risk, 417

Inflammatory Bowel Disease, Pain Control and Skin Care, 1156

Intestinal Obstruction, 1124

Intraoperative Positioning, Prevention of Complications, 267

Kidney Test or Procedure Using Contrast Medium, 1338

LGBTQ Patients, TJC Recommendations for Creating Safe Environment, 1495

Lumbar Spinal Surgery, Assessment and Management of Complications, 907

Magnetic Resonance Imaging Preparation, 1013

Malignant Hyperthermia, 260

Mechanical Ventilation Care, 630

Meningitis, 882

Minimally Invasive Inguinal Hernia Repair (MIIHR), 1139

Musculoskeletal Injury Prevention, 908

Musculoskeletal Injury, Neurovascular Status Assessment, 1037

Myasthenia Gravis, Improving Nutrition, 921

Myelosuppression and Neutropenia, 397

Myxedema Coma, 1274

Nosebleed, Anterior, 557

Nutrition Screening Assessment, 1213

Ocular Irrigation, 981

Ophthalmic Ointment Instillation, 970

Opioid Overdose, 285

Oral Cavity Problems, 1077

Oxygen Therapy, 530

Pain, Reducing Postoperative and Promoting Comfort, 285

Paracentesis, 1177

Parkinson Disease, 870

Pericarditis, 713

Peritoneal Dialysis Catheter, 1420

Phlebostatic Axis Identification, 780

Plasmapheresis, Preventing and Managing Complications, 915
Postmortem Care, 114
Postoperative Hand-off Report, 271
Post-Traumatic Stress Disorder Prevention in Staff Following a Mass Casualty Event, 156
Pressure Injuries and Wound Management, 457
Pressure Injury Prevention, 449
Primary Osteoporosis, Risk Assessment, 1017
Prostatectomy, Open Radical, 1484
Pulmonary Embolism Prevention, 617
Pulmonary Embolism, 619
Radioactive Sealed Implants, 389
Relocation Stress in Older Adults, 33
Reproductive Health Problem Assessment, 1432
Restraint Alternatives, 42
Seizures, Tonic-Clonic or Complete Partial, 878
Sickle Cell Crisis, 811
Skin Problem, Nursing History, 435
Sports-Related Injuries, 1056
Surgical Wound Evisceration, 283
Systemic Sclerosis and Esophagitis, 330
Thrombocytopenia and Prevention of Injury, 398
Thrombocytopenia, 825
Thyroid Storm, 1270
Total Parenteral Nutrition, Care and Maintenance, 1224
Tracheostomy Care, 542
Transfusion in Older Adults, 834
Transfusion Therapy, 833
Transurethral Resection of the Prostate, 1480
Tube-Feeding Care and Maintenance, 1221
Urinary Incontinence, Bladder Training and Habit Training to Reduce, 1351
Venous Catheters, Placement of Short Peripheral, 203
Vertebroplasty and Kyphoplasty, 1050
Viral Hepatitis Prevention in Health Care Workers, 1182
Vision Reduction, 975
Wandering, Prevention in Hospitalized Patients, 864
Wound Care, Perineal, 1133
Wound Monitoring, 460

COMMON EXAMPLES OF DRUG THERAPY

Acute Coronary Syndrome (Nitrates, Beta Blockers, Antiplatelets), 776
Adrenal Gland Hypofunction, 1255
Antidysrhythmic Medication, 677
Asthma, 569
Biologic Disease-Modifying Antirheumatic Drugs (DMARDs), 370
Biological Response Modifiers for Rheumatoid Arthritis and Other Connective Tissue Diseases, 323
Burn Wounds, 501
Diabetes Mellitus, 1292
Glaucoma, 976
HIV Infection, 351
Hypertension Management, 725
Hyperthyroidism, 1268
Hypovolemic Shock, 759
Inhalation Anthrax, Prophylaxis and Treatment, 612
Intravenous Vasodilators and Inotropes, 783
Kidney Disease, 1410
Nausea and Vomiting, Chemotherapy-Induced, 399

Osteoporosis, 1021
Pain, Postoperative, 284
Peptic Ulcer Disease, 1106
Plaque Psoriasis, 466
Pulmonary Embolism, 621
Transplant Rejection, 302
Tuberculosis, First-Line Treatment, 608
Urinary Incontinence, 1350
Urinary Tract Infections, 1360

CONCEPT MAP

Benign Prostatic Hyperplasia, 1478
Chronic Kidney Disease, 1406
Chronic Obstructive Pulmonary Disease, 575
Cirrhosis, 1176
Community-Acquired Pneumonia (CAP), 602
Diabetes Mellitus Type 2, 1290
Hypertension, 724
Hypovolemic Shock, 757
Multiple Sclerosis, 893
Pressure Injury, 456
Primary Open-Angle Glaucoma, 973

KEY FEATURES

Acidosis, 193
Acute Leukemia, 819
Adrenal Insufficiency, 1254
AIDS, 346
Alkalosis, 196
Alzheimer's Disease, 860
Anaphylaxis, 364
Anemia, 814
Angina and Myocardial Infarction, 773
Asthma Control Levels, 566
Asthma Control, Step System for Medication Use, 566
Autonomic Dysreflexia, 896
Bowel Obstructions, Small and Large, 1123
Brain Tumors, Common, 951
Celiac Disease, 1164
Cervical Diskectomy and Fusion Complications, 910
Cholecystitis, 1193
Compartment Syndrome, 1034
Cor Pulmonale, 574
Diabetes Insipidus, 1250
Esophageal Tumors, 1096
Fluid Overload, 172
Gastric Cancer, Early Versus Advanced, 1116
Gastritis, 1105
Gastroesophageal Reflux Disease, 1088
Gastrointestinal Bleeding, Upper, 1109
Guillain-Barré Syndrome, 914
Heat Stroke, 134
Hiatal Hernias, 1093
Hypercortisolism (Cushing's Disease/Syndrome), 1257
Hyperthyroidism, 1265
Hypothermia, 143
Hypothyroidism, 1271
Infective Endocarditis, 711
Inhalation Anthrax, 612
Intracranial Pressure (ICP), Increased, 936

Kidney Disease, Severe Chronic and End-Stage, 1403
Liver Trauma, 1186
Meningitis, 881
Migraine Headaches, 874
Multiple Sclerosis, 889
Myasthenia Gravis, 917
Nephrotic Syndrome, 1379
Oral Cancer, 1080
Osteomyelitis, Acute and Chronic, 1023
Pancreatic Cancer, 1206
Pancreatitis, Chronic, 1203
Peripheral Arterial Disease, Chronic, 732
Peritonitis, 1145
Pituitary Hyperfunction, 1248
Pituitary Hypofunction, 1246
Polycystic Kidney Disease, 1381
Pressure Injuries, 452
Pulmonary Edema, 702
Pulmonary Emboli: Fat Embolism Versus Blood Clot
    Embolism, 1034
Pulmonary Embolism, 618
Pyelonephritis, Acute, 1374
Pyelonephritis, Chronic, 1374
Renovascular Disease, 1384
Rheumatoid Arthritis, 318
Shock, 752
Skin Conditions, Inflammatory, 463
Skin Infections, Common, 467
Stroke Syndromes, 933
Strokes, Left and Right Hemisphere, 933
Sustained Tachydysrhythmias and Bradydysrhythmias, 672
Systemic Lupus Erythematosus (SLE) and Systemic
    Sclerosis (SSc), 326
Transient Ischemic Attack, 928
Traumatic Brain Injury, Mild, 945
Ulcers, Lower-Extremity, 734
Uremia, 1398
Urinary Tract Infection, 1358
Valvular Heart Disease, 706
Ventricular Failure, Left, 695
Ventricular Failure, Right, 696

EVIDENCE-BASED PRACTICE

Ambulation and Ambulation Protocol Effectiveness, 24
Benign Prostatic Hyperplasia Surgery and
    Quality of Life, 1481
Bone Loss, Risk Factors in Men, 1017
Central Venous Access Device, Best Method for Securing, 213
Chronic Pain Management in Older Adults, 56
Dementia Caregivers and Telephone Support, 867
End-of-Life Care for Prisoners, 106
Hearing Loss in Combat, 997
Heat Stroke and On-Site Treatment, 135
Hepatitis C, Care of Military Veterans, 1183
Hip Fracture, Resources for Caregivers, 1049
HIV Self-Management and mHealth Technology Among
    African-American Women, 345
Hysterectomy and Sexuality, 1462
Noninvasive Ventilation (NIV) Effectiveness, 535
Opioid Usage, 279
Oral Care, Preoperative and Postsurgical Outcomes, 1082

Preoperative Assessment, 239
Pressure Injury Reduction Using Skin Integrity
    Care Bundle, 449
Sickle Cell Disease and Self-Care in Young Adults, 813
Traumatic Brain Injury (TBI) and Mannitol to Reduce
    Mortality, 948
Veterans with Dementia, Reducing Hospital Admissions and
    Emergency Department Visits, 126

FOCUSED ASSESSMENT

AIDS, 356
Diabetic Foot, 1306
Diabetic Patient, Home or Clinic Visit, 1318
Hearing, 998
Hypophysectomy for Hyperpituitarism, 1249
Infection Risk, 821
Kidney Transplant, 1425
Oral Cancer and the Postoperative Older Adult, 1082
Pneumonia Recovery, 605
Postanesthesia Care Unit Discharge to
    Medical-Surgical Unit, 272
Preoperative Patient, 238
Pressure Injuries, 461
Seizures, Nursing Observations and Documentation, 878
Sexually Transmitted Infection, 1507
Thyroid Dysfunction, 1274
Total Abdominal Hysterectomy, Postoperative Care, 1462
Tracheostomy, 542
Urinary Incontinence, 1346

HOME CARE ASSESSMENT

Amputation, Lower-Extremity, 1056
Breast Cancer Surgery Recovery, 1453
Cataract Surgery, 971
Chronic Obstructive Pulmonary Disease, 581
Colostomy, 1134
Heart Failure, 704
Inflammatory Bowel Disease, 1158
Laryngectomy, 554
Myocardial Infarction, 790
Peripheral Vascular Disease, 737
Pulmonary Embolism, 624
Sepsis Risk, 766
Ulcer Disease, 1115

LABORATORY PROFILE

Acid-Base Assessment, 188
Acid-Base Imbalances (Uncompensated), 193
Adrenal Gland Assessment, 1255
Anticoagulation Therapy and Monitoring With
    Blood Tests, 622
Blood Glucose Values, 1288
Burn Assessment During the Resuscitation Phase, 493
Cardiovascular Assessment, 656
Connective Tissue Disease, 320
Gastrointestinal Assessment, 1069
Hematologic Assessment, 804
Hypovolemic Shock, 758
Kidney Disease, 1395

Kidney Function Blood Studies, 1332
Musculoskeletal Assessment, 1012
Parathyroid Function, 1276
Reproductive Assessment, 1434
Respiratory Assessment, 522
Thyroid Function for Adults, 1267
Urinalysis, 1333
Urine Collections, 24-Hour, 1336

NURSING FOCUS ON THE OLDER ADULT

Acid-Base Imbalance, 191
Burn Injury Complications, 490
Cancer Assessment, 380
Cardiovascular System, 647
Cerumen Impaction, 995
Coronary Artery Bypass Graft Surgery, 790
Coronary Artery Disease, 779
Diverticulitis, 1163
Dysrhythmias, 682
Ear and Hearing Changes, 987
Electrolyte Values, 165
Endocrine System Changes, 1241
Eye and Vision Changes, 961
Fecal Impaction Prevention, 1126
Fluid Balance, 165
Gastrointestinal System Changes, 1064
Heat-Related Illness Prevention, 134
Hematologic Assessment, 800
Immune Function, 291
Infection, Factors That May Increase Risk, 415
Integumentary System, 434
Intraoperative Nursing Interventions, 264
Low Back Pain, 904
Malnutrition Risk Assessment, 1216
Musculoskeletal System Changes, 1007
Nervous System, 845
Nutrition Intake Promotion, 1219
Pain, 59
Preoperative Considerations for Care Planning, 236
Renal System Changes, 1328
Reproductive System Changes, 1431
Respiratory Disorder, Chronic, 564
Respiratory System, 513
Shock, Risk Factors, 764
Skin Care, Postoperative, 281
Spinal Cord Injury, 902
Surgical Risk Factors, 234
Thyroid Problems, 1274
Total Hip Arthroplasty, 311
Traumatic Brain Injury, 944
Urinary Incontinence, Contributing Factors, 1346
Vision Impairment, Promoting Independent Living, 974

PATIENT AND FAMILY EDUCATION: PREPARING FOR SELF-MANAGEMENT

Arthritis and Energy Conservation, 324
Arthropod Bite/Sting Prevention, 137
Asthma Management, 568
Bariatric Surgery, Discharge Teaching, 1231
Beta Blocker/Digoxin Therapy, 705

Bleeding Risk, 827
Brain Injury, Mild, 949
Breast Cancer Surgery Recovery, 1453
Breathing Exercises, 578
Cancer Risk, Dietary Habits to Reduce, 379
Cardioverter/Defibrillator, 688
Caregiver Stress Reduction, 866
Cast Removal and Extremity Care, 1045
Central Venous Catheter Home Care, 826
Cerumen Removal and Self–Ear Irrigation, 987
Cervical Ablation Therapies, 1470
Cervical Biopsy Recovery, 1437
Chest Pain Management at Home, 792
Cirrhosis, 1179
Condom Use, 1508
Coronary Artery Disease and Activity, 791
Coronary Artery Disease Prevention, 771
Cortisol Replacement Therapy, 1260
Death, Emotional Signs of Approaching, 108
Death, Physical Manifestations, 113
Death, Physical Signs and Symptoms of Approaching, 107
Dry Powder Inhaler (DPI) Use, 571
Dry Skin Prevention, 462
Dysrhythmias Prevention, 682
Ear Infection or Trauma Prevention, 1000
Ear Surgery Recovery, 993
Epilepsy and Health Teaching, 880
Epinephrine Injectors, Care and Use of Automatic, 364
Exercise, 1301
Eyedrops Use, 962
Foot Care Instructions, 1307
Gastritis Prevention, 1104
Gastroenteritis, Preventing Transmission, 1150
Glucosamine Supplements, 309
Halo Device, 899
Hearing Aid Care, 999
HIV Testing and One-Time Screening, CDC Recommendations, 341
Hyperkalemia, Nutritional Management, 179
Hypoglycemia, Home Management, 1310
Hysterectomy, Total Vaginal or Abdominal, 1463
Ileostomy Care, 1157
Infection Prevention, 351
Infection Prevention, 397
Infection Prevention, 827
Inhaler, Correct Use, 570
Injury and Bleeding Prevention, 398
Injury and Bleeding Prevention, 623
Insulin Administration, Subcutaneous, 1297
Joint Protection Instructions, 317
Kidney and Genitourinary Trauma Prevention, 1387
Kidney and Urinary Problem Prevention, 1402
Laparoscopic Nissen Fundoplication (LNF) and Paraesophageal Repair via Laparoscope, Postoperative Instructions, 1094
Laryngectomy Home Care, 554
Leg Exercises, Postoperative, 245
Lightning Strike Prevention, 141
Low Back Pain and Injury Prevention, 904
Low Back Pain Exercises, 906
Lupus Erythematosus and Skin Protection, 328
Lyme Disease Prevention and Early Detection, 333

Migraine Attack Triggers, 876
MRSA, Preventing Spread, 469
Mucositis and Mouth Care, 400
Myasthenia Gravis and Drug Therapy, 922
Oral Cancer and Home Care, 1083
Oral Cavity Maintenance, 1076
Osteoarthritis and Rheumatoid Arthritis Exercises, 317
Pacemakers, Permanent, 676
Pancreatitis, Chronic, Enzyme Replacement, 1203
Pancreatitis, Chronic, Prevention of Exacerbations, 1204
Peak Flow Meter Use, 568
Pelvic Muscle Exercises, 1347
Peripheral Neuropathy, Chemotherapy-Induced, 401
Peripheral Vascular Disease and Foot Care, 737
Pneumonia Prevention, 600
Polycystic Kidney Disease, 1382
Polycythemia Vera, 817
Post-Mastectomy Exercises, 1449
Radiation Therapy and Skin Protection, 390
Radioactive Isotope Safety Precautions, 1269
Reflux Control, 1090
Respiratory Care, Perioperative, 244
Sexually Transmitted Infections and Oral
    Antibiotic Therapy, 1516
Sick-Day Rules, 1314
Sickle Cell Crisis Prevention, 812
Skin Cancer Prevention, 476
Smoking Cessation, 515
Snakebite Prevention, 136
Sperm Banking, 1488
Stretta Procedure, Postoperative Instructions, 1091
Stroke and Modifiable Risk Factors, 930
Supraglottic Method of Swallowing, 553
Testicular Self-Examination, 1486
Total Hip Arthroplasty, 312

Toxic Shock Syndrome Prevention, 1471
Urinary Calculi, 1366
Urinary Catheter Care at Home, 1486
Urinary Incontinence, 1353
Urinary Tract Infection Prevention, 1357
Valvular Heart Disease, 710
Venous Insufficiency, 747
Viral Hepatitis, 1185
Viral Hepatitis, Health Practices to Prevent, 1182
Vulvovaginitis Prevention, 1471
Warfarin (Coumadin) and Interference of
    Food and Drugs, 746
Wellness Promotion Through Lifestyles and Practices, 30
West Nile Virus Protection, 884

QUALITY IMPROVEMENT

Core Measure and Interprofessional Collaboration, 601
Diabetes and Increasing Blood Glucose Control and
    Insulin-Mealtime Match, 1310
Electrode Placement and Proper Skin Preparation, 668
Improving Medication Reconciliation With a Nurse-Led
    Protocol, 4
Joint Replacement and Shortening Hospital
    Length of Stay, 314
Opioid-Induced Respiratory Depression, Reducing with
    Capnography, 524
Oral Anticancer Agents, Text Message Reminders Improve
    Adherence, 394
Safe Handling Practices and Protection of
    Health Care Staff, 93
Sepsis, Early Recognition and Intervention, 763
Surgical Site Infection Prevention, 786
Tracheostomies and Reducing Caregiver Anxiety, 555
Urinary Tract Infections, Reducing Catheter-Associated, 415

CHAPTER | 1

Overview of Professional Nursing Concepts for Medical-Surgical Nursing

Donna D. Ignatavicius

http://evolve.elsevier.com/Iggy/

PRIORITY AND INTERRELATED CONCEPTS

The priority concepts for this chapter are:
- PATIENT-CENTERED CARE
- SAFETY
- TEAMWORK AND INTERPROFESSIONAL COLLABORATION
- EVIDENCE-BASED PRACTICE
- QUALITY IMPROVEMENT

- INFORMATICS AND TECHNOLOGY
- CLINICAL JUDGMENT
- ETHICS
- HEALTH CARE ORGANIZATIONS
- HEALTH CARE DISPARITIES

LEARNING OUTCOMES

Safe and Effective Care Environment
1. Briefly describe the scope of medical-surgical nursing.
2. Explain the current priority focus on patient SAFETY and quality of care.
3. Identify the purpose and function of the Rapid Response Team (RRT).
4. Differentiate the six core Quality and Safety Education for Nurses (QSEN) competencies that interprofessional health care team members need to provide safe, PATIENT-CENTERED CARE.
5. Identify six major ETHICS principles that help guide decision making and CLINICAL JUDGMENT.
6. Communicate patient values, preferences, and expressed needs to other members of the INTERPROFESSIONAL health care team for effective COLLABORATION.
7. Outline the five rights of the delegation and supervision process.

8. Describe the SBAR procedure for successful hand-off communication in health care agencies.
9. Describe the nurse's role in the systematic QUALITY IMPROVEMENT process.
10. Identify three ways that INFORMATICS AND TECHNOLOGY are used in health care.
11. Outline the major differences in types of HEALTH CARE ORGANIZATIONS.

Psychosocial Integrity
12. Explain why many minority populations such as members of the LGBTQ community are at risk for HEALTH CARE DISPARITIES.
13. Identify the role of the nurse when communicating with LGBTQ patients.

Medical-surgical nursing, sometimes called *adult health nursing,* is a specialty practice area in which nurses promote, restore, or maintain optimal health for patients from 18 to older than 100 years of age (Academy of Medical-Surgical Nurses [AMSN], 2012). A separate chapter on care of older adults is part of this textbook because the majority of medical-surgical patients in most health care settings are older than 65 years (see Chapter

3). In addition, special features throughout the book highlight the unique needs of older adults.

To be consistent with the most recent health care literature, the authors use the term *patient* rather than *client* (except in NCLEX Examination Challenge questions where *client* is used to reflect that licensure examination). To be patient-centered, be sure to refer to individuals according to the policy of the health care organization and the individual's preference. The *family* refers to the patient's relatives and significant others in the patient's life whom the patient identifies and values as important.

Medical-surgical nursing is practiced in many types of settings, such as acute care agencies, skilled nursing facilities, ambulatory care clinics, and the patient's home, which could be either a single residence or group setting such as an assisted living facility. The role of the nurse in these settings includes care coordinator and transition manager, caregiver, patient educator, leader, and patient and family advocate. To function in these various roles, nurses need to have the knowledge, skills, attitudes, and abilities (KSAs) to keep patients and their families safe.

This chapter reviews 10 nursing concepts needed for effective professional practice. Six of the 10 concepts are Quality and Safety Education for Nurses core competencies. The additional four concepts are also essential to nursing practice and are typically introduced in foundations or fundamentals of nursing courses. For more information about these concepts, see your foundations or fundamentals of nursing textbook.

QUALITY AND SAFETY EDUCATION FOR NURSES CORE COMPETENCIES

The Institute of Medicine (IOM, now the National Academy of Medicine [NAM]), a highly respected U.S. organization that monitors health care and recommends health policy, published many reports during the past 20 years suggesting ways to improve patient safety and quality care. One of its reports, *Health Professions Education: A Bridge to Quality,* identified five broad core competencies for health care professionals to ensure patient safety and quality care (Institute of Medicine [IOM], 2003). All of these competencies are interrelated and include:

- Provide *patient-centered care.*
- *Collaborate* with the interdisciplinary health care team.
- Implement *evidence-based practice.*
- Use *quality improvement* in patient care.
- Use *informatics* in patient care.

Several years later, the QSEN initiative, now called the *QSEN Institute,* validated the IOM (NAM) competencies for nursing practice and added *safety* as a sixth competency to emphasize its importance. More information about the QSEN Institute can be found on its website at www.qsen.org.

In addition to emphasizing these six QSEN competency concepts, the authors selected four professional nursing concepts to integrate throughout the text. This chapter reviews these 10 nursing concepts, and includes the concept definition, scope, and attributes (characteristics) for each one. Each concept review then ends with examples of how the concept is used in practice. The 10 concepts reviewed in this chapter are:

- Patient-centered care
- Safety
- Teamwork and interprofessional collaboration
- Evidence-based practice
- Quality improvement
- Informatics and technology
- Clinical judgment
- Ethics
- Health care organizations
- Health care disparities

PATIENT-CENTERED CARE

Definition of Patient-Centered Care

To be competent in patient-centered, the nurse recognizes "the patient or designee as the source of control and full partner in providing compassionate and coordinated care based on respect for [the] patient's preferences, values, and needs" (Quality and Safety Education for Nurses [QSEN], 2011). Implied in this widely used definition is the need for the nurse to be culturally competent when caring for diverse patients and their families. The Joint Commission, a major accrediting organization for health care agencies, uses the term *family-centered care* to emphasize the importance of including the patient's support system as part of interprofessional collaboration.

Scope of Patient-Centered Care

Patient-centered care has been a focus of health professions' education and research for several decades. Prior to this period of time, patients in inpatient facilities and their families often had little to no input into their health care. Many health care professionals believed that they were better-prepared than patients to make care decisions and did not consistently include the patient and family in this process. The Joint Commission and other organizations called for the rights of patients or their designees (e.g., family members, guardians) to make their own informed decisions. The IOM (now NAM) further emphasized the need for all health care agencies to place patients and their families at the center of the interprofessional team to make mutual decisions based on patient preferences and values.

Attributes of Patient-Centered Care

The attributes, or characteristics, of patient-centered care were identified by researchers as a result of a classic medical study (Frampton, et al., 2008). These attributes include:

- Respect for patients' values, preferences, and expressed needs
- Coordination and integration of care
- Information, communication, and education
- Physical comfort
- Emotional support and alleviation of fear and anxiety
- Involvement of family and friends
- Transition and continuity
- Access to care

Showing respect for the patient and family's preferences and needs is essential to ensure a holistic or "whole person" approach to care. To help illustrate the importance of culture and spirituality, and prepare nursing students for a multicultural society, this text includes *Cultural/Spiritual Considerations* features to highlight this important information. Additional features that focus on the culture and needs of special populations include:

- *Considerations for Older Adults*
- *Gender Health Considerations*
- *Veterans' Health Considerations*

Canadian nursing practice includes culture from a safety perspective. Promoting safety requires nursing practice that respects and nurtures the unique and dynamic characteristics of patients and families to meet their needs, preferences, values, and rights (Doane & Varcoe, 2015). Cultural safety is part of relational inquiry and practice and is valued in Canada as a major attribute in professional nursing.

TABLE 1-1 Examples of Integrative (Complementary and Alternative) Therapies Used in Health Care Organizations

- Pet therapy
- Massage therapy
- Guided imagery
- Biofeedback
- Exercise and fitness programs
- Nutritional supplements
- Massage therapy
- Health-focused television
- Music therapy
- Acupuncture
- Acupressure
- Disease management programs

Examples of Context of Patient-Centered Care to Nursing and Health Care

Patient-centered care is a major emphasis in all health care settings. For example, many health care organizations integrate complementary and alternative medicine (CAM) as a supplement to traditional health care to meet the preferences of patients and their families. This *integrative care* model is in response to the increasing use of these therapies by consumers to maintain health and help manage chronic health issues, such as joint pain, back pain, and anxiety or depression (Halm & Katseres, 2015). Integrative care reflects nursing theories of caring, compassion, and holism to *respect the diverse preferences and needs* of patients and their families. Examples of these therapies are listed in Table 1-1. Specific complementary and integrative therapies are highlighted throughout this text as appropriate.

Patients want to have their *basic physical care and comfort needs* met. For example, patients in a variety of settings often experience acute and/or chronic pain. Nurses continually assess the patient's pain management needs and implement interventions to relieve or reduce pain in a timely manner. Chapter 4 describes pain assessment and interventions in detail.

After discharge from a hospital or other inpatient setting, patients also have a need for individualized coordinated care. Many patients discharged from a hospital, especially older adults, are readmitted within 30 days at a cost of more than $4 billion due to lack of coordinated care (Polster, 2015; Stubenrauch, 2015). Care coordination is the deliberate organization of and communication about patient care activities between two or more members of the health care team (including the patient) to facilitate appropriate and continuous health care to meet that patient's needs (Lamb, 2014). One of the most important members of the health care team who assists with care coordination is the case manager (CM) or discharge planner, who is typically a nurse or social worker in health care agencies.

The purpose of the case management process is to provide quality and cost-effective services and resources to achieve positive patient outcomes. In collaboration with the nurse, the CM coordinates inpatient and community-based care before discharge from a hospital or other facility. Part of that process may involve communicating with other CMs who are employed by third-party health care payers (e.g., Medicare) to keep patients from being readmitted to the hospital.

In addition to coordination and access of care following hospital discharge, transitions of care (also called transition management) are essential to prevent adverse events and hospital readmissions. Transition management involves safe and seamless movement of patients among health care settings, health care providers, and the community for ongoing care to meet patient needs. The Joint Commission (2013) recommends these components for effective care coordination and transition management:

- Understandable discharge instructions for the patient and family
- Explanation of self-care activities
- Ongoing or emergency care information
- List of community and outpatient (ambulatory care) resources and referrals
- Knowledge of the patient's language, culture, and health literacy
- Medication reconciliation (also a Joint Commission National Patient Safety Goal)

Medication reconciliation is a formal evaluative process in which the patient's actual current medications are compared to his or her prescribed medications at time of admission, transfer, or discharge to identify and resolve discrepancies. The types of information that clinicians use to reconcile medications include drug name, dose, frequency, route, and purpose. This comparison addresses duplications, omissions, and interactions and the need to continue current medications. Medication discrepancies can cause negative patient outcomes, including rehospitalizations for medical complications. A quality improvement project by Ruggerio et al. (2015) demonstrated the effectiveness of a medication reconciliation process by increasing the accuracy of information provided to patients at discharge in a large metropolitan hospital system (see the Quality Improvement box).

In this text the authors use the heading *Care Coordination and Transition Management* to describe the specific activities, including medication reconciliation and discharge health teaching that are essential for patients with selected health problems and their families. Nurses play a major role in coordinating this care with the interprofessional team to promote safe, quality care.

SAFETY

Definition of Safety

Safety is the ability to keep the patient and staff free from harm and minimize errors in care. Health care errors by providers, nurses, and other professionals have been widely reported for the past 20 years. Many of these errors resulted in patient injuries or deaths, and increased health care costs. A number of national and international organizations implemented new programs and standards to combat this growing problem.

Scope of Safety

Safety is essential for patients, staff members, and health care organizations. Although most literature discusses safety for patients, safety for members of the staff and interprofessional team is equally important. The scope of safety can be described as *unsafe*, possibly causing harm or even death, or *safe* to prevent harm or negative outcomes. Nurses have accountability for and play a key role in promoting safety and preventing errors, including "missed nursing care," the necessary care that should have been provided by one or more nurses.

Patient harm and errors generally occur as a result of (Benner et al., 2010):

- Lack of clear or adequate communication among patient, family, and members of the interprofessional health care team

QUALITY IMPROVEMENT ⟨QSEN⟩

Improving Medication Reconciliation With a Nurse-Led Protocol

Ruggerio, J., Smith, J., Copeland, J., & Boxer, B. (2015). Discharge time out: An innovative nurse-driven protocol for medication reconciliation. *MEDSURG Nursing*, *24*(3), 165–172.

Medication reconciliation is a requirement for agencies accredited by The Joint Commission to ensure consistency between admission medications and those prescribed at discharge. A retrospective medical record review by nurse leaders at a large East Coast metropolitan hospital found a 77.9% discrepancy rate between admission and discharge medication reconciliation forms. Physician staff, most often residents, completed these forms before patient discharge. Three problem areas were identified: medication omissions, changes in doses at discharge without prescriptions, and omission of core measures requirements.

An oversight interprofessional team was formed to decrease these problems; the Define Measure Analyze Improve Control (DMAIC) methodology was used to guide the improvement process. A decision was made to transfer the responsibility of medication reconciliation from physician staff to nursing staff. All nurses on the pilot unit were educated on how to complete the reconciliation forms accurately during a patient discharge time-out. As a result of implementation and follow-up for 20 months, the discharge discrepancies decreased from 77.9% to 21.2%. These data showed the benefit of the new nurse-led protocol for discharge medication reconciliation.

Commentary: Implications for Practice and Research

In 2011 the Institute of Medicine (now the National Academy of Medicine) called on nurses to lead and coordinate collaborative improvement initiatives to transform their practice and the health care systems in which they work. This project was consistent with this goal by empowering nurses to identify and improve problems that affect patient safety. But the limitation of this project is that it is unknown whether the decrease in errors was the result of awareness of the issue or if using nurses rather than medical residents improved accuracy. More research is needed to answer this question.

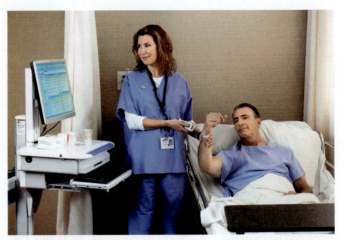

FIG. 1-1 Example of a bar-code medication administration (BCMA) system. (Courtesy Zebra Technologies).

Three types of *Nursing Safety Priority* boxes are found throughout this text to emphasize its importance in daily practice. These features delineate safety based on patient and/or staff need. For example, *Nursing Safety Priority: Critical Rescue* emphasizes the need for action for potential or actual life-threatening problems. *Nursing Safety Priority: Action Alert* boxes focus on the need for action but not necessarily for life-threatening situations. But safety alerts are essential to ensure optimal outcomes. As the name implies, *Nursing Safety Priority: Drug Alert* boxes specify actions needed to ensure safety related to drug administration, monitoring, or related patient and family education.

Examples of Context of Safety to Nursing and Health Care

In 2002 The Joint Commission (TJC) published its first annual National Patient Safety Goals (NPSGs). These goals require health care organizations to focus on specific priority safety practices, many of which involve establishing nursing and health system approaches to safe care. Since that time, TJC continues to add new goals each year. NPSGs address high-risk issues such as safe drug administration, prevention of health care–associated infections, and communication effectiveness among the interprofessional team. When appropriate, this textbook highlights related NPSGs. A complete list of the latest goals can be found on the TJC website at www.jointcommission.org.

The Joint Commission (TJC) requires that health care organizations create a culture of safety. A culture of safety provides a blame-free approach to improving care in high-risk, error-prone health care organizations using interprofessional collaboration. Patients and families are encouraged to become safety partners in protecting patients from harm. In this environment, nurses and other interprofessional health team members should not hesitate to report and document errors or missed care using appropriate internal organizational documents for risk management, quality improvement, and staff education purposes. These variations in the standard of care are often referred to as adverse events. The Joint Commission requires that health care organizations report serious adverse events, known as *sentinel events*. A sentinel event is a severe variation in the standard of care that is caused by

- Lack of attentiveness and patient monitoring
- Lack of clinical judgment
- Inadequate measures to prevent health complications
- Errors in medication administration
- Errors in interpreting authorized provider prescriptions
- Lack of professional accountability and patient advocacy
- Inability to carry out interventions in an appropriate and timely manner
- Lack of mandatory reporting

Attributes of Safety

Patient and staff safety is a major priority for professional nurses. Best safety practices reduce error and harm through established protocols, memory checklists, and systems such as bar-code medication administration (BCMA) (Fig. 1-1). Maintaining safety requires that nurses and other health care professionals use these systems and practices consistently and as specified to achieve positive outcomes. Working around these systems (often called *work-arounds)* is not acceptable and can increase the risk of error to patients and/or staff.

human or system error and results in an avoidable patient death or major harm.

TEAMWORK AND INTERPROFESSIONAL COLLABORATION

Definition of Teamwork and Interprofessional Collaboration

To provide patient- and family-centered care, the nurse "functions effectively within nursing and interprofessional teams, fostering open communication, mutual respect, and shared decision-making to achieve quality patient care" (QSEN, 2011). Therefore the knowledge and skills needed for this competency are effective communication and team functioning. Communication is an essential process for evaluating patient care together using an interprofessional (IP) plan of care. To help meet this purpose, health care organizations have frequent and regular IP meetings and conduct IP patient care rounds.

Scope of Teamwork and Interprofessional Collaboration

In this textbook the interprofessional health care team includes the patient, family, nurses, unlicensed assistive personnel (UAP such as nursing assistants), and other health professionals and their assistants needed to provide appropriate and safe, evidence-based care. Other older terms used for these members include the *interdisciplinary* or multidisciplinary team, depending on health care organization, context, or setting. Although there are many health care team members, some health care professionals work more closely with nurses than others. For example, the physician or other health care provider and medical-surgical nurse collaborate frequently in a given day regarding patient care. The occupational therapist may not work as closely with the nurse unless the patient is receiving rehabilitation services. Collaboration with the rehabilitation team is discussed in Chapter 6.

Attributes of Teamwork and Interprofessional Collaboration

In 2011 the Interprofessional Education Collaborative (IPEC) Expert Panel published competencies to guide health professionals in education and practice; these competencies were updated in 2016. The four general competencies include:

- *Values/Ethics for Interprofessional Practice:* Work with individuals of other professions to maintain a climate of mutual respect and shared values.
- *Role-Responsibilities:* Use the knowledge of one's own role and those of other professions to appropriately assess and address the health care needs of patients and populations served.
- *Interprofessional Communication:* Communicate with patients, families, communities, and other health professionals in a responsive and responsible manner that supports a team approach to the maintenance of health and the treatment of disease.
- *Teams and Teamwork:* Apply relationship-building values and the principles of team dynamics to perform effectively in different team roles to plan and deliver patient-/population-centered care that is safe, timely, efficient, effective, and equitable.

Specific competencies for each of these general statements are delineated in the IPEC report. Examples of *Interprofessional Communication* are listed in Table 1-2.

TABLE 1-2 Interprofessional Communication Competencies

CC1. Choose effective communication tools and techniques, including information systems and communication technologies, to facilitate discussions and interactions that enhance team function.

CC2. Organize and communicate information with patients, families, and health care team members in a form that is understandable, avoiding discipline-specific terminology when possible.

CC3. Express one's knowledge and opinions to team members involved in patient care with confidence, clarity, and respect, working to ensure common understanding of information and treatment and care decisions.

CC4. Listen actively and encourage ideas and opinions of other team members.

CC5. Give timely, sensitive, instructive feedback to others about their performance on the team, responding respectfully as a team member to feedback from others.

CC6. Use respectful language appropriate for a given difficult situation, crucial conversation, or interprofessional conflict.

CC7. Recognize how one's own uniqueness, including experience level, expertise, culture, power, and hierarchy within the health care team, contributes to effective communication, conflict resolution, and positive interprofessional working relationships.

CC8. Communicate consistently the importance of teamwork in patient-centered and community focused care.

Data from Interprofessional Education Collaborative Expert Panel. (2016). *Core competencies for interprofessional collaborative practice: Report of an expert panel* (2nd ed.). Washington, D.C.: Interprofessional Education Collaborative.

Examples of Context of Teamwork and Interprofessional Collaboration to Nursing and Health Care

Electronic mail (e-mail) allows for quick communication among health care professionals to enhance collaboration and coordination of care. *However, it should not replace face-to-face and phone communication.*

Communication

Poor communication between professional caregivers and health care agencies causes many medical errors and patient safety risks. In 2006 The Joint Commission began to require systematic strategies for improving communication. Two years later, another National Patient Safety Goal mandated that nurses communicate continuing patient care needs such as pain management or respiratory support to post-discharge caregivers for safe transition management.

To improve communication between staff members and health care agencies, procedures for hand-off communication were established. An effective procedure used in many agencies today is called *SBAR* (pronounced S-Bar) or similar method. SBAR is a formal method of communication between two or more members of the health care team. The SBAR process includes these four steps:

- **S**ituation: Describe what is happening at the time to require this communication.
- **B**ackground: Explain any relevant background information that relates to the situation.
- **A**ssessment: Provide an analysis of the problem or patient need based on assessment data.
- **R**ecommendation/**R**equest: State what is needed or what the desired outcome is.

Several modifications of SBAR include I-SBAR, I-SBAR-R, and SBARQ. In these methods the "I" reminds the individual to *identify* himself or herself. The last "R" stands for the *response* that the receiver provides based on the information given. The "Q" represents any additional questions that need to be answered. Be sure to follow the established documentation and reporting protocols in your health care organization.

TeamSTEPPS is also a systematic communication approach for interprofessional teams that was designed to improve safety and quality. STEPPS stands for **S**trategies and **T**ools to **E**nhance **P**erformance and **P**atient **S**afety. Adapted from the aviation industry, this model reminds professionals that mistakes can cause negative outcomes, including death (Haynes & Strickler, 2014). In addition to SBAR, these common communication tools as part of TeamSTEPPS are very effective for promoting patient safety and teamwork:

- *CUS words:* State "I'm **c**oncerned; I'm **u**ncomfortable; I don't feel like this is **s**afe."
- *Check backs:* Restate what a person said to verify understanding by all team members.
- *Call outs:* Shout out important information (such as vital signs) for all team members to hear at one time.
- *Two-challenge rule:* State a concern twice as needed; if ignored, follow the chain of command to get the concern addressed.

Delegation and Supervision

As a nursing leader you will delegate certain nursing tasks and activities to unlicensed assistive personnel (UAP) such as patient care technicians (PCTs) or nursing assistants (NAs). **Delegation** is the process of transferring to a competent person the authority to perform a selected nursing task or activity in a selected patient care situation. This process requires precise and accurate communication. *The nurse is always accountable for the task or activity that is delegated!*

An important process that is sometimes not consistently performed by busy medical-surgical nurses is supervision of the UAP to whom the task or activity has been delegated. **Supervision** is guidance or direction, evaluation, and follow-up by the nurse to ensure that the task or activity is performed appropriately. Examples of delegated tasks are turning and positioning, vital signs, and intake and output measurements.

Be sure to follow these five rights when you delegate and supervise a nursing task or activity to a UAP:

- *Right task:* The task is within the UAP's scope of practice and competence.
- *Right circumstances:* The patient care setting and resources are appropriate for the delegation.
- *Right person:* The UAP is competent to perform the delegated task or activity.
- *Right communication:* The nurse provides a clear and concise explanation of the task or activity, including limits and expectations.
- *Right supervision:* The nurse appropriately monitors, evaluates, intervenes, and provides feedback on the delegation process as needed.

Other activities or patient care responsibilities may be assigned by a registered nurse (RN) to another RN or to a licensed practical or vocational nurse (LPN/LVN). Each state designates which tasks may be safely delegated and assigned to nursing team members. Interventions that you can typically delegate or assign in any state are indicated throughout this text. Some of the *Clinical Judgment and NCLEX Examination Challenges* throughout this book will test your understanding of the delegation and supervision process.

EVIDENCE-BASED PRACTICE

Definition of Evidence-Based Practice

Evidence-based practice (EBP) is the integration of the best current evidence and practices to make decisions about patient care. It considers the patient's preferences and values and one's own clinical expertise for the delivery of optimal health care (Melnyk & Fineout-Overholt, 2015; QSEN, 2011).

Scope of Evidence-Based Practice

The best source of evidence is research. Fig. 1-2 shows the level of evidence (LOE) pyramid that is commonly used to rate the quality (strength) or scope of available evidence. The highest levels of evidence are systematic reviews and integrative or meta-analysis studies. In these studies the researcher conducts a thorough literature search for appropriate studies and then analyzes findings of those studies to determine which best practices answer the research question. The types of research in nursing may be limited in some areas and may not reflect the highest or best level of evidence. Some nursing research is designed as small, descriptive studies to explore new concepts. The findings of these studies cannot be generalized, but they provide a basis for future larger and better-designed research.

Evidence-Based Practice boxes are found throughout the text to provide the most current research that serves as a basis for nursing practice. Each of these features presents a brief summary

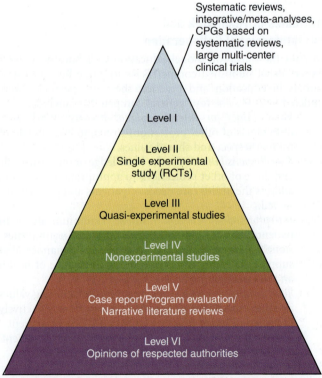

Systematic reviews, integrative/meta-analyses, CPGs based on systematic reviews, large multi-center clinical trials

Level I

Level II
Single experimental study (RCTs)

Level III
Quasi-experimental studies

Level IV
Nonexperimental studies

Level V
Case report/Program evaluation/ Narrative literature reviews

Level VI
Opinions of respected authorities

FIG. 1-2 Levels (strength) of evidence. Level 1 is the strongest evidence. (©2010. Rona F. Levin & Jeffrey M. Keefer.)

of the research, identifies the LOE using the scale in Fig. 1-2, and concludes with a "Commentary: Implications for Practice and Research" discussion to help you apply the findings of the study to daily nursing practice.

Attributes of Evidence-Based Practice

EBP promotes safety for patients, families, staff, and health care systems because it is based on reliable studies, guidelines, consensus, and expert opinion. However, recall that a best practice identified through research or clinical practice guideline may not be consistent with the patient's or family's personal preferences or beliefs. Nurses must respect the values of the patient or designee at all times even if those values differ from their own or those of the interprofessional health care team.

Examples of Context of Evidence-Based Practice to Nursing and Health Care

Health care organizations receiving Medicare and/or Medicaid funding are obligated to follow the evidence-based interprofessional Core Measures to ensure that best practices are followed for selected health problems. Examples of Core Measures are highlighted throughout this textbook, such as those related to heart failure, stroke, venous thromboembolism, and acute myocardial infarction.

In addition to complying with federal mandates and those outlined by The Joint Commission (TJC), many hospitals have achieved or are on the path to achieve the American Nurses Credentialing Center's Magnet Recognition. This highly desired recognition requires nurses to demonstrate how best current evidence guides their practice. Many hospitals have nursing research departments with experts to facilitate this process. Using research to guide practice is a way to continuously improve the quality of care, as described as part of the following concept.

QUALITY IMPROVEMENT

Definition of Quality Improvement

Quality improvement (QI), sometimes referred to as *continuous quality improvement (CQI)*, is a process in which nurses and the interprofessional health care team use indicators (data) to monitor care outcomes and develop solutions to change and improve care. This process is also sometimes called the *evidence-based practice improvement (EBPI)* process because the best sources of evidence are used to support the improvement or change in practice.

Scope of Quality Improvement

When a patient care or system issue is identified as needing improvement, specific systematic QI models such as the Plan-Do-Study-Act (PDSO) or the FOCUS-PDCA are typically used. The steps of the PDSO model include (Sutton & Suhayda, 2015):

1. Identify and analyze the problem (Plan).
2. Develop and test an evidence-based solution (Do).
3. Analyze the effectiveness of the test solution, including possible further improvement (Study).
4. Implement the improved solution to positively impact care (Act).

The steps of the more specific FOCUS-PDCA model are:
- **F**ind a process to improve.
- **O**rganize a team.
- **C**larify the current process.
- **U**nderstand variations in current process.
- **S**elect the process to improve.
- **P**lan the improvement.
- **D**o the improvement.
- Check for results.
- **A**ct to hold the gain.

A QI project using the FOCUS-PDCA model was successfully conducted by a group of nurses to improve communication during morning rounds on a medical-surgical unit. The QI team developed a written communication tool for each patient that included a place for the staff nurse to list primary concerns for the patient. The physicians and other primary health care providers used the same tool to outline the goals and plan of care for the day. The results of this project improved daily communication between nurses and physicians, which led to improved patient care and safety (Perry et al., 2016).

Another method called the DMAIC model is gaining popularity as it more clearly delineates each QI step and includes the need to continue the new intervention or change over time. The steps of this model are:

1. **D**efine the issue or problem.
2. **M**easure the key aspects of the current process for the issue (collect data).
3. **A**nalyze the collected data.
4. **I**mprove or optimize the current process by implementing an evidence-based intervention/solution.
5. **C**ontrol the future state of the intervention to ensure continuity of the process.

Attributes of Quality Improvement

As a medical-surgical nurse, you will be expected to be involved in the QI process on your unit or in your agency. You will need the knowledge and skills to:
- Identify indicators to monitor quality and effectiveness of health care.
- Access and evaluate data to monitor quality and effectiveness of health care.
- Recommend ways to improve care processes.
- Implement activities to improve care processes.

Examples of Context of Quality Improvement to Nursing and Health Care

This textbook features *Quality Improvement* boxes that summarize articles on QI projects and end with a "Commentary: Implications for Practice and Research" discussion. These features will help you learn how nurses get involved in QI and the benefits to patients, staff, and health care systems or patient care units. An example of how one hospital unit improved practice using the DMAIC model to improve medication reconciliation is summarized in the *Quality Improvement* box in this chapter. Additional information about the QI process can be found in nursing leadership and management resources.

INFORMATICS AND TECHNOLOGY

Definition of Informatics and Technology

Informatics and technology are the access and use of information and electronic technology to communicate, manage knowledge, prevent error, and support decision making (QSEN, 2011).

Scope of Informatics and Technology

Most health care settings have information technology (IT) departments. The largest application of health care informatics is use of the electronic health record (EHR) (also called *electronic patient record [EPR]* or *electronic medical record [EMR]*) for documenting nursing and interprofessional care. Computers may be located at the nurses' work station, at the patient's bedside (point of care [POC]), or near the nurses' station. Handheld mobile devices or laptops are also popular because of their ease of use and portability.

Attributes of Informatics and Technology

Although safety and quality of health care are the major purposes of informatics and technology, patient and family privacy may be at risk unless precautions are implemented. For example, staff and students may take photos of patients to show their family and friends about the health problems for which they care. In some cases these photos are posted on social media such as Facebook. *This action is a violation of patient privacy and confidentiality.*

Examples of Context of Informatics and Technology for Nursing and Health Care

Another major purpose of informatics is for retrieval of data for evidence-based practice and quality improvement. The Internet provides ways to search for multiple sources of information very efficiently. However, all data sources must be evaluated for their credibility and reliability.

New technologies for patient, staff, and resource (inventory) management are used in health care agencies to promote patient safety and improve efficiency. An example of these technologies is radiofrequency identification (RFID). RFID allows any person or object to be tracked electronically. Bar-code medication administration (BCMA) systems (see Fig. 1-1) and Smart IV pumps are other examples of systems used to ensure safety through technology.

Nurses need to be involved in decisions about introducing new or advanced health care technologies into the health care agency. They should also be included in designing technology that improves the effectiveness and efficiency of health care while providing for patient and staff privacy.

CLINICAL JUDGMENT

Definition of Clinical Judgment

Clinical judgment is the process that nurses and other members of the interprofessional team use to make decisions based on interpretation of the patient's needs or problems. The nursing process, critical thinking, and a variety of reasoning patterns help the medical-surgical nurse make clinical decisions while being respectful of the patient's and family's cultural diversity, age, gender, and lifestyle choices. This textbook presents many *Clinical Judgment Challenges* and *NCLEX Examination Challenges* to help you practice how to use clinical judgment to make appropriate decisions based on current evidence as available.

Scope of Clinical Judgment

Appropriate or "sound" clinical judgment (also referred to as *sound judgment*) leads to positive patient or staff outcomes. By contrast, inappropriate or "poor" judgment results in negative outcomes that can pose a risk to patient or staff safety. In her classic systematic review, Tanner (2006) concluded that sound clinical judgment is influenced by how well the nurse knows the patient's typical response pattern and the situational context or culture of the nursing care unit. Reflection on nursing practice is often triggered by poor clinical judgment and is essential for developing knowledge and improving reasoning.

The worst result of poor judgment is a growing health care crisis referred to as *failure to rescue.* Failure to rescue is the inability of nurses or other interprofessional health team members to save a patient's life in a timely manner when a health care issue or medical complication occurs. Patients often have beginning or subtle signs and symptoms 2 to 3 days before cardiopulmonary arrest or multiple organ failure. Failure to rescue occurs when those signs and symptoms are not noticed or accurately interpreted and therefore action to improve the patient's condition is not implemented (Garvey, 2015).

Attributes of Clinical Judgment

According to Tanner, clinical judgment involves specific reasoning and critical thinking skills. In this edition of the text, each of these skills is paired with the steps of the nursing process for all exemplar health problems as follows:

- Assessment: Noticing
- Analysis: Interpreting
- Planning and Implementation: Responding
- Evaluation: Reflecting

Examples of Context of Clinical Judgment to Nursing and Health Care

To improve patient safety and prevent failure to rescue, most hospitals have a Rapid Response Team (RRT), also called the *Medical Emergency Team (MET).* Rapid Response Teams save lives and decrease the risk for harm by providing care *before* a medical emergency occurs by intervening rapidly when needed for patients who are *beginning* to clinically decline. Members of an RRT are critical care experts who are on-site and available at any time. Although membership varies among agencies, the team may consist of an intensive care unit (ICU) nurse, respiratory therapist, intensivist (physician who specializes in critical care), and/or hospitalist (family practice physician or internist employed by the hospital). In other hospitals acute care nurse practitioners or medical residents may be part of the team. The team responds to emergency calls, usually from clinical nurses, according to established agency protocols and policies (Allen et al., 2015). Patient families may also activate the RRT.

The Joint Commission's National Patient Safety Goals also include the need for early intervention for patients who are clinically changing. They require each health care organization to establish criteria for patients, families, or staff to call for additional assistance in response to an actual or perceived change in the patient's condition.

ETHICS

Definition of Ethics

According to the American Nurses Association (ANA), ethics is "a theoretical and reflective domain of human knowledge that addresses issues and questions about morality in human choices, actions, character, and ends (ANA, 2015, p. xii). *Applied*

TABLE 1-3 Examples of Provisions of the ANA Code of Ethics

- The nurse practices with compassion and respect for the inherent dignity, worth, and unique attributes of every person.
- The nurse promotes, advocates for, and protects the rights, health, and safety of the patient.
- The nurse has authority, accountability, and responsibility for nursing practice; makes decisions; and takes action consistent with the obligation to promote health and to provide optimal care.
- The nurse owes the same duties to self as to others, including the responsibility to promote health and safety, preserve wholeness of character and integrity, maintain competence, and continue personal and professional growth.
- The nurse collaborates with other health professionals and the public to protect human rights, promote health diplomacy, and reduce health disparities.

professional nursing ethics is about considering what is right and wrong when using clinical judgment to make clinical decisions.

Scope of Ethics

Clinical decisions are either ethical or not ethical and are based on one or more of six principles described under Attributes of Ethics. Ethics is also described by the type of ethics or setting in which these decisions are made. For example, *organizational* ethics refers to the ethical practices of health care organizations. Applied nursing ethics is a type of *professional* ethics that are used in practice by individual nurses. Examples of the provisions of the ANA Code of Ethics are listed in Table 1-3.

Attributes of Ethics

Respect for people is the basis for six essential *ethical principles* that nurses and other health care professionals should use as a guide for clinical decision making. Respect implies that patients are treated as autonomous individuals capable of making informed decisions about their care. This patient **autonomy** is also referred to as *self-determination* or *self-management*. When the patient is not capable of self-determination, you are ethically obligated to protect him or her as an advocate within the professional scope of practice, according to the American Nurses Association (ANA) Code of Ethics for Nurses (ANA, 2015).

The second ethical principle is **beneficence**, which promotes positive actions to help others. In other words, it encourages the nurse to do good for the patient. **Nonmaleficence** emphasizes the importance of preventing harm and ensuring the patient's well-being. Harm can be avoided only if its causes or possible causes are identified. As described earlier in this chapter, patient safety is currently a major national focus to prevent deaths and injuries.

Fidelity refers to the agreement that nurses will keep their obligations or promises to patients to follow through with care. **Veracity** is a related principle in which the nurse is obligated to tell the truth to the best of his or her knowledge. If you are not truthful with a patient, his or her respect for you will diminish, and your credibility as a health care professional will be damaged.

Social justice, the last principle, refers to equality and fairness; that is, all patients should be treated equally and fairly, regardless of age, gender identity, sexual orientation, religion, race, ethnicity, or education. For example, a patient who cannot afford health care receives the same quality and level of care as one who has extensive insurance coverage. An older patient with dementia is shown the same respect as a younger patient who can communicate. A Hispanic patient who can communicate only in Spanish receives the same level of care as a Euro-American patient whose primary language is English. More information on ethics and ethical principles can be found in your fundamentals textbook.

Examples of Context of Ethics to Nursing and Health Care

Nurses and other members of the interprofessional team are involved in many ethical decisions and dilemmas in daily practice. Examples of these dilemmas include issues surrounding advance directives and aggressive treatment options. Some of the *Clinical Judgment Challenges* in this book relate to common ethical issues in medical-surgical nursing.

HEALTH CARE ORGANIZATIONS

Definition of Health Care Organizations

Health care organizations (HCOs) are purposely designed and structured systems in which health care is provided by members of nursing and interprofessional teams (Giddens, 2016).

Scope of Health Care Organizations

HCOs are classified by their ownership (e.g., private versus public), financial purpose, and mission. For example, public HCOs are owned by county, state, provincial, and federal governments; they are usually nonprofit and supported by tax revenue. Private institutions are typically owned by companies or organizations. Many of these agencies are for-profit HCOs, but others are nonprofit or not-for-profit. Some HCOs are large research and teaching institutions such as Johns Hopkins in Baltimore, MD. Others are rural or small community hospitals.

HCOs can be single institutions or part of larger systems. For example, a single nursing home or assisted-living facility may be privately owned and not part of a network. By contrast, a large hospital system may house acute care, chronic care, rehabilitative care, ambulatory care, and skilled care in one or multiple locations.

HCOs also vary by mission or purpose; some offer generalized services, whereas others offer more specialized services. For example, free-standing rehabilitation facilities limit their services to care of patients with rehabilitative needs. Critical Care Access Hospitals (CAHs) are specially designated HCOs that must meet the following criteria:

- Be located in a rural area at least 35 miles away from any other hospital
- Have no more than 25 inpatient beds
- Maintain an annual average patient length of stay of no more than 96 acute inpatient hours
- Offer 24-hour, 7 day–a-week emergency care

Patients served by a CAH either have common stable health problems or are referred to larger hospitals once their conditions are stabilized.

In some cases HCOs restrict the population they serve based on mission or purpose. For example, Veterans Administration

(VA) hospital systems provide services only for active or retired military patients. U.S. Indian Health Services HCOs provide care for American Indians.

Attributes of Health Care Organizations

An HCO is characterized by its:
- Mission and philosophy
- Organizational structure
- Workforce (health care and ancillary)
- Patients
- Services provided

These characteristics allow the agency to provide safe, quality patient care that the public or local community can trust.

Examples of Context of Health Care Organizations to Nursing and Health Care

Nurses often choose to work in an HCO based on its characteristics. For example, if a nurse prefers working with specialized populations such as veterans, he or she usually seeks employment in the VA system. If the nurse desires to work in a large teaching institution, he or she would need to work in an urban area where these HCOs are located. Opportunities for career advancement and continuing education may also be more readily available in larger institutions.

HEALTH CARE DISPARITIES

Definition of Health Care Disparities

Health care disparities are differences in patient access to or availability of appropriate health care services.

Scope of Health Care Disparities

A major focus of the U.S. *Healthy People 2020* initiative is to decrease health care disparities caused by poor communication, health care access, health literacy, and health care provider biases and discrimination. Although progress has been made over the past few decades, many minority populations have a high incidence of chronic disease and mortality as a result of health care disparities (Neumayer & Plumper, 2016). The National Center on Minority Health and Health Disparities of the National Institutes of Health leads and coordinates the efforts to reduce these disparities in the United States. Similar organizations in other countries exist for this same purpose.

Attributes of Health Care Disparities

Many factors affect patient access to quality health care services, including geographic location, cultural variables, and resources. For instance, some individuals live in very rural areas that do not have quality health care services. In other cases the care is available, but the individual may not have transportation to get to the provider or value the need for regular preventive health care. Language barriers may also prevent the individual from accessing services. For example, many older individuals in Hispanic communities do not speak English, and most health care professionals do not speak Spanish. This communication barrier and possible mistrust of primary care providers can prevent access to needed health services.

Some individuals remain uninsured or underinsured and cannot afford health care services. "Working poor" patients may have health insurance but their copayments are too high to seek services. Copayments for a health care provider office visit may be as high as $50 or more. Medication copayments can range from $5 to over $100 per prescription, depending on which type of insurance the patient has. These expenses are usually not a priority over other personal financial needs such as food and rent.

Examples of Context of Health Care Disparities to Nursing and Health Care

Entire groups of people are vulnerable or likely to experience an inability to access available health care for a variety of reasons. Health care professionals may have biases and beliefs about certain cultures and groups that prevent them from being effective in developing an appropriate individualized plan of care. Examples of these groups include older adults, ethnic minorities, and the lesbian, gay, bisexual, transgender, and queer and/or questioning (LGBTQ) population.

Special Needs of Older Adults

Older adults are a growing subset of the adult population as the baby boomers turn 60 to 70. This group of young older adults is different from previous generations as they aged. Many are working well past 65 years of age and have very active social lives. Chapter 3 in this text is dedicated to the special health care needs of older adults, especially those between 70 and over 100 years old.

Special Needs of Ethnic Minorities

Early health care research focused on promoting health or managing health problems among affluent Euro-Americans. More recent research has included implications for or differences in care based on ethnicity or gender. Health care disparities have been identified as they affect various groups and populations. As mentioned earlier in this chapter, many *Cultural/Spiritual Considerations* features are integrated throughout this textbook to highlight differences in care needed to meet the special health needs of individuals from a variety of racial and ethnic groups.

Special Needs of the LGBTQ Population

Nurses today have been made aware of cultural variations and learned how to incorporate these differences to individualize patient care. However, one group that is seldom addressed in the nursing literature is the LGBTQ population (Pettinato, 2012). This terminology is widely accepted by the LGBTQ community and is commonly used, although *LGBT* may be seen more often in health care literature. Queer and/or questioning individuals prefer not having strict labels on their sexualities or genders. Another term that may also be used is *LGBTQI* to include intersex individuals. Intersex individuals have sexual or reproductive organs that are not clearly male or female or may have a combination of both male and female organs.

Many studies provide evidence that LGBTQ individuals do not feel comfortable with or trust health care professionals because of previous discrimination (IOM, 2011). The *Healthy People 2020* initiative added a category for these individuals because of health disparities in this population and the need to improve LGBTQ health. The complete document can be found on www.healthypeople.gov/2020. This textbook includes special health needs of this population as part of its *Gender Health Considerations* features. A separate chapter in this book on transgender health helps students learn about the special needs of transgender patients.

The health care system, like other facets of society, often overlooks sexualities and genders that are alternative to the standard of heterosexuality and clearly delineated maleness or femaleness. As a health care professional, it is essential to not be restricted by rigid standards of identity. A good way of rethinking concepts of sexuality and gender is to think of each as existing along a spectrum rather than categorizing people into heterosexual/homosexual and male/female.

To begin to gain trust and show respect for the LGBTQ patient, health care professionals need to know their patient's sexual orientation and gender identity. Do not assume that every patient is heterosexual or clearly gendered. *Include questions about gender identity and sexual activity as part of your patient's health assessment.* Table 1-4 lists recommended patient interview questions about sexual orientation, gender identity, and health care.

TABLE 1-4   Recommended Patient Interview Questions About Sexual Orientation, Gender Identity, and Health Care

- Do you have sex with men, women, both, or neither?
- Does anyone live with you in your household?
- Are you in a relationship with someone who does not live with you?
- If you have a sexual partner, have you or your partner been evaluated about the possibility of transmitting infections to each other?
- If you have more than one sexual partner, how are you protecting both of you from infections such as hepatitis B, hepatitis C, or HIV?
- Have you disclosed your gender identity and sexual orientation to your health care provider?
- If you have not, may I have your permission to provide that information to members of the health care team who are involved in your care?
- Whom do you consider to be your closest family members?

HIV, Human immune deficiency virus.

GET READY FOR THE NCLEX® EXAMINATION!

KEY POINTS

Review these Key Points for each NCLEX Examination Client Needs Category.

Safe and Effective Care Environment

- Medical-surgical nursing is a specialty practice that requires a broad knowledge base and clinical skills to meet the needs of adult patients in a variety of settings.
- Medical-surgical nurses help meet human needs of adult patients such as mobility and gas exchange in a caring, respectful relationship.
- **The Joint Commission requires that health care organizations create a culture of safety by following the National Patient Safety Goals (NPSGs).**
- Rapid Response Teams (RRTs) save lives and decrease the risk for patient harm before a respiratory or cardiac arrest occurs. **QSEN: Safety**
- Remember to always observe for slow and sudden changes in patient condition, especially changes in vital signs and mental status.
- A vital role of the nurse is as an advocate to empower patients and their families to have control over their health care and function as safety partners. **QSEN: Safety**
- Examples of the provisions of the ANA Code of Ethics for Nurses are listed in Table 1-3.
- Six essential ethical principles to consider when making clinical decisions are autonomy, beneficence, nonmaleficence, fidelity, veracity, and social justice. **Ethics**
- Nurses collaborate by communicating patient's needs and preferences with members of the interprofessional health care team to establish an individualized approach to care. **QSEN: Teamwork and Collaboration**
- The SBAR procedure or similar established method is used for successful hand-off communication between caregivers and between health care agencies.

- When delegating a nursing task to unlicensed assistive personnel (UAP), the nurse is always accountable to ensure that the task was performed safely and accurately. **QSEN: Safety**
- Evidence-based practice (EBP) is the integration of best current evidence to make decisions about patient care. It considers the patient's preferences and values and one's own clinical expertise.
- Nurses are active participants in the systematic quality improvement (QI) process in their health care agency and used one of several QI models to improve care and promote patient safety. **QSEN: Quality Improvement**
- Informatics and technology are used for patient documentation, electronic data access, and health care resource tracking. **QSEN: Informatics**
- Health care organizations vary by size, mission, financial goal, and purpose; some are single agencies and others are part of large networks in multiple locations. **Health Care Organizations**

Psychosocial Integrity

- Nurses must show respect and compassion for the uniqueness of every individual to ensure patient-centered and family-centered care.
- Health care disparities are differences in the access or availability of health care; members of minority groups and other vulnerable populations are particularly at risk for health disparities. **Health Care Disparities**
- The lesbian, gay, bisexual, transgender, queer and/or questioning (LGBTQ) population typically does not trust health care professionals; use sensitive questioning about sexual orientation and gender identity as part of your interview with patients in this group (see Table 1-4). **QSEN: Patient-Centered Care**

SELECTED BIBLIOGRAPHY

Asterisk indicates a classic or definitive work on this subject.

*Academy of Medical-Surgical Nurses (AMSN) (2012). *Scope and standards of medical-surgical nursing practice* (5th ed.). Pitman, NJ: Author.

Alfaro-LeFevre, R. (2016). *Critical thinking, clinical reasoning, and clinical judgment: A practical approach to outcome-focused thinking* (6th ed.). Philadelphia: Saunders.

Allen, D., Weinhold, M., Miller, J., Joswiak, M. E., Bursiek, A., Rubin, A., et al. (2015). Nurses as champions for patient safety and interdisciplinary problem solving. *Medsurg Nursing, 24*(2), 107–110.

American Nurses Association (ANA) (2015). *Code of ethics for nurses with interpretive statements.* Silver Spring, MD: Author.

*Benner, P. E., Malloch, K., & Sheets, V. (2010). *Nursing pathways for patient safety.* St. Louis: Mosby.

Doane, G. H., & Varcoe, C. (2015). *How to nurse: Relational inquiry with individuals and families in changing health and health care contexts.* Philadelphia: Wolters Kluwer.

*Frampton, S., Guastello, S., Brady, C., Hale, M., Horowitz, S., Smith, S. B., et al. (2008). *Patient-centered care improvement guide.* Derby, CT: Planetree.

Furst, C. M., Finto, D., Malouf-Todaro, N., Moore, C., Orr, D., Santos, J., et al. (2013). Changing times: Enhancing clinical practice through evolving technology. *Medsurg Nursing, 22*(2), 131–134.

Garvey, P. K. (2015). Failure to rescue: The nurse's impact. *Medsurg Nursing, 24*(3), 145–149.

Giddens, J. F. (2016). *Concepts for nursing practice* (2nd ed.). St. Louis: Elsevier.

Halm, M. A., & Katseres, J. (2015). Integrative care: The evolving landscape in American hospitals. *The American Journal of Nursing, 115*(10), 22–30.

Haynes, J., & Strickler, J. (2014). TeamSTEPPS makes strides for better communication. *Nursing, 44*(1), 62–63.

Henderson, M., & Dahnke, M. (2015). The ethical use of social media in nursing practice. *Medsurg Nursing, 24*(1), 62–64.

*Institute of Medicine (IOM) (2003). *Health professions education: A bridge to quality.* Washington, DC: National Academies Press.

*Institute of Medicine (IOM) (2011). *The health of lesbian, gay, bisexual, and transgender people: Building a foundation for better understanding.* Washington, DC: National Academies Press.

*Interprofessional Education Collaborative Expert Panel (2016). *Core competencies for interprofessional collaborative practice: Report of an expert panel* (2nd ed.). Washington, D.C.: Interprofessional Education Collaborative.

Lamb, G. (2014). *Care coordination: The game changer.* Silver Spring, MD: American Nurses Association.

Melnyk, B. M., & Fineout-Overholt, E. (2015). *Evidence-based practice in nursing and healthcare* (2nd ed.). Philadelphia: Lippincott Williams & Wilkins.

Neumayer, E., & Plumper, T. (2016). Inequalities of income and inequalities of longevity: A cross-country study. *American Journal of Public Health, 106*(1), 160–165.

Perry, V., Christiansen, M., & Simmons, A. (2016). A daily goals tool to facilitate indirect nurse-physician communication during morning rounds on a medical-surgical unit. *Medsurg Nursing, 25*(2), 83–87.

*Pettinato, M. (2012). Providing care for LGBTQ patients. *Nursing, 42*(12), 22–27.

Polster, D. (2015). Patient discharge information: Tools for success. *Nursing, 45*(5), 43–50.

*Quality and Safety Education for Nurses (QSEN) (2011). *Competency KSAs (pre-licensure).* www.qsen.org.

Robert, R. R., & Petersen, S. (2013). Critical thinking at the bedside. *Medsurg Nursing, 22*(2), 85–93.

Roller, C. G., Sedlak, C., & Draucker, C. B. (2015). Navigating the system: How transgender individuals engage in health care services. *Journal of Nursing Scholarship, 47*(5), 417–424.

Ruggerio, J., Smith, J., Copeland, J., & Boxer, B. (2015). Discharge time out: An innovative nurse-driven protocol for medication reconciliation. *MEDSURG Nursing, 24*(3), 165–172.

Schneider, M. A., & Kuth-Sahd, L. A. (2015). Fundamentals: Still the building blocks of safe patient care. *Nursing, 44*(6), 60–63.

Shafer, L., & Aziz, M. G. (2013). Shaping a unit's culture through effective nurse-led quality improvement. *Medsurg Nursing, 22*(4), 229–236.

*Sherwood, G., & Barnsteiner, J. (2012). *Quality and safety in nursing: A competency approach to improving outcomes.* Hoboken, NJ: Wiley-Blackwell.

Stubenrauch, J. M. (2015). Project RED reduces hospital admissions. *The American Journal of Nursing, 115*(10), 18–19.

Sutton, K., & Suhayda, R. (2015). Outcomes achieved through implementation of interdisciplinary plans of care. *Medsurg Nursing, 24*(5), 304–308.

*Tanner, C. A. (2006). Thinking like a nurse: A research-based model of clinical judgment in nursing. *Journal of Nursing Education, 45*(6), 204–211.

The Joint Commission. (2013). *Transitions of care: The need for a more effective approach to continuing patient care.* www.jointcomission.org/assets/1/18/Hot_Topics_Transitions_of_Care.pdf.

CHAPTER 2

Overview of Health Concepts for Medical-Surgical Nursing

Donna D. Ignatavicius and Kristin Oneail

http://evolve.elsevier.com/Iggy/

PRIORITY AND INTERRELATED CONCEPTS

The priority concepts for this chapter are:

- ACID-BASE BALANCE
- CELLULAR REGULATION
- CLOTTING
- COGNITION
- COMFORT
- ELIMINATION
- FLUID AND ELECTROLYTE BALANCE
- GAS EXCHANGE

- GLUCOSE REGULATION
- IMMUNITY
- MOBILITY
- NUTRITION
- PERFUSION
- SENSORY PERCEPTION
- SEXUALITY
- TISSUE INTEGRITY

LEARNING OUTCOMES

Safe and Effective Care Environment

1. Collaborate with the nursing and interprofessional team to help patients meet selected physiologic health needs.

Health Promotion and Maintenance

2. Develop an evidence-based teaching plan to enable adults to meet selected health needs and promote health.
3. Assess unsafe or unhealthy behaviors that could prevent the patient from meeting physiologic health needs.
4. Plan health promotion strategies to promote sensory perception in adults and maintain safety.

Psychosocial Integrity

5. Differentiate delirium and dementia as common cognitive impairments.

Physiological Integrity

6. Review the definition and scope of selected physiologic health needs of adults.
7. Describe common physiologic consequences when basic health needs are not met.
8. Document essential assessments to determine if basic health needs are met.
9. Plan patient-centered nursing interventions to help patients meet selected physiologic health needs.

Nurses care for adults in a variety of settings to help them meet a multitude of biopsychosocial needs. When these needs are not met, the nurse plans and implements care in collaboration with the interprofessional health team. This chapter reviews the 15 health concepts that are emphasized and built on in this text, and are presented alphabetically for easy access. For more information about these basic concepts, see your foundations or fundamentals of nursing textbook. Each chapter in the body systems units applies appropriate health concepts to patient assessment or interventions for selected health problems, identified as exemplars.

ACID-BASE BALANCE

Definition of Acid-Base Balance

Acid-base balance is the maintenance of arterial blood pH between 7.35 and 7.45 through control of hydrogen ion production and elimination. Blood pH represents a delicate balance between hydrogen ions (acid) and bicarbonate (base) and is largely controlled by the lungs and kidneys.

Scope of Acid-Base Balance

If the arterial blood pH is either below 7.35 or above 7.45, the patient has a type of acid-base *imbalance* (Fig. 2-1). *Acidosis* occurs if the arterial blood pH level falls below 7.35 and is caused by either too many hydrogen ions in the body (respiratory acidosis) or too little bicarbonate (metabolic acidosis). Conversely, *alkalosis* occurs if the pH is greater than 7.45 and is caused by either too few hydrogen ions in the body (respiratory alkalosis) or too much bicarbonate (metabolic alkalosis). Both severe acidosis and alkalosis can lead to death if the patient is not diagnosed accurately and treated quickly.

Common Risk Factors for Acid-Base Imbalance

Any individual is at risk for an acid-base imbalance, but it occurs most commonly as a complication of many acute and

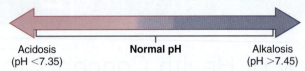

Acidosis
(pH <7.35)

Normal pH

Alkalosis
(pH >7.45)

FIG. 2-1 Scope of acid-base balance.

chronic health problems. The most common risk factors include poisoning such as excessive salicylate ingestion; medical conditions such as chronic obstructive pulmonary disease (COPD), uncontrolled diabetes mellitus (especially type 1), and chronic kidney disease; excessive emesis, diarrhea, or intravenous (IV) infusions; and fluid and electrolyte imbalances. A more thorough discussion of acid-base imbalances by specific type may be found in Chapter 12 of this text.

Physiologic Consequences of Acid-Base Imbalance

When the body has an impaired acid-base balance, several mechanisms are activated in an attempt to correct the imbalance, a process referred to as *compensation*. For example, if the patient is acidotic (pH lower than 7.35), the kidneys typically decrease the amount of bicarbonate ions (base) that is excreted through the urine. The lungs may try to rid the body of carbon dioxide (source of carbonic acid) through increased and deeper respirations. In this case, both compensatory mechanisms aim to restore acid-base balance by increasing the blood pH to greater than 7.35. These actions can only occur if the individual has healthy lungs and kidneys.

Assessment of Acid-Base Balance

Take a patient health history for chronic illnesses such as diabetes mellitus or COPD and any past experiences of acid-base imbalance. Ask about the presence or recent history of signs and symptoms that could predispose the patient to acidosis or alkalosis such as excessive vomiting or diarrhea. The patient's current or recent use of medications, including over-the-counter drugs and herbal supplements, should be reviewed to determine if they could cause acid-base imbalance.

Arterial blood gas monitoring gives the health care team an understanding of the type of acid-base imbalance the patient is experiencing. Assessing the pH determines whether the patient has an imbalance and, if so, how severe it is. The $PaCO_2$ level (normal value is 35-45 mm Hg), or partial pressure of carbon dioxide, indicates how well the lungs are functioning in blowing off or retaining carbon dioxide as needed to help correct the acid-base imbalance. The bicarbonate level, or HCO_3 (normal value is 21-28 mEq/L [21-28 mmol/L ✦]), indicates how well the kidneys are excreting or reabsorbing base as needed.

Interventions to Promote Acid-Base Balance and Prevent Acid-Base Imbalance

The best way for an individual to maintain acid-base balance is to practice health promotion measures, including living a healthy lifestyle. For example, most cases of COPD can be prevented by avoiding or quitting smoking. Regular exercise and a healthy diet can decrease the incidence of type 2 diabetes mellitus and help control blood glucose in all types of diabetes.

Teach patients who are at risk for acute or chronic vomiting or diarrhea to be monitored carefully by a primary health care provider to assess for fluid, electrolyte, and acid-base imbalances. (See discussion of fluid and electrolyte balance later in this chapter.)

Interventions for Patients With Acid-Base Imbalances

Managing a patient with an acid-base imbalance depends on which type of imbalance is present. When possible, the health care team aims to diagnose and treat the underlying cause(s) of the imbalance. Chapter 12 describes the pathophysiology and management of common types of acid-base imbalance in detail.

CELLULAR REGULATION

Definition of Cellular Regulation

Cellular regulation is the process to control cellular growth, replication, and differentiation to maintain homeostasis. Cellular *growth* refers to division and continued growth of the original cell. Cell *replication* refers to making a copy of a specific cell. Cell *differentiation* refers to the process of the cell becoming specialized to accomplish a specific task.

Scope of Cellular Regulation

Cellular function can have both positive and negative effects within the body. Positive aspects of cellular function include cell development and reproduction of healthy cells, whereas negative aspects include cell replication and growth of unhealthy cells that represent tumors or neoplasms.

Common Risk Factors for Impaired Cellular Regulation

Risk factors that increase the probability of impaired cellular regulation include:

- Older age (55 years and older, with significant potential for abnormal cell development at ages >70)
- Smoking
- Poor nutrition
- Physical inactivity
- Environmental pollutants (such as air, water, soil)
- Radiation
- Selected medications (such as chemotherapy)
- Genetic predisposition or risk

Physiologic Consequences of Impaired Cellular Regulation

It is important to differentiate benign and malignant cell growth. *Benign* cell growth mirrors the original cell, but excessive cells are present. Benign cells do not have the capability to spread to other tissues or organs. However, benign masses can cause health risks because of the ability to obstruct or compress organs in the body, causing significant discomfort or high risk to the individual. For example, a meningioma (benign mass) can compress the brain and lead to increased intracranial pressure (ICP), a potentially fatal complication.

Malignant (cancerous) cells, over time, have no comparison to the original cells from which they are derived. Replication of abnormal cells leads to significant invasion of healthy cells, tissues, and organs through tumor formation and invasion.

Assessment of Cellular Regulation

Perform a thorough patient history, extensive family history, and a psychosocial history. Completing a thorough and detailed physical examination may identify any visible or palpable masses, pain, or difficulty breathing. Diagnostic tests such as radiographic examination, computed tomography (CT), or magnetic resonance imaging (MRI) may identify the location of any mass. More invasive tests such as a colonoscopy or endoscopy give the primary health care provider an opportunity to actually see the mass. Laboratory tests can provide additional information regarding the overall health of the patient and the composition of any mass. For example, tissue biopsies and cell cytology are essential to identify the type of abnormal cell that is present. Grading and staging to identify the extent and severity of the growth are a necessity to diagnose, treat, and offer a prognosis for the patient.

Interventions to Promote Cellular Regulation and Prevent Impaired Cellular Regulation

Interventions include primary and secondary prevention techniques. *Primary prevention* includes minimizing the risk of developing impaired cellular regulation. Teach patients to:

- Minimize exposure to sunlight or other source of ultraviolet light such as tanning beds (to prevent skin cancers).
- Stop smoking or other tobacco use if applicable (to prevent many cancer types, including lung, oral, and bladder cancers).
- Consume a diet low in saturated fat and high in fiber (to prevent breast and colon cancer).
- Increase physical activity and regular exercise (to prevent all cancer types).
- Avoid exposure to environmental hazards (to prevent all cancer types).

Healthy People 2020 addresses goals for reducing cancer risk and includes maintaining a healthy weight, managing proper oral health, and being aware of one's family history or genetic makeup.

Secondary prevention includes proper and regular screening to identify early any risks or hazards that could be present. Screening also enables the primary health care provider to diagnose cancer early, which often increases the patient's chance for a cure or long-term survival.

Interventions for Patients With Impaired Cellular Regulation

Collaborative interventions for the patient with impaired cellular regulation can include surgery, radiation therapy, chemotherapy, hormonal therapy, targeted therapy, biologic therapy, and bone marrow or hemapoietic stem cell transplants. The type and course of interprofessional management depends on the type and severity of cellular regulation impairment. The two chapters on cancer in this textbook discuss the pathogenesis of cancer and its patient-centered management.

CLOTTING

Definition of Clotting

Clotting is a complex, multi-step process by which blood forms a protein-based structure (clot) in an appropriate area of tissue injury to prevent excessive bleeding while maintaining whole body blood flow (perfusion). A major component of this process involves specialized cells called *platelets* (thrombocytes) that circulate in the blood until they are needed. When injury occurs, platelets are activated to become sticky, causing them to

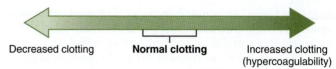

FIG. 2-2 Scope of clotting.

aggregate (clump together) to form a temporary semi-solid plug. The platelet aggregation triggers a rapid complex process, known as the *clotting cascade,* in which multiple clotting factors (enzymes and plasma proteins) work together to create a fibrin clot and local blood coagulation (clotting). Another pathway, known as the *fibrinolytic system,* is triggered to cause clot lysis (breakdown) (McCance et al., 2014). Chapter 40 describes these processes in more detail.

Scope of Clotting

An inability to form adequate clots can result in bleeding and threaten a person's life. In some cases an excess of platelets or excessive platelet stickiness can lead to hypercoagulability (increased clotting ability), which can impair blood flow. Therefore the scope of clotting can range from increased or excessive clotting to an inability to adequately clot, either locally at the site of an injury or systemically. Fig. 2-2 illustrates the potential scope of clotting.

Common Risk Factors for Inadequate Clotting

When taking a patient and family history, be aware that impaired clotting may result in either excessive or inadequate clotting. Common risk factors for *increased* clotting include immobility or decreased mobility, health problems such as polycythemia, and smoking. Immobility slows venous blood flow to the heart and can result in venous stasis and venous thromboembolism (VTE), described later in this text. Certain chronic health problems such as diabetes mellitus are also associated with decreased blood flow, making patients more likely than healthy adults to develop VTE. Polycythemia causes an excessive production of red blood cells, which can lead to multiple clots. Atrial fibrillation causes pooling of blood in the atria (stasis) and often leads to embolic stroke. As people age and smoke, platelets typically become stickier and therefore tend to aggregate more easily. In addition, venous valves that normally prevent the backflow of blood become weak and often inadequate as adults age. The result is venous stasis and an increased risk for VTE.

Decreased clotting most often occurs when there is an inadequate number of circulating platelets (thrombocytopenia). For example, chemotherapeutic drugs and corticosteroids cause bone marrow suppression where platelets and other blood cells are produced. Patients with cirrhosis of the liver also have a decreased production of clotting factors, including prothrombin, causing them to be at an increased risk for bleeding. Some rare genetic diseases such as recessive sex-linked hemophilia A and B are the result of defective clotting factors that also increase the risk for bleeding.

Physiologic Consequences of Inadequate Clotting

For patients at risk for *increased* or excessive clotting, recognize that clots can occur in either venous or arterial blood vessels. Venous thrombosis is a clot formation in either superficial or deep (most often) veins, usually in the leg. If a thrombus becomes dislodged, it is known as an embolus. Emboli may travel to the brain (causing a stroke) or lung (pulmonary embolus).

For patients with a *decreased* ability to clot, prolonged internal (systemic) or external (localized) bleeding may occur. Internal bleeding may occur in the brain (hemorrhagic stroke), gastrointestinal (GI) tract (frank or occult blood in the stool), and/or urinary tract (hematuria). It may also occur under the skin (purpura). External bleeding often manifests as epistaxis (nose bleeds) or prolonged bleeding at the site of soft tissue trauma.

Assessment of Clotting

Observe patients for signs and symptoms of *decreased* clotting, especially purpural lesions such as ecchymosis (bruising) and petechiae (pinpoint purpura). Notice if bleeding is prolonged as a result of injury or trauma. Check urine and stool for the presence of occult or frank blood. Observe for frank bleeding from the gums or nose.

For patients with *increased* risk for clotting or excessive clotting, observe for signs and symptoms of *venous* thrombosis such as localized redness, swelling, and warmth.

> ### ⚠ NURSING SAFETY PRIORITY QSEN
> #### *Critical Rescue*
>
> An *arterial* thrombosis is not locally observable and is typically manifested by decreased blood flow (PERFUSION) to a distal extremity or internal organ. For example, a femoral arterial clot causes an occlusion (blockage) of blood to the leg. In this case the distal leg becomes pale and cool; distal pulses may be weak or absent; *this is an emergent problem requiring immediate intervention*. If these changes are present, notify the primary health care provider or Rapid Response Team immediately. If this condition continues, the leg may become gangrenous and require amputation. A mesenteric artery thrombosis can cause small bowel ileus and gangrene if not treated in a timely manner. A renal artery thrombosis can cause acute kidney injury.

A number of serum laboratory tests are available to measure clotting factor levels and bleeding time. The most common tests are prothrombin time (PT) and activated partial thromboplastin time (aPTT). An international normalized ratio (INR) indicating a derived measure of prothrombin is used to monitor the effectiveness of warfarin (Coumadin, Warfilone ♣).

Interventions to Promote Adequate Clotting and Prevent Inadequate Clotting

Teach patients with *decreased* clotting ability to report unusual bleeding or bruising immediately.

Be sure to teach patients at risk for *increased* clotting to:
- Drink adequate fluids to prevent dehydration.
- Avoid crossing the legs.
- Ambulate frequently and avoid prolonged sitting.
- Refer patients for smoking cessation programs as needed.
- Call a health care provider if redness, swelling, and warmth occur in a lower extremity.

Interventions for Patients With Inadequate Clotting

In addition to the previous interventions, for many adults at increased risk for clotting, *anticoagulants or antiplatelet drugs*

(also called *blood thinners* by many patients) are prescribed either in community or inpatient settings. Examples of medications that require frequent laboratory testing are sodium heparin and warfarin. *Teach adults the importance of obtaining these tests and monitor results to ensure that they are within the desired range to ensure patient safety.*

Newer anticoagulants called *direct thrombin inhibitors* may be given to decrease the risk of stroke in patients with atrial fibrillation. Monitor patients receiving any of these drugs for signs of bleeding, including bruising and blood in the urine or stool. Continued bleeding can lead to anemia or hemorrhage.

COGNITION

Definition of Cognition

Cognition is the complex integration of mental processes and intellectual function for the purposes of reasoning, learning, memory, and personality. *Reasoning* is a high-level thinking process that allows an individual to make decisions and judgments. *Memory* is the ability of an individual to retain and recall information for learning or recall of past experiences. *Personality* refers to the way an individual feels and behaves, often based on how he or she thinks.

Scope of Cognition

An adult may have either intact or adequate cognitive functioning or inadequate cognitive functioning. Examples of inadequate cognition include delirium (acute fluctuating confusion) and dementia (chronic confusion). Table 2-1 compares these two major cognitive disorders that are most common in older adults. Chapter 3 describes these health problems in detail. Adults may also have delayed intellectual functioning or amnesia (loss of memory) caused by brain trauma, congenital disorders, or acute health problems such as a stroke.

TABLE 2-1 **Differences in the Characteristics of Delirium and Dementia**

VARIABLE	DEMENTIA	DELIRIUM
Description	A chronic, progressive cognitive decline	An acute, fluctuating confusional state
Onset	Slow	Fast
Duration	Months to years	Hours to less than 1 month
Cause	Unknown, possibly familial, chemical	Multiple, such as surgery, infection, drugs
Reversibility	None	May be possible
Management	Treat signs and symptoms	Remove or treat the cause
Nursing interventions	Reorientation is not effective in the late stages; use validation therapy (acknowledge the patient's feelings and do not argue); provide a safe environment; observe for associated behaviors such as delusions and hallucinations	Reorient the patient to reality; provide a safe environment

Common Risk Factors for Inadequate Cognition

Inadequate cognition is complex and includes a variety of signs and symptoms. They may be short term and reversible or long term and not reversible. Common risk factors include:

- Advanced age (although dementia is *not* a normal physiologic change of aging)
- Brain trauma at any age, including at birth
- Disease or disorder such as brain tumor, hypoxia, or stroke (infarction)
- Environmental exposure to toxins such as lead
- Substance use disorder
- Genetic diseases such as Down syndrome
- Depression
- Opioids, steroids, psychoactive drugs, and general anesthesia, especially in older adults
- Fluid and electrolyte imbalances

Physiologic Consequences of Inadequate Cognition

Common signs and symptoms of inadequate cognition include:

- Loss of short- and/or long-term memory
- Disorientation to person, place, and/or time
- Impaired reasoning and decision-making ability
- Impaired language skills
- Uncontrollable or inappropriate emotions such as severe agitation and aggression
- Delusions and hallucinations

These manifestations often result in patient safety and communication issues. For example, an adult with impaired short-term memory may forget to turn off a stove burner that could result in a fire. A person who has impaired reasoning and decision-making ability may decide to drive a motor vehicle or operate machinery. Communication with a patient who is disoriented, aggressive, and/or delusional may not be possible.

Assessment of Cognition

Taking a thorough history is essential to determine potential or actual cognitive impairment. Conduct a mental status assessment using one of several available mental health/behavioral health screening tools such as the Confusion Assessment Method (CAM). Other tools also assess memory, speech and language, judgment, thought processes, calculation, and abstract reasoning. Discussion of assessment tools to screen for specific cognitive problems may be found throughout this text and in mental health textbooks.

Diagnostic testing includes brain imaging procedures such as magnetic resonance imaging (MRI) to determine the presence of brain abnormalities such as trauma, tumors, and infarction. Neuropsychological testing by a licensed clinical psychologist may be performed to diagnose the cause and severity of specific changes associated with cognitive problems.

Interventions to Promote Cognition and Prevent Inadequate Cognition

Teach adults to avoid risk factors such as substance use and lifestyle behaviors such as motorcycle driving without protective headgear. Teach older adults to stimulate the intellectual part of their brain through new learning activities such as taking music lessons, mastering a new language, or completing crossword puzzles or other "brain teasers."

Interventions for Patients With Inadequate Cognition

Nursing interventions focus on *safety* to prevent injury and foster communication. For adults with delirium or mild dementia, provide orientation to person, time, and place. Collaborate with the interprofessional team to determine the underlying cause of delirium, such as psychoactive drugs or hypoxia. Patients with moderate or severe dementia cannot be oriented to reality because they have chronic confusion.

> **! NURSING SAFETY PRIORITY** QSEN
> *Action Alert*
>
> Teach families and caregivers to provide a safe environment for the individual with cognitive impairment living in the community! Adults who are confused or cannot follow instructions may be injured by operating machinery or driving a motor vehicle. For those in inpatient facilities, provide a safe environment, depending on the patient's specific cognitive deficit. For example, implement fall precautions for those who need help getting out of bed. Adults with delirium or dementia may wander outside and be injured. Be sure they wear an alarm and identification bracelet.

In some cases the primary health care provider may prescribe psychoactive drug therapy for specific cognitive disorders. Some of these drugs are described later in this text but are discussed in more detail in mental health/behavioral health textbooks.

COMFORT

Definition of Comfort

Comfort is a state of physical well-being, pleasure, and absence of pain or stress. This definition implies that comfort has physical and emotional dimensions. A primary role of the nurse is to promote basic care and comfort.

Scope of Comfort

The desired outcome for optimal health and well-being of any individual is to have comfort or be comfortable. Many health problems can cause decreased comfort, also called *discomfort*. Most often patients report pain or other sensation that disrupts their ability to function, either physically or mentally.

Common Risk Factors for Decreased Comfort

Risk factors can be divided into physical causes and emotional, or psychosocial, causes. In some cases patients have risk factors for both physical and emotional discomfort. For example, patients who are having surgery are often anxious and feel stressed about the procedure. They may worry about who will care for them or their family after the surgery. This emotional stress is uncomfortable and can affect the outcomes of surgery. In addition, patients who have surgery typically have acute pain. This unpleasant sensation causes more emotional stress and discomfort. Some postoperative patients also have nausea or light-headedness as a result of the anesthesia used during the surgical procedure. All of these symptoms are causes of discomfort.

Physiologic Consequences of Decreased Comfort

Physical causes of decreased comfort (discomfort) such as pain, nausea, and itching can result in emotional stress and discomfort. The body's "fight or flight" mechanism helps the individual cope with the source and manifestations of the discomfort. If this response is not successful in reducing stress, the individual may develop chronic pain and anxiety.

Assessment of Comfort

Ask patients if they are comfortable. If pain is the source of discomfort, assess the level of pain and plan interventions to manage it. See Chapter 4 of this text for pain assessment. If emotional stress is the source of discomfort, be sure to help the patient describe the nature and cause of stress. Once the underlying cause(s) of discomfort is identified, coordinate with the interprofessional health care team to treat or remove it if possible.

Interventions to Prevent Impaired Comfort

Pain and emotional stress are the most common sources of decreased comfort. To prevent these sensations, anticipate which patient may experience them and provide preplanned interventions. For example, for postoperative pain control, ensure that the patient receives a basal dose of patient-controlled analgesia for continuous pain control.

Interventions for Patients With Decreased Comfort

Assess patients at risk for discomfort and plan interventions to alleviate it, depending on its source and cause. Collaborate care with members of the interprofessional health care team as needed. For example, refer the patient to a counselor, social worker, or other qualified mental health professional to manage emotional stress. Consult with the primary health care provider and pharmacist to manage acute and chronic pain.

ELIMINATION

Definition of Elimination

Elimination is the excretion of waste from the body by the gastrointestinal (GI) tract (as feces) and by the urinary system (as urine). *Bowel* elimination occurs as a result of food and fluid intake and ends with passage of feces (stool) or solid waste products from food into the rectum of the colon. The fecal material remains in the rectum until the urge to defecate occurs. Bowel elimination control depends on multiple factors, including muscle strength and nerve function.

Urinary elimination occurs as a result of multiple kidney processes and ends with the passage of urine through the urinary tract. When the urge to void occurs, urine is passed from the bladder through the urinary sphincter, urethra, and meatus. Urine consists of water and waste products (toxins) from many chemical processes in the body. Urinary elimination control also depends on multiple factors, including muscle strength and nerve function.

Scope of Elimination

Adults desire voluntary control of both bowel and urinary elimination, a normal condition called *continence*. However, a number of factors can cause *incontinence* (lack of bowel or bladder control) or *retention* (an inability to expel stool or excrete urine).

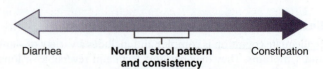

Diarrhea   **Normal stool pattern and consistency**   Constipation

FIG. 2-3 Scope of bowel elimination.

Bowel elimination may also be categorized by the consistency of fecal material, which is shown in Fig. 2-3. At one end of the continuum the stool can be watery and without solid form, a condition called diarrhea. At the other end of the continuum, the stool can be hard, dry, and difficult to pass through the rectum, a condition called constipation. The inability to pass stool is known as obstipation.

Common Risk Factors for Changes in Elimination

Incontinence of either the bowel or bladder can occur as a result of aging when pelvic floor muscles become weaker. It may also occur in adults who have neurologic disorders such as stroke, dementia, and multiple sclerosis. Excessive use of laxatives may also cause fecal (diarrheal) incontinence. *Diarrhea* also results from acute GI infections such as gastroenteritis and chronic inflammatory bowel diseases such as Crohn's disease. Irritable bowel syndrome causes frequent diarrhea, constipation, or intermittent episodes of diarrhea and constipation.

Urinary retention is often a problem in older men who have benign prostatic hyperplasia (overgrowth). This overgrowth blocks the bladder neck and prevents urination or complete bladder emptying. *Retention of stool*, or constipation, is also common in older adults who have decreased peristalsis and/or lack of adequate dietary fiber and fluids to promote fecal passage. Lack of exercise and use of certain medications such as opioids, diuretics, and psychoactive drugs can contribute to constipation in adults of any age. Spinal cord and brain injuries or diseases often cause involuntary control or retention of both bowel and bladder.

Renal and urinary health problems can alter urinary elimination, depending on the type of disease or disorder. For example, urinary tract obstructions such as ureteral stones may prevent urine from reaching the bladder. Chronic kidney disease can cause changes in the amount of urinary output, depending on the stage of the disease. In the end stage the patient experiences oliguria (scant urine) or anuria (absence of urine) because the kidneys have lost their ability to make urine.

Physiologic Consequences of Changes in Elimination

Adults who have urinary or bowel *incontinence* are at risk for damage to tissue integrity. If not removed promptly from the skin, stool and urine can cause skin irritation, fungal infection, and/or skin breakdown, which are very uncomfortable. Loss of bladder and bowel control can also lead to depression and anxiety. Older adults in both health care and community settings may wear undergarments or briefs to prevent soiling their clothes. Many older adults perceive these protective garments as "diapers" and are embarrassed or feel humiliated when wearing them.

If not treated, patients with prolonged *diarrhea* may develop fluid and electrolyte imbalances, especially dehydration and hypokalemia (decreased serum potassium). These problems are serious and can be life-threatening because hypokalemia often causes cardiac rhythm abnormalities (dysrhythmias).

Urinary or bowel *retention* can result in a buildup of toxins and waste products in the body. Although not common, a large amount of retained urine can cause rupture of the bladder. A large amount of stool can lead to bowel impaction and result in partial or total intestinal obstruction. These conditions can be life threatening.

Assessment of Elimination

Take a patient history to determine risk factors or the underlying cause for impaired or altered elimination. Ask the patient or designated family member if incontinence or retention is or has been a problem. Assess the perineal area and buttocks for skin breakdown, redness, and fungal infection in patients who have incontinence.

Monitor the frequency, amount, consistency, and characteristics of urine and stool. Listen to bowel sounds in all four quadrants for presence of adequate bowel sounds. Expect overactive bowel sounds in a patient who has diarrhea; anticipate hypoactive bowel sounds in patients who have constipation. Palpate the bladder and bowel for distention.

For some patients laboratory testing of urine or stool may be useful in determining the cause of elimination changes. For example, a urinalysis and culture and sensitivity are appropriate for the patient with suspected urinary stones, retention, and infection. Radiologic testing and ultrasonography for stones or other structural abnormalities may also be performed.

A stool culture and sensitivity may be done for patients suspected of have methicillin-resistant *Staphylococcus aureus* (MRSA) infection. This infection often causes severe diarrhea in older adults who have received antibiotic therapy.

Interventions to Prevent Changes in Elimination

Maintaining normal elimination requires adequate nutrition and hydration. Teach adults to ensure a diet high in fiber, including eating fruits, vegetables, and whole grains, and drinking 8 to 12 glasses of water each day unless medically contraindicated. Remind them to promptly toilet or void when the urge occurs. Patients at risk for *constipation* may need to take bulk-forming agents or stool softeners in addition to a high-fiber diet and fluids. Remind adults who have or are at risk for constipation to exercise frequently to stimulate peristalsis.

Interventions for Patients With Changes in Elimination

Adults with *diarrhea* need medical attention to determine the underlying cause of the problem. Monitor the patient for signs and symptoms of fluid and electrolyte imbalances. These problems can be treated to help the patient return to more normal elimination patterns and restore lost fluids and electrolytes. Chart 2-1 outlines nursing best practices for care of the patient experiencing diarrhea.

Nursing care for patients with *constipation* includes health teaching and collaboration with the interprofessional health care team. In addition to teaching about measures to prevent worsening of constipation as described previously, recommend that the patient take stool softeners, bulk-forming agents, and/or mild laxatives as needed to restore normal elimination patterns. In some cases enemas are needed to stimulate peristalsis and empty the rectum.

Adults who experience urinary *incontinence* need frequent toileting every 1 to 2 hours. This routine can prevent incontinence and train the bladder to empty at more regular intervals. A similar toileting schedule, especially after a meal,

---

> ◎ **CHART 2-1   Best Practice for Patient Safety and Quality Care** [QSEN]
>
> ### Patient With Diarrhea
>
> - Protect the perineal and buttock area with zinc oxide or other barrier cream to prevent skin irritation and excoriation, especially for patients who are incontinent.
> - Wash and dry skin where stool and urine have made contact, especially for patients who are incontinent.
> - Encourage fluid intake and ensure that the patient consumes foods high in potassium such as oranges and potatoes.
> - Document food and fluid intake and urinary/stool output.
> - Check the patient's weight each day for weight loss.
> - Collaborate with the primary health care provider for prescribing an antifungal cream if needed.

can help train the bowel to evacuate at about the same time each day.

Patients with short-term urinary *retention* require one or more straight urinary catheterizations to empty the bladder until the usual voiding pattern returns. For those with long-term retention, especially retention caused by lack of nerve stimuli, teach the patient or family/caregiver how to perform catheterizations on a daily routine schedule.

FLUID AND ELECTROLYTE BALANCE

Definition of Fluid and Electrolyte Balance

Fluid and electrolyte balance is the regulation of body fluid, fluid osmolality, and electrolytes by processes such as filtration, diffusion, and osmosis. To maintain balance or homeostasis in the body, fluid and electrolyte balance must be as close to normal as possible. Water makes up 55% to 60% of total body weight. Older adults have less body fluid than younger adults.

Fluid occupies the inside of the cell (intracellular fluid) and the outside of the cell (extracellular fluid). Extracellular fluid is found in the vascular space (plasma) and interstitial space (fluid between cells, often referred to as *third space fluid*). *Electrolytes* are chemicals in the body needed for normal body functioning, especially the heart and brain. Examples of electrolytes are sodium, potassium, calcium, and magnesium.

Scope of Fluid and Electrolyte Balance

Fluid imbalances range from decreased fluid (deficit), often causing dehydration, to excessive fluid (overload), often causing edema. *Electrolyte imbalances* may also occur as deficits such as hypokalemia (low serum potassium) and excesses such as hyperkalemia (high serum potassium). Table 2-2 lists common fluid and electrolyte imbalances.

Common Risk Factors for Fluid and Electrolyte Imbalance

Risk factors that can alter a person's fluid and electrolyte balance include acute illnesses (e.g., vomiting and diarrhea), severe burns, serious injury or trauma, chronic kidney disease, surgery, and poor nutritional intake. Older adults are especially at risk for imbalances in fluids and electrolytes because they have less body water and are most likely to experience acute and chronic illnesses.

TABLE 2-2	Common Fluid and Electrolyte Imbalances	
Common Fluid Imbalances	**Common Electrolyte Imbalances**
Fluid volume deficit (dehydration)	Hyponatremia (low serum sodium)
Fluid volume excess (overload)	Hypernatremia (high serum sodium)
	Hypokalemia (low serum potassium)
	Hyperkalemia (high serum potassium)
	Hypocalcemia (low serum calcium)
	Hypercalcemia (high serum calcium)
	Hypomagnesemia (low serum magnesium)
	Hypermagnesemia (high serum magnesium)

Physiologic Consequences of Fluid and Electrolyte Imbalance

Physiologic consequences of *fluid deficit* are the result of lack of blood flow and oxygen to all parts of the body. A decrease in blood volume leads to hypotension (low blood pressure). In an attempt to compensate for hypotension and perfuse major organs, the heart rate increases (tachycardia). Peripheral pulses become weak and thready. For patients with severe dehydration, fever may occur due to inadequate body water. Older adults may also experience delirium due to lack of blood flow to the brain. If fluid deficit is not adequately managed, the kidney function diminishes, as evidenced by a decrease in urinary output. Recall that the minimum hourly urinary output should be at least 30 mL per hour.

Patients with *fluid excess* (overload) usually have an increase in blood pressure due to increased blood volume. Peripheral pulses are often strong and bounding. Many patients experience peripheral edema due to fluid excess. Fluid from the vascular space shifts to the interstitial space (third spacing).

The physiologic consequences of *electrolyte deficit* depend on which electrolyte is decreased. For example, a decrease in serum potassium level (hypokalemia) can result in cardiac dysrhythmias (abnormal heart rhythms) and muscle weakness. A decreased sodium level (hyponatremia) can result in changes in mental status and generalized weakness.

The consequences of *electrolyte excess* also depend on which electrolyte is increased. For example, an increase in serum potassium (hyperkalemia) or calcium (hypercalcemia) can cause cardiac dysrhythmias. In addition, skeletal muscle spasms are likely. An increased calcium level can also result in kidney or urinary tract calculi (stones). Chapter 11 describes specific fluid and electrolyte imbalances in detail.

Assessment of Fluid and Electrolyte Balance

Take a complete health history for past experiences of fluid and electrolyte imbalance and for any risk factors that can lead to an imbalance. Ask about any current episodes of nausea, vomiting, or diarrhea. Inquire about the current use of medications, including over-the-counter and herbal supplements.

Monitor vital signs, especially blood pressure and pulse rate and quality, fluid intake and output, and weight. *Changes in weight are the best indicator of fluid volume changes in the body.* Assess skin and mucous membranes for dryness and decreased skin turgor. Monitor and interpret laboratory tests to determine fluid or electrolyte imbalance. Examples of common tests are measurements of serum electrolyte concentration, blood urea nitrogen (BUN), and serum osmolality. Chapter 11 discusses each of these assessments in detail.

Interventions to Promote Fluid and Electrolyte Balance and Prevent Fluid and Electrolyte Imbalance

Maintaining fluid and electrolyte balance in the body is essential for normal body functioning. Teach patients to drink adequate fluids to remain hydrated. Eight glasses or more of water a day are often recommended unless medically contraindicated. Older adults may not feel thirsty or want to limit their fluid intake to prevent urinary incontinence. Teach them the importance of drinking adequate fluids to prevent dehydration and potential urinary tract infection.

Remind all adults about the need to eat a well-balanced diet that promotes electrolyte balance. Certain foods contain high concentrations of essential vitamins, minerals, and electrolytes. For instance, milk and other dairy products are a good source of calcium. Bananas and potatoes are good sources of potassium.

Interventions for Fluid and Electrolyte Imbalances

Priority nursing interventions include maintenance of patient safety and comfort measures when managing fluid or electrolyte imbalances. For patients with a *fluid deficit,* the primary collaborative intervention is fluid replacement, either orally or parenterally. Depending on the cause of *fluid overload,* patients may require a fluid restriction (e.g., for those with chronic kidney disease). Diuretic therapy is often used for patients with fluid overload caused by chronic heart failure to prevent pulmonary edema, a potentially life-threatening complication. If lower extremity edema is present, teach patients the importance of elevating the legs above the heart to promote venous return.

Interprofessional collaborative management of electrolyte imbalance depends on which electrolyte balance is impaired. In general, electrolyte deficits are treated by replacing them, usually parenterally as intravenous (IV) fluids. Electrolyte excesses are managed by restricting additional electrolytes or using a medication or fluids that can help eliminate the excess. For example, sodium polystyrene sulfonate (Kayexalate) may be used for patients with hyperkalemia to eliminate excess potassium via the GI system.

GLUCOSE REGULATION

GLUCOSE REGULATION is the process of maintaining optimal blood glucose levels. Though this concept is not a primary concept of this title, it is discussed in connection to multiple interrelated concepts with the GLUCOSE REGULATION concept exemplar Diabetes Mellitus in Chapter 64.

GAS EXCHANGE

Definition of Gas Exchange

Gas exchange is the process of oxygen transport to the cells and carbon dioxide transport away from the cells through ventilation and diffusion. This process begins with ventilation triggered by neurons in the brain sensing the need for gas exchange. These neurons stimulate contraction of skeletal muscles that expand the chest cavity, causing inhalation of oxygen-containing air into the airways and lungs. From the lung alveoli, oxygen diffuses into blood and red blood cells, and the waste gas carbon dioxide diffuses from the blood into the alveoli. Once in the alveoli, carbon dioxide is exhaled from the body as a result of recoil of lung elastic tissues and contraction of skeletal muscles that constrict the chest cavity. The oxygen in red blood cells bound to hemoglobin is transported through the blood by cardiac effort to tissue cells (perfusion), where low oxygen concentration allows release of oxygen from hemoglobin and diffusion or cell metabolism. The high concentration of carbon dioxide waste resulting from cellular metabolism allows diffusion of this gas into the blood and red blood cells. The waste gas is then transported back to the lungs to diffuse into the alveoli for removal during exhalation.

Scope of Gas Exchange

Gas exchange is either normal to allow for adequate perfusion and removal of waste gas (carbon dioxide) or decreased. Decreased gas exchange can range from minimal to severe.

Common Risk Factors for Decreased Gas Exchange

Adequate ventilation requires normal functioning central (brain and spinal cord) neurons, normal diaphragm function, adequate skeletal muscle contractility (especially the intercostal muscles between the ribs), and an intact chest thorax. Any acute or chronic problems that affect these functions can result in decreased ventilation, which impairs gas exchange. For example, pneumonia or lung abscess prevents adequate ventilation and gas exchange. A patient who experienced a cervical spinal cord injury often has decreased ventilation ability due to damage to spinal nerves that control the diaphragm.

As adults age, pulmonary alveoli lose some of their elasticity, causing a decrease in gas exchange. Health problems can also affect lung functioning. Any condition that decreases ventilation such as asthma can impair gas exchange. Asthma causes bronchospasm and narrowed airways, which diminishes the amount of oxygen available for gas exchange. Other lung diseases such as chronic obstructive pulmonary disease (COPD) directly damage the alveoli, decreasing both oxygen and/or carbon dioxide diffusion (Fig. 2-4). Risk factors for developing these diseases include smoking and environmental pollutants.

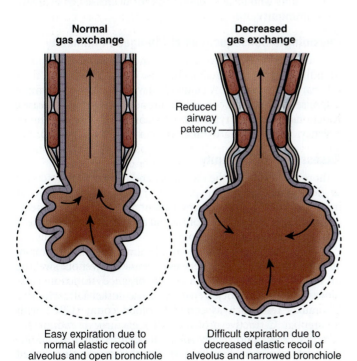

Normal gas exchange

Decreased gas exchange

Reduced airway patency

Easy expiration due to normal elastic recoil of alveolus and open bronchiole

Difficult expiration due to decreased elastic recoil of alveolus and narrowed bronchiole

FIG. 2-4 Damaged inelastic alveoli common in patients with COPD cause decreases in oxygen and carbon dioxide diffusion.

In addition, prolonged immobility can decrease gas exchange as a result of inadequate pulmonary ventilation.

Physiologic Consequences of Decreased Gas Exchange

Decreased gas exchange results in (1) inadequate transportation of oxygen to body cells and organs; and/or (2) retention of carbon dioxide. Inadequate oxygen results in cell dysfunction (ischemia) and possible cell death (necrosis or infarction) (Fig. 2-5). An excessive buildup of carbon dioxide combines with water to produce carbonic acid. This increase in acid causes respiratory acidosis and lowers the pH of blood. See the previous discussion of acid-base imbalance earlier in this chapter and in Chapter 12.

Assessment of Gas Exchange

Take a complete health history and perform a focused respiratory assessment. Ask the patient about current or history of lung disease or trauma. Assess the patient's breathing effort, oxygen saturation, capillary refill, thoracic expansion, and lung sounds anteriorly and posteriorly. Monitor for the presence of a cough; sputum; report of shortness of breath; dizziness; chest pain; presence of cyanosis; or adventitious lung sounds such as wheezing, rhonchi, or crackles. Interpret associated laboratory results, including arterial blood gases (ABGs) and complete blood count (CBC). When necessary, a chest x-ray, chest computerized tomography (CT), or $\dot{V}/\dot{Q}$ scan may be performed to determine the presence and severity of lung disease. Pulmonary function tests can determine the extent of airway disease in the small and large airways of the lungs and their structures. Bronchoscopy can provide direct visualization into the bronchus and its extending structures.

Interventions to Promote Gas Exchange and Prevent Decreased Gas Exchange

Teach patients the importance of using infection control measures (primarily proper handwashing), smoking cessation to prevent COPD, and getting vaccinations as recommended to prevent influenza and pneumonia. Instruct them to be aware of exposure to specific respiratory conditions, including tuberculosis and influenza.

Interventions for Decreased Gas Exchange

Managing decreased gas exchange requires finding the underlying cause and treating it, often with drug therapy. Examples of drugs used to treat respiratory health problems include antihistamines, decongestants, glucocorticoids, bronchodilators, mucolytics, and antimicrobials.

Chest expansion is improved when the patient is sitting or is in a semi-Fowlers position. Teach the patient about the need for deep breathing and coughing to further enhance lung expansion and decrease breathing effort. Teach him or her how to correctly use incentive spirometry and inhalers if indicated. Administer oxygen therapy and monitor pulse oximetry to determine its effectiveness.

IMMUNITY

Definition of Immunity

Immunity is protection from illness or disease that is maintained by the body's physiologic defense mechanisms. *Natural active* immunity occurs when an antigen enters the body and the body creates antibodies to fight off the antigen. *Artificial active* immunity occurs via a vaccination or immunization.

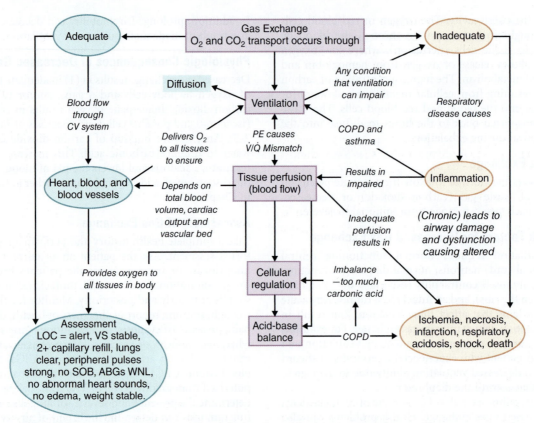

FIG. 2-5 Concept map showing comparison of adequate and inadequate gas exchange with consequences of impaired gas exchange. (*ABG*, Arterial blood gas; *COPD*, chronic obstructive pulmonary disease; *CV*, cardiovascular; *LOC*, level of consciousness; *PE*, pulmonary embolism; *SOB*, shortness of breath; *V̇/Q̇*, ventilation-perfusion; *VS*, vital signs; *WNL*, within normal limits.)

Natural passive immunity occurs when antibodies are passed from a mother to the fetus through the placenta or using colostrum or the breast milk; *artificial passive* immunity occurs via a specific transfusion such as immunoglobulins.

Multiple organs and cells in the body are involved in the immune response. *Antibody-mediated immunity* (humoral immunity) includes the antigens and antibodies interacting in an attempt to slow down or destroy the foreign body. B-cells play a major role in this activity, together with the macrophages, T-lymphocytes (T-cells), and spleen. *Cell-mediated immunity* involves the functions of numerous cells to fight off the antigen, including white blood cells (WBCs), T-cells, natural killer (NK) cells, and multiple cytokines. The thymus and lymph nodes also play a role in this immune process.

Scope of Immunity

Immunity has the potential to be decreased (suppressed or weakened) or excessive (exaggerated or heightened).

Common Risk Factors for Changes in Immunity

Adult populations at risk for impaired immunity include but are not limited to:

- Older adults (diminished immunity due to normal aging changes)
- Low socioeconomic groups (inability to obtain proper immunizations)
- Nonimmunized adults
- Adults with chronic illnesses that weaken the immune system

- Adults on chronic drug therapy such as corticosteroids and chemotherapeutic agents
- Adults experiencing substance use disorder
- Adults who have a genetic risk for decreased or excessive immunity

Physiologic Consequences of Changes in Immunity

An individual with a decreased immune response is susceptible to multiple types of infections because of the inability to "fight off" particular antigens. An individual with an excessive immune response has allergies or autoimmune reactions or diseases. Reactions are graded types I to IV and have varying degrees of urgency. These types are discussed in detail in Chapter 20.

Assessment of Immunity

A thorough history of the individual and the family is necessary to determine any of the previous risks associated with an immune problem. Identify any patient allergies, current medications, and history of environmental exposures. Ask the patient about an immunization history.

Assess weight, adequate wound healing, cognitive function, allergic responses (red, watery eyes; nasal congestion; swelling or rashes), and potential or actual organ dysfunction (cardiovascular, respiratory, renal or musculoskeletal). Monitor laboratory tests such as complete blood count (CBC) with differential, C-reactive protein (CRP), erythrocyte sedimentation rate (ESR), and allergy testing to identify any susceptibilities that may exist. Specific tests such as the enzyme-linked immunosorbent assay (ELISA) and Western blot tests may be performed to identify the presence of human immune deficiency virus (HIV) antibodies. A complete immune panel, including antinuclear antibody (ANA) and rheumatoid factor (RF) testing, helps to detect autoimmune disease.

Interventions to Promote Immunity and Prevent Changes in Immunity

Avoiding infections, handwashing, and having recommended immunizations are essential for promoting healthy immune function. Teach patients to practice a healthy lifestyle, including eating a well-balanced diet to ensure adequate vitamins and minerals, getting at least 7 to 8 hours of sleep each day, and having regular primary health care provider physical examinations. Remind them to avoid environmental hazards such as potential allergens (if sensitive) and people with contagious infections such as influenza.

Interventions for Changes in Immunity

Patients with a *decreased* immune system for any reason are very prone to infection. Teach them to avoid large crowds or anyone with a transmittable infectious disease or illness. Remind them to wash their hands frequently and use hand sanitizer when water and soap are not available.

Patients with an *excessive* immune function have hypersensitivity reactions. Interprofessional collaborative management of these adults depends on the type and severity of the reaction. The expected outcome of treatment is to decrease symptoms and promote a quality of life. In some cases remission of the health problem can be achieved, but not a cure. Examples of autoimmune diseases that typically have remissions and exacerbations (flare-ups) are rheumatoid arthritis and lupus erythematosus (see Chapter 18).

MOBILITY

Definition of Mobility

Mobility is the ability of an individual to perform purposeful physical movement of the body. When a person is able to move, he or she is usually able to perform activities of daily living (ADLs) such as eating, dressing, and walking. This ability depends primarily on the function of the central and peripheral nervous system and the musculoskeletal system and is sometimes referred to as *functional ability*.

Scope of Mobility

The scope of mobility can be best understood as continuum of a person's ability to move, with high-level (normal) mobility on one end of the continuum and total immobility on the other end. Many patients have varying degrees of impaired or altered physical mobility. *Decreased* physical mobility is the inability to move purposefully within the environment because of multiple factors, such as severe fatigue, decreased muscle strength, pain, or advanced dementia.

Common Risk Factors for Decreased Mobility

Patients who have dysfunction of the musculoskeletal or nervous system are most at risk for decreased mobility or immobility. For example, a patient with a fractured hip is not able to walk because of pain and hip joint instability until the hip is surgically repaired and healed. Patients who have severe brain or spinal cord injuries have decreased mobility or total immobility caused by lack of neuronal communication or damaged nerve tissues

TABLE 2-3 Common Complications of Decreased Mobility and Causes
Physiologic Complications (Occur Most Often in Older Adults)
• Pressure injuries (pressure on skin over bony prominences)
• Disuse osteoporosis (increased bone resorption)
• Constipation (decreased gastrointestinal [GI] motility)
• Weight loss or gain (decreased appetite and movement)
• Muscle atrophy (catabolism)
• Atelectasis/hypostatic pneumonia (decreased lung expansion)
• Venous thromboembolism (e.g., deep venous thrombosis and pulmonary embolus [decreased blood circulation])
• Urinary system calculi (stones) (urinary stasis)
Psychosocial Complications
• Depression (isolation, inability to provide self-care)
• Changes in sleep-wake cycle (especially if confined to bed)
• Sensory deprivation (especially if confined to bed)

that enable body movement. Any person who is bedridden or on prolonged bedrest is at risk for immobility issues, regardless of health problem or medical diagnosis (Crawford & Harris, 2016).

Physiologic Consequences of Decreased Mobility

Decreases in mobility or total immobility for even a few days can cause serious and often life-threatening complications (Teodoro et al., 2016). Table 2-3 lists the most common complications seen in adult patients.

Assessment of Mobility

Observe patients within the environment to determine their mobility level. The mobility level of the patient is adequate if he or she can move purposely to walk with an erect posture and coordinated gait and perform ADLs without assistance. Several functional assessment tools are available to measure the level at which a patient can perform ADLs (see Chapter 6). Assessment of muscle strength and joint range of motion (ROM) can also be measured using a scale of 0 to 5, with 5 being normal and 0 indicating no muscle contractility.

Interventions to Prevent Decreased Mobility

The nurse has a major role in promoting mobility and preventing immobility. First assess the patients who are most at risk for decreased mobility. In general, to maintain a high level of mobility or prevent decreased mobility in high-risk patients, perform these priority interventions for the patient at home or in a health care facility:

• Teach patients to do active ROM exercises every 2 hours. Assess and manage pain to promote more comfortable movement.
• Teach patients to perform "heel pump" activities and drink adequate fluids to help prevent venous thromboembolism (VTE) such as deep vein thrombosis (DVT).
• In collaboration with the occupational therapist, evaluate the patient's need for assistive devices to promote ADL independence such as a plate guard or splint; encourage self-care.
• Evaluate the patient's need for ambulatory aids such as a cane or walker; encourage ambulation; collaborate with the physical therapist if needed.

A study by Teodoro et al. (2016) found that a practical nurse–led ambulation program designed for hospitalized patients significantly improved mobility (see the Evidence-Based Practice box).

Interventions for Patients With Decreased Mobility

For patients who are immobile or have decreased mobility, perform these nursing interventions in collaboration with the interprofessional team at home or in a health care agency:

- Perform passive ROM exercises for patients who are immobile or have severe impaired mobility.
- Turn and reposition the patient every 1 to 2 hours; assess for skin redness and intactness.
- Keep the patient's skin clean and dry; use pressure-relieving or pressure-reducing devices as indicated.
- In collaboration with the registered dietitian, teach the patient and family the need for adequate nutrition, including high-fiber and protein-rich foods to promote elimination and slow muscle loss.
- Teach the patient to eat high-calcium foods to help prevent bone loss; avoid excessive high-calorie foods to prevent obesity.
- Encourage deep-breathing and coughing exercises; teach the patient how and when to use incentive spirometry.

- Teach the patient and family the need for adequate hydration to prevent renal calculi (stones) and constipation.
- Teach the patient and family to report signs and symptoms of complications of immobility such as pressure injuries; swollen, reddened lower leg; and excessive respiratory secretions.
- Collaborate with the physical therapist to ambulate the patient with mobility aids (e.g., walker, cane) if needed.

NUTRITION

Definition of Nutrition

Nutrition is the process of ingesting and using food and fluids to grow, repair, and maintain optimal body functions. Nutrients from food and fluids are used for optimal cellular metabolism and health promotion. Examples of nutrient groups are proteins, carbohydrates, fats, vitamins, and minerals.

Scope of Nutrition

An optimal nutritional status means that the individual has adequate nutrients for body functioning. However, some adults have decreased or poor nutritional status because of lack of available nutrients or inadequate use of nutrients. *Malnutrition* occurs in adults who are underweight or overweight/obese. Some individuals have *generalized* malnutrition; others have specific nutrient deficiencies such as lack of vitamin D, iron, or protein.

Common Risk Factors for Decreased Nutrition

Older adults are the largest population at risk for malnutrition as a result of acute and chronic diseases, poor oral health, and social isolation. Obesity is a common problem in people who have type 2 diabetes mellitus and metabolic syndrome.

In addition to these high-risk populations, other common risk factors for decreased nutrition in adults include lack of money to purchase healthy food and substance use. Adults with anorexia or bulimia nervosa are also malnourished. These disorders are discussed in textbooks on mental and behavioral health. Table 2-4 summarizes common risk factors for decreased nutrition.

Physiologic Consequences of Decreased Nutrition

The physiologic changes that occur as a result of decreased nutrition depend on whether the individual has generalized malnutrition or a lack of specific nutrients such as vitamin D,

---

EVIDENCE-BASED PRACTICE QSEN

Is a Nurse-Initiated Ambulation Protocol Effective in Promoting Patient Ambulation?

Teodoro, C. R., Breault, K., Garvey, C., Klick, C., O'Briend, J., Purdue, T., et al. (2016). STEP-UP: Study of the effectiveness of a patient ambulation protocol. *MEDSURG Nursing, 25*(2), 111–116.

Impaired mobility or immobility in hospitalized patients can cause multiple complications, many of which are life-threatening (e.g., deep vein thrombosis, hospital-acquired pneumonia). The authors assigned 48 patients on a 30-bed medical-surgical unit in a community hospital to one of two randomly assigned matched groups: 22 patients participated in the formal ambulation protocol (STEP-UP group), and 26 patients received usual care. All patients in the study sample were in the hospital for at least 3 days and had orders for ambulation. All patients were alert and oriented and able to be ambulated with the assistance of one or two staff members. Each patient in the sample viewed a short educational video on the importance of ambulation. Each participant wore a pedometer to track the number of steps taken for 2 consecutive study days. The participants in the STEP-UP group had significantly higher numbers of steps when compared to the group who received usual care.

Level of Evidence: 3
The study used a quasi-experimental design.

Commentary: Implications for Practice and Research
This study illustrates the need for staff nurses to ensure that hospitalized patients who are able continue to ambulate using a systematic approach or protocol to prevent impaired mobility and its associated complications. Complications of immobility are often life threatening and costly. In addition, third-party payers such as Medicare do not pay for acquired complications resulting from inadequate care.

More research is needed to follow a larger group of patients for a longer period of time in multiple settings to increase the generalizability of the findings this study. Additional studies are also needed to compare the incidence of complications from impaired mobility in both groups of patients.

TABLE 2-4 Risk Factors for Decreased Nutrition

- Familial predisposition or genetic risk
- High stress level
- Depression and social isolation, especially among older adults
- Consuming fad diets that do not provide adequate nutrients
- Obesity
- Substance use
- Lack of money to purchase food
- Impaired food intake caused by dysphagia, poor appetite, or poor oral health
- Thyroid disorders
- Chronic diseases such as chronic obstructive pulmonary disease (COPD) and cancer
- Gastrointestinal (GI) distress such as excessive diarrhea or vomiting
- Anorexia or bulimia nervosa

iron, and protein. For example, an individual who is lactose intolerant may not ingest adequate amounts of vitamin D in the diet. This deficit can cause bone demineralization such as osteoporosis. An adult who does not eat meat or other sources of iron can develop iron-deficiency anemia. Most of these patients have low serum protein, especially albumin and prealbumin, resulting in generalized edema. Serum proteins exert an osmotic pull to keep fluid within the vascular space. When they are decreased, fluid leaves the vascular system and moves into the interstitial space (third spacing).

Assessment of Nutrition

Conduct a complete patient and family history for risk factors that could cause impaired nutrition. Ask about current or recent GI symptoms such as nausea, vomiting, constipation, and diarrhea. Obtain the patient's height and weight and calculate body mass index (BMI). Assess the patient's skin, hair, and nails. Malnutrition often causes very dry skin and brittle hair and nails.

Serum laboratory testing depends on which nutrients are inadequate. For example, older women often have vitamin D and calcium testing to determine risk for bone demineralization risk. Low serum iron levels and anemia indicate an iron deficiency. The most common assessment for generalized malnutrition is prealbumin and albumin measurement. Albumin is a major serum protein that is below normal in patients who have had inadequate nutrition for weeks. Prealbumin assessment is preferred because it decreases more quickly when nutrition is not adequate. Monitor and interpret these laboratory data to assess the patient's nutritional status.

Interventions to Promote Nutrition and Prevent Decreased Nutrition

Teach adults to follow a healthy lifestyle that includes regular exercise and adequate nutrients to promote optimal nutrition and a BMI between 19 and 24.9. Remind them to avoid high-calorie, high-fat foods with no nutritive value. For patients at risk for decreased nutrition, collaborate with the interprofessional team to implement the appropriate interventions discussed in the following section.

Interventions for Patients With Decreased Nutrition

Collaborative interventions to improve nutrition depend on the cause of decreased nutrition. For those with weight loss or low weight, common interventions include high-protein oral supplements, enteral supplements (either oral or by feeding tube), or parenteral nutrition. Collaborate with the registered dietitian for specific instructions regarding enteral feedings; consult with the pharmacist to administer parenteral therapy. Drug therapy such as iron or vitamin D to replace selected nutrients may also be given. To determine effectiveness of these interventions, weigh the patient at least once a week or as prescribed, using the same scale at the same time of day and preferably before breakfast.

Patients experiencing obesity may be prescribed drug therapy to help them lose weight. In some cases bariatric surgical procedures are needed to restrict the volume of food that can be ingested and/or decrease the absorptive area for nutrients. These procedures have the potential to cause multiple complications and require an interprofessional team approach for success. Chapter 60 describes these surgeries in detail and their associated nursing and interprofessional collaborative care.

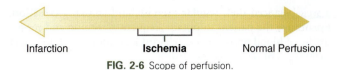

Infarction   **Ischemia**   Normal Perfusion

FIG. 2-6 Scope of perfusion.

PERFUSION

Definition of Perfusion

Perfusion is adequate arterial blood flow through the peripheral tissues (*peripheral* perfusion) and blood that is pumped by the heart to oxygenate major body organs (*central* perfusion). Perfusion is a normal physiologic process of the body; without adequate perfusion, cell death can occur.

Scope of Perfusion

The scope of perfusion can best be understood as a continuum of the heart's ability to adequately supply blood to the body and the patency of arteries to adequately supply blood to peripheral tissues. *Ischemia* refers to impaired perfusion, whereas *infarction* is complete tissue death (Fig. 2-6).

Common Risk Factors for Decreased Perfusion

Risk factors for decreased perfusion can be either modifiable (can be changed) or nonmodifiable (cannot be changed). *Nonmodifiable* factors include age, gender, and family history (genetics). Older adults are at the most risk for impaired perfusion. Examples of *modifiable* risk factors are smoking, lack of physical activity, and obesity. Patients with hyperlipidemia, diabetes mellitus, peripheral vascular disease, and arteriosclerosis are at a very high risk for both decreased central and peripheral perfusion.

Physiologic Consequences of Decreased Perfusion

Decreased *peripheral* perfusion most often occurs in the lower extremities. The distal legs become cool and pale or cyanotic. Pedal pulses may be diminished or absent. If not treated, inadequate perfusion can result in skin ulcers (see tissue integrity later in this chapter) or cell death such as gangrene. Decreased *central* perfusion can result in life-threatening systemic events such as acute myocardial infarction, stroke, and shock as a result of decreased blood flow to major organs.

Assessment of Perfusion

Conduct a complete patient and family history for risk factors and existing problems with perfusion. Assess for signs and symptoms of inadequate central perfusion, including dyspnea, dizziness or syncope, and chest pain. Signs and symptoms of decreased cardiac output include hypotension, tachycardia, diaphoresis, anxiety, decrease in cognitive function, and dysrhythmias. Assess for signs and symptoms of decreased *peripheral* perfusion, including decreased hair distribution, pallor, coolness, and/or cyanosis of the extremities. Document the presence and quality of distal peripheral pulses.

Interventions to Promote Perfusion and Prevent Decreased Perfusion

The nurse plays a vital role in promoting adequate perfusion and preventing any impairment. Help the patient identify modifiable risk factors such as poor nutrition and smoking. Teach the importance of a heart-healthy lifestyle that includes a well-balanced diet, regular exercise, and smoking cessation. Encourage the patient to obtain frequent screening and monitoring of blood pressure and relevant laboratory work to detect early signs of decreased perfusion.

Interventions for Decreased Perfusion

Inadequate perfusion can cause serious and life-threatening consequences. For patients who have decreased perfusion, the primary health care provider may prescribe vasodilating drugs to promote blood flow. However, for many patients a vascular intervention to open the occluded or narrowed artery is performed. This type of procedure can be done to open coronary arteries (central perfusion) or peripheral arteries such as the femoral or pelvic arteries in the leg.

SENSORY PERCEPTION

Definition of Sensory Perception

Sensory perception is the ability to perceive and interpret sensory input into one or more meaningful responses. Sensory input is usually received through the five major senses of vision, hearing, smell, taste, and touch.

Scope of Sensory Perception

The most likely cause of changes in smell and taste for adults is a dry mouth, which is a common side effect of drug therapy. Examples of drugs that can cause dry mouth include antidepressants, chemotherapeutic agents, antihistamines, and antiepileptic drugs (AEDs). When the causative drug is discontinued, the problem typically subsides. Touch (peripheral sensation loss) is most often affected in patients who have acute and chronic neurologic problems such as stroke, traumatic brain injury, or spinal cord injury. For many patients this sensory deficit is permanent. These health problems are discussed elsewhere in this text.

Problems of sensory perception that occur in the adult population largely affect vision and hearing. Therefore the following discussion is limited to these two sensory functions.

Vision and hearing abilities (acuity) vary from person to person, depending on a number of factors. Acuity of vision and hearing ranges from optimum through a continuum to complete blindness (vision) and deafness (hearing). Many adults have visual or hearing deficits but are able to function independently.

Common Risk Factors for Changes in Sensory Perception

As adults age, they are at an increased risk for decreased visual and hearing acuity. Older adults typically have *presbyopia* (farsightedness) and *presbycusis* (sensorineural type) caused by the aging process. Chronic diseases such as diabetes mellitus and hypertension can lead to decreased visual acuity. Although these health problems can occur in any age-group, they most commonly occur in older adults. The older population is also more at risk for glaucoma, cataracts, and macular degeneration, all of which can cause loss of vision.

Other causes for changes in or loss of vision include direct mechanical or chemical trauma, genetic risk, cranial nerve II (optic) damage, and drug therapy such as antihistamines and antihypertensives. Hearing loss may be caused by direct physical trauma, cranial nerve VIII (acoustic, or auditory) damage, occupational factors (e.g., consistent loud noises), genetic risk, and drugs that are ototoxic. Examples of drugs that can cause ototoxicity are salicylates, diuretics, AEDs, and antibiotics, especially aminoglycosides.

Physiologic Consequences of Changes in Sensory Perception

Adults with visual and hearing acuity loss that cannot be corrected are at risk for physical injury, including falls and other accidents. They may not be able to perform ADLs or ambulate independently and may require assistance. Those with hearing loss may not be able to rely solely on verbal communication. Visually impaired adults may not be able to use written communication.

Assessment of Sensory Perception

Conduct a thorough patient and family history to determine risk factors for vision or hearing loss. Ask the patient about the use of eyeglasses, contacts, or a magnifier to improve vision. Inquire if he or she uses one or more hearing aids or amplifier. If any of these corrective aids are used, determine their effectiveness.

Ask the patient to read from a written text source such as a newspaper. Assess the patient to determine reading ability before requesting this screening. In the community setting a Snellen chart is often used to assess visual acuity. Use a whisper test to determine if the patient can hear. More extensive testing of the eyes and ears, including physical assessment, is performed by the health care provider or other qualified health professional.

Interventions to Promote Sensory Perception and Prevent Changes in Sensory Perception

Primary and secondary preventive interventions are used to promote vision and hearing and prevent sensory deficits. *Primary* measures focus on avoiding risk factors that cause vision and hearing loss or using protective devices to minimize risk. For example, safety goggles help prevent eye injury when working with materials that can get into the eye. Ear plugs or other ear protective devices can minimize the exposure to loud noises such as that caused by machinery. A healthy lifestyle can help prevent the risk for diseases such as diabetes mellitus and hypertension, thus reducing the chance for decreased visual acuity from chronic disease.

The purpose of secondary prevention is to perform screening and diagnostic tests for early detection of beginning sensory loss. Examples of these strategies include regular eye examinations (annually for older adults) and physical examinations to diagnose and manage any chronic diseases early.

Interventions for Patients With Changes in Sensory Perception

For patients who have glaucoma, drug therapy (local or systemic) may decrease intraocular pressure and prevent loss of vision. For some patients, corrective lenses or eye surgery (LASIK) can improve refractory vision problems. Adults with visual changes may have correction with eyeglasses or contact lenses; those with hearing loss may benefit from one or two hearing aids (Fig. 2-7). Adults who are totally blind may use guide dogs and/or braille. Those who are deaf may use closed-caption television, assistive listening devices, and sign language.

Assess patients with vision and hearing loss for self-image and anxiety, especially those with a new onset of one of these deficits. Consult with or refer those who are having

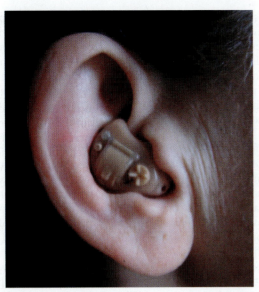

FIG. 2-7 Example of a hearing aid. (From Touhy, T. A., & Jett, K. (2012). *Ebersole & Hess' toward healthy aging* (8th ed.). St. Louis: Mosby. Courtesy Kathleen Jett.)

psychological distress to a qualified member of the interprofessional health team.

SEXUALITY

Definition of Sexuality

Sexuality is a complex integration of physiologic, emotional, and social aspects of well-being related to intimacy, self-concept, and role relationships. It is not the same as *reproduction,* which is the process of conceiving and having a child. Sexuality involves sex, sexual acts, and sexual orientation; these terms are *not* the same as gender identity, which is discussed later in Chapter 73.

Scope of Sexuality

The concept of sexuality ranges from positive sexual health and function to negative sexual health, impairment, or dysfunction (Giddens, 2016). Men and women often define sexuality, sex, and sexual health differently. Women usually view sexuality as defined previously; men often associate the term sexuality only with the act of sexual intercourse (Giddens, 2016). Therefore the concept of sexuality may be perceived differently by different individuals.

Common Risk Factors for Changes in Sexuality

For some adults, changes in sexuality may be equated with poor sexual health or lack of sexual intercourse. During menopause some women perceive more positive sexuality, but others feel that changes such as vaginal atrophy and moodiness cause a more negative sexual experience. Men who have problems with erection or deal with prostate problems often feel sexually inadequate and have a poor self-concept when they are unable to satisfy their partners. As men get older, the risk of erectile dysfunction (ED) increases.

Physiologic Consequences of Changes in Sexuality

Depending on the individual, the major consequence of sexuality changes or sexual dysfunction may not be physiologic. Rather, the adult experiencing changes in sexuality often has a poor self-image and self-concept. Being able to be intimate with another person is an important human need for most people. Sexual intimacy shows a deep sense of caring for another person.

Assessment of Sexuality

Discussing sexuality, sexual health, and sexual intercourse is often difficult for both the patient and nurse. Ask patients about their perception of their sexuality, including both sexual activity and intimacy behaviors. Determine if they have sex and/or intimacy with one or more partners. Ask about protection measures and any history of sexually transmitted infections (STIs) or problems during sexual intercourse.

Interventions to Promote Sexuality and Prevent Changes in Sexuality

Interventions include STI screening and physical examinations to determine any physical cause of changes in sexuality. For example, a man may have ED, and a woman may have decreased libido due to menopause. Assess patients for self-concept related to these issues or other intimacy concerns. Encourage patients at risk for STIs to be evaluated for their occurrence.

Interventions for Patients With Changes in Sexuality

Interventions depend on the cause of the sexual impairment. Physical causes such as ED or STIs can be managed by drug therapy and other measures. Refer the patient whose impaired sexuality is caused by emotional or psychological factors to a qualified health care provider.

TISSUE INTEGRITY

Definition of Tissue Integrity

Tissue integrity is the intactness of the structure and function of the integument (skin and subcutaneous tissue) and mucous membranes. The skin is the largest organ of the body and has multiple functions, including protection from infection, fluid preservation, and temperature control.

Scope of Tissue Integrity

Tissue integrity can vary from intact (normal) to impaired tissue integrity, often referred to as a wound or ulcer, depending on its cause. Tissue integrity changes can occur as a result of infections, burns, local skin reactions, injury/trauma, growths or lesions, and inadequate peripheral perfusion (decrease in oxygenated blood to a specific area of the body). The degree of tissue damage is referred to as partial- or full-thickness loss. A *partial-thickness* wound extends through the epidermis and dermis. *Full-thickness* wounds extend into the subcutaneous tissue and can expose muscle or bone.

Common Risk Factors for Tissue Integrity Changes

Changes in tissue integrity can occur at any age, but older adults are at an increased risk. The skin and underlying tissues of older adults become thinner, drier, and more likely to bruise because of increased capillary fragility. Arterial blood flow is often decreased. Certain medical conditions also increase the risk of impaired tissue integrity and include malnutrition, neurologic disorders, diabetes mellitus, peripheral vascular disease, urinary and bowel incontinence, and immune suppression. The most common tissue impairment is *pressure injuries,* which account for a significant number of hospital and long-term care admissions.

Physiologic Consequences of Tissue Integrity Changes

Alterations in tissue integrity can lead to localized (cellulitis) or systemic (sepsis) infection. Both partial- and full-thickness wounds can be very painful and difficult to heal, especially for patients with diabetes and other diseases in which arterial perfusion is diminished.

Assessment of Tissue Integrity

Take a thorough health history of previous and current chronic health problems and current medications (prescribed and over-the-counter [OTC]). Assess for change in skin color, moles or lesions, excessive skin dryness, bruising, and hair loss or brittle nails (indicating decreased tissue perfusion). Document any existing tissue impairment in detail, including wound size, color, depth, and drainage. Monitor serum albumin and prealbumin levels to ensure that the patient has adequate protein for preventing tissue impairment or healing any existing wounds.

Interventions to Promote Tissue Integrity and Prevent Tissue Integrity Changes

The primary health promotion focus is on proper hygiene and nutrition to enhance tissue health. Teach patients at risk for impaired tissue integrity to inspect the skin every day. Keep the skin clean and dry; when needed, moisturize the skin to prevent excessive dryness. For patients who are confined to a bed or chair, ensure that pressure is relieved by changing body position every 1 to 2 hours. Be sure that patients sit or lie on pressure-reducing surfaces such as mattress overlays or chair gel pads. Assess patients at risk for pressure injuries with evidence-based screening tools such as the Braden Scale, discussed elsewhere in this text.

Interventions for Tissue Integrity Changes

Provide preventive interventions as described previously to prevent further skin and tissue breakdown. Ensure that patients eat an adequate diet and receive supplements as needed for healing. Protein and vitamin C are especially important for preventing skin breakdown and promoting healing of existing wounds. Protein shakes and powders can be added to the daily diet.

Interprofessional collaborative management of any tissue integrity alteration may include drug therapy (e.g., antibiotics, topical steroids, and creams). Chemical and/or surgical wound débridement for necrotic tissue is essential to allow healing. In some cases, the primary health care provider may need to perform an interventional procedure to open arteries that are narrowed or obstructed to increase blood flow and promote wound healing.

GET READY FOR THE NCLEX® EXAMINATION!

KEY POINTS

Review these Key Points for each NCLEX Examination Client Needs Category.

Safe and Effective Care Environment

- Collaborate with members of the interprofessional health care team as needed to meet the patient's physiologic needs. For example, consult with the registered dietitian for patients who have impaired nutrition; consult with the physical therapist for patients with impaired mobility. **QSEN: Teamwork and Collaboration**

Health Promotion and Maintenance

- Provide patient education/health teaching to promote physiologic health, including nutrition, mobility, and gas exchange.
- Assess patient lifestyle behaviors and other factors to determine risks for impairments in basic physiologic needs such as mobility, gas exchange, and perfusion (see Tables 2-3 and 2-4). **Clinical Judgment**

Psychosocial Integrity

- Differentiate the assessment findings associated with dementia versus delirium (see Table 2-1).
- Plan interventions to promote sensory perception, especially in older adults. **QSEN: Patient-Centered Care**

Physiological Integrity

- Provide evidence-based nursing interventions to manage impairments in physiologic needs such as impaired nutrition and mobility to maintain patient safety (see Chart 2-1). **QSEN: Evidence-Based Practice; Safety**

SELECTED BIBLIOGRAPHY

Crawford, A., & Harris, H. (2016). Caring for adults with impaired physical mobility. *Nursing, 46*(12), 36–42.

Frasier, D., Spiva, L., Forman, W., & Hallen, C. (2015). Original research: Implementation of an early mobility program in an ICU. *American Journal of Nursing, 115*(12), 49–58.

Giddens, J. F. (2016). *Concepts for nursing practice* (2nd ed.). St. Louis: Elsevier.

McCance, K., Huether, S., Brashers, V., & Rote, N. (2014). *Pathophysiology: The biologic basis for disease in adults and children* (7th ed.). St. Louis: Mosby.

Pagana, K. D., Pagana, T. J., & Pagana, T. N. (2017). *Mosby's diagnostic and laboratory test reference* (13th ed.). St. Louis: Elsevier.

Pagana, K. D., Pagana, T. J., & Pike-MacDonald, S. A. (2013). *Mosby's Canadian manual of diagnostic and laboratory tests.* Toronto, ON: Elsevier Canada.

Potter, P. A., Perry, A. G., Stockert, P. A., & Hall, A. (2017). *Basic nursing* (8th ed.). St. Louis: Elsevier.

Teodoro, C. R., Breault, K., Garvey, C., Klick, C., O'Briend, J., Purdue, T., et al. (2016). STEP-UP: Study of the effectiveness of a patient ambulation protocol. *MEDSURG Nursing, 25*(2), 111–116.

CHAPTER 3

Common Health Problems of Older Adults

Donna D. Ignatavicius

http://evolve.elsevier.com/Iggy/

PRIORITY AND INTERRELATED CONCEPTS

The priority concepts for this chapter are:
- MOBILITY
- NUTRITION
- COGNITION

The interrelated concepts for this chapter are:
- ELIMINATION
- SENSORY PERCEPTION
- TISSUE INTEGRITY

LEARNING OUTCOMES

Safe and Effective Care Environment

1. Collaborate with the interprofessional team to help the patient, family, and caregivers achieve positive health outcomes.
2. Identify risk factors for falls and impaired driving ability, including decreased MOBILITY and SENSORY PERCEPTION, in older adults who live in the community or are hospitalized.
3. Explain evidence-based falls risk and prevention interventions for older adults in the hospital and community.
4. Summarize best practices to promote patient safety when using restraints.

Health Promotion and Maintenance

5. Teach selected evidence-based lifestyle practices to promote health in older adults.
6. Identify health disparities for subgroups within the older-adult population.
7. Conduct a medication assessment for potential risks for adverse drug events in older adults.

Psychosocial Integrity

8. Assess the older patient's risk for and signs of neglect and abuse.
9. Select valid and reliable assessment tools to document inadequate COGNITION in the older adult.
10. Compare characteristics of common problems of COGNITION: depression, delirium, and dementia.
11. Develop interprofessional collaborative interventions to assist the older adult to cope with relocation stress syndrome.

Physiological Integrity

12. Identify the four major subgroups of older adults.
13. Explain factors that contribute to decreased NUTRITION and ELIMINATION changes among older adults in the community and inpatient facilities.
14. Describe the effects of drugs on the older adult.
15. Identify key interventions to prevent TISSUE INTEGRITY changes in older adults.

About 13% of the people in the United States are currently older than 65 years, but this number is expected to grow to 20% by 2030 and 25% by 2050 (Ortman et al., 2014). Although Euro-Caucasians are the majority of the current older population, the ethnic and racial makeup of this group is expected to change over the next few decades. In general, women live longer than men, although the exact reason for this difference is not known. Most patients on adult acute care and nursing home units are older than 65 years; many of these patients are discharged for home health services. Therefore nurses and other interprofes-sional team members need to know about the special needs of older adults to care for them in a variety of settings.

This chapter describes the major health issues, sometimes referred to as geriatric syndromes, associated with late adulthood in community and inpatient settings (Brown-O'Hara, 2013). The care of older adults (sometimes referred to as *elders*) with specific acute and chronic health problems is discussed as appropriate throughout this text. *Nursing Focus on the Older Adult* charts and *Considerations for Older Adults* boxes highlight the most important information. A brief review of major physiologic changes of aging is listed in the Assessment chapter of each body system unit. A number of gerontologic nursing textbooks and journals are available for additional information about older adult care.

OVERVIEW

Late adulthood can be divided into four major subgroups:
- 65 to 74 years of age: the young old
- 75 to 84 years of age: the middle old
- 85 to 99 years of age: the old old
- 100 years of age or older: the elite old

The fastest growing subgroup is the old old, sometimes referred to as the advanced older-adult population. Members of this subgroup are sometimes referred to as the *frail elderly,* although a number of 85- to 95-year-olds are very healthy and do not meet the criteria for being frail. *Frailty* is actually a geriatric syndrome in which the older adult has unintentional weight loss; weakness and exhaustion; and slowed physical activity, including walking. Frail older adults are also at high risk for adverse outcomes (Brown-O'Hara, 2013).

The vast majority of older adults live in the community at home, in assisted-living facilities, or in retirement or independent living complexes. Of all older adults, only about 5% live in long-term care (LTC) facilities (mostly nursing homes), and another 10% to 15% are ill but are cared for at home. Older adults from any setting usually experience one or more hospitalizations in their lifetime. Many older adults will likely be admitted at some time during their life for short-term stays in a skilled unit of a LTC facility, usually for rehabilitation or complex medical-surgical follow-up care.

Other institutions also have an increase in aging adults. For example, men older than 50 years are the fastest growing group of prisoners today. Like the rest of the older population, older prisoners have multiple chronic health problems. However, these problems are often complicated by a history of substance use and poor NUTRITION that require specific management strategies. Nurses who work in these settings must have expertise in care of older adults.

The number of homeless people older than 60 years is also growing. The inability to pay for housing and family/partner relationship problems are primary factors that contribute to this trend. Most homeless adults have one or more chronic health problems, including mental health/behavioral health disorders (Gerber, 2013). A growing number are veterans of recent wars.

HEALTH ISSUES FOR OLDER ADULTS IN COMMUNITY-BASED SETTINGS

Health is a major concern for many older adults. Health status can affect the ability to perform ADLs and to participate in social activities. A failure to perform these activities may increase dependence on others and may have a negative effect on morale and life satisfaction. If older adults lose the ability to function independently, they often feel empty, bored, and worthless. Loss of autonomy is a painful event related to the physical and mental changes of aging and/or illness.

Older adults may also experience a number of losses that can affect a sense of control over their lives such as the death of a spouse and friends or the loss of social and work roles. Nurses need to support older adults' self-esteem and feelings of

---

CHART 3-1 Patient and Family Education: Preparing for Self-Management

Lifestyles and Practices to Promote Wellness

Health-Protecting Behaviors
- Have yearly influenza vaccinations (preferably after October 1).
- Obtain a pneumococcal vaccination.
- Obtain a shingles vaccination.
- Have a tetanus immunization and get a booster every 10 years.
- Wear seat belts when you are in an automobile.
- Use alcohol in moderation or not at all.
- Avoid smoking; if you do smoke, do not smoke in bed.
- Install and maintain working smoke detectors and/or sprinklers.
- Create a hazard-free environment to prevent falls; eliminate hazards such as scatter rugs and waxed floors.
- Use medications, herbs, and nutritional supplements according to your primary health care provider's prescription.
- Avoid over-the-counter medications unless your primary health care provider directs you to use them.

Health-Enhancing Behaviors
- Have a yearly physical examination; see your primary health care provider more often if health problems occur.
- Reduce dietary fat to not more than 30% of calories; saturated fat should provide less than 10% of your calories.
- Increase your daily dietary intake of complex carbohydrate– and fiber-containing food to five or more servings of fruits and vegetables and six or more servings of grain products.
- Increase calcium intake to between 1000 and 1500 mg daily; take a vitamin D supplement every day if not exposed daily to sunlight.
- Allow at least 10 to 15 minutes of sun exposure two or three times weekly for vitamin D intake; avoid prolonged sun exposure.
- Exercise regularly three to five times a week.
- Manage stress through coping mechanisms that have been successful in the past.
- Get together with people in different settings to socialize.
- Reminisce about your life through reflective discussions or journaling.

---

independence by encouraging them to maintain as much control as possible over their lives, to participate in decision making, and to perform as many tasks as possible.

Like younger and middle-age adults, older adults need to practice health promotion and illness prevention to maintain or achieve a high level of wellness. Teach them the importance of promoting wellness and strategies for meeting this outcome (Chart 3-1).

Common health issues and geriatric syndromes that often affect older adults in the community include:
- Decreased NUTRITION and hydration
- Decreased MOBILITY
- Stress, loss, and coping
- Accidents
- Drug use and misuse
- Inadequate COGNITION
- Substance use
- Elder neglect and abuse

Decreased Nutrition and Hydration

Chapter 2 includes a concept review of NUTRITION. The minimum nutritional requirements of the human body remain consistent from youth through old age, with a few exceptions. Older adults need an increased dietary intake of calcium and vitamins D, C, and A because aging changes disrupt the ability to store, use, and absorb these substances. For older adults who have a sedentary lifestyle and decreased metabolic rate, a reduction in total caloric intake to maintain an ideal body weight is needed. Decreased NUTRITION, either underweight or overweight/obesity, can occur in older adults when these needs are not met.

Many physical aging changes influence nutritional status or the ability to consume needed nutrients. For example, diminished senses of taste and smell often result in a loss of desire for food. Older adults often have less ability to taste sweet and salt than to taste bitter and sour. This aging change may result in an overuse of table sugar and salt to compensate. Some older adults consume numerous desserts and other sweet foods, which can cause them to become overweight or obese. Teach older adults how to balance their diets with healthy food selections. Remind them to substitute herbs and spices to season food and vary the textures of food substances to feel satisfied.

Tooth loss and poorly fitting dentures from inadequate dental care or calcium loss can also cause the older adult to avoid important nutritious foods. Unlike today, dental preventive programs were not readily available or stressed as being important when today's older adults were younger. Older people with dentition problems may eat soft, high-calorie foods such as ice cream and mashed potatoes, which lack roughage and fiber. Unless the person carefully chooses more nutritious soft foods, vitamin deficiencies, constipation, and other problems can result. The extensive use of prescribed and over-the-counter (OTC) drugs, including herbal supplements, may decrease appetite, affect food tolerances and absorption, and cause constipation.

Constipation can reduce quality of life for older adults and cause pain, depression, anxiety, and decreased social activities. In some cases it leads to a small or large bowel obstruction, a potentially life-threatening event. Constipation is common among older adults and can be caused by multiple risk factors, including foods, drugs, and diseases.

> **! NURSING SAFETY PRIORITY** QSEN
> *Action Alert*
>
> Teach older adults to increase fiber and fluid intake, exercise regularly, and avoid risk factors that contribute to constipation. Older adults should consume 35 to 50 g of fiber each day and drink at least 2 liters a day unless medically contraindicated. Some people may also add a "colon cocktail" of equal parts of prune juice, applesauce, and psyllium (e.g., Metamucil) to their daily diet. Remind older adults to take 1 to 2 tablespoons of the mixture daily. If these measures do not prevent constipation, teach them to take a stool softener. For opioid-induced constipation (OIC), drug therapy may be prescribed.

Reduced income, chronic disease, fatigue, and decreased ability to perform ADLs are other factors that contribute to decreased NUTRITION and constipation among older adults. "Fast food" is often inexpensive and requires no preparation. However, it is usually high in fat, carbohydrates, and calories but lacking in healthy nutrients. Older adults can become overweight or obese when they consume a diet high in fast food.

Other older adults may reduce their intake of food to near-starvation levels, even with the availability of programs such as food stamps (Supplemental Nutritional Assistance Program [SNAP]), community food banks, and Meals on Wheels. Many senior centers and homeless shelters offer meals and group

social activities. The lack of transportation, the necessity of traveling to obtain such services, and the inability to carry large or heavy groceries prevent some older adults from taking advantage of food programs. Others are too proud to accept free services.

Decreased NUTRITION may also be related to loneliness. Older adults may respond to loneliness, depression, and boredom by not eating, which can lead to weight loss. Many who live alone lose the incentive to prepare or eat balanced diets, especially if they do not "feel well." Men who live at home alone are especially at risk for undernutrition.

> **! NURSING SAFETY PRIORITY** QSEN
> *Action Alert*
>
> Perform nutritional screening for older adults in the community who are at risk for decreased NUTRITION—either weight loss or obesity. Ask the person about unintentional weight loss or gain, eating habits, appetite, prescribed and OTC drugs, and current health problems. Determine contributing factors for older adults who have or are at risk for poor NUTRITION such as transportation issues or loneliness. Based on these assessment data, develop and implement a plan of care in collaboration with the registered dietitian, pharmacist, and/or case manager to manage these problems. Chapter 60 describes nutritional assessment and management of NUTRITION problems in more detail.

Some older adults are at risk for **geriatric failure to thrive (GFTT)**—a complex syndrome including under-nutrition, impaired physical functioning, depression, and cognitive impairment (Rocchiccioli & Sanford, 2009). However, drug therapy, chronic diseases, major losses, and poor socioeconomic status can cause these same health problems. Be sure to consider these factors when screening for GFTT. For those at risk for or who have GFTT, collaborate with the older adult and family to plan referral to his or her primary health care provider for extensive evaluation. Early supportive intervention can help prevent advanced levels of deterioration.

People older than 65 years are also at risk for dehydration because they have less body water content than younger adults. In severe cases they require emergency department visits or hospital stays.

> **! NURSING SAFETY PRIORITY** QSEN
> *Action Alert*
>
> Older adults sometimes limit their fluid intake, especially in the evening, because of decreased MOBILITY, prescribed diuretics, and urinary incontinence. *Teach older adults that fluid restrictions make them likely to develop dehydration and electrolyte imbalances (especially sodium and potassium) that can cause serious illness or death.*

Incontinence may actually increase because the urine becomes more concentrated and irritating to the bladder and urinary sphincter. Teach older adults the importance of drinking 2 liters of water a day plus other fluids as desired. Remind them to avoid excessive caffeine and alcohol because they can cause dehydration. Chapter 11 discusses fluid and electrolyte imbalances in detail.

Decreased Mobility

Chapter 2 provides a concept review of MOBILITY. Exercise and activity are important for older adults as a means of promoting

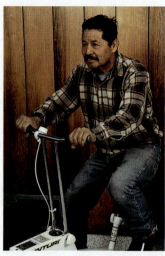

FIG. 3-1 Exercise is important to older adults for health promotion and maintenance.

💡 NCLEX EXAMINATION CHALLENGE 3-1

Health Promotion and Maintenance

Which statement by the older adult indicates a need for further teaching about meeting nutrition and hydration needs?
A. "I will make sure I eat plenty of fruits and vegetables and avoid red meat."
B. "I will stop drinking liquids after dinner to prevent getting up at night."
C. "I'm going to check if I can get food stamps to help me afford better food."
D. "I've got to increase more fiber in my diet to help my bowels work better."

---

and maintaining mobility and overall health (Fig. 3-1). Physical activity can help keep the body in shape and maintain an optimal level of functioning. Regular exercise has many benefits for older adults in community-based settings. The major advantages of maintaining appropriate levels of physical activity include:
- Decreased risk for falls
- Increased muscle strength and balance
- Increased MOBILITY
- Increased sleep
- Reduced or maintained weight
- Improved sense of well-being and self-esteem
- Improved longevity
- Reduced risks for diabetes, coronary artery disease, and dementia

Assess older adults in any setting regarding their history of exercise and any health concerns they may have. For independent older adults, remind them to check with their health care provider to implement a supervised plan for regular physical activity. Teach older adults about the value of physical activity.

For people who are homebound, focus on functional ability such as performing ADLs. For those who are not homebound, teach the importance of exercise. For example, resistance exercise maintains muscle mass. Aerobic exercise such as walking improves strength and endurance. One of the best exercises is walking at least 30 minutes, 3 to 5 times a week. During the winter indoor shopping centers and other public places can be used. In addition, many senior centers and community centers offer exercise programs for older adults. For those who have limited MOBILITY, chair exercises are provided.

Swimming is also a good way to exercise but does not offer the weight-bearing advantage of walking. Weight bearing helps build bone, an especially important advantage for older women to prevent osteoporosis (see Chapter 50). Teach older adults who have been sedentary to start their exercise programs slowly and gradually increase the frequency and duration of activity over time under the direction of their primary health care provider.

Stress, Loss, and Coping

Stress can speed up the aging process over time, or it can lead to diseases that increase the rate of degeneration. It can also impair the reserve capacity of older adults and lessen their ability to respond and adapt to changes in their environment.

Although no period of the life cycle is free from stress, the later years can be a time of especially high risk. Frequent sources of stress and anxiety for the older population include:
- Rapid environmental changes that require immediate reaction
- Changes in lifestyle resulting from retirement or physical incapacity
- Acute or chronic illness
- Loss of significant others
- Financial hardships
- Relocation

How people react to these stresses depends on their personal coping skills and support networks. For instance, losses leave many older adults without friends for support and help. As a result, many must rely solely on their personal resources to maintain their mental health/behavioral health. A combination of poor physical health and social problems can leave older adults susceptible to stress overload, which can result in illness and premature death.

The ways in which people adapt to old age depend largely on the personality traits and coping strategies that have characterized them throughout their lives. Establishing and maintaining relationships with others throughout life are especially important to the older person's happiness. Even more important than having friends is the nature of the friendships. People who have close, intimate, stable relationships with others in whom they confide are often more likely to cope with crisis.

Some older adults choose to return to work at least on a part-time basis to increase their income and socialize with other people. If a person retired between the ages of 55 and 65 years and lives into his or her 80s, retirement funds can deplete. As one ages, additional income is needed to meet basic needs, including money for prescription drugs. Although US government Medicare Part A pays for inpatient hospital care, older adults pay for Medicare Part B to reimburse for 80% of most ambulatory care services, Medicare Part D for prescription drugs, and a private Medi-Gap insurance (e.g., United Health or Blue Cross/Blue Shield) to cover the costs not paid for by Medicare. The premiums for these insurances are very expensive and may still require that older adults pay out-of-pocket copayments for health care services and prescription drugs.

In other developed countries part of or all older-adult care is provided for publicly by the federal government. For example, in Canada all acute and primary health care provider care is paid for publicly. In Germany all older-adult care, including long-term care, is paid for by the government.

CHART 3-2 Best Practice for Patient Safety & Quality Care QSEN

Minimizing the Effects of Relocation Stress in Older Adults

- Provide opportunities for the patient to assist in decision making.
- Carefully explain all procedures and routines to the patient before they occur.
- Ask the family or significant other to provide familiar or special keepsakes to keep at the patient's bedside (e.g., family picture, favorite hairbrush).
- Reorient the patient frequently to his or her location.
- Ask the patient about his or her expectations during hospitalization or assisted-living or nursing home stay.
- Encourage the patient's family and friends to visit often.
- Establish a trusting relationship with the patient as early as possible.
- Assess the patient's usual lifestyle and daily activities, including food likes and dislikes and preferred time for bathing.
- Avoid unnecessary room changes.
- If possible, have a family member, significant other, staff member, or volunteer accompany the patient when leaving the unit for special procedures or therapies.

Fortunately most older adults are relatively healthy and live in and own their own homes. Physical and/or mental health/ behavioral health problems may force some to relocate to a retirement center or an assisted-living facility, although these facilities can be very expensive. Others move in with family members or to apartment buildings funded and designated for seniors. Older adults usually have more difficulty adjusting to major change when compared with younger and middle-age adults. Being admitted to a hospital or nursing home is a particularly traumatic experience. Older adults often suffer from relocation stress syndrome, also known as *relocation trauma.* **Relocation stress syndrome** is the physical and emotional distress that occurs after the person moves from one setting to another. Examples of physiologic behaviors are sleep disturbance and increased physical symptoms such as GI distress. Examples of emotional manifestations are withdrawal, anxiety, anger, and depression. Chart 3-2 lists nursing interventions that may help decrease the effects of relocation.

Family members and facility staff need to be aware that older adults need personal space in their new surroundings. Older adults need to participate in deciding how the space will be arranged and what they can keep in their new home to help offset potential feelings of powerlessness. Suggest that the patient or family bring in personal items such as pictures of relatives and friends, favorite clothing, and valued knickknacks to help make the new setting seem more familiar and comfortable. This same intervention can be carried out in a hospital setting.

Accidents

Accidents are very common among older adults; falls are the most common. Motor vehicle crashes increase as well because of physiologic changes of aging or chronic diseases such as Alzheimer's disease or peripheral neuropathy.

Fall Prevention

Most accidents occur at home. Teach older adults about the need to be aware of safety precautions to prevent accidents such as falls. Incapacitating accidents are a primary cause of decreased MOBILITY and chronic pain in old age. Some people develop **fallophobia** (fear of falling) and avoid leaving their homes. This reaction is particularly common for those who have previously fallen and/or have osteoporosis (bone tissue loss). Osteoporosis is especially common in older thin Euro-Caucasian women who typically have a stooped posture (kyphosis), which can cause problems with balance (see Ch. 50).

Home modifications may help prevent falls (Saccomano & Ferrara, 2015). Collaborate with the older adult, family, and significant others when recommending useful changes to prevent injury. Safeguards such as handrails, slip-proof pads for rugs, and adequate lighting are essential in the home. Avoiding scatter rugs, slippery floors, and clutter is also important to prevent falls. Installing grab bars and using nonslip bathmats can help prevent falls in the bathroom. Raised toilet seats are also important, especially for those who have hip and knee arthritis. Remind older adults to avoid going out on days when steps are wet or icy and to ask for help when ambulating. To minimize sensory overload, advise the older adult to concentrate on one activity at a time.

Changes in SENSORY PERCEPTION and MOBILITY can create challenges for older adults in any environment. For example, **presbyopia** (farsightedness that worsens with aging) may make walking more difficult; the person is less aware of the location of each step. In addition, the older adult may have disorders that affect visual acuity such as macular degeneration, cataracts, glaucoma, or diabetic retinopathy. Teach the person to look down at where he or she is walking and have frequent eye examinations to update glasses or contact lenses to improve vision. Drug therapy or surgery may be needed to correct glaucoma or cataracts.

A reduced sense of touch decreases the awareness of body orientation (e.g., whether the foot is squarely on the step). The decreased reaction time that commonly results from age-related changes in the neurologic system may also impair the ability to recognize or move from a dangerous setting. Chronic diseases such as peripheral neuropathy and arthritis can affect MOBILITY and SENSORY PERCEPTION in the older adult as well. If needed, encourage the use of visual, hearing, or ambulatory assistive devices. High costs and a fear of appearing old sometimes prevent older adults from obtaining or using hearing aids, eyeglasses, walkers, or canes.

Once an older person has been identified as being at high risk for falls, choose interventions that help prevent falls and possible serious injury. For example, for those in the community, tai chi exercise or yoga for seniors is very helpful to improve balance and MOBILITY and decrease the fear of falling, especially among older women (Saccomano & Ferrara, 2015).

? NCLEX EXAMINATION CHALLENGE 3-2

Safe and Effective Care Environment

The nurse performs an initial assessment for an older adult being admitted to an assisted-living facility. Which nursing findings indicate that the client is at risk for falls? **Select all that apply.**

A. Uses a roller walker
B. Has had arthritis for 20 years
C. Is oriented to person, place, and time
D. Wears eyeglasses
E. Has bilateral cataracts
F. Has severe osteoporosis

Driving Safety

Motor vehicle crashes are a major cause of accidents and death among the older-adult population. Increased national concerns about this growing problem have prompted many states to require more frequent testing for older drivers. As one ages, reaction time and the ability to multitask decrease. Sleep disturbances, especially insomnia, are also common in older adults but are *not* part of normal aging. Some crashes occur because the person falls asleep while driving.

The older the person, the more likely that he or she will have chronic diseases and the drugs needed to manage them. These health problems and treatments can contribute to motor vehicle crashes. For instance, peripheral neuropathy may prevent a driver from feeling whether his or her foot is on the brake or accelerator. Drugs used for hypertension can cause orthostatic hypotension (low blood pressure when changing body position from a supine to sitting or standing position).

Primary health care providers play a major role in identifying driver safety issues. Yet many are reluctant to intervene because older patients think they will lose their independence if they cannot drive. They may also be angry and resistant to the idea of giving up perhaps their only means of transportation. As an alternative, health care professionals can recommend driving refresher courses and suggest that high-risk driving conditions such as wet roads be avoided. Newer vehicles have safety features to help older adults such as large-print digital readouts for speed and rear cameras to see behind the vehicle. Chart 3-3 lists additional ways to improve older-adult driver safety.

Drug Use and Misuse

Drug therapy for the older population can be another major health issue. Because of the multiple chronic and acute health problems that occur in this age-group, drugs for older adults account for about one third of all prescription drug costs. The term **polymedicine** has been used to describe the use of many drugs to treat multiple health problems for older adults. **Polypharmacy** is the use of multiple drugs, duplicative drug therapy,

high-dosage medications, and drugs prescribed for too long a period of time.

Older adults commonly take multiple nonprescription or over-the-counter (OTC) drugs such as analgesics, antacids, cold and cough preparations, laxatives, and herbal/nutritional supplements, often without consulting a health care provider. Therefore this population is at high risk for adverse drug events (ADEs) directly related to the number of drugs taken and the frequency with which they are taken. Drug-drug, food-drug, drug-herb, and drug-disease interactions are common ADEs that often lead to hospital admission.

Effects of Drugs on Older Adults

Older adults often do not tolerate the standard dosage of drugs traditionally prescribed for younger adults. The physiologic changes related to aging make drug therapy more complex and challenging. These changes affect the absorption, distribution, metabolism, and excretion of drugs from the body. Even common antibiotics can lead to temporary memory loss or acute confusion. More commonly, antibiotic therapy can cause a *Clostridium difficile* infection, as discussed in Chapter 23.

Age-related changes that can potentially affect drug *absorption* from an oral route include an increase in gastric pH, a decrease in gastric blood flow, and a decrease in GI motility. Despite these changes, older adults do not have major absorption difficulties because of age-related changes alone.

Age-related changes that affect drug *distribution* include smaller amounts of total body water, an increased ratio of adipose tissue to lean body mass, a decreased albumin level, and a decreased cardiac output. Increased adipose tissue in proportion to lean body mass can cause increased storage of lipid-soluble drugs. This leads to a decreased concentration of the drug in plasma but an increased concentration in tissue.

Drug *metabolism* often occurs in the liver. Age-related changes affecting metabolism include a decrease in liver size, a decrease in liver blood flow, and a decrease in serum liver enzyme activity. These changes can result in increased plasma concentrations of a drug. Monitor liver function studies and teach older adults to have regular physical examinations.

Changes in the kidneys can also result in high plasma concentrations of drugs. The *excretion* of drugs usually involves the renal system. Age-related changes of the renal system include decreased renal blood flow and reduced glomerular filtration rate. These changes result in a decreased creatinine clearance and thus a slower excretion time for medications. Consequently serum drug levels can become toxic, and the patient can become extremely ill or die. *Monitor renal studies, especially serum creatinine and creatinine clearance, when giving drugs to older adults!*

A creatinine clearance test measures the glomerular filtration rate of the kidneys. A commonly used formula for calculating creatinine clearance for men rather than directly measuring it is:

$$\frac{(140 - \text{Age in years}) \times \text{Lean body weight in kg}}{\text{Serum creatinine in mg/dL} \times 72}$$

For women, use this formula and multiply the answer by 0.85. A normal creatinine clearance for men is 107 to 139 mL/min and for women 87 to 107 mL/min. Values decrease as a person ages.

When chronic disease is added to the physiologic changes of aging, drug reactions have a more dramatic effect and take

---

 CHART 3-3 **Best Practice for Patient Safety & Quality Care** **QSEN**

Recommendations for Improving Older Adult Driver Safety

- Discuss driving ability with the patient to assess his or her perception.
- Assess physical and mental deficits that could affect driving ability.
- Consult with appropriate primary health care providers to treat health problems that could interfere with driving.
- Suggest community-based transportation options, if available, instead of driving.
- Discuss driving concerns with patients and their families.
- Remind the patient to wear glasses and hearing aids if prescribed.
- Encourage driver-refresher classes, often offered by AARP (formerly the American Association of Retired Persons).
- Consult a certified driving specialist for an on-road driving assessment.
- Encourage avoiding high-risk driving locations or conditions such as busy urban interstates and wet or icy weather conditions.
- Report unsafe drivers to the state department of motor vehicles if they continue to drive.

TABLE 3-1 **Common Adverse Drug Events (ADEs) in Older Adults**	
• Edema	• Dizziness
• Severe nausea and vomiting	• Syncope
• Anorexia	• Urinary retention
• Dehydration	• Diarrhea
• Dysrhythmias	• Constipation/impaction
• Fatigue	• Hypotension
• Weakness	• Acute confusion

Data from Berryman, S. N., Jennings, J., Ragsdale, S., Lofton, T., Huff, D. C., & Rooker, J. S. (2012). Beers criteria for potentially inappropriate medication use in older adults. *MEDSURG Nursing, 21*(3), 129-133.

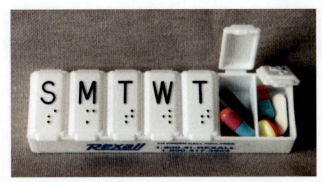

FIG. 3-2 A medication system for safe self-administration.

longer to correct. Often a lower dose of a drug is necessary to prevent ADEs. The policy of "start low, go slow" is essential when health care providers prescribe drugs for older adults. The physiologic changes of aging are highly individual. Alterations in drug therapy should always be individualized according to the actual physiologic changes present and the occurrence and severity of chronic disease. Common ADEs are listed in Table 3-1.

Self-Administration of Drugs

Most people older than 65 years take their own medications. Because the risk for drug toxicity is considerably increased in the older population, help patients assume this task responsibly. Teach patients and their caregivers, providing clear and concise directions and developing ways to help them overcome difficulties with self-administration.

Older adults may make errors in self-administration or do not adhere to the drug regimen for several reasons. First they may simply forget. In the rush of daily activities, they may not take their drugs or may take them too often because they cannot remember when or whether they have taken the medications. It is often helpful if they associate pill taking with daily events (e.g., meals) or keep a simple chart or calendar. Pill boxes are available for a daily, weekly, or monthly supply of medicine that can be placed in small compartments (Fig. 3-2). Egg cartons can be very cost-effective pill boxes. Large print on the drug label helps patients who have poor vision. Writing the drug regimen on the top of the bottle with large letters and numbers is helpful for some older adults. Colored labels or dots can also be applied. Easy-open bottle caps help older adults with limited hand mobility or strength.

A second reason for drug errors is poor communication with health care professionals. These problems result from poor explanations that are not understood because of educational limitations, language barriers, or difficulty with hearing and vision. Health care professionals often presume that their patients have learned the information if they have taught them about the drugs. Help older adults plan their drug therapy schedules as needed.

A third reason for errors is the varying ways that older adults take their medications. Many people older than 65 years use a multitude of complementary and integrative therapies. Some add to their drug regimen by taking OTC drugs, which can interact with prescription drugs and cause serious problems. For example, a patient receiving warfarin (Coumadin, Warfilone) for anticoagulation may take ibuprofen (Motrin) regularly for arthritis or garlic for hypertension. Because ibuprofen

and garlic can inhibit clotting, this combination can cause serious bleeding. When obtaining a drug history, ask patients about all OTC drugs, including herbal and food supplements.

Some older adults avoid taking their prescribed drugs. The fear of dependency or the cost of the drugs may cause many to discontinue their drug therapy too soon or not begin taking the drug. In addition, the actions or side effects of some drugs may not be desirable. For example, diuretics may cause incontinence when patients cannot get to the bathroom quickly enough. Others may think that two pills are twice as effective and therefore it is better to take two rather than just one. Some older adults take drugs that are left over from a previous illness or one that is borrowed from someone else. Teach patients to take their medications exactly as prescribed by their health care providers.

Medication Assessment and Health Teaching

The *Healthy People 2020* initiative recommends that older adults be interviewed regarding their medication use and include these questions:

- Do you take five or more prescription medications?
- Do you take herbs, vitamins, other dietary supplements, or OTC medications?
- Do you have your prescriptions filled at more than one pharmacy?
- Is more than one health care practitioner prescribing your medications?
- Do you take your medications more than once a day?
- Do you have trouble opening your medication bottles?
- Do you have poor eyesight or hearing?
- Do you live alone?
- Do you have a hard time remembering to take your medications?

The Beers Criteria for Potentially Inappropriate Medication Use in Older Adults assessment tool, simply known as the *Beers criteria*, is also very useful in screening for medication-related risks in older adults who have chronic health problems (Berryman et al., 2012). The tool lists multiple medications and related concerns. Examples of these "at-risk" drugs are listed in Table 3-2.

Inadequate Cognition

Chapter 2 reviews the concept of cognition. Older adults are usually mentally sound and competent. Some changes in COGNITION have been identified as age related and are linked to specific cognitive functions rather than intellectual capacity. These changes include a decreased reaction time to stimuli and

TABLE 3-2 Examples of Beers Criteria for Potentially Inappropriate Medication Use in Older Adults

- meperidine (Demerol)
- cyclobenzaprine (Flexeril)
- digoxin (Lanoxin) (Should not exceed 0.125 mg daily except for atrial fibrillation)
- ticlopidine (Ticlid)
- fluoxetine (Prozac)
- amitriptyline (Elavil)
- diazepam (Valium)
- promethazine (Phenergan)
- ketorolac (Toradol)
- short-acting nifedipine (e.g., Procardia)
- ferrous sulfate (Iron) (Should not exceed 325 mg daily)
- chlorpropamide (Diabinese)
- diphenhydramine (Benadryl)

Data from Berryman, S. N., Jennings, J., Ragsdale, S., Lofton, T., Huff, D. C., & Rooker, J. S. (2012). Beers criteria for potentially inappropriate medication use in older adults. *MEDSURG Nursing, 21*(3), 129-133.

! NURSING SAFETY PRIORITY QSEN

Drug Alert

To reduce drug-related risks in older adults, perform a medication assessment every 6 months or more often if an acute illness or exacerbation of a chronic disease occurs. Be sure to:

- Obtain a list of all medications taken on a regular and as-needed basis; include OTC and prescribed drugs, herbs, and nutritional supplements. If a list is not available, ask the older adult or family to gather all ointments, pills, lotions, eyedrops, inhalers, injectable solutions, vitamins, minerals, herbs, and other OTC medications and place into a bag for review.
- Highlight all medications that are part of the Beers criteria; highlight any medication for which the indication for its use is not clear, is inappropriate, or could be discontinued (e.g., duplicative drug).
- Collaborate with the older adult, family, pharmacist, and primary health care provider if appropriate to determine the need for medication changes. Suggest once-a-day dosing if possible.
- Give older adults verbal and written information (at the appropriate reading level) regarding any change or new medication prescribed.
- Promote adherence to the drug therapy regimen exactly as prescribed; remind older adults to check with their primary care provider if they want to change their regimen or add an OTC medication or natural product (nutritional or herbal supplement, or probiotic).
- Encourage lifestyle changes and other nonpharmacologic interventions to help manage or prevent health problems.
- Remind older adults not to share or borrow medications.

? NCLEX EXAMINATION CHALLENGE 3-3

Physiological Integrity

A nurse conducts an assessment of an older adult's medications and herbal/nutritional supplements. Which supplement is **most** likely to cause an interaction with prescribed medications?
A. Probiotics
B. Echinacea
C. Vitamin D
D. Vitamin C

an impaired memory for recent events. *However, severe cognitive impairment and psychosis are not common.*

Two forms of competence exist: legal competence and clinical competence. A person is **legally competent** if he or she is:

- 18 years of age or older
- Pregnant or a married minor

- A legally emancipated (free) minor who is self-supporting
- Not declared incompetent by a court of law

If a court determines that an older adult is not legally competent, a **guardian** is appointed to make health care decisions. Guardians may be family members or a person who is not related to the patient. When no one is available, a guardian may be appointed from a local Area Agency on Aging, an organization with comprehensive services and resources for older adults.

A person is **clinically competent** if he or she is legally competent and can make clinical decisions. Decisional capacity is determined by a person's ability to identify problems, recognize options, make decisions, and provide the rationale supporting the decisions. Selected behavioral/mental illnesses often affect both legal and clinical competence.

Nurses are in a unique position to teach older adults about ways to promote cognitive health. Cognitive training (e.g., learning a new skill), physical activity, social engagement, and NUTRITION are the most helpful interventions to prevent cognitive changes in older adults. In some communities online cognitive training is playing a role in helping to improve memory in older adults (Haesner at al., 2015).

As older adults age, they are at increasing risk for cognitive impairments—depression, delirium, and dementia, often referred to as the *3Ds*. The 3Ds are discussed briefly here; more comprehensive discussions can be found in mental health/behavioral health textbooks.

♥ VETERANS' HEALTH CONSIDERATIONS

Patient-Centered Care QSEN

Many older veterans of the Korean and Vietnam wars also suffer from chronic pain, depression, post-traumatic stress disorder (PTSD), and severe anxiety. Substance use, especially alcoholism, is common among young and older veterans. Alcoholism can contribute to cognitive decline and may be used as a coping mechanism for loss. As a result, many of today's homeless population are veterans of previous and more recent wars.

Depression

Depression is the most common mental health/behavioral health problem among older adults in the community. It increases in incidence when older adults are admitted to the hospital or nursing home. **Depression** is broadly defined as a mood disorder that can have cognitive, affective, and physical manifestations. It can be primary or secondary and can range from mild to severe or major. As a *primary* problem, depression is thought to result from a lack of the neurotransmitters *norepinephrine* and *serotonin* in the brain. *Secondary* depression, sometimes called *situational* depression, can result when there is a sudden change in the person's life such as an illness or loss. Common illnesses that can cause secondary depression include stroke, arthritis, and cardiac disease. It is often underdiagnosed by primary health care providers and is therefore undertreated.

Families and nurses are in the best position to suspect depression in an older adult. Several screening tools are available to help determine if the patient has clinical depression. The **Geriatric Depression Scale—Short Form (GDS-SF)** is a valid and reliable screening tool and is available in multiple languages. The patient selects "yes" or "no" to 15 questions, or a nurse or

Geriatric Depression Scale—Short Form

Choose the best answer for how you have felt over the past week:

1. Are you basically satisfied with your life? YES / **NO**

2. Have you dropped many of your activities and interests? **YES** / NO

3. Do you feel that your life is empty? **YES** / NO

4. Do you often get bored? **YES** / NO

5. Are you in good spirits most of the time? YES / **NO**

6. Are you afraid that something bad is going to happen to you? **YES** / NO

7. Do you feel happy most of the time? YES / **NO**

8. Do you often feel helpless? **YES** / NO

9. Do you prefer to stay at home, rather than going out and doing new things? **YES** / NO

10. Do you feel you have more problems with memory than most? **YES** / NO

11. Do you think it is wonderful to be alive now? YES / **NO**

12. Do you feel pretty worthless the way you are now? **YES** / NO

13. Do you feel full of energy? YES / **NO**

14. Do you feel that your situation is hopeless? **YES** / NO

15. Do you think that most people are better off than you are? **YES** / NO

Answers in bold indicate depression. Score 1 point for each bolded answer.

A score > 5 points is suggestive of depression.
A score ≥ 10 points is almost always indicative of depression.
A score > 5 points should warrant a follow-up comprehensive assessment.

FIG. 3-3 The Geriatric Depression Scale—Short Form. (From the Aging Clinical Research Center (ACRC), a joint project of Stanford University and the VA Palo Alto Health Care System, Palo Alto, CA, funded by the National Institute of Aging and the Department of Veterans Affairs.)

other health care professional can ask the patient the questions. A score of 10 or greater is consistent with a possible diagnosis of clinical depression (Fig. 3-3). These patients are then evaluated more thoroughly by the health care provider for treatment. Without diagnosis and treatment, depression can result in:

- Worsening of medical conditions
- Risk for physical illness
- Alcoholism and drug use
- Increased pain and disability
- Delayed recovery from illness
- Suicide (especially in Euro-Caucasian men between 75 and 85 years of age)

Older adults with depression may have early-morning insomnia, excessive daytime sleeping, poor appetite, a lack of energy, and an unwillingness to participate in social and recreational activities. The primary treatment for depression usually includes drug therapy and psychotherapy, depending on the severity of the problem. Selective serotonin reuptake inhibitors (SSRIs) are the first choice for drug therapy but take 2 to 3 weeks to work. They act by increasing the amount of serotonin and norepinephrine at nerve synapses in the brain.

Reminiscence or reflective therapies also help older adults overcome feelings of depression and despair. More information about depression, including strategies for preventing depres-

! NURSING SAFETY PRIORITY **QSEN**

Drug Alert

Tricyclic antidepressants should not be used for older adults because they have anticholinergic properties that can cause acute confusion, severe constipation, and urinary incontinence. For older adults who may be prescribed this group of drugs, question the primary health care provider and request an SSRI or other treatment.

sion, is available in mental health/behavioral health nursing textbooks.

Dementia

Dementia is a broad term used for a syndrome that involves a slowly progressive cognitive decline, sometimes referred to as *chronic confusion*. This syndrome represents a global impairment of intellectual function and is generally chronic and progressive. There are many types of dementia, the most common being Alzheimer's disease. Multi-infarct dementia, the second most common dementia, results from a vascular disorder. Chapter 42 discusses dementias in detail, with a focus on Alzheimer's disease.

Delirium

Whereas dementia is a chronic, progressive disorder, delirium has an *acute* and fluctuating onset. It is often seen among older adults in a setting with which they are unfamiliar, including both acute and long-term care (Kalish et al., 2014). Delirium is characterized by the patient's inattentiveness, disorganized thinking, and altered level of consciousness (either hypoalert or hyperalert). In addition to cognitive changes, some patients have physical and emotional manifestations and may become psychotic.

The types of delirium are *hyperactive, hypoactive,* and *mixed. Hyperactive* patients may try to climb out of bed or become agitated, restless, and aggressive. *Hypoactive* patients are quiet, apathetic, lethargic, unaware, and withdrawn. They often move very slowly and stare. Patients with hypoactive dementia are often not diagnosed. *Mixed* delirium patients have a combination of hyperactive and hypoactive manifestations.

Identify patients who are at risk for delirium; high-risk patients are usually the late old and those with alcoholism and/or disorders of major body organs. Some hospitals offer programs to prevent delirium and loss of function in high-risk patients such as the Hospital Elder Life Program (HELP) (Kalish et al., 2014).

Some of the many factors that can cause delirium are:
- Drug therapy (especially anticholinergics, opioids, and psychoactive drugs)
- Fluid and electrolyte imbalances
- Infections, especially urinary tract, pneumonia, and sepsis
- Fecal impaction or severe diarrhea
- Surgery (especially fracture hip repair and post-transplant)
- Metabolic problems such as hypoglycemia
- Neurologic disorders such as tumors
- Circulatory, renal, and pulmonary disorders
- Nutritional deficiencies
- Hypoxemia (decreased arterial oxygen level)
- Mechanical ventilation
- Relocation
- Major loss
- Critical care setting

Many patients have more than one of these factors as causes for their delirium.

! NURSING SAFETY PRIORITY (QSEN)

Action Alert

Delirium is a major predictor of morbidity and mortality (Kalish et al., 2014). For example, acutely confused patients who are discharged from the hospital are at an increased risk for functional decline, falls, and incontinence at home. Therefore carefully assess older patients in any setting for acute confusion so it can be managed.

A number of tools have been developed for point-of-care screening for delirium, including the Confusion Assessment Method (CAM), Delirium Index (DI), NEECHAM Confusion Scale, and Mini-Cog. The CAM is a short and easy-to-use tool that consists of nine open-ended questions and a diagnostic algorithm for determining delirium (Table 3-3). This screening tool is easily adaptable for computerized point-of-care charting.

TABLE 3-3   The Confusion Assessment Method (CAM)

1. Acute onset and fluctuating course (e.g., Is there evidence of an acute change in mental status from the patient's baseline?)
2. Inattention (e.g., Does the patient have difficulty focusing attention or keeping track of what is being said?)
3. Disorganized thinking (e.g., Is the patient's thinking and conversation disorganized or incoherent?)
4. Altered level of consciousness (e.g., Is the patient lethargic, hyperalert, or difficult to arouse?)

The diagnosis of delirium by the CAM is the presence of features 1 and 2 *and* either 3 *or* 4.

Data from Sendelbach, S., & Guthrie, P. F. (2009). Evidence-based guideline—Acute confusion/delirium: Identification, assessment, treatment, and prevention. *Journal of Gerontological Nursing, 35*(11), 11-17.

Collaborate with the interprofessional health care team to remove or treat risk or causative factors for acute confusion. For example, if the patient has a low oxygen saturation level, provide supplemental oxygen therapy to increase oxygen to the brain. If the patient has a urinary tract infection (UTI), it is treated. The primary sign of a UTI in older adults is acute confusion.

To help prevent and manage delirium, use a calm voice to frequently reorient the patient. For example, playing tapes of soothing music may have a calming effect. Providing a doll or stuffed animal with which to "fidget" may prevent the patient from removing important medical tubes or equipment. Some nurses believe that providing dolls and stuffed animals is treating the adult like a child, but this intervention can sometimes be very effective when used for therapeutic purposes. If the patient has a favorite item such as an afghan blanket or a picture, ask the family or significant others to provide it for the same purpose.

Table 2-1 in Chapter 2 highlights the major differences between delirium and dementia and lists the major nursing considerations for each. The most difficult challenge is caring for a patient who is experiencing both problems at the same time.

Substance Use

Excessive substance use (both alcohol and illicit drugs) increases the risk for falls and other accidents; affects mood and COGNITION; and leads to complications of chronic diseases such as diabetes mellitus, hypertension, and heart disease. Isolation, depression, and delirium can result from substance use. The National Institute on Aging (NIA) recommends that people older than 65 years have no more than one alcoholic drink a day or seven drinks in a week (NIA, 2012). Illicit drugs such as cannabis (marijuana) should be avoided unless they are needed for therapeutic use.

The Short Michigan Alcoholism Screening Test—Geriatric Version (SMAST-G) is often used by nurses and other health care professionals in ambulatory care settings to detect alcohol use or alcoholism. The 10 yes/no question test is available in English and Spanish and can be either self-administered or administered by a clinician. Examples of questions on the tool are:
- Do you drink to take your mind off your problems?
- When you feel lonely, does having a drink help?

A "yes" answer is worth one point. A total score of two or more points indicates that the person has a problem with alcohol.

Other screening tools for alcohol use in older adults include the CAGE questionnaire, the Alcohol-Related Problems Survey (ARPS), and the Short ARPS (shARPS). The acronym *CAGE* comes from four questions:

- Have you ever tried to **c**ut down on your drinking?
- Have people **a**nnoyed you by criticizing your drinking?
- Have you ever felt bad or **g**uilty about your drinking?
- Have you ever had a drink first thing in the morning to settle your nerves to get rid of a hangover (**e**ye-opener)?

Elder Neglect and Abuse

Another problem for some older adults is neglect and abuse, both verbal and physical. Some older adults are more vulnerable to these problems than others, especially widows who may have difficulty being assertive. Elder abuse and neglect is a serious problem that affects many older adults each year. Older people who are neglected or abused are often physically dependent from one or more disabilities. The abuser is often a family member who becomes frustrated or distraught over the burden of caring for the older adult. Unfortunately only a few cases of elder abuse are reported.

Prolonged caregiving by a family member is a common new role for adult children, usually women. This new role may result in role fatigue, conflict, and strain. As a result, neglect can occur when a caregiver fails to provide for an older adult's basic needs such as food, clothing, medications, or assistance with ADLs. The caregiver refuses to let other people such as nursing assistants or home care nurses into the home. Whether intentional or unintentional, neglect accounts for almost half of all cases of actual elder abuse.

Physical abuse is the use of physical force that results in bodily injury, especially in the "bathing suit" zone (abdomen, buttocks, genital area, upper thighs). Examples of physical abuse are hitting, burning, pushing, and molesting the patient. Sedating the older adult is also abusive. Financial abuse occurs when the older adult's property or resources are mismanaged or misused; this is more common than physical abuse. Emotional abuse is the intentional use of threats, humiliation, intimidation, and isolation toward older adults.

Carefully assess the patient for signs of abuse such as bruises in clusters or regular patterns; burns, commonly to the buttocks or the soles of the feet; unusual hair loss; or multiple injuries, especially fractures. If the older adult is too weak or has no other resources or support systems, he or she may not admit that abuse is occurring. Neglect may be manifested by pressure injuries, contractures, dehydration or malnutrition, urine burns, excessive body odor, and listlessness. Depression and dementia are common in community older adults who are abused or neglected.

Be sure to screen for abuse and neglect of older adults using an appropriate assessment tool. Table 3-4 lists tools that can be used by nurses and other health care professionals to screen for elder abuse and neglect. The older adult should be referred to the appropriate service when there is:

- Evidence of mistreatment without sufficient clinical explanation
- Report by an older adult of being abused or neglected
- A belief by the health care professional that there is a high risk for or probable abuse, neglect, abandonment, or exploitation

All states in the United States and other Western countries have laws requiring health care professionals to report suspected

TABLE 3-4   **Examples of Elder Abuse Screening Tools**
• Elder Abuse Suspicion Index • Elder Assessment Instrument • Indicators of Abuse Screen • Questions to Elicit Elder Abuse • Hwalek-Sengstock Elder Abuse Screening Tool • Caregiver Abuse Screen • Brief Abuse Screen for the Elderly • Vulnerability to Abuse Screening Scale

elder abuse. In the community, if physical abuse or neglect is suspected, notify the local Adult Protective Services agency or other advocate organization. In a hospital or nursing home, notify the social worker or ombudsman, who then will investigate the case and report the problem to the appropriate agency.

HEALTH ISSUES FOR OLDER ADULTS IN HOSPITALS AND LONG-TERM CARE SETTINGS

Forty percent of adults in critical care settings are over 65 years of age; 60% of medical-surgical patients in hospitals are also over 65 (Ellison et al., 2015). Older adults who are admitted to hospitals and long-term care settings such as nursing homes have special needs and potential health problems. Many of these problems are similar to those seen among community older adults as discussed in this chapter. Since 1996 the Hartford Institute for Gerontological Nursing has worked to ensure that all hospitalized patients 65 years of age and older be given quality care.

⊕ CULTURAL/SPIRITUAL CONSIDERATIONS

Patient-Centered Care QSEN

The health of Hispanic older adults continues to lag behind that for non-Hispanic whites due to a number of factors such as language barriers, inadequate health insurance, and lack of health care access. To add to this health disparity, most nurses and other health care professionals are not educated in the language or culture of Hispanic older adults. Some older Hispanic patients may have beliefs and values that conflict with traditional Western health care views. Many have strong religious and spiritual beliefs. For example, traditional Catholicism is practiced among most Hispanic elders in the Southwestern United States. Be respectful of these differences and incorporate them into your patient's plan of care. Become educated about the Hispanic culture and learn to speak basic medical Spanish to foster communication and trust (Strunk et al., 2013).

Nurses may not be aware that the needs of older adults differ from those of younger adults. Some health care systems have designated Acute Care of the Elderly (ACE) units with geriatric resources nurses and geriatric clinical nurse specialists. The patients are cared for by geriatricians who specialize in the care of older adults.

Other hospitals have developed interprofessional health programs system-wide to meet the special needs of older patients. The incentive for these new programs is the Nurses Improving Care for Healthsystem Elders (NICHE) project, which continues to generate evidence-based practice guidelines for older adult care.

GENDER HEALTH CONSIDERATIONS
Patient-Centered Care (QSEN)

Significant health disparities are also associated with the lesbian, gay, bisexual, transgender, and questioning (LGBTQ) older-adult population. Compared with heterosexual adults, LGBTQ older adults are at an elevated risk for disability from chronic disease and mental distress (Fredriksen-Goldsen, 2011). When admitted to the hospital or nursing home, they may hide their gender identity and/or sexual orientation from the nurse and primary health care providers because of fear of rejection or discrimination or lack of adequate health care.

Do not assume that your older patients or visitors are heterosexual. Establish a safe and trusting relationship with the patient and discuss sexual orientation and gender identity in a private setting to emphasize confidentiality. Do not force patients to answer any questions with which they feel uncomfortable. Teach direct caregivers such as nursing assistants that they may observe patients with sexual organs that conflict with the patient's gender identity. If this situation occurs, remind them not to be offensive or judgmental but, rather, to carry out the task as planned. Chapter 73 in this text describes care of transgender patients in detail.

The purpose of all of these programs and units is to focus on the special health care issues or geriatric syndromes seen in the older population (Brown-O'Hara, 2013). The **Fulmer SPICES** framework was developed as part of the NICHE project and identifies six serious "marker conditions" that can lead to longer hospital stays, higher medical costs, and even deaths. These conditions are:

- Sleep disorders
- Problems with eating or feeding
- Incontinence
- Confusion
- Evidence of falls
- Skin breakdown

Each of these problems is described briefly here and also is discussed in more detail in other parts of this chapter and the textbook. Other problems such as depression and constipation are also common in older hospitalized patients. Rather than being fully comprehensive, this classic, well-known SPICES framework is intended to be an easy tool that has been called *geriatric vital signs* (Fulmer, 2007).

Problems of Sleep, Nutrition, and Continence

Sleep disorders are common in hospitalized patients, especially older adults. Adequate rest is important for healing and for physical and mental functioning. Pain, chronic disease, environmental noise and lighting, and staff conversations are a few of the many contributing factors to insomnia in the acute and long-term care setting. Assess the patient and ask how he or she is sleeping. If the patient is not able to answer, observe for restlessness and other behaviors that could indicate lack of adequate rest. Manage the patient's pain by giving pain medication before bedtime. Attempt to keep patients awake during the day to prevent insomnia. Keep staff conversations as quiet as possible and away from patients' rooms. Dim the lights to make the patient area as dark as possible. Avoid making loud noises such as slamming doors. Postpone treatments until waking hours or early morning if they can be delayed safely. If possible, place a "Do Not Disturb" sign on the patient's door to avoid unnecessary interruptions in sleep.

Problems with eating and feeding prevent the older patient from receiving adequate NUTRITION. Malnutrition is common among older adults and is associated with poor clinical outcomes, including death. Nurses need to perform nutritional screenings on the first day of patient admission, including a thorough nutritional history and weight, height, and body mass index (BMI) calculation. Chapter 60 describes nutritional screening in more detail.

Collaborate with the registered dietitian about the patient's nutritional status as needed to achieve health goals. Consider cultural preferences and determine which foods the patient likes. Manage symptoms such as pain, nausea, and vomiting. If the patient has difficulty chewing or swallowing, coordinate a plan of care with the speech-language pathologist and dietitian. If there are no dietary restrictions, encourage family members or friends to bring in food that the patient might enjoy. Additional interventions to prevent nutrition-related problems are discussed in Chapter 60.

Urinary and bowel ELIMINATION issues vary in type and severity and may be caused by many factors, including acute or chronic disease, ADL ability, and available staff. Assess the patient to identify causes for incontinence or retention. *These problems are not physiologic changes of aging but are very common in both the hospital and long-term care setting.* Place the patient on a toileting schedule or a bowel or bladder training program, if appropriate. Delegate this activity to unlicensed assistive personnel and supervise them. Chapter 6 discusses bowel and bladder training in detail; constipation was described earlier in this chapter.

Confusion, Falls, and Skin Breakdown

Acute and chronic confusion affect many older patients in both the hospital and nursing home. Whereas chronic confusion states such as dementia are not reversible, acute confusion, or delirium, may be avoidable and is often reversible when the causes are resolved or removed (see Table 2-1). For example, avoiding multiple drugs and promoting adequate sleep can help prevent acute confusion. Help the patient by reorienting him or her to reality as much as needed. Keep the patient as comfortable as possible (e.g., provide interventions to control pain). Delirium is discussed earlier in this chapter. Chapter 42 describes dementia in detail.

 NCLEX EXAMINATION CHALLENGE 3-4
Physiological Integrity

An older adult has been taking furosemide 20 mg daily for the past 6 months. The family reports that the client suddenly became confused, weak, and very agitated. What is the nurse's **best** action?
A. Begin intravenous fluid therapy.
B. Draw blood to assess electrolyte levels.
C. Start oxygen via mask at 6 L/min.
D. Place the patient on strict intake and output.

The most common accident among older patients in a hospital or nursing home setting is falling. A **fall** is an unintentional change in body position that results in the patient's body coming to rest on the floor or ground. Some falls result in serious injuries such as fractures and head trauma. **The Joint Commission's National Patient Safety Goals (NPSGs) require** that all inpatient health care settings use admission and daily fall risk assessment tools and a fall reduction program for patients who are at high risk.

Assess all older patients for risk for falls. Many evidence-based assessment tools such as the Morse Fall Scale, STRATIFY, and the Hendrich II Fall Risk Model (HIIFRM) have been developed to help the nurse focus on factors that increase an older person's risk for falling. Some of these tools also recommend selected interventions, depending on the patient's fall risk score (Swartzell et al., 2013). Chart 3-4 lists some of the common risk factors that should be assessed and evidence-based, collaborative interventions for preventing falls in high-risk patients. *A recent history of falling is the single most important predictor for falls.*

Toileting-related falls are very common, especially at night. Older patients often have **nocturia** (urination at night) and get out of bed to go to the bathroom. They may forget to ask for assistance and may subsequently fall as a result of disorientation in the darkness in an unfamiliar environment. In some cases they may crawl over the side rail, which can make the fall more serious. Because of this, side rails are used far less often in both hospitals and nursing homes. In both settings side rails are classified as restraints unless the use of rails helps patients increase mobility.

A **restraint** is any device or drug that prevents the patient from moving freely and must be prescribed by a health care provider. In 1990 the US government enforced a law that gives nursing home residents the right to be restraint free. Removing physical restraints from nursing home residents has reduced serious injuries, although falls and minor injuries have increased in some cases. Mattresses placed on floors next to patient beds or "low beds" have helped reduce injury.

Hospitals have also reduced the use of physical restraints. The Joint Commission has specific standards that limit the use of physical restraints in hospitals and nursing homes. Although not appropriate, chemical restraints (psychoactive drugs) such as haloperidol (Haldol) have sometimes been used in place of physical restraints.

Experts agree that older adults should not be placed in a physical restraint or sedated just because they are old. Use alternatives before applying any type of restraint (Chart 3-5). However, if all other interventions (e.g., reminding patients to call for assistance when needed; asking a family member to stay with patients) are not effective in fall prevention, a physical restraint may be required for a limited period. Applying a restraint is a serious intervention and should be analyzed for its risk versus its benefit. Check the patient in a restraint every 30 to 60 minutes and release the restraint at least every 2 hours for turning, repositioning, and toileting. Physical restraints such as vests have caused serious injury and even death. *If restraint is needed, use the least restrictive device first. Be sure to follow your facility policy and procedure for using restraints.*

Chemical restraints are often overused in hospital settings. Examples include:

- Antipsychotic drugs
- Antianxiety drugs
- Antidepressant drugs
- Sedative-hypnotic drugs

The most potent group of psychoactive drugs is the antipsychotics. These drugs are appropriate only for the control of certain behavioral problems such as delusions, acute psychosis, and schizophrenia. Typical antipsychotic drugs include haloperidol (Haldol, Peridol) and thiothixene (Navane). These drugs should not be used to treat anxiety or induce sedation.

CHART 3-4 Best Practice for Patient Safety & Quality Care QSEN

Assessing Risk Factors and Preventing Falls in Older Adults

Assess for the presence of these risk factors:
- History of falls
- Advanced age (>80 years)
- Multiple illnesses
- Generalized weakness or decreased mobility
- Gait and postural instability
- Disorientation or confusion
- Use of drugs that can cause increased confusion, mobility limitations, or orthostatic hypotension
- Urinary incontinence
- Communication impairments
- Major visual impairment or visual impairment without correction
- Alcohol or other substance use
- Location of patient's room away from the nurses' station (in the hospital or nursing home)
- Change of shift or mealtime (in the hospital or nursing home)

Implement these nursing interventions for all patients, regardless of risk:
- Monitor the patient's activities and behavior as often as possible, preferably every 30 to 60 minutes.
- Teach the patient and family about the fall prevention program to become safety partners.
- Remind the patient to call for help before getting out of bed or a chair.
- Help the patient get out of bed or a chair if needed; lock all equipment such as beds and wheelchairs before transferring patients.
- Teach patients to use the grab bars when walking in the hall without assistive devices or when using the bathroom.
- Provide or remind the patient to use a walker or cane for ambulating if needed; teach him or her how to use these devices.
- Remind the patient to wear eyeglasses or a hearing aid if needed.
- Help the incontinent patient to toilet every 1 to 2 hours.
- Clean up spills immediately.
- Arrange the furniture in the patient's room or hallway to eliminate clutter or obstacles that could contribute to a fall.
- Provide adequate lighting at all times, especially at night.
- Observe for side effects and toxic effects of drug therapy.
- Orient the patient to the environment.
- Keep the call light and patient care articles within reach; ensure that the patient can use the call light.
- Place the bed in the lowest position with the brakes locked.
- Place objects that the patient needs within reach.
- Ensure that adequate handrails are present in the patient's room, bathroom, and hall.
- Have the physical therapist assess the patient for mobility and safety.

For patients at a high risk for falls:
- Implement all assessments and interventions listed previously.
- Relocate the patient for best visibility and supervision.
- Encourage family members or significant other to stay with the patient.
- Collaborate with other members of the health care team, especially the rehabilitative services.
- Use technologic devices such as mattress sensor pads and chair alarms to alert staff to patients getting out of bed.
- Use low beds or futon-type beds to prevent injury if the patient is at risk for falling out of bed.

CHART 3-5   Best Practice for Patient Safety & Quality Care QSEN

Using Restraint Alternatives

- If the patient is acutely confused, reorient him or her to reality as often as possible.
- If the patient has dementia, use validation to reaffirm his or her feelings and concerns.
- Check the patient often, at least every hour.
- If the patient pulls tubes and lines, cover them with roller gauze or another protective device; be sure that IV insertion sites are visible for assessment.
- Keep the patient busy with an activity, pillow or apron, puzzle, or art project.
- Provide soft, calming music.
- Place the patient in an area where he or she can be supervised. (If the patient is agitated, do not place him or her in a noisy area.)
- Turn off the television if the patient is agitated.
- Ask a family member or friend to stay with the patient at night.
- Help the patient to toilet every 2 to 3 hours, including during the night.
- Be sure that the patient's needs for food, fluids, and comfort are met.
- If agency policy allows, provide the patient with a pet visit.
- Provide familiar objects or cherished items that the patient can touch.
- Document the use of all alternative interventions.
- If a restraint is applied, use the least restrictive device (e.g., mitts rather than wrist restraints, a roller belt rather than a vest).

! NURSING SAFETY PRIORITY QSEN

Drug Alert

Closely monitor older adults receiving antipsychotics for adverse drug events (ADEs). Assess patients for:
- Anticholinergic effects, the most common problem, causing constipation, dry mouth, and urinary retention
- Orthostatic hypotension, which increases the patient's risk for falls and fractures
- Parkinsonism, including tremors, bradycardia, and a shuffling gait
- Restlessness and the inability to stay still in any one position
- Hyperglycemia and diabetes mellitus, which occur more with drugs such as risperidone (Risperdal) and quetiapine (Seroquel)

If any of these ADEs occur, notify the primary health care provider immediately.

Skin breakdown, especially pressure injuries, is a major TISSUE INTEGRITY problem among older adults in hospitals and nursing homes. In some cases these wounds cause death from infection. Therefore prevention is the best approach. **The Joint Commission's NPSGs require that all health care agencies have a program to prevent agency-associated pressure injuries. The program should include these evidence-based interventions:**
- **Nutritional support**
- **Avoidance of skin injury from friction or shearing forces**
- **Repositioning and support surfaces**

- **A plan to increase mobility and activity level when appropriate**
- **Skin cleaning and use of moisture barriers**

Assess older adults for their risk for pressure injuries, using an assessment tool such as the Braden Scale for Predicting Pressure Sore Risk (see Chapter 25). Implement evidence-based interventions to prevent agency-acquired pressure injuries and maintain TISSUE INTEGRITY. Coordinate these interventions with members of the interprofessional health care team, including the dietitian and wound care specialist.

! NURSING SAFETY PRIORITY QSEN

Action Alert

Supervise unlicensed assistive personnel (UAP) for frequent turning and repositioning for the patient who is immobile. Assess the skin every 8 hours for reddened areas that do not blanch. Remind UAP to keep the skin clean and dry. Use pressure-relieving mattresses and avoid briefs or absorbent pads that can cause skin irritation and excess moisture. Chapter 25 describes in detail additional interventions for prevention and management of pressure injuries.

Skin tears are also common in older adults, especially the old-old group and those who are on chronic steroid therapy. Teach UAP to use extreme caution when handling these patients. Use a gentle touch and report any open areas. Avoid bruising because older adults have increased capillary fragility.

Care Coordination and Transition Management

Some older adults and their families experience a breakdown in communication and coordination of care when transitioning from the hospital or long-term care (LTC) setting (nursing home) to the home setting. If the transition is not optimal, older adults experience high readmission rates and an increase in visits to the emergency department or primary health care provider's office.

A qualitative study by Dossa et al. (2012) showed that health care professionals, especially nurses, did not communicate effectively when they prepared for the discharge of older adults. Care was not coordinated among health care professionals, which led to confusion for the older adult and family caregivers. To help prevent these problems, the authors recommended that a system be in place to address patients' communication needs. The system should include follow-up phone calls after discharge to home and having one case manager to coordinate care during and after the transition from the inpatient agency to home. A home care nurse or other health care professional can serve as a "health coach" to ensure understanding of discharge instructions, consistent follow-up appointments, and a designated emergency contact for the patient and family. Discharge instructions should be easy to read, in large print, and accurate. Continuity of care for high-quality transition between settings is essential to achieve positive outcomes for older adults.

GET READY FOR THE NCLEX® EXAMINATION!

KEY POINTS

Review these Key Points for each NCLEX Examination Client Needs Category.

Safe and Effective Care Environment

- Collaborate with the interprofessional team when providing care to older adults in the community or inpatient setting. For example, consult with the registered dietitian for problems with NUTRITION; consult with the pharmacist to discuss the patient's drug regimen. **Health Care Organizations; QSEN: Teamwork and Collaboration**
- Assess all older adults for risk factors for impaired driving ability such as decreased MOBILITY, SENSORY PERCEPTION, and COGNITION (see Chart 3-3).
- Assess older adults in the community and inpatient settings for falls risk factors (e.g., cognitive decline and vision impairment) and implement interventions as delineated in Chart 3-4. **QSEN: Safety**
- Physical and chemical restraints should not be used for older adults until all other alternatives have been tried (see Chart 3-5). **QSEN: Evidence-Based Practice**
- **Follow The Joint Commission's National Patient Safety Goals and federal/state standards when using patient restraints to maintain patient safety. QSEN: Safety**

Health Promotion and Maintenance

- Teach older adults about the benefits of regular physical exercise.
- Provide information regarding community resources for older adults to help them meet their basic needs. **Clinical Judgment**
- Be aware that nonwhite subgroups such as Hispanics and elders who identify as LGBTQ often are afraid or unable to obtain adequate health services. **Health Care Disparities**
- Teach health promotion practices as listed in Chart 3-1.
- Conduct a medication assessment for potential risks in older adults using the Beers criteria. **QSEN: Safety**

Psychosocial Integrity

- Depression is the most common yet most underdiagnosed and undertreated mental health/behavioral health disorder among older adults.

- Delirium is acute confusion that has a sudden onset and fluctuating course; dementia is chronic confusion (see Table 2-1). Confusion is not part of the normal aging process.
- Screen older adults for alcohol abuse or alcoholism and refer those with identified problems to appropriate resources. **QSEN: Evidence-Based Practice**
- Screen older adults for neglect and abuse, which are serious problems; family caregivers are usually the abusers (see Table 3-4). **QSEN: Safety**
- Relocation stress syndrome is the reaction of an older adult when transferred to a different environment; ways to minimize this problem are listed in Chart 3-2.

Physiological Integrity

- The four subgroups of the older-adult population are the young old, middle old, old old, and elite old.
- The biggest concern regarding accidents among older adults in both the community and inpatient setting is falls. **QSEN: Safety**
- Physiologic changes of aging predispose older adults to toxic effects of medication; drugs are absorbed, metabolized, and distributed more slowly than in younger people. They are also excreted more slowly by the kidneys. **QSEN: Safety**
- Medication use in older adults is often a problem when they commit errors when self-medicating, avoid needed medications, or have problems understanding their medication regimen. **QSEN: Evidence-Based Practice**
- **Follow The Joint Commission's National Patient Safety Goals and best practice guidelines to prevent agency-acquired pressure injuries.**
- Promote sleep and rest for older adults to decrease the incidence of delirium and to prevent falls. **QSEN: Evidence-Based Practice**
- Use the SPICES assessment tool for identifying serious health problems that can be prevented or managed early.

SELECTED BIBLIOGRAPHY

Asterisk indicates a classic or definitive work on this subject.

Beach, P. R., & White, B. E. (2015). Applying the evidence to help caregivers torn in two. *Nursing*, *45*(6), 30–37.

*Berryman, S. N., Jennings, J., Ragsdale, S., Lofton, T., Huff, D. C., & Rooker, J. S. (2012). Beers criteria for potentially inappropriate medication use in older adults. *MEDSURG Nursing*, *21*(3), 129–133.

Brown-O'Hara, R. (2013). Geriatric syndromes and their implications for nursing. *Nursing*, *43*(1), 1–3.

Chu, R. Z. (2017). Preventing in-patient falls: The nurse's pivotal role. *Nursing2017*, *47*(3), 24–31.

*Dossa, A., Bokhour, B., & Hoenig, H. (2012). Care transitions from the hospital to home for patients with mobility impairments: Patient and family caregiver experiences. *Rehabilitation Nursing*, *37*, 277–285.

Ellison, D., White, D., & Farrar, F. C. (2015). Aging population. *Nursing Clinics of North America*, *50*(1), 185–213.

Faught, D. D. (2014). Delirium: The nurse's role in prevention, diagnosis, and treatment. *Medsurg Nursing*, *23*(5), 301–305.

*Fredriksen-Goldsen, K. I. (2011). Resilience and disparities among lesbian, gay, bisexual, and transgender older adults. *Public Policy and Aging Report*, *21*(3), 3–7.

*Fulmer, T. (2007). How to try this: Fulmer SPICES. *American Journal of Nursing*, *107*(10), 40–48.

Gerber, L. (2013). Bringing home effective nursing care for the homeless. *Nursing*, *43*(3), 32–38.

*Graham, B. C. (2012). Examining evidence-based interventions to prevent inpatient falls. *Medsurg Nursing*, *21*, 267–270.

*Greenberg, S. A. (2007). How to try this: The Geriatric Depression Scale—Short Form. *American Journal of Nursing, 107*(10), 60–69.

Haesner, M., Steinert, A., O'Sullivan, J. L., & Weichenberger, M. (2015). Evaluating an online cognitive training platform for older adults: User experience and implementation requirements. *Journal of Gerontological Nursing, 41*(8), 22–31.

Hastings, S. N., Sloane, R., Morey, M. C., Pavon, J. M., & Hoenig, H. (2014). Assisted early mobility for hospitalized older veterans: Preliminary data from the STRIDE program. *Journal of the American Geriatric Society, 62*(11), 2180–2184.

Kalish, V. B., Gillham, J. E., & Unwin, B. K. (2014). Delirium in older persons: Evaluation and management. *American Family Physician, 90*(3), 150–158.

Layne, T., Haas, S. A., Davidson, J. E., & Klopp, A. (2015). Postoperative delirium prevention in the older adult: An evidence-based process improvement project. *Medsurg Nursing, 24*(4), 256–262.

*Lee, L. Y., Lee, D. T., & Woo, J. (2010). The psychosocial effect of Tai Chi on nursing home residents. *Journal of Clinical Nursing, 19*(7–8), 927–938.

Lyons, D. L. (2014). Implementing a comprehensive functional model of care in hospitalized older adults. *Medsurg Nursing, 23*(6), 379–385.

*National Institute on Aging (NIA) (2012). *Alcohol use in older people.* Washington, DC: US Department of Health and Human Services.

Ortman, J. M., Velkoff, V. A., & Hogan, H. (2014). *The aging nation: The older population in the United States,* Current Population Reports. Washington DC: US Census Bureau.

Phillips, L. A. (2013). Delirium in geriatric patients: Identification and prevention. *Medsurg Nursing, 22,* 9–12.

*Rocchiccioli, J. T., & Sanford, J. T. (2009). Revisiting geriatric failure to thrive. *Journal of Gerontological Nursing, 35*(1), 18–24.

Saccomano, S. J., & Ferrara, L. R. (2015). Fall prevention in older adults. *Nurse Practitioner, 40*(6), 40–47.

*Sendelbach, S., & Guthrie, P. F. (2009). Evidence-based guideline— Acute confusion/delirium: Identification, assessment, treatment, and prevention. *Journal of Gerontological Nursing, 35*(11), 11–17.

*Stark, S. (2012). Elder abuse: Screening, intervention, and prevention. *Nursing, 42*(10), 24–29.

Strunk, J., Townsend-Rocchiccioli, J., & Sanford, J. T. (2013). The aging Hispanic in America: Challenges for nurses in a stressed health care environment. *Medsurg Nursing, 22,* 45–50.

Swartzell, K. L., Fulton, J. S., & Friesth, B. M. (2013). Relationship between occurrence of falls and fall-risk scores in an acute care setting using the Hendrich II Fall Risk Model. *Medsurg Nursing, 22*(3), 180–187.

*Toner, F., & Claros, E. (2012). Preventing, assessing, and managing constipation in older adults. *Nursing, 42*(12), 32–38.

*Tzeng, H. M., & Yin, C. Y. (2012). Toileting-related inpatient falls in adult acute care settings. *Medsurg Nursing, 21,* 372–377.

*Volkert, D., Saegitz, C., Gueldenzoph, H., Sieber, C. C., & Stehle, P. (2010). Underdiagnosed malnutrition and nutrition-related problems in geriatric patients. *Journal of Nutrition, Health & Aging, 14*(5), 387–392.

Zisberg, A., & Syn-Hershko, A. (2016). Factors related to the mobility of hospitalized older adults: A prospective cohort study. *Geriatric Nursing, 37*(2), 96–100.

CHAPTER 4

Assessment and Care of Patients With Pain

Melanie H. Simpson and Donna D. Ignatavicius

e http://evolve.elsevier.com/Iggy/

PRIORITY AND INTERRELATED CONCEPTS

The priority concept for this chapter is COMFORT.

❋ The COMFORT concept exemplar for this chapter is Pain, below.

The interrelated concepts for this chapter are:
- COGNITION
- SENSORY PERCEPTION

LEARNING OUTCOMES

Safe and Effective Care Environment

1. Identify the role of the nurse as an advocate for patients with acute pain or chronic cancer or noncancer pain.
2. Collaborate with members of the interprofessional team to develop the pain management plan of care.

Health Promotion and Maintenance

3. Develop a teaching plan for patients to include complementary and integrative therapies for pain management and promotion of COMFORT.
4. Incorporate special considerations for older adults and veterans of war related to pain assessment and management.
5. Describe how to provide patient-centered care by respecting patients' preferences, values, and beliefs regarding pain and COMFORT management.

Psychosocial Integrity

6. Discuss the attitudes and knowledge of patients and their families regarding pain assessment and management.

Physiological Integrity

7. Document a complete pain assessment per agency policy.
8. Compare and contrast the characteristics of the major types of pain and give examples of each.
9. Explain the role of the three analgesic groups in pain management.
10. Prioritize evidence-based nursing interventions to prevent common side effects of opioid analgesics, including the effects on COGNITION and SENSORY PERCEPTION.
11. Compare the advantages and disadvantages of drug administration routes.
12. Describe the benefits and limitations of selected safety-enhancing technologies used in pain management.
13. Use clinical judgment to prioritize care for the patient receiving patient-controlled analgesia.
14. Outline care for a patient receiving epidural analgesia.
15. Incorporate nonpharmacologic interventions into the patient's plan of care as needed to control pain and promote COMFORT.

❋ OVERVIEW of COMFORT CONCEPT EXEMPLAR Pain

Pain is a universal, complex, and personal experience that everyone has at some point in life. It is the most common reason people seek medical care and the number-one reason people take medication. Pain causes impaired COMFORT and can lead to poor health for many millions of people. Unrelieved pain can alter or diminish quality of life more than any other single health-related problem. Despite more than 30 years of education and dissemination of guideline recommendations, the failure to adequately manage pain remains a major health problem worldwide.

In response to mandates by multiple organizations and The Joint Commission (TJC), many hospitals and other health care agencies have implemented interprofessional pain initiatives to help ensure that patients receive the best possible treatment.

Some hospitals address this mandate by establishing pain resource nurse (PRN) programs. As the name implies, one or more nurses per clinical unit are educated to serve as a resource to other members of the health care team in managing pain and promoting COMFORT. Other hospitals have a formal team or pain service consisting of one or more nurses, pharmacists, case managers, and/or primary health care providers. In larger facilities, pain services may specialize by type of pain (e.g., acute pain service or pain and palliative care team). Although a large part of the interprofessional team's plan may center on drug therapy, these groups also recommend nonpharmacologic measures when appropriate.

Scope of the Problem

Pain is a major economic problem and a leading cause of disability that changes the lives of many people, especially older adults. Chronic noncancer pain such as osteoarthritis, rheumatoid arthritis, and diabetic neuropathy is the most common cause of long-term disability, affecting millions of Americans and others throughout the world.

 CONSIDERATIONS FOR OLDER ADULTS
Patient-Centered Care QSEN

> Pain is treated inadequately in almost all health care settings. Populations at the highest risk in medical-surgical nursing are older adults, patients with substance use disorder, and those whose primary language differs from that of the health care professional. Older adults in nursing homes are at especially high risk because many residents are unable to report their pain. In addition, there often is a lack of staff members who have been educated to manage pain in the older-adult population.

Inadequate pain management can lead to many adverse consequences affecting the patient and family members (Table 4-1). Therefore nurses have a legal and ethical responsibility to promote COMFORT and ensure that patients receive adequate pain control. Many professional organizations, including the American Society for Pain Management Nursing (ASPMN), the American Pain Society (APS), and TJC state that patients in all health care settings, including home care, have a right to effective pain management.

Patients rely on nurses and other health care professionals to adequately assess and manage their pain. As the coordinator of patient care, be sure to accurately document your assessments and actions, including patient and caregiver teaching. Communication and collaboration among the patient and members of the interprofessional health team about the patient's pain, expectations, and progress toward control are equally important.

Definitions of Pain

Pain is defined as an unpleasant sensory and emotional experience associated with actual or potential tissue damage. McCaffery (1968) offered the more classic and personal definition when she stated that pain is whatever the experiencing person says it is and exists whenever he or she says it exists. This has become the clinical definition of pain worldwide and reflects an understanding that the patient is the authority and the *only* one who can describe the pain experience. *In other words, self-report is always the most reliable indication of pain.* Nurses who

approach pain from this perspective can help the patient achieve effective management by advocating for proper control. If the patient cannot provide self-report, a variety of other methods such as observation of behavioral indicators are used for pain assessment (see later in this chapter).

Categorization of Pain by Duration

Pain is often described as being acute or chronic based on its duration (Table 4-2). *Acute pain* is usually short-lived, whereas *chronic pain* can last a person's lifetime. *Acute pain* often results from sudden, accidental trauma (e.g., fractures, burns, lacerations) or from surgery, ischemia, or acute inflammation. *Chronic pain* or *persistent pain* is further divided into two subtypes. *Chronic cancer pain* is pain associated with cancer and is usually the result of tissue changes from tumor growth. *Chronic noncancer pain* is associated with past or ongoing tissue damage such as chronic back or neck pain or osteoarthritis pain. *Noncancer pain is the most common type of chronic pain.*

Acute Pain

Almost everyone experiences acute pain at some time. Brief acute pain serves a biologic purpose in that it acts as a warning signal by activating the sympathetic nervous system and causing various physiologic responses. Although not consistent in all people, when acute pain is severe, you may see responses similar to those found in "fight-or-flight" reactions such as increased vital signs, sweating, and dilated pupils. Most people protect themselves by drawing away from the painful stimulus. Behavioral signs may include restlessness (especially among cognitively impaired older adults who sometimes fidget and pick at clothing), an inability to concentrate, apprehension, and overall distress of varying degrees. These heightened physiologic and behavioral responses are often referred to as the *acute pain model*. It is important to remember that the response to pain is highly individual and that humans quickly adapt physiologically and behaviorally to pain. Be careful not to expect certain responses when assessing any type of pain. *The absence of the*

TABLE 4-1   Impact of Unrelieved Pain

Physiologic Impact	Quality-of-Life Impact
• Prolongs stress response	• Interferes with ADLs
• Increases heart rate, blood pressure, and oxygen demand	• Causes anxiety, depression, hopelessness, fear, anger, and sleeplessness
• Decreases GI motility	• Impairs family, work, and social relationships
• Causes immobility	
• Decreases immune response	**Financial Impact**
• Delays healing	• Costs Americans billions of dollars per year
• Poorly managed acute pain increases risk for development of chronic pain	• Increases length of hospital stay
	• Leads to lost income and productivity

TABLE 4-2   Characteristics of Acute Pain and Chronic Pain

ACUTE	CHRONIC* (OR PERSISTENT)
• Has short duration	• Usually lasts longer than 3 months
• Usually has a well-defined cause	• May or may not have well-defined cause
• Decreases with healing	• Usually begins gradually and persists
• Is usually reversible	• Serves no useful purpose
• Initially serves a biologic purpose (warning sign to withdraw from painful stimuli or seek help)	• Ranges from mild-to-severe intensity
• When prolonged, serves no useful purpose	• Often accompanied by multiple quality-of-life and functional adverse effects, including depression; fatigue; financial burden; and increased dependence on family, friends, and the health care system
• Ranges from mild-to-severe intensity	
• May be accompanied by anxiety and restlessness	
• When unrelieved can increase morbidity and mortality and prolong length of hospital stay	• Can impact the quality of life of family members and friends

*Includes chronic cancer pain and chronic noncancer pain.

physiologic and behavioral responses does not mean the absence of pain.

Acute pain is usually temporary, has a sudden onset, and is easily localized. The pain is typically confined to the injured area and may subside with or without treatment. As the injured area heals, the SENSORY PERCEPTION of pain changes and, in most cases, diminishes and resolves. Both the caregiver and the patient can see an end to the pain, which usually makes coping somewhat easier.

Pain that accompanies surgery is one of the most common examples of acute pain, but it is not always well managed. *The response to pain after surgery is highly individual and variable.* There is no evidence that shows that one type of surgery is consistently more or less painful than another. Usually poorly managed postoperative pain is a result of inadequate drug (analgesic) therapy. Poorly managed and prolonged acute pain serves no useful purpose and has many adverse effects, including inability of the patient to participate in the recovery process with subsequent increased disability. The severity of early postoperative pain may be a predictor of long-term pain. Those who experience unrelieved severe postoperative pain are at high risk for the development of chronic persistent postsurgical pain (Wright, 2015).

Chronic Pain

Chronic pain (also called *persistent pain)* is often defined as pain that lasts or recurs for an indefinite period, usually for more than 3 months. The onset is gradual, and the character and quality of the pain often change over time. *Chronic pain serves no biologic purpose.* Because it persists for an extended period, it can interfere with personal relationships and performance of ADLs. Chronic pain can also result in emotional and financial burdens, depression, and hopelessness for patients and their families. It is important to remember that the body adapts to persistent pain; thus vital signs such as pulse and blood pressure may actually be lower than normal in people with chronic pain. *Although many characteristics of chronic pain are similar in different patients, be aware that each patient is unique and requires a highly individualized plan of care.*

Chronic Cancer Pain. Many patients with cancer report pain at the time of diagnosis, which increases in advanced stages of the disease. Most cancer pain can be managed successfully by giving adequate amounts of oral opioids around the clock, yet patients with cancer are often treated inadequately for what can be persistent, excruciating pain and suffering.

Most cancer pain is the result of tumor growth, including nerve compression; invasion of tissue; and/or bone metastasis, an extremely painful condition. Cancer treatments also can cause *acute pain* (e.g., from repetitive blood draws and other procedures, surgery, and toxicities from chemotherapy and radiation therapy).

Patients with cancer pain generally have pain in two or more areas of the body but usually talk about only the primary area. Be sure to perform a complete pain assessment to ensure an effective plan of care.

Chronic Noncancer Pain. Chronic noncancer pain is a global health problem, occurring most often in people older than 65 years. This type of pain was formerly called *chronic nonmalignant* pain. However, most experts, and certainly patients who suffer daily, believe that all pain is malignant. There are many sources and types of chronic noncancer pain. Among the most common are neck, shoulder, and low back pain following injury.

Chronic conditions such as diabetes, rheumatoid arthritis, Crohn's disease, and interstitial cystitis often are associated with chronic pain. People who have had a stroke or trauma or are paralyzed may report persistent pain as a result of central nervous system (CNS) damage. Sometimes the exact cause of the pain is unclear, as with fibromyalgia.

> ### ♥ VETERANS' HEALTH CONSIDERATIONS
> #### *Patient-Centered Care* QSEN
>
> Over half of the veterans of recent wars such as those in Iraq and Afghanistan have chronic noncancer pain, mostly due to musculoskeletal disorders (MSDs) from either trauma or arthritis. Research shows that pain-related MSD causes or exacerbates depression, post-traumatic stress disorder (PTSD), and a decreased sense of well-being in this young to middle-age population (Matthias et al., 2014). Some of these patients are managed through Veterans Administration Medical Centers in ambulatory care clinics in the United States. Unfortunately others are jobless and homeless and therefore receive no care to manage their physical or psychological health problems.

Categorization of Pain by Underlying Mechanisms

Pain is more commonly categorized as either nociceptive (normal pain processing) or neuropathic (abnormal pain processing) (Table 4-3). The duration of nociceptive and neuropathic pain can be either acute (short lived) or chronic (persistent), and a person can have both types.

Nociceptive Pain

Nociception is the term that is used to describe how pain becomes a conscious experience. It involves the *normal functioning of physiologic systems* that process noxious stimuli, with the ultimate result being that the stimuli are perceived to be painful. In short, nociception means "normal" pain transmission and is generally discussed in terms of four processes: transduction, transmission, perception, and modulation (Fig. 4-1). Although it is helpful to consider nociception in the context of these four processes, it is important to understand that they do not occur as four separate and distinct entities. They are continuous, and the processes overlap as they flow from one to another.

Transduction is the first process of nociception and refers to the means by which noxious events activate neurons that exist throughout the body (skin, subcutaneous tissue, and visceral [or somatic] structures) and have the ability to respond selectively to specific noxious stimuli. These neurons are called *nociceptors.* When they are stimulated directly, a number of excitatory compounds (e.g., serotonin, bradykinin, histamine, substance P, and prostaglandins) are released that further activate more nociceptors (see Fig. 4-1).

Transmission is the second process involved in nociception. Nociceptors have small-diameter axons—either A-delta or C fibers (see Fig. 4-1). Effective transduction generates an electric signal (action potential) that is transmitted in these nerve fibers from the periphery toward the CNS. *A-delta fibers* are lightly myelinated and conduct faster than unmyelinated C fibers. The endings of A-delta fibers detect thermal and mechanical injury. The SENSORY PERCEPTION accompanying A-delta fiber activation is sharp and well localized and leads to an appropriately rapid protective response such as reflex withdrawal from the painful stimuli. *C fibers* are unmyelinated or poorly myelinated

TABLE 4-3 **Physiologic Sources of Nociceptive Pain and Neuropathic Pain**

PHYSIOLOGIC STRUCTURE	CHARACTERISTICS OF PAIN	SOURCES OF ACUTE POSTOPERATIVE PAIN	SOURCES OF CHRONIC PAIN SYNDROMES
Nociceptive Pain (Normal Pain Processing)			
Somatic Pain			
Cutaneous or superficial: skin and subcutaneous tissues	Well localized	Incisional pain, pain at insertion sites of tubes and drains, wound complications, orthopedic procedures, skeletal muscle spasms	Bony metastases, osteoarthritis and rheumatoid arthritis, low back pain, peripheral vascular diseases
	Sharp, throbbing		
Deep somatic: bone, muscle, blood vessels, connective tissues	Dull, aching, cramping		
Visceral Pain			
Organs and the linings of the body cavities	Poorly localized	Chest tubes, abdominal tubes and drains, bladder distention or spasms, intestinal distention	Pancreatitis, liver metastases, colitis, appendicitis
	Diffuse, deep cramping or pressure, sharp, stabbing		
Neuropathic Pain (Abnormal Pain Processing)			
Peripheral or central nervous system: nerve fibers, spinal cord, and higher central nervous system	Poorly localized	Phantom limb pain, postmastectomy pain, nerve compression	HIV-related pain, diabetic neuropathy, postherpetic neuralgia, chemotherapy-induced neuropathies, cancer-related nerve injury, radiculopathies
	Shooting, burning, fiery, shocklike, tingling, painful numbness		

HIV, Human immune deficiency virus.

slow conductors and respond to mechanical, thermal, and chemical stimuli. Activation after acute injury yields a poorly localized (more widely distributed) typically aching or burning pain. In contrast to the intermittent nature of A-delta sensations, C fibers usually produce more continuous pain.

Perception is the third broad process involved in nociception. Perception, which may be viewed as the end result of the neural activity associated with transmission of information about noxious events, involves the conscious awareness of pain (see Fig. 4-1). It requires the activation of higher brain structures, including the cortex, and involves both awareness and the occurrence of emotions and drives associated with pain. The physiology of pain perception is very poorly understood but presumably can be targeted by therapies that activate higher cortical functions and COGNITION to achieve pain control or coping. Cognitive-behavioral therapy and specific approaches such as distraction and imagery (discussed later in the chapter) have been developed based on evidence that brain processes can strongly influence pain perception.

Modulation of afferent input generated in response to noxious stimuli happens at every level from the periphery to the cortex (see Fig. 4-1). The neurochemistry of modulation is complex and not yet fully understood, but it is known that multiple peripheral and central systems and dozens of neurochemicals are involved. For example, the endogenous opioids (endorphins) are found throughout the peripheral nervous system (PNS) and CNS and, like the exogenous opioids administered therapeutically, they inhibit neuronal activity by binding to opioid receptors. Other central inhibitory neurotransmitters important in the modulation of pain include serotonin and norepinephrine, which are released in the spinal cord and brainstem by the descending fibers of the modulatory system to inhibit pain.

Nociceptive pain is the result of actual or potential tissue damage or inflammation and is often categorized as being somatic or visceral. *Somatic pain* arises from the skin and musculoskeletal structures, and *visceral pain* arises from organs.

Examples include pain-associated trauma, surgery, burns, and tumor growth.

Neuropathic Pain

Neuropathic pain is a descriptive term used to refer to pain that is believed to be sustained by a set of mechanisms driven by damage to or dysfunction of the PNS and/or CNS. In contrast to nociceptive pain, which is sustained by ongoing activation of essentially *normal* neural systems, neuropathic pain is sustained by the *abnormal* processing of stimuli. Whereas nociceptive pain involves tissue damage or inflammation, neuropathic pain may occur in the absence of either.

It is not clear why noxious stimuli result in neuropathic pain in some people and not in others and why some treatments work in some and not in others. Neuropathic pain is difficult to treat and often resistant to first-line analgesics. Asking patients to describe it is the best way to identify the presence of neuropathic pain. Common distinctive descriptors include "burning," "shooting," "tingling," and "feeling pins and needles." Much is unknown about what causes and maintains neuropathic pain; it is the subject of intense ongoing research.

❖ INTERPROFESSIONAL COLLABORATIVE CARE
◆ Assessment: Noticing

All accepted guidelines identify the patient's self-report as the gold standard for assessing the existence and intensity of pain (Pasero & McCaffery, 2011). Because pain is such a private and personal experience, it may be difficult for the person to describe or explain it to others. However, subjective descriptions of the experience and measurement of pain intensity are more reliable and accurate than observable qualities of pain. The amount of pain and responses to it vary from person to person; therefore interpreting it solely on actions or behaviors can be misleading and is not recommended. Patients may report pain in the absence of any observable or documented physiologic changes.

Although nurses and other members of the interprofessional team are entitled to their doubts and opinions about a patient's

Refer the patient and family to self-help groups such as the American Chronic Pain Association (http://theacpa.org), which provides the "10-Step Program from Patient to Person."

CULTURAL/SPIRITUAL CONSIDERATIONS
Patient-Centered Care QSEN

If the chronic pain is associated with a progressive disease such as cancer, rheumatoid arthritis, or peripheral vascular disease, the patient may have worries and concerns about the consequences of the illness. People with cancer-related pain may fear death or body mutilation. Some may think they are being punished for some wrongdoing in life. Others may attach a religious or spiritual significance to lingering pain.

Ask open-ended questions (e.g., "Tell me how your pain has affected your job or your role as a mother.") to allow the patient to describe personal attitudes about pain and its influence on life. This opportunity can help someone whose life has been changed by pain. However, some patients choose not to share their private information or fears. As a patient-centered nurse, always respect patients' preferences and values.

❓ NCLEX EXAMINATION CHALLENGE 4-1
Physiological Integrity

A client who had a total knee replacement 2 weeks ago reports severe pain at the surgical site. Which responses by the nurse are **most** appropriate for the client at this time? **Select all that apply.**
A. "Please rate your pain on a 0-10 scale, with 10 being the worst possible pain."
B. "Could you describe the pain in your knee?"
C. "By now your pain should be a lot less than it was 2 weeks ago."
D. "Which positions make the pain feel worse or better?"
E. "Having your joint replaced should have decreased your knee pain."

Assessment Challenges. Patients who are unable to report their pain using the customary self-report assessment tools are at higher risk for undertreated pain than those who can report. These include patients who are cognitively impaired, critically ill (intubated, unresponsive), comatose, or imminently dying. Patients who are receiving neuromuscular blocking agents or are sedated from general anesthetics and other drugs given during surgery are also among this at-risk population.

The *Hierarchy of Pain Measures* is recommended by many professional organizations today as a framework for assessing pain in patients who cannot self-report. The key components of the Hierarchy require the nurse to (1) attempt to obtain self-report; (2) consider underlying pathology or conditions and procedures that might be painful (e.g., surgery); (3) observe behaviors; (4) evaluate physiologic indicators; and (5) conduct an analgesic trial. See Table 4-5 for detailed information on each component of the Hierarchy of Pain Measures.

Patients with problems of COGNITION are among those at highest risk for undertreated pain because they are unable to report or have difficulty reporting their pain. The Hierarchy of Pain Measures lists several strategies to use when obtaining self-report is a challenge. When these are ineffective, the Hierarchy suggests that a number of behaviors have been shown to be indicators of pain. Behavioral pain assessment tools are often

TABLE 4-5	**Hierarchy of Pain Measures**

1. Attempt to obtain the patient's self-report, the single most reliable indicator of pain. Do not assume that a patient cannot provide a report of pain; many cognitively impaired patients are able to use a self-report tool if simple actions are taken.
   - Try using a standard pain assessment tool (see Fig. 4-3).
   - Ensure that eyeglasses and hearing aids are functioning.
   - Increase the size of the font and other features of the scale.
   - Present the tool in vertical format (rather than the frequently used horizontal).
   - Try using alternative words such as "ache," "hurt," and "sore" when discussing pain.
   - Ask about pain in the present.
   - Repeat instructions and questions more than once.
   - Allow ample time to respond.
   - Remember that head nodding and eye blinking or squeezing the eyes tightly can also be used to signal presence of pain and sometimes to rate intensity.
   - Ask awake and oriented ventilated patients to point to a number on the numeric scale if they are able.
   - Repeat instructions and show the scale each time pain is assessed.
2. Consider the patient's condition or exposure to a procedure that is thought to be painful. If appropriate, *assume pain is present* (APP) and document APP when approved by institution policy and procedure. As an example, pain should be assumed to be present in an unresponsive, mechanically ventilated, critically ill trauma patient. Nurses should assume that certain procedures are painful and premedicate based on that assumption.
3. Observe behavioral signs (e.g., facial expressions, crying, restlessness, and changes in activity). A pain behavior in one patient may not be in another. Try to identify pain behaviors that are unique to the patient ("pain signature"). Many behavioral pain assessment tools are available that will yield a pain behavior score and may help determine if pain is present. However, it is important to remember that a behavioral score is not the same as a pain intensity score. Behavioral tools are used to help identify the presence of pain and whether an intervention is effective, but the pain intensity is unknown if the patient is unable to provide it.
   - A surrogate who knows the patient well (e.g., parent, spouse, or caregiver) may be able to provide information about underlying painful pathology or behaviors that may indicate pain.
   - Although surrogates may be helpful in identifying behaviors that may indicate pain, research has shown that they commonly underestimate or overestimate the intensity of the pain. Therefore they should not be asked to rate the patient's pain intensity.
4. Evaluate physiologic indicators with the understanding that they are the *least* sensitive indicators of pain and may signal the existence of conditions other than pain or a lack of it (e.g., hypovolemia, blood loss). Patients quickly adapt physiologically despite pain and may have normal or below-normal vital signs in the presence of severe pain. The overriding principle is that the absence of an elevated blood pressure or heart rate does not mean the absence of pain.
5. Conduct an analgesic trial to confirm the presence of pain and to establish a basis for developing a treatment plan if pain is thought to be present. An analgesic trial involves administering a low dose of analgesic and observing patient response. The initial low dose may not be enough to illicit a change in behavior and should be increased if the previous dose was tolerated, or another analgesic may be added. If behaviors continue despite optimal analgesic doses, other possible causes should be investigated.
   - In patients who are unresponsive, no change in behavior will be evident, and the optimized analgesic dose should be continued.

From Pasero, C., & McCaffery, M. (2011). *Pain assessment and pharmacologic management.* St. Louis: Mosby.

used to systematically evaluate behaviors to help determine the presence of pain. Improvement in the behavioral pain score helps confirm suspicions that pain is present and provides a reference point for assessing the effectiveness of interventions.

It is important for nurses to remember that *a score obtained from the use of a behavioral tool is not the same as a self-reported pain intensity score.* Although it may seem logical to assume that the higher the behavioral score, the more intense the pain, this cannot be proven without the patient's report. Some patients remain nonverbal and lie completely still (which would yield a low behavioral score) despite having severe pain. The reality is that, if a patient cannot report the intensity of pain, the exact intensity is unknown. Two of the most commonly used behavioral assessment tools that are used for patients with problems of COGNITION such as delirium (acute confusion) or dementia (chronic confusion) are:

- Checklist of Nonverbal Pain Indicators (CNPI) has been tested in the acute care setting in patients with varying levels of cognitive impairment. The tool groups behavioral indicators of pain into six categories. Each category allows a score of 0 if the behavior is not observed and a 1 if the behavior occurred even briefly during activity or rest:
  - Facial expression (e.g., grimacing, crying)
  - Verbalizations or vocalizations (e.g., screaming)
  - Body movements (e.g., restlessness)
  - Changes in interpersonal interactions
  - Changes in activity patterns or routines
  - Mental status changes (e.g., confusion, increased confusion)
- Pain Assessment in Advanced Dementia (PAINAD) scale has been tested in patients with severe dementia (Herr et al., 2011). The tool groups behavioral indicators into five categories for scoring using a graduated scale of 0 (least intense behaviors) to 2 (most intense behaviors) per category for a maximum behavioral score of 10:
  - Breathing (independent of vocalization)
  - Negative vocalization
  - Facial expression
  - Body language
  - Consolability (ability to calm the patient)

For patients who are mechanically ventilated or may not be able to use other tools for communication, try these interventions:

- Establish a reliable yes-no signal (e.g., thumbs up or down, head nods, or eye blinks) to determine the presence of pain.
- Use communication boards, alphabet boards, computer, or picture boards with word labels for patients with COGNITION problems.
- Correctly interpret lip reading by maintaining eye contact, encouraging the patient to speak slowly, and using dentures if required.

◆ *Interventions: Responding*

Pain is managed using nonpharmacologic interventions, drug therapy, or both. Although nonpharmalogic interventions are commonly used, they are most often combined with drug therapy as complementary or supplemental therapies. Because drug therapy is the most often used approach to pain management, it is presented first in this chapter.

Drug Therapy. Safe and effective use of analgesics requires the development of an individualized treatment plan based on

a comprehensive assessment. This plan includes clarifying the desired outcomes of treatment and discussing options and preferences with the patient and family. Desired outcomes are periodically re-evaluated, and changes made, depending on patient response and in some cases disease progression.

Multimodal Analgesia. Pain is complex, which explains why there is no single, universal treatment for it. Its complexity is also the basis for the widespread recommendation that a multimodal analgesic approach be used, regardless of the type of pain (American Society of Anesthesiologists [ASA], 2012; Pasero & McCaffery, 2011). Multimodal treatment involves the use of two or more classes of analgesics or interventions to target different pain mechanisms in the PNS or CNS. It relies on the thoughtful and rational combination of analgesics to maximize relief and prevent analgesic gaps that may lead to worsening pain or unnecessary episodes of uncontrolled pain.

A multimodal approach may allow lower doses of each of the drugs in the treatment plan. Lower doses have the potential to produce fewer side effects. Further, multimodal analgesia can result in comparable or greater relief than can be achieved with any single analgesic. For postoperative pain the use of combination therapy to prevent both inflammatory and neuropathic pain is likely to yield the best immediate results. It also offers the promise of reducing the incidence of prolonged or persistent postsurgical pain.

The multimodal strategy also has a role in the management of persistent pain. The complex nature of the many chronic conditions indicates the need for appropriate combinations of analgesics such as anticonvulsants, antidepressants, and local anesthetics to target differing underlying mechanisms.

Preemptive analgesia involves the administration of local anesthetics, opioids, and other drugs (multimodal analgesia) in anticipation of pain along the continuum of care during the preoperative, intraoperative, and postoperative periods. This continuous approach is designed to decrease pain severity in the postoperative period, reduce analgesic dose requirements, prevent morbidity, shorten hospital stay, and avoid complications after discharge. Continuous multimodal analgesia may inhibit changes in the spinal cord that can lead to changes in the PNS and CNS that initiate and sustain chronic persistent postsurgical pain (see Nociception earlier in the chapter).

Routes of Administration. The oral route is the *preferred* route of analgesic administration. It should be used whenever feasible because it is generally the least expensive, best tolerated, easiest to administer, and replicable at home once the patient is discharged. Other routes of administration are used when the oral route is not possible such as in patients who are NPO, nauseated, or unable to swallow. For example, early postoperative pain and pain that is severe and escalating are managed with the IV route of administration. Then patients are transitioned to oral analgesics when they are able to tolerate oral intake.

Around-the-Clock Dosing. Two basic principles of providing effective interprofessional collaborative care are (1) preventing pain and (2) maintaining a level of pain control that allows the patient to function and have an acceptable quality of life. Accomplishment of these desired outcomes may require the mainstay analgesic to be administered on a scheduled around-the-clock (ATC) basis rather than PRN ("as needed") to maintain stable analgesic levels. *ATC dosing regimens are designed to control pain for patients who report it being present 12 hours or more during a 24-hour period,* such as that associated with most chronic syndromes and pain during the first 24 to 48 hours after surgery or other tissue injury. PRN dosing of analgesics is appropriate for intermittent pain such as before painful procedures and breakthrough pain (additional pain that "breaks through" the pain being managed by the mainstay analgesic), for which supplemental doses of analgesic are provided.

Patient-Controlled Analgesia. Patient-controlled analgesia (PCA) is an interactive method of management that allows patients to treat their pain by self-administering doses of analgesics. It is used to manage all types of pain and given by multiple routes of administration, including IV, subcutaneous, epidural, and perineural. A PCA infusion device ("pump") is used when PCA is delivered by invasive routes of administration and is programmed so the patient can press a button ("pendant") to self-administer a set dose of analgesic ("PCA dose") at a set time interval ("demand" or "lockout") as needed. *Patients who use PCA must be able to understand the relationships among pain, pressing the PCA button and taking the analgesic, and pain relief. They must also be cognitively and physically able to use any equipment that is used to administer the therapy.*

PCA may be given with or without a basal rate (continuous infusion). The use of a basal rate is common when patient-controlled epidural analgesia (PCEA) is used. For IV PCA, a basal rate may be added for opioid-tolerant patients to replace their home analgesic regimen. Basal rates should be used with great caution and only in special circumstances for opioid-naïve patients receiving IV PCA. Remember that the patient has no control over the delivery of a continuous infusion. Essential to the safe use of a basal rate is prompt discontinuation of the basal rate if increased sedation or respiratory depression occurs.

> ## ⚠ NURSING SAFETY PRIORITY QSEN
> ### *Action Alert*
>
> Teach patients how to use the PCA device and to report side effects such as dizziness, nausea and vomiting, and excessive sedation. As with all opioids, monitor the patient's sedation level and respiratory status at least every 2 hours. Promptly decrease the opioid dose (i.e., discontinue basal rate) if increased sedation is detected.

The primary benefit of PCA is that it recognizes that only the patient can feel the pain and only the patient knows how much analgesic will relieve it. This fact reinforces that *PCA is for patient use only and that unauthorized activation of the PCA button (called "PCA by proxy") can be very dangerous.* Instruct staff, family, and other visitors to contact the nurse if they have concerns about pain control rather than pressing the PCA button for the patient.

The Three Analgesic Groups. Analgesics are categorized into three main groups: (1) nonopioid analgesics, which include acetaminophen and the NSAIDs; (2) opioid analgesics such as morphine, hydrocodone, hydromorphone, fentanyl, and oxycodone; and (3) adjuvant analgesics (sometimes referred to as *co-analgesics*), which make up the largest group and include a variety of agents with unique and widely differing mechanisms of action. Examples are local anesthetics, muscle relaxants, and some anticonvulsants and antidepressants.

Nonopioid Analgesics. Acetaminophen and NSAIDs make up the nonopioid analgesic group. *Acetaminophen* is thought to relieve pain by underlying mechanisms in the CNS. It has analgesic and antipyretic properties but is not effective for treating inflammation. In contrast, *NSAIDs* have analgesic, antipyretic, and anti-inflammatory properties. These drugs produce pain relief by blocking prostaglandins through inhibition of the enzyme *cyclooxygenase (COX)* in the peripheral nervous system (see Nociception and Fig. 4-1 earlier in the chapter).

Nonopioids are available in a variety of formulations and given by multiple routes of administration. They are also flexible analgesics used for a wide range of conditions. Nonopioid drugs are appropriate alone for mild-to-moderate nociceptive pain (e.g., from surgery, trauma, or osteoarthritis) or are added to opioids, local anesthetics, and/or anticonvulsants as part of a multimodal analgesic regimen for more severe nociceptive pain. *However, they have limited benefit for neuropathic pain.*

Acetaminophen and an NSAID may be given together, and there is no need for staggered doses. Unless contraindicated, all surgical patients should routinely be given acetaminophen and an NSAID in scheduled doses as the foundation of the pain treatment plan throughout the postoperative course, preferably initiated before surgery.

The nonopioids are often combined in a single tablet with opioids such as oxycodone (Percocet) or hydrocodone (Vicodin, Norco, Vicoprofen) and are very popular for the treatment of mild-to-moderate acute pain. Many people with persistent pain also take a combination nonopioid/opioid analgesic. However, it is important to remember that these combination drugs are not appropriate for severe pain of any type because the maximum daily dose of the nonopioid limits the escalation of the opioid dose.

Oral *acetaminophen* (Tylenol, Abenol) has a long history of safety in recommended doses in all age-groups and most patient populations. It is recommended as first line for musculoskeletal pain (e.g., osteoarthritis) in older adults but has no inflammatory properties. Therefore acetaminophen is less effective than NSAIDs for chronic inflammatory pain (e.g., rheumatoid arthritis). IV acetaminophen (Ofirmev) is approved for treatment of pain and fever in adults and is given by a 15-minute infusion in single or repeated doses. It can be given alone for mild-to-moderate pain or in combination with opioid analgesics for more severe pain.

The most serious complication of acetaminophen is hepatotoxicity (liver damage) as a result of overdose. Patient's hepatic risk factors must always be considered before administration of acetaminophen. In the healthy adult a maximum daily dose below 4000 mg is rarely associated with liver toxicity. Many experts recommend reducing the daily dose (e.g., 2500 to 3000 mg daily) when used for *long-term* treatment in older adults. Acetaminophen does not increase bleeding time and has a low incidence of GI adverse effects, making it the analgesic of choice in many people in pain, especially older adults (see Evidence-Based Practice box).

A benefit of the *NSAID* group is the availability of a wide variety of agents for administration via noninvasive routes. Ibuprofen (Motrin, Novo-Profen), naproxen (Naprosyn, Nu-Naprox), and celecoxib (Celebrex) are the most widely used oral NSAIDs in the United States and Canada. Diclofenac (Voltaren) is prescribed in patch and gel form for topical administration. An intranasal patient-controlled formulation of ketorolac (Sprix) has been approved for short-term treatment of acute pain. IV formulations of ketorolac (Toradol), ibuprofen (Caldolor), and diclofenac (Dyloject) are also used to manage acute pain. Each have been shown to produce excellent analgesia

EVIDENCE-BASED PRACTICE QSEN

What Are the Best Practices for Managing Chronic Pain in Older Adults?

Makris, U. E., Adams, R. C., Gurland, B., & Reid, M. C. (2014). Management of persistent pain in the older patient: A clinical review. *JAMA, 312*(8), 825-836.

The researchers conducted an extensive review of 92 meta-analysis studies, Cochrane reviews, systematic reviews, consensus statements, and clinical guidelines to determine best practices for managing chronic (persistent) pain in older adults. Of the reviewed studies and reviews, 35 focused on drug therapy for pain control; 57 focused on nonpharmacologic strategies. Fifty of the 92 studies discussed pain management for older adults with osteoarthritis, the most common cause of chronic musculoskeletal pain in this population. The authors concluded that acetaminophen is the primary drug of choice, followed by a trial of topical NSAIDs or tramadol if acetaminophen is not effective. Further, the researchers found no support for long-term use of oral NSAIDs due to toxicities and common adverse effects of these drugs among the older-adult population. Nonpharmacologic measures should be used based on the patient's preference to supplement the drug therapy regimen.

Level of Evidence: 1

This research presents the results of an in-depth clinical review of multiple published meta-analyses and systematic reviews. In addition, the authors examined guidelines and consensus statements.

Commentary: Implications for Practice and Research

This study reinforced the need to teach older adults to avoid the long-term use of NSAIDs and use acetaminophen for pain control because it is a safer drug. In addition, teach patients about the value of topical NSAIDs and nonpharmacologic modalities that may supplement the drug therapy. More research is needed on which nonpharmacologic strategies are best practice measures for chronic pain associated with osteoarthritis in older adults.

! NURSING SAFETY PRIORITY QSEN

Drug Alert

Teach patients to tell their primary health care provider about the amounts of acetaminophen and NSAIDs they take each day. Remind patients of the importance of being alert to the adverse effects of the medications they take and to complete any prescribed laboratory tests (e.g., liver enzymes) to identify early indicators of adverse effects.

! NURSING SAFETY PRIORITY QSEN

Drug Alert

NSAIDs can cause GI disturbances and decrease platelet aggregation (clotting), which can result in bleeding. Therefore observe the patient for gastric discomfort or vomiting and for bleeding or bruising. Tell the patient and family to stop taking these drugs and report these effects to the primary health care provider immediately if any of these problems occur. Celecoxib has no effect on bleeding time and produces less GI toxicity compared with other NSAIDs.

CONSIDERATIONS FOR OLDER ADULTS

Patient-Centered Care QSEN

Older adults are at increased risk for NSAID-induced GI toxicity. Acetaminophen should be used for mild pain. If an NSAID is needed for inflammatory pain or additional analgesia, the least ulcer-causing NSAID is recommended. The addition of a proton pump inhibitor (e.g., lansoprazole, omeprazole) to NSAID therapy or use of opioid analgesics rather than an NSAID is recommended for high-risk patients. Topical NSAIDs may be used as needed, especially for musculoskeletal disorder pain (Makris et al., 2014).

? NCLEX EXAMINATION CHALLENGE 4-2

Physiological Integrity

An older client takes ibuprofen 1600 mg daily for osteoarthritis. Which health teaching will the nurse provide for the client related to this medication? **Select all that apply.**
A. "Be sure and take your medication with food to prevent stomach ulcers."
B. "Take your medication only when you need it for chronic pain."
C. "Avoid any over-the-counter medications that may contain ibuprofen."
D. "Take your blood pressure often because ibuprofen can cause it to go up."
E. "You might want to take acetaminophen because it has fewer side effects than ibuprofen."

---

alone for mild-to-moderate nociceptive pain and significant opioid dose-sparing effects when administered as part of a multimodal analgesic plan for more severe pain.

NSAIDs have more adverse effects than acetaminophen, with gastric toxicity and ulceration being the most common. Risk factors for NSAID adverse effects include being older than 60 years or having a history of peptic ulcer or cardiovascular (CV) disease. An important principle of NSAID use is to administer the lowest dose for the shortest time necessary.

All NSAIDs carry a risk for CV adverse effects through prostaglandin inhibition. The US Food and Drug Administration (FDA) cautions against the use of any NSAIDs after high-risk open-heart surgery because of an elevated CV risk with NSAIDs in this population. Prostaglandins also affect renal function. Be sure that the patient is adequately hydrated when administering NSAIDs to prevent acute renal failure.

Opioid Analgesics. Opioid analgesics are the mainstay in the management of moderate-to-severe nociceptive types of pain such as postoperative, surgical, trauma, and burn pain. Although it is often used, the term *narcotic* is considered obsolete and inaccurate when discussing the use of opioids for pain management. "Narcotic" is used loosely by law enforcement and the media to refer to a variety of substances of potential abuse. Legally controlled substances classified as narcotics include opioids, cocaine, and others. *The preferred term is "opioid analgesics" when discussing these agents in the context of pain management.* Some patients prefer the term *pain medications* or *pain medicine.*

Opioids produce their effects by interacting with opioid receptor sites located throughout the body, including in the peripheral tissues, the GI system, and the spinal cord and brain. When an opioid binds to the opioid receptor sites, it produces analgesia and unwanted effects such as constipation, nausea, sedation, and respiratory depression. There are three classifications of opioids:

- Full or *mu agonists* ("morphine-like") bind primarily to the mu-type opioid receptors in the CNS and, among

🧬 **GENETIC/GENOMIC CONSIDERATIONS**
Patient-Centered Care **QSEN**

It has long been known that the cytochrome (CY) *P450* enzyme system is important to the metabolism of some opioids. Interethnic variations in phenotypes of the *CYP450* enzymes are common, causing decreased metabolism of selected analgesics in a small percentage of Caucasians and Asians. These variations have clinical implications when the opioid *codeine*, which is metabolized by the *CYP450* enzyme system, is administered. Slow metabolizers may not respond well to codeine, and ultra-rapid metabolizers may have an exaggerated response. Current research is focused on other genetic variables that may explain an individual's response to opioids to manage pain (Wright, 2015).

other actions, block the release of the neurotransmitter *substance P*, which prevents the opening of calcium channels and the transmission of pain (Wright, 2015). A major benefit of the mu opioid agonists is that they have no ceiling on analgesia. This means that increases in dose produce increases in pain relief and that there is no maximum dose (see Physical Tolerance later in the chapter). This property makes the mu opioid agonists the first-line opioid analgesics for moderate-to-severe nociceptive pain. Examples are morphine, fentanyl, hydromorphone, oxycodone, oxymorphone, and hydrocodone.

- *Mixed agonists antagonists* bind to more than one type of opioid receptor. They bind as agonists to the kappa opioid receptors to produce analgesia and other effects and to the mu opioid receptors as antagonists. This antagonistic property explains why these drugs can trigger severe pain and opioid withdrawal syndrome characterized by rhinitis, abdominal cramping, nausea, agitation, and restlessness in patients who have been taking regular daily doses of a mu agonist opioid for several days. Another undesirable effect of these drugs is that they produce a dose-ceiling effect, which means that further increases in dose will not produce further relief. This latter property limits their usefulness in pain management. Occasionally these drugs are used in very low doses to antagonize (in hopes of relieving) opioid-induced side effects such as pruritus. However, this approach risks reversing analgesia; therefore patients must be assessed frequently to ensure that adequate pain control and COMFORT are maintained. Examples are butorphanol (Stadol) and nalbuphine (Nubain).

- *Partial agonists* have some kappa and mu opioid receptor activity but produce an analgesia plateau and are not easily reversed by opioid antagonists such as naloxone (Narcan). These properties limit their role in pain management. Buprenorphine is a partial agonist opioid, available in a transdermal patch (Butrans) for stable pain management. The drug has been formulated alone (Subutex) and with naloxone (Suboxone) for the treatment of the disease of addiction.

Opioid antagonists (e.g., naloxone [Narcan], naltrexone [Revia]) are drugs that also bind to opioid receptors but produce no analgesia. If an antagonist is present, it competes with opioid molecules for binding sites on the opioid receptors and has the potential to block analgesia and other effects. They are used most often to reverse opioid effects such as excessive sedation and respiratory depression.

Key Principles of Opioid Administration. Many factors are considered when determining the appropriate opioid analgesic for the patient with pain. These include the unique characteristics of the various opioids and patient factors such as type of pain, pain intensity, age, gender, coexisting disease, current drug regimen and potential drug interactions, prior treatment outcomes, and patient preference.

🔬 **GENDER HEALTH CONSIDERATIONS**
Patient-Centered Care **QSEN**

Research has identified differences between females and males in a number of factors that influence the pharmacokinetics (absorption, distribution, metabolism, and excretion) and pharmacodynamics (effects on the body) of drugs. Some of these factors are organ physiology, body composition, gastric emptying time, enzyme activity, and drug clearance (Wright, 2015). Research also shows that women are at substantially greater risk for more pain conditions than men and that they may experience more postoperative and procedural pain than men (Fillingim et al., 2009). In the immediate postoperative period women seem to have a higher opioid requirement, but men demonstrate higher opioid consumption after the initial recovery period. This difference may be partly explained by the faster recovery after general anesthesia in women. Side effects and complications associated with opioid and nonopioid analgesics appear to be more prevalent in women than in men. Creatinine clearance (drug excretion) is generally higher in men than in women because of increased muscle mass, and clearance varies with the menstrual cycle in women. Additional research is needed to better understand the effects of gender on the pain experience.

Titration (dose increases or decreases) of the opioid dose is usually required at the start and throughout the course of treatment when opioids are administered. Whereas patients with cancer pain most often are titrated upward over time for progressive pain, patients with acute pain, particularly postoperative pain, are eventually titrated downward as pain resolves. Although the dose and analgesic effect of mu agonist opioids have no ceiling, the dose may be limited by side effects. The absolute dose administered is unimportant as long as a balance between pain relief and side effects is favorable. *The desired outcome of titration is to use the smallest dose that provides satisfactory pain relief with the fewest side effects.*

When an increase in the opioid dose is necessary and safe, the increase can be titrated by percentages. When a slight improvement in analgesia is needed, a 25% increase in the opioid dose may be sufficient; a 50% increase for moderate improvement; and a 100% increase may be indicated for strong improvement such as when treating severe, escalating pain (Pasero & McCaffery, 2011). The time at which the dose can be increased is determined by the onset and peak effects of the opioid and its formulation. For example, the frequency of IV opioid doses during initial titration may be as often as every 5 to 15 minutes (see later discussion of specific opioids). In contrast, at least 24 hours should elapse before the dose of transdermal fentanyl is increased after the first patch application.

In some cases, needed drug therapy for older adults experiencing pain may not be provided. A study by Platts-Mills et al. (2013) found that among the prehospital population, older adults received analgesia less often than younger adults. Adults older than 85 years of age were the least likely to receive any analgesia. When reporting mild-to-moderate pain, they were

CONSIDERATIONS FOR OLDER ADULTS

Patient-Centered Care (QSEN)

Although the patient's weight is not a good indicator of analgesic requirement, *age is considered an important factor to consider when selecting an opioid dose.* For older adults the guideline is to "start low and go slow" with all drug dosing. For example, the starting opioid dose may need to be reduced by 25% to 50% in older adults because they are more sensitive to opioid side effects than are younger adults. The subsequent doses are based on patient response, which should be evaluated frequently. Monitor sedation level and respiratory status and promptly reduce the drug dose if sedation occurs or the respiratory rate is markedly decreased, depending on agency policy. Chart 4-1 describes best practices for pain assessment and management in the older adult.

less likely to be given analgesics than younger adults with the same pain intensity. However, older women reporting a pain level of 8 or greater (on a pain scale of 0 to 10) were treated for their pain more often than their younger counterparts reporting the same level of pain. Clearly a consistent pain assessment and management protocol is needed for all patients, starting with prehospital and emergency department (ED) care. Many older adults are admitted to the ED with fractures of the hip, pelvis, and spine, which are very painful and require prompt and adequate pain management to promote patient COMFORT.

Physical Dependence, Tolerance, and Addiction. The terms *physical dependence* and *tolerance* often are confused with *addiction;* thus clarification of definitions is important. The most widely accepted definitions of these terms are:

- *Physical dependence is a normal response* that occurs with repeated administration of an opioid for several days. It is manifested by the occurrence of withdrawal symptoms when the opioid is stopped suddenly or rapidly reduced or an antagonist such as naloxone is given. Withdrawal symptoms may be suppressed by the natural, gradual reduction of the opioid as pain decreases or by gradual, systematic reduction, referred to as *tapering. Physical dependence is not the same as addictive disease.*
- *Tolerance is also a normal response* that occurs with regular administration of an opioid and consists of a decrease in one or more effects of the opioid (e.g., decreased analgesia, sedation, or respiratory depression). Like physical dependence, *tolerance is not the same as addictive disease.* Tolerance to analgesia usually occurs in the first days to 2 weeks of opioid therapy but is uncommon after that. It may be treated with increases in dose or rotation to a different opioid. However, disease progression, not tolerance to analgesia, appears to be the reason for most dose escalations. Stable pain usually results in stable opioid doses. With the exception of constipation, tolerance to the opioid side effects develops with regular daily dosing of opioids over several days.
- *Opioid addiction is a chronic neurologic and biologic disease.* The development and characteristics of addiction are influenced by genetic, psychosocial, and environmental factors. No single cause of addiction such as taking an opioid for pain relief has been found. It is characterized by one or more of these behaviors: impaired control over drug use, compulsive use, continued use despite harm, and craving. *The disease of addiction is a treatable disease; as for any other suspected disease, refer the patient to an expert for diagnosis and treatment.*

- *Pseudoaddiction* is a mistaken diagnosis of addictive disease. When a patient's pain is not well controlled, the patient may begin to manifest symptoms suggestive of addictive disease. For example, in an effort to obtain adequate pain relief, the patient may respond with demanding behavior, escalating demands for more or different medications, and repeated requests for opioids on time or before the prescribed interval between doses has elapsed. Pain relief typically eliminates these behaviors and is often accomplished by increasing opioid doses or decreasing intervals between doses.

Opioid Naïve Versus Opioid Tolerant. Patients are often characterized as being either opioid naïve or opioid tolerant. An *opioid-naïve* person has not recently taken enough opioid on a regular basis to become tolerant to the effects of an opioid. An *opioid-tolerant* person has taken an opioid long enough at doses high enough to develop tolerance to many of the effects, including analgesia and the undesirable effects such as nausea and sedation. There is no set time for the development of tolerance, with wide individual variation among people. Some patients do not develop tolerance at all. Opioid tolerance can be defined as regularly taking opioids for about 7 days or longer.

Equianalgesia. The term *equianalgesia* means approximately "equal analgesia." An equianalgesic chart provides a list of analgesic doses, both oral and parenteral (IV, subcutaneous, and IM), that are approximately equal to one another in ability to provide pain relief (Table 4-6). Equianalgesic conversion of doses is used to help ensure that patients receive approximately the same pain relief when they are switched from one opioid or route of administration to another. It requires a series of calculations based on the daily dose of the current opioid to determine the equianalgesic dose of the opioid to which the patient is to be switched. Consult and collaborate with the pharmacist whenever equianalgesic conversion is indicated.

Relative potency is the ratio of drug doses required to produce the same effect. For example, note in Table 4-6 that a single dose of 1.5 mg of parenteral hydromorphone produces approximately the same analgesia as 10 mg of parenteral morphine. This means that hydromorphone is more potent than morphine, but increased potency does not mean that the drug is therapeutically superior or that it provides any advantage. Safe and effective pain management requires nurses to appreciate the differences in the potencies of the various opioids and apply the principles of equianalgesia when administering opioids.

Drug Formulation Terminology. The terms *short acting, fast acting, immediate release (IR),* and *normal release* have been used interchangeably to describe oral opioids that have an onset of action of about 30 minutes and a relatively short duration of 3 to 4 hours. The term *immediate release* is misleading because none of the oral analgesics have an immediate or even a fast onset of analgesia. The term *short acting* is preferred to reflect the short duration of oral opioids. Oral transmucosal and intranasal formulations are appropriately referred to as *ultra-fast acting* because they have a peak effect of 5 to 15 minutes, depending on formulation.

The terms *modified release, extended release (ER), sustained release (SR),* and *controlled release (CR)* are used to describe opioids that are formulated to release over a prolonged period of time. For the purposes of this chapter, the term *modified release* will be used when discussing these opioid formulations. *Long acting* is applied to drugs with a long *half-life* such as methadone. The half-life of a drug provides an estimate of how fast the drug leaves the body. By definition, half-life is the time

CHART 4-1 Nursing Focus on the Older Adult

Pain

Prevalence of Pain

- Recognize that older adults are at high risk for undertreated pain and those with cognitive impairment are at even higher risk.
- Common caregiver and health care team misconceptions such as that pain sensitivity decreases with aging and older adults cannot tolerate analgesics without significant adverse effects contribute to the undertreatment of pain in older adults.

Beliefs About Pain

- Older adults tend to report pain less often than younger adults, which frequently results in members of the health care team administering suboptimal analgesics and doses. The failure of older adults to report pain may be related to common beliefs and concerns they have about pain and reporting it such as:
  - Pain is an inevitable consequence of aging and little can be done to relieve it.
  - Expressing pain is unacceptable or is a sign of weakness.
  - Reporting pain will result in being labeled as a "bad" patient or a "complainer."
  - Nurses and physicians are too busy to listen to reports of pain.
  - Pain signifies a serious illness or impending death.
- Be aware of the common beliefs of older patients regarding pain and its management and correct misconceptions to help prevent barriers to achieving optimal pain relief.
- Nurses and other caregivers can overcome their reluctance to administer prescribed analgesics in adequate doses by following the principles of pain management in older people (see *Management of Pain section*).

Assessment of Pain

- Ask the patient to provide his or her own report of pain; even mild to some moderate cognitively impaired older adults are able to provide self-report if nurses and caregivers take the time to obtain it.
  - Offer various self-report pain tools.
  - Always show tools in hard copy with large lettering, adequate space between lines, nonglossy paper, and color for increased visualization.
  - Be sure that the patient is wearing glasses and hearing aids if needed and available.
  - Provide adequate lighting and privacy to avoid distracting background noise.
  - Repeat questions more than once and allow adequate time for response.
  - Use verbal descriptions such as "ache," "sore," and "hurt" if the patient seems to have difficulty relating to the word "pain."
  - Ask about present pain only.
  - If the patient is able to use a self-report tool, use the same tool and reteach the tool each time pain is assessed.

Considerations for Cognitively Impaired Patients (also see Table 4-5)

- Remember to "assume that pain is present" in patients with diseases and conditions or procedures commonly associated with pain (see discussion below on *analgesic trial*).

- If the patient is unable to provide self-report, look for behaviors that may indicate the presence of pain.
  - Someone who knows the patient well such as a family member or caregiver may be helpful in identifying behaviors that might indicate pain. Do not ask others to rate pain intensity and do not attempt to rate it yourself. Only the patient knows how severe the pain is; if he or she cannot rate or describe the intensity, the exact intensity is unknown.
- Assess using a reliable and valid behavioral pain assessment tool.
  - Remember that behavioral tools tell us that pain might be present and provide a reference point to help determine the effectiveness of interventions, but the scores on behavioral tools have not been correlated with the ratings on pain intensity scales. A behavioral score is not a pain intensity rating.
  - Use the same behavioral assessment tool each time pain is assessed.
- Consider an analgesic trial to help determine the presence of pain and to establish an ongoing treatment plan in patients who are thought to have pain. This involves the administration of a low-dose analgesic; changes or decreases in the intensity of behaviors indicate that pain may be the cause of the behaviors. Doses should be increased, or additional analgesics added as appropriate.

Management of Pain

- Use a multimodal approach that combines analgesics with different underlying mechanisms with the desired outcome of achieving optimal pain relief with lower doses than would be possible with a single analgesic; lower doses result in fewer side effects.
- Consider the type of pain and begin therapy with the first-line analgesics that are recommended for that type of pain.
- Do not give meperidine to older adults because most have decreased renal function and are unable to efficiently eliminate its central nervous system (CNS)–toxic metabolite *normeperidine*.
- Use around-the-clock (ATC) dosing of analgesics for pain that is of a continuous nature (e.g., chronic osteoarthritis or cancer pain; chronic neuropathic pain, first 24 to 48 hours after surgery).
- Use as needed (PRN) dosing for intermittent pain and before painful activities such as before ambulation and physical therapy.
- Be aware of the main side effects of the analgesics that are administered and that they may be more likely to occur or be more severe in older than in younger adults.
- *Start low and go slow* with drug dosing; increase doses to achieve adequate analgesia based on patient's response to the previous dose.
- Teach the patient and family or other caregiver about the pain management plan (analgesics and nonpharmacologic strategies) and when to notify the primary health care provider for unrelieved pain or unmanageable or intolerable drug side effects.
- To promote adherence to the pain management plan in the home setting, suggest using a pillbox to organize each day's medications and keeping a diary to identify times of the day or activities that increase pain. The diary can be presented to the primary health care provider who can use it to make necessary adjustments in the treatment plan.

---

it takes for the amount of drug in the body to be reduced by 50%.

Selected Opioid Analgesics. Morphine is the standard against which all other opioid drugs are compared. It is the most widely used opioid throughout the world, particularly for cancer pain, and its use is established by extensive research and clinical experience. Morphine is a *hydrophilic* drug (readily absorbed in aqueous solution), which accounts for its slow onset and long duration of action when compared with other opioid analgesics. It is available in a wide variety of short-acting and

! NURSING SAFETY PRIORITY QSEN

Drug Alert

Modified-release opioids should never be crushed, broken, or chewed because doing so alters the formulation of the drug and can result in adverse events, including death from respiratory depression if consumed. Teach the patient to swallow the drug whole and allow the "time-release" function of the drug to take effect. Intact modified-release tablets may be administered rectally in some patients who cannot swallow.

TABLE 4-6 Equianalgesic Dose Chart for Common Mu Opioid Analgesics

- *Equianalgesic* means approximately the same pain relief.
- The equianalgesic chart is a guideline for selecting doses for opioid-naïve patients. Doses and intervals between doses are titrated according to each person's responses.
- The equianalgesic chart is helpful when switching from one drug or route of administration to another.

OPIOID	ORAL	PARENTERAL	COMMENTS
Morphine	30 mg	10 mg	Standard for comparison; first-line opioid via multiple routes of administration; once-daily and twice-daily oral formulations; clinically significant metabolites
Fentanyl	No formulation	100 mcg IV 100 mcg/hr of transdermal fentanyl is approximately equal to 4 mg/hr of IV morphine; 1 mcg/hr of transdermal fentanyl is approximately equal to 2 mg/24 hr of oral morphine	First-line opioid via IV, transdermal, and intraspinal routes; available in oral transmucosal and buccal formulations for breakthrough pain in opioid-tolerant patients; no clinically relevant metabolites
Hydrocodone	30 mg	No formulation	Available in combination with nonopioid, short-acting, and twice-daily formulations
Hydromorphone (Dilaudid)	7.5 mg	1.5 mg	First-line opioid via multiple routes of administration; once-daily oral formulation; clinically significant metabolites noted with long-term, high-dose infusion
Oxycodone	20 mg	No formulation in the United States	Short-acting and twice-daily oral formulations
Oxymorphone	10 mg	1 mg	Parenteral, short-acting, and twice-daily oral formulations

Data from Pasero, C., & McCaffery, M. (2011). *Pain assessment and pharmacologic management.* St. Louis: Mosby.

modified-release oral formulations and is given by multiple other routes of administration, including rectal, subcutaneous, and IV.

Fentanyl (Sublimaze) differs from morphine significantly in characteristics. It is a *lipophilic* (readily absorbed in fatty tissue) opioid and, as such, has a fast onset and short duration of action. These characteristics make it the most commonly used IV opioid when rapid analgesia is desired such as for the treatment of severe, escalating acute pain and for procedural pain when a short duration of action is desirable. Fentanyl is the recommended opioid for patients with end-organ failure because it has no clinically relevant metabolites. It also produces fewer hemodynamic adverse effects than other opioids; therefore it is often preferred in patients who are hemodynamically unstable such as the critically ill.

Its lipophilicity makes fentanyl ideal for drug delivery by transdermal patch (Duragesic) for long-term opioid therapy, and by the oral transmucosal (Actiq), sublingual (Subsys), and buccal (Fentora) routes for breakthrough pain treatment in opioid-tolerant patients. After application of the transdermal patch, a subcutaneous depot of fentanyl is established in the skin near the patch. After absorption from the depot into the systemic circulation, the drug distributes to fat and muscle. When the first patch is applied, 12 to 18 hours are required for clinically significant analgesia to be obtained. Be aware that the patient may need adequate supplemental analgesia during that time. Change the patch every 48 to 72 hours, depending on patient response.

! NURSING SAFETY PRIORITY QSEN

Drug Alert

Teach patients using transdermal fentanyl not to apply heat (e.g., hot packs, heating pads) directly over the patch because heat increases absorption of the drug and can result in adverse events, including death from fentanyl-induced respiratory depression. Ask patients about the presence of patches on admission and document and communicate this information to other members of the interdisciplinary health care team.

Hydromorphone (Dilaudid) is less hydrophilic than morphine but less lipophilic than fentanyl, which contributes to an onset and duration of action that is intermediate between morphine and fentanyl. The drug is often used as an alternative to morphine, especially for acute pain, most likely because the two drugs produce similar analgesia and have comparable side effects. It is a first- or second-choice opioid (after morphine) for postoperative management via IV patient-controlled analgesia (PCA) and is available in a once-daily modified-release oral formulation (Exalgo) for long-term opioid treatment.

? NCLEX EXAMINATION CHALLENGE 4-3

Physiological Integrity

A client has a one-time prescription for morphine 1 mg IV push. The drug is available as 5 mg/mL. The nurse administers _____ mL of morphine for one dose.

Oxycodone is available in the United States for administration by the oral route only and is used to treat all types of pain. In combination with acetaminophen or ibuprofen, it is appropriate for mild-to–some moderate pain. Single-entity, short-acting (OxyIR) and modified-release (OxyContin) oxycodone formulations are used in patients with moderate-to-severe chronic pain. It has been used successfully as part of a multimodal treatment plan for postoperative pain as well. Like morphine, it is available in liquid form for patients who are unable to swallow tablets.

Hydrocodone in combination with nonopioids (Norco, Vicodin) limits its use to the treatment of mild-to–some moderate pain. It is the most commonly prescribed opioid analgesic in the United States and Canada, but its prescription for treatment of persistent pain (except for breakthrough dosing) should be evaluated carefully because of its ceiling on efficacy and safety related to the nonopioid constituent (ingredient). It is also available as a modified-release formulation (Zohydro, Hysingla) for chronic pain.

Methadone (Dolophine) is a unique opioid analgesic that may have advantages over other opioids in carefully selected patients. In addition to being a mu opioid, it is an antagonist at the NMDA (*N*-methyl-D-aspartate) receptor site and thus has the potential to produce analgesic effects as a second- or third-line option for some neuropathic pain states.

Although it has no active metabolites, methadone has a very long and highly variable half-life (5 to 100+ hours; average is 20 hours). Patients must be watched closely for excessive sedation—a sign of drug accumulation during the titration period. Other limitations are its tendency to interact with a large number of medications and prolong corrected QT (QTc) interval. Methadone should be prescribed only by providers who are familiar with its unique properties.

Dual Mechanism Analgesics. The dual mechanism analgesics *tramadol* (Ultram) and *tapentadol* (Nucynta) have been useful additions to the pain management arena. These drugs bind weakly to the mu opioid-receptor site and block the reuptake (resorption) of the inhibitory neurotransmitters *serotonin* and/or *norepinephrine* in the spinal cord and brainstem of the modulatory descending pain pathway (see Nociception earlier in this chapter). This makes these neurotransmitters more available to fight pain. Because they have the opioid receptor-binding property, they are discussed in the Opioid Analgesics section of this chapter. However, they are usually referred to as dual mechanism or mixed analgesics rather than opioid analgesics.

Tramadol is used for both acute and chronic pain and is available in oral short-acting (Ultram) and modified-release (Ultram ER) formulations, including a short-acting tablet in combination with acetaminophen (Ultracet). It is appropriate for acute pain and has been designated as a second-line analgesic for the treatment of neuropathic pain. Side effects are similar to those of opioids. The drug can lower seizure threshold and interact with other drugs that block the reuptake of serotonin such as the selective serotonin reuptake inhibitor (SSRI) antidepressants. Although rare, this combination can have an additive effect and result in serotonin syndrome, characterized by agitation, diarrhea, heart and blood pressure changes, and loss of coordination.

The newer dual-mechanism analgesic *tapentadol* is also available in short-acting (Nucynta) and modified-release (Nucynta ER) formulations and is appropriate for both acute and chronic pain. Major benefits of tapentadol are that it has no active metabolites and a significantly more favorable side effect profile (particularly GI effects) compared with opioid analgesics.

Opioids to Avoid. *Meperidine* (Demerol) was once the most widely used opioid analgesic in the inpatient setting. In recent years it has either been removed from or severely restricted on US hospital formularies for the treatment of pain in an effort to improve patient safety. A major drawback to the use of meperidine is its active metabolite, *normeperidine*, a CNS stimulant that can cause delirium, irritability, tremors, myoclonus, and generalized seizures. It is a particularly poor choice in older adults because they have decreased renal function, which prevents the elimination of the toxic metabolite. Meperidine has no advantages over any other opioid, and it has no place in the treatment of persistent pain or in delivery systems such as PCA. If prescribed, meperidine should not be used for more than 48 hours or at doses exceeding 600 mg/24 hours.

Codeine in combination with nonopioids (e.g., with acetaminophen in Tylenol No. 3) has been used for many years for the management of mild-to-moderate pain; however, it has largely been replaced by analgesics that are more efficacious and better tolerated (e.g., Percocet, Vicodin). Research has shown that codeine/acetaminophen is less effective and associated with more adverse effects than NSAIDs such as ibuprofen and naproxen for acute pain.

Intraspinal Analgesia. Intraspinal analgesia involves the administration of analgesics via a needle or catheter placed in the epidural space or the intrathecal (subarachnoid) space by an anesthesia provider (see Fig. 4-4). The intraspinal routes of administration are used to manage both acute pain such as postoperative pain and some chronic cancer and noncancer pain.

Epidural analgesia can be delivered by intermittent bolus technique, continuous infusion, or patient-controlled epidural analgesia (PCEA) with or without continuous infusion. The most commonly administered analgesics by the epidural route are the opioids *morphine, hydromorphone,* and *fentanyl* in combination with a long-acting local anesthetic such as bupivacaine (Marcaine) or ropivacaine (Naropin). This multimodal approach allows lower doses of both the opioid and local anesthetic and produces fewer side effects. A single epidural injection of preservative-free morphine (Duramorph) is effective for about 24 hours. An extended-release formulation of preservative-free epidural morphine (DepoDur) is effective for 48 hours.

Intrathecal (spinal) analgesia is usually delivered via single bolus technique for patients with acute pain (e.g., hysterectomy) or continuous infusion via an implanted device (pump) for the treatment of chronic pain. Because the drug is delivered directly into the aqueous cerebrospinal fluid (CSF), morphine with its hydrophilic nature is used most often for intrathecal

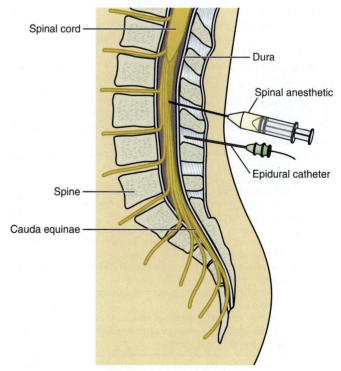

FIG. 4-4 Intraspinal analgesia.

analgesia. Extremely small amounts of drug are administered by the intrathecal route (about 10 times less than by the epidural route) because the drug is so close to the spinal action site.

The side effects of intraspinal analgesia depend on the type of drug administered. In other words, if opioids are administered, the same opioid-induced side effects that occur with other routes of administration can occur with intraspinal administration. If local anesthetics are administered, common side effects are urinary retention, hypotension, and numbness and weakness of lower extremities. The latter can occur on a continuum (mild and localized) to a complete block (undesirable and requires prompt anesthesia evaluation). In most cases the side effects that occur during continuous infusion or PCEA can be managed by decreasing the dose.

Complications of intraspinal analgesia are rare but can be life threatening. Complications from the intrathecal pump can be surgical, pump related, or catheter related (Textor, 2016). Chart 4-2 summarizes best practices needed when caring for a patient who has an intrathecal pump. Perform frequent neurologic assessments and promptly report abnormal findings to the anesthesiologist or nurse anesthetist.

> ## ◎ CHART 4-2 Best Practice for Patient Safety & Quality Care QSEN
>
> ### Care of the Patient Who Has an Intrathecal Pump for Managing Cancer Pain
>
> Provide postoperative care and health teaching to include:
> - Carefully monitor respiratory status, including respiratory rate, oxygen saturation, and level of consciousness every 1 to 2 hours after surgery for at least 12 hours or as per surgeon or agency protocol.
> - Apply an abdominal binder in place as prescribed to hold the pump in a flat position.
> - Teach the patient that a burning sensation may occur around the pump area. Cold packs and topical lidocaine may provide COMFORT; do *not* use heat over the lumbar pump site.
> - Teach the patient to avoid lifting more than 5 lb or twisting/bending at the waist for 6 weeks or as instructed by the surgeon.
>
> Monitor for and teach the patient and family to report these potential complications:
> - Surgical complications
>   - Infection: Observe for fever and localized redness or hematoma at the lumbar site.
>   - Cerebrospinal (CSF) fluid leak: Ask about headache; observe for swelling without redness at the lumbar site.
> - Catheter-related complications
>   - Structural damage, including kinks, occlusion, or disconnection; note change in pain control or signs of opioid withdrawal.
> - Pump-related complications (not common)
>   - Malfunction or displacement: Observe for opioid overdose or underdosing, causing a change in pain control or opioid withdrawal.
>
> Keep these safety and care precautions in mind when caring for the patient:
> - Be sure that the pump is shielded if the patient received external beam radiation.
> - Be sure that the patient does not have an abrupt discontinuation of baclofen (can cause respiratory depression) or clonidine (can cause hypertension and stroke).

Data adapted from Textor, L. (2016). Intrathecal pumps for cancer pain. *AJN, 116*(5), 36-41.

> ## ! NURSING SAFETY PRIORITY QSEN
> ### Drug Alert
>
> Assess patients receiving epidural local anesthetic for their ability to bend their knees and lift their buttocks off the mattress (if not prohibited by surgical procedure). Ask them to point to any areas of numbness and tingling. Mild, transient lower-extremity motor weakness and orthostatic hypotension may be present, necessitating assistance with ambulation. Most undesirable effects can be managed with a reduction in local anesthetic dose. Promptly report areas of numbness outside of the surgical site, inability to bear weight, and severe hypotension to the anesthesia provider. *Do not delegate assessment of local anesthetic effects to unlicensed assistive personnel!*

SENSORY PERCEPTION manifestations (e.g., increasing numbness and tingling of extremities), decreasing ability to bear weight, and/or changes in bowel or bladder function can indicate the development of an epidural hematoma or abscess. If not detected, a hematoma or abscess can cause spinal cord compression and paralysis.

Nurses have an extensive role in the management and monitoring of intraspinal techniques, including infusion device operation, replacing empty drug reservoirs, checking and protecting infusion sites and systems, treating side effects, preventing complications, discontinuing therapy, and removing catheters.

Adverse Effects of Opioid Analgesics. The most common side effects of opioid analgesics are constipation, nausea, vomiting, pruritus, and sedation. Respiratory depression is less common but the most feared of the opioid side effects. *Most of the opioid side effects are dose related; therefore simply decreasing the opioid dose is sufficient to eliminate or make the most of the side effects tolerable for most patients.* Table 4-7 lists interventions to prevent and manage opioid-induced side effects.

Most patients experience sedation at the beginning of opioid therapy and whenever the opioid dose is increased significantly. *If undetected or left untreated, excessive sedation can progress to clinically significant respiratory depression.* Like most of the other opioid side effects, sedation and respiratory depression are dose related. Preventing clinically significant opioid-induced respiratory depression begins with administering the lowest effective opioid dose (multimodal analgesia with a nonopioid foundation), careful titration, and closely monitoring sedation and respiratory status throughout therapy. *Unless the patient is at the end of life, promptly reduce opioid dose or stop titration whenever increased sedation is detected to prevent respiratory depression.* In some patients (e.g., those with obstructive sleep apnea, pulmonary dysfunction, multiple comorbidities), mechanical monitoring such as capnography (to measure exhaled carbon dioxide) and pulse oximetry (to measure oxygen saturation) is needed.

Occasionally drugs that produce significant sedation are used to treat side effects and other conditions that accompany the pain experience. For example, *antianxiety agents* (anxiolytics) such as alprazolam (Xanax) and lorazepam (Ativan) are prescribed to reduce anxiety. Many of the drugs used to treat opioid side effects are sedating, such as the antihistamines (diphenhydramine) for pruritus and the antiemetics *promethazine (Phenergan)* and *hydroxyzine (Vistaril)* for nausea. It is important to recognize that administration of these drugs together has an additive sedating effect. If administered,

TABLE 4-7 Nursing Interventions to Prevent and Treat Selected Opioid Side Effects

Constipation

- Assess previous bowel habits.
- Keep a record of bowel movements.
- Remind patients that tolerance to this side effect does not develop, so *a preventive approach must be used;* administer a stool softener plus mild stimulant laxative for duration of opioid therapy; do not give bulk laxatives because these can result in obstruction in some patients.
- Provide privacy, encourage adequate fluids and activity, and give foods high in roughage.
- If ineffective, try suppository or Fleet's enema.
- For long-term opioid-induced constipation (OIC) in patients with chronic pain, drug therapy may be used (e.g., lubiprostone [Amitiza], methylnaltrexone [Relistor]).

Nausea and Vomiting (N/V)

- Use a multimodal antiemetic preventive approach (e.g., dexamethasone plus ondansetron in moderate- to high-risk patients).
- Assess cause of nausea and eliminate contributing factors if possible.
- Reduce opioid dose if possible.
- Reassure patients taking long-term opioid therapy that tolerance to this side effect develops with regular daily opioid doses.
- Treat with antiemetic drug as prescribed.
- Consider switching to another opioid for unresolved N/V.

Sedation

- Remember that sedation precedes opioid-induced respiratory depression; identify patient and iatrogenic risk factors and monitor sedation level and respiratory status frequently during the first 24 hours of opioid therapy.
- Use a simple sedation scale to monitor for unwanted sedation (see Table 4-8).

- If excessive sedation is detected, reduce opioid dose to prevent respiratory depression.
- Eliminate unnecessary sedating drugs such as antihistamines, anxiolytics, muscle relaxants, and hypnotics. If it is necessary to administer these drugs during opioid therapy, monitor sedation and respiratory status closely.
- Reassure patients taking long-term opioid therapy that tolerance to this side effect develops with regular daily opioid doses.
- Be aware that stimulants such as caffeine may counteract opioid-induced sedation.
- Consider switching to another opioid for unresolved excessive sedation during long-term opioid therapy.

Respiratory Depression

- Be aware that counting respiratory rate alone does not constitute a comprehensive respiratory assessment. Proper assessment of respiratory status includes observing the rise and fall of the patient's chest to determine depth and quality in addition to counting respiratory rate for 60 seconds.
- Recognize that *snoring is respiratory obstruction* and an ominous sign (see text).
- Remember that sedation precedes opioid-induced respiratory depression; identify patient and iatrogenic risk factors and monitor sedation level and respiratory status frequently during the first 24 hours of opioid therapy (see Sedation section).
- Stop opioid administration immediately for clinically significant respiratory depression, stay with patient, continue attempts to arouse patient, support respirations, call for help (consider Rapid Response Team or Code Blue), and consider giving naloxone.
- Reassure patients taking long-term opioid therapy that tolerance to this side effect develops with regular daily opioid doses.

---

closely monitor for sedation and assess respiratory status frequently.

To assess sedation, use a simple, easy-to-understand sedation scale developed for assessment of *unwanted* sedation that includes what should be done at each level of sedation. Table 4-8 presents a widely used sedation scale. The key to assessing sedation is to determine how easy it is to arouse the patient. Assess each person's response to the first dose of an opioid. If opioids are administered by bolus technique, assess sedation level and respiratory status at the opioid's peak time after each bolus.

Respiratory depression is assessed on the basis of what is normal for a particular person and is usually described as clinically significant when there is a significant decrease in the rate, depth, and regularity of respirations from baseline, rather than just by a specific number of respirations per minute. Risk factors for opioid-induced respiratory depression include age 55 years or older, obesity, obstructive sleep apnea, and pre-existing pulmonary dysfunction or other comorbidities.

Adjuvant Analgesics. Adjuvant analgesics (sometimes called *co-analgesics*) are drugs that have a primary indication other than pain but are analgesic for some painful conditions (see Table 4-6). For example, the primary indication for antidepressants is depression, but some antidepressants help relieve some types of pain. The adjuvant analgesics are the largest and most diverse of the three analgesic groups. Drug selection and dosing

⚠ NURSING SAFETY PRIORITY QSEN

Critical Rescue

Watch the rise and fall of the patient's chest to determine depth and regularity of respirations in addition to counting the respiratory rate for 60 seconds. For accuracy, respiratory assessment is done before arousing the sleeping patient. *If a patient is difficult to arouse, always stop the opioid, stay with the patient, continue vigorous attempts to arouse, and call for help!*

Listening to the sound of the patient's respiration is critical as well—*snoring indicates airway obstruction and must be attended to promptly* with repositioning, including placing the patient in a sitting position. Depending on severity, collaborate with the respiratory therapist for consultation and further evaluation.

are based on both experience and evidence-based practice guidelines.

Anticonvulsants and Antidepressants. Anticonvulsants (also called *antiepileptic drugs [AEDs]* when used for seizure management) produce analgesia by blocking sodium and calcium channels in the CNS, thereby diminishing the transmission of pain. The gabapentinoids *gabapentin (Neurontin)* and *pregabalin (Lyrica)* are recommended as first-line analgesics for persistent neuropathic pain. Gabapentin may also be administered as an epidural injection. These drugs are increasingly being added

TABLE 4-8 **Pasero Opioid-Induced Sedation Scale (POSS) With Interventions***

S = Sleep, easy to arouse
Acceptable; no action necessary; may increase opioid dose if needed.

1 = Awake and alert
Acceptable; no action necessary; may increase opioid dose if needed.

2 = Slightly drowsy, easily aroused
Acceptable; no action necessary; may increase opioid dose if needed.

3 = Frequently drowsy, arousable, drifts off to sleep during conversation
Unacceptable; monitor respiratory status and sedation level closely until sedation level is stable at less than 3 and respiratory status is satisfactory; decrease opioid dose 25% to 50%[1] or notify primary[2] or anesthesia provider for orders; consider administering a nonsedating, opioid-sparing nonopioid such as acetaminophen or a NSAID if not contraindicated; ask patient to take deep breaths every 15-30 minutes.

4 = Somnolent; minimal or no response to verbal and physical stimulation
Unacceptable; stop opioid; consider administering naloxone[3,4]; call Rapid Response Team (code blue); stay with patient, stimulate, and support respiration as indicated by patient status; notify primary[2] or anesthesia provider; monitor respiratory status and sedation level closely until sedation level is stable at less than 3 and respiratory status is satisfactory.

From Pasero, C., & McCaffery, M. (2011). *Pain assessment and pharmacologic management.* St. Louis: Mosby. Copyright 1994. Used with permission.
*Appropriate action is given in italics at each level of sedation.
[1]Opioid analgesic prescriptions or a hospital protocol should include the expectation that a nurse will decrease the opioid dose if a patient is excessively sedated.
[2]For example, the physician, nurse practitioner, advanced practice nurse, or physician assistant responsible for the pain management prescription.
[3]For adults experiencing respiratory depression, administer dilute solution (0.4 mg of naloxone in 10 mL of normal saline) very slowly (0.5 mL over 2 minutes) while observing the patient's response (titrate to effect).
[4]Hospital protocols should include the expectation that a nurse will administer naloxone to any patient suspected of having life-threatening opioid-induced sedation and respiratory depression.

! NURSING SAFETY PRIORITY **QSEN**

Drug Alert

Unless the patient is at the end of life, promptly administer the opioid antagonist naloxone (Narcan) IV to reverse clinically significant opioid-induced respiratory depression, usually when the respiratory rate is less than 8 breaths per minute or according to agency protocol. When giving the opioid antagonist naloxone, administer it slowly until the patient is more arousable and respirations increase to an acceptable rate. The desired outcome is to reverse just the sedative and respiratory depressant effects of the opioid but not the analgesic effects. Giving too much naloxone too fast not only can cause severe pain but also can lead to ventricular dysrhythmias, pulmonary edema, and even death. Continue to closely monitor the patient after giving naloxone because its duration is shorter than that of most opioids and respiratory depression can recur. Sometimes more than one dose of naloxone is needed.

CONSIDERATIONS FOR OLDER ADULTS

Patient-Centered Care **QSEN**

The incidence of opioid side effects in the older-adult population varies, depending on the side effect. Older adults are sensitive to the sedating effects of opioids, making them higher risk for respiratory depression than in younger adults.

? NCLEX EXAMINATION CHALLENGE 4-4
Physiological Integrity

A nursing technician reports that a client who is receiving IV PCA morphine is very drowsy, unable to complete a sentence without falling asleep, and has a respiratory rate of 10 breaths per minute. What is the nurse's **priority** action at this time?
A. Wake the client and raise the head of the bed to a 90-degree angle.
B. Promptly call the primary health care provider to reduce the opioid dose.
C. Document the assessment findings and take vital signs in an hour.
D. Give naloxone according to agency protocol.

---

to postoperative treatment plans to address the neuropathic component of surgical pain. Primary side effects are sedation and dizziness, which are usually transient and most notable during the titration phase of treatment.

Antidepressants relieve pain on the descending modulatory pathway by blocking the body's reuptake of the inhibitory neurochemicals *norepinephrine* and *serotonin*. Antidepressant adjuvant analgesics are divided into two major groups: the *tricyclic antidepressants* (TCAs) and the newer *serotonin and norepinephrine reuptake inhibitors* (SNRIs). Evidence-based guidelines recommend the TCAs *desipramine (Norpramin)* and *nortriptyline (Aventyl, Pamelor)* and the SNRIs *duloxetine (Cymbalta)* and *venlafaxine (Effexor)* as first-line options for neuropathic pain treatment (D'Arcy, 2014).

The most common side effects of the TCAs are dry mouth, sedation, dizziness, mental clouding, weight gain, and constipation. Orthostatic hypotension is a potentially serious TCA side effect, making TCAs a poor choice for older adults. The most serious adverse effect is cardiotoxicity, especially for patients with existing significant heart disease. The SNRIs have a more favorable side effect profile and are better tolerated than the TCAs. The most common SNRI side effects are nausea, headache, sedation, insomnia, weight gain, impaired memory, sweating, and tremors.

CONSIDERATIONS FOR OLDER ADULTS

Patient-Centered Care **QSEN**

Older adults are often sensitive to the effects of the adjuvant analgesics that produce sedation and other CNS effects such as anticonvulsants and antidepressants. Therapy should be initiated with low doses, and titration should proceed slowly with systematic assessment of patient response. Caregivers in the home setting must be taught to take preventive measures to reduce the likelihood of falls and other accidents. A home safety assessment is highly recommended and can be arranged by social services before discharge.

Local Anesthetics. Local anesthetics relieve pain by blocking the generation and conduction of the nerve impulses necessary to transmit pain. The local anesthetic effect is dose related. A high enough dose of local anesthetic can produce complete anesthesia, and a low enough dose (subanesthetic) can produce analgesia.

Local anesthetics have a long history of safe and effective use for the treatment of all types of pain. Allergy to local anesthetics is rare, and side effects are dose-related. CNS signs of systemic toxicity include ringing in the ears, metallic taste, irritability, and seizures. Signs of cardiotoxicity include tingling and numbness, bradycardia, cardiac dysrhythmias, and cardiovascular collapse.

The *lidocaine patch 5%* (Lidoderm) is 10 cm by 14 cm and contains 700 mg of lidocaine. The patch is placed directly over or adjacent to the painful area for absorption into the tissues directly below. A major benefit of the drug is that it produces minimal systemic absorption and side effects. The patch is left in place for 12 hours and then removed for 12 hours (12-hours-on, 12-hours-off regimen). This application process is repeated as needed for continuous analgesia.

Topical local anesthetic creams for superficial procedures such as IV insertion include *EMLA* (eutectic mixture of local anesthetics) *and LMX-4-* EMLA contains a combination of lidocaine 2.5% and prilocaine 2.5% and is applied to intact skin for 60 to 120 minutes before the procedure. *LMX-4* contains 4% lidocaine and is applied 30 minutes before the procedure. EMLA has a longer duration of action (2 hours) than LMX-4 (30 minutes) after cream removal. Topical local anesthetic side effects are rare and usually transient, with local skin reactions being the most common.

Liposomal bupivacaine (Exparel) for postoperative wound infiltration is a sustained-release formulation injected as a single dose into the surgical site by the surgeon. The sustained-release formulation has been shown to produce prolonged analgesia, which decreases the need for potent opioids.

For many years *regional anesthesia* has been administered by single-injection peripheral nerve blocks using a long-acting local anesthetic such as bupivacaine or ropivacaine to target a specific nerve or nerve plexus. This technique is highly effective in producing pain relief, but the effect is temporary (4-12 hours). *Continuous peripheral nerve block* (also called *perineural regional analgesia*) offers an alternative with longer-lasting analgesia. A continuous peripheral nerve block involves establishment by an anesthesia provider of an initial block followed by placement of a catheter through which an infusion of local anesthetic is administered continuously, with or without PCA capability. When PCA capability is added, this is referred to as patient-controlled regional analgesia *(PCRA)*. Just as with epidural and intrathecal analgesia, nurses are responsible for monitoring and managing the therapy.

Use of Placebos. A **placebo** is defined as any medication or procedure, including surgery, which produces an effect in a patient because of its implicit or explicit intent, not because of its specific physical or chemical properties. A saline injection is one example of a placebo. Administration of a medication at a known subtherapeutic dose (e.g., 0.05 mg of morphine in an adult) is also considered a placebo.

Placebos are appropriately used as controls in research evaluating the effects of a new medication. Patients or volunteers who participate in placebo-controlled research must be able to give informed consent or have a guardian who can provide informed consent. Unfortunately occasionally placebos are used clinically in a deceitful manner and without informed consent. This is often done when the clinician does not accept the patient's report of pain. Pain relief resulting from a placebo, should it occur, is mistakenly believed to invalidate a patient's report of pain. This typically results in the patient being deprived of pain-relief measures despite research showing that many patients who have obvious physical stimuli for pain (e.g.,

abdominal surgery) report pain relief after placebo administration. The use of placebos has both ethical and legal implications, violates the nurse-patient relationship, and deprives patients of more appropriate methods of assessment or treatment.

> **! NURSING SAFETY PRIORITY** (QSEN)
> *Drug Alert*
>
> Deceitful administration of a placebo violates informed consent law and jeopardizes the nurse-patient therapeutic relationship. Never administer a placebo to a patient. Promptly contact your nursing supervisor if you are given an order to do so.

Nonpharmacologic Management. Most people use self-management and nonpharmacologic strategies to deal with their health issues and promote well-being. Nonpharmacologic methods are appropriate alone for mild- and some moderate-intensity pain and should be used to complement, not replace, pharmacologic therapies for more severe pain. The effectiveness of nonpharmacologic methods can be unpredictable. Although not all have been shown to relieve pain, they offer many benefits to some patients of all ages. For example, research has shown that nonpharmacologic methods can facilitate relaxation and reduce anxiety, stress, and depression, which often accompany the pain experience (Bruckenthal, 2010; Wright, 2015). Many patients find that the use of nonpharmacologic methods helps them cope better and feel greater control over the pain experience. Nurses play an important role in providing and teaching their patients about nonpharmacologic strategies. Many of the methods are relatively easy for nurses to incorporate into daily clinical practice and may be used individually or in combination with other nonpharmacologic therapies.

Nonpharmacologic interventions are categorized as being body-based (physical) modalities; mind-body (cognitive-behavioral) methods; biologically based therapies; and energy therapies. Biologically based and energy therapies are used most often in the ambulatory care setting and are beyond the scope of this chapter. Body-based and mind-body therapies are often used by patients to self-manage their pain and enhance COMFORT.

Physical Modalities. In the acute care setting the physical modalities are used most often because of their ease in implementation and their role in postoperative recovery. In the ambulatory care setting or at home, sustained physical regimens such as regular low-impact exercise, in combination with analgesics and other interventions, improve outcomes for people with chronic pain. Many of the physical modalities require a prescription for use and reimbursement. Some require a trained expert to administer the technique (e.g., acupuncture). Among the most effective physical modalities used to manage or prevent pain are:

- Physical therapy
- Occupational therapy
- Aquatherapy
- Functional restoration (also has cognitive-behavioral components)
- Acupuncture
- Low-impact exercise programs such as slow walking and yoga

The physical modalities are often administered using an interprofessional collaborative approach. The assistance of physical and occupational therapists to help design and implement an individualized plan with realistic goal setting promotes effectiveness of these methods. Coordinate with the therapist to implement strategies to decrease pain before therapy sessions with the purpose of increasing function and preventing further deterioration. Teach patients to adhere to their drug regimen to maximize effectiveness of the treatment plan. Expected patient outcomes include an increase in the range of motion, strength, and function of the affected area and an improved quality of life. The occupational therapist may also help decrease pain by making one or more splints to rest severely inflamed joints.

A number of *cutaneous (skin) stimulation* strategies, which apply mild stimulation to the skin and subcutaneous tissues, have been used for many years to relieve pain. Examples of cutaneous stimulation include:

- Application of heat, cold, or pressure
- Therapeutic massage
- Vibration
- Transcutaneous electrical nerve stimulation (TENS)

Cold applications (ice) are especially helpful for inflamed areas such as for patients with rheumatoid arthritis and those who have knee surgery. Heat is appropriate when an increased blood flow is desired such as for patients with osteoarthritis pain. Paraffin dips for the hands can be helpful to increase movement for those patients as well. Warm showers and compresses that can be done at home are useful in reducing stiffness and promoting movement in patients with arthritis, especially after awakening. Local short-acting gels and creams may provide *cryotherapy (cold treatment)* to relieve muscle aches and pains. These products can often be bought over the counter (OTC) (e.g., Bengay, Icy Hot). The effects of this type of application can last up to 2 hours. Discuss this information with the patient before the use of a cutaneous method.

The benefits of cutaneous stimulation are highly unpredictable and may vary from application to application. Despite these potential drawbacks, it can be effective in the management of both acute and chronic pain in selected patients. A major benefit of these methods is that many are easy for patients to self-administer.

TENS is used as an adjunctive treatment for pain. Although there are several types of **transcutaneous electrical nerve stimulation (TENS)** units, each involves the use of a battery-operated device capable of delivering small electrical currents through electrodes applied to the painful area (Fig. 4-5). The voltage or current is regulated by adjusting a dial to the point at which the patient perceives a prickly "pins-and-needles" SENSORY PERCEPTION rather than the pain. The current is adjusted based on the degree of desired relief. Newer, smaller, and less expensive TENS units are easy for anyone to apply and are often used at home or other community-based setting. The cost for a single unit usually ranges between $100 to $300 per unit, depending on the number of settings and leads.

Spinal cord stimulation is an *invasive* stimulation technique that provides pain control by applying an electrical field over the spinal cord. A trial with a percutaneous epidural stimulator is conducted to determine whether permanent placement of the device is appropriate. If the trial is successful, electrodes are surgically placed in the epidural space and connected to an external or implanted programmable generator. The patient is taught to program and adjust the device to maximize comfort. Spinal cord stimulation can be extremely effective in selected patients but is reserved for intractable neuropathic pain syndromes that have been unresponsive to less invasive methods.

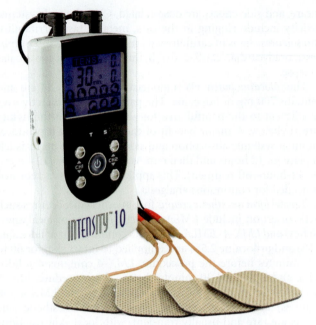

FIG. 4-5 TENS unit used in the home by the patient. (Courtesy Compass Health Brands, Middleburg Heights, Ohio.)

Care for the patient with an implanted spinal cord stimulator is the same as that for anyone who has back surgery and epidural anesthesia.

Cognitive-Behavioral Strategies. Cognitive-behavioral strategies, sometimes referred to as *cognitive-behavioral therapy (CBT),* is facilitated by a licensed psychologist or other qualified mental health professional. These strategies are referred to by some psychologists as third-wave interventions or treatments (Morley & Williams, 2015). Cognitive-behavioral strategies are useful in reducing the patient's focus on pain but do not physiologically block pain transmission. Instead they help the patient adapt to challenges presented by the pain experience such as anxiety and distress (Morley & Williams, 2015). They are most appropriate as an adjunct to pharmacologic therapy.

Cognitive-behavioral methods range from simple (e.g., prayer, relaxation breathing, artwork, reading, and watching television) to more complex (e.g., mindfulness, meditation, guided imagery, hypnosis, biofeedback, and virtual reality). It is important to recognize that many of the methods require patient teaching and subsequent patient participation. Many patients use these methods as part of their self-management and COMFORT promotion. Not all patients are receptive to the use of these methods. To respect their wishes, values, and preferences as part of patient-centered care, do not insist that patients use any one particular method.

Distraction is probably the most commonly used cognitive-behavioral method. All of us use simple distraction measures in our daily life when we watch television or read a book. Nurses often observe that patients request less pain medication when family members are present and when talking on the phone. After visiting hours it is not unusual for patients to request pain medication because they are no longer distracted.

Visual distracters (e.g., looking at a picture, watching television, playing a video game) can divert the attention to something pleasant or interesting. Auditory distracters (e.g., listening to music or relaxation tapes) can have a calming effect. Changing the environment involves removing or reducing unpleasant stressors that can interfere with the patient's ability to cope with pain such as loud noise and bright lights.

Imagery is a more complex form of distraction in which the patient is encouraged to visualize or think about a pleasant or desirable feeling, sensation, or event. The person is encouraged to sustain a sequence of thoughts aimed at diverting attention away from the pain. Patients who practice this technique can mentally and vividly experience sights, sounds, smells, events, or other sensations. Intense concentration is required to visualize images; therefore patients must have fairly well-controlled pain to participate.

Before suggesting imagery, assess the patient's level of concentration to determine whether he or she can sustain a particular thought or thoughts for a desired time. The time interval for mental imagery can vary from 5 to 60 minutes. Behaviors that may be helpful in assessing whether a patient is a candidate for teaching guided imagery include that the patient is able to:
- Read and comprehend a newspaper or magazine article
- Tap to a rhythm or sing while listening to music
- Follow the logic and participate in sustained conversation
- Have an interest in environmental surroundings

When the patient has demonstrated ability to concentrate, help him or her identify a pleasant or favorable thought. Encourage the patient to focus on this thought to divert attention away from painful stimuli. CDs or other audio recordings, either commercial or created by the patient and family, may help form and maintain images. Internet-based technology can be used to help patients whose language differs from that of the facilitating practitioner (Morley & Williams, 2015; Wilson et al., 2015).

Mindfulness is similar to imagery except that the patient focuses on his or her actual environment rather than imagining it. For example, in the fall in an area where tree leaves change colors, the patient focuses on the beauty of the colors to appreciate them.

Patients may also use *relaxation techniques* to reduce anxiety, tension, and emotional stress, all of which can exacerbate pain. For example, before and during a painful procedure, patients can be reminded to breathe slowly, deeply, and rhythmically to divert attention and promote relaxation. Relaxation techniques can be both physical and psychological. Physical relaxation techniques include:
- Relaxation breathing
- Receiving a body massage, back rub, or warm bath
- Modifying the environment to reduce distractions
- Moving into a comfortable position

Psychological relaxation techniques include:
- Pleasant conversation
- Laughter and humor
- Music (provide a range of choices)
- Relaxation tapes

Care Coordination and Transition Management

Before patients are discharged from any health care setting, collaborate with members of the interprofessional health care team to optimize pain control. Before discharge or transfer ensure that the patient, especially one who will receive opioid analgesia, has appropriate prescriptions and enough doses to last at least until the first follow-up visit with the primary health care provider.

Home Care Management. Fatigue exacerbates pain. If physical modifications in the home (e.g., installing a downstairs

♥ VETERANS' HEALTH CONSIDERATIONS
Patient-Centered Care (QSEN)

Veterans of recent wars with chronic pain can benefit from CBT strategies. A recent randomized clinical trial of veterans with chronic noncancer pain (musculoskeletal) evaluated a stepped-care pain management approach in a randomized clinical trial of 241 veterans (Bair et al., 2015). These young veterans were randomly assigned to one of two groups: 121 were assigned to the treatment group to receive 12 weeks of analgesia and self-management techniques followed by 12 weeks of CBT. The other 120 veterans were assigned to the usual chronic-care group for the same period of time. A 9-month follow-up showed that the treatment group receiving the drug therapy, self-management, and CBT had significantly lower pain-related disability, pain interference with daily life, and pain intensity when compared with the usual care group. All interventions were facilitated by nurse care managers.

This large study demonstrates the value of nonpharmacologic methods in managing pain in this vulnerable population. In addition, it shows that nurses play a key role in pain management as part of the interprofessional health care team.

☗ CLINICAL JUDGMENT CHALLENGE 4-1
Patient-Centered Care; Safety (QSEN)

A 79-year-old woman had a femur fracture for which she had an open reduction with internal fixation (ORIF) surgery 6 weeks ago. She has been going to physical therapy (PT) but finds that her pain and anxiety prevent her from following the instructions provided by PT. She continues to take her oral opioid on an as-needed basis and believes that she cannot function without it. Her physical therapist suggests that she look into nonpharmacologic methods of pain management, including improving her spiritual health. Today she is having her follow-up with the orthopedic surgeon. She asks you, the office nurse, for advice on what she should do. The surgeon wants her to discontinue the opioid medication immediately.

1. Which questions will you ask the patient at this time in preparation for teaching?
2. What are the concerns about her current pain management regimen?
3. Which nonpharmacologic methods might benefit her? How will you determine if they are appropriate for her values and beliefs?
4. Who else on the interprofessional team might be able to help this patient and how?

bathroom) are unrealistic, suggest changes in schedules, role responsibilities, and daily routines to help prevent or reduce it.

At home, patients may require a referral for physical therapy, especially to start or continue exercise regimens, treatment with cutaneous stimulation, or heat or cold techniques. Patients may need a social worker to help them develop coping strategies or maintain adequate family dynamics. A hospice or palliative care referral (hospital- or community-based) can help maintain continuity of care in the management of terminally ill patients and those who require treatment of some chronic conditions.

Home infusion therapy programs provide a wide variety of services to patients who require technology-supported pain management at home. Many of these services depend on approval by the insurance carrier, usually before analgesic options are considered and therapy is started. Case managers can be helpful in answering insurance and other payment questions. Well-defined home agency practices and professional support at home are required if patients leave the hospital with infusion therapy for pain management. Often family members are taught to assume the responsibilities of home infusion therapy.

Self-Management Education. Teach the patient and family about analgesic regimens, including any technical skills needed to administer the analgesic; the purpose and action of various drugs, their side effects, and complications; and the importance of correct dosing and dosing intervals. Explain how to prevent or treat the constipation commonly associated with taking opioid analgesics and other medications. Inform the patient about what to do and who to contact if the prescribed management regimen is not controlling pain well or when side effects are intolerable or unmanageable.

Help the patient establish an analgesic regimen that does not interfere with sleep, rest, appetite, and level of physical mobility. Ensure that patients are aware of any dangers associated with driving or operating mechanical equipment. Tell patients to ask their primary health care provider when these activities are safe to perform. Older patients and others at risk for falls or accidents in the home setting may benefit from a home safety assessment.

In patients with pain from advanced cancer, all efforts are directed toward maximizing relief and symptom control at home and eliminating unnecessary hospital re-admissions. This may mean that the primary health care provider prescribes a flexible analgesic schedule that allows the patient to adjust analgesics according to the amount of pain. Teach the patient and family how to safely treat breakthrough pain and increase drug doses within the prescribed dosing guidelines. If painful ambulatory care treatments or procedures are expected, tell the patient how important it is to talk with his or her primary health care provider to determine available options for preventing procedural pain (e.g., premedicating).

Evaluate family support systems to help the patient adhere to and continue the proposed medical treatment and nursing plan of care. Inform and include family members in activities during and after hospitalization. To achieve a reasonable level of involvement in life activities for the patient, suggest ways to continue participation in household, social, sexual, and work-oriented activities after discharge. Help the patient identify important activities and plan to do them with adequate rest periods.

The patient with chronic pain needs continued support to cope with the anxiety, fear, and powerlessness that often accompany this type of pain. Help the patient and family or significant others identify coping strategies that have worked in the past. Outside support systems are often extremely helpful (e.g., organizations such as the *American Chronic Pain Association* [http://theacpa.org]). This organization has the "10-Step Program from Patient to Person," provides numerous educational materials, and facilitates the establishment of local support groups for people with chronic pain. Teach patients about the value of nonpharmacologic methods, including mindfulness as part of CBT.

Health Care Resources. Ask the prescriber for a home health care or hospice referral, as appropriate, for patients who require assistance or supervision with the pain management regimen at home. Important information to provide to the home health care nurse includes the patient's condition, level of sedation, weakness or fatigue, possible constipation or nutritional problem, sleep patterns, and functional status. Detailed information about the patient's current pain management regimen and how well it has been tolerated is essential. Use a structured procedure such as SBAR (**s**ituation, **b**ackground, **a**ssessment, **r**ecommendations) to communicate this information.

In addition to explaining the patient's physical status to the home health care nurse, describe his or her level of anxiety and general expectations about pain after discharge. Close relationships and available support networks are important factors in providing ongoing support for effective pain intervention strategies.

Referral to an advanced practice nurse pain specialist, social worker, or psychologist may be necessary for some patients and families to provide continued support, reinforce instructions for complex pharmacologic or nonpharmacologic strategies, or evaluate overall physical and emotional adaptation after discharge. When severe chronic or intractable pain exists, health care professionals should direct the patient and family to appropriate resources such as pain centers or primary health care providers who specialize in long-term pain management.

GET READY FOR THE NCLEX® EXAMINATION!

▌ KEY POINTS

Review these Key Points for each NCLEX Examination Client Needs Category.

Safe and Effective Care Environment
- The nurse is legally and ethically responsible for acting as an advocate for patients experiencing pain.
- Collaborate with the interprofessional team as needed to provide adequate analgesia and nonpharmacologic pain management methods. **QSEN: Teamwork and Collaboration**

Health Promotion and Maintenance
- Provide information to the patient and family about non-pharmacologic physical modalities such as ice, heat, and the use of TENS units.
- Teach the value of cognitive-behavioral strategies such as mindfulness, distraction, and imagery. **QSEN: Evidence-Based Practice**

- Consider the special needs of older adults when assessing and managing their pain (see Chart 4.1). **QSEN: Patient-Centered Care**
- Recognize that many veterans of war have chronic pain caused by trauma; some are managed in Veterans Administration Medical Centers, whereas many others are homeless and do not receive care. **Health Care Disparities**
- Assess and meet the patient's need for pain management promptly to promote relief; be sensitive to the cultural preferences and values of the patient and family. **QSEN: Patient-Centered Care**

Psychosocial Integrity
- Be aware that some nurses and physicians may have biases about pain assessment and management; be objective when caring for patients with pain. **Clinical Judgment**
- Assess and document the patient's and family's expectations for management of pain and promotion of COMFORT. **QSEN: Patient-Centered Care**

- Provide accurate information to patients who have misconceptions and misunderstandings about pain management to prevent these from becoming barriers. **Ethics**

Physiological Integrity

- Remember that pain is what the patient says it is; self-report is always the most reliable indicator of pain. **QSEN: Patient-Centered Care**
- Perform and document a complete pain assessment, including duration, location, intensity, and quality of pain (see Tables 4.4 and 4.5). **QSEN: Informatics**
- Never use placebos to assess the presence of pain; their deceitful use is prohibited by state boards of nursing and numerous professional organizations. **Ethics**
- Factors that can affect pain and its management include age, gender, genetics, and culture. **QSEN: Patient-Centered Care**
- The two major types of pain are nociceptive pain and neuropathic pain. Pain is also classified by its duration as acute or chronic. Chronic pain is further classified as cancer or noncancer chronic pain (see Tables 4-2 and 4-3).
- Examples of causes for acute pain include surgery and trauma; arthritis and cancer are common causes of chronic pain.
- Multimodal analgesia is the evidence-based approach for the management of all types of pain. Multimodal analgesia combines different drugs with different underlying mechanisms of action with the goal of producing better pain relief at lower analgesic doses than would be possible with any single analgesic alone. **QSEN: Evidence-Based Practice**
- Assess patients on acetaminophen for signs and symptoms of hepatotoxicity and nephrotoxicity; these adverse drug effects may occur when the medication is taken in higher than recommended daily doses. **QSEN: Safety**
- Recall that NSAIDs should be used with caution in older adults because of adverse effects such as GI toxicity, bleeding, and fluid retention, for which they are at higher risk than younger adults. **QSEN: Safety**
- The mu opioid agonists are first-line therapy for moderate-to-severe nociceptive pain. Morphine, fentanyl, hydromorphone, and oxycodone are the most commonly used mu opioid agonists and are available in a wide variety of formulations for administration by a variety of routes of administration for both acute and chronic pain. **QSEN: Evidence-Based Practice**
- Meperidine is not recommended for the treatment of any type of pain. Its toxic metabolite (normeperidine) can accumulate and cause confusion, seizures, and even death. **QSEN: Evidence-Based Practice**
- Physical dependence is a normal response that occurs with repeated administration of an opioid for several days. It is manifested by the occurrence of withdrawal symptoms when the opioid is suddenly stopped or rapidly reduced or an antagonist such as naloxone is given.

- Tolerance is a normal response that occurs with regular administration of an opioid and consists of a decrease in one or more effects of the opioid (e.g., decreased analgesia, sedation, or respiratory depression). It cannot be equated with addictive disease.
- Opioid addiction is a chronic neurologic and biologic disease. The development and characteristics of addiction are influenced by genetic, psychosocial, and environmental factors. It is characterized by one or more of these behaviors: impaired control over drug use, compulsive use, continued use despite harm, and craving.
- Use an equianalgesic chart (see Table 4-6 when changing from one opioid or route of administration to another to help ensure that the patient receives about the same relief with the new opioid or route as with the previous. **QSEN: Evidence-Based Practice**
- Be aware of the advantages and disadvantages of the various routes of analgesic administration.
- Observe for and prevent common side effects of analgesics (see Table 4-7). Remember that the single most effective treatment of most side effects is to decrease the dose of the drug causing the side effect. **Clinical Judgment**
- Remember that sedation precedes opioid-induced respiratory depression; assess sedation using a sedation scale and decrease the opioid dose if excessive sedation is detected (see Table 4-8). **QSEN: Safety**
- The intraspinal routes include the intrathecal (also called *spinal*) and epidural routes of administration. Intrathecal analgesia is given by single injection of opioid (most often) into the subarachnoid space for acute pain or implanted device for chronic pain; epidural analgesia is given by single injection or continuous infusion with or without PCA capability for all types of pain and usually combines an opioid with a local anesthetic.
- Adjuvant analgesics are drugs that have a primary indication other than pain but are analgesic for some painful conditions. The most commonly used are antidepressants, anticonvulsants, and local anesthetics. Examples are listed in Table 4-6.
- Nonpharmacologic therapies may be effective alone for mild pain and are used to complement, not replace, pharmacologic interventions for moderate-to-severe pain. **QSEN: Evidence-Based Practice**
- Pain can be managed in any setting, including the home. All patients require teaching with regard to their pain management regimen to ensure continuity of care. Patients or family members will require specialized training when infusion therapy is used in the home setting.
- Request referral or consultation with pain specialists and/or pain centers for patients with pain that cannot be managed with customary methods. **QSEN: Teamwork and Collaboration**

SELECTED BIBLIOGRAPHY

Asterisk indicates a classic or definitive work on this subject.

*Allred, K. D., Byers, J., & Sole, M. L. (2010). The effect of music on postoperative pain and anxiety. *Pain Management Nursing, 11*, 15–25.

*American Society of Anesthesiologists (ASA) Task Force on Acute Pain Management. (2012). Practice guidelines for acute pain management in the perioperative setting: An updated report by the

American Society of Anesthesiologists Task Force on Acute Pain Management. *Anesthesiology, 116*(2), 248–273.

Bair, M. J., Ang, D., Wu, J., Outcalt, S. D., Sargent, C., Kempf, C., et al. (2015). Evaluation of stepped care for chronic pain (ESCAPE) in veterans of the Iraq and Afghanistan conflicts: A randomized clinical trial. *JAMA Internal Medicine, 175*(5), 682–689.

*Bruckenthal, P. (2010). Integrating nonpharmacologic and alternative strategies into a comprehensive management approach for older adults with pain. *Pain Management Nursing, 11*(2), S23–S31.

Costello, M. (2015). Prescription opioid analgesics: Promoting patient safety with better patient education. *AJN, 115*(11), 50–56.

D'Arcy, Y. (2014). Living with the nightmare of neuropathic pain. *Nursing, 44*(6), 38–44.

*Fillingim, R. B., King, C. D., Ribeiro-Dasilva, M. C., Rahim-Williams, B., & Riley, J. L. (2009). Sex, gender, and pain: A review of recent clinical and experimental findings. *Journal of Pain, 10*(5), 447–485.

*Fouladbakhsh, J. M., Szczesny, S., Jenuwine, E. S., & Vallerand, A. H. (2011). Nondrug therapies for pain management among rural older adults. *Pain Management Nursing, 12*(2), 70–81.

*Herr, K., Coyne, P. J., McCaffery, M., Manworren, R., & Merkel, S. (2011). *American Society for Pain Management Nursing position statement with clinical practice recommendations: Pain assessment in the patient unable to self report* (revised). http://aspmn.org/Organization/documents/UPDATED_NonverbalRevisionFinalWEB.pdf.

*Institute of Medicine (IOM) (June 2011). *Relieving pain in America: A blueprint for transforming prevention, care, education, and research.* www.iom.edu/~/media/Files/Report%20Files/2011/Relieving-Pain-in-America-A-Blueprint-for-Transforming-Prevention-Care-Education-Research/Pain%20Research%202011%20Report%20Brief.pdf.

Kubes, L. F. (2015). Imagery for self-healing and integrative nursing practice. *American Journal of Nursing, 115*(11), 36–43.

Makris, U. E., Adams, R. C., Gurland, B., & Reid, M. C. (2014). Management of persistent pain in the older patient: A clinical review.

JAMA: The Journal of the American Medical Association, 312(8), 825–836.

Matthias, M. S., Miech, E. J., Myers, L. J., Sargent, C., & Blair, M. J. (2014). A qualitative study of chronic pain in Operation Enduring Freedom/Operation Iraqi Freedom veterans: "A burden on my soul.". *Military Medicine, 179*(1), 26–30.

*McCaffery, M. (1968). *Nursing practice and theories related to cognition, bodily pain, and man-environment interactions.* Los Angeles: University of California at Los Angeles Students' Store.

Morley, S., & Williams, A. (2015). New developments in the psychological management of chronic pain. *Canadian Journal of Psychiatry, 60*(4), 168–175.

*Pasero, C., & McCaffery, M. (2011). *Pain assessment and pharmacologic management.* St. Louis: Mosby.

Platts-Mills, T. F., Hunold, K. M., Weaver, M. A., Dickey, R. M., Fernandez, A. R., Fillingim, R. B., et al. (2013). Pain treatment for older adults during prehospital emergency care: Variations by patient gender and pain severity. *Journal of Pain, 14*(9), 966–974.

*Snidvongs, S. (2008). Gender differences in responses to medications and side effects of medications. *Pain Clinical Updates, 16*(5), 1–6.

Textor, L. (2016). Intrathecal pumps for cancer pain. *AJN, 116*(5), 36–41.

Wilson, M., Roll, J. M., Corbett, C., & Barbosa-Leiker, C. (2015). Empowering patients with persistent pain using an Internet-based self-management program. *Pain Management Nursing, 16*(4), 503–514.

Wright, S. (2015). *Pain management in nursing practice.* Los Angeles: Sage.

CHAPTER 5

Principles of Genetics and Genomics for Medical-Surgical Nursing

M. Linda Workman

ⓔ http://evolve.elsevier.com/Iggy/

PRIORITY AND INTERRELATED CONCEPTS

The priority concept for this chapter is CELLULAR REGULATION.

The interrelated concepts for this chapter are:
- ETHICS
- PATIENT-CENTERED CARE

LEARNING OUTCOMES

Safe and Effective Care Environment

1. Collaborate with the interprofessional team to coordinate high-quality PATIENT-CENTERED CARE to adults who may have a genetic-based increased risk for a health problem.
2. Ensure that appropriate informed consent procedures are followed before a patient undergoes genetic testing.

Health Promotion and Maintenance

3. Teach the patient and family who are at increased genetic risk for a disease or disorder to implement environmental modifications to reduce the risk and to participate in early detection screening programs.
4. Identify resources for patients who have an increased genetic risk for a health problem.

Psychosocial Integrity

5. Implement patient-centered nursing interventions to decrease the psychosocial impact caused by genetic assessment and genetic testing.

Physiological Integrity

6. Apply knowledge of anatomy and physiology and genetic/genomic principles when performing an evidence-based genetic assessment and generating a three-generation pedigree for adult health problems that have a potential increased genetic risk.
7. Ensure the use of professional ETHICS when integrating genomic health into medical-surgical nursing practice.
8. Ensure PATIENT-CENTERED CARE by helping the patient and family who undergo genetic testing receive an appropriate level of genetic counseling to interpret the findings.

The purpose of genes and genetics is to provide cellular regulation in all cells throughout the lifespan. CELLULAR REGULATION are the processes that control cellular growth, replication, and differentiation to maintain homeostasis. Thus the turning on and off of specific genes determines everything that a cell does, including what it produces, how it functions within a group, when it reproduces, and even when it dies. Chapter 2 provides a summary discussion of cellular regulation.

Genetic and genomic influences are part of today's comprehensive PATIENT-CENTERED CARE and form the basis for "precision health care" (precision medicine) in which therapies are tailored to an adult's specific genetic makeup. These influences have become especially important in determining the exact drug therapy for best patient responses. It is important for nurses to understand the genetic basis of disease because most of the serious, common adult-onset disorders have a genetic component (Cheek and Howington, 2017; Paz De Jesus & Mitchel, 2016; Quigley, 2015).

Although the terms genetics and genomics often are used interchangeably, there are some differences. Genetics is concerned with the general mechanisms of heredity and the variation of inherited traits. Thus how genetic traits are transmitted from one generation to the next composes genetics. The definition of genomics is both broader and more specific, focusing on the *function* of all of the human DNA, including genes and noncoding DNA regions. Thus how a gene is expressed and its effects on CELLULAR REGULATION within a person or family constitute genomics.

Many adult-onset health problems have a genetic basis, meaning that variation of gene sequences and expression contributes to an adult's risk for disease development. Some of these health problems also demonstrate heritability, meaning that the risk for developing the disorder can be transmitted to one's children in a recognizable pattern. Some adult-onset disorders such as Huntington disease are unavoidable when a person inherits a specific genetic mutation that causes the disorder. For other health problems, the risk is increased but is not absolute, indicating a *predisposition* or *susceptibility* toward the problem when a specific genetic mutation is inherited, but such a disorder may never occur. For example, certain gene variations increase the risk for type 2 diabetes; however, the disease is more likely to develop only when the adult with the genetic variations has a sedentary lifestyle and is overweight. One outcome of genomic health care is to identify personal risk for disease development and help the adult reduce the risk by modifying his or her environment (Manuck & McCaffery, 2014).

Specific discoveries regarding each adult's genetic differences are being used to assess disease risk, enhance disease prevention strategies, and personalize disease management approaches (Bielinski et al., 2014). As a result, all health care professionals, including registered nurses, are expected to have at least a minimum knowledge of basic genetics to provide the best possible care for patients and families (Calzone et al., 2013). Table 5-1 lists selected genetic competencies important in medical-surgical nursing. Nurses are expected to know enough about basic genetics to recognize when a patient or family has a possible genetic risk for a health problem and to coordinate the attention of health care team members to ensure appropriate care.

GENETIC BIOLOGY REVIEW

Genes are the coded instructions for the CELLULAR REGULATION of all the proteins the human body produces. For every hormone, enzyme, and other proteins the human body makes, it is the specific genes that tell each cell which protein to make, how to make it, when to make it, and how much to make. Think of each gene as a specific "recipe" for making a protein.

Every human somatic cell with a nucleus contains the entire set of human genes, known as the genome. The human genome contains between 20,000 and 25,000 genes. For example, all cells have the gene for insulin. However, the only cell type that allows the insulin gene to be expressed (turned on, activated) for CELLULAR REGULATION and make insulin is the beta cell of the pancreas. So although the insulin gene is present in skin cells, heart cells, brain cells, and other cells, only in the beta cells is this gene selectively expressed when insulin is needed.

Genes are composed of DNA, which is present as 46 separate large chunks within the nucleus (Fig. 5-1). During cell division each large chunk of DNA replicates and then organizes into a chromosome form to ensure precise delivery of the genetic information to each of the two new daughter cells. Thus DNA, chromosomes, and genes refer to different structures of the same materials.

Each chromosome has many genes within it. Humans have 23 pairs of chromosomes—46 individual chromosomes. The Y chromosome is small and has fewer than 100 genes. Larger chromosomes such as the number 1 chromosome contain thousands of genes.

TABLE 5-1 Selected Essential Genetic Competencies for Medical-Surgical Nursing Practice

- Use appropriate genetic terminology.
- Recognize that a person/family with an identified genetic variation is a full member of society deserving of the same quality of health care as that provided to all others.
- Differentiate between genetic predisposition to a health problem and the actual expression or diagnosis of the health problem.
- Recognize the genetic and environmental influences on development of common adult-onset health problems.
- Be aware of genetic-based individual variation in responses to drug therapy.
- Consider genetic transmission patterns when performing a detailed patient and family history assessment.
- Ask appropriate questions during assessment to obtain information relevant to potential genetic risk or predisposition to a specific health problem(s).
- Construct a family pedigree, using standard symbols, that encompasses at least three generations.
- Identify patients/families at increased genetic risk for potential disease development.
- Ensure that patients/families identified to be at increased genetic risk for potential disease development are referred to the appropriate level of genetics professional.
- Individualize patient teaching about genetic issues using terminology and language the patient/family understands.
- Inform patients/families about potential risks and benefits of genetic testing.
- Advocate for patients with regard to their rights of accurate information, informed consent, competent counseling, refusal of genetic testing, freedom from coercion, and sharing of testing results.
- Help patients/families find credible resources regarding a specific genetic issue.
- Maintain patient/family confidentiality regarding any issue related to genetic testing, genetic predisposition, or genetic diagnosis, including whether genetic testing is even being considered.
- Support the patient's/family's decisions regarding any aspect of genetic testing or genetic diagnosis.

Data from competencies identified by American Association of Colleges of Nursing. (2008). *The essentials of baccalaureate education for nursing practice.* Washington, DC: Author; and Jenkins, J., Calzone, K., Caskey, S., Culp, S., Weiner, M., & Badzek, L. (2015). Methods of genomic competency integration in practice. *Journal of Nursing Scholarship, 47*(3), 200-210.

One way to think of it is to consider all the DNA in the genome of any cell to be a giant "cookbook" containing all the recipes needed for total CELLULAR REGULATION to make all the proteins, hormones, enzymes, and other substances your body needs. The chromosome pairs are the different book chapters (so the human genome cookbook has 23 chapters), and the genes are the individual recipes contained within the chapters.

There is a specific chromosome location (locus) for every gene. For example, the locus of the gene for blood type is on chromosome 9. The location and the exact DNA sequence for many, but not all, genes is now known.

DNA

DNA Structure

In humans DNA is a linear, double-stranded structure composed of multiple units of four different nitrogenous bases, each attached to a sugar molecule. The bases in each strand are linked together by phosphate groups. These two individual strands are

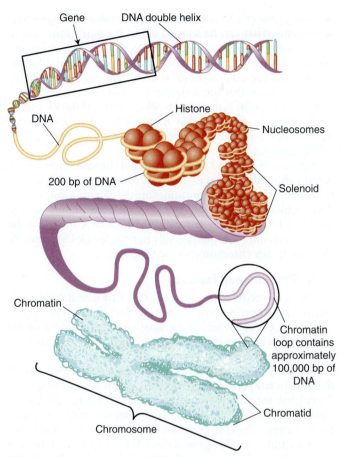

FIG. 5-1 The various forms of DNA from a loose double helix to coiled tightly into a chromosome. *bp,* Base pair.

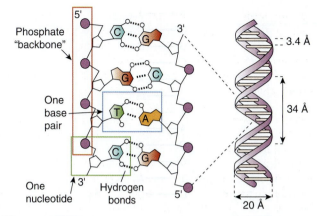

FIG. 5-2 The structure of DNA. (Modified from Nussbaum, R., McInnes, R., & Willard, H. (2007). *Thompson & Thompson: Genetics in medicine* (7th ed.). Philadelphia: Saunders.)

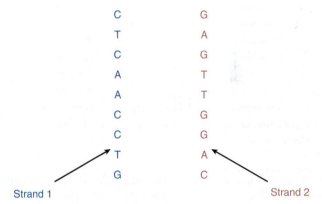

FIG. 5-3 Complementary strands of DNA.

held together loosely. This double-stranded DNA is arranged like a long set of railroad tracks. The "backbones" of the track are the two long steel rails. For DNA these backbones are the phosphate groups that hold the bases in place. The bases are the individual railroad ties. Think of each tie as having two pieces—one piece attached to the right rail and one piece attached to the left rail.

Fig. 5-2 shows a very small piece of double-stranded DNA on the left (containing only four base pairs) taken from the larger piece of DNA on the right. The phosphate groups that hold the nucleotides together as a strand are in the red box. The green box in the lower left section shows a whole nucleotide (a base with the sugar and the phosphate group) in place in the left DNA strand. The blue box in the middle of the two strands shows how the base from the left strand lines up with and pairs to a complementary base in the right strand.

Bases are the essential parts of DNA. Many trillions of bases in the DNA are found in the nucleus of just one cell. The four bases in DNA are adenine (A), guanine (G), cytosine (C), and thymine (T). Each base becomes a complete **nucleotide** when a five-sided sugar (known as a *deoxyribose sugar*) and a phosphate group are attached (see Fig. 5-2). Nucleotides form the DNA strands with the phosphate groups holding the bases in place.

Base pairs are the linked bases in the two opposite strands of DNA. The bases always link together across from each other in a very specific way. Thymine always forms a pair with adenine,

and cytosine always forms a pair with guanine. Thus the bases of each pair are *complementary* to each other. Because these complementary base pairs in DNA are specific, if the base sequence of one strand of DNA is known, the opposite strand's sequence could be accurately predicted. For example, if the left section of DNA (strand 1 in Fig. 5-3) had the sequence C-T-C-A-A-C-C-T-G, the corresponding (complementary) right section (strand 2 in Fig. 5-3) of DNA would have the sequence G-A-G-T-T-G-G-A-C.

When the two strands of DNA are lined up properly, they twist into a loose helical shape (see Fig. 5-1). In this shape the DNA is so fine that it can be seen only with electron microscopes. Only when a cell undergoes mitosis does the DNA super-coil tightly into dense pieces called *chromosomes* (Fig. 5-1), which can be seen with standard microscopes.

DNA Replication

DNA must reproduce itself (**replicate**) every time a cell divides (undergoes mitosis). The purpose of mitosis is for one cell to reproduce into two new daughter cells, each of which is identical to the parent cell that started mitosis. For each new cell to have exactly the right amount of DNA and genes, the DNA in the dividing cell must replicate exactly. This process involves having the double strands of DNA separate and then build two new strands that are perfectly complementary to the original strands (Fig. 5-4). The result is two sets of double-stranded

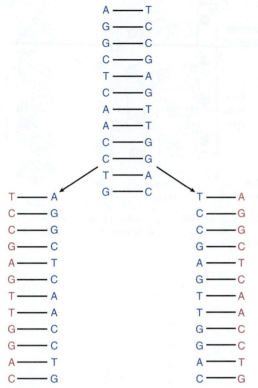

FIG. 5-4 DNA replication. *Blue type,* Original DNA; *red type,* newly replicated DNA.

DNA. At the time of actual cell division with the separation into two new cells, one set of DNA will move into one of the two new cells made during mitosis, and the second set will move into the other new cell. In this way every new cell ends up with exactly the right amount of DNA with all the genes for appropriate CELLULAR REGULATION.

Chromosomes

As shown in Fig. 5-1, a chromosome is a specific large chunk of highly condensed double-stranded DNA, with each chunk containing billions of bases and hundreds (and sometimes thousands) of genes. Each chromosome forms and moves to the center of the cell that is about to divide. Just before the cell splits into two cells, each chromosome is pulled apart so half of each chromosome goes into one new cell and the other half goes into the other new cell. Thus chromosomes are temporary structures to ensure the precise delivery of DNA to the two new cells. Humans have 46 chromosomes divided into 23 pairs.

Some things about an adult can be known by examining his or her chromosomes, but limited information can be obtained by chromosomal analysis because each chromosome is composed of a large chunk of DNA. Only very large deletions, additions, or rearrangements of DNA show up at the level of the chromosome. Losses or gains of even tens of thousands of bases cannot be detected by chromosome analysis.

A karyotype is an organized arrangement of all of the chromosomes present in a cell during the metaphase section of mitosis (Fig. 5-5). A picture of the chromosomes is made. Chromosomes are first paired up and then arranged according to size (largest first) and centromere position. This gross organization of DNA can be used to determine missing or extra whole chromosomes and some large structural rearrangements.

A missing gene or a mutated gene would not show up at this level of analysis. What can be learned about the adult from whom the karyotype in Fig. 5-7 was made is that she is human and euploid (has the correct number of chromosome pairs for the species). She is chromosomally "normal," although she probably has some genes that are different (variant from or mutated) compared with the same gene in other people. If the karyotype is abnormal in any way (has more or less than the normal number or has broken chromosomes), the karyotype would be called aneuploid.

Autosomes are the 22 pairs of human chromosomes (numbered 1 through 22) that do not code for the sexual differentiation of a human. Sex chromosomes are the pair of chromosomes that include the genes for the sexual differentiation of the human. Chromosomally normal males have an X and a Y as the sex chromosomes. Chromosomally normal females have two Xs (XX) as the sex chromosomes (see Fig. 5-5).

Gene Structure and Function

A gene is a specific segment(s) of DNA that contains the code (recipe) for a specific protein (see Fig. 5-1) involved in CELLULAR REGULATION. Genes are the smallest functional unit of the DNA. Each chromosome is a large segment of DNA that contains hundreds of genes.

For many human traits, one gene controls the expression of that trait in any person. Such traits are known as *single gene traits (monogenic traits).* For each single gene we have two alleles. An allele (pronounced "ah-**lee**-el") is an alternate form (or variation) of a gene. For example, there is one gene for blood type but there are three possible gene alleles (A, B, and O). Each person has only two of the three specific gene alleles for blood type. One of these alleles is on one chromosome 9 of the pair; the other allele is located on the other number 9 chromosome. Because each person only has two number 9 chromosomes, he or she can have only two of the three possible alleles for blood type. One gene allele was inherited from the person's mother, and the other gene allele was inherited from the person's father. *Some traits have even more than three possible alleles, but each person has only two.* Which blood type-gene alleles are inherited from a person's parents determines which blood type he or she expresses.

If a person has inherited a blood-type A allele from his or her mother and a blood-type B allele from his or her father, he or she has the A and B alleles; the blood type expressed when the blood bank determines type is type AB. Fig. 5-6 shows this concept. In Fig. 5-6 a woman is about to become pregnant with the help of a specific adult man. What are the possibilities for this baby to have a specific type of ear shape (pointy, rounded, square, triangular)? The gene for ear shape is trait 1, and it (for the purposes of this explanation) is on chromosome number 6.

Each of the father's sperm contains only one number 6 chromosome, and each of the mother's eggs contains only one number 6 chromosome (so when the sperm fertilizes the egg, the resulting person conceived will have only one pair of chromosome number 6 instead of two pairs of chromosome number 6).

Half the father's sperm have the 1a allele for ear shape, and the other half have allele 1b for ear shape. Half the mother's eggs have 1c for ear shape, and the other half have 1d. The baby can inherit only either a 1a or a 1b from the father, not both; and this same baby can inherit only a 1c or a 1d from the mother—again, not both. The lower part of Fig. 5-6 shows all the combinations possible for each ear shape gene alleles for any child these two adults have.

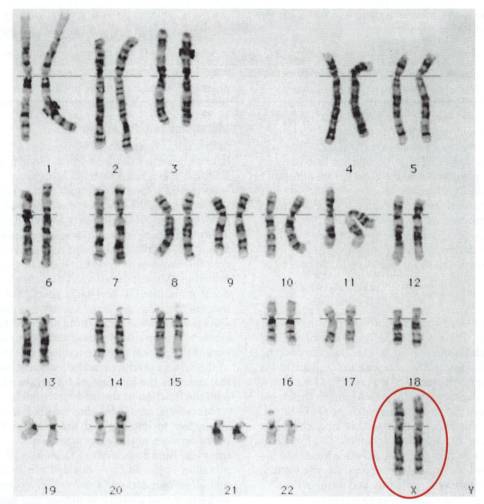

FIG. 5-5 A karyotype of a chromosomally normal female. (The sex chromosomes are *circled in red.*) (Modified from Jorde, L., Carey, J., Bamshad, M., & White, R. (2000). *Medical genetics* (2nd ed.). St. Louis: Mosby.)

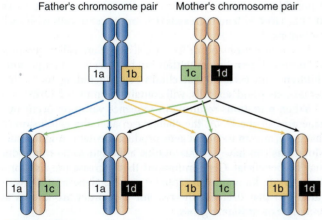

FIG. 5-6 Inheritance of four possible alleles for the single gene trait 1. (Any one person can have only two alleles for a single gene trait.)

If a person has two identical alleles for a single gene trait, that person is said to be *homozygous* for that trait. Thus if a person has an A blood-type gene allele on one number 9 chromosome and an A blood-type gene allele on the other number 9 chromosome, he or she is homozygous for that trait and will express the A blood type.

If a person has two different alleles for a single gene trait, he or she is *heterozygous* for that trait. So if a person has an A blood-type gene allele on one number 9 chromosome and a B blood-type gene allele on the other number 9 chromosome, that person is heterozygous for that trait and will express the AB blood type. Because the A and B alleles are equally dominant (*codominant*), they will both be expressed in the actual blood type.

There are differences in expression of the alleles for a trait depending on whether an allele is dominant or recessive. If a person has an A blood-type gene allele on one number 9 chromosome and an O blood-type gene allele on the other number 9 chromosome, that person is heterozygous for that trait and expresses only the A blood type. Because the A allele is dominant and the O allele is recessive, they will not both be expressed in the actual blood type. Only the dominant allele is expressed, and the recessive allele is "silent." More information about dominant, recessive, and co-dominant expression is presented later in the Patterns of Inheritance section.

Phenotype

The **phenotype** of any gene for a person is which characteristic can actually be observed or, in some cases, determined by a laboratory test. For example, the person who has the AO gene alleles for blood type has the phenotype of type A blood. A person with curly hair has a curly-hair phenotype, regardless of whether he or she has two alleles for curly hair or one allele for curly hair and one allele for straight hair.

Genotype

The genotype for a person's single gene trait is what the actual alleles are for that trait—not just what can be observed. A person with a phenotype of type A blood could have either an AA genotype or an AO genotype. The person who has type O blood would have an OO genotype. When a person has homozygous alleles for a trait, we would expect the genotype and phenotype to be the same. When a person has heterozygous alleles for a trait, the phenotype and the genotype are not always the same. *Recessive traits are expressed only when the person is homozygous for the alleles.* Thus for expressed recessive traits phenotype and genotype are the same. Dominant traits are expressed whether the person is homozygous for the gene alleles or heterozygous for the gene alleles. Thus for dominant traits phenotype and genotype can be the same but do not have to be the same.

Gene Expression

Genes control CELLULAR REGULATION by coding for the making of a specific protein. For example, the hormone *insulin* is a protein. When an adult's blood glucose level starts to rise, the beta cells of the pancreas rapidly make insulin to maintain his or her blood glucose homeostasis.

To continue the cookbook analogy, each gene is the recipe needed to make a specific protein for CELLULAR REGULATION. All the hormones, enzymes, growth factors, and chemicals needed to keep an adult functioning are proteins. These proteins are *gene products* because they are produced when the right gene is *expressed.* Just a few examples of gene products are insulin, hemoglobin, erythropoietin, angiotensin, and estrogen.

Protein Synthesis

Protein synthesis is the process by which genes are used to make the proteins needed for physiologic function and CELLULAR REGULATION. Proteins are made up of individual amino acids hooked together like beads on a string. There are 22 different amino acids. Every protein has a specific number of each of the amino acids and a specific order in which they are placed. *If even one amino acid is out of order or completely deleted from the sequence, the protein may be less functional or perhaps nonfunctional and unable to assist with cellular regulation.*

For example, the hormone *insulin* is a protein that contains 51 amino acids in a specific sequence. If some of the amino acids are missing or are in the wrong position, the protein made would be different from real insulin and could not reduce blood glucose levels. *Thus the actual order of the amino acids is critical for cellular regulation and the final function of any protein.*

Within the DNA there is a three-nucleotide (base) code for each amino acid. A gene for a specific protein contains all the amino acid codes in exactly the right order for that protein. For example, the final active form of the protein *insulin* has 51 amino acids. Thus the minimum number of bases needed in the gene for insulin would be 153 (three bases per amino acid × 51 amino acids). Fig. 5-7 shows an example of a short protein made up of only seven amino acids.

The key for making a functional protein is accurate placement of all the amino acids in the order specified by the gene. When problems exist in the base sequence of a gene, its expression may not result in a functional protein. In addition, the

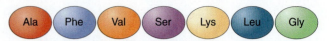

FIG. 5-7 A sample protein composed of seven amino acids.

process of protein synthesis involves many steps. A problem at any step could cause failure to produce a functional protein.

Mutations and Variations

Many human genes have been sequenced, meaning that their base sequence is known and so is the sequence of their amino acids in the expressed proteins. Most people have the same base sequence for a specific gene such as the gene for insulin. When this sequence is the most common one found in a large population of humans, it is referred to as the *wild-type* gene sequence. Think of the term wild-type as meaning "normal" or "expected." When a person has a different sequence for a gene compared with the known wild-type sequence, the gene has a variation or mutation. Mutations as small variations in gene sequences occur more often in very large genes, and the significance of some of these changes is not known. It is these variations in the sequences of some genes from the wild-type that are being examined more closely. Some variations can reduce the function of the protein produced, some can eliminate the function of the protein produced, and a few variations have been found that enhance the function of the produced protein compared with the function of the wild-type protein.

Mutations are DNA changes that are passed from one generation to another and thus are *inherited.* An inherited mutation does not have to mean that the mutation is passed from one human generation to another. It can mean that the mutation is passed from one *cell* generation to another and may affect only certain tissues within a person rather than be a problem within a family. Mutations that occur in general body cells (somatic cells) are known as *somatic mutations.* Because these mutations occur in a person's cells after conception, the adult cannot pass a somatic mutation on to his or her children. A possible outcome of somatic mutations is a loss of CELLULAR REGULATION with an increased risk for cancer in cells with such mutations.

When mutations occur in sex cells, they are called *germline mutations.* A germline mutation *can* be passed on to a person's children; and each of that child's cells, including his or her somatic cells and sex cells, will contain the mutated DNA.

When mutations resulting in sequence variation occur in a gene area of the DNA, the change can alter the expression of that gene, and an incorrect gene product (protein) might result. Mutations can have serious results, although some mutations may be beneficial. Gene mutations that increase the risk for a disorder are known as *susceptibility* genes. Gene mutations or variations that decrease the risk for a disorder are known as *protective* or *resistance* genes.

The gene sequences for most proteins are generally the same in all people. Sometimes a base in one person's gene for a specific protein is not the same as that in the wild-type. Either this difference can be a variation known as a *single nucleotide polymorphism, or SNP* ("snip"), or it can be a mutation. When a base difference allows the protein to be made but there are differences in how well the protein works, the difference is called a *gene variation* or a polymorphism. When a base difference causes a loss of protein function leading to impaired CELLULAR REGULATION, it is called a mutation.

Clinically many SNPs exist within different people in the genes of a large family of enzymes involved in drug metabolism. These enzymes are the cytochrome P-450 family, coded for by at least ten separate extremely large genes, with as many as 100 subsets of genes. Cytochrome p is abbreviated as CYP (pronounced "sip"). SNPs in these genes can make the resulting enzyme less active than normal or more active than normal. Either way, a change in activity of any one of these enzymes can affect a person's response to drug therapy. For example, the drug warfarin (Coumadin) is metabolized for elimination primarily by two enzymes from this system, CYP2C9 and CYP2C19. About 17% to 37% of white adults have an SNP variation in CYP2CP that slows the metabolism of warfarin. This means that warfarin remains in the patient's system longer, greatly increasing the risk for bleeding and other side effects. For adults who have this gene mutation, warfarin doses need to be much lower than those for the general population (Cheek et al., 2015).

Another example of changes in patient responses to drugs is codeine, an opioid analgesic. When taken orally or given parenterally, codeine is an inactive prodrug that must be metabolized by the CYP2D6 enzyme in the tissues to morphine, which is the active drug. Patients who have nonfunctional or poorly functional CYP2D6 because of a gene variation obtain no pain relief from codeine but do obtain pain relief from morphine (Kelly, 2013).

? NCLEX EXAMINATION CHALLENGE 5-1

Safe and Effective Care Environment

What therapy outcome does the nurse expect for a client receiving warfarin therapy who has a variant of the CYP2C9 that makes the enzyme have **greater** activity?

A. Having an increased risk for drug side effects
B. Having excessive bleeding from minor trauma
C. Requiring a higher dose to achieve the desired anticoagulation level
D. Requiring a lower dose to achieve the desired anticoagulation level

---

🌐 CULTURAL/SPIRITUAL CONSIDERATIONS

Patient-Centered Care QSEN

Many adults of Ethiopian heritage have a variation of the CYP2D6 gene that results in much higher levels of the enzyme produced and are known as "ultrametabolizers." This enzyme deactivates and helps eliminate many drugs, including metoprolol, which is often used to control blood pressure. An adult who ultrametabolizes this drug does not achieve a high enough blood level of the drug for it to be effective. They eliminate the drug too quickly. Thus any adult of Ethiopian heritage who needs antihypertensive therapy is not likely to respond to metoprolol or any other beta blockers. When patients do not respond to beta-blocker therapy as expected, be sure to ask about their cultural and ethnic heritage.

The most devastating gene mutations are the ones that change the amino acid codes so a proper protein is not made or does not function at all. Other changes may impair CELLULAR REGULATION by altering how often or how well a group of cells divides. Gene mutations or variations may cause one adult to have a greater-than-normal risk for developing a disease. A different variation in the same gene may cause another adult to have a smaller-than-normal risk for developing the same disease.

Microbiome

A current issue in precision health care and genomics is the microbiome. The microbiome for an adult is genomes of all the microorganisms that coexist in and on him or her and can affect CELLULAR REGULATION (Abbas et al., 2015). This includes the organisms that live in the mouth, the rest of the GI tract, the nose and sinuses, the vagina, and on the skin. The number of microbial cells in the body outnumber human cells by about ten to one. Most of these organisms are part of our "normal flora," which differ somewhat from person to person. These organisms are mostly nonpathogenic (non–disease causing) when they remain confined to the expected area. However, when they manage to escape their normal human habitat and move elsewhere, they may be pathogenic in the new environment. For example, when gut organisms get into the urinary tract or the blood, serious infections can occur.

Adults start acquiring their microbiomes from birth, and their specific microbiome profiles change almost daily over time. The interaction between an adult and his or her microbiome is complex and represents all the lifelong experiences of the foods eaten, the drugs taken, and the touching of other people and animals, along with the specific human genes inherited. To a large extent an adult's microbiome is protective in nature and is important for good health such as helping with food digestion and keeping some pathogenic organisms in check (Abbas et al., 2015). Recent discoveries indicate that the types of gut organisms an adult has can even change how well he or she responds to immunotherapy for cancer.

When the types of organisms that compose the microbiome in an area change, health can suffer. For example, when natural "gut" organisms are reduced or eliminated by antibiotic therapy, *Clostridium difficile* (C. diff) can overgrow and cause chronic severe, bloody diarrhea. A very successful therapy for this problem is the reconstitution of the "healthy" microbiome through fecal transplantation or transfer from one person to another.

PATTERNS OF INHERITANCE

For every single gene trait, a person inherits one allele for that gene from his or her mother and one allele from his or her father. How these traits are expressed depends on whether one or both alleles are "dominant" or "recessive." Expression also depends on whether the gene for the trait is located on an autosome or on a sex chromosome.

It is possible to determine how the gene for a specific trait is passed from one human generation to the next *(transmitted)*. By looking at how that trait is expressed through several generations of a family, patterns emerge that indicate whether the gene for the trait is dominant or recessive and whether it is located on an autosomal chromosome or on one of the sex chromosomes. This information can be determined through *pedigree analysis*. Determining inheritance patterns for a specific trait makes it possible to predict the relative risk for any one person to have a trait or transmit that trait to his or her children.

Pedigree

A pedigree is a graph of a family history for a specific trait or health problem over several generations. Its use by nurses is important for assessing certain PATIENT-CENTERED CARE needs

(Lough & Seidel, 2015). Fig. 5-8 shows common symbols used when creating a pedigree. Fig. 5-9 shows a typical three-generation pedigree. Although the term *pedigree* is the correct genetic term, it can offend some patients. Use the term *family tree* in place of pedigree when talking with patients. Construct a pedigree that includes at least three generations when taking the family history. When analyzing a pedigree, note the answers to these:

- Is any pattern of inheritance recognized, or does the trait appear sporadic?
- Is the trait expressed equally among male and female family members or unequally?
- Is the trait present in every generation, or does it skip one or more generations?
- Do only affected adults have children who are affected with the trait, or do unaffected adults also have children who express the trait?

The four types of inheritance patterns associated with single gene—controlled traits are autosomal dominant, autosomal recessive, sex-linked dominant, and sex-linked recessive. Each inheritance pattern has specific defining criteria. Table 5-2 lists the patterns of inheritance for some disorders that occur in adults or may be identified in children who live to adulthood.

Autosomal Dominant Pattern of Inheritance

Autosomal dominant (AD) single gene traits require that the gene alleles controlling the trait be located on an autosomal chromosome. A dominant gene allele is usually expressed, even when only one allele of the pair is dominant. Other criteria for AD inheritance include:

- The trait appears in every generation with no skipping.
- The risk for an affected adult to pass the trait to a child is 50% with each pregnancy.

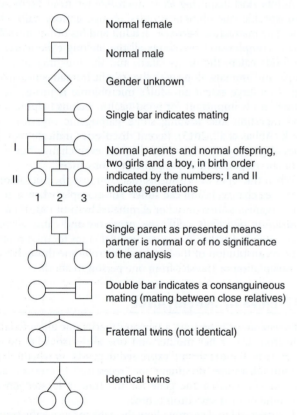

FIG. 5-8 Standard pedigree symbols. (Modified from Jorde, L., Carey, J., & Bamshad, M. (2010). *Medical genetics* (4th ed.). St. Louis: Mosby.)

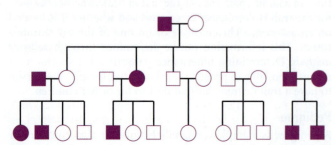

FIG. 5-9 A three-generation pedigree showing an autosomal dominant pattern of inheritance.

TABLE 5-2	**Patterns of Inheritance for Genetic Disorders Among Adults**
PATTERN OF INHERITANCE	**DISORDER**
Autosomal dominant	Breast cancer* (mutation of *BRCA1* or *BRCA2* genes)
	Diabetes mellitus type 2*
	Familial adenomatous polyposis
	Familial melanoma
	Familial hypercholesterolemia
	Hereditary nonpolyposis colon cancer (HNPCC)
	Huntington disease
	Long QT syndrome and sudden cardiac death
	Malignant hyperthermia (MH)
	Marfan syndrome
	Myotonic dystrophy
	Neurofibromatosis (types 1 and 2)
	Ovarian cancer* (mutation of *BRCA1* genes)
	Polycystic kidney disease† (types 1 and 2)
	Retinitis pigmentosa†
	von Willebrand's disease
Autosomal recessive	Albinism
	Alpha₁-antitrypsin deficiency
	Beta thalassemia
	Bloom syndrome
	Cystic fibrosis
	Hereditary hemochromatosis
	Sickle cell disease
	Xeroderma pigmentosum
Sex-linked recessive	Glucose-6-phosphate dehydrogenase deficiency
	Hemophilia
	Red-green color blindness
Complex disorders/ familial clustering	Alzheimer's disease
	Autoimmune disorders
	Bipolar disorder
	Parkinson disease
	Schizophrenia
	Hypertension
	Rheumatoid arthritis

*Some disorders have both a genetic and nongenetic form.
†Some disorders have more than one genetic form and can also be autosomal recessive.

- Unaffected adults do not have affected children; therefore their risk is essentially 0%.
- The trait is found about equally in males and females.

An example of an AD trait is blood type A. If a person is homozygous for the blood-type A allele, he or she will express type A blood (with genotype being identical to the phenotype). If a person is heterozygous for the blood-type A allele with the other allele being type O (which is a recessive trait), he or she will also express type A blood. However, in this case the phenotype is **not** identical to the genotype. *When a dominant allele is paired with a recessive allele, only the dominant allele is expressed.* The blood-type B allele is a dominant allele. When a B allele is paired with an O allele, B blood type is expressed. However, when a person has one blood-type A allele and a blood-type B allele, both alleles are expressed because they are equally dominant (co-dominant), and the person has type AB blood.

Some health problems inherited as autosomal dominant (AD) single gene traits are not apparent at birth but develop as the person ages (see Table 5-2). Two factors that affect the expression of some AD single gene traits are penetrance and expressivity.

Penetrance

Penetrance is how often or how well, within a population, a gene is expressed when it is present. Some genes are more penetrant than others. For example, the gene for Huntington disease (HD) has an autosomal dominant pattern of transmission. This gene is "highly penetrant" (sometimes called *fully penetrant*). This means that, if a person has the HD gene allele, his or her risk for expressing the gene and developing the disease is about 99.99%. Therefore a person who has one HD allele is at high risk for developing HD.

Some dominant gene alleles have "reduced" penetrance. So a person who has the gene mutation has a lower risk for this gene being expressed and actually developing the disorder.

Penetrance has been calculated by examining a population of people known to have the gene mutation and assessing the percentage that go on to express the gene by developing the disorder. For example, the *BRCA2* gene mutation increases a person's risk for breast cancer. This gene is not fully penetrant; so some women (and men) who have the gene do not develop breast cancer. The penetrance rate for this gene mutation is calculated to be between 60% and 80%, meaning that an adult who has the gene mutation has a 60% to 80% risk for developing breast cancer. Although this risk is far higher than among adults who do not have the mutated gene, the risk is not 100%. Having the gene mutation does not absolutely predict that the adult will develop breast cancer—just that the risk is high. However, the adult with the mutation can pass on this genetic mutation to his or her children, who will then have an increased risk for breast cancer development.

Expressivity

Expressivity is the degree of expression a person has when a dominant gene is present. So it is a personal issue, not a population issue. The gene is *always* expressed, but some people have more severe problems than other people. For example, the gene mutation for one form of neurofibromatosis (NF1) is dominant. Some people with this gene mutation have only a few light brown skin tone areas known as *café au lait spots*. Other people with the same gene mutation develop hundreds of tumors (neurofibromas) that protrude through the skin.

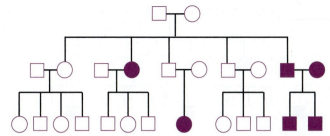

FIG. 5-10 A typical pedigree showing an autosomal recessive pattern of inheritance.

Expressivity accounts for some variation in genetic disease severity.

Autosomal Recessive Pattern of Inheritance

Autosomal recessive (AR) single gene traits require that the gene controlling the trait be located on an autosomal chromosome. Normally the trait can be expressed *only* when both alleles are present. Table 5-2 lists some AR adult disorders. Fig. 5-10 shows a typical pedigree for an AR disorder. Criteria for AR patterns of inheritance include:

- The trait may not appear in all generations of any one branch of a family.
- The trait often first appears only in siblings rather than in parents and children.
- About 25% of a family will be affected and express the trait.
- The children of two affected parents will *always* be affected (risk is 100%).
- Unaffected adults who are carriers (heterozygous for the trait) and do not express the trait themselves *can* transmit the trait to their children if their partner either is also a carrier or is affected.
- The trait is found about equally in male and female members of the same family.

An example of an AR trait is type O blood. The blood-type O allele is recessive, and both alleles must be type O (homozygous) for the person to express type O blood. If only one allele is a type O allele and the other allele is either type A or type B, the dominant allele will be expressed, and the O allele, although present, is not expressed. For AR single gene traits, phenotype and genotype are always the same.

An adult who has one mutated allele for a recessive genetic disorder is a carrier. A carrier, even though he or she may have one mutated allele, may not have any signs or symptoms of the disorder but can pass this mutated allele on to his or her children. For some autosomal recessive disorders, a carrier may have mild symptoms. One example is sickle cell trait. A patient with two sickle cell alleles has the disease and many associated health problems. A carrier with one sickle cell allele (has "sickle cell trait") may be healthy most of the time and have symptoms only under conditions of severe hypoxia.

Sex-Linked Recessive Pattern of Inheritance

Some genes are present only on the sex chromosomes. The Y chromosome has only a few genes that are not also present on the X chromosome. These genes are important for male sexual development. The X chromosome has many single genes that are not present on the Y or elsewhere in the genome. Some of

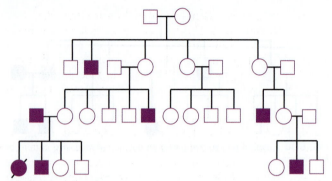

FIG. 5-11 A typical pedigree showing a sex-linked (X-linked) recessive pattern of inheritance.

NCLEX EXAMINATION CHALLENGE 5-2

Health Promotion and Maintenance

Which type pattern of inheritance does the nurse determine is probably present when reviewing the pedigree of a client diagnosed with a health problem in which the problem is present in both males and females, unaffected parents have affected children, and the problem appears mostly in siblings in about 25% of the three familial generations?
A. Autosomal dominant
B. Autosomal recessive
C. Sex-linked recessive
D. Familial clustering

these genes are specific for female sexual development, but there are also several hundred genes on the X chromosome that code for other functions. Few disorders have X-linked dominant expression and are not discussed in this chapter.

Because the number of X chromosomes in males and females is not the same (1:2), the number of X-linked chromosome genes in the two genders is also unequal. Males have only one X chromosome. As a result, X-linked recessive genes have dominant expression in males and recessive expression in females. This difference in expression is because males do not have a second X chromosome to balance the presence of a recessive gene on the first X chromosome.

Sex-linked (X-linked) recessive single gene traits require that the gene allele be present on both of the X chromosomes for the trait to be expressed in females (homozygous) and on only one X chromosome for the trait to be expressed in males. Fig. 5-11 shows a typical pedigree for a sex-linked recessive disorder. Features of a sex-linked recessive pattern of inheritance are:

- The incidence of the trait is much higher among males in a family than among females.
- The trait cannot be passed down (transmitted) from father to son.
- Transmission of the trait is from father to all daughters (who will be carriers).
- Female carriers have a 50% risk (with each pregnancy) of passing the gene to their children.

Complex Inheritance and Familial Clustering

Some health problems appear in families at a rate higher than normal and greater than can be accounted for by chance alone; however, no specific pattern occurs within a family. Although clusters suggest a genetic influence, it is likely that additional factors such as gender and the environment also influence disease development or severity. Such disorders include Alzheimer's disease, type 1 diabetes, and many others. These disorders are often called *complex* and *multifactorial,* because, although an increased genetic risk may be present, the risk is changed by diet, lifestyle, exposure to toxins, infectious agents, and other factors.

GENETIC TESTING

Purpose of Genetic Testing

Many adults are eager to have genetic testing but also are fearful of it. The lay public often believe that a single genetic test can "tell everything about you." Although genetic testing has the potential to be that informative, this is not currently how testing is conducted. *It is important to remember that no single adult is genetically perfect.*

Genetic testing can be performed with many different techniques. Some genetic tests are specific for a disorder. Others may show a gene variation, but the significance of the variation may not be known. Unexpected information can be found during genetic testing. Some ordinary tests such as blood typing and tissue typing provide genetic information. Tests that measure the amount of an enzyme or protein also provide genetic information.

Testing for the purpose of assessing genetic information can be performed at many levels. Cellular or biochemical tests provide information about gene products made by a cell, tissue, or organ. Chromosomes and chromosome segments can be assessed for missing, extra, broken, or rearranged chromosomes. The sequence of a gene can be examined to determine variation or mutation. At present not all genes can be analyzed, and the analysis of even one gene may be limited by expense and availability. Specific base pairs can be evaluated for mutations (Conley et al., 2013). Many tests are expensive, and the results may not be conclusive (Fisco et al., 2015). Table 5-3 lists purposes of genetic testing for adults.

Benefits and Risks of Genetic Testing

Genetic testing is different from any other type of testing. Informed consent is required before genetic testing is performed. The adult tested is the one who gives consent, even though genetic testing *always* gives information about family members—not just the patient (Badzek et al., 2013). Thus genetic testing is a unique and personal aspect of PATIENT-CENTERED CARE.

Benefits of genetic testing include the ability to confirm a diagnosis or to test adults who are at risk for a health problem but do not have any symptoms (presymptomatic testing). The information can help an adult, family, and their primary health care provider develop a specific plan for care or provide early detection (Fisco et al., 2015). For example, in the case of a strong genetic predisposition for colon cancer, identifying a patient before symptoms appear allows interventions to prevent the disease or to diagnosis it earlier, when cure is more likely.

Risks are associated with genetic testing that are not associated with other types of tests. Genetic testing results do not change. Thus a positive test result cannot be "taken back." Other risks may include psychological or social risks, as well as a risk for family disruption. Often genetic tests are expensive and may not be covered by insurance. Some genetic tests have limited value for predicting future risk. Testing may identify a patient

TABLE 5-3	Purposes of Genetic Testing for Adults
PURPOSE/TYPE	**DEFINITION**
Carrier testing	Determining whether a patient without symptoms has an allele for a recessive disorder that could be transmitted to his or her children. Disorders for which carrier testing is common include sickle cell disease, hemophilia, hereditary hemochromatosis, cystic fibrosis, beta thalassemia, and Tay-Sachs disease.
Diagnostic testing	Determining whether a patient has or does not have a mutation that increases the risk for a specific disorder.
Symptomatic	Patient has symptoms; test results confirm a diagnosis.
Presymptomatic	Patient has no symptoms but is at high risk for inheriting a specific genetic disorder for which there is no known prevention or treatment. A disorder for which presymptomatic testing is commonly performed is Huntington disease.
Predisposition	Family history or genetic testing indicates that risk is high for a known genetic disorder. The patient does not have any symptoms but wants to know whether he or she has the specific mutation and what the chances are that it will be expressed. Disorders for which predisposition testing is often performed include hereditary breast/ovarian cancer and hereditary colorectal cancers. The advantage of predisposition testing is that the patient can then engage in heightened screening activities or medical and surgical interventions that reduce risk.

at great risk for the future development of a serious health problem that cannot be prevented or managed. Such a disorder is Huntington disease (HD), which currently has no treatment. Knowing positive test results in this case can lead to depression, blame, and guilt.

Another risk of genetic testing is that positive results may be used to discriminate against an adult or a family. Some protection is in place to prevent health insurance companies from failing to insure a person or dropping the coverage of a person who is at high risk for developing a serious illness (e.g., breast or ovarian cancer). However, there are no protections against rate hikes or exclusions of specific treatments. Patients often fear workplace and personal discrimination if positive test results become known. This problem is less common since the 2008 passage of federal legislation in the Genetic Information and Nondiscrimination Act (GINA), which provides federal protection against employment and insurance discrimination.

Genetic Counseling

Genetic testing is not a standard test that any adult should have performed without knowing the benefits and risks. Counseling patients before, during, and after testing is critical and required by the professional ETHICS governing genetic medicine. Entire families may be a part of the genetic evaluation and follow-up. For example, a 45-year-old woman has breast cancer. In her family her mother, grandmother, brother, and one sister have

all had breast cancer. Genetic testing indicates that she has a *BRCA1* gene mutation. This woman's older daughter wonders whether she has a gene mutation for breast cancer and asks to be tested. When she and her younger sister are tested, the older daughter does not have the mutation, but the younger sister does. Even a negative test result requires PATIENT-CENTERED CARE considerations.

Genetic counseling is a process—not a single session or a single recommendation. This process should begin when the patient or family is first identified as potentially having a genetic problem. The process continues through actual testing if the decision to test is made, and it continues through interpretation of results and follow-up. Chart 5-1 lists the steps in the process.

As a nurse and patient advocate providing PATIENT-CENTERED CARE, it is your professional duty to determine whether the patient understands the consequences of testing. Often a patient may request genetic testing even when there is no indication of an increased risk for a genetic disorder. Counseling and evaluation can help patients understand whether any useful information could be obtained from testing.

Counseling should be a collaborative effort performed by an interprofessional team with members who have defined expertise in interpretation of genetic testing results. Such professionals include advanced practice nurses with specialization in genetics, certified genetic counselors, clinical geneticists, and medical geneticists. Each profession has a different level of preparation in genetics and different skills or roles in the counseling process. For example, an advanced practice genetic nurse may counsel a patient about the Huntington disease gene mutation because this test is not ambiguous and the gene is highly penetrant. When a genetic test shows a variation or mutation in an unusual gene region or when penetrance is reduced, the patient may best be served by counseling from a certified genetic counselor or a clinical or medical geneticist.

No matter which professional is involved in genetic counseling, a key feature of this counseling is to be "nondirective" in ensuring PATIENT-CENTERED CARE. When using a nondirective approach, the counselor provides as much information as possible about the risks and benefits but does not influence the patient's decision to test or not to test. Once the patient has made the decision, the counselor supports the patient and the decision.

Ethical Issues

ETHICS and ethical issues are involved at every level of genetic testing. Some of the most important issues focus on the patient's right to know versus the right to not know his or her gene status, confidentiality, coercion, and sharing of information.

The right to know genetic risk versus the right to not know is the individual patient's choice. Sometimes a patient's right to know has an impact on the right of another family member to not know.

Confidentiality is crucial to genetic counseling. *The results of a genetic test must remain confidential to the patient. The results cannot be given to a family member, other primary health care provider, or insurance carrier without the patient's permission.*

Coercion is possible by other family members and health care professionals. *The final decision to have genetic testing or not to have genetic testing rests with the patient.* Other people may believe it is important for the patient to have the test; however, the patient must make the decision without such pressures. As a patient advocate ensuring PATIENT-CENTERED CARE, professional ETHICS require you to assess whether the patient is freely

CHART 5-1 Best Practice for Patient Safety & Quality Care QSEN

Steps for Genetic Testing and Counseling

Pretesting Assessment and Patient Education (May Take Multiple Sessions)

- Determining patient understanding and why testing or counseling is being sought
- Determining whether testing is reasonable (considering cost of the test, specificity, probable risk, accuracy of testing)
- Establishing a trusting professional relationship
- Ensuring privacy and confidentiality
- Reviewing informed consent procedures
- Assessing the patient's ability to communicate accurately (including language issues, cognitive function, sensory perception)
- Assessing the patient's psychosocial status and availability of social support
- Taking a detailed patient health history (including drugs, diet, exercise, hormonal history, lifestyle issues)
- Obtaining physical assessment data relevant to the at-risk disorder
- Taking a detailed family history and constructing a three-generation pedigree (minimum)
- Obtaining and verifying information obtained from:
  - Patient
  - Family members
  - Medical records
  - Pathology reports
  - Death certificates
- Interpreting the family history
- Discussing the consequences of testing
- Discussing patient rights and obligations regarding disclosure of information
- Discussing testing options
- Assessing to determine whether coercion is occurring
- Obtaining material to be tested (usually blood)

Test Result Presentation

- Re-assessing the patient's wish to know or not know the test results
- Respecting the patient's decision to not know the test results
- Ensuring privacy and confidentiality
- Presenting the test results
- Interpreting the test results
- Assessing the patient's perception of the test results

Follow-Up

- Supporting the patient's decision to disclose or not disclose the information to other family members
- Discussing the potential risks for other family members
- Ensuring privacy and confidentiality
- Addressing the patient's concerns
- Discussing prevention, early detection, and treatment options
- Discussing family concerns
- Addressing psychosocial issues
- Discussing available resources for information, support, and further counseling
- Providing summary of results and consultation to the patient

Adapted from Beery, T., & Workman, M. L. (2012). *Genetics and genomics in nursing and health care*. Philadelphia: F.A. Davis.

making the decision to have genetic testing or whether someone else is urging him or her to test. This important issue can be difficult to assess. Ask the patient who in the family wants to know the results of testing.

Sharing test result information, negative or positive, can be stressful. The patient makes the final decision whether to share the information with family members. Some patients choose not to share this information, even when other family members may also be at risk. This can be difficult for the health care provider who knows that the patient has a positive test result for a serious inherited condition and that the patient chooses not to tell other family members who may be at risk (Berkman & Hull, 2014). For example, hereditary nonpolyposis colon cancer (HNPCC) has an autosomal dominant inheritance pattern, and each child of the patient has a 50% risk for having the gene. If the patient chooses not to tell his or her grown children, they then do not have the opportunity for increased screening to find the cancer at an early stage when cure is possible. Ethical dilemmas arise when the primary health care provider wants to inform the children of their risk.

THE ROLE OF THE MEDICAL-SURGICAL NURSE IN GENETIC COUNSELING

Medical-surgical nurses providing PATIENT-CENTERED CARE help patients during the assessing, testing, and counseling processes, although they do not provide in-depth genetic counseling. Patients often feel most comfortable sharing information with nurses and asking nurses to clarify information.

Nurses may be the first health care professionals to identify a patient at specific genetic risk. Some of the "red flags" that a patient may have a genetic risk for a disease or disorder are:

- The disease or disorder occurs at a higher incidence within the family compared with the general population.
- The patient or close family members have another identified genetic problem.
- The incidence of a specific disease or disorder occurs in the patient or in family members at an unusually early age.
- A rare disease is present in two or more family members.
- More than one type of cancer is present in any one adult.
- The specific physical characteristic is associated with one or more genetic disorders (e.g., unusual freckling or skin pigmentation, bicuspid aortic valve, deafness).

The nurse may be the health care professional who first verifies information to bring a genetic problem to light. For example, during an assessment a patient reveals that her mother died of bone cancer when she was 40 years old. Bone cancer is quite rare among adults; thus the nurse might then ask, "Did your mother ever have any other type of cancer?" Often the patient may then reveal that her mother had breast cancer some years before ("bone cancer" was actually breast cancer that had spread to the bones). Breast cancer at an early age can indicate a genetic predisposition.

Patients may ask questions that indicate they have an interest in genetic testing. These are examples of questions that may be cues that the patient has genetic concerns:

- Will my children get this disease?
- Because my sister has this problem, what are the chances I might also develop it?
- Is there a way to test and see whether my chances of getting this disease or problem are high or low?

There are many areas of responsibility for any medical-surgical nurse providing PATIENT-CENTERED CARE when working with a patient who is considering or having genetic testing. These areas include communication, privacy and confidentiality, information accuracy, patient advocacy, and support.

Communication

Using professional ETHICS, act as a patient advocate by ensuring that communication between the patient and whoever is providing the genetic information is clear. First assess the patient's ability to receive and process information. Can he or she see and hear clearly, or are assistive devices needed? Does the patient understand English, or will an interpreter be needed? Does the patient have adequate cognition at the time of meeting with the genetics professional, or is it impaired by medication, disease, anxiety, or fear?

If the patient appears not to understand terms or jargon during a discussion between him or her and a genetics professional, ask the professional to use common terms and examples for the patient. Verify with the patient that he or she understands or does not understand.

After any discussion about genetic risk or genetic testing, assess the patient's understanding of what was said. Ask the patient to explain, in his or her own words, what the issue means and what his or her expectations are.

Privacy and Confidentiality

Professional ETHICS require that all conversations regarding potential diagnoses or genetic testing need to occur in a private environment. The patient has the right to determine who may be a part of the discussion and can decide to exclude the primary physician and any family member from the discussion with a genetics professional. It is important that health care professionals who may be present during such discussion do not disclose information, formally or informally, without the patient's permission. It is the nurse's ethical duty and responsibility in providing PATIENT-CENTERED CARE to protect this information from improper disclosure to family members, other health care professionals, other patients, insurance providers, or anyone not specified by the patient.

Information Accuracy

Correct myths about genetic disorders and teach patients about the nature of genetic testing. In addition, help patients find accurate and helpful resource materials or websites. Medical-surgical nurses are not genetics experts and would not be expected to be the final source of definitive information; however, with interprofessional collaboration they can help ensure that the patient is referred to the correct level of genetic counseling. If you are present during the patient's discussions with a genetics professional, assess whether he or she understands the issues regarding the health problem.

Patient Advocacy and Support

Professional ETHICS require you to ensure that the patient's rights are not neglected or ignored. Ask the patient privately what his or her wishes are regarding genetic testing. Ask whether another adult or agency is insisting on the testing. Remind the patient that he or she does not have to agree to be tested. Verify that he or she has signed an informed consent statement for the test.

Considering or having genetic testing is a stressful experience. The patient and family require support and may need help with coping. Ethically genetic testing should be performed only after genetic counseling has occurred and should be followed with more counseling.

Patients may feel anger, depression, guilt, or hopelessness. Patients who have positive results (results indicating that a specific mutation is present) from genetic testing may have issues of risk for early death or disability and the possibility of having passed the risk for a health problem on to their children. Patients who have an ambiguous test result or one of unknown significance may believe that they have agonized over a decision

and spent money and still have no clear answer. Even patients who have negative genetic test results (results indicating that a specific mutation is not present) need counseling and support as part of PATIENT-CENTERED CARE. Some patients may have an unrealistic view of what a negative result means for their general health. Others may feel guilty that they were "spared" when other family members were not.

Assess the patient's response to genetic test results. Determine which coping methods were used successfully in the past. If the patient has disclosed information to family members, assess whether they can help provide support or need support themselves. Assess whether the information about positive test results has strained family relationships. Refer the patient to appropriate support groups and interprofessional counseling services.

For some positive genetic test results such as having a *BRCA1* gene mutation, the risk for developing breast cancer is high but is not a certainty. With high risk the patient needs a plan for prevention and risk reduction. One form of prevention is early detection. Thus a patient who tests positive for a *BRCA1* mutation should have at least annual mammograms and ovarian ultrasounds to detect cancer at an early stage when it is more easily cured. Provide PATIENT-CENTERED CARE by teaching the patient who has positive test results that indicate an increased risk for a specific health problem about the types of screening procedures that are available and how often screening should occur. For example, some patients at known high genetic risk for breast cancer and ovarian cancer choose the primary prevention methods of bilateral prophylactic mastectomies (surgical removal of the breasts) and oophorectomies (surgical removal of the ovaries). Although these strategies are severe, they are effective, and the patient should be informed about their availability.

Teach patients at known high risk for a specific disorder how to modify the environment to reduce risk. For example, a patient who has a specific mutation in the $\alpha 1AT$ (alpha$_1$-antitrypsin) gene is at increased risk for early-onset emphysema. The onset of emphysema is even earlier when the patient smokes or is chronically exposed to inhalation irritants. By modifying his or her environment, the disease can be delayed, or the symptoms reduced.

❓ NCLEX EXAMINATION CHALLENGE 5-3
Psychosocial Integrity

Which action(s) performed by a nurse with a client who is at increased genetic risk for a health problem is/are consistent with a "nondirective manner?" **Select all that apply.**
A. Providing only the information the client or family specifically requests
B. Skillfully directing the client and family toward the best choice that is supported by evidence-based research
C. Being present (at the client's request) when the client discloses his or her specific status to other family members
D. Presenting all facts and available options in a manner that neither promotes nor excludes any legally permitted decision or action.
E. Clarifying the client's misconception that being positive for the BRCA1 gene guarantees that the client will develop breast or ovarian cancer.
F. Filtering management options and focusing on the information that will support the decision the nurse believes is right for the individual client and family.

CLINICAL JUDGMENT CHALLENGE 5-1

Ethical and Legal; Teamwork and Collaboration QSEN

You are caring for a patient who is 48 years old and dying from ovarian cancer. Her daughter tells you that she is afraid she may be at risk for ovarian cancer because her gynecologist told her that some forms of this disease are inherited. She would like to be tested but only if her mother is positive for a BRCA1 mutation, and her mother has not been tested. She does not want to ask her mother to be tested because her mother is already in pain and would worry that she has passed on a risk for cancer. The daughter asks you if you would obtain a cheek swab from her mother without her mother's knowledge so the daughter can take it and have it tested.

1. Is the daughter's concern that she may be at risk for ovarian cancer justified? If so, how? (You may need to look up information on BRCA1 and BRCA2 mutations and ovarian cancer risk and on cost of testing.)
2. How should you respond to this request? Provide a rationale for your response.
3. Review the ethical principles in Chapter 1. Which principle(s) are in play here, and are there any unique factors? Explain your choices.
4. Which other members of the interprofessional team would be helpful in this situation to the patient, the daughter, and to you? Explain your choices.

GET READY FOR THE NCLEX® EXAMINATION!

KEY POINTS

Review these Key Points for each NCLEX Examination Client Needs Category.

Safe and Effective Care Environment

- Ensure that an adult or family with indications of an increased genetic risk for a disease or disorder is referred to an appropriate genetics professional. **QSEN: Teamwork and Collaboration**
- Advocate for the patient with regard to whether or not to have genetic testing, informed consent before testing, and sharing of test results. **QSEN: Patient-Centered Care**
- Ensure that confidentiality of genetic test results is maintained by all health care team members. **QSEN: Safety**
- Determine whether an informed consent statement was obtained before any genetic test is performed. **QSEN: Safety**

Health Promotion and Maintenance

- Identify patients and families at increased genetic risk for disease or disorder. **QSEN: Patient-Centered Care**
- Teach patients and families at known increased genetic risk for disease or disorder which types of screening procedures and schedules are most appropriate (check specific disorder chapters for the appropriate screening guidelines). **QSEN: Evidence-Based Practice**
- Teach patients and families at known increased genetic risk for disease or disorder which types of environmental modifications can reduce risk, delay disease onset, or reduce symptom severity (check specific disorder chapters for appropriate modifications). **QSEN: Evidence-Based Practice**

Psychosocial Integrity

- Assess patients who have received results of genetic testing for responses such as anger, guilt, or depression. **QSEN: Patient-Centered Care**
- Allow the patient and family who have been identified as being at increased genetic risk for serious health problems to express concerns and feelings. **QSEN: Patient-Centered Care**

- Ensure that the patient who undergoes genetic testing is appropriately counseled before testing, while waiting for test results, and after test results are obtained. **QSEN: Teamwork and Collaboration**
- Support the decision of the patient and family to have or not to have genetic counseling or testing. **QSEN: Patient-Centered Care**
- When a serious health problem with a genetic basis is found, help the patient and family locate appropriate community or Internet support groups and resources. **QSEN: Patient-Centered Care**

Physiological Integrity

- Be aware that mutations or variations in gene sequences can change the activity of a protein and have adverse effects on health.
- Keep in mind that many common adult diseases or disorders have a genetic basis (hypertension, diabetes, cancer), although some of these diseases also may occur among adults with no genetic risk.
- Remind the patient that having a gene variation that increases the risk for a disorder does not necessarily mean that the disorder will ever develop.
- Ensure that patients understand that genetic testing reveals information about their family members, as well as about themselves.
- Construct a three-generation pedigree from data obtained during the family history section of patient assessment.
- Remind patients that the results of genetic testing cannot be "taken back."
- Be prepared to assume the accepted roles of the medical-surgical nurse in genetic counseling, which include examining assessment data for indications of genetic risk, acting as a patient advocate, correcting myths about genetic disorders and genetic testing, protecting the patient's privacy and rights, and helping to ensure that the patient and family at increased genetic risk are referred to a genetics professional.

BIBLIOGRAPHY

Abbas, A., Lichtman, A., & Pillai, S. (2015). *Cellular and molecular immunology* (8th ed.). Philadelphia: Elsevier.

Badzek, L., Henaghan, M., Turner, M., & Monsen, R. (2013). Ethical, legal, and social issues in the translation of genomics into health care. *Journal of Nursing Scholarship, 45*(1), 15–24.

Berkman, B., & Hull, S. (2014). The right not to know in the genomic era: Time to break from tradition? *The American Journal of Bioethics: AJOB, 14*(3), 28–31.

Bielinski, S., Olson, J., Pathak, J., et al. (2014). Preemptive genotyping for personalized medicine: Design of the right drug, right dose, right time—using genomic data to individualize treatment protocol. *Mayo Clinic Proceedings, 89*(1), 25–33.

Blix, A. (2014). Personalized medicine, genomics, and pharmacogenomics: A primer for nurses. *Clinical Journal of Oncology Nursing, 18*(4), 437–441.

Boucher, J., Habin, K., & Underhill, M. (2014). Cancer genetics and genomics: Essentials for oncology nurses. *Clinical Journal of Oncology Nursing, 18*(3), 355–359.

Calzone, K. A., Jenkins, J., Nicol, N., Skirton, H., Feero, W. G., & Green, E. D. (2013). Relevance of genomics to healthcare and nursing practice. *Journal of Nursing Scholarship, 45*(1), 1–2.

Cheek, D., & Howington, J. (2017). Patient care in the dawn of the genomic age. *Am Nurse Today, 12*(3), 16–21.

Cheek, D., Bashore, L., & Brazeau, D. (2015). Pharmacogenomics and implications for nursing practice. *Journal of Nursing Scholarship, 47*(6), 496–504.

Conley, Y. P., Biesecker, L. G., Gonsalves, S., Merkle, C. J., Kirk, M., & Aouizerat, B. E. (2013). Current and emerging technology approaches in genomics. *Journal of Nursing Scholarship, 45*(1), 5–14.

Fisco, J., Soltis-Vaughan, B., Atwood, J., Reiser, G., & Schaefer, G. B. (2015). Adults' perceptions of genetic counseling and genetic testing. *Applied Nursing Research, 28*(1), 25–30.

Jarvis, C. (2016). *Physical examination & health assessment* (7th ed.). St. Louis: Elsevier Saunders.

Jenkins, J., Calzone, K., Caskey, S., Culp, S., Weiner, M., & Badzek, L. (2015). Methods of genomic competency integration in practice. *Journal of Nursing Scholarship, 47*(3), 200–210.

Jorde, L., Carey, J., & Bamshad, M. (2016). *Medical genetics* (5th ed.). Philadelphia: Elsevier.

Kelly, P. (2013). Pharmacogenomics: Why standard codeine doses can have serious toxicities or no therapeutic effect. *Oncology Nursing Forum, 40*(4), 322–324.

Kisor, D., Bright, D., Manion, C., & Smith, T. (2016). Pharmacogenomics: Overview of applications and relation to infusion therapy. *Journal of Infusion Nursing, 39*(3), 139–148.

Knisely, M., Carpenter, J., & Von Ah, D. (2014). Pharmacogenomics in the nursing literature: An integrative review. *Nursing Outlook, 63*(2), 285–296.

Lough, M., & Seidel, G. (2015). Legal and clinical issues in genetics and genomics. *Clinical Nurse Specialist CNS, 29*(2), 68–70.

Manuck, S., & McCaffery, J. (2014). Gene environment interaction. *Annual Review of Psychology, 65*(1), 41–70.

McCance, K., Huether, S., Brashers, V., & Rote, N. (2014). *Pathophysiology: The biologic basis for disease in adults and children* (7th ed.). St. Louis: Elsevier.

Munroe, T., & Loerzel, V. (2016). Assessing nursing students' knowledge of genomic concepts and readiness for use in practice. *Nurse Educator, 41*(2), 86–89.

Paz De Jesus, M., & Mitchel, M. (2016). Today's nurses need genetics education. *Nursing, 46*(10), 68.

Plavskin, A. (2016). Genetics and genomics of pathogens: Fighting infections with genome-sequencing technology. *Medsurg Nursing, 25*(2), 91–96.

Quigley, P. (2015). Mapping the human genome: Implications for practice. *Nursing, 45*(9), 27–33.

Williams, J., & Cashion, A. (2015). Using clinical genomics in health care: Strategies to create a prepared workforce. *Nursing Outlook, 63*(5), 607–609.

6 | CHAPTER

Rehabilitation Concepts for Chronic and Disabling Health Problems

Michelle Camicia and Donna D. Ignatavicius

e http://evolve.elsevier.com/Iggy/

PRIORITY AND INTERRELATED CONCEPTS

The priority concepts for this chapter are:
- MOBILITY
- ELIMINATION
- COGNITION

The interrelated concepts for this chapter are:
- TISSUE INTEGRITY
- NUTRITION
- SENSORY PERCEPTION
- HEALTH CARE ORGANIZATIONS

LEARNING OUTCOMES

Safe and Effective Care Environment

1. Identify the roles of each member of the collaborative interprofessional rehabilitation team.
2. Identify HEALTH CARE ORGANIZATIONS where rehabilitation care is provided.
3. Delegate and supervise selected nursing tasks as part of care for the rehabilitation patient.
4. Coordinate recommendations for home modifications and care coordination/transition management with the patient, family, occupational therapist, and case manager.
5. Explain how to use safe patient handling practices based on current evidence to prevent self-injury.

Health Promotion and Maintenance

6. Develop a teaching plan to prevent complications for the rehabilitation patient who has decreased MOBILITY, including impaired TISSUE INTEGRITY.

Psychosocial Integrity

7. Assess the patient's response to chronic or disabling health problems.

8. Identify special considerations for older adults undergoing rehabilitative care, including assessment of cognition.

Physiological Integrity

9. Interpret health assessment findings to plan appropriate collaborative care for the rehabilitation patient in the acute or long-term care setting.
10. Assess the ability of patients to use assistive/adaptive devices to promote MOBILITY and SENSORY PERCEPTION.
11. Identify the role of NUTRITION in the care of the patient in a rehabilitation setting.
12. Plan interventions to prevent impaired TISSUE INTEGRITY for rehabilitation patients.
13. Differentiate retraining methods for a patient with a spastic versus flaccid bladder and bowel to promote ELIMINATION.

Rehabilitation is a philosophy of practice and an attitude toward caring for people with disabilities and chronic health problems (Larsen, 2011). The practice of rehabilitation nursing is recognized as the specialty of managing the care of people with disabilities and chronic health conditions across the lifespan. A **disabling health condition** is any physical or mental health/behavioral health problem that can cause disability. A **chronic health condition** is one that has existed for at least 3 months. This text focuses primarily on physical health problems; psychosocial health problems are integrated throughout the text as

needed to describe whole-person care. They are discussed in more detail in textbooks on mental health/behavioral health nursing.

Patients with chronic and disabling health conditions need the integration of rehabilitation nursing concepts into their care, regardless of setting, to prevent further disability, maintain function, and restore individuals to optimal functioning in their community. This desired outcome requires care coordination and collaboration with the interprofessional health care team.

OVERVIEW

Chronic and Disabling Health Conditions

Chronic diseases and conditions are among the most common, costly, and preventable of all health problems in the United States. Eighty-six percent of all health care spending in 2010 was for people with one or more chronic health conditions (Gerteis et al., 2014). The rate of chronic and disabling conditions is expected to increase as more "baby boomers" approach late adulthood.

Stroke, coronary artery disease, cancer, chronic obstructive pulmonary disease (COPD), asthma, and arthritis are common chronic diseases that can result in varying degrees of disability. Most occur in people older than 65 years. However, younger adults are living longer with potentially disabling genetic disorders that in the past would have shortened life expectancy. Some of these more common disorders are discussed throughout this text.

Chronic and disabling conditions are not always illnesses (e.g., heart disease); they may also result from accidents. Accidents are a leading cause of trauma and death among young and middle-age adults. Increasing numbers of people survive accidents with severe injuries because of advances in medical technology and safety equipment such as motor vehicle airbags. As a result, they are often faced with chronic, disabling neurologic conditions such as traumatic brain injury (TBI) and spinal cord injury (SCI). Because people are living longer with chronic and disabling health problems, the need for rehabilitation is increasing!

♥ VETERANS' HEALTH CONSIDERATIONS

Patient-Centered Care QSEN

Combat in war is another major source of major disability. Many military men and women who served in recent wars such as those in Iraq and Afghanistan have one or more physical or mental health/behavioral health disabilities, most commonly TBI, single or multiple limb amputations, and post-traumatic stress disorder (PTSD). There is also a large population of veterans living with disabilities from wars of the past. These disabilities require months to years of follow-up rehabilitation after returning to the community. *Physical* veteran disabilities are described in this text; PTSD is discussed in your mental health/behavioral health book.

Rehabilitation Settings

Many people with chronic and disabling conditions live independently or with assistance in the community. For example, a new-onset illness such as a stroke may require post-acute care (PAC) following the initial hospitalization for rehabilitation. This continuing care can be in an acute inpatient rehabilitation facility (IRF), skilled nursing facility (SNF), long-term acute care (LTAC) facility, or home health agency (HHA). Rehabilitation in each of these HEALTH CARE ORGANIZATIONS seeks to maximize the function of the individual impacted by the injury or chronic condition. Each of these care settings varies in the amount and type of rehabilitation and the nursing, health care provider, and other services offered.

Individuals requiring rehabilitation are referred to as *clients, patients,* or *residents,* depending on the setting. For the purpose of consistency within this text, the term *patient* is used throughout this chapter. *However, be sure to refer to individuals in rehabilitation programs by the term that is consistent with the setting and according to patient preference to be patient centered.*

The determination of the right level of PAC for an individual must be based on the individual's biopsychosocial and ecological assessment (Camicia et al., 2014). Factors that are considered include biological, social, financial, environmental, and systems factors. Biological factors include the individual's medical needs, pre-injury or pre-illness level of function, and tolerance of rehabilitation. Social factors include psychological, informal, and formal community supports. Other important considerations are financial resources and stressors and the physical environment of the community living setting. Systems factors include the components of care and services, the intensity of service provision (e.g., number of hours of nursing care or therapy), and the structure and process of the program. The PAC setting must be matched to the patients' needs. The nurse coordinates care from acute through community-based care to ensure the person's optimal function and participation in the community.

Rehabilitation care occurs on a continuum. The intensity of services decreases across the continuum from the inpatient rehabilitation facility (IRF) or skilled nursing facility (SNF) to home health to comprehensive ambulatory care (outpatient) programs. The most resource-intensive level of PAC is the IRF. These HEALTH CARE ORGANIZATIONS are freestanding rehabilitation hospitals or rehabilitation units within hospitals. **Skilled nursing facilities (SNFs)** are part of either a hospital or long-term care (nursing home) setting (Fig. 6-1). For older adults in the United States, rehabilitation services for the first 100 days of inpatient care are paid by Medicare A.

Individuals in skilled nursing facilities, custodial nursing homes, and assisted-living facilities are called *residents.* The term **resident** implies that the person lives in the facility and has all the rights of anyone living in his or her home. Residents wear street clothes rather than hospital gowns and have choices in what they eat and how they plan each day.

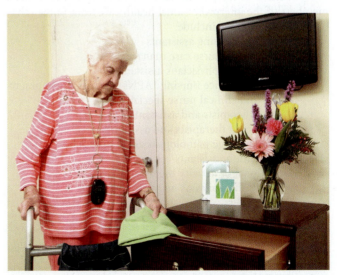

FIG. 6-1 Patient (resident) in a skilled nursing facility rehabilitation unit. (From Kostelnick, C. [2015]. *Mosby's textbook for long-term care nursing assistants* [7th ed.]. St. Louis: Mosby.)

Ambulatory care rehabilitation departments and home rehabilitation programs may be needed for continuing less-intensive services. Some agencies have specialized clinics focused on rehabilitation of patients with specific health problems such as those that care for individuals with strokes; amputations; and large, chronic, and/or nonhealing wounds.

People who are able to rehabilitate to independence or who have a caregiver and a home without environmental barriers are able to return home following a disabling medical event. Home for older adults is often in senior citizens' housing units, their family's home, or assisted-living facilities. Part-time rehabilitation services may be provided in any of these home settings by a variety of health care professionals. These services may be reimbursed by Medicare B or other private health insurance.

Alternative living settings include a board-and-care facility or transitional living apartment. Group homes are facilities in which individuals live independently together with other people with disabilities. Each patient or group of patients has a care provider such as a personal care aide to assist with ADLs. The patients may or may not be actively employed. In some cases the care home offers employment opportunities to the residents. The purpose of these homes is to provide independent living arrangements outside an institution, especially for younger people with TBI or SCI.

The desired outcome of rehabilitation is that the patient will return to the best possible physical, mental, social, vocational, and economic capacity. Rehabilitation is not limited to the return of function in post-traumatic situations. It also includes education and therapy for any chronic conditions characterized by a change in a body system function or body structure. Rehabilitation programs related to respiratory, cardiac, and musculoskeletal health problems are common examples that do not involve trauma.

The Rehabilitation Interprofessional Team

Successful rehabilitation depends on the coordinated team effort of the patient, family, and health care professionals in planning, implementing, and evaluating care. The focus of the interprofessional rehabilitation team is to restore and maintain the patient's function to the greatest extent possible.

In addition to the patient, family, and/or significant others, members of the interprofessional health care team in the rehabilitation setting may include:

- Nurses and nursing assistants
- Rehabilitation nurse case managers
- Physicians and physicians assistants
- Advanced practice nursing (APNs) such as nurse practitioners and clinical nurse specialists
- Physical therapists and assistants
- Occupational therapists and assistants
- Speech-language pathologists and assistants
- Rehabilitation assistants/restorative aides
- Recreational or activity therapists
- Cognitive therapists or neuropsychologists
- Social workers
- Clinical psychologists
- Vocational counselors
- Spiritual care counselors
- Registered dietitians (RDs)
- Pharmacists

Not all settings that offer rehabilitation services have all of these members on their team. Not all patients require the services of

all health care team members. The team should be comprised of providers who are clinically indicated for each patient.

Rehabilitation nurses in the inpatient setting coordinate the collaborative plan of care and therefore function as the patient's case manager. Nurses also create a rehabilitation milieu, which includes:

- Allowing time for patients to practice self-management skills
- Encouraging patients and providing emotional support
- Protecting patients from embarrassment (e.g., bowel training)
- Making the inpatient unit a more homelike environment

Table 6-1 summarizes the nurse's role as part of the rehabilitation team. Because of an increase in the need for older-adult rehabilitation, some nurses specialize in gerontologic rehabilitation. Nurses and other health care professionals may be designated as *rehabilitation case managers. Advanced practice nurses (APNs)* are masters- and doctorate-prepared nurses who function independently or under the supervision of a physician, depending on the rules and regulations of the state or province.

As their name implies, *nursing assistants* or *nursing technicians* assist in the physical care of patients. These members of the rehabilitation team function under the direct supervision of the registered nurse (RN) or licensed practical or vocational nurse (LPN or LVN).

A physician who specializes in rehabilitative medicine is called a **physiatrist**. Physiatrists oversee the rehabilitation medical plan of care from the emergency department, intensive care unit, telemetry unit, and medical surgical unit into the community. The physiatrist is the attending physician at the IRF with consultation from general practitioners. They may also provide consultation in the SNF. *Physician assistants (PAs)* work under the supervision of the physician.

Physical therapists (PTs), also called *physiotherapists,* intervene to help the patient achieve self-management by focusing on *gross* MOBILITY skills (e.g., by facilitating ambulation and teaching the patient to use an assistive device such as a walker) (Fig. 6-2). They may also teach techniques for performing activities such as transferring (e.g., moving into and out of bed),

TABLE 6-1   Nurse's Role in the Rehabilitation Team

- Advocates for the patient and family
- Creates a therapeutic rehabilitation milieu
- Provides and coordinates whole-person patient care in a variety of health care settings, including the home
- Collaborates with the rehabilitation team to establish expected patient outcomes to develop a plan of care
- Coordinates rehabilitation team activities to ensure implementation of the plan of care
- Acts as a resource to the rehabilitation team who has specialized knowledge and clinical skills needed to care for patient with chronic and disabling health problems
- Communicates effectively with all members of the rehabilitation team, including the patient and family
- Plans continuity of care when the patient is discharged from the health care facility
- Evaluates the effectiveness of the interprofessional plan of care for the patient and family

Adapted from Association of Rehabilitation Nurses. (2008). *Standards and scope of rehabilitation nursing practice,* Glenview, IL: Author.

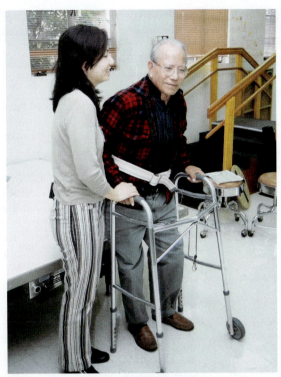

FIG. 6-2 A physical therapist helping a patient ambulate with a walker.

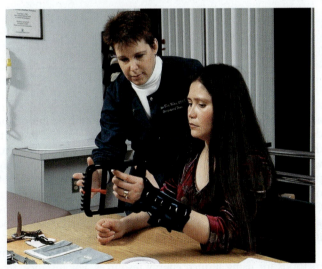

FIG. 6-3 A registered occupational therapist working with a patient on improving hand strength.

ambulating, and toileting. In some settings PTs play a major role in providing wound care and cognitive retraining. Physical therapy assistants (PTAs) may be employed to help the PT.

Occupational therapists (OTs) work to develop the patient's *fine* motor skills used for ADL self-management such as those required for eating, hygiene, grooming, and dressing. They also teach patients how to perform independent living skills such as cooking and shopping. To accomplish these outcomes, OTs teach skills related to coordination (e.g., hand movements) and cognitive retraining (Fig. 6-3). Occupational therapy assistants (OTAs) may be available to help the OT.

Speech-language pathologists (SLPs) evaluate and retrain patients with speech, language, or swallowing problems. *Speech* is the ability to say words, and *language* is the ability to understand and put words together in a meaningful way. Some patients, especially those who have experienced a head injury or stroke, have difficulty with both speech and language. Those who have had a stroke also may have dysphagia (difficulty with swallowing). SLPs provide screening and testing for dysphagia. If the patient has this problem, the SLP recommends appropriate foods and eating techniques. Speech-language pathology assistants (SLPAs) may be employed to help the SLP.

PTs, OTs, and SLPs are collectively referred to as **rehabilitation therapists**. Assistants to PTs, OTs, and SLPs are called **rehabilitation assistants**. In long-term care settings, *restorative aides* may enhance the therapy team to continue the rehabilitation therapy plan of care when therapists are not available.

Recreational or *activity therapists* work to help patients continue or develop hobbies or interests. These activities may also contribute to strengthening fine motor skills.

Cognitive therapists, usually neuropsychologists, work primarily with patients who have experienced a stroke, brain injury, brain tumor, or other condition resulting in cognitive impairment. Computer programs are often used to assist with cognitive retraining.

Various professionals promote community reintegration of the patient and acceptance of the disability or chronic conditions. For example, *social workers* help patients identify support services and resources, including financial assistance. *Clinical psychologists* assess and diagnose mental health/behavioral health or COGNITION issues resulting from the disability or chronic condition and help both the patient and family identify strategies to foster coping. *Spiritual counselors* specialize in spiritual assessments and care and are able to address the needs of a wide array of patient preferences and beliefs.

Vocational counselors help with job placement, training, or further education. Work-related skills are taught if the patient needs to change careers because of the disability. If the patient has not yet completed high school, tutors may help with completion of the requirements for graduation.

Registered dietitians (RDs) help ensure that patients meet their needs for NUTRITION. For example, for patients who need weight reduction, a restricted-calorie diet can be planned. For patients who need additional calories or other nutrients, including vitamins, dietitians can plan a patient-specific diet.

Pharmacists collaborate with the other members of the health care team to ensure that the patient receives the most appropriate drug therapy, if required. They oversee the prescription and preparation of medications and provide the interprofessional team with essential information regarding drug safety, interactions, and side effects.

Depending on the patient's health care needs, additional team members may be included in the rehabilitation program such as the geriatrician, respiratory therapist, and prosthetist. Interprofessional team conferences for planning care and evaluating the patient's progress are held regularly with the patient, family and significant others, and the health care team.

❖ INTERPROFESSIONAL COLLABORATIVE CARE
◆ Assessment: Noticing

History. Collect the history of the patient's present condition, any current medications (prescribed and over the counter [OTC]), and any treatment programs in progress. Begin by obtaining general background data about the patient and family. This information includes cultural and spiritual

NCLEX EXAMINATION CHALLENGE 6-1

Psychosocial Integrity

A client who can't move his right leg or arm tells the nurse: "Life is over for me. I don't want to live if I'm going to be a burden to everyone." What is the nurse's **best** action?
A. Report the client's concern to the primary health care provider.
B. Consult with the clinical psychologist or social worker.
C. Share the client's feelings with the family.
D. Refer the client to the vocational counselor.

practices and the patient's home environment and support system. In collaboration with the occupational therapist, the nurse or case manager assesses the physical layout of the home and determines whether the layout, including stairs or the width of doorways, will present architectural barriers for the patient after discharge.

Assess the patient's usual daily schedule and habits of everyday living. These data include hygiene practices, nutrition, elimination, sexual activity, and sleep. Ask about the patient's preferred method and time for bathing and hygiene. In assessing dietary patterns, note food likes and dislikes. Also obtain information about the patient's bowel and bladder function and the usual pattern of elimination.

In assessing sexuality patterns, ask about changes in sexual function since the onset of the disability. The patient's current and previous sleep habits, patterns, usual number of hours of sleep, and use of hypnotics are also determined. Question whether the patient feels well rested after sleep. Sleep patterns have a significant impact on activity patterns. The assessment of activity patterns focuses on work, exercise, and recreational activities.

CONSIDERATIONS FOR OLDER ADULTS

Patient-Centered Care QSEN

Older adults who need rehabilitation often have other chronic diseases that need to be managed, including diabetes mellitus, coronary artery disease, osteoporosis, and arthritis. These health problems, added to the normal physiologic changes associated with aging, predispose older adults to secondary complications such as falls, pressure injuries, and pneumonia. When discharged from the acute care setting, some older patients are undernourished, which causes weakness and fatigue. The longer the hospital stay, the more debilitated the older adult can become. For some patients severe undernutrition results in decreased serum albumin and prealbumin, causing third spacing. Assess the older adult for generalized edema, especially in the lower extremities. Be sure to collaborate with the RD to improve the patient's nutritional status, with a focus on increasing protein intake that is needed for healing and decreasing edema.

Health teaching may be challenging because some older patients may have beginning changes in COGNITION, including short-term memory loss. Sensory loss, like vision and hearing, may also affect their ability to give an accurate history or grasp new information.

Physical Assessment/Signs and Symptoms. On admission for baseline and at least daily (depending on agency policy and type of setting), collect physical assessment data systematically according to major body systems (Table 6-2). The primary focus of the assessment related to rehabilitation and chronic disease is the *functional* abilities of the patient.

Cardiovascular and Respiratory Assessment. An alteration in cardiac status may affect the patient's cardiac output or cause

TABLE 6-2	Assessment of Patients in Rehabilitation Settings	
BODY SYSTEM	**RELEVANT DATA**
Cardiovascular system	Chest pain Fatigue Fear of heart failure
Respiratory system	Shortness of breath or dyspnea Activity tolerance Fear of inability to breathe
Gastrointestinal system and nutrition	Oral intake, eating pattern Anorexia, nausea, and vomiting Dysphagia Laboratory data (e.g., serum prealbumin level) Weight loss or gain Bowel elimination pattern or habits Change in stool (constipation or diarrhea) Ability to get to toilet
Renal-urinary system	Urinary pattern Fluid intake Urinary incontinence or retention Urine culture and urinalysis
Neurologic system	Motor function Sensation Perceptual ability Cognitive abilities
Musculoskeletal system	Functional ability Range of motion Endurance Muscle strength
Integumentary system	Risk for skin breakdown Presence of skin lesions

activity intolerance. Assess associated signs and symptoms of decreased cardiac output (e.g., chest pain, fatigue). If present, determine when the patient experiences these symptoms and what relieves them. The primary health care provider may prescribe a change in drug therapy or a prophylactic dose of nitroglycerin to be taken before the patient resumes activities. Collaborate with the primary health care provider and appropriate therapists to determine whether activities need to be modified.

For the patient showing fatigue, the nurse and patient plan methods for using limited energy resources. For instance, frequent rest periods can be taken throughout the day, especially before performing activities. Major tasks might be performed in the morning because most people have the most energy at that time. The nurse must communicate needs for breaks in the therapy schedule for rest as needed. Schedule nursing care according to the patient's need for rest.

Ask the patient whether he or she has shortness of breath, chest pain, or severe weakness and fatigue during or after activity. *Determine the level of activity that can be accomplished without these symptoms.* For example, can the patient climb one flight of stairs without shortness of breath, or does shortness of breath occur after climbing only two steps?

Gastrointestinal and Nutritional Assessment. Monitor the patient's oral intake and pattern of eating. Assess for the presence of anorexia, dysphagia, nausea, vomiting, or discomfort that may interfere with oral intake. Determine whether the patient wears dentures and, if so, assess the fit. Review the patient's height, weight, hemoglobin and hematocrit levels, serum prealbumin and albumin, and blood glucose levels. (See Chapter 60 for discussion of how to perform a screening for NUTRITION status and Chapter 2 for a description of basic nutritional assessments.) Weight loss or weight gain is particularly significant and may be related to an associated disease or to the conditions that caused the disability.

Bowel ELIMINATION habits vary from person to person. They are often related to daily job or activity schedules, dietary patterns, age, and family or cultural background. Ask about usual bowel patterns before the injury or the illness. Note any changes in the patient's bowel routine or stool consistency. The most common problem for rehabilitation patients is constipation.

If the patient reports any alteration in ELIMINATION pattern, try to determine whether it is caused by a change in diet, activity pattern, or medication use. Always assess bowel habits on what is normal for that person.

Ask whether the patient can manage bowel function independently. Independence in bowel elimination requires adequate cognition, manual dexterity, sensation, muscle control, and mobility. If the patient requires help, determine whether someone is available at home to provide it. Also assess the patient's and family's ability to cope with any dependency in bowel elimination. Assessment of ELIMINATION is summarized in Chapter 2.

Renal and Urinary Assessment. Ask about the patient's baseline urinary ELIMINATION patterns, including the number of voidings. Determine whether he or she routinely awakens during the night to empty the bladder (nocturia) or sleeps through the night. Record fluid intake patterns and volume, including the type of fluids ingested and the time they were consumed.

Question whether the patient has ever had any problems with urinary incontinence or retention. Monitor laboratory reports, especially the results of the urinalysis and culture and sensitivity, if needed. *Urinary tract infections (UTIs) among older adults are often missed because acute confusion may be the only indicator of the infection.* Unfortunately some health care professionals expect older patients to be confused and may not detect this problem. If untreated, UTIs can lead to kidney infection and possible failure.

Neurologic and Musculoskeletal Assessment. The neurologic assessment includes motor function (MOBILITY), SENSORY PERCEPTION, and COGNITION. Chapter 2 reviews general assessment of these concepts. Assess the patient's pre-existing problems, general physical condition, and communication abilities. Patients may have dysphasia (slurred speech) because of facial muscle weakness or aphasia (inability to speak or comprehend) because of brain damage commonly occurring in those with a stroke or traumatic brain injury (TBI). These communication problems are discussed in detail in the chapters on problems of the nervous system.

Determine if the patient has paresis (weakness) or paralysis (absence of movement). Observe the patient's gait. Identify changes in SENSORY PERCEPTION such as visual acuity that could contribute to risk for injury. Assess his or her response to light touch, hot or cold temperature, and position change in each extremity and on the trunk. For a perceptual assessment, evaluate the patient's ability to receive and understand what is heard and seen and the ability to express appropriate motor and verbal responses. During this part of the assessment, begin to assess short-term and long-term memory.

Assess the patient's cognitive abilities, especially if there is a head injury or stroke. Several tools are available to evaluate COGNITION. One of the most commonly used tools in rehabilitation and long-term care settings is the Brief Interview for Mental Status (BIMS), which is described in Chapter 41. The Confusion Assessment Method (CAM) is used to determine if the patient has delirium, an acute confusional state. (See Chapter 3 for description of the CAM tool.)

As with other body systems, nursing assessment of the musculoskeletal system focuses on function. Assess the patient's musculoskeletal status; response to the impairment; and demands of the home, work, or school environment. Determine his or her endurance level and measure active and passive joint range of motion (ROM). Review the results of manual muscle testing by physical therapy, which identifies the patient's ROM and resistance against gravity. In this procedure the therapist determines the degree of muscle strength present in each body segment.

Skin and Tissue Integrity Assessment. Identify actual or potential interruptions in skin and TISSUE INTEGRITY. Chapter 2 reviews the general assessment of this concept. To maintain healthy skin, the body must have adequate food, water, and oxygen intake; intact waste-removal mechanisms; sensation; and functional MOBILITY. Changes in any of these variables can lead to rapid and extensive skin breakdown.

If a pressure injury or other change in TISSUE INTEGRITY develops, accurately assess the problem and its possible causes. In the inpatient setting inspect the skin every 8 to 12 hours. Teach the patient or caregiver to inspect the skin daily at home. Measure the depth and diameter of any open skin areas in inches or centimeters, depending on the policy of the facility or country. Assess the area around the open lesion to determine the presence of cellulitis or other tissue damage. Chapter 25 includes several widely used classification systems for assessing skin breakdown. Determine the patient's knowledge about the cause and treatment of skin breakdown and his or her ability to inspect the skin and participate in maintaining TISSUE INTEGRITY.

In most health care agencies the skin assessment is documented on a special form or part of the electronic health record to keep track of each area of skin breakdown. A baseline assessment is conducted on admission and updated periodically, depending on organization policy, and more frequently as indicated. In most long-term care, acute care, and rehabilitation settings and with the patient's (or family's if the patient cannot communicate) permission, photographs of the skin are taken on admission and at various intervals to pictorially document the appearance of the wound.

❓ NCLEX EXAMINATION CHALLENGE 6-2
Physiological Integrity

The nurse performs an admission assessment for an older adult following a fractured hip repair. Which priority client assessment findings will require the nurse to collaborate with members of the interprofessional health team? **Select all that apply.**

A. Mild dependent edema in both ankles when sitting
B. Chest pain when ambulating with the walker
C. Lack of appetite and weight loss
D. Report of joint pain at a 8 on a 0-10 intensity scale
E. Dry and itchy skin over legs and arms

Assessment of Functional Ability. *Functional ability* refers to the ability to perform activities of daily living (ADLs) such as bathing, dressing, eating, using the toilet, and ambulating. Instrumental activities of daily living (IADLs) refer to activities necessary for living in the community such as using the telephone, shopping, preparing food, and housekeeping. Functional assessment tools are used to assess a patient's abilities. Rehabilitation nurses, physiatrists, or rehabilitation therapists complete assessment tools to document functional levels. The Centers for Medicare and Medicaid (CMS) require cross-setting assessment measures to evaluate a patient's function, regardless of the post-acute care (PAC) setting where they receive rehabilitation. These tools include functional assessment items for self-care and mobility on the Inpatient Rehabilitation Facility Patient Assessment Instrument (IRF-PAI) used in the IRF, the Minimum Data Set (MDS) used in the SNF (Table 6-3), and the Outcome and Assessment Information Set (OASIS) used in home health agencies. These assessments are also used for reimbursement from the CMS in the United States.

Another commonly used classic assessment tool is the Functional Independence Measure (FIM) developed by Granger and Gresham (1984). This tool is intended to measure the burden of care for a patient, not what a person should do or how the person would perform under different circumstances. Categories for assessment are self-care, sphincter control, MOBILITY and locomotion, communication, and COGNITION. Scoring is a 1-to-7 scale, in which 1 is dependent and 7 is independent. Each score has a definition for every item. The patient is evaluated when he or she is admitted to and discharged from a rehabilitation provider and at other specified times to determine progress toward desired outcomes (also referred to as *goals)*. The FIM system has also been adapted for use in across-care settings, including acute care and home care, and is available in multiple languages.

Psychosocial Assessment. In addition to determining COGNITION, assess the patient's body image and self-esteem through verbal indicators and descriptions of self-care. Encourage the family to allow the patient to perform as many functions as possible independently to build feelings of self-worth.

Assess the patient's use of defense mechanisms and manifestations of anxiety. If indicated, ask him or her to describe feelings concerning the loss of a body part or function. Assess for the presence of any stress-related physical problem. Some patients have symptoms of depression such as fatigue, a change in appetite, or feelings of powerlessness. See Chapter 7 for a thorough discussion of loss and grieving and Chapter 3 for a brief discussion of depression among the older-adult population.

⊕ CULTURAL/SPIRITUAL CONSIDERATIONS
Patient-Centered Care

> Determine the availability of support systems for the patient. The major support system is typically the family or significant others; those who do not have these support systems are more likely to develop depression. Ask patients what is important to them and gives meaning to their lives. Identify the patient's cultural, spiritual, and/or religious needs and refer to an appropriate health care team member as needed. Assess sexuality and intimacy needs.

Vocational Assessment. Patients in the United States should be informed about the Americans with Disabilities Act, which was passed by Congress in 1991 to prevent employer discrimination against people with disabilities. The employer must offer *reasonable* assistance to an employee with a disability to allow him or her to perform the job. For example, if an employee has a severe hearing loss, the employer may need to hire a sign language interpreter.

The rehabilitation team assesses the cognitive and physical demands of the patient's job to determine whether he or she can return to the position or if retraining in another field is necessary. The physical demands of jobs range from light in sedentary occupations (0 to 10 lb [4.54 kg] often lifted) to heavy (more than 100 lb [45.45 kg] often lifted). The nurse must also consider other required aspects of the job such as MOBILITY or SENSORY PERCEPTION (e.g., hearing).

Job analysis also involves assessing the work environment of the patient's former or current job. Collaborate with the vocational counselor to determine whether the environment is conducive to the patient's return to work because job modifications may be needed. If an injured worker requires vocational rehabilitation, refer him or her to vocational rehabilitation personnel to evaluate skills and necessary skill development. In most states Workers' Compensation insurance helps support vocational rehabilitation.

◆ Analysis: Interpreting

Regardless of age or specific disability, these priority patient problems are common. Additional problems depend on the patient's specific chronic condition or disability. The priority collaborative problems for patients with chronic and disabling health conditions typically include:

1. Decreased mobility due to neuromuscular impairment, sensory-perceptual impairment, and/or chronic pain
2. Decreased functional ability due to neuromuscular impairment and/or impairment in perception or cognition
3. Risk for pressure injury due to altered sensation and/or altered nutritional state
4. Urinary incontinence or urinary retention due to neurologic dysfunction and/or trauma or disease affecting spinal cord nerves
5. Constipation due to neurologic impairment, inadequate nutrition, or decreased mobility

---

TABLE 6-3 Assessment Components of the Minimum Data Set (MDS) 3.0

- Hearing, Speech, and Vision
- Cognitive Patterns
- Mood
- Behavior
- Preferences for Customary Routines and Activities
- Functional Status
- Bowel and Bladder
- Active Disease Diagnoses
- Health Conditions (e.g., pain, fall history)
- Swallowing and Nutritional Status
- Oral/Dental Status
- Skin Condition
- Medications
- Special Treatments and Procedures
- Restraints
- Participation in Assessment and Goal Setting
- Supplemental Therapies

Data from Centers for Medicare and Medicaid Services (CMS). *MDS 3.0 for nursing homes and swing bed providers*, 2013, http://www.cms.gov/Medicare/Quality-Initiatives-Patient-Assessment-Instruments/NursingHomeQualityInits/NHQIMDS30.html.

◆ Planning and Implementation: Responding

Increasing Mobility

Planning: Expected Outcomes. The patient with chronic conditions or a disability is expected to reach the highest level of physical MOBILITY that can be obtained with or without assistive devices. The patient is also expected to be free of complications of immobility.

Interventions. Most problems requiring rehabilitation relate to decreased or impaired physical MOBILITY. For example, patients with neurologic disease or injury, amputations, arthritis, and cardiopulmonary disease usually experience some degree of mobility impairment. Coordinate care with physical and occupational therapists as the key rehabilitation team members in helping patients meet their mobility outcomes. Complications of decreased MOBILITY or immobility and how to help prevent them are described in Chapter 2.

Safe Patient Handling and Mobility Practices. Before they learn to become independent, patients with decreased MOBILITY in any health care setting or at home often need assistance with positioning in bed and transfers such as from a bed to a chair, commode, or wheelchair. Patients may not be able to bear full weight, may have inadequate balance, and/or may be very obese. For many years nurses relied on "body mechanics" to prevent staff injury when moving patients or helping them move. This traditional, but outdated, approach was based on the belief that correct body positioning by staff members would protect them from the force of lifting and moving.

Heavy lifting and dependent transfers by staff members have resulted in a very high incidence of **work-related musculoskeletal disorders (MSDs)**, most often chronic back and shoulder injuries, which can be prevented (see the Quality Improvement box). As a response to this costly problem, the National Institute for Occupational Safety and Health (NIOSH) established evidence-based guidelines for safe patient handling. Based on this document, the American Nurses Association, in partnership with NIOSH and the Veterans Health Administration, developed a curriculum for all nursing students and practicing nurses on how to safely handle and move patients in any health care setting or home environment (American Nurses Association, 2012). In addition, the Association of Rehabilitation Nurses (ARN), in collaboration with the American Physical Therapy Association (APTA), the American Occupational Therapy Association (AOTA), and the Veteran's Health Administration, outlined strategies that improve patient and health care provider safety in patient handling and movement tasks. In collaboration with other interprofessional team members, nurses must assess patient mobility and use best practices for safe patient handling and mobility (SPHM).

Because each patient has unique needs and characteristics, assess his or her mobility level using a standardized tool to plan interventions for SPHM. An example of an appropriate assessment tool for this purpose is shown in Fig. 6-4. Before moving the patient, assess his or her environment for potential hazards that could cause injury such as a slippery or uneven floor.

Use these general SPHM practices and teach staff members to:

- Maintain a wide, stable base with your feet
- Put the bed at the correct height—waist level while providing direct care and hip level when moving patients

QUALITY IMPROVEMENT QSEN

Do Safe Handling Practices Protect Health Care Staff from Personal Injury?

Kennedy, B. & Kopp, T. (2015). Safe handling protects employees too. *Nursing, 45*(8), 65–67.

During clinical rounds the nursing leaders of a large southeastern acute care hospital identified problems related to employee injuries, patient falls, and hospital-acquired pressure injuries. An interprofessional team was formed to develop an improvement process to decrease these problems and reduce workers' compensation costs. Using the American Nurses Association's best practice guidelines, a proposal to purchase over $1 million of equipment such as ceiling-mounted mechanical lifts and friction-reducing slides and aids was approved. The equipment vendor worked with the improvement team to create a culture of safety and establish transfer mobility coaches to support the culture change. All nursing staff members were educated on how to use the new equipment correctly, and ongoing continuing education was provided each month.

As a result of implementing these interventions, the average number of monthly employee injuries decreased from 4.58 to 1.9. The monthly cost for workers' compensation decreased by more than $2000. In addition, patient falls declined, and the number of pressure injuries was reduced by 50% in the first year of the new program as a result of less shearing and skin tears.

Commentary: Implications for Research and Practice

This change project was very successful at improving patient outcomes and reducing staff injuries. Strong administrative, financial, and interprofessional support was essential in meeting the project's outcomes. This QI project needs to be implemented in other health care organizations for comparison with the reported positive outcomes.

- Keep the patient or work directly in front of you to prevent your spine from rotating
- Keep the patient as close to your body as possible to prevent reaching

The Veterans Health Administration and many other health care systems follow a no-lift or limited-lift policy for all of their facilities. This means that nurses and therapists either rely on the patient to independently move and transfer or use a powered, mechanical full-body lift that is either ceiling- or wall-mounted or portable (mobile) (Fig. 6-5). Most lifts use slings that are comfortable, safe, and easy to apply. Electric-powered, portable sit-to-stand devices are also available. Mechanical lifts are also available for home use.

For patients who are learning to become independent in transfer or bed MOBILITY skills, the physical or occupational therapist usually specifies the procedure for these maneuvers. For example, a patient with quadriplegia may use a sliding board for transfer, whereas a patient with paraplegia may be able to transfer when the wheelchair arms are removed. A patient may be taught to turn independently using the side rails. In any case, for safety always plan or teach the patient to plan the transfer technique before initiating it. The desired outcome is that the patient will eventually be able to transfer safely, providing their maximum effort while assistance is provided by equipment and caregivers as needed.

Weight gain is another potential problem when rehabilitation patients have decreased MOBILITY. Excessive weight hinders transfers both for the nurse or the therapist who is assisting and for the patient who is learning to transfer independently. Weight

Assessment Tool and Care Plan for Safe Patient Handling and Movement

I. Patient's Level of Assistance
_____Independent—Patient performs task safely, with or without staff assistance, with or without assistive devices.
_____Partial Assist—Patient requires no more help than standby, cueing, or coaxing, or caregiver is required to lift no more than 35 lb of a patient's weight.
_____Dependent—Patient requires nurse to lift more than 35 lb of the patient's weight, or patient is unpredictable in the amount of assistance offered. In this case, assistive devices should be used.

An assessment should be made before each task if the patient has a varying level of ability to assist because of medical reasons, fatigue, medications, etc. When in doubt, assume the patient cannot assist with the transfer/repositioning.

II. Weight-Bearing Capability
_____Full
_____Partial
_____None

III. Bilateral Upper-Extremity Strength
_____Yes
_____No

IV. Patient's Level of Cooperation and Comprehension
_____Cooperative—May need prompting; able to follow simple commands.
_____Unpredictable or variable (patient whose behavior changes frequently should be considered unpredictable)—Not cooperative or unable to follow simple commands.

V. Weight_____   Height _____

Body Mass Index (BMI) (needed if patient's weight is over 300 lb)*
If BMI exceeds 50, institute Bariatric Algorithms.

The presence of the following conditions is likely to affect the transfer/repositioning process and should be considered when identifying equipment and techniques needed to move the patient.

VI. Check Applicable Conditions Likely to Affect Transfer/Repositioning Techniques

_____Hip/knee/shoulder replacements	_____ Respiratory/cardiac compromise	_____Fractures
_____History of falls	_____ Wounds affecting transfer/positioning	_____Splints/traction
_____Paralysis/paresis	_____ Amputation	_____Severe osteoporosis
_____Unstable spine	_____ Urinary/fecal stoma	_____Severe pain/discomfort
_____Severe edema	_____ Contractures/spasms	_____Postural hypotension
_____Very fragile skin	_____ Tubes (IV, chest, etc.)	

Comments: _____

_____

_____

_____

_____

VII. Appropriate Lift/Transfer Devices Needed
Vertical Lift:
Horizontal Lift:
Other Patient-Handling Devices Needed:

Sling Type

_____Seated	_____ Seated (Amputee)	_____ Standing
_____Supine	_____ Ambulation	_____ Limb Support

Sling Size_____

Signature _____   Date _____

*If patient weighs more than 300 lb, the BMI is needed. For online BMI table and calculator, see http://www.nhlbi.nih.gov/guidelines/obesity/bmi_tbl.htm.

FIG. 6-4 Example of a tool to assess physical mobility.

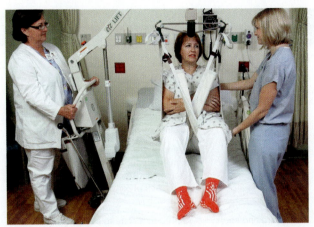

FIG. 6-5 Example of powered, mechanical full-body lift. (From Potter, P., Perry, A., Stockert, P., & Hall, A. [2017]. *Fundamentals of nursing* [9th ed.]. St. Louis: Mosby.)

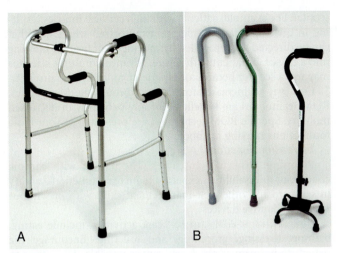

FIG. 6-6 Assistive devices for ambulation. Assistive devices vary in the amount of support they provide. A straight (single-point) cane provides less support than a walker (**A**) or quadripod cane (**B**).

⚠ NURSING SAFETY PRIORITY QSEN

Action Alert

Assess the patient and the situation before any transfer. Orthostatic, or postural, hypotension is a common problem and may contribute to falls. If the patient moves from a lying to a sitting or standing position too quickly, his or her blood pressure may drop; as a result, he or she can become dizzy or faint. This problem is worsened by antihypertensive drugs, especially in older adults. To prevent this situation, help the patient change positions slowly, with frequent pauses to allow the blood pressure to stabilize. If needed, measure blood pressure with the patient in the lying, sitting, and standing positions to examine the differences. Orthostatic hypotension is indicated by a drop of more than 20 mm Hg in systolic pressure or 10 mm Hg in diastolic pressure between positions. Notify the health care provider and the therapists about this change.

If the patient has problems maintaining blood pressure while out of bed, the physical therapist may start him or her on a tilt table to gradually increase tolerance. A low blood pressure is a particularly common problem for patients with quadriplegia because they have a delayed blood flow to the brain and upper part of the body.

◎ CHART 6-1 Best Practice for Patient Safety & Quality Care QSEN

Gait Training With Selected Ambulatory Aids

Walker-Assisted Procedure
- Apply a transfer belt around the patient's waist.
- Guide the patient to a standing position.
- Remind the patient to place both hands on the walker.
- Ensure that the patient's body is well balanced.
- Teach the patient repeatedly to perform this sequence:
  - Lift the walker.
  - Move the walker about 2 feet forward and set it down on all legs.
  - While resting on the walker, take small steps.
  - Check balance.
  - Repeat the sequence.

Cane-Assisted Procedure
- Apply a transfer belt around the patient's waist.
- Guide the patient to a standing position.
- Be sure the cane is at the height of the patient's wrist when the arm is placed at his or her side. (Many canes can be adjusted to the required height.)
- Remind the patient to place his or her strong hand on the cane.
- Ensure that the patient's body is well balanced.
- Teach the patient to perform this sequence repeatedly:
  - Move the cane and weaker leg forward at the same time.
  - Move the stronger leg one step forward.
  - Check balance and repeat the sequence.

is usually checked every week to monitor gains or losses. If needed, collaborate with the dietitian to plan a weight-reduction diet.

Gait Training. The physical therapist works with patients for gait training if ambulation is a realistic goal. While regaining the ability to ambulate, patients may need to use assistive devices such as a variety of canes or walkers (Fig. 6-6). The specific device selected for each patient depends on the amount of weight bearing that is allowed or tolerated. For example, a stroke patient who has problems with maintaining balance or a steady gait when walking might need a cane that provides greater steadying. Some patients use walkers with rollers made of tennis-ball materials; others who tire easily may need a walker with a built-in seat to rest at intervals (sometimes referred to as a *rollator*). A patient who had a total hip replacement 6 weeks ago may be able to use a straight (also called *single-point*) cane.

When working with patients who are using these devices, also known **as** ambulatory aids, the physical therapist ensures that there is a level surface on which to walk. The therapist or nurse should use a gait belt to guide him or her during

ambulation to help prevent falls. Use of transfer belts is recommended as one of the best practices for safe patient handling (ANA, 2012).

Reinforce the physical therapist's instructions and encourage practice, with the outcome being optimal mobility for the individual. Chart 6-1 outlines best practices for patient safety when teaching patients how to use ambulatory aids.

Some patients never regain the ability to walk because of their impairment such as advanced multiple sclerosis or complete high spinal cord injury. They may require the use of a wheelchair and need to learn wheelchair or motorized-scooter mobility skills. With the help of physical and occupational therapy, most patients can learn to move anywhere in a wheelchair or electric scooter. For example, patients with high cervical injuries resulting in quadriplegia may require a motorized wheelchair that can be directed and propelled by moving their head or blowing into a device. A patient with severe, advanced multiple sclerosis may use a scooter because of fatigue or mobility impairment.

One way to increase MOBILITY is through ROM exercises. ROM techniques are beneficial for any patient with decreased mobility. Specific ROM techniques are presented in your basic foundations nursing textbook.

Increasing Functional Ability

Planning: Expected Outcomes. The patient with chronic conditions or disability is expected to increase functional ability in self-care and other self-management skills with or without assistive/adaptive devices.

Interventions. ADLs, or self-care activities, include eating, bathing, dressing, grooming, and toileting. Encourage the patient to perform as much self-care as possible. Allow time to complete the task as independently as possible. Collaborate with the occupational therapist (OT) to identify ways in which self-care activities can be modified so the patient can perform them as independently as possible and with minimal frustration. For example, teach a patient with hemiplegia to put on a shirt by first placing the affected arm in the sleeve, followed by the unaffected arm. Slip-on shoes or shoes with Velcro straps may be recommended for some patients. Encourage patients to practice and allow them time to try to be independent in ADLs.

In SNF settings federal regulations require that residents not lose their functional skills while they are in the facility. Most facilities have developed *restorative nursing* programs and have coordinated these programs with rehabilitation therapy and activities therapy. The focus of this coordinated effort includes:

- Bed mobility
- Walking
- Transfers
- Dressing
- Grooming
- Active range of motion
- Communication

A variety of devices are available for patients with chronic conditions and disability for *assisting with self-care*. An **assistive/ adaptive device** is any item that enables the patient to perform all or part of an activity independently and safely. Examples include long-handled shoehorns and "reachers" to prevent bending and losing one's balance. Table 6-4 identifies common devices and describes their use.

Many medical equipment stores and large pharmacies carry clothing and assistive/adaptive devices designed for patients with disabilities. The occupational therapist determines the specific needs for this equipment. Collaborate with the occupational therapist to look for creative and inexpensive alternatives to meeting these needs. For example, barbecue tongs may be used as "reachers" for pulling up pants or obtaining items on high shelves. A foam curler with the plastic insert removed may be placed over a pencil or eating utensil to make a built-up device. The patient might use an extended shoehorn to operate light switches from wheelchair height. Hook-and-loop fasteners (Velcro) sewn on clothes can prevent the frustrations caused by buttons and zippers.

Assistive technology has further increased the ability for people with disabilities to care for themselves. For example, mobile devices, telephones, and computer keyboards can be operated by voice-activation devices. **Robotic technology**

TABLE 6-4 **Examples and Uses of Common Assistive/Adaptive Devices**

DEVICE	USE
Buttonhook	Threaded through the buttonhole to enable patients with weak finger mobility to button shirts Alternative uses include serving as pencil holder or cigarette holder
Extended shoehorn	Assists in the application of shoes for patients with decreased mobility Alternative uses include turning light switches off or on while patient is in a wheelchair
Plate guard and spork (spoon and fork in one utensil)	Applied to a plate to assist patients with weak hand and arm mobility to feed themselves; spork allows one utensil to serve two purposes
Gel pad	Placed under a plate or glass to prevent dishes from slipping and moving Alternative uses include placement under bathing and grooming items to prevent them from moving
Foam buildups	Applied to eating utensils to help patients with weak hand grasps feed themselves Alternative uses include application to pens and pencils to assist with writing or over a buttonhook to assist with grasping the device
Hook and loop fastener (Velcro) straps	Applied to utensils, a buttonhook, or a pencil to slip over the hand and provide a method of stabilizing the device when the patient's hand grasp is weak
Long-handled reacher	Assists in obtaining items located on high shelves or at ground level for patients who are unable to change positions easily
Elastic shoelaces or Velcro shoe closure	Eliminates the need for tying shoes

provides mechanical parts for the extremities when they are not functional or have been amputated. However, the cost of these aids has prevented their widespread use.

Fatigue often occurs with chronic and disabling conditions. Therefore collaborate with the OT to assess the patient's self-care abilities and determine possible ways of *conserving energy*. Preparation for ADLs can help reduce effort and energy expenditure (e.g., gathering all necessary equipment before starting grooming routines). If a patient has high energy levels in the morning, he or she can be taught to schedule energy-intensive activities in the morning rather than later in the day or evening. Spacing activities is also helpful for conserving energy. In addition, allowing time to rest before and after eating and toileting decreases the strain on energy level.

Preventing Pressure Injury

Planning: Expected Outcomes. The patient with chronic conditions or disability is expected to have intact skin and TISSUE INTEGRITY.

Interventions. *The best intervention to prevent pressure injury and maintain TISSUE INTEGRITY is frequent position changes in*

(See Chapter 25 for a complete discussion of skin care interventions.)

CLINICAL JUDGMENT CHALLENGE 6-1

Teamwork and Collaboration; Safety QSEN

An 81-year-old widow is admitted to a skilled nursing facility (SNF) for rehabilitation and reconditioning after emergent abdominal surgery as part of a 30-day acute care stay. After surgery she was out of bed only a few times in a chair and has not ambulated. Before her hospitalization she was able to walk independently with a walker and lived alone. The patient has a history of advanced rheumatoid arthritis, osteoarthritis, diabetes mellitus, and peripheral vascular disease. As her nurse you complete her admission assessment. She is alert and oriented and has no history of cognitive impairment.

1. What are this resident's priority problems? How might they affect the course of her rehabilitation?
2. With which health care team members will you need to collaborate and why?
3. Which safe patient handling practices would you need to use?
4. Which type of ambulatory assistive device would be most appropriate for her at this time?
5. What health teaching does the resident need regarding her mobility and functional ability?

combination with adequate skin care and sufficient nutritional intake. Teach staff to assist with turning and repositioning at least every 2 hours if patients are unable to perform this activity independently. This time frame may not be sufficient for people who are frail and have thin skin, especially older adults. To determine the best turning schedule, assess the patient's skin condition during each turning and repositioning. For example, if the patient has been sleeping and the nursing assistant decides to postpone turning and repositioning, reddened areas over the bony prominences may be present. If reddened areas do not fade within 30 minutes after pressure relief or do not blanch, they may be classified as pre–pressure injury areas, or stage I pressure areas (see Chapter 25).

Patients who sit for prolonged periods in a wheelchair need to be repositioned at least every 1 to 2 hours. Each patient is evaluated by the physical or occupational therapist for the best seating pad or cushion that is comfortable yet reduces pressure on bony prominences. Patients who are able are taught to perform pressure relief by using their arms to lift their buttocks off the wheelchair seat for 20 seconds or longer every hour or more often if needed (sometimes referred to as wheelchair push-ups). The PT or OT helps them strengthen their arm muscles in preparation for performing pressure relief.

Many patients with neurologic problems have decreased or absent sensation and may not be able to feel the discomfort of increased pressure. Check any areas where there may be pressure, including places such as the lower legs where the leg of the wheelchair could rub against the skin.

Adequate skin care is an essential component of prevention. Perform or help patients complete skin care each time they are turned, repositioned, or bathed. Delegate and supervise skin care to unlicensed assistive personnel (UAP), including cleaning soiled areas, drying carefully, and applying a moisturizer. If a patient is incontinent, use topical barrier creams or ointments to help protect the skin from moisture, which can contribute to skin breakdown. To prevent damage to the already fragile capillary system, teach UAP to avoid rubbing reddened areas. Instead carefully observe the areas for further breakdown and relieve pressure on the areas as much as possible. Bed pillows are often

good pressure-relieving devices. (See Chapter 25 for a complete discussion of skin care interventions.)

Sufficient NUTRITION is needed both to repair wounds and to prevent pressure injuries. Collaborate with the dietitian to assess the patient's food selection and ensure that it contains adequate protein and carbohydrates. Both the nurse and the dietitian closely monitor the patient's weight and serum prealbumin levels. If either of these indices decreases significantly, he or she may need high-protein, high-carbohydrate food supplements (e.g., milkshakes) or commercial preparations. Chapter 60 describes nutritional supplementation in detail.

Pressure-relieving or pressure-reducing devices include waterbeds, gel mattresses or pads, air mattresses, low–air loss overlays or beds, and air-fluidized beds. Mattress overlays such as air and gel types and replacement mattresses are often effective in reducing pressure. The use of any mechanical device (except air-fluidized beds) does not eliminate the need for turning and repositioning.

Specialty beds are categorized as either "low air loss" or "air fluidized." Air-fluidized therapy provides the most effective pressure relief by distributing the patient's weight to prevent pressure in any one area. These beds are not often used to prevent skin breakdown because insurers may not reimburse the agency for the use of the bed. Therefore they are reserved for severe skin problems that have not healed with the use of a conventional bed or other mechanical device. The primary disadvantage of this therapy is its expense, which may exceed several hundred dollars for each day of use. Patients also report discomfort from the heat generated by the bed. Although air-fluidized beds are heavy to move, lighter and more portable versions are available for home use. The cost of air-fluidized therapy is reimbursed by some health insurance providers if the bed is deemed medically necessary to treat the patient's skin problem.

Establishing Urinary Continence

Planning: Expected Outcomes. Most patients with chronic conditions or disability are expected to have normal patterns of urinary ELIMINATION without retention, infection, or incontinence.

Interventions. Neurologic disabilities often interfere with successful bladder control. These disabilities result in two basic functional types of neurogenic bladder: overactive (e.g., reflex or spastic bladder) and underactive (e.g., hypotonic or flaccid bladder).

An overactive spastic (upper motor neuron) bladder causes incontinence with sudden voiding. The bladder does not usually empty completely, and the patient is at risk for urinary tract infection. Neurologic problems affecting the upper motor neuron typically occur in patients with strokes or with high-level spinal cord injuries (cervical) or those above the mid-thoracic region. These injuries result in a failure of impulse transmission from the lower spinal cord areas to the cortex of the brain. When the bladder fills and transmits impulses to the spinal cord, the patient cannot perceive the sensation. Because there is no injury to the lower spinal cord and the voiding reflex arc is intact, the efferent (motor) impulse from a distended bladder is relayed, and the bladder contracts.

Nonpharmacologic Management. An underactive flaccid or areflexic (lower motor neuron) bladder results in urinary retention and overflow (dribbling). Injuries that damage the lower motor neuron at the spinal cord level of S2-4 (e.g., multiple sclerosis, spinal cord injury or tumor below T12) may directly interfere with the reflex arc or may result in inaccurate interpretation of impulses to the brain. The bladder fills, and afferent (sensory) impulses conduct the message via the spinal cord to the brain cortex. Because of the injury, the impulse is not interpreted correctly by the bladder center of the brain, and there is a failure to respond with a message for the bladder to contract.

Patients who cannot completely empty their bladder are at risk for post-void residual urine and subsequent possible urinary tract infection. Post-void residual (PVR) is the amount of urine remaining in the bladder after voiding. PVR assessments using a noninvasive ultrasound device called the *BladderScan* are performed by nurses at the bedside. The residual amount measured is accurate if the device is used correctly. Obesity may interfere with accuracy. The outcome of bladder ultrasonography is to prevent the unnecessary use of an indwelling urinary catheter. Long-term urinary catheters cause urinary tract infections that are often chronic. A picture of the BladderScan device is in Chapter 65.

The nurse can teach a variety of techniques to assist the patient in bladder management, including (Table 6-5):
- Facilitating, or triggering, techniques
- Intermittent catheterization
- Consistent scheduling of toileting routines ("timed void")

These techniques may not be as effective in patients with physiologic changes associated with aging, including stress incontinence in women with weak pelvic floor muscles and overflow incontinence in men with enlarged prostate glands.

Facilitating (triggering) techniques are used to stimulate voiding. If there is an upper motor neuron problem but the reflex arc is intact (reflex bladder pattern), the voiding response can be initiated by any stimulus that sends the message to the spinal cord level S2-4 that the bladder might be full. Such techniques include stroking the medial aspect of the thigh, pinching the area above the groin, massaging the peno-scrotal area, pinching the posterior aspect of the glans penis, and providing digital anal stimulation.

When the patient has a lower motor neuron problem, the voiding reflex arc is not intact (flaccid bladder pattern), and additional stimulation may be needed to initiate voiding. Two techniques used to facilitate voiding are the Valsalva maneuver and the Credé maneuver. For the Valsalva maneuver, teach the patient to hold his or her breath and bear down as if trying to defecate. This technique should not be used by a spinal cord–injured patient who is at risk for bradycardia as a result of loss of vagus nerve control. Help the patient perform the Credé maneuver by placing his or her hand in a cupped position directly over the bladder area. Then instruct him or her to push inward and downward gently as if massaging the bladder to empty.

Intermittent catheterization may be needed for a flaccid or spastic bladder. Initially a urinary catheter is inserted to drain urine every few hours—after the patient has attempted voiding and has used the Valsalva and Credé maneuvers. If less than 100 to 150 mL of post-void residual is obtained, the nurse typically increases the interval between catheterizations. *The patient should not go beyond 8 hours between catheterizations.* If intermittent self-catheterization is needed at home after discharge from the rehabilitation facility, the patient may use a specialized appliance to help perform the procedure, especially if he or she has problems with manual dexterity. For those who cannot catheterize themselves, a family member or significant other may need to be taught how to perform the procedure.

Most patients who need intermittent catheterization have chronic bacteriuria (bacteria in the urine with a positive culture), especially those with spinal cord injury (SCI). Unless the patient has symptoms of a urinary tract infection (UTI) such as fever or burning when voiding, the infection is not treated. *Older adults may become acutely confused as the only indication of a UTI.*

Consistent toileting routines may be the best way to re-establish voiding continence when the patient has an overactive bladder. Assess the patient's previous voiding pattern and determine his or her daily routine. At a minimum the nurse or nursing staff helps the patient voiding after awakening in the morning, before and after meals, before and after physical activity, and at bedtime. *Remind the staff to toilet the patient every 2 hours during the day and every 3 to 4 hours at night.*

Consider the patient's bladder capacity, which may range from 100 to 500 mL, MOBILITY limitations, and restrictive clothing. Bladder capacity is determined by measuring urine output. Ensure that the patient is aware of nearby bathrooms at all times or has a call system to contact the nurse or unlicensed assistive personnel for assistance. Chapter 66 also describes methods of achieving bladder control.

Drug Therapy. Drugs are not commonly used for urinary ELIMINATION problems. Mild overactive bladder problems may be treated with antispasmodics such as oxybutynin (Ditropan XL, Apo-Oxybutynin), solifenacin (VESIcare), or tolterodine (Detrol LA) to prevent incontinence on a short-term basis.

Patients with symptomatic UTIs are managed with short-term antibiotics such as trimethoprim (Trimpex) or trimethoprim/sulfamethoxazole (Septra, Bactrim). Patients who have frequent UTIs may be placed on pulse antibiotic therapy in which they alternate 1 week of antibiotic therapy with 3 weeks without antibiotics. Report progress in bladder training to the rehabilitation team so the best decision regarding drug therapy can be made.

TABLE 6-5	Management of Neurogenic Bladder		
FUNCTIONAL TYPE	**NEUROLOGIC DISABILITY**	**DYSFUNCTION**	**RE-ESTABLISHING VOIDING PATTERNS**
Reflex (spastic)	Upper motor neuron spinal cord injury above T12	Urinary frequency, incontinence but may not empty completely	Triggering or facilitating techniques Drug therapy, as appropriate Bedside bladder ultrasound Intermittent catheterization Consistent toileting schedule Indwelling urinary catheter (as last resort) Increased fluids
Flaccid	Lower motor neuron spinal cord injury below T12 (affects S2-4 reflex arc)	Urinary retention, overflow	Valsalva and Credé maneuvers Increased fluids Intermittent or indwelling urinary catheterization

CONSIDERATIONS FOR OLDER ADULTS

Patient-Centered Care QSEN

> When urinary antispasmodic drugs are used in older adults, observe for, document, and report hallucinations, delirium, or other acute cognitive changes caused by the anticholinergic effects of the drugs.

Establishing Bowel Continence

Planning: Expected Outcomes. The patient with chronic conditions or disability is expected to have regular evacuation of stool without constipation. If possible, patients control their bowel ELIMINATION schedule.

Interventions. Neurologic problems often affect the patient's bowel pattern by causing a reflex (spastic) bowel, a flaccid bowel, or an uninhibited bowel. Bowel retraining programs are designed for each patient to best meet the expected outcomes (Table 6-6). Pardee et al. (2012) found that establishing a successful bowel program can also enhance the quality of life for patients, especially those who have a spinal cord injury (SCI).

Upper motor neuron diseases and injuries such as a cervical or mid-level spinal cord injury (e.g., quadriplegia) may result in a reflex (spastic) bowel pattern, with defecation occurring suddenly and without warning. With this intact reflex pattern, any facilitating or triggering mechanism may lead to defecation if the lower colon contains stool. An example of facilitating or triggering techniques is digital stimulation. For this technique, use a lubricated glove or finger cot and massage the anus in a circular motion for no less than 1 full minute.

! NURSING SAFETY PRIORITY QSEN

Action Alert

> Do not use digital stimulation for patients with cardiac disease because of the risk for inducing a vagal nerve response. This response causes a rapid decrease in heart rate (bradycardia).

Lower motor neuron diseases and injuries (e.g., paraplegia) interfere with transmission of the nervous impulse across the reflex arc and may result in a flaccid bowel pattern, with defecation occurring infrequently and in small amounts. The use of manual disimpaction may get the best results. Some patients also need oral laxatives and/or stool softeners. Digital stimulation or suppositories are usually unsuccessful because of loss of the reflex for elimination.

Neurologic injuries that affect the brain may cause an uninhibited bowel pattern, with frequent defecation, urgency, and reports of hard stool. Patients may manage uninhibited bowel patterns through a consistent toileting schedule, a high-fiber diet, and the use of stool softeners.

In some cases patients are not able to regain their previous level of control over their bowel function. The rehabilitation team assists in designing a bowel ELIMINATION program that accommodates the disability.

Collaborate with patients to schedule bowel ELIMINATION as close as possible to their previous routine. For example, a patient who had stools at noon every other day before the illness or injury should have the bowel program scheduled in the same way. An exception is the patient who prefers another time that best fits into his or her daily routine. If he or she is employed during the day, a time-consuming bowel elimination program in the morning may not work. The bowel protocol can then be changed to the evening when there is more time.

Bowel retraining programs for patients with neurologic problems are often designed to include a combination of methods. Although drug therapy should not be a first choice when formulating a bowel training program, consider the need for a suppository if the patient cannot re-establish defecation habits through a consistent toileting schedule, dietary modification, or digital stimulation.

Bisacodyl (Dulcolax), a commonly used laxative, may be prescribed either rectally or orally as part of a bowel training program. Suppositories must be placed against the bowel wall to stimulate the sacral reflex arc (if intact) and promote rectal emptying. Results occur in 15 to 30 minutes. Administer the suppository when the patient expects to defecate (e.g., after a meal) to coincide with the gastrocolic reflex. Using the suppository every second or third day is usually effective in re-establishing defecation patterns for patients with upper motor neuron problems where the reflex arc is not damaged.

Care Coordination and Transition Management

Care coordination and transition management begin at the time of the patient's admission. If the patient is transferred from a hospital to an IRF or SNF, orient him or her to the change in routine and emphasize the importance of self-care. When the patient is admitted, a case manager and/or OT/PT assess his or her current living situation at home. Together with the patient

TABLE 6-6 Management of Neurogenic Bowel

FUNCTIONAL TYPE	NEUROLOGIC DISABILITY	DYSFUNCTION	RE-ESTABLISHING DEFECATION PATTERNS
Reflex (spastic)	Upper motor neuron spinal cord injury above T12	Defecation without warning, but may not empty completely	Triggering mechanisms Facilitation techniques High-fiber diet Increased fluids Laxative use (for some patients) Consistent toileting schedule Manual disimpaction
Flaccid	Lower motor neuron spinal cord injury below T12 (affects S2-4 reflex arc)	Usually absent stools for patients with complete lesions	Triggering or facilitating techniques Increased fluids High-fiber diet Suppository use Consistent toileting schedule Manual disimpaction

♲ **CONSIDERATIONS FOR OLDER ADULTS**

Patient-Centered Care **QSEN**

Many rehabilitation patients are at high risk for constipation, especially older adults. Encourage fluids (at least eight glasses a day) and 20 to 35 g of fiber in the diet. Teach patients to eat two to three daily servings of whole grains, legumes, and bran cereals and five daily servings of fruits and vegetables. Do not offer a bedpan when toileting. Instead be sure that the patient sits upright on a bedside commode or bathroom toilet to facilitate defecation. Additional information regarding managing constipation can be found in Chapter 2.

💡 **NCLEX EXAMINATION CHALLENGE 6-3**

Physiological Integrity

Which statement by a patient with complete paraplegia indicates a need for the nurse to provide further teaching about bowel retraining?

A. "I'll eat high-fiber foods each day to help prevent constipation."
B. "I'll drink at least 8 to 10 glasses of water every day."
C. "I'll do my daily bowel training routine after I eat breakfast."
D. "I'll use a suppository to help empty my rectum."

---

and family or significant others, they determine the adequacy of the current situation and the potential needs after discharge to home. The patient with chronic conditions and disability may require home care, assistance with ADLs, nursing care, or physical or occupational therapy after discharge.

Other health care professionals may be necessary to meet the patient's needs. For example, patients with traumatic brain injury (TBI) may benefit from life planning—a process that examines and plans to meet lifelong needs. External case managers specializing in life planning may be part of the interprofessional rehabilitation team.

Home Care Preparation. Before the patient returns home, the nurse assesses his or her readiness for discharge from the institutional setting. The home may be assessed in multiple ways and points in time.

Predischarge Assessment. Before discharge the home must be assessed to ensure accessibility for the patient, given a new mobility impairment. This may be completed by having the family videotape or photograph the home and provide measurements to the PT or OT. Some facilities use live stream such as Skype or Face Time to "walk through" the home with the patient's family. Other programs provide a PT or OT visit to the home to assess its layout, accessibility, and potential barriers or environmental risks. For example, a patient with a fractured hip who is ambulating well with a walker may neglect to explain to the nurse that the bathroom in the home is accessible by stairway only. The patient may not consider that it is important to mention that throw rugs, which can cause falls, are scattered throughout the apartment. Fall prevention strategies in the home environment for older adults are discussed in Chapter 3.

The accessibility of bathrooms, bedrooms, and kitchen is assessed. If the patient will use a wheelchair after discharge from the facility, home modifications such as ramps to replace steps may be needed. Doorways should be checked for adequate width. A doorway width of 36 to 38 inches (slightly less than 1 meter [m]) is usually sufficient for a standard-size wheelchair. Obese patients require bariatric wheelchairs and furniture and therefore need a wider door opening. Any room that the patient needs to use is assessed. The bedroom should have sufficient space for the patient to maneuver transfers to and from the wheelchair and the bed, if needed. The bathroom may need a toilet seat raised to at least 17 inches (43 cm).

Space requirements depend on the patient's need to use a wheelchair, walker, or cane. In the bathroom, grab bars may need to be installed before the patient comes home. Bathtub benches can provide support for the individual who has difficulty with mobility and, when used in combination with a handheld showerhead, can provide easily accessible bathing facilities. Assessment of the kitchen may or may not be critical, depending on whether the patient has help with cooking and preparing meals. If the patient will be cooking after discharge, the kitchen may need to be assessed for wheelchair or walker accessibility, appliance accessibility, and the need for adaptive equipment.

Therapeutic Leave-of-Absence Visit. A second method of assessing the patient's home is through a brief home visit, also called a *leave-of-absence (LOA) visit,* before discharge. Explain the need for the trial home visit and assess the patient's comfort level with this idea. The patient who has been hospitalized for a lengthy period may feel intense anxiety about returning home. The nurse may allay such anxieties with careful preparation. Before the visit the rehabilitation nurse meets with the patient and family members or significant others to set goals for the visit and identify specific tasks to be attempted while at home. After the home visit interview the patient to determine the success of the visit and to assess additional education or training needs before final discharge and transition of care.

Going home may not be an option for everyone. Some patients may not have a support network of family members or significant others. For example, many older adults have no spouse or close friends living nearby. Children may live far away, which can make home care difficult. If no caregiver is available, the family must decide whether care can be provided in the home by an outside resource. The patient may need to be admitted to a 24-hour supervised health care setting such as a transitional living apartment, board and care facility, assisted-living facility, or nursing home. The least restrictive, least institutional discharge environment is the desired outcome for all patients.

Self-Management Education. The OT and PT teach the patient to perform ADLs and IADLs independently. The patient's learning potential and cognitive capacity are assessed. He or she is asked to perform or direct each skill or technique independently to verify understanding. Written material explaining the steps in the procedure is provided to the patient and family members to reinforce learning and provide support with the technique after discharge. Before distributing written material the rehabilitation team assesses the reading level of the material and determines whether it is appropriate for the patient's reading ability and language skills.

Any chronic conditions or disability necessitates changes in lifestyle and body image. Help the patient deal with such changes by encouraging verbalization of feelings and emotions. A focus on existing capabilities instead of disabilities is emphasized.

The patient may fail to relate psychologically to the disability during hospitalization. For example, he or she may display anger or frustration in attempting to perform self-care routines before discharge from the rehabilitation facility. Encourage the patient to be open about such feelings and to talk about ways to prevent worries from becoming realities after discharge. If needed, refer the patient to a mental health/behavior health care professional to help with adjustment and coping strategies.

The LOA home visit assists the patient and family members or significant others in psychosocial preparation for discharge. It allows the experience of the home situation while being able to return to the hospital environment after a few hours. Often the patient finds new problems in the home that must be addressed before discharge. Review this information in preparation for transition to the home.

Health Care Resources. After discharge to the home, various health care resources (e.g., physical therapy, home care nursing, vocational counseling) are available to the patient with chronic conditions and disabilities. Assess the need for additional care and support throughout the hospitalization and coordinate with the case manager and health care provider in arranging for home services. A newer process using technology called *tele-health* or *telerehabilitation* allows for care coordination in the home setting. Through the use of various electronic devices, phone, or computer software, a health care team member can monitor the patient's vital signs, weight, and other assessment data. Other programs such as Rehab@Home allow patients to perform therapeutic exercises at home using Wii, a webcam, and a computer.

◆ *Evaluation: Reflecting*

The patient and rehabilitation team evaluate the effectiveness of interdisciplinary interventions based on the common patient problems. Expected outcomes may include that the patient will:

- Reach a level of mobility that allows him or her to function independently with or without assistive devices
- Prevent complications of decreased MOBILITY
- Perform self-care and other self-management skills independently or with minimal assistance, possibly using assistive/adaptive devices
- Have intact skin and underlying tissues.
- Establish urinary ELIMINATION without infection, incontinence, or retention
- Have regular evacuation of stool without constipation or incontinence

GET READY FOR THE NCLEX® EXAMINATION!

▌ KEY POINTS

Review these Key Points for each NCLEX Examination Client Needs Category.

Safe and Effective Care Environment

- Recall that rehabilitation is the process of learning to live with chronic and disabling conditions; the role of the rehabilitation nurse is outlined in Table 6-1.
- Collaborate with members of the interprofessional rehabilitation team, including physicians, nurse practitioners, staff nurses, physiotherapists, occupational therapists, dietitians, and speech/language pathologists; the patient and family are the center of and members of the team. **QSEN: Teamwork and Collaboration**
- Know that acute (short-term) rehabilitation care occurs in a variety of settings, including inpatient rehabilitation facilities (IRFs) and skilled nursing facilities (SNFs) in either a nursing home or hospital. **Health Care Organizations**
- Delegate and supervise selected nursing tasks such as reporting reddened skin areas as part of quality care for the rehabilitation patient.
- After assessing the home environment, the case manager, OT, and/or rehabilitation nurse make recommendations to the patient and family about home modifications. **QSEN: Teamwork and Collaboration**
- Use evidence-based safe patient handling practices such as using mechanical lifts and working with other team members when assessing and moving patients to prevent injury and improve mobility. **QSEN: Evidence-Based Practice; Safety**
- Recall that the rehabilitation therapists teach patients transfer, bed mobility, and gait training techniques (see Chart 6-1).
- Encourage the patient to be as independent as possible when performing ADLs and safe mobility skills.

Health Promotion and Maintenance

- In coordination with the PT and OT, assess the patient's ability to perform ADLs, IADLs, and MOBILITY skills using a functional assessment process. **QSEN: Teamwork and Collaboration**
- Prevent complications of immobility for clients, and teach them how to prevent complications by using interventions discussed in Chapter 2. Examples include pressure injuries, urinary calculi, constipation, and venous thromboembolism. **QSEN: Evidence-Based Practice**

Psychosocial Integrity

- Assess the patient's self-esteem and changes in body image caused by chronic or disabling health problems.
- Assess the patient's COGNITION to screen for depression, delirium, and dementia using tools such as the Confusion Assessment Method (CAM), especially for older adults. **QSEN: Safety**
- Assess the patient's and family's response to chronic and disabling conditions, including feelings of loss and grief.
- Assist patients in coping with their loss and assess the availability of support systems, especially for older adults. **QSEN: Patient-Centered Care**

Physiological Integrity

- Assess rehabilitation patients as outlined in Table 6-2 to help plan appropriate collaborative care.
- Review the Functional Independence Measure (FIM) system as one tool used to assess functional ability of the patient in rehabilitation, including the need for assistive/adaptive devices.
- Assess patients in rehabilitation for risk factors that make them likely to develop skin breakdown; interventions to

prevent skin problems include repositioning and adequate NUTRITION. **QSEN: Quality Improvement**
- Patients with neurogenic bladder and bowel ELIMINATION problems are managed by training programs; overactive (spastic or reflex) and underactive (hypotonic or flaccid) elimination problems are managed differently (see Tables 6-5 and 6-6).

- In collaboration with the rehabilitation therapists, evaluate the ability of clients to use assistive/adaptive devices to promote independence. **QSEN: Teamwork and Collaboration**
- Determine patient and family needs regarding discharge to home or other community-based setting.

SELECTED BIBLIOGRAPHY

Asterisk indicates a classic or definitive work on this subject.

*American Nurses Association. (2012). *Safe patient handling and mobility: Interprofessional standards across the care curriculum.* Silver Spring, MD: Author.

*Association of Rehabilitation Nurses. (2008). *Standards and scope of rehabilitation nursing practice.* Glenview, IL: Author.

Camicia, M., Black, T., Farrell, J., Waites, K., Wirt, S., & Lutz, B. (2014). The essential role of the rehabilitation nurse in facilitating care transitions: a white paper by the association of rehabilitation nurses. *Rehabilitation Nursing*, 39(1), 3–15. doi:10.1002/rnj.135.

Kennedy, B., & Kopp, T. (2015). Safe handling protects employees too. *Nursing*, 45(8), 65–67.

Gerteis, J. I. D., Deitz, D., LeRoy, L., Ricciardi, R., Miller, T., & Basu, J. (2014). *Multiple chronic conditions chartbook.* http://www.ahrq.gov/sites/default/files/wysiwyg/professionals/prevention-chronic-care/decision/mcc/mccchartbook.pdf.

*Larsen, P. D. (2011). *The specialty practice of rehabilitation nursing: A core curriculum* (C. Jacelon Ed 6th ed.). Glenview, IL: Association of Rehabilitation Nurses.

*Pardee, C., Bricker, D., Rundquist, J., MacRae, C., & Tebben, C. (2012). Characteristics of neurogenic bowel in spinal cord injury and perceived quality of life. *Rehabilitation Nursing*, 37(3), 128–135.

Vaughn, S., Mauk, K. L., Jacelon, C. S., Larsen, P. D., Rye, J., Wintersgill, W., et al. (2015). The Competency Model for Professional Rehabilitation Nursing. *Rehabilitation Nursing*, doi:10.1002/rnj.225.

CHAPTER 7

End-of-Life Care Concepts

Mary K. Kazanowski

e http://evolve.elsevier.com/Iggy/

PRIORITY AND INTERRELATED CONCEPTS

The priority concept for this chapter is COMFORT.

❊ The COMFORT concept exemplar for this chapter is End of Life, p. 104.

The interrelated concepts for this chapter are:
- COGNITION
- PERFUSION
- ETHICS

LEARNING OUTCOMES

Safe and Effective Care Environment

1. Collaborate with members of the interprofessional health care team when caring for the dying patient and family or other caregivers.
2. Discuss the legal and ETHICS obligations of the nurse with regard to end-of-life (EOL) care.

Health Promotion and Maintenance

3. Explain to patients and their families the purpose and procedure for advance directives.

Psychosocial Integrity

4. Assess the patient's and family's ability to cope with the dying process.
5. Assess and plan interventions to meet the dying patient's spiritual needs.

6. Incorporate the patient's cultural practices and beliefs when promoting COMFORT and providing care during the dying process and death.

Physiological Integrity

7. Explain the difference between palliative care consultations and hospice.
8. Assess patients for signs and symptoms related to the end of life.
9. Explain how to promote COMFORT and provide evidence-based end-of-life care to the dying patient, including managing symptoms that may result from impaired COGNITION and PERFUSION.
10. Describe best practice guidelines for performing postmortem care.

OVERVIEW OF DEATH, DYING, AND END OF LIFE

Although dying is part of the normal life cycle, it is often feared as a time of pain and suffering. For the family, death of a member is a life-altering loss that can cause significant and prolonged suffering. As sad and difficult as the death may be, the experience of dying need not be physically painful for the patient or emotionally agonizing for the family. The dying process can be an opportunity to change a difficult situation into one that is tolerable, peaceful, comfortable, and meaningful for the patient and the family left behind.

Because nurses spend more time with patients than do any other members of the interprofessional health care team, it is the nurse who often has the greatest impact on an adult's experience with death. A nurse can affect the dying process to prevent death without dignity (sometimes referred to as a *bad death*) from occurring while striving to promote a peaceful and meaningful death (sometimes referred to as a *good death*). A **peaceful death** is one that is free from avoidable distress and suffering for patients and families, in agreement with patients' and families' wishes, and consistent with clinical practice standards.

Table 7-1 lists the most common causes of death in the United States. Of all people who die, only a small percentage of them die suddenly and unexpectedly. Most people die after a long period of illness (e.g., cardiac, renal, respiratory disease), with gradual deterioration until a significant decline preceding death. Most people who die are older than 65 years. In most

TABLE 7-1   Leading Causes of Death in the United States
• Heart disease
• Cancer (malignant neoplasms)
• Chronic lower respiratory disease
• Accidents (intentional injuries)
• Stroke
• Alzheimer's disease
• Diabetes mellitus
• Influenza and pneumonia
• Kidney disease (nephritis, nephrotic syndrome, and nephrosis)
• Suicide (intentional self-harm)

Data from National Vital Statistics Bureau. (2013). *10 Leading causes of death by age-group, United States—2013.* www.cdc.gov/injury/wisqars/pdf/leading_causes_of_death_in_the_United_States_2013-a.pdf.

countries family and other lay caregivers provide the majority of long-term home care. In some countries such as Canada, these caregivers may be compensated by the local or provincial government for the health care they provide.

The U.S. health care system continues to be based on the acute care model, which is focused on prevention, early detection, and cure of disease. This focus and advances in survival rates for once deadly diseases have made it difficult for patients and providers to accept death as an outcome. Many health care providers view death as a failure. These views have led to a major deficiency in the quality of care provided to many at the end of life. In 1995 a landmark study highlighted the poor quality of dying experienced by hospitalized patients. The Study to Understand Prognoses and Preferences for Outcomes and Risks of Treatment (SUPPORT) showed that more than 50% of a sample of 9105 hospitalized patients with a life-threatening disease had moderate-to-severe pain during the last days of their lives. It was also learned that they did not have their wishes met, even when their wishes were known.

Since the SUPPORT study, some progress has been made in improving the dying process in the United States. However, multiple barriers remain, often related to the reluctance of the patient, family, or health care provider to stop treatment when the end of life is near.

PATHOPHYSIOLOGY OF DYING

Death is defined as the cessation of integrated tissue and organ function, manifested by lack of heartbeat, absence of spontaneous respirations, or irreversible brain dysfunction. It generally occurs as a result of an illness or trauma that overwhelms the compensatory mechanisms of the body, eventually leading to cardiopulmonary failure/arrest. Direct causes of death include:

- Heart failure secondary to cardiac dysrhythmias, myocardial infarction, or cardiogenic shock
- Respiratory failure secondary to pulmonary embolism, heart failure, pneumonia, lung disease, or respiratory arrest caused by increased intracranial pressure
- Shock secondary to infection, blood loss, or organ dysfunction, which leads to lack of blood flow (i.e., PERFUSION) to vital organs

Inadequate PERFUSION to body tissues deprives cells of their source of oxygen, which leads to anaerobic metabolism with acidosis, hyperkalemia, and tissue ischemia. Dramatic changes in vital organs lead to the release of toxic metabolites and destructive enzymes, referred to as *multiple organ dysfunction syndrome (MODS)*. As illness or organ damage progresses, the syndrome occurs with renal and liver failure. Renal or liver failure can also *start* the dying process.

When the body is hypoxic and acidotic, a lethal dysrhythmia such as ventricular fibrillation or asystole can occur, which ultimately leads to lack of cardiac output and PERFUSION. Shortly after cardiac arrest, respiratory arrest occurs. When respiratory arrest occurs first, cardiac arrest follows within minutes.

❈ COMFORT CONCEPT EXEMPLAR End of Life

In 1991 the U.S. Congress passed the Patient Self-determination Act (PSDA), which granted Americans the right to determine the medical care they wanted if they became incapacitated. Documentation of self-determination is accomplished by completing an advance directive (AD). The PSDA requires that a representative in every health care agency ask patients when admitted if they have written advance directives. Patients who do not have ADs should be provided with information on the value of having an AD in place and given the opportunity to complete the state-required forms. Ideally advance directives should be completed long before a medical crisis.

Advance directives vary from state to state but are readily available through Caring Connections, an online program of the National Hospice and Palliative Care Organization (www.caringinfo.org). Anyone can complete the forms without legal consultation. Titles for ADs vary from state to state. Generally speaking, most have a section in which one names a durable power of attorney for health care (DPOAHC) (Fig. 7-1). The DPOAHC is not the same as durable power of attorney for one's finances. It may or may not be the same person, depending on who the patient designates.

The DPOAHC, often referred to as a *health care proxy, health care agent,* or *surrogate decision maker,* does not make health care decisions until a physician states that the person lacks capacity to make his or her own health care decisions. This is usually the result of impairment in COGNITION.

To have decision-making ability, a person must be able to perform three tasks:
- Receive information (but not necessarily be totally oriented)
- Evaluate, deliberate, and mentally manipulate information
- Communicate a treatment preference

By definition, the comatose patient does not have decisional ability.

The second part of the advance directive is a living will (LW), which identifies what one would (or would not) want if he or she were near death. Treatments that are discussed include cardiopulmonary resuscitation (CPR), artificial ventilation, and artificial nutrition or hydration. The third type of advance directive is a do-not-resuscitate (DNR) or do-not-attempt-to-resuscitate (DNAR) order, signed by a physician or other authorized primary health care provider, which instructs that CPR not be attempted in the event of cardiac or respiratory arrest. DNRs/DNARs are intended for people with life-limiting conditions, for whom resuscitation is not prudent. Depending on the state of residence, people who have made the decision not to be resuscitated may have portable DNR documents and or bracelets to identify themselves as having directions not to

INSTRUCTIONS

INSTRUCTIONS

PRINT YOUR NAME

PRINT THE NAME AND
ADDRESS OF YOUR
AGENT

INSTRUCTION
STATEMENTS

CIRCLE AND INITIAL THE
RESPONSES THAT
REFLECT YOUR WISHES

TERMINAL ILLNESS

PERMANENTLY
UNCONSCIOUS

ARTIFICIAL NUTRITION
AND HYDRATION

ADD PERSONAL
INSTRUCTIONS (IF ANY)

ALTERNATE AGENT

PRINT THE NAME AND
ADDRESS OF YOUR
ALTERNATE AGENT

LOCATION OF THE
ORIGINAL AND COPIES

DATE AND SIGN THE
DOCUMENT HERE

WITNESSING PROCEDURE

WITNESSES MUST SIGN
AND PRINT THEIR
ADDRESSES

AND A NOTARY PUBLIC
OR JUSTICE OF THE
PEACE MUST COMPLETE
THIS SECTION

©2005 National Hospice and
Palliative Care Organization
2014 Revised

NEW HAMPSHIRE ADVANCE DIRECTIVE
PART I: NEW HAMPSHIRE DURABLE POWER OF ATTORNEY FOR HEALTH CARE

I,_____, hereby appoint _____
(name)   (name of agent)
of _____
(address)

as my agent to make any and all health care decisions for me, except to the extent I state otherwise in this directive or as prohibited by law. This durable power of attorney for health care shall take effect in the event I lack the capacity to make my own health care decisions.

In the event the person I appoint above is unable, unwilling or unavailable, or ineligible to act as my health care agent, I hereby appoint _____ of _____
(name of an alternate agent)   (address)
as alternate agent.

When making health care decisions for me, my agent should think about what action would be consistent with past conversations we have had, my treatment preferences as expressed in this advance directive, my religious and other beliefs and values, and how I have handled medical and other important issues in the past. If what I would decide is still unclear, then my health care agent should make decisions for me that my health care agent believes are in my best interest, considering the benefits, burdens, and risks of my current circumstances and treatment option.

STATEMENT OF DESIRES, SPECIAL PROVISIONS, AND LIMITATIONS REGARDING HEALTH CARE DECISIONS.

For your convenience in expressing your wishes, some general statements concerning the withholding or removal of life-sustaining treatment are set forth below. (Life-sustaining treatment is defined as procedures without which a person would die, such as but not limited to the following: mechanical respiration, kidney dialysis or the use of other external mechanical and technological devices, drugs to maintain blood pressure, blood transfusions, and antibiotics.) There is also a section which allows you to set forth specific directions for these or other matters. If you wish, you may indicate your agreement or disagreement with any of the following statements and give your agent power to act in those specific circumstances.

A. LIFE-SUSTAINING TREATMENT.
1. If I am near death and lack the capacity to make health care decisions, I authorize my agent to direct that:
    (Initial beside your choice of (a) or (b).)
    _____(a) life-sustaining treatment not be started, or if started, be discontinued.
OR _____(b) life-sustaining treatment continue to be given to me.
2. Whether near death or not, if I become permanently unconscious I authorize my agent to direct that:
    (Initial beside your choice of (a) or (b).)
    _____(a) life-sustaining treatment not be started, or if started, be discontinued.
OR _____(b) life-sustaining treatment continue to be given to me.

B. MEDICALLY ADMINISTERED NUTRITION AND HYDRATION.
1. I realize that situations could arise in which the only way to allow me to die would be to not start or to discontinue medically administered nutrition and hydration. In carrying out any instructions I have given in this document, I authorize my agent to direct that: (Initial beside your choice of (a) or (b).)
    _____(a) medically administered nutrition and hydration not be started or, if started, be discontinued.
OR _____(b) even if all other forms of life-sustaining treatment have been withdrawn, medically administered nutrition and hydration continue to be given to me.

INITIAL THE RESPONSES THAT REFLECT YOUR WISHES

C. ADDITIONAL INSTRUCTIONS. Here you may include any specific desires or limitations you deem appropriate, such as when or what life-sustaining treatment you would want used or withheld, or instructions about refusing any specific types of treatment that are inconsistent with your religious beliefs or are unacceptable to you for any other reason. You may leave this question blank if you desire.

_____
_____
_____
(attach additional pages as necessary)

I hereby acknowledge that I have been provided with a disclosure statement explaining the effect of this directive. I have read and understand the information contained in the disclosure statement. The original of this document will be kept at:
_____, and the following persons and institutions will have signed copies:
_____ Name _____ Name
_____ Address _____ Address

ADD OTHER INSTRUCTIONS, IF ANY, REGARDING YOUR ADVANCE CARE PLANS
THESE INSTRUCTIONS CAN FURTHER ADDRESS YOUR HEALTH CARE PLANS, SUCH AS YOUR WISHES REGARDING HOSPICE TREATMENT, BUT CAN ALSO ADDRESS OTHER ADVANCE PLANNING ISSUES, SUCH AS YOUR BURIAL WISHES

PART II. NEW HAMPSHIRE DECLARATION
Declaration made this _____ day of _____. (day) (month, year)
I, _____, (name) being of sound mind, willfully and voluntarily make known my desire that my dying shall not be artificially prolonged under the circumstances set forth below, do hereby declare:

If at any time I should have an incurable injury, disease or illness and I am certified to be near death or in a permanently unconscious condition by 2 physicians or a physician and an ARNP, and two physicians or a physician and an ARNP have determined that my death is imminent whether or not life-sustaining treatment is utilized and where the application of life-sustaining treatment would serve only to artificially prolong the dying process, or that I will remain in a permanently unconscious condition, I direct that such procedures be withheld or withdrawn, and that I be permitted to die naturally with only the administration of medication, the natural ingestion of food or fluids by eating or drinking, or the performance of any medical procedure deemed necessary to provide me with comfort care. I realize that situations could arise in which the only way to allow me to die would be to discontinue medically administered nutrition and hydration.

In carrying out any instruction I have given under this section, I authorize that:
(Initial beside your choice of (a) or (b).)
    _____(a) medically administered nutrition and hydration not be started or, if started, be discontinued,
OR _____(b) even if other forms of life-sustaining treatment have been withdrawn, medically administered nutrition and hydration continue to be given to me.
Other directions:

FIG. 7-1 An example of a durable power of attorney for health care (DPOAHC). (©2005. National Hospice and Palliative Care Organization, 2007 Revised. All rights reserved. Reproduction and distribution by an organization or organized group without the written permission of the National Hospice and Palliative Care Organization is expressly forbidden. Visit caringinfo.org for more information.)

resuscitate. Some states also have directives referred to as *POLST* (physician orders for life-sustaining treatment), which document additional instructions in case of cardiac or pulmonary arrest. Like portable DNRs/DNARs, POLST follow the patient across health care settings.

By law all primary health care providers in the United States must initiate CPR for a person who is not breathing or is pulseless unless that person has a DNR order. The problem with performing CPR is that it can be a violent and likely painful intervention that prevents a peaceful death. CPR may also be unsuccessful or result in the patient being more compromised than they were before the event, perhaps for life. Many patients and families do not understand the limitations of CPR and do not realize that it was never intended to be performed on patients with end-stage disease.

Hospice and Palliative Care

The concept of hospice in the United States and other countries came about from a grassroots effort in response to the unmet needs of terminally ill people. As both a philosophy and a system of care, hospice is considered to be the model for quality, compassionate care for people facing a life-limiting illness or injury. Hospice uses a team-oriented approach to providing expert medical care, pain management, and emotional and spiritual support expressly tailored to the person's needs and wishes. Support is also provided to the person's loved ones. Hospice systems of care are provided in a variety of settings. They are often affiliated with home care agencies, providing services to patients at home or in a long-term care or assisted-living facility. Some communities also have hospice houses, which provide care to patients in the terminal phase of their lives.

Hospice services may also be provided in non–health-related institutions such as prisons. In their recent systematic review, Wion and Loeb (2016) described end-of-life and hospice care for prisoners who were older and/or had terminal illness (see Evidence-Based Practice box).

The *Medicare Hospice Benefit* serves as a guide for hospice care in the United States. This benefit pays for hospice services for Medicare recipients who have a prognosis of 6 months or less to live and who agree to forego curative treatment for their terminal illness. Historically those with terminal cancer made up the majority of patients receiving hospice care. However, the proportion of patients with terminal cancer has decreased, with increases in numbers of patients with other terminal illnesses, (e.g., dementia, end-stage chronic obstructive pulmonary disease [COPD], cardiac disease, or neurologic disease).

Guidelines are available to help primary health care providers and families identify who is entitled to hospice care under Medicare. Patients who do not qualify for Medicare may have benefits through private insurance or government medical assistance programs (e.g., Medicaid).

Palliative care is a philosophy of care for people with life-threatening disease that helps patients and families identify their outcomes for care, assists them with informed decision making, and facilitates quality symptom management. Unlike hospice, *palliation* is provided by a physician, nurse practitioner, or team of providers as a consultation visit, with one or more follow-up visits. Palliative care consultations are provided in a large number of hospitals and on an ambulatory care basis in some communities. Table 7-2 compares palliative care to hospice care. Classic research has demonstrated the benefits of early initiation of palliative care consultation (Campbell

EVIDENCE-BASED PRACTICE QSEN
Is End-of-Life Care Provided for Prisoners?

Wion, R. K., & Loeb, S. J. (2016). End-of-life care behind bars: A systematic review. *AJN, 116*(3), 24–36.

As the population ages, prisoners with long-term sentences are also aging and developing life-threatening and terminal health conditions. This study was conducted as a systematic review of the published research on end-of-life (EOL) care in prisons in the United States and the United Kingdom. Nineteen articles published between 2002 and 2014 met the inclusion criteria for review. While criteria varied across settings, hospice services were provided in many prisons, with a daily average census of three hospice patients. Care was provided by prison staff, interprofessional health care team members, and inmates. In many cases the number and types of health care disciplines caring for prisoners were higher than those provided in community hospice settings. Inmate caregiving and training varied, but many inmates found that providing end-of-life care was a transformational experience.

Level of Evidence: 1
This research presents the results of an in-depth review of multiple research articles published in the United States (18 studies) and the United Kingdom (1 study).

Commentary: Implications for Practice and Research
Nurses who work in prisons are in a unique position to increase awareness of and information about available end-of-life care for inmates. Nurses in other settings often provide care for dying inmates and can facilitate care transition for follow-up when the inmate returns to the prison setting. All people deserve to have a dignified death regardless of their setting or circumstance.

CONSIDERATIONS FOR OLDER ADULTS
Patient-Centered Care QSEN

In the last 15 years, twice as many older adults died in hospice care as in a hospital or nursing home compared to the previous decade. Despite increase in use, hospice is often a last resort after aggressive critical care. Earlier referrals to hospice care would be a benefit for older adults and their families.

et al., 2012). Despite these benefits, palliative care is often not implemented until late in the patient's illness (Institute of Medicine [IOM], 2014). Because of their proximity to patients, nurses are in an excellent position to identify individuals who would benefit from palliative consultation. To accomplish this desired outcome, nurses need to have knowledge of end-of-life (EOL) care, compassion, advocacy, and therapeutic communication skills.

❖ INTERPROFESSIONAL COLLABORATIVE CARE
◆ Assessment: Noticing

Obtain information about the patient's diagnosis, past medical history, and recent state of health to identify the risks for symptoms of distress at the end of life. People with lung cancer, heart failure, or chronic respiratory disease are at high risk for respiratory distress and dyspnea as they decline. Those with brain tumors are at risk for seizure activity. Patients with tumors near major arteries (e.g., head and neck cancer) are at risk for hemorrhage. Those who have been experiencing pain often continue to have pain at the end of life, which may increase, decrease, or remain at the same level of intensity.

TABLE 7-2   Comparison of Hospice and Palliative Care

HOSPICE CARE	PALLIATIVE CARE
Patients have a prognosis of six (6) months or less to live.	Patients can be in any stage of serious illness.
Care is provided when curative treatment such as chemotherapy has been stopped.	A consultation is provided that is concurrent with curative therapies or therapies that prolong life.
Care is provided in 60- and 90-day periods with an opportunity to continue if eligibility criteria are met.	Care is not limited by specific time periods.
Ongoing care is provided by RNs, social workers, chaplains, and volunteers.	Care is in the form of a consult visit by a primary health care provider who makes recommendations; follow-up visits may be provided.

Physical Assessment/Signs and Symptoms. As death nears, patients often have signs and symptoms of decline in physical function, manifested as weakness; sleeping more; anorexia; and changes in cardiovascular function, breathing patterns, and genitourinary function. Level of consciousness often declines to lethargy, unresponsiveness, or coma. Cardiovascular dysfunction leads to decreases in peripheral circulation and poor tissue PERFUSION manifested as cold, mottled, and cyanotic extremities. Blood pressure decreases and often is only palpable. The dying person's heart rate may increase, become irregular, and gradually decrease before stopping. Changes in breathing pattern are common, with breaths becoming very shallow and rapid. Periods of apnea and Cheyne-Stokes respirations (apnea alternating with periods of rapid breathing) are also common. Death occurs when respirations and heartbeat stop.

As the patient's level of consciousness decreases, he or she may lose the ability to speak. When caring for those who are unable to communicate their distress or needs, identify alternative ways to assess symptoms of distress. Teach family caregivers to watch closely for objective signs of impaired COMFORT (e.g., restlessness, grimacing, moaning) and identify when these symptoms occur in relation to positioning, movement, medication, or other external stimuli. Teach them how to perform interventions that can help relieve discomfort and stress as described in Chart 7-1.

Although the patient's point of view is the most valid indicator of comfort or distress, the family's perception of symptoms and COMFORT level is also important. Family caregivers, health care providers, and dying patients may differ in their perceptions of symptoms in terms of intensity, significance, and meaning. Whereas primary health care providers are often able to identify symptoms of distress, families are often more knowledgeable about the patient's habits and preferences. Incorporate all pertinent information into the plan for symptom management and work with patients and families toward a common outcome.

Assess any symptom of distress in terms of intensity, frequency, duration, quality, exacerbating (worsening) and relieving factors, and effect on the patient's comfort when awake or

CHART 7-1   Patient and Family Education: Preparing for Self-Management

Common Physical Signs and Symptoms of Approaching Death With Recommended Comfort Measures

Coolness of Extremities

Circulation to the extremities is decreased; the skin may become mottled or discolored.
- Cover the person with a blanket.
- Do not use an electric blanket, hot water bottle, electric heating pad, or hair dryer to warm the person.

Increased Sleeping

Metabolism is decreased.
- Spend time sitting quietly with the person.
- Do not force the person to stay awake.
- Talk to the person as you normally would, even if he or she does not respond.

Fluid and Food Decrease

Metabolic needs have decreased.
- Do not force the person to eat or drink.
- Offer small sips of liquids or ice chips at frequent intervals if the person is alert and able to swallow.
- Use moist swabs to keep the mouth and lips moist and comfortable.
- Coat the lips with lip balm.

Incontinence

The perineal muscles relax.
- Keep the perineal area clean and dry. Use disposable underpads (Chux) and disposable undergarments.
- Offer a Foley catheter for comfort.

Congestion and Gurgling

The person is unable to cough up secretions effectively.
- Position the patient on his or her side. Use toothette to gently clean mouth of secretions.
- Administer medications to decrease the production of secretions.

Breathing Pattern Change

Slowed circulation to the brain may cause the breathing pattern to become irregular, with brief periods of no breathing or shallow breathing.
- Elevate the person's head.
- Position the person on his or her side.

Disorientation

Decreased metabolism and slowed circulation to the brain.
- Identify yourself whenever you communicate with the person.
- Reorient the patient as needed.
- Speak softly, clearly, and truthfully.

Restlessness

Decreased metabolism and slowed circulation to the brain.
- Play soothing music and use aromatherapy.
- Do not restrain the person.
- Massage the person's forehead.
- Reduce the number of people in the room.
- Talk quietly.
- Keep the room dimly lit.
- Keep the noise level to a minimum.
- Consider sedation if other methods do not work.

Adapted from the Hospice of North Central Florida, Inc.

asleep. A method for rating the intensity of symptoms should be used to facilitate ongoing assessments and evaluate treatment response. A rating scale of 0 to 10 is commonly used, with 0 indicating no distress and 10 indicating the worst possible distress. The intensity of the symptom before and after an intervention (e.g., medication) is documented by the nurse or the family caregiver and is used daily to evaluate the patient's overall COMFORT.

Psychosocial Assessment. People facing death may have fear and/or anxiety about their impending death with difficulty coping. Assess cultural considerations, values, and religious beliefs of the patient and family for their influence on the dying experience, control of symptoms, and family bereavement.

🌐 CULTURAL/SPIRITUAL CONSIDERATIONS

Patient-Centered Care QSEN

Be aware that patients differ in their needs at the end of life, depending on their culture and spiritual beliefs. If possible, ask the patient what to tell the family about the patient's condition. In some cultures, families may not want to know about the terminal conditions of their loved ones. This decision may be based on respect for older family members. Ask the family what they want to know and if they desire the assistance of a language interpreter.

At the end of life adults may feel challenged about their spirituality or want spirituality to become a bigger part of their lives (Finocchiaro, 2016). Many patients reaffirm their faith and/or spirituality with hope that they have a peaceful death and eternal hope and life. Other patients who do not believe in an afterlife may still experience hope for a cure and a comfortable death.

When assessing a patient's spirituality at the end of life, use this classic HOPE mnemonic as a guide. Determine the patient's:

H: Sources of hope and strength

O: Organized religion (if any) and role that it plays in one's life

P: Personal spirituality, rituals, and practices

E: Effects of religion and spirituality on care and end-of-life decisions (Finocchiaro, 2016)

Families of people near death often manifest fear, anxiety, and knowledge deficits regarding the process of death and their role in providing care. Assess the patient and family for fear and anxiety and their expectations of the death experience. Provide them with information about the process itself, emphasizing that symptoms of distress do not always occur and, if they occur, can be treated and controlled. Ask them if they want to talk to a bereavement (grief) counselor or want guidance from clergy. Explain the common emotional signs of approaching death as described in Chart 7-2.

◆ Interventions: Responding

The desired outcomes for a patient near the end of life (EOL) are that the patient will have:

- Needs and preferences met
- Control of symptoms of distress
- Meaningful interactions with family
- A peaceful death

Interventions are planned to meet the physical, psychological, social, and spiritual needs of patients using a coordinated interprofessional health team approach to end-of-life care.

👤 CHART 7-2 Patient and Family Education: Preparing for Self-Management

Common Emotional Signs of Approaching Death

Withdrawal

The person is preparing to "let go" from surroundings and relationships.

Vision-Like Experiences

The person may talk to people you cannot see or hear and see objects and places not visible to you. These are not hallucinations or drug reactions.

- Do not deny or argue with what the person claims.
- Affirm the experience.

Letting Go

The person may become agitated or continue to perform repetitive tasks. Often this indicates that something is unresolved or is preventing the person from letting go. As difficult as it may be to do or say, the dying person takes on a more peaceful demeanor when loved ones are able to say things such as, "It's okay to go. We'll be alright."

Saying Goodbye

When the person is ready to die and you are ready to let go, saying "goodbye" is important for both of you. Touching, hugging, crying, and saying "I love you," "Thank you," "I'm sorry," or "I'll miss you so much" are all natural expressions of sadness and loss. Verbalizing these sentiments can bring comfort both to the dying person and to those left behind.

Adapted from the Hospice of North Central Florida, Inc.

Although the perception of hospice is that it provides care for the dying, the major focus of hospice care is on quality of life.

When developing a plan of care for people nearing the end of their lives, consideration should be given for where the person wants to die. A large percentage of Americans would like to die at home. If this is the patient's preference, work with the patient, family, and health care provider to determine if this desired outcome is possible. Arrange for patients and families to meet with hospice representatives who are educated in end-of-life care in a variety of settings.

Managing Symptoms of Distress. The most common end-of-life symptoms that can cause the patient distress are:

- Pain
- Weakness
- Breathlessness/dyspnea
- Nausea and vomiting
- Agitation and delirium
- Seizures

Interventions to relieve symptoms of distress include positioning, administration of medications, and a variety of complementary and integrative therapies. When medications are used, they are often scheduled around the clock to maintain COMFORT and prevent recurrence of the symptom.

Managing Pain. *Pain is the symptom that dying patients fear the most.* Diseases such as cancer often cause tumor pain as a result of the infiltration of cancer cells into organs, nerves, and bones. Other causes of impaired COMFORT in dying patients include osteoarthritis, muscle spasms, and stiff joints secondary to immobility.

Both nonopioid and opioid analgesics play a role in pain management near the end of life. Patients who have had their pain controlled with either short- or long-acting opioids should continue their scheduled doses to prevent recurrence of the pain. However, as patients get closer to death, they often lose the ability to swallow. Long-acting oral opioids generally cannot be crushed; and rotation to rectal, transdermal, intravenous, or a subcutaneous route may be necessary. Short-acting nonopioids such as acetaminophen or opioids such as morphine sulfate oxycodone, or hydromorphone elixir can be given sublingually. They may also be given rectally if the patient and family are receptive to this route. Short-acting analgesics are quick acting; effective; and safe to administer, even to comatose patients.

CONSIDERATIONS FOR OLDER ADULTS
Patient-Centered Care QSEN

Pain in older adults is often underreported and undertreated. Do not withhold opioid drugs from older adults at the end of their lives. Instead give low doses of opioids initially, with slow increases, monitoring for changes in mental status or excessive sedation.

Some experts in symptom management at the end of life (EOL) recommend discontinuing routine doses of opioids such as morphine when patients become oliguric or anuric. The rationale for this decision is to decrease the risk for delirium that may occur as the result of the inability of a failing kidney to excrete morphine metabolites from the body. If delirium is causing distress for the patient, consider changing the opioid to fentanyl, which does not have active metabolites. The delirium may improve. For patients with known renal failure, fentanyl should ideally be used from the start of opioid administration. When it cannot be easily obtained (i.e., when not available by sublingual or IV route), oxycodone may be a better choice than morphine. Chapter 4 describes in detail the management of chronic pain.

Complementary and Integrative Health. Nonpharmacologic interventions are often integrated into the pain management plan. Some common approaches are presented here and in Chapter 4.

Massage may decrease pain in people with cancer and is one of the most popular complementary interventions used for patients at the end of life. This technique involves manipulating the patient's muscles and soft tissue, which improves circulation and promotes relaxation. Patients who are severely weak, are arthritic, or have advanced age may not tolerate extensive massage but may benefit from a short treatment to sites of their choice. In working with patients with cancer, use light pressure and avoid deep or intense pressure. Massage should not be performed over the site of tissue damage (e.g., open wounds, tissue undergoing radiation therapy), in patients with bleeding disorders, and in those who are uncomfortable with touch (Westman & Blaisdell, 2016).

Music therapy is another complementary therapy used by people near the end of life that has been shown to decrease pain by promoting relaxation. Select music based on patient preferences and values.

Therapeutic Touch involves moving one's hands through the patient's energy field to relieve pain. Reiki therapy is another type of energy therapy being evaluated for its role in pain and symptom management. Use of Reiki requires a Reiki practitioner who is trained in the method.

Aromatherapy can be used in conjunction with other treatments to relieve pain near the end of life. It is thought to decrease pain by promoting relaxation and reducing anxiety. Lavender, capsicum, bergamot, chamomile, rose, ginger, rosemary, lemongrass, sage, and camphor have been used in end-of-life care (Allard & Katseres, 2016).

NCLEX EXAMINATION CHALLENGE 7-1
Physiological Integrity

An older client with advanced dementia and severe osteoarthritis is unresponsive but grimaces and moans when repositioned. Which intervention is the **most** appropriate for the nurse to implement for this client?
A. Administer acetaminophen 650 mg by mouth PRN.
B. Start an intravenous with 5% D/W solution.
C. Provide range of motion once a shift.
D. Obtain an order for transdermal fentanyl.

Managing Weakness. Patients commonly experience weakness and fatigue as death nears. At this point they are generally advised to remain in bed to avoid falls and injuries. Mechanical or electric beds are often obtained to elevate the patient's head to promote air exchange and facilitate administration of medications, food, or fluids. Insertion of a long-term urinary (e.g., Foley) catheter to avoid the need for exertion with voiding should be offered as a COMFORT measure. Risk for infection should not be a consideration when a person is near death.

Weakness combined with decreased neurologic function may impair the ability to swallow (dysphagia). Once the patient has difficulty swallowing, oral intake should be limited to soft foods and sips of liquids, offered but not forced. Teach families about the risk for aspiration and reassure them that anorexia is normal at this stage. Families often have difficulty accepting that their loved ones are not being fed and may request that IV fluids be started. With great sensitivity, reinforce that having no appetite or desire for food or fluids is expected. Inform families that giving fluids can actually increase discomfort in a person with multisystem slowdown. Impaired COMFORT from fluid replacement could lead to respiratory secretions (and distress), increased GI secretions, nausea, vomiting, edema, and ascites. Most experts believe that dehydration in the last hours of life (i.e., terminal dehydration) does not cause distress and may stimulate endorphin release that promotes the patient's sense of well-being. To avoid a dry mouth and lips, moisten them with soft applicators and apply an emollient to lips.

Managing Breathlessness/Dyspnea. Dyspnea is a subjective experience in which the patient has an uncomfortable feeling of breathlessness, often described as terrifying. It is a common symptom of distress near the end of life, especially among older adults because of decreased oxygen reserves associated with aging. Patients, families, and health care providers often consider it the major cause of suffering at the end of life. Dyspnea can be:
- Directly related to the primary diagnosis (e.g., lung cancer, breast cancer, coronary artery disease, chronic obstructive pulmonary disease [COPD])
- Secondary to the primary diagnosis (e.g., pleural effusion)

! NURSING SAFETY PRIORITY (QSEN)

Drug Alert

Dysphagia near death presents a problem for oral drug therapy. Although some tablets may be crushed, drugs such as sustained-release capsules should not be taken apart. Reassess the need for each medication. Collaborate with the prescriber about discontinuing drugs that are not needed to control pain, dyspnea, agitation, nausea, vomiting, cardiac workload, or seizures. In collaboration with a pharmacist experienced in palliation, identify alternative routes and/or alternative drugs to promote COMFORT and maintain control of symptoms. Choose the least invasive route such as oral, buccal mucosa (inside cheek), transdermal (via the skin), or rectal. Some oral drugs can be given rectally. Depending on patient needs, the subcutaneous or IV route may be used if access is available. The intramuscular (IM) route is almost never used at the end of life because it is considered painful and drug distribution varies among patients.

do not respond promptly to morphine or other drugs should be tried on oxygen (2 to 6 L by nasal cannula) to assess its effect. Patients often feel more comfortable when the oxygen saturation is greater than 90%. If possible, provide oxygen by nasal cannula (NC) because masks can be frightening. If oxygen is not effective, discontinue it.

! NURSING SAFETY PRIORITY (QSEN)

Action Alert

Offer oxygen to any patient with dyspnea near death, regardless of his or her oxygen saturation, because COMFORT is the desired outcome. If the patient is feeling dyspneic even though the oxygen saturation is above 90%, be sure that he or she receives oxygen to relieve respiratory distress. In addition, offer an electric fan directed toward the patient's face. Some patients find the circulating air more helpful than oxygen therapy.

- Related to treatment of the primary disease (e.g., heart failure caused by chemotherapy, pneumonitis, or constrictive pericarditis caused by radiation therapy, anemia related to chemotherapy)
- Unrelated to the primary disease (e.g., pneumonia or congestive heart failure [CHF]).

Depending on the cause, the pathophysiology of dyspnea can involve:
- Obstructive, restrictive, or vascular disturbances in the airways with tumor or lymph node involvement
- Pulmonary congestion secondary to fluid overload and/or cardiac dysfunction
- Bronchoconstriction and bronchospasm as seen with respiratory infection, COPD, or airway blockage by a tumor
- Decreased hemoglobin-carrying capacity as with anemia
- Hyperventilation secondary to neuromuscular disease with limited movement of the diaphragm

Perform a thorough assessment of the patient's dyspnea. Include onset, severity (e.g., 0-to-10 scale), and precipitating factors. Precipitating factors may include time of day, position, anxiety, pain, cough, or emotional distress. *Pharmacologic interventions should begin early in the course of dyspnea.* Nonpharmacologic interventions are used in conjunction with but not in place of drug therapy.

Opioids such as morphine sulfate are the standard treatment for dyspnea near death. They work by (1) altering the perception of air hunger, reducing anxiety and associated oxygen consumption, and (2) reducing pulmonary congestion. Patients who have not been receiving opioids are given starting doses of morphine 5 to 6 mg (or less for patients of advanced age) orally every 4 hours during the day and 10 mg at bedtime. If dyspnea occurs only with activity, give morphine before the activity up to every 2 hours. Those who are taking morphine or other opioids for pain may need higher doses for breathlessness, at times up to 50% more than their usual dose.

If a patient is having severe respiratory distress and poor oxygenation, morphine by mouth may need to be repeated as often as every 30 minutes and an IV or subcutaneous route may need to be established. Subcutaneous or IV doses of 1 to 2 mg of morphine may be given every 5 to 10 minutes until dyspnea is relieved.

Oxygen therapy for dyspnea near death has not been established as a standard of care for all patients. However, those who

Bronchodilators such as albuterol (Proventil) or ipratropium bromide (Atrovent, Apo-Ipravent) via a metered-dose inhaler (MDI) or nebulizer may be given for symptoms of bronchospasm (heard as wheezes). *Corticosteroids* such as prednisone (Deltasone, Winpred) may also be given for bronchospasm and inflammatory problems within and outside the lung. Superior vena cava syndrome and cancer-related lymphangitis causing dyspnea may also respond to corticosteroids (also see Chapter 22).

People who have fluid overload with dyspnea, crackles on auscultation, peripheral edema, and other signs of chronic congestive heart failure (CHF) may be given a *diuretic* such as furosemide (Lasix, Uritol) to decrease blood volume, reduce vascular congestion, and reduce the workload of the heart. Furosemide can be administered by mouth, IV, or subcutaneously. IV push administration, which is effective within minutes, may be preferred for heart failure and pulmonary edema.

Antibiotics may be indicated for dyspnea related to a respiratory infection. A trial of an appropriate antibiotic may be considered to make the patient comfortable.

Secretions in the respiratory tract and oral cavity may also contribute to dyspnea near death. Loud, wet respirations (referred to as **death rattle**) are disturbing to family and caregivers even when they do not seem to cause dyspnea or respiratory distress. Reposition the patient onto one side to reduce gurgling and place a small towel under his or her mouth to collect secretions. *Anticholinergics* such as atropine (ophthalmic) solution 1% given sublingually every 4 hours as needed or hyoscyamine (Levsin) every 6 hours are commonly given to dry up secretions. Scopolamine may also be given transdermally to reduce secretion production. Oropharyngeal suctioning is not recommended for loud secretions in the bronchi or oropharynx because it is often not effective and may only agitate the patient.

Fear and anxiety may be components of respiratory distress at the end of life. For this reason benzodiazepines are commonly given when morphine does not fully control the person's dyspnea. Low-dose lorazepam (Ativan) is administered orally, sublingually, or IV every 4 hours as needed or around the clock.

Other nonpharmacologic interventions include:
- Limiting exertion to avoid exertional dyspnea
- Inserting a long-term urinary (Foley) catheter to avoid dyspnea on exertion

- Positioning the patient with the head of the bed up either in a hospital bed or a reclining chair to increase chest expansion
- Applying wet cloths to the patient's face
- Encouraging imagery and deep breathing

Managing Nausea and Vomiting. Although not as common a problem as pain or dyspnea, nausea and vomiting occur frequently among terminally ill patients during the last week of life. It is particularly common in patients with acquired immune deficiency syndrome (AIDS) and with breast, stomach, or gynecologic cancers.

Other causes of nausea and vomiting at the end of life include:

- Uremia (increased serum urea nitrogen)
- Hypercalcemia
- Increased intracranial pressure
- Constipation or impaction
- Bowel obstruction

If constipation is identified as the cause of nausea and vomiting, give the patient a biphosphate enema (e.g., Fleet) to remove stool quickly. If stool in the rectum cannot be evacuated, a mineral oil enema followed by gentle disimpaction may relieve the patient's distress. Nausea and vomiting related to other causes can be controlled by one or more antiemetic agents such as prochlorperazine (Compazine), ondansetron (Zofran), dexamethasone (Decadron, Deronil, Dexasone), or metoclopramide (Reglan, Maxeran). Based on a patient's response, one or more of these drugs may be combined and compounded into rectal suppositories or oral troches. In addition to providing medications, be sure to remove sources of odors and keep the room temperature at a level that the patient desires.

Complementary and Integrative Health. Aromatherapy using chamomile, camphor, fennel, lavender, peppermint, and rose may reduce or relieve vomiting. However, some patients may have worse nausea with aroma. Ask the patient and family about their preferences and respect culturally established practices.

Managing Agitation and Delirium. Agitation at the end of life first requires assessing for pain or urinary retention, constipation, or another reversible cause. If pain, urinary retention, and constipation are ruled out as causes, delirium (acute confusion) is suspected. Delirium is an acute and fluctuating change in mental status and is accompanied by inattention, disorganized thinking, and/or an altered level of consciousness. It can be hyperactive, hypoactive, or mixed (both). *Hypoactive (quiet)* delirium is probably not uncomfortable for patients. *Agitated (noisy)* delirium with psychotic and behavioral symptoms (e.g., yelling, hallucinations) can be uncomfortable, especially for family. Chapter 3 discusses delirium in more detail.

When delirium occurs in the week or two before death, it is referred to as *terminal delirium*. Possible causes include the adverse effects of opioids, benzodiazepines, anticholinergics, or steroids. If medications are suspected causes, they may be decreased or discontinued. Ideally antipsychotic drugs are given only to control psychotic symptoms such as hallucinations and delusions. However, if they are needed to facilitate COMFORT, they should be available.

Benzodiazepines generally are not used as a first choice for older adults with agitation because of their risk for causing delirium. Development of increased agitation after receiving a benzodiazepine could represent a paradoxical reaction—the opposite of what is expected.

⚠ NURSING SAFETY PRIORITY (QSEN)
Drug Alert

Do not give the patient more than one antipsychotic drug at a time because of the risk for adverse drug events (ADEs). A neuroleptic drug such as a low dose of haloperidol (Haldol, Peridol) 0.5-2 mg orally, IV, subcutaneously, or rectally is commonly used at the end of life. Although haloperidol has the potential to cause extrapyramidal symptoms or adverse cardiovascular events and death in older adults with dementia, the benefits of treating psychosis associated with delirium usually outweigh the risks.

Complementary and Integrative Health. Music therapy may produce relaxation by quieting the mind and promoting a restful state. Aromatherapy with chamomile may also help overcome anxiety, anger, tension, stress, and insomnia in dying patients.

Managing Seizures. Seizures are not common at the end of life but may occur in patients with brain tumors, advanced AIDS, and pre-existing seizure disorders. Around-the-clock drug therapy is needed to maintain a high seizure threshold for patients who can no longer swallow antiepileptic drugs (AEDs). Benzodiazepines such as diazepam (Valium) and lorazepam (Ativan) are the drugs of choice. For home use rectal diazepam gel or sublingual lorazepam oral solution (2 mg/mL) may be preferred. As a second choice, barbiturates such as phenobarbital may be given rectally or IV.

Managing Refractory Symptoms of Distress. Patients receiving opioids for pain or dyspnea and other drugs such as antiemetics or antianxiety agents may experience mild sedation as a side effect to therapy. Depending on the patient and how soon death is expected, sedation may decrease with time. What is important to understand is that drug therapy for symptoms of distress at the end of life are guided by protocols, using medications believed to be safe, with the intent of alleviating suffering. *There is no evidence that administering medications for symptoms of distress using established protocols hastens death.* The ethical responsibility of the nurse in caring for patients near death is to follow guidelines for drug use to manage symptoms and to facilitate prompt and effective symptom management until death.

A small percentage of patients have refractory symptoms of distress that do not respond to treatment near the end of life. These patients may be candidates for **proportionate palliative sedation**—a care management approach involving the administration of drugs such as benzodiazepines (e.g., midazolam [Versed]), neuroleptics, barbiturates, or anesthetic agents (e.g., propofol [Diprivan]) for the purpose of decreasing suffering by lowering patient consciousness. *The intent of proportionate palliative sedation to promote comfort and not hasten death distinguishes it from euthanasia (discussed later in this chapter).*

Meeting Psychosocial Needs. The personal experience of dying or of losing a loved one through death is life altering. Unexpected deaths, particularly in young people, tend to be most traumatic. When a person has a chronic life-threatening disease, he or she and the family may have some knowledge of the expected outcome. However, others may have never considered their illness to be potentially terminal. It is important to first assess what patients and family understand about the illness and then help them identify the desired outcomes for care in its context.

CLINICAL JUDGMENT CHALLENGE 7-1

Patient-Centered Care **QSEN** *; Clinical Judgment*

An 88-year-old woman has been in a Memory Care unit of a long-term care facility for the past 2 years because of advanced Alzheimer's disease. She does not recognize her family and stopped communicating or providing self-care about 6 months ago. Last week she developed a urinary tract infection and was transferred to the skilled unit in the same facility for IV antibiotics. She has a durable power of attorney for health care (her daughter) and a living will, which her family supports. For the past 2 days, the resident has refused to drink or eat anything. She is barely responsive when the staff attempts to arouse her but moans at times.

1. Why is the resident receiving antibiotic therapy in view of the fact that Alzheimer's disease is considered a terminal health problem?
2. With which members of the interprofessional health care team will you consult and collaborate and why?
3. Is the resident a candidate for hospice at this time? Why or why not?
4. Which symptoms of distress do you anticipate that she may have based on your clinical judgment?

Whereas death is the termination of life, dying is a process. People facing death may demonstrate emotional signs and symptoms of their response to the dying process through behaviors that equate to saying goodbye or through actual withdrawal. Some patients attempt to make families feel better by reassuring them that everything will be fine. Teach families that such behaviors are normal (see Chart 7-2).

Assisting Patients During the Grieving Process. Grief is the emotional feeling related to the perception of the loss. Patients who are dying suffer not only from the anticipated death but also from the loss of the ability to engage with others and in the world. Mourning is the outward social expression of the loss. Interventions to help patients and families grieve and mourn are based on cultural beliefs, values, and practices. Some patients and their families express their grief openly and loudly, whereas others are quiet and reserved. Table 7-3 lists basic beliefs regarding death, dying, and afterlife for some of the major religions.

Nursing interventions are aimed at providing appropriate emotional support to allow patients and their families verbalize their fears and concerns. Support includes keeping the patient and family involved in health care decisions and emphasizing that the goal is to keep the patient as comfortable as possible until death.

Intervene with those grieving an impending death by "being with" as opposed to "being there." "Being with" implies that you are physically and psychologically with the grieving patient, empathizing to provide emotional support. Listening and acknowledging the legitimacy of the patient's and/or family's impending loss are often more therapeutic than speaking; this concept is often referred to as **presence**. Nurses facilitate the expression of grief by giving the person who is mourning permission to express himself or herself. Your manner and words show that these expressions of grief are acceptable and expected. An example of therapeutic communication might be "This must be very difficult for you" or "I'm sorry this is happening."

Do not minimize a patient's or family member's reaction to an impending loss/death. Avoid trite assurances such as "Things will be fine. Don't cry," "Don't be upset. She wouldn't want it that way," or "In a year you will have forgotten." Such comments can be barriers to demonstrating care and concern. Accept whatever

TABLE 7-3   Basic Beliefs Regarding Care at End of Life and Death Rituals for Selected Religions

Christianity
- There are many Christian denominations, which have variations in beliefs regarding medical care near the end of life.
- Roman Catholic tradition encourages people to receive Sacrament of the Sick, administered by a priest at any point during an illness. This sacrament may be administered more than once. Not receiving this sacrament will NOT prohibit them from entering heaven after death.
- People may be baptized as Roman Catholics in an emergency situation (e.g., person is dying) by a layperson. Otherwise they are baptized by a priest.
- Christians believe in an afterlife of heaven or hell once the soul has left the body after death.

Judaism
- The dying person is encouraged to recite the confessional or the affirmation of faith, called the *Shema*.
- According to Jewish law, a person who is extremely ill and dying should not be left alone.
- The body, which was the vessel and vehicle to the soul, deserves reverence and respect.
- The body should not be left unattended until the funeral, which should take place as soon as possible (preferably within 24 hours).
- Autopsies are not allowed by Orthodox Jews, except under special circumstances.
- The body should not be embalmed, displayed, or cremated.

Islam
- Based on belief in one God Allah and his prophet Muhammad. Qur'an is the scripture of Islam, composed of Muhammad's revelations of the Word of God (Allah).
- Death is seen as the beginning of a new and better life.
- God has prescribed an appointed time of death for everyone.
- Qur'an encourages humans to seek treatment and not to refuse treatment. Belief is that only Allah cures but that Allah cures through the work of humans.
- On death the eyelids are to be closed, and the body should be covered. Before moving and handling the body, contact someone from the person's mosque to perform rituals of bathing and wrapping body in cloth.

Data from Giger, J. N. (2013). *Transcultural nursing: Assessment and intervention* (6th ed.). St. Louis: Mosby.

the grieving person says about the situation. Remain present, be ready to listen attentively, and guide gently. In this way you can help the bereaved family and significant others prepare for the necessary reminiscence and integration of the loss.

Storytelling through reminiscence and life review can be an important activity for patients who are dying. Life review is a structured process of reflecting on what one has done through his or her life. This is often facilitated by an interviewer. Reminiscence is the process of randomly reflecting on memories of events in one's life. The benefits of storytelling through either method provide the ability to attain perspective and enhance meaning. Suggest that the patient and family record autobiographic stories (print or video), write memories in a journal, or develop a scrapbook. Young dying parents often write letters or record videos for their children when they are older.

Perform a spiritual assessment to identify the patient's spiritual needs and facilitate open expression of his or her beliefs and needs. A spiritual assessment could start with questions such as "What is important to you?" or "What gives you meaning or purpose in your life?"

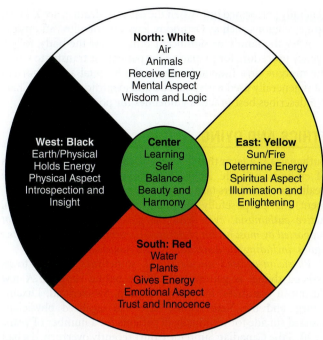

FIG. 7-2 An example of a medicine wheel used by indigenous people to provide harmony and balance in life and transition into the spirit worlds after death.

North: White
Air
Animals
Receive Energy
Mental Aspect
Wisdom and Logic

West: Black
Earth/Physical
Holds Energy
Physical Aspect
Introspection and
Insight

Center
Learning
Self
Balance
Beauty and
Harmony

East: Yellow
Sun/Fire
Determine Energy
Spiritual Aspect
Illumination and
Enlightening

South: Red
Water
Plants
Gives Energy
Emotional Aspect
Trust and Innocence

🌐 CULTURAL/SPIRITUAL CONSIDERATIONS
Patient-Centered Care QSEN

Spirituality is whatever or whoever gives ultimate meaning and purpose in one's life that invites particular ways of being in the world in relation to others, oneself, and the universe. A person's spirituality may or may not include belief in God. **Religions** are formal belief systems that provide a framework for making sense of life, death, and suffering and responding to universal spiritual questions. Religions often have beliefs, rituals, texts, and other practices that are shared by a community. Spirituality and religion can help some patients cope with the thought of death, contributing to quality of life during the dying process.

When assessing the spiritual needs of the dying patient, consider end-of-life preferences based on ethnic beliefs and practices. For example, the medicine wheel represents the spiritual journey to find one's own path for indigenous people in many countries, including American Indians (e.g., Cherokee, Navajo, Lakota) and Aboriginal people (e.g., Inuit, First Nations) in Canada and Alaska (also known as *Canada or Alaska Natives*). The medicine wheel helps people in these groups maintain balance and harmony within four life dimensions (Fig. 7-2). Depending on specific tribal practices and beliefs, the dimensions may be represented by colors, seasons, or directions.

As part of the dying process, certain tribal ceremonies must take place for patients to have a peaceful transition into the Spirit World and experience a "good death." One special ceremony involves smudging: Selected tribal medicines are burned, and the smoke is passed over the patient's body to cleanse it.

Regardless of whether a person has had an affiliation with a religion or a belief in God or other Supreme Being, he or she

---

👤 CHART 7-3 Patient and Family Education: Preparing for Self-Management
Physical Manifestations Indicating That Death Has Occurred

- Breathing stops.
- Heart stops beating.
- Pupils become fixed and dilated.
- Body color becomes pale and waxen.
- Body temperature drops.
- Muscles and sphincters relax.
- Urine and stool may be released.
- Eyes may remain open, and there is no blinking.
- The jaw may fall open.
- Observers may hear trickling of fluids internally.

can experience what is referred to as *spiritual* or *existential distress*. Existential distress is brought about by the actual or perceived threat to one's continued existence. Terminal illness and facing death can pose a profound threat to one's personhood. The main task for a person at the end of life is coming to terms with one's losses, which may include loss of meaning, loss of relationships, and facing the unknown. Acknowledge the patient's spiritual pain and encourage verbalization. Use a family tree to discuss relationships, fears, hopes, and unfinished business. If the patient or family prefers, arrange for counseling with chaplains, spiritual leaders, or others trained in end-of-life care. *Do not try to explain the loss in philosophic or religious terms.* Statements such as "Everything happens for the best" or "God sends us only as much as we can bear" are not helpful when the person has yet to express feelings of anguish or anger.

Although emotionally challenging, witnessing the death of a loved one may help facilitate the family to accept death. Witnessing how ill a person is makes the event real and enhances an understanding of how disease affects bodily function and decline. Describe the physical signs in detail—realistic enough to be unmistakable yet not so graphic as to alarm the listeners (see Chart 7-1). Booklets with this information should be provided to families to help them see what is expected and "normal" to the dying process.

Families witnessing the dying process often have difficulty distinguishing what is a normal finding of decline from signs and symptoms of distress. Instructing families about signs and symptoms of pain (e.g., grimacing, moaning, guarding behaviors) or dyspnea is essential. Emphasize that, in the absence of dyspnea or pain, patients often die very peacefully with cessation of breathing. Nurses and family members know that a person has died when he or she stops breathing. Chart 7-3 lists other manifestations of death.

Nurses, patients, and families may benefit from written information about the dying process and what is known about the patient experience and needs. *Fast Facts and Concepts* are a group of evidence-based summaries on key palliative care topics available on the Palliative Care Network of Wisconsin (2016) website (http://www.mypcnow.org). They provide concise, practical, peer-reviewed information on topics common to patients facing serious illness.

In Canada, the Canadian Hospice Care Association provides information for patients, families, lay caregivers/volunteers, and members of the interprofessional health care team. A number of documents on palliative care and hospice services are available on the website (www.chpca.net).

 NCLEX EXAMINATION CHALLENGE 7-2

Psychosocial Integrity

A client receiving palliative care asks the nurse, "Why is this happening to me?" What is the nurse's **best** response?
A. "I don't know. God only knows when your time is up on this earth."
B. "I'm sorry. I know that this is a difficult time for you."
C. "It's going to be OK; at least you aren't leaving any family behind."
D. "We'll make sure that all of your needs are met, so don't worry."

POSTMORTEM CARE

If the death was in the home and expected, emergency assistance (911) should *not* be called. If the person was a patient in a hospice program, the family calls hospice. If a death is unexpected or suspicious, the medical examiner is notified. Otherwise the nurse or primary health care provider performs the pronouncement and completes a death certificate (Chart 7-4). Most states allow nurses to pronounce death in nursing homes and other long-term care facilities, but only a few states permit nurses to pronounce in acute care facilities such as hospitals. Be sure to check your health care agency policies for who can pronounce death and the specific procedure to follow.

After the patient dies, ask the family or other caregivers if they would like to spend time with the patient to help them cope with what has happened and say their good-byes. Even if the death has been anticipated, no one knows how he or she will feel until it occurs. It may take hours to days to weeks or months for each person to realize the full effect of the event. Some family members may find it therapeutic to bathe and prepare the person's body for transfer to the funeral home or the hospital morgue. Offer families this opportunity if it is culturally acceptable.

Before preparing the body for transfer, ask the primary health care provider whether an autopsy will be required. When the death is expected, an autopsy is not likely. An autopsy is

generally performed only when the cause of death is not known. Some religions such as Orthodox Jews do not allow autopsies.

After the family or significant others view the body, follow agency procedure for preparing the patient for transfer to either the morgue or a funeral home. In the hospital a postmortem kit is generally used with a shroud and identification tags. Chart 7-5 describes best practice guidelines for postmortem care.

ETHICS AND DYING

Euthanasia is a term that has been used to describe the process of ending one's life. *Active euthanasia* implies that primary health care providers take action (e.g., give medication or treatment) that purposefully and directly causes the patient's death. *Active euthanasia, even with the patient's permission, is not supported by most health professional organizations in the United States, including the American Nurses Association.*

Physician-assisted suicide (PAS), sometimes referred to as assisted dying, is gaining worldwide public support. A few European countries, including Belgium, Switzerland, Luxembourg, and the Netherlands, have had legalized physician-assisted suicide for terminally ill patients for a number of years. In 2015 the Canadian Supreme Court recently overturned a ban on physician-assisted suicide. In the United States PAS is now legally approved in Oregon, Washington, Vermont, Montana, and New Mexico. Twenty-six other states and the District of Columbia are considering legislation on end-of-life options. At this time nurses are generally not involved in physician-assisted suicide but need to be knowledgeable about the legislation in the state where they practice.

Withdrawing or withholding life-sustaining therapy, formerly called *passive euthanasia,* involves discontinuing one or more

 CHART 7-4 **Best Practice for Patient Safety & Quality Care** **QSEN**

Pronouncement of Death

- Note time of death that the family or staff reported the cessation of respirations.
- Identify the patient by identification (ID) tag if in facility. Note the general appearance of the body.
- Ascertain that the patient does not rouse to verbal or tactile stimuli. Avoid overtly painful stimuli, especially if family members are present.
- Auscultate for the absence of heart sounds; palpate for the absence of carotid pulse.
- Look and listen for the absence of spontaneous respirations.
- Document the time of pronouncement and all notifications in the medical record (i.e., to attending physician). Document if the medical examiner needs to be notified (may be required for unexpected or suspicious death). Document if an autopsy is planned per the attending primary health care provider and family.
- If your state and agency policy allows an RN to pronounce death, document as indicated on the death certificate.

 CHART 7-5 **Best Practice for Patient Safety & Quality Care** **QSEN**

Postmortem Care

- Provide all care with respect to communicate that the person was important and valued.
- Ask the family or significant others if they wish to help wash the patient or comb his or her hair; respect and follow their cultural practices for body preparation.
- If no autopsy is planned, remove or cut all tubes and lines according to agency policy.
- Close the patient's eyes unless the cultural/religious practice is for a family member or other person to close the eyes.
- Insert dentures if the patient wore them.
- Straighten the patient and lower the bed to a flat position.
- Place a pillow under the patient's head.
- Wash the patient as needed and comb and arrange the patient's hair unless the family desires to perform bathing and body preparation.
- Place waterproof pads under the patient's hips and around the perineum to absorb any excrement.
- Clean the patient's room or unit.
- Allow the family or significant others to see the patient in private and to perform any religious or cultural customs they wish (e.g., prayer).
- Assess that all who need to see the patient have done so before transferring to the funeral home or morgue.
- Notify the hospital chaplain or appropriate religious leader if requested by the family or significant others.
- Ensure that the nurse or physician has completed and signed the death certificate.
- Prepare the patient for transfer to either a morgue or funeral home; wrap the patient in a shroud (unless the family has a special shroud to use), and attach identification tags per agency policy.

therapies that might prolong the life of a person who cannot be cured by the therapy. Another phrase sometimes used is "letting the person die naturally" or "allowing natural death (AND)," as discussed earlier in this chapter. *In this situation, the withdrawal of the intervention does not directly cause the patient's death.* The progression of the patient's disease or poor health status is the cause of death. Professional health care organizations and some religious communities support the right of patients and their surrogate decision makers to refuse or stop treatment when patients are close to death and interventions are considered medically futile or capable of causing harm. The U.S. court system also supports withdrawal of aggressive treatment and the rights of surrogate decision makers to refuse or stop treatment.

A newer concept as the legal alternative method for death in all 50 states is *voluntary stopping of eating and drinking (VSED)*, also called *terminal dehydration* (Lachman, 2015). With VSED, competent patients with a terminal or incurable disease or illness refuse to eat or drink to hasten their death. Many patients want control over their lives and wish to die rather than continue experiencing severe pain and suffering. In addition, patients often want to end the caregiver burden that is often assumed by the family or significant other for their care. As described earlier in this chapter, terminal dehydration is not painful when discomfort is managed with palliative measures (Lachman, 2015).

Nurses are usually in the best and most immediate position to discuss these issues. To do this, they must be knowledgeable about terminology and ethical issues related to death and dying. In all cases the principles of informed consent must be met: the patient is competent, the death is voluntary, and the patient understands the benefit, burden, and consequences of the death.

GET READY FOR THE NCLEX® EXAMINATION!

KEY POINTS

Review these Key Points for each NCLEX Examination Client Needs Category.

Safe and Effective Care Environment

- Hospice care uses an interprofessional team-oriented approach to expert medical care, pain management, and emotional and spiritual support expressly tailored to the person's needs and wishes. Support is also provided to the person's family, friends, and lay caregivers. **QSEN: Teamwork and Collaboration**
- The decision by DPOAHC to withdraw or withhold life-sustaining therapy is supported by the US Supreme Court and other professional/religious organizations.
- Be aware that physician-assisted suicide is legal in several countries and five states in the United States. However, legislation for the right to die has been introduced in 26 other states and the District of Columbia. **Ethics**
- Be aware that nurses have an ethical obligation to provide timely information about expected care outcomes so patients and families can make the best end-of-life decisions. **Ethics**

Health Promotion and Maintenance

- Assess the patient and family to determine if they have written advance directives such as a durable power of attorney for health care (DPOAHC), a living will, or portable DNR/DNAR.
- Stress the importance of having a DPOAHC to inform health care providers of your wishes if you lack capacity.
- Teach the patient and family that an advance directive is a written document that specifies what, if any, extraordinary actions the patient would want if he or she could no longer make decisions about care.

Psychosocial Integrity

- Assess the patient's emotional signs of impending death; assess coping ability of the patient and family or other caregiver (see Chart 7-2).
- Incorporate the patient's personal cultural practices and spiritual beliefs regarding death and dying (see Table 7-3). **QSEN: Patient-Centered Care**

- Be aware that people facing death may experience fear and anxiety about their impending death and have difficulty coping.
- Provide psychosocial interventions to support the patient and family during the dying process.

Physiological Integrity

- Death is defined as the cessation of integrated tissue and organ function, manifested by cessation of heartbeat, absence of spontaneous respirations, or irreversible brain dysfunction.
- Hospice and palliative care are different, as described in Table 7-2.
- Assess the patient for pain, dyspnea, agitation, nausea, and vomiting, which are common problems at the end of life. **QSEN: Evidence-Based Practice**
- Recognize that older adults are often undertreated for pain or other symptoms at the end of life.
- Assess for the common physical signs of approaching death, as listed in Chart 7-1.
- Medications are frequently given to control dyspnea, pain, nausea, vomiting, delirium, and seizures in patients near death.
- Because of the risk for delirium, particularly in older adults, providers may avoid use of benzodiazepines for treatment of anxiety, even at the end of life. Development of increased agitation after receiving benzodiazepine could represent a paradoxical reaction. **QSEN: Safety**
- Terminal delirium may occur in a week or two before death. Haloperidol given orally or IV is the drug of choice to manage psychosis associated with delirium.
- Assessment of oxygen saturation for patients at the end of life is not necessary. Oxygen should be provided based on comfort. **QSEN: Evidence-Based Practice**
- Common complementary and integrative therapies used for symptom management at the end of life include aromatherapy, music therapy, and energy therapies such as Therapeutic Touch.
- Follow Chart 7-5 for best-practice guidelines for performing postmortem care; incorporate the patient's cultural and religious beliefs in body preparation and burial (see Table 7-3). **QSEN: Patient-Centered Care**

SELECTED BIBLIOGRAPHY

Asterisk indicates a classic or definitive work on this subject.

Abrahm, J. L. (2014). *A physician's guide to pain and symptom management in cancer patients* (3rd ed.). Baltimore: John Hopkins University Press.

Allard, M. E., & Katseres, J. (2016). Using essential oils to enhance nursing practice and for self-care. *AJN, 116*(2), 42–51.

American Association of Colleges of Nursing (2016). *Palliative CARES: Competencies and recommendations for educating undergraduate nursing students preparing nurses to care for the seriously ill and their families.* Washington, DC: AACN.

Bodtke, S., & Ligon, K. (2016). *Hospice and palliative medicine handbook: A clinical guide.* San Diego: Authors.

*Campbell, M. L., Weissman, D. E., & Nelson, J. E. (2012). Palliative care consultation in the ICU. *Journal of Palliative Medicine, 15*(6), 715–716.

Coyle, N. (2016). Legal and ethical aspects of care. In B. Ferrell (Ed.), *HPNA Palliative nursing manuals.* New York: Oxford University Press.

*Doka, K. J., & Tucci, A. S. (Eds.), (2011). *Spirituality and end-of-life care.* Washington, DC: Hospice Foundation of America.

*Ferrell, B. (2010). Palliative care research: Nursing response to emergent society needs. *Nursing Science Quarterly, 23*(3), 221–225.

Finocchiaro, D. N. (2016). Supporting the patient's spiritual needs at the end of life. *Nursing, 46*(5), 57–59.

Giger, J. N. (2013). *Transcultural nursing: Assessment and intervention* (6th ed.). St. Louis: Mosby.

Institute of Medicine. *Dying in America: Improving quality and honoring individual preferences near the end of life.* http://www.iom.edu/Reports/2014/Dying-in America-Improving-and Honoring-Individual-Preferences-Near-the-End-of-Life.aspx. Released Sept 17, 2014.

Lachman, V. (2015). Voluntary stopping of eating and drinking: An ethical alternative to physician-assisted suicide. *Medsurg Nursing, 24*(1), 56–59.

Matzo, M. L., & Sherman, D. W. (Eds.), (2015). *Palliative care nursing: Quality care to the end of life* (4th ed.). New York: Springer.

National Consensus Project for Quality Palliative Care. (2013). *Clinical practice guidelines for quality palliative care* (3rd ed.). Pittsburgh.

*National Hospice and Palliative Care Organization. (2012). *NHPCO Facts and figures: Hospice care in America*: Author.

National Vital Statistics Bureau. (2013). *10 Leading causes of death by age-group, United States—2013.* www.cdc.gov/injury/wisqars/pdf/leading_causes_of_death_in_the_United_States_2013-a.pdf.

Paice, J. A. (2016). Care of the imminently dying. In B. Ferrell (Ed.), *HPNA Palliative nursing manuals.* New York: Oxford University Press.

Paice, J. A. (2016). Physical aspects of care. In B. Ferrell (Ed.), *HPNA Palliative nursing manuals.* New York: Oxford University Press.

*Perrin, K. (2012). Ethical responsibilities and issues in palliative care. In K. Perrin, C. Sheehan, M. Potter, & M. Kazanowski (Eds.), *Palliative care nursing: Caring for suffering patients* (pp. 77–117). New York: Springer.

Perrin, K. (2015). Communicating with seriously ill and dying patients, their families, and their healthcare practitioners. In M. Matzo & D. W. Sherman (Eds.), *Palliative care nursing* (4th ed.). New York: Springer.

Perrin, K. (2016). Caring for the ICU patient at the end of life. In K. Perrin & C. E. MacLeod (Eds.), *Understanding the essentials of critical care nursing.* Upper Saddle River, NJ: Pearson.

Perrin, K., & Kazanowski, M. (2015). Overcoming barriers to palliative care consultation. *Critical Care Nurse, 35*(5), 44–51.

Quill, T., Bower, K. A., Holloway, R., Shah, M. S., Caprio, T. V., Olden, A. M., et al. (2014). *Primer of palliative care* (6th ed.). Glenview, IL: American Academy of Hospice and Palliative Medicine.

Ramenofsky, D. H., & Weissman, D. E. CPR Survival in the hospital setting. S Marks. (Ed.). (July 2015.) *Fast facts and concepts # 179.* http://www.mypcnow.org.

*Support Study Principal Investigators. (1995). A controlled trial to improve care for seriously ill hospitalized patients: The Study to Understand Prognoses and Preferences for Outcomes and Risks for Treatments (SUPPORT). *Journal of the American Medical Association, 274*, 1591–1598.

Teno, J. M., Gozalo, P. L., Bynum, J. P., Leland, N. E., Miller, S., Morden, N. E., et al. (2013). Change in end-of-life care for Medicare beneficiaries' site of death, place of care, and health care transitions in 2000, 2005, and 2009. *Journal of the American Medical Association, 309*(5), 470–477.

*Tian, J., Kaufman, D., Zarich, S., Ong, P., Amoateng-Adjepong, Y., & Manthous, C. (2010). Outcomes of critically ill patients who received cardiopulmonary resuscitation. *American Journal of Respiratory Critical Care Medicine, 182*(4), 501–506.

Westman, K. F., & Blaisdell, C. (2016). Many benefits, little risk: The use of massage in nursing practice. *AJN, 116*(1), 34–41.

CHAPTER 8

Principles of Emergency and Trauma Nursing

Linda Laskowski-Jones and Karen L. Toulson

 http://evolve.elsevier.com/Iggy/

PRIORITY AND INTERRELATED CONCEPTS

The priority concepts for this chapter are:
- SAFETY
- TEAMWORK AND INTERPROFESSIONAL COLLABORATION
- COMMUNICATION

LEARNING OUTCOMES

Safe and Effective Care Environment

1. Describe the emergency department (ED) environment, including vulnerable populations seen.
2. Engage in TEAMWORK AND INTERPROFESSIONAL COLLABORATION with interprofessional team members in the ED.
3. Implement strategies to maintain staff and patient SAFETY in the ED.
4. Explain selected core competencies required of ED nurses.
5. Prioritize order of ED care delivery via triage.
6. Prioritize resuscitation interventions based on assessment of the injured patient.

Psychosocial Integrity

7. Implement nursing interventions to support survivors after the death of a loved one.

Physiological Integrity

8. Describe the expected sequence of events from admission through disposition of a patient treated in the ED.

The health care needs of individuals within the United States continue to see a rise in the demand for emergency care. Functioning as safety nets for communities of all sizes, emergency departments (EDs) provide services to insured and uninsured patients seeking medical care. They are also responsible for SAFETY through public health surveillance and emergency disaster preparedness. Some hospital-based EDs also provide observation, procedural care, and employee or occupational health services. Other hospital-based EDs have interprofessional specialty teams who take part in TEAMWORK AND INTERPROFESSIONAL COLLABORATION to provide first-line care for patients with stroke and cardiac problems (The Joint Commission [TJC], 2017b). The role of the ED is so vital that the Centers for Medicare and Medicaid Services (2013) has a process for designating small rural facilities of 25 inpatient beds or fewer as critical access hospitals if they provide around-the-clock emergency care services 7 days a week. Critical access hospitals are considered *necessary providers of health care* to community residents that are not close to other hospitals in a given region.

Emergency departments play a unique role within the US health care system because of the multi-specialty nature of the environment. More than 136.3 million people visit the ED each year, or 44.5 visits per 100 people (Centers for Disease Control and Prevention [CDC], 2017). The demand for emergency care has greatly increased over the past 15 years, and the health care consumer has higher expectations. However, the capacity to provide necessary resources has not kept pace in many systems. Emergency department crowding occurs when the need for care exceeds available resources in the department, hospital, or both (Bellow & Gillespie, 2014). The Joint Commission (TJC, 2017c) has established a set of metrics (Core Measure Sets) based on ED length of stay (LOS) that hospitals are required to submit.

The longer the ED length of stay for admitted patients, the more overcrowded the ED becomes. That, in turn, limits access to other patients who are in need of ED beds for emergency care. A prolonged LOS also indicates problems with inpatient bed availability and poor overall hospital throughput.

In 2010, the Affordable Care Act became the impetus for health care initiatives that impacted emergency services; the full spectrum of that impact has continued to evolve and may change again if this Act is repealed. Continued or changed availability, as well as the cost, of health insurance will influence how patients use emergency departments, primary care networks, disease management programs, home care services, and community resources. The widespread availability of health insurance may produce an increase in the number of patients who use the ED because they now have greater access to the necessary financial resources. Emergency department use may actually decrease for some types of patients as hospitals and providers partner in Accountable Care Organization models. This will better control costs by managing patient outcomes through primary care networks and disease management programs. Emergency departments may also experience a shift in focus from admitting the majority of acutely ill patients to the hospital for care to use of more TEAMWORK AND INTERPROFESSIONAL COLLABORATION with home care services and community access to resources that enable patients to be safely discharged home from the ED when possible.

THE EMERGENCY DEPARTMENT ENVIRONMENT OF CARE

In the emergency care environment rapid change is expected. The typical ED is fast paced and, at the height of activity, might even appear chaotic. Patients seek treatment for a number of physical, psychological, spiritual, and social reasons. Many nurses work in this environment because they thrive in challenging, stimulating work settings. Although most EDs have treatment areas that are designated for certain populations such as patients with trauma or cardiac, psychiatric, or gynecologic problems, care can actually take place almost anywhere. In a crowded ED patients may receive initial treatment outside of the usual treatment rooms, including the waiting room and hallways.

The ED is typically alive with activity and noise, although the pace decreases at times because arrivals are random. Emergency nurses can expect background sounds that include ringing telephones, monitor alarms, vocal patients, crying children, and radio transmissions between staff and incoming ambulance or helicopter personnel. Interruptions and distractions are the norm, and the nurse must ensure to the best degree possible that these events do not impact patient SAFETY.

Demographic Data and Vulnerable Populations

Staff members in the ED provide care for people across the life span with a broad spectrum of issues, illnesses, and injuries and various cultural and religious values. Especially vulnerable populations who visit the ED include the homeless, the poor, patients with mental health/behavioral health and substance abuse issues and older adults. During a given shift the emergency nurse may function as a cardiac nurse, a geriatric nurse, a psychiatric nurse, a pediatric nurse, and a trauma nurse. Patient acuity ranges from life-threatening emergencies to minor symptoms that could be addressed in a primary care

office or community clinic. Some of the most common reasons that people seek ED care are:

- Abdominal pain
- Chest pain
- Breathing difficulties
- Injuries (especially falls in older adults)
- Headache
- Fever
- Pain (the most common symptom)

CONSIDERATIONS FOR OLDER ADULTS
Patient-Centered Care QSEN

Older adults often visit the ED because of worsening of an existing chronic condition or because the condition affects their ability to perform ADLs. Older adults are also sometimes admitted from nursing homes or assisted-living facilities for procedures (e.g., insertion of a percutaneous endoscopic gastrostomy [PEG] tube or peripherally inserted central catheter [PICC]) or treatments (e.g., blood transfusions). Some hospitals plan direct admission of the patient to same-day surgery or hold a bed for the procedure or treatment to bypass the ED. This arrangement decreases the patient's wait time and therefore decreases the risks for adverse events such as pressure injury development or hospital-acquired infection. Incorporating family members or caregivers of older adults into the ED care process can aid in overall patient evaluation, decision making, and satisfaction with the ED experience.

Special Nursing Teams—Members of the Interprofessional Team

Many EDs have specialized nursing teams that deal with high-risk populations of patients. One example is the forensic nurse examiner team. Forensic nurse examiners (RN-FNEs) are educated to obtain patient histories; collect forensic evidence; and offer counseling and follow-up care for victims of rape, child abuse, and domestic violence—also known as *intimate partner violence (IPV)* (International Association of Forensic Nurses, 2016). They recognize evidence of abuse and when to intervene on the patient's behalf. Forensic nurses who specialize in helping victims of sexual assault are called *sexual assault nurse examiners (SANEs)* or *sexual assault forensic examiners (SAFEs)*.

Interventions performed by forensic nurses may include providing information about developing a SAFETY plan or how to escape a violent relationship. Forensic nurse examiners document injuries and collect physical and photographic evidence. They may also provide testimony in court as to what was observed during the examination and information about the type of care provided.

The psychiatric crisis nurse team is another example of an ED specialty team. Many patients who visit the ED for their acute problems also have chronic mental health disorders. Patients who are experiencing an acute psychiatric crisis situation as their primary problem such as a suicide attempt secondary to severe depression or a new onset of psychosis may also arrive in the ED. The availability of mental health/behavioral health nurses can improve the quality of care delivered to these patients who require specialized interventions in the ED and can offer valuable expertise to the emergency health care staff. This team evaluates patients with emotional behaviors or mental illness and facilitates the follow-up treatment plan, including possible admission to an appropriate psychiatric facility. These nurses also interact with patients and families when sudden illness, serious injury, or death of a loved one may have caused a crisis. On-site interventions can help patients and families cope with these unexpected changes in their lives.

Some EDs have a specialized area to treat patients with psychiatric disorders that is designed to promote optimal safety. Features may include closed-circuit video monitoring, access-control door locks, solid ceilings (to prevent patients from climbing into the ceiling), a secured area to retain patient belongings, metal detectors, panic alarms, and elimination of any items or room features that could pose a safety risk to patients or staff.

Interprofessional Team Collaboration

The emergency nurse is one member of the large interprofessional team who provides care for patients in the ED. A team approach to emergency care using TEAMWORK AND INTERPROFESSIONAL COLLABORATION is considered a standard of practice (Fig. 8-1). In this setting the nurse coordinates care with all levels of health care team providers, from prehospital emergency medical services (EMS) personnel to physicians, hospital technicians, and professional and ancillary support staff.

Prehospital care providers are typically the first caregivers that patients see before transport to the ED by an ambulance or helicopter (Fig. 8-2). Local protocols define the skill level of the EMS responders dispatched to provide assistance.

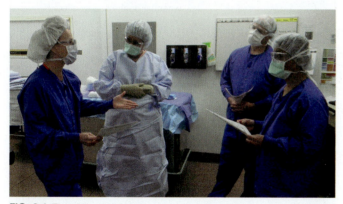

FIG. 8-1 The ability to work as part of an interprofessional team is crucial to positive outcomes for emergency department (ED) patients. (From Rothrock, J. C. (2015). *Alexander's Care of the Patient in Surgery.* (15th ed.) St. Louis: Mosby.)

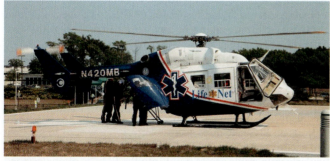

FIG. 8-2 Advanced life support helicopter arriving at emergency department landing zone. Helicopters are used to rapidly transport critically ill and injured patients to the hospital for emergent care.

Emergency medical technicians (EMTs) offer basic life support (BLS) interventions such as oxygen, basic wound care, splinting, spinal immobilization, and monitoring of vital signs. Some units carry automatic external defibrillators (AEDs) and may be authorized to administer selected drugs such as an EpiPen, intranasal naloxone (Narcan), or nitroglycerin based on established medical protocols. For patients who require care that exceeds BLS resources, paramedics are usually dispatched. Paramedics are advanced life support (ALS) providers who can perform advanced techniques, which may include cardiac monitoring, advanced airway management and intubation, needle chest decompression, establishing IV or intraosseous access, and administering drugs en route to the ED (Fig. 8-3).

The prehospital provider is a key source for valuable patient data. Emergency nurses rely on these providers to be the "eyes and ears" of the health care team in the prehospital setting and to ensure COMMUNICATION of this information to other staff members for continuity of care.

Another integral member of the emergency health care team is the emergency medicine physician. These medical professionals receive specialized education and training in emergency patient management. As emergency care has become increasingly complex and specialized, emergency medicine is a recognized physician specialty practice.

The emergency nurse interacts with a number of staff and community physicians involved in patient care but is involved in closest collaboration with emergency medicine physicians. Even though other physician specialists may be involved in ED patient treatment, the emergency medicine physician typically directs the overall care in the department. Many EDs also employ nurse practitioners (NPs) and physician assistants (PAs) to assume designated roles in patient assessment and treatment. Teaching hospitals have resident physicians who train in the ED. They act in collaboration with or under the supervision of the emergency medicine physician to assist with emergency care delivery.

The emergency nurse interacts and regularly takes part in TEAMWORK AND INTERPROFESSIONAL COLLABORATION with *professional and ancillary staff* who function in support roles. These personnel include radiology and ultrasound technicians, respiratory therapists, laboratory technicians, social workers, case managers, nursing assistants, and clerical staff. Each

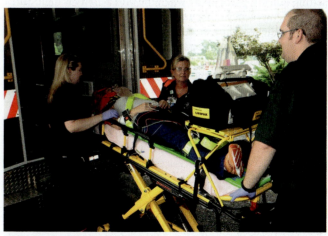

FIG. 8-3 Prehospital providers take a patient from the ambulance to be brought into the emergency department.

support staff member is essential to the success of the emergency health care team. For example, the respiratory therapist can help the nurse troubleshoot mechanical ventilator issues. Laboratory technicians can offer advice regarding best practice techniques for specimen collection. During the discharge planning process, social workers or case managers can be tremendous patient advocates in locating community resources, including temporary housing, durable medical equipment (DME), drug and alcohol counseling, health insurance information, follow-up care, and prescription services. The ED nurse is accountable for COMMUNICATION of pertinent staff considerations, patient needs, and restrictions to support staff (e.g., physical limitations, safety concerns, Transmission-Based Precautions) to ensure that ongoing patient and staff safety issues are addressed.

The emergency nurse's interactions extend beyond the walls of the ED. Communication with nurses from the inpatient units is necessary to ensure continuity of patient care. Providing a concise but comprehensive report of the patient's ED experience is essential for the *hand-off communication* process and patient SAFETY. Information should include the patient's:

- Situation (reason for being in the ED) and admitting diagnosis
- Pertinent medical history, including implantable devices and any history of organ transplant
- Assessment and diagnostic findings, particularly critical results
- Transmission-Based Precautions and safety concerns (e.g., fall risk, allergies) as indicated
- Interventions provided in the ED and response to those interventions

The Joint Commission's National Patient Safety Goals (NPSGs) (The Joint Commission [TJC], 2017a) advocate that hospitals and other health care agencies use a standardized approach to hand-off communications to prevent errors caused by poor or inadequate communication. Many agencies use the SBAR method (situation, background, assessment, response) or some variation of that method to ensure complete and clearly understood COMMUNICATION. Chapter 1 discusses the SBAR technique in more detail.

Both emergency nurses and nurses on inpatient units need to understand the unique aspects of their two practice environments to prevent conflicts. For example, nurses on inpatient units may be critical of the push to move patients out of the ED setting quickly, particularly when the unit activity is high. Similarly the emergency nurse may be critical of the inpatient unit's lack of understanding or enthusiasm for accepting admissions rapidly. Effective interpersonal COMMUNICATION skills and respectful negotiation can optimize TEAMWORK AND INTERPROFESSIONAL COLLABORATION between the emergency nurse and the inpatient unit nurse. For instance, when ED patient volume or acuity is overwhelming, the unit nurse can volunteer to assist the ED nurse by moving a monitored patient to the hospital bed. Whenever possible, the emergency nurse may decide to delay sending admitted patients to inpatient units during change of shift or crisis periods such as a cardiac arrest on the unit.

STAFF AND PATIENT SAFETY CONSIDERATIONS

In the emergency department (ED) setting, staff and patient SAFETY are major concerns (Chart 8-1).

 CHART 8-1   Best Practice for Patient Safety & Quality Care QSEN

Maintaining Patient and Staff Safety in the Emergency Department

SAFETY CONSIDERATION	INTERVENTIONS TO MINIMIZE RISK
Patient identification	Provide an identification (ID) bracelet for each patient.
	Use two unique identifiers (e.g., name, date of birth).
	If patient identity is unknown, use a special identification system.
Injury prevention for patients	Keep rails up on stretcher.
	Keep stretcher in lowest position.
	Remind the patient to use call light for assistance.
	Reorient confused patient frequently.
	If patient is confused, ask a family member or significant other to remain with him or her.
	Implement measures to protect skin integrity for patients at risk for skin breakdown.
Risk for errors and adverse events	Obtain a thorough patient and family history.
	Check the patient for a medical alert bracelet or necklace.
	Search the patient's belongings for weapons or other harmful items such as drugs and drug paraphernalia when he or she has an altered mental status.
Injury prevention for staff	Use Standard Precautions at all times.
	Anticipate hostile, violent patient, family, and/or visitor behavior.
	Plan and practice options if violence occurs, including assistance from the security department.

Staff Safety

Staff safety concerns center on the potential for transmission of disease and on personal safety when dealing with aggressive, agitated, or violent patients and visitors. The emergency nurse uses Standard Precautions at all times when a potential for contamination by blood or other body fluids exists. Patients with tuberculosis or other airborne pathogens are preferentially placed in a negative-pressure room if available. The nurse wears a powered air-purifying respirator (PAPR) or a specially fitted facemask before engaging in any close interaction with these patients (see Chapter 23).

Emergency departments use several methods of ensuring SAFETY. Many EDs have at least one security guard present at all times for immediate assistance with these situations. Metal detectors may be used as a screening device for individuals who are suspected of having weapons. Strategically located panic buttons and remote door access controls allow staff to get help and secure major entrances. The triage reception area—a particularly vulnerable access point into the ED—is often designed to serve as a security barrier with bullet-proof glass and staff-controlled door entry into the treatment area. Hospitals may

! NURSING SAFETY PRIORITY QSEN
Action Alert

Hostile patient and visitor behaviors also pose injury risks to staff members. Be alert for volatile situations or people who demonstrate aggressive or violent tendencies through verbal abuse or acting out. Be sure to follow the hospital security plan, including identifying the nearest escape route, attempting de-escalation strategies before harm can occur, and notifying security and supervisory staff of the situation. Emergency visits resulting from gang or domestic violence can produce particularly hazardous conditions. Report all episodes of assaultive or violent behaviors through the hospital event documentation process so leaders and risk managers are aware of the scope of the problem and can plan safety strategies, including staff education, accordingly.

! NURSING SAFETY PRIORITY QSEN
Action Alert

Help patients move slowly from a supine to an upright position and when ambulating, if needed. In addition, confirm that side rails are up and locked on stretchers, that the call light is within reach, and that a patient's fall risk is communicated clearly to visitors and staff members who may assume responsibility for care.

Older adults who are on beds or stretchers should *always* have all side rails up and the bed or stretcher in the lowest position. Access to a call light is especially important; instruct the patient to call for the nurse if assistance is needed rather than attempt independent ambulation. Many older adults have difficulty adjusting to the noise and pace of the ED and/or have illnesses or injuries that cause delirium, an acute state of confusion. Reorient the patient frequently and re-assess mental status. Undiagnosed delirium increases the risk for mortality for older adults who are admitted to the hospital. Assess the need for a family member, significant other, or sitter to stay with the patient to prevent falls and help with reorientation. Additional safety strategies are listed in Chart 8-1.

even employ canine units made up of specially trained officers and dogs to patrol high-risk areas and respond to handle threatening situations.

Patient Safety

In addition to concerns about staff safety, some of the most common *patient* SAFETY issues are:

- Patient identification
- Fall risk
- Skin breakdown in vulnerable populations
- High risk for medical errors or adverse events

Hospital emergency departments have unique factors that can affect patient SAFETY. These factors include the provision of complex emergency care, constant interruptions, and the need to interact with the many providers involved in caring for one patient.

Correct *patient identification* is critical in any health care setting. All patients are issued an identification bracelet at their point of entry in the ED—generally at the triage registration desk or at the bedside if emergent needs exist. For patients with an unknown identity and those with emergent conditions that prevent the proper identification process (e.g., unconscious patient without identification, emergent trauma patient), hospitals commonly use a "Jane/John Doe" or another identification system. **Whatever method is used, always verify the patient's identity using two unique identifiers before each intervention and before medication administration per The Joint Commission's 2017 National Patient Safety Goals. Examples of appropriate identifiers include the patient's name, birth date, agency identification number, home telephone number or address, and/or Social Security number.**

Fall prevention starts with identifying people at risk for falls and then implementing appropriate fall precautions and SAFETY measures. Patients can enter the ED without apparent fall risk factors, but because of interventions such as pain medication, sedation, or lower-extremity cast application, they can develop a risk for falls. Falls can also occur in patients with medical conditions or drugs that cause syncope ("blackouts"). Many older adults experience orthostatic (postural) hypotension as a side effect of cardiovascular drugs. In this case patients become dizzy when changing from a lying or sitting position (see Chapter 3).

Some patients spend a lengthy time on stretchers while awaiting unit bed availability—possibly as long as 1 to 2 days in some hospitals, especially during high census periods such as flu season. During that time basic health needs require attention, including providing nutrition, hygiene, SAFETY, and privacy for all ED patients. Waiting in the ED can cause increased pain in patients with back pain or arthritis.

Protecting skin integrity also begins in the ED. Emergency nurses need to assess the skin frequently and implement preventive interventions into the ED plan of care, especially when caring for older adults or those of any age who are immobilized. Interventions that promote clean, dry skin for incontinent patients, mobility techniques that decrease shearing forces when moving the immobile patient, and routine turning help prevent skin breakdown. Chapter 25 describes additional nursing interventions for preventing skin breakdown.

A significant SAFETY risk for all patients who enter the emergency care environment is the *potential for medical errors or adverse events*, especially those associated with medication administration. The episodic and often chaotic nature of emergency management in an environment with frequent interruptions can easily lead to errors.

To reduce error potential, the emergency nurse makes every attempt to obtain essential and accurate medical history information from the patient, family, or reliable significant others as necessary. When working with patients who arrive with an altered mental status, a quick survey to determine whether the individual is wearing a medical alert bracelet or necklace is important to gain medical information. In addition, a two-person search of patient belongings may yield medication containers; the name of a physician, pharmacy, or family contact person; or a medication list. Some EDs employee pharmacists or pharmacy technicians to help gather medication history to improve timeliness and accuracy of the information recorded. Through these processes the nurse may find information that promotes SAFETY, help determine the diagnosis, and influence the overall emergency treatment plan.

Automated electronic tracking systems are also available in some EDs to help staff identify the location of patients at any given time and monitor the progress of care delivery during the visit. These valuable safety measures are especially important in large or busy EDs with a high population of older adults (Laskowski-Jones, 2008).

In addition to falls and pressure injury development, another adverse event that can result from a prolonged stay in the ED is a *hospital-acquired infection*. Older adults in particular are at risk for urinary tract or respiratory infections. Patients who are immune suppressed, especially those on chronic steroid therapy or immune modulators, are also at a high risk. Nurses and other ED personnel must wash their hands frequently and thoroughly or use hand sanitizers to help prevent pathogen transmission.

? CLINICAL JUDGMENT CHALLENGE 8-1

Safety QSEN

The emergency department manager has created a nursing task force to focus on fall prevention for patients who are seen in the ED. The task force created a list of questions about fall prevention and then discussed appropriate nursing interventions.

1. Which populations are at highest risk for falls while in the emergency department?
2. Which specific interventions can nurses implement to decrease falls?
3. Which actions can be appropriately delegated to unlicensed personnel to decrease fall risk?
4. How can the nursing staff reduce the risk for falls for patients who are confused (from dementia, medication side effects, or delirium)?

SCOPE OF EMERGENCY NURSING PRACTICE

The scope of emergency nursing practice encompasses management of patients across the life span from birth through death and all health conditions that prompt a person of any age to seek emergency care.

Core Competencies

Emergency nursing practice requires that nurses be skilled in patient assessment, priority setting and clinical decision making, multitasking, documentation, and COMMUNICATION; a sound cognitive knowledge base is also essential (Harding et al., 2013). Flexibility and adaptability are vital traits because situations within the ED and individual patients can change rapidly.

Like that of any practicing nurse, the foundation of the emergency nurse's skill base is *assessment* (also known as *noticing*). He or she must be able to rapidly and accurately interpret assessment findings according to acuity and age. For example, mottling of the extremities may be a normal finding in a newborn, but it may indicate poor peripheral perfusion and a shock state in an adult.

Another skill for the emergency nurse is *priority setting*, which is essential in the triage process. Priority setting depends on accurate assessment and good critical thinking and clinical decision-making skills. These skills are generally gained through hands-on clinical experience in the ED. However, discussion of case studies and the use of human patient simulation and simulation software and aids can help prepare nurses to acquire this skill base in a nonthreatening environment and then apply it in the actual clinical situation (Jeffries et al., 2015).

The knowledge base for emergency nurses is broad and ranges from critical care emergencies to less common problems such as snakebites and hazardous materials contamination (see Chapters 9 and 10). ED nurses also learn to recognize and manage the legal implications of societal problems such as

---

🧓 CONSIDERATIONS FOR OLDER ADULTS

Patient-Centered Care QSEN

Some older adults may not be able to provide an accurate history because of memory loss or acute delirium. If possible, review their prior hospitalization records to obtain complete histories or ask a family member or friend for pertinent information. Older adults usually have many pre-existing diseases (comorbidities) that must be considered as part of the assessment. *Knowing the history is vital because these conditions might adversely affect or complicate the cause for the ED visit.* For example, a patient who has rib fractures but has a history of severe chronic obstructive pulmonary disease (COPD) may not be able to maintain adequate gas exchange without endotracheal intubation and mechanical ventilatory support in the ED.

Another consideration for older-adult assessment is that the presenting symptoms of older adults are often different or less specific than those of younger adults. For example, increasing weakness, fatigue, and confusion may be the only admission concerns. These vague symptoms can be caused by serious illnesses such as an acute myocardial infarction (MI), urinary tract infection, or pneumonia. Diagnosing older adults often keeps them in the ED for extended periods, which can lead to patient safety concerns as discussed in the Patient Safety section.

---

domestic violence, child maltreatment, elder abuse, and sexual assault.

Although most EDs have physicians available around the clock who are physically located within the ED, the nurse often initiates collaborative interprofessional protocols for lifesaving interventions such as cardiac monitoring, oxygen therapy, insertion of IV catheters, and infusion of appropriate parenteral solutions. In many EDs nurses function under clearly defined medical protocols that allow them to initiate drug therapy for emergent conditions such as anaphylactic shock and cardiac arrest. Emergency care principles extend to knowing which essential laboratory and diagnostic tests may be needed and, when necessary, obtaining them.

The emergency nurse must be proficient in performing a variety of technical skills (multitasking), sometimes in a stressful, high-pressure environment such as a cardiac or trauma resuscitation. In addition to basic skills, he or she may also need to be proficient with critical care equipment such as invasive pressure-monitoring devices and mechanical ventilators. This type of equipment is commonly found in EDs that are part of Level I and Level II trauma centers.

The nurse also collaborates with and assists the ED provider of care with a number of procedures. Knowledge and skills related to procedural setup, patient preparation, teaching, and postprocedure care are key aspects of emergency nursing practice. Common ED procedures include:

- Simple and complex suturing for wound closure
- Foreign body removal
- Central line insertion
- Endotracheal intubation and initiation of mechanical ventilation
- Lumbar puncture
- Pelvic examination
- Chest tube insertion
- Paracentesis
- Fracture management

More than one nurse may be necessary to assist with some procedures. For example, if deep or moderate sedation is used to produce amnesia and relaxation during fracture reduction, one nurse assists the physician with the actual procedure while the other nurse monitors the patient before, during, and after the moderate-sedation medications are administered.

Finally an essential aspect of the emergency nurse's skill base is COMMUNICATION. The ED environment is complex; therefore multiple barriers to effective communication are likely. One common barrier is the patient's cultural beliefs and practices, especially if they differ from those of the health care team. Assess each patient as an individual and be careful not to stereotype anyone based on ethnicity, socioeconomic status, gender identity, or religion.

CULTURAL/SPIRITUAL CONSIDERATIONS
Patient-Centered Care QSEN

Be aware of the various cultural and religious values of patients that may influence care. Many people have distinct beliefs that must be respected in the health care setting. For example, individuals from some cultures are modest and do not like to have their bodies exposed.

Patients with language barriers can present a challenge. The population of non–English-speaking people is rapidly increasing in the United States. When a patient who is not proficient in English arrives to the ED seeking care, access available resources such as telephone language lines and dedicated interpreters contracted by the hospital to ensure an understanding of all aspects of care. Similarly deaf interpreters are essential when providing care for patients who are hearing impaired.

A religious belief system can also affect the delivery of care. For example, Jehovah's Witness patients do not accept blood transfusions and may not accept certain medications that are derived from human blood components.

Be aware that not all patients identify themselves as male or female. Some patients may be in the process of changing their gender identity from male to female or female to male (transgender people), whereas others identify as gender neutral or gender fluid. Ask the patient which pronoun (he, she, or other term) the person prefers. Demonstrate professional behaviors that promote trust. Chapter 73 discusses the special care for this population in detail.

ED crowding and insufficient nursing personnel to meet the demand for services also create difficulties with COMMUNICATION of pertinent patient information and quality of written documentation. The high-stress ED environment can negatively affect effective interpersonal behaviors, particularly when nurses must deal with angry, violent, or demanding patients.

Training and Certification

Two general types of certification are referred to in emergency nursing practice: the "certification" that marks successful completion of a particular course of study and emergency nursing specialty certification (Table 8-1). As part of the orientation and employment requirements for staff nurses in most US EDs, successful completion of the Basic Life Support (BLS) for Healthcare Providers, Advanced Cardiac Life Support (ACLS), and Pediatric Advanced Life Support (PALS) provider courses through the American Heart Association is necessary. These courses provide instruction in fundamental, evidence-based management theory and techniques for cardiopulmonary resuscitation (CPR). Course participants include physicians,

TABLE 8-1 Descriptions of Training and Certifications for Emergency Nursing

CERTIFICATION	DESCRIPTION
Basic Life Support (BLS) (required)	Noninvasive assessment and management skills for airway maintenance and cardiopulmonary resuscitation (CPR)
Advanced Cardiac Life Support (ACLS) (usually required)	Invasive airway-management skills, pharmacology, and electrical therapies; special resuscitation situations
Pediatric Advanced Life Support (PALS) (may be required)	Neonatal and pediatric resuscitation
Trauma Nursing Core Course (may be required)	Trauma nursing priorities, interventions, diagnostic studies, injury management
Certified Emergency Nurse (CEN) (optional)	Validates core emergency nursing knowledge base

nurses, and prehospital personnel. The ACLS course builds on the BLS content to include:
- Advanced concepts in cardiac monitoring
- Invasive airway-management skills
- Pharmacologic and electrical therapies
- Intravascular access techniques
- Special resuscitation situations
- Post-resuscitation management considerations

Additional certification may be required through successful completion of trauma continuing education courses.

EMERGENCY NURSING PRINCIPLES

Triage

Emergency department triage is an organized system for sorting or classifying patients into priority levels, depending on illness or injury severity. The organization of emergency care and the ED is structured through triage principles. The key concept is that patients who present to the ED with the highest acuity needs receive the quickest evaluation; treatment; and prioritized resource utilization such as x-rays, laboratory work, and computed tomography (CT) scans. These patients also have priority for hospital service areas such as the operating room or cardiac catheterization laboratory. An individual with a lower-acuity problem may wait longer in the ED because a high-acuity patient is moved to the "head of the line." The staff may need to communicate information about this system to the patient and family who may not understand why other patients are treated first.

The triage nurse is the gatekeeper in the emergency care system. When patients present to the ED, regulatory standards dictate that a registered nurse (RN), physician, or physician assistant (PA) perform a rapid assessment to determine triage priority. The RN is typically assigned to perform the triage function in most hospitals. The triage nurse requires appropriate training and experience in both emergency nursing and triage decision-making concepts to develop an expert knowledge base and provide ongoing mentoring and quality improvement feedback (Dateo, 2013). In some instances the triage

TABLE 8-2 Three-Tiered Triage System and Examples of Patients Triaged in Each Tier

TIER LEVEL	EXAMPLES OF PATIENTS TRIAGED IN EACH TIER
Emergent (life threatening)	Respiratory distress Chest pain with diaphoresis Stroke Active hemorrhage Unstable vital signs
Urgent (needs quick treatment, but not immediately life threatening)	Severe abdominal pain Renal colic Displaced or multiple fractures Complex or multiple soft tissue injuries New-onset respiratory infection, especially pneumonia in older adults
Nonurgent (could wait several hours if needed without fear of deterioration)	Skin rash Strains and sprains "Colds" Simple fracture

nurse may seek the input of an emergency physician, advanced practice nurse (e.g., nurse practitioner [NP] or clinical nurse specialist [CNS]), or PA to help establish the acuity level if the patient's presentation is highly unusual.

Based on the triage priority, patients may be rushed into a treatment room, directed to a lower-acuity area within the ED, or asked to sit in the waiting room. Variations on this theme include:

- Triage nurse–initiated protocols for laboratory work or diagnostic studies that may be performed before the patient is actually evaluated by an ED provider of care
- Initiation of care while the patient is on a stretcher in the hallway of a crowded ED

These protocols are especially beneficial for certain populations who require rapid diagnosis and collaborative treatment within a defined time frame from ED arrival to meet established standards of care. Examples are patients with chest pain or those with a clinical presentation indicative of stroke, sepsis, or pneumonia.

Emergent, Urgent, and Nonurgent Categories

Many triage systems can be used by a hospital ED. Any system must be applied consistently by triage nursing staff and endorsed by the emergency medicine physician staff. Based on the severity of the patient's condition, a well-known triage scheme used in the United States is the three-tiered model of "emergent, urgent, and nonurgent" (Table 8-2). In this system, for example, a patient experiencing crushing substernal chest pain, shortness of breath, and diaphoresis would be classified as emergent and triaged immediately to a treatment room within the ED. Similarly a critically injured trauma patient or an individual with an active hemorrhage would also be prioritized as emergent. The emergent triage category implies that a condition exists that poses an immediate threat to life or limb.

The urgent triage category indicates that the patient should be treated quickly but that an immediate threat to life does not exist at the moment. Reassessment is needed if a health care provider cannot evaluate the patient in a timely manner. In people with evidence of clinical deterioration, triage priority

may be upgraded from urgent to emergent. Examples of patients who typically fall into the urgent category are those with a new onset of pneumonia (as long as respiratory failure does not appear imminent), renal colic, complex lacerations not associated with major hemorrhage, displaced fractures or dislocations, and temperature greater than 101°F (38.3°C). Those categorized as nonurgent can generally tolerate waiting several hours for health care services without a significant risk for clinical deterioration. Conditions within this classification include patients with sprains and strains, simple fractures, "cold" symptoms, and general skin rashes.

Other Multi-Tiered Models

To further sort patient conditions within an acuity classification or triage priority system, four- and five-tier triage models also exist. Such models are based either on comprehensive lists of conditions that indicate the particular triage priority to which a patient should be assigned or on the nature of resources that a patient will use in the ED setting. A patient situation may generate various triage classifications in different hospitals, depending on the triage priority system used at that particular institution. Some schemes may even take into account the presence of pre-existing conditions such as a history of anticoagulant use, diabetes, heart disease, and organ transplantation.

It is surprising that there is no universally accepted triage system recognized in the United States. Thus there is no standardization of triage acuity data to compare patient acuity among hospitals. Medical providers, health insurance companies, and patients often disagree on the definition of an emergent versus a nonurgent ED visit, making it essential to use a practical triage system to maintain department efficiency and allocation of resources. The Emergency Nurses Association in collaboration with the American College of Emergency Physicians studied the available research literature on acuity scales and concluded that two standardized five-level systems, the Emergency Severity Index (ESI) and the Canadian Triage Acuity Scale (CTAS), are the most reliable (Shelton, 2010). The ESI model uses an algorithm that fosters rapid, reliable, and clinically pertinent categorization of patients into five groups, from Level 1 (emergent) to Level 5 (nonurgent). The CTAS model differs from ESI in that lists of descriptors are used to establish the triage level.

Whatever triage model is used, triage nurses must use a systematic approach, apply solid clinical decision-making skills, and maintain a caring ethic. Compassion fatigue, or burnout, can hinder objectivity in dealing with patients who present to the ED. A biased approach threatens the ED nurse's ability to triage patients accurately. Mistriage is a patient SAFETY risk that can be the "root cause" of delayed or inadequate treatment with potentially deadly consequences.

Disposition

At the conclusion of the assessment the physician must make a decision regarding patient disposition (i.e., where the patient should go after being discharged from the ED). Should he or she be admitted to the hospital, transferred to a specialty care center, or be discharged to home with instructions for continued care and follow-up? Usually the answer is straightforward. A patient who has an evolving myocardial infarction, sepsis, stroke, or acute surgical need is admitted.

Sometimes, though, the ED disposition decision is less clear. Often the ED provider of care discusses this decision in

? NCLEX EXAMINATION CHALLENGE 8-1

Safe and Effective Care Environment

The ED nurse who is just beginning a shift is assigned to care for four clients. Which client does the nurse assess **first**?

A. 19-year-old with a closed femur fracture who received pain medication 15 minutes earlier

B. 24-year-old with nausea, vomiting, and diarrhea who has infusing IV fluids and is resting

C. 33-year-old who cut hand while working in a kitchen and is awaiting suturing

D. 41-year-old awaiting transport to the operating room for an emergency appendectomy

CONSIDERATIONS FOR OLDER ADULTS

Patient-Centered Care QSEN

If discharge from the ED to home is possible, ensure that safety issues are considered. For example, collaborate with the ED physician to evaluate the patient's current prescriptions and over-the-counter medications to determine if the drug regimen should be continued. Involve the ED-based pharmacist if one is available for consultation when necessary. If the medication regimen needs to be changed, be sure that the patient and family member or significant other has the new information in writing and that it is explained verbally. If needed, assess whether the patient has someone who can presort and place medications into a medication dispenser to ensure accuracy and prevent adverse drug events. Consider a social services or case-management referral for patients in need of financial resources to obtain prescribed medications.

To prevent future ED visits, screen older adults per agency policy for functional assessment, cognitive assessment, and risk for falls. Depression screening is also important because suicide rates are two times higher among older adults when compared with younger adults. White men older than 85 years are at the highest risk (Touhy & Jett, 2015).

Older patients are often admitted to the hospital directly from the ED. If hospitalization is needed, determine if the patient has advance directives or is able to make decisions about advance directives before admission. If the patient was admitted from a nursing home, contact the facility to let them know the patient's status. If the patient was receiving home health care services, notify the agency about the hospital admission. Contact the patient's primary physician and designated family member if he or she is not present with the patient.

collaboration with the emergency nurse. The nurse may have a greater sense of how well a patient will manage in a home setting, depending on whether other family members or caregivers are available to assist and are reliable. For example, in the event that a patient with a minor head injury has suffered a loss of consciousness, someone is typically expected to remain with that person for the first 12 to 24 hours to be sure that he or she does not show any evidence of neurologic deterioration. Another common scenario involves the potential risk to the patient in cases of actual or suspected domestic violence. If discharge to home is not deemed safe, the patient may be admitted to the hospital in an observation status until resources can be organized to provide for a safe environment. Coordinate the discharge plan and continuing care with the social worker or case manager.

Case Management

Some EDs employ registered nurse case managers who screen ED patients and intervene when necessary to arrange appropriate

referral and follow-up. This is an evolving role in the ED setting that can be beneficial in providing comprehensive care and as a strategy to avoid inappropriate use of resources.

ED case managers, supported by electronic information systems, can review the ED census on both a "real-time" and a retrospective basis to determine which patients have visited the ED frequently in a given period. The case manager can then determine the reasons they sought emergency services such as lack of a primary health care provider, exacerbation ("flare-up") of a chronic condition, a lack of health education, or lack of the financial resources necessary to manage the health condition. Collaborative case-management interventions include facilitating referrals to primary care providers or to subsidized community-based health clinics for patients or families in need of routine services.

For those with needs related to chronic conditions, the case manager can arrange referral into appropriate disease management programs in the community if available. Disease management programs are specific to a particular condition such as asthma, COPD, diabetes, hypertension, heart failure, and renal failure. They help patients learn how to manage their condition on a day-to-day basis to prevent exacerbations or clinical deterioration. The desired outcome is to keep the person out of the hospital as long as possible. Health teaching is a key component of these programs. For other health teaching needs, the ED case manager directs the patient to the appropriate educational resources such as a health educator, registered dietitian, or community organization (e.g., the American Cancer Society, the American Heart Association).

Other functions of the ED case manager might include working in collaboration with staff to plan disposition for homeless people or veterans, locating a safe environment for victims of domestic violence or elder abuse, or providing information on resources for low-cost or free prescriptions. Homeless adults often have multiple chronic medical illnesses for which they visit EDs frequently. A large study of homeless adults with chronic medical illnesses demonstrated a decrease in ED visits and hospital admissions as a result of an organized follow-up system for housing and ongoing case-management support (Popovich et al., 2012). Another study demonstrated a decrease in ED visits and admissions for veterans based on a care-coordination program partnership between Veterans Affairs (VA) medical centers and Alzheimer's Association chapters (Bass et al., 2015). (See the Evidence-Based Practice box.)

Patient and Family Education

A key role of the emergency nurse is health teaching. At the most basic level nurses review discharge instructions with the patient and family before signing them out of the department.

In addition to discharge instructions, the ED environment and community-at-large present many opportunities for health education. Emergency nurses are in an ideal position to educate the public about wellness and injury prevention strategies. If the patient presented after a motor vehicle crash, for instance, the nurse can reinforce the need to wear seat belts or use child safety seats correctly. ED visits that result from mishaps in the home provide an excellent opportunity to discuss home SAFETY issues (e.g., the need for smoke detectors and carbon monoxide detectors) and fall prevention tips (e.g., the need for proper lighting, removal of throw rugs). Injury is not the only topic that affords a teaching opportunity. A new onset or an exacerbation of a medical condition also allows for education, such as how to

EVIDENCE-BASED PRACTICE [QSEN]

Community Partnerships to Decrease Hospital Admissions and ED Visits for Veterans With Dementia

Bass, D., et al. (2015). Impact of the care coordination program "Partners in Dementia Care" on veterans' hospital admissions and emergency department visits. *Alzheimer's & Dementia: Translational Research & Clinical Interventions, 1*(1), 13–22.

This study sought to determine whether "Partners in Dementia Care" (PDC), a care coordination partnership between Veterans Affairs (VA) medical centers and Alzheimer's Association chapters, would reduce the emergency department (ED) visits and hospital admissions for veterans with dementia, especially those with more profound behavioral and cognitive symptoms.

The sample included 328 veterans with dementia and their primary caregiver from five matched sites—two of which were randomly selected treatment sites. Veterans who were eligible received primary health care from the VA, resided outside a residential care facility at enrollment time, lived within an area where a partnering Alzheimer's Association chapter existed, were over the age of 60, and had at least one ICD-9 dementia diagnostic code. After initial assessment an action plan of approximately seven personalized activities—the core of PDC—was put in place for each veteran and caregivers. Action steps were easy-to-accomplish processes that were targeted to provide necessary services and answers for veterans and caregivers such as calling to inquire about service availability, creating a list of questions to ask the health care provider, and contacting other family members to assist with a caregiving task.

Data on VA and non-VA hospital and ED use (including the use of urgent care facilities) were collected electronically for 1 year after initial assessment. Caregivers were surveyed at 6-month intervals to report services used between months 1 and 6 and months 7 and 12. Logistic regression was used with dichotomous-dependent variables to analyze the data.

Data showed that just over one third of veterans had at least one hospital admission and over half had at least one ED visit. One hundred and eighteen veterans experienced at least one hospital admission. PDC veterans with more cognitive symptoms at the 6-month interval, and those with behavioral difficulties at baseline had fewer admissions.

Level of Evidence: 2

This quasi-experimental study provided for control at baseline and randomization of two of the five matched sites. It was built on the Stress Hospital Model, which further strengthens its credibility.

Commentary: Implications for Practice and Research

Cost and resource utilization for patients with dementia is substantial because of the nature of the disease, which requires progressive supervision and intervention as the patient's condition deteriorates over time. This study demonstrated that PDC did decrease the number of hospital admissions and ED visits for veterans with dementia but did not impact the likelihood of an initial admission. Nurses can use this information in practice by recognizing that partnerships and collaborations between community resource groups and hospital services may favorably impact the frequency of subsequent admissions and ED visits for patients with dementia, particularly as symptoms progress, which often leads to high resource utilization and cost of care. Further research is ongoing in the form a replication study that is being conducted in Ohio, with the support of Administration for Community Living (grant 90DS0001), Ohio Department of Aging, Benjamin Rose Institute on Aging, Louis Stokes Cleveland VA Medical Center, the Western Reserve Area Agency on Aging, and the Greater East Ohio Area Alzheimer's Association Chapter.

CULTURAL/SPIRITUAL CONSIDERATIONS

Patient-Centered Care [QSEN]

Most discharge instructions are either preprinted or computer generated and can be customized to address the patient's needs. Consider his or her reading level, primary language, and visual acuity. Educational materials and instructions should be available at no higher than the sixth-grade reading level. For patients with English as a second language, many hospitals have educational materials available in Spanish and other regional languages. However, interpreters may be necessary to help the health care provider customize the information appropriately. For older adults and others with vision deficits, large-print materials may be helpful.

measure blood glucose and ways to control blood pressure or reduce the risk for heart disease.

Death in the Emergency Department

Not all critically ill or injured patients who come to the ED can be saved. Sometimes a patient's death is expected by family members, typically when they have dealt with a loved one's terminal condition or age-related decline. Usually, however, a death in the ED is a sudden and unexpected event that produces a state of crisis and chaos for family and significant others. Emergency department staff members need to address the needs of the family members in this overwhelming time.

If resuscitation efforts are still under way when the family arrives, one or two family members may be given the opportunity to be present during lifesaving procedures. Family presence during resuscitation is gaining wider acceptance in the health care community; however, a significant number of hospitals still have not devised clear policies or guidelines to facilitate family-witnessed resuscitation (Porter et al., 2014).

If the patient dies before family members arrive, ED staff members try to prepare the body and the room for viewing by the family. However, certain types of ED deaths may require forensic investigation or become medical examiner's cases. Therefore ED staff may not be able to remove IV lines and indwelling tubes or clean the patient's skin if these actions could potentially damage evidence. Trauma deaths, suspected homicide, or abuse cases always fall into this category. In these situations cover the body with a sheet or blanket while leaving the patient's face exposed and dim the lights before family viewing.

When dealing with family members in crisis, simple and concrete COMMUNICATION is best. Words such as *death* or *died*, although seemingly harsh, create less confusion than terms such as *expired* or *passed away*. Demonstrate caring, compassion, and empathy during all interactions, even in periods of heightened emotions. Intense grief can provoke a range of family reactions from silence to violence. If available, coordinate with crisis staff (social workers or psychiatric nurses) to assist families and maintain SAFETY during this time. Offer the family the option of speaking with clergy or calling someone of their choice for additional support. A family member may need to be admitted to the ED to be treated for anxiety or physical manifestations of stress such as chest pain, difficulty breathing, or severe headache.

Dealing with death is often difficult for ED personnel, especially during busy periods when the ability to console family members may be limited. In response, some EDs have developed bereavement committees that focus on meeting the needs of grieving families. Actions such as sending sympathy cards, attending funerals, making follow-up phone calls, and creating memory boxes are common. These actions facilitate COMMUNI-CATION of caring and compassion after the moment of crisis.

THE IMPACT OF HOMELESSNESS

Homelessness affected 564,708 people on any given night in January 2015; one quarter of all homeless people were under the age of 18 (United States Department of Housing and Urban Development, 2015). The homeless population is made up of both adults and children who live from day to day in a state of fear, chaos, and confusion (Gerber, 2013). People become homeless as a result of a crisis or persistent poverty (Gerber, 2013). They have a high incidence of acute and chronic health conditions, psychiatric illnesses, physical disabilities or limitations, and problems with substance abuse (Gerber, 2013). They are vulnerable to physical trauma, weather exposure, sexually transmitted diseases, infestation, and infectious diseases such as tuberculosis and influenza.

Homeless patients often seek ED care for a variety of reasons. Because the ED is open 24 hours per day and is mandated by federal law to perform an emergency medical screening examination on all of its patients, patients who are homeless know that they will gain entry despite their inability to pay for services. The ED represents a safe place to go for shelter in poor weather and for food, medical care, pain relief, and human interaction. Some homeless patients simply seek a temporary respite from their current living conditions, which may be a park, homeless shelter, car, abandoned building, or cardboard box. People who have been persistently homeless may assimilate into the homeless culture, learn to take great pride in their survival skills, and fiercely protect their few belongings and their living space. They may develop a distrust of outsiders, including members of the health care profession, and are especially sensitive to any perceived bias or stereotyping (Gerber, 2013).

Patients who are homeless bring special challenges to their ED evaluation, treatment, and disposition. Some visit the ED frequently and do not adhere to treatment recommendations or follow up with community referrals. Those with mental illness or substance abuse may act out or become disruptive, posing a SAFETY risk to staff and patients.

To best care for homeless patients in the ED setting, nurses must first maintain their situational awareness and attend to their own needs for personal safety. These include not only anticipating the potential for violent behavior but also using Standard Precautions and assessing the need to isolate the patient in a negative-pressure room if airborne disease such as tuberculosis is a concern. The key nursing action is to demonstrate behaviors that promote trust. These include making eye contact (if culturally appropriate), speaking calmly, avoiding any prejudicial or stereotypical remarks, being patient, showing genuine care and concern by listening, following through on promises, and exercising caution when there is a need to enter into the patient's personal space (Gerber, 2013). Clear professional boundaries must be stated if the patient becomes disruptive, profane, or sexually inappropriate. While collaborating with the emergency care provider to ensure that the patient's emergency medical needs are identified and treated, consult a social worker or case manager to work with the patient to identify safety needs, referral options, and community resources. It is also important to develop an individual care plan with the interprofessional health care team if the patient uses the ED frequently. This type of care plan is extremely beneficial in establishing a consistent approach to patient management,

especially when the patient has complex conditions or exhibits drug-seeking and disruptive behavior.

TRAUMA NURSING PRINCIPLES

The general public tends to use the term *trauma* to mean any type of crisis, ranging from a heart attack to psychological stress. Among health care professionals, though, trauma refers to bodily injury. More than 192,000 people in the United States die each year as a result of injuries; and over 2.4 million are hospitalized, often with permanent and disabling consequences (National Center for Injury Prevention and Control [NCIPC], 2017). Injuries can be categorized as either intentional (i.e., assault, homicide, suicide) or unintentional (i.e., accidents). *Unintentional injury* such as a motor vehicle crash is the leading cause of death for Americans younger than 35 years and is one of today's most significant public health problems (NCIPC, 2017).

Injury management is a key component of ED services. Over 30 million people in the United States visit the ED each year to receive treatment for injuries (NCIPC, 2017). Therefore a core competency in general trauma care is an important part of emergency nursing practice. For emergency nurses who work in accredited trauma centers, opportunities typically exist to further develop expertise in trauma nursing through ongoing clinical practice, specialty training programs, and continuing education. Trauma nursing is a field that encompasses the continuum of care from injury prevention and prehospital services to acute care, rehabilitation, and ultimately community reintegration.

Trauma Centers and Trauma Systems

Trauma centers have their roots in military medicine. Injured soldiers who received rapid transport from the battlefield and treatment from skilled health care personnel had a survival advantage in the mobile army surgical hospital (MASH) units first deployed in the Korean and Vietnam wars. Consequently the MASH unit became the original model for the development of civilian trauma centers. In modern society the trauma center in the United States is a specialty care facility that provides competent and timely trauma services to patients, depending on its designated level of capability.

Trauma Centers

Not all EDs that offer around-the-clock emergency services are trauma centers. The American College of Surgeons Committee on Trauma (2014) has set forth national standards for trauma center accreditation and categorizes the resource requirements necessary for the highest capability trauma center (Level I) to the lowest (Level IV) (Table 8-3).

A *Level I trauma center* is a regional resource facility that is capable of providing leadership and total collaborative care for every aspect of injury, from prevention through rehabilitation. These centers also have a responsibility to offer professional and community education programs, conduct research, and participate in system planning. Because a significant resource and experience commitment is required to maintain strict accreditation standards, Level I trauma centers are usually located in large teaching hospitals and serve dense population areas (Fig. 8-4).

Level II trauma centers are usually located in community hospitals and are capable of providing care to the vast majority of injured patients. However, a Level II trauma center may not be able to meet the resource needs of patients who require very complex or multi-system injury management. These people are generally transferred to a Level I trauma center for specialty

TABLE 8-3	Levels and Functions of Trauma Centers

LEVELS OF TRAUMA CENTER	FUNCTIONS OF TRAUMA CENTER
Level I	Usually located in large teaching hospital systems in densely populated areas Provides a full continuum of trauma services for adult and/or pediatric patients Conducting research is a requirement for trauma center verification
Level II and Level III	Both typically located in community hospitals **Level II** Provides care to most injured patients Transfers patient if needs exceed resource capabilities **Level III** Stabilizes patients with major injuries Transfers patient if needs exceed resource capabilities
Level IV	Usually located in rural and remote areas Provides basic trauma patient stabilization and advanced life support within resource capabilities Arranges transfer to higher trauma center levels as necessary

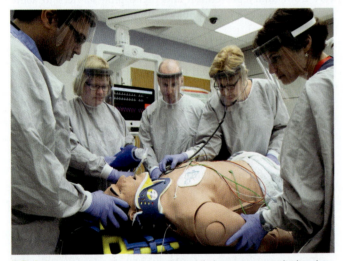

FIG. 8-4 A trauma team participates in a realistic trauma resuscitation simulation. This type of training ensures that staff remain proficient in skills and able to care for any situation that might present to the emergency department.

care. In communities without a Level I trauma center, Level II centers play a significant leadership role in injury management, education, prevention, and emergency preparedness planning.

A *Level III trauma center* is a critical link to higher-capability trauma centers in communities that do not have ready access to Level I or II centers. The primary focus is initial injury stabilization and patient transfer. Level III trauma centers are often found in smaller, rural hospitals and serve areas with lower population density. Because Level III trauma centers have general surgeons and orthopedic surgeons immediately available, patients with some major injuries may be admitted for care. However, if the injuries are severe or critical, transfer to a Level I or II trauma center occurs after ED assessment,

resuscitation, and stabilization—sometimes after emergent, lifesaving surgery. Patients are typically transported out in either an advanced life support ambulance or helicopter with critical care transport personnel in attendance.

The function of a *Level IV trauma center* is to offer advanced life support care in rural or remote settings that do not have ready access to a higher-level trauma center such as a ski area. Patients are stabilized to the best degree possible before transfer, using available personnel such as advanced practice nurses, physician assistants, nurses, and paramedics. Resources, including the consistent availability of a physician, may be extremely limited. Transport time to the final care center can be prolonged because of both distance and bad weather conditions that may prevent transfer by air.

Level III and Level IV trauma centers establish close collaborative relationships with Level I and Level II trauma centers. Based on accreditation standards, care providers at Levels I and II trauma centers have a responsibility to readily accept injured patients in transfer. They provide timely feedback to trauma personnel at referring hospitals and share expertise by offering educational opportunities to advance trauma care delivery in the region. In addition, personnel from all levels of trauma centers participate in focused system improvement and patient safety initiatives that enhance quality of care and solve identified problems.

Trauma Systems

Trauma centers save lives, but a trauma center is only as good as the overall trauma system that supports it. A **trauma system** is an organized and integrated approach to trauma care designed to ensure that all critical elements of trauma care delivery are aligned to meet the injured patient's needs. These elements include (Cooper & Laskowski-Jones, 2006):

- Access to care through COMMUNICATION technology (e.g., an enhanced 911 service)
- Timely availability of prehospital emergency medical care
- Rapid transport to a qualified trauma center
- Early provision of rehabilitation services
- System-wide injury prevention, research, and education initiatives

The overall desired outcome of an organized trauma system is to enable an injured patient not only to recover from trauma but also to return to a productive role in society.

A well-functioning trauma system is also essential to general public health and SAFETY. It provides the structure necessary for disaster readiness and community emergency preparedness (see Chapter 10). Although most states in the United States now have at least some basic elements of a trauma system in place, significant gaps still exist in many regions.

Mechanism of Injury

The **mechanism of injury (MOI)** describes how the patient's traumatic event occurred, such as a high-speed motor vehicle crash, a fall from a standing height, or a gunshot wound to the torso. Knowing key details about the MOI can provide insight into the energy forces involved and may help trauma care providers predict injury types, and in some cases, patient outcomes. Prehospital care providers report the MOI as a COMMUNICATION standard when handing off care to ED and trauma personnel. Similarly, patients who present to the ED for medical care will often relate the MOI by describing the particular chain of events that caused their injuries.

Two of the most common injury-producing mechanisms are blunt trauma and penetrating trauma. **Blunt trauma** results from impact forces such as those sustained in a motor vehicle crash; a fall; or an assault with fists, kicks, or a baseball bat. **Blast effect** from an exploding bomb also causes blunt trauma. The energy transmitted from a blunt-trauma mechanism, particularly the rapid **acceleration-deceleration** forces involved in high-speed crashes or falls from a great height, produces injury by tearing, shearing, and compressing anatomic structures. Trauma to bones, blood vessels, and soft tissues occurs.

Penetrating trauma is caused by injury from sharp objects and projectiles. Examples are wounds from knives, ice picks, other comparable implements, and bullets (gunshot wounds [GSWs]) or pellets. Fragments of metal, glass, or other materials that become airborne in an explosion (shrapnel) can also produce penetrating trauma. Each mechanism has the risk for specific injury patterns and severity that the trauma team considers when planning diagnostic evaluation and management strategies. Certain injury mechanisms such as a gunshot wound to the chest or abdomen or a stab wound to the neck are so highly associated with life-threatening consequences that they automatically require trauma team intervention for a rapid and coordinated resuscitation response.

 NCLEX EXAMINATION CHALLENGE 8-2

Safe and Effective Care Environment

The nurse is caring for a client who was attacked on a rooftop. The client was repeatedly kicked and then shot in the leg, which contributed to a fall from the five-story building. Which mechanism of injury will the nurse document? **Select all that apply.**
A. Blunt
B. Blast
C. Penetration
D. Acceleration-deceleration
E. Laceration

Primary Survey and Resuscitation Interventions

A basic tenet of emergency care in any environment is scene SAFETY. In the prehospital setting emergency care providers must ensure that they are aware of any hazards that might pose a threat to rescuers and take actions to decrease or eliminate the risk. This same concept applies to the hospital ED setting. Before engaging in trauma resuscitation as a nurse member of the trauma team, keep in mind that there is a high risk for contamination with blood and body fluids. For this reason use Standard Precautions in *all* resuscitation situations and at other times when exposure to blood and body fluids is likely. Proper attire consists of an impervious cover gown, gloves, eye protection, a facemask, surgical cap, and shoe covers (if *significant* blood loss is anticipated such as during an ED procedure).

The initial assessment of the trauma patient is called the **primary survey**, which is an organized system to rapidly identify and effectively manage immediate threats to life. The primary survey is typically based on a standard "ABC" mnemonic plus a "D" and "E" for trauma patients: airway/cervical spine (**A**); breathing (**B**); circulation (**C**); disability (**D**); and exposure (**E**). Resuscitation efforts occur simultaneously with each element of the primary survey (Gurney & Westergard, 2014). Even though the resuscitation team may encounter multiple clinical problems or injuries, issues identified in the primary survey are managed before the team engages in interventions of lower priority such as splinting fractures and dressing wounds.

There is one notable exception to the standard ABCDE trauma resuscitation approach. Lessons learned from the military have made it clear that in the presence of massive, uncontrolled external bleeding, hemorrhage control techniques are the highest priority intervention (Gurney & Westergard, 2014). In this situation the sequence of priorities shifts to CAB, whereby the initial focus of resuscitation is to effectively stop the active bleeding (Gurney & Westergard, 2014).

A: Airway/Cervical Spine

Even minutes without an adequate oxygen supply can lead to brain injury that can progress to anoxic brain death. Establishing a patent airway is the highest-priority intervention when managing a trauma patient unless massive, life-threatening external hemorrhage as described previously is present.

! NURSING SAFETY PRIORITY QSEN

Critical Rescue

Recognize that you must clear the airway of any secretions or debris either with a suction catheter or manually if necessary. Respond by protecting the trauma patient's cervical spine by manually aligning the neck in a neutral, in-line position and using a jaw-thrust maneuver when establishing an airway. Provide supplemental oxygen for patients who require resuscitation.

In general a nonrebreather mask is best for the spontaneously breathing patient. Bag-valve-mask (BVM) ventilation with the appropriate airway adjunct and a 100% oxygen source is indicated for the person who needs ventilatory assistance during resuscitation. A patient with significantly impaired consciousness (Glasgow Coma Scale [GCS] of 8 or less) requires an endotracheal tube and mechanical ventilation (Gurney & Westergard, 2014).

B: Breathing

After the airway is successfully secured, breathing becomes the next priority in the primary survey. *This assessment determines whether or not ventilatory efforts are effective—not only whether or not the patient is breathing.* Listen to breath sounds and evaluate chest expansion, respiratory effort, and any evidence of chest wall trauma or physical abnormalities. Both apneic patients and those with poor ventilatory effort need BVM ventilation for support until endotracheal intubation is performed and a mechanical ventilator is used. If cardiopulmonary resuscitation (CPR) becomes necessary, the mechanical ventilator is disconnected, and the patient is manually ventilated with a BVM device. Lung compliance can be assessed through sensing the degree of difficulty in ventilating the patient with the BVM.

C: Circulation

When effective ventilation is ensured, the priority shifts to circulation. The adequacy of heart rate, blood pressure, and overall perfusion becomes the focus of the assessment. Common threats to circulation include cardiac arrest, myocardial dysfunction, and hemorrhage leading to a shock state. Interventions are targeted at restoring effective circulation through cardiopulmonary resuscitation, hemorrhage control, IV vascular access with fluid and blood administration as necessary, and drug therapy. *External* hemorrhage is usually quite obvious and best controlled with firm, direct pressure on the bleeding site with thick, dry dressing material. This method is effective in decreasing blood flow for most wounds. *Tourniquets that occlude arterial blood flow distal to the injury should be used to manage severe, compressible bleeding from extremity trauma when direct pressure fails to achieve hemorrhage control; hemostatic dressings (e.g., dressings impregnated with substances that speed the formation of a blood clot) are another essential tool to apply directly over the bleeding site in the management of life-threatening hemorrhage).* Internal hemorrhage is a more hidden complication that must be suspected in injured patients or those who present in a shock state.

In a resuscitation situation blood pressure (BP) can be quickly and easily estimated before a manual cuff pressure can be obtained by palpating for the presence or absence of peripheral and central pulses:

- Presence of a radial pulse: BP at least 80 mm Hg systolic
- Presence of a femoral pulse: BP at least 70 mm Hg systolic
- Presence of a carotid pulse: BP at least 60 mm Hg systolic

By the time hypotension occurs, compensatory mechanisms used by the body in an attempt to maintain vital signs in a shock state have been exhausted. Timely, effective intervention is critical to preserve life and vital organ function.

IV access is best achieved initially with insertion of large-bore (16-gauge) peripheral IV lines in the antecubital area (inside bend of the elbow). Additional access can be obtained via central veins in the femoral, subclavian, or jugular sites using large-bore (8.5 Fr) central venous catheters. Intraosseous access is an excellent initial approach for critically ill patients when veins cannot be rapidly accessed by the resuscitation team (see Chapter 13 for discussion of intraosseous infusion therapy). Ringer's lactate and 0.9% normal saline (NS) are the crystalloid solutions of choice for resuscitation; hypertonic saline may also be prescribed in some situations, particularly in the case of head trauma. Fluids and blood products should be warmed before administration to prevent hypothermia. Anticipate the need for rapid blood component administration in a hemorrhagic shock state using packed red blood cells, fresh frozen plasma, and platelets to both replace blood loss and prevent coagulopathy. However, the priority intervention is always to stop the bleeding.

D: Disability

The disability examination provides a rapid baseline assessment of neurologic status. A simple method to evaluate level of consciousness is the "AVPU" mnemonic:

- A: **A**lert
- V: Responsive to **v**oice
- P: Responsive to **p**ain
- U: **U**nresponsive

Another common way of determining and documenting level of consciousness is the Glasgow Coma Scale (GCS), an assessment that scores eye opening, verbal response, and motor response. The lowest score is 3, which indicates a totally unresponsive patient; a normal GCS score is 15. Metabolic abnormalities (e.g., severe hypoglycemia), hypoxia, neurologic injury, and illicit drugs or alcohol can impair level of consciousness. Frequent reassessment is needed for rapid intervention in the event of neurologic compromise or deterioration.

E: Exposure

The final component of the primary survey is exposure.

! **NURSING SAFETY PRIORITY** QSEN

Action Alert

Remove all clothing to allow for thorough assessment. Always carefully cut away clothing with scissors:

- During resuscitation when rapid access to the patient's body is critical
- When manipulating a patient's limbs to remove clothing could cause further injury
- When thermal or chemical burns have caused fabrics to melt into the patient's skin

If evidence preservation is an issue, handle items per institutional policy. Evidence may include articles of clothing, impaled objects, weapons, drugs, and bullets. Emergency nurses are often called on to provide testimony in court regarding their recall of the presentation and treatment of patients in the ED. Examples of types of cases in which evidence collection is vital are rape, elder abuse, domestic violence, homicide, suicide, drug overdose, and assault.

Once clothing is removed, hypothermia (body temperature less than or equal to 95°F [36°C]) poses a risk to injured patients (Weaver et al., 2014), especially those with burns and traumatic shock states. Hypothermia is discussed in detail in Chapter 9.

Table 8-4 highlights the primary survey and associated resuscitation interventions.

? **NCLEX EXAMINATION CHALLENGE 8-3**

Safe and Effective Care Environment

A flight nurse is preparing to care for a client who has been involved in a serious motor vehicle crash. When the helicopter lands, what is the nurse's **priority** action?
A. Apply oxygen.
B. Assess airway and stabilize cervical spine.
C. Start two large-bore IVs and infuse normal saline.
D. Apply pressure to any small bleeding wounds.

The Secondary Survey and Resuscitation Interventions

After the ED resuscitation team addresses the immediate life threats, other activities that the emergency nurse can anticipate include insertion of a gastric tube for decompression of the GI tract to prevent vomiting and aspiration, insertion of a urinary catheter to allow careful measure of urine output, and preparation for diagnostic studies. The resuscitation team also performs a more comprehensive head-to-toe assessment, known as the secondary survey, to identify other injuries or medical issues that need to be managed or that might affect the course of treatment. Splints will be applied to fractured extremities, and temporary dressings will be placed over wounds while the patient undergoes diagnostic testing or preparation for more definitive management.

Disposition

The patient may be transported immediately to the operating room or interventional radiology suite directly from the ED, depending on the nature of the injury. When no immediate procedural intervention is indicated, patients are admitted to inpatient units for management and nursing care based on the nature and severity of their injuries and any other pre-existing

TABLE 8-4 The Primary Survey and Resuscitation Interventions

PRIORITIES OF THE PRIMARY SURVEY	EXAMPLES OF SPECIFIC INTERVENTIONS
A: Airway/cervical spine	Establish a patent airway by positioning, suctioning, and oxygen as needed. Protect the cervical spine by maintaining alignment; use a jaw-thrust maneuver if there is a risk for spinal injury. If the Glasgow Coma Scale (GCS) score is 8 or less or the patient is at risk for airway compromise, prepare for endotracheal intubation and mechanical ventilation.
B: Breathing	Assess breath sounds and respiratory effort. Observe for chest wall trauma or other physical abnormality. Prepare for chest decompression if needed. Prepare to assist ventilations if needed.
C: Circulation	Monitor vital signs, especially blood pressure and pulse. Maintain vascular access with a large-bore catheter. Use direct pressure for external bleeding; anticipate need for a tourniquet for severe, uncontrollable extremity hemorrhage and use of a hemostatic dressing.
D: Disability	Evaluate the patient's level of consciousness (LOC) using the GCS. Re-evaluate the patient's LOC frequently.
E: Exposure	Remove all clothing for a complete physical assessment. Prevent hypothermia (e.g., cover the patient with blankets, use heating devices, infuse warm solutions).

medical conditions that could complicate trauma care. However, if the facility does not have the resource capabilities to manage the injured patient, the physician arranges for transfer to a higher level of care.

It is during this time that you should also assess for any signs of human trafficking, which affects more than 20 million people globally, with up to 80% of the victims being seen by a health care provider while under the trafficker's control (Byrne et al., 2017). This practice of sexual exploitation is a type of modern-day slavery in which the victim is forced or coerced to provide sex to others in exchange for money or valuables that are given to the trafficker. Nurses must be aware that patients seen for recurrent sexually transmitted infections (STIs), pregnancy tests, and abortions may be victims of human trafficking. Physical signs of trafficking include headaches, dizziness, back pain, missing patches of hair (where it has been pulled out), burns, bruises, vaginal or rectal trauma, jaw problems, and head injuries. The victim may also have unusual tattooing or "branding" marks, which are a sign of trafficker ownership. Psychosocial symptoms experienced by victims include stress, paranoia, fear, suicidal ideation, depression, anxiety, shame, and self-loathing (Byrne et al., 2017). You can assess the patient by asking questions such as, "Do you feel free to come and go anywhere as you please?", "Does anyone you work for make you feel unsafe?", and "Have you ever felt like you cannot leave your employer?" If you suspect that a patient is a trafficking victim,

follow agency policy, contact local authorities, and report to the National Human Trafficking Resource Center.

Work in collaboration with the interprofessional team to address the trauma patient's complex health care needs, including early consultation with social services and the rehabilitation team. Coordinate with other support services as necessary such as pastoral care, nutrition support, psychiatry, mental health/behavioral health specialists, and substance abuse counselors. Trauma centers are required to incorporate systems to identify patients with high-risk alcohol use (American College of Surgeons Committee on Trauma, 2014). An effective strategy is to implement a SBIRT (**s**creening, **b**rief **i**ntervention, and **r**eferral to **t**reatment) program in which interprofessional trauma team members, including emergency and trauma nurses, are educated to assess patients for problem drinking. The typical interaction involves a brief, respectful conversation that offers feedback, counsel, and motivation to reduce alcohol consumption.

Consider the needs of family members in crisis and address them when planning nursing care. A trauma advanced practice nurse, if available, can help coordinate trauma care by offering clinical expertise; facilitating COMMUNICATION among caregivers; and serving as an educator for the patient, staff, and family. He or she can organize family meetings with the interprofessional team and arrange for necessary resources. If this resource is not available, a case manager or specially educated direct-care nurse may perform these functions.

GET READY FOR THE NCLEX® EXAMINATION!

KEY POINTS

Review these Key Points for each NCLEX Examination Client Needs Category.

Safe and Effective Care Environment

- Understand that emergency departments (EDs) are fast-paced, often crowded environments where care occurs for patients with a variety of health problems across the life span.
- Recognize that vulnerable populations who seek care in the ED include patients who may be uninsured or

underinsured, poor, homeless, and older adults. **Health Care Disparities**
- Anticipate that the most common reasons that patients seek ED care include chest pain, abdominal pain, difficulty breathing, injury, headache, fever, and pain.
- Collaborate with members of the interprofessional team in the ED and at subsequent points of care, which includes prehospital providers, physicians, nurses, specialty teams, and support staff. **QSEN: Teamwork and Collaboration**

- Review Chart 8-1 to plan and implement best practices to maintain staff and patient SAFETY in the ED. **QSEN: Safety**
- Explain core competencies needed for ED nurses, including assessment, priority setting, knowledge, technical skills, and COMMUNICATION.
- Understand that the three-level triage model categorizes patients as emergent, urgent, and nonurgent (see Table 8-2). The Emergency Severity Index is a five-tier triage system that uses both acuity and the prediction of necessary resources to rapidly categorize the priority of patients.
- Recall that trauma centers are categorized as Levels I through IV, based on their resource capabilities as listed in Table 8-3.
- Remember that the mechanism of injury describes the manner in which the traumatic event occurred.
- Recall that the two most common injury-producing mechanisms are blunt trauma and penetrating trauma.
- Prioritize resuscitation interventions based on the primary survey of the injured patient by implementing the steps of the primary survey and trauma resuscitation as outlined in Table 8-4. **QSEN: Safety**

- Recall that ED nurses always include patient education as an important part of discharge planning.

Psychosocial Integrity

- Implement TEAMWORK AND COLLABORATION strategies with the psychiatric crisis team as needed. **QSEN: Teamwork and Collaboration**

Physiological Integrity

- Remember that the expected sequence of events from admission through discharge in the ED includes treatment, stabilization, and discharge to their homes or admission for observation or inpatient care.
- Recall that older adults who visit the ED are frequently admitted to the hospital. **QSEN: Patient-Centered Care**
- Understand that ED nurses are accountable for preventing or reducing risks such as falls, medication errors, pressure injuries, and hospital-acquired infections.
- Remember that communication with the older adult may be challenging if the patient has memory loss or acute delirium while in the ED. **QSEN: Patient-Centered Care**

SELECTED BIBLIOGRAPHY

Asterisk indicates a classic or definitive work on this subject.

Alexander, D., Kinsley, T. L., & Waszinski, C. (2013). Journey to a safe environment: Fall prevention in an emergency department at a level I trauma center. *JEN: Journal of Emergency Nursing, 39*(4), 346–352.

American College of Surgeons Committee on Trauma (2014). *Resources for optimal care of the injured patient 2014.* Chicago: Author.

Bass, D., et al. (2015). Impact of the care coordination program "Partners in Dementia Care" on veterans' hospital admissions and emergency department visits. *Alzheimer's & Dementia: Translational Research & Clinical Interventions, 1*(1), 13–22.

Bellow, A. A., & Gillespie, G. L. (2014). The evolution of ED crowding. *Journal of Emergency Nursing, 40*(2), 153–160.

Byrne, M., Parsh, B., & Ghilain, C. (2017). Victims of human trafficking: Hiding in plain sight. *Nursing, 47*(3), 49–52.

Centers for Disease Control and Prevention (CDC) (2017). FastStats: *Emergency department visits.* https://www.cdc.gov/nchs/fastats/emergency-department.htm.

Centers for Medicare and Medicaid Services (2013). *Critical access hospitals.* www.cms.gov/Medicare/Provider-Enrollment-and-Certification/CertificationandComplianc/CAHs.html.

*Cooper, G., & Laskowski-Jones, L. (2006). Development of trauma care systems. *Prehospital Emergency Care, 10*(3), 328–331.

Dateo, J. (2013). What factors increase the accuracy and inter-rater reliability of the emergency severity index among emergency nurses in triaging adult patients? *Journal of Emergency Nursing, 39*(2), 203–207.

Gerber, L. (2013). Bringing home effective nursing care for the homeless. *Nursing, 43*(3), 32–38.

Gurney, D., & Westergard, A. M. (2014). Chapter 5: Initial assessment. In D. Gurney (Ed.), *TNCC: Trauma nursing core course provider manual* (7th ed.). Des Plaines, IL: Emergency Nurses Association.

Harding, A. D., Walker-Cillo, G. E., Duke, A., Campos, G. J., & Stapleton, S. J. (2013). A framework for creating and evaluating competencies for emergency nurses. *Journal of Emergency Nursing, 39*, 252–264.

International Association of Forensic Nurses. (2016). http://www.forensicnurses.org.

Jeffries, P., Rodgers, B., & Adamson, K. (2015). NLN Jeffries Simulation Theory: Brief narrative description. *Nursing Education Perspectives, 36*(5), 292–293.

*Laskowski-Jones, L. (2008). Change management at the hospital front door: Integrating automatic patient tracking in a high volume emergency department and Level I trauma center. *Nurse Leader, 6*(2), 52–57.

National Center for Injury Prevention and Control (NCIPC) (2017). *Injury prevention and control: Data & statistics (WISQARS).* www.cdc.gov/injury/wisqars/index.html.

Popovich, M. A., Boyd, C., Dachenhaus, T., & Kusler, D. (2012). Improving stable patient flow through the emergency department by utilizing evidence-based practice: One hospital's journey. *Journal of Emergency Nursing, 38*(5), 474–478.

Porter, J. E., Cooper, S. J., & Sellick, K. (2014). Family presence during resuscitation (FPDR): Perceived benefits, barriers and enablers to implementation and practice. *International Emergency Nursing, 22*(2), 69–74.

*Shelton, R. (2010). ESI: A better triage system? *Nursing Critical Care, 5*(6), 34–37.

The Joint Commission (TJC) (2017a). *2016 National Patient Safety Goals.* www.jointcommission.org.

The Joint Commission (TJC) (2017b). *Certification for primary stroke centers.* http://www.jointcommission.org/certification/primary_stroke_centers.aspx.

The Joint Commission (TJC) (2017c). *Core measures set.* https://www.jointcommission.org/core_measure_sets.aspx.

Touhy, T. A., & Jett, K. (2015). *Ebersole & Hess' toward healthy aging: Human needs and nursing response* (9th ed.). St. Louis: Mosby.

U.S. Department of Housing and Urban Development (2015). *The 2015 annual homeless assessment report (HAR) to Congress.* https://www.hudexchange.info/resources/documents/2015-AHAR-Part-1.pdf.

Weaver, M., Rittenberger, J., Patterson, D., McEntire, S., Corcos, A., Ziembicki, J., et al. (2014). Risk factors for hypothermia in EMS-treated burn patients. *Prehospital Emergency Care, 18*(3), doi:10.3109/10903127.2013.864354.

Care of Patients With Common Environmental Emergencies

Linda Laskowski-Jones

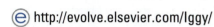
http://evolve.elsevier.com/Iggy/

PRIORITY AND INTERRELATED CONCEPTS

The priority concept for this chapter is TISSUE INTEGRITY.

The interrelated concept for this chapter is COMFORT.

LEARNING OUTCOMES

Safe and Effective Care Environment
1. Collaborate with the interprofessional health care team when providing care for patients with environmental emergencies.

Health Promotion and Maintenance
2. Teach people at risk how to prevent environmental emergencies.

Physiological Integrity
3. Prioritize first aid/prehospital interventions for patients who have thermoregulation problems, arthropod bites or stings, or venomous snake bites affecting TISSUE INTEGRITY and COMFORT.
4. Apply knowledge of pathophysiology to identify best practices for care of patients with environmental emergencies.
5. Create an evidence-based plan of care for patients who have experienced an environmental emergency.

Every day people leave their homes to enjoy recreational activities. Although seemingly harmless, there are activities that can have environmental risks, especially for older adults. Some bites, stings, and environmental conditions also pose concerns indoors. This chapter provides an overview of selected environmental emergencies, their initial emergency management (first aid), and acute care interventions.

HEAT-RELATED ILLNESSES

The most common environmental factors causing heat-related illnesses are high environmental temperature (above 95°F [35°C]) and high humidity (above 80%). These thermoregulation-related illnesses include heat exhaustion and heat stroke. Some of the most vulnerable, at-risk populations for these problems are older adults (who have less body fluid volume and can easily become dehydrated), people with mental health/behavioral health conditions, those who work outside, homeless individuals, users of illicit drugs, athletes who engage in outdoor sports, and members of the military stationed in hot climates.

A patient's health status can also increase the risk for heat-related illness, especially obesity, heart disease, fever, infection, strenuous exercise, seizures, mental health disorders, and all degrees of burns (even sunburn). The use of prescribed drugs such as lithium, neuroleptics, beta-adrenergic blockers, anticholinergics, angiotensin-converting enzyme (ACE) inhibitors, and diuretics can also increase the risk for heat-related illness.

Health Promotion and Maintenance
Teach older adults before participating in any hot weather activity how to take steps to eliminate or minimize risks whenever possible. Ask them to have a family member, friend, or neighbor check on them several times each day to ensure that there are no signs of heat-related illness. Chart 9-1 lists other essential heat-related illness prevention strategies for older adults, many of which apply to adults of any age.

HEAT EXHAUSTION

❖ PATHOPHYSIOLOGY

Heat exhaustion is a syndrome resulting primarily from dehydration. It is caused by heavy perspiration and inadequate fluid and electrolyte intake during heat exposure over hours to days. Profuse diaphoresis can lead to profound, even fatal, dehydration and hyponatremia caused by excessive sodium lost in perspiration. *If untreated, heat exhaustion can lead to heat*

CHART 9-1   Nursing Focus on the Older Adult

Heat-Related Illness Prevention

- Avoid alcohol and caffeine.
- Prevent overexposure to the sun; use a sunscreen with an SPF of at least 30 with UVA and UVB protection.
- Rest frequently and take breaks from being in a hot environment. Plan to limit activity at the hottest time of day.
- Wear clothing suited to the environment. Lightweight, light-colored, and loose-fitting clothing is best.
- Pay attention to your personal physical limitations; modify activities accordingly.
- Take cool baths or showers to help reduce body temperature.
- Stay indoors in air-conditioned buildings if possible.
- Ask a neighbor, friend, or family member to check on the older adult at least twice a day during a heat wave.

SPF, Sun protection factor; *UVA,* ultraviolet A; *UVB,* ultraviolet B.

CHART 9-2   Key Features

Heat Stroke

- Body temperature more than 104°F (40°C)
- Hot and dry skin; may or may not perspire
- Mental status changes such as:
  - Acute confusion
  - Bizarre behavior
  - Anxiety
  - Loss of coordination
  - Hallucinations
  - Agitation
  - Seizures
  - Coma
- Vital sign changes, including:
  - Hypotension
  - Tachycardia
  - Tachypnea (increased respiratory rate)
- Electrolyte imbalances, especially sodium and potassium
- Decreased renal function (oliguria)
- Coagulopathy (abnormal clotting)
- Pulmonary edema (crackles)

---

stroke, which is a true emergency condition that has a very high mortality rate.

❖ INTERPROFESSIONAL COLLABORATIVE CARE

Patients with heat exhaustion usually have flu-like symptoms with headache, weakness, nausea, and/or vomiting. Body temperature may not be significantly elevated in this condition. The patient may continue to perspire despite dehydration.

! NURSING SAFETY PRIORITY QSEN

Action Alert

Patients should be assessed for orthostatic hypotension and tachycardia, especially the older adult who can dehydrate quickly. Older adults with dehydration often experience acute confusion and are at risk for falls.

Instruct the patient to immediately stop physical activity and move to a cool place. Use cooling measures such as placing cold packs on the neck, chest, abdomen, and groin. Soak the victim in cool water or fan while spraying water on the skin. Remove constrictive clothing. Sports drinks or an oral rehydration-therapy solution can be provided. Mistakenly drinking plain water can worsen the sodium deficit. *Do not give salt tablets,* which can cause stomach irritation, nausea, and vomiting. If signs and symptoms persist, call an ambulance to transport the patient to the hospital.

In the clinical setting, monitor vital signs. Rehydrate the patient with IV 0.9% saline solution if nausea or vomiting persists. Draw blood for serum electrolyte analysis. Hospital admission is indicated only for patients who have other health problems that are worsened by the heat-related illness or for those with severe dehydration and evidence of physiologic compromise. The management of hypovolemic dehydration is discussed in more detail in Chapter 11.

HEAT STROKE

❖ PATHOPHYSIOLOGY

Heat stroke is a *true medical emergency* in which body temperature may exceed 104°F (40°C). It has a high mortality rate if not treated in a timely manner. The victim's thermoregulation mechanisms fail and cannot adjust for a critical elevation in body temperature. If the condition is not treated or the patient does not respond to treatment, organ dysfunction and death can result.

Exertional heat stroke has a sudden onset and is often the result of strenuous physical activity (especially when wearing too heavy clothing) in hot, humid conditions. Classic heat stroke, also referred to as *nonexertional heat stroke,* occurs over a period of time as a result of chronic exposure to a hot, humid environment such as living in a home without air conditioning in the high heat of the summer.

❖ INTERPROFESSIONAL COLLABORATIVE CARE

◆ Assessment: Noticing

Victims of heat stroke have a profoundly elevated body temperature (above 104°F [40°C]). *Although the patient's skin is hot and dry, the presence of sweating does not rule out heat stroke—people with heat stroke may continue to perspire.*

Mental status changes occur as a result of thermal injury to the brain and are the hallmark findings in heat stroke. Symptoms can include confusion, bizarre behavior, seizures, or even coma (Chart 9-2). The patient may have hypotension, tachycardia, and tachypnea. Cardiac troponin I (cTnI) is frequently elevated during nonexertional heat-related illnesses; research indicates that this test can be used to cost effectively predict severity and organ damage at the beginning of heat stroke, even in a remote setting (Audet et al., 2015).

◆ Planning and Implementation: Responding

Coordinate care with the health care team to recognize and treat immediately and aggressively to achieve optimal patient outcomes. Chart 9-3 lists evidence-based emergency care of patients with heat stroke.

First Aid/Prehospital Care. Do not give food or liquid by mouth because vomiting and aspiration are risks in patients with neurologic impairment. Immediate medical care using advanced life support is essential (see the Evidence-Based Practice box).

Hospital Care. The first priority for collaborative care is to monitor and support the patient's airway, breathing, and circulatory status. Provide high-concentration oxygen therapy, start several IV lines with 0.9% saline solution, and insert an indwelling urinary catheter. Continue aggressive interventions to cool the patient until the rectal temperature is 102°F (38.9°C). External continuous cooling methods include using cooling blankets and applying ice packs in the axillae and groin and on the neck and head. Internal cooling methods

CHART 9-3   Best Practice for Patient Safety & Quality Care QSEN

Emergency Care of the Patient With Heat Stroke: Restoring Thermoregulation

At the Scene
- Ensure a patent airway.
- Remove the patient from the hot environment (into air-conditioning or into the shade).
- Remove the patient's clothing.
- Pour or spray cold water on the patient's body and scalp.
- Fan the patient (not only the person providing care, but all surrounding people should fan the patient with newspapers or whatever is available).
- If ice is available, place ice in cloth or bags and position the packs on the patient's scalp, in the groin area, behind the neck, and in the armpits.
- Contact emergency medical services to transport the patient to the emergency department.

At the Hospital
- Give oxygen by mask or nasal cannula; be prepared for endotracheal intubation.

- Start at least one IV with a large-bore needle or cannula.
- Administer normal saline (0.9% sodium chloride) as prescribed, using cooled solutions if available.
- Use a cooling blanket.
- Do not give aspirin or any other antipyretics.
- Insert a rectal probe to measure core body temperature continuously or use a rectal thermometer and assess temperature every 15 minutes.
- Insert an indwelling urinary drainage catheter.
- Monitor vital signs frequently as clinically indicated.
- Obtain baseline laboratory tests as quickly as possible: serum electrolytes, cardiac enzymes, liver enzymes, and complete blood count (CBC).
- Assess arterial blood gases.
- Administer muscle relaxants (benzodiazepines) if the patient begins to shiver.
- Measure urine output and specific gravity to determine fluid needs.
- Stop cooling interventions when core body temperature is reduced to 102°F (39°C).
- Obtain urinalysis and monitor urine output.

EVIDENCE-BASED PRACTICE QSEN

What Does Evidence Say About On-Site Treatment of Exertional Heat Stroke?

Sloan, B. K., Kraft, E. M., Clark, D., Schmeissing, S., Byrne, B. C., & Rusyniak, D. E. (2015). On-site treatment of exertional heat stroke. *The American Journal of Sports Medicine*, 43(4), 823-829.

Exertional heat stroke can lead to morbidity and mortality if untreated or undertreated. The authors conducted a descriptive epidemiological study of people over an 8-year period who developed exertional heat stroke when participating in the Indianapolis half marathon. They identified signs of heat stroke, methods of treatment at the marathon site, and eventual outcomes whether treatment concluded on-site or the runner was sent to the hospital.

Of the 696 runners who received medical care on-site at the half marathon, 32 were diagnosed with heat stroke, 22 of whom were successfully treated on-site with cold-water immersion. Only 10 others, who did not undergo cold-water immersion, were transported from the site to a hospital; 4 of these were then discharged to go home.

Level of Evidence: 4
This is a descriptive epidemiological study.

Commentary: Implications for Practice and Research
This study demonstrates that rapid cooling is cost reasonable and is effective in decreasing morbidity and mortality of patients with heat stroke. The major nursing implication from this study is that nurses working at community events such as a 5K, half, or full marathon should be aware of and prepared to administer appropriate methods of rapid cooling for individuals who have heat stroke. Strengths of the study included the large sample size collected over a long period of time. A weakness might be the level of evidence, but this is likely outweighed by the sampling method and the time factor of review. Nurses are in a key position to advocate for individuals in the community and to implement interventions that can help treat heat stroke. Chart 9-1 lists best practices for decreasing the risk for heat-related illnesses in older adults.

! NURSING SAFETY PRIORITY QSEN

Critical Rescue

After ensuring that the patient has a patent airway, effective breathing, and adequate circulation, recognize that you must use rapid cooling as the first priority for care. Respond by implementing methods for rapid cooling, which include removing clothing; placing ice packs on the neck, axillae, chest and groin; immersing the patient or wetting the patient's body with cold water; and fanning rapidly to aid in evaporative cooling.

? NCLEX EXAMINATION CHALLENGE 9-1

Physiological Integrity

The nurse is caring for an older-adult client with heat exhaustion. Which assessment finding indicates to the nurse that the client may need hospitalization?
A. Alert and oriented
B. Reports nausea and weakness
C. Continues to sweat while being cooled
D. Mucous membranes are dry and sticky

may include iced gastric and bladder lavage. Use a continuous core temperature–monitoring device (e.g., rectal or esophageal probe) or a temperature-monitoring urinary bladder catheter to prevent hypothermia.

If shivering occurs during the cooling process, give a parenteral benzodiazepine such as diazepam (Valium). Lorazepam (Ativan) is an alternative agent. Seizure activity can further elevate body temperature and is also treated with an IV benzodiazepine. Once the patient is stabilized, admission to a critical care unit is warranted to monitor for complications such as multi-system organ dysfunction syndrome and severe electrolyte imbalances; these problems increase mortality risk.

SNAKEBITES AND ARTHROPOD BITES AND STINGS

Most snakes fear humans and attempt to avoid contact with them. Sudden, unexpected confrontations at close range often lead to defensive strikes. Awareness is the key to snakebite prevention. Although most snake species are nonvenomous (nonpoisonous) and harmless, there are two families of poisonous snakes in North America: pit vipers (*Crotalidae*) and coral snakes (*Elapidae*). Chart 9-4 provides common-sense actions to avoid being bitten by a poisonous snake.

CHART 9-4 Patient and Family Education: Preparing for Self-Management

Snakebite Prevention

- Do not keep venomous snakes as pets.
- Be extremely careful in locations where snakes may hide such as tall grass, rock piles, ledges and crevices, woodpiles, brush, boxes, and cabinets. Snakes are most active on warm nights.
- Don protective attire such as boots, heavy pants, and leather gloves. When walking or hiking, use a walking stick or trekking poles.
- Inspect suspicious areas before placing hands and feet in them.
- Do not harass any snakes you may encounter. Striking distance can be up to two thirds the length of the snake. Even young snakes pose a threat; they are capable of envenomation from birth.
- Be aware that newly dead or decapitated snakes can inflict a bite for up to an hour after death because of persistence of the bite reflex.
- Do not transport the snake with the victim to the medical facility for identification purposes; instead, take a digital photo of the snake at a safe distance if possible.

! NURSING SAFETY PRIORITY QSEN

Critical Rescue

Recognize that the first priority is to move the person to a safe area away from the snake and encourage rest to decrease venom circulation. Respond (when in the safe area) by removing jewelry and constricting clothing before swelling worsens. Call for immediate emergency assistance. Do not attempt to capture or kill the snake, but do take digital photographs at a safe distance if possible to aid in snake identification.

Pit vipers are named for the characteristic depression or pit between each eye and nostril that serves as a heat-sensitive organ for locating warm-blooded prey. They include various species of rattlesnakes, copperheads, and cottonmouths and account for the majority of the poisonous snakebites in the United States (Figs. 9-1 and 9-2). Management of a patient who has a snakebite from a pit viper depends on the severity of envenomation (venom injection), as noted in Table 9-1.

Coral snakes (Fig. 9-3) are found from North Carolina to Florida and in the Gulf states through Texas and the southwestern United States. They have broad bands of red and black rings separated by yellow or cream rings. Several harmless snake species closely resemble the coral snake. If a black band lies between the red and yellow bands, the snake is usually nonvenomous. If the red band touches the yellow band, the snake is venomous. A helpful memory aid for identifying coral snakes is "red on yellow can kill a fellow" and "red on black, venom lack." *Be aware that this saying applies only to coral snakes found in the United States!* These nonaggressive snakes have short, fixed fangs and inject highly neurotoxic venom into prey.

! NURSING SAFETY PRIORITY QSEN

Critical Rescue

Recognize that the most significant risk to the snakebite victim is airway compromise and respiratory failure. Respond by ensuring that the patient's IV lines are patent and that resuscitation equipment is immediately available.

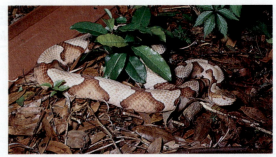

FIG. 9-1 Southern copperhead (*Agkistrodon contortrix*) has markings that make it almost invisible when lying in leaf litter. (From Auerbach, P. S. [2017]. *Wilderness medicine* [7th ed.]. Philadelphia: Mosby; courtesy Michael Cardwell & Carl Barden Venom Laboratory.)

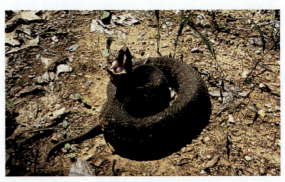

FIG. 9-2 Cottonmouth water moccasin (*Agkistrodon piscivorus*). The open-mouthed threat gesture is characteristic of this semiaquatic pit viper. (From Auerbach, P. S. [2017]. *Wilderness medicine* [7th ed.]. Philadelphia: Mosby; courtesy Sherman Minton, MD.)

TABLE 9-1 Grades of Pit Viper Envenomation

ENVENOMATION	CHARACTERISTICS
None	Fang marks, but no local or systemic reactions
Minimal	Fang marks, local swelling and pain, but no systemic reactions
Moderate	Fang marks and swelling progressing beyond the site of the bite; systemic signs and symptoms such as nausea, vomiting, paresthesias, or hypotension.
Severe	Fang marks present with marked swelling of the extremity; subcutaneous ecchymosis; severe symptoms, including manifestations of coagulopathy

From Auerbach, P. S., Donner, H. J., & Weiss, E. A. (2013). *Field guide to wilderness medicine* (4th ed.). St. Louis: Mosby.

Arthropods include spiders, scorpions, bees, and wasps. Unlike snakes, almost all species of spiders are venomous to some degree—most are not harmful to humans either because their mouth is too small to pierce human skin or the quantity or quality of their venom is inadequate to produce major health problems. Brown recluse (Figs. 9-4 and 9-5) and black widow spiders, scorpions (Fig. 9-6), bees, and wasps are examples of venomous arthropods that can cause toxic reactions in humans.

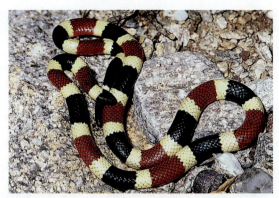

FIG. 9-3 Sonoran coral snake *(Micruroides euryxanthus)* is also known as the *Arizona coral snake.* No documented fatality has followed a bite by this species. (From Auerbach, P. S. [2017]. *Wilderness medicine* [7th ed.]. Philadelphia: Mosby; courtesy Michael Cardwell & Jude McNally.)

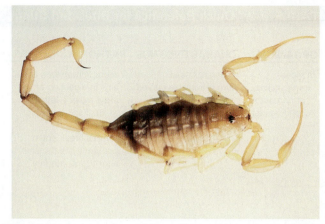

FIG. 9-6 The bark scorpion of Arizona *(Centruroides sculpturatus).* (From Auerbach, P. S. [2012]. *Wilderness medicine* [6th ed.] Philadelphia: Mosby.)

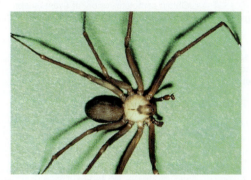

FIG. 9-4 Brown recluse spider *(Loxosceles reclusa).* (From Auerbach, P. S. [2017]. *Wilderness medicine* [7th ed.]. Philadelphia: Mosby; courtesy Indiana University Medical Center.)

👤 CHART 9-5 **Patient and Family Education: Preparing for Self-Management**

Arthropod Bite/Sting Prevention

- Wear protective clothing, including gloves and shoes, when working in areas known to harbor venomous arthropods such as spiders, scorpions, bees, and wasps.
- Cover garbage cans. Bees and wasps are attracted to uncovered garbage.
- Use screens in windows and doors to prevent flying insects from entering buildings.
- Inspect clothing, shoes, and gear for insects before putting on these items.
- Shake out clothing and gear that have been on the ground to prevent arthropod "stowaways" and inadvertent bites and stings.
- Consult an exterminator to control arthropod populations in and around the home. Eliminating insects that are part of the arthropod's food source may also limit their presence.
- Identify nesting areas such as yard debris and rock piles; remove them whenever possible.
- Do not place unprotected hands where the eyes cannot see.
- Avoid handling insects or keeping them as "pets."
- Do not swat insects, wasps, and Africanized bees because they can send chemical signals that alert others to attack.
- Carry a prescription epinephrine autoinjector and antihistamines if known to be allergic to bee and wasp stings. Ensure that at least one family member is also able to use the autoinjector.

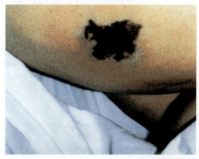

FIG. 9-5 Brown recluse spider bite after 24 hours, with central ischemia and rapidly advancing cellulitis. (From Auerbach, P. S. [2017]. *Wilderness medicine* [7th ed.]. Philadelphia: Mosby; courtesy Paul S. Auerbach, MD.)

Chart 9-5 lists actions that help prevent arthropod bites and stings.

Bees and wasps are also venomous arthropods. Stings can produce a wide range of reactions from mild changes in levels of COMFORT at the sting site to severe pain, multi-system problems, and life-threatening anaphylaxis in allergic people. Bumblebees, hornets, and wasps are capable of stinging repeatedly when disturbed. They have a smooth stinger that may or may not become lodged in the victim. Honeybees can sting just once. When a honeybee stings a person, the stinger and venom sac pull away from the bee. The bee dies, but venom injection continues because the stinger and sac remain in the victim.

"Africanized" bees, also called "killer bees," are a very aggressive species that are found in the southwestern United States. They are known to attack in groups and can remain agitated for several hours. People under attack should attempt to outrun the bees, if possible, and keep their mouth and eyes protected from the swarm. A person should never go into a body of water because the bees will attack when he or she comes up for air. When a person sustains multiple stings, reactions are more severe and may be fatal because multiple venom doses have cumulative toxic effects.

Table 9-2 provides detailed information about each of these organisms, their characteristics, pathophysiology of the bite/sting, first aid and prehospital care, and interprofessional collaborative care that takes place in an acute care setting. Chart 9-5 lists actions that may help prevent arthropod bites and stings.

TABLE 9-2   Quick Reference for Bites and Stings

ORGANISM	CHARACTERISTICS	PATHOPHYSIOLOGY	FIRST AID/PRE-HOSPITAL CARE	INTERPROFESSIONAL COLLABORATIVE CARE
Pit viper (rattlesnakes, cottonmouths, copperheads)	Triangular head Two retractable curved fangs Rattlesnakes have vibrating horny rings in their tails	Venom immobilizes and aids in digestion of prey; may be lethal Has local and systemic effects Enzymes break down human tissue proteins, alter tissue integrity	Move to safety, away from snake. Call for immediate emergency assistance. Encourage rest to decrease venom circulation. Remove jewelry and constrictive clothing. Take photos of snake from a safe distance to aid in identification. Immobilize affected extremity in position of function—maintain at level of heart. Keep patient warm, provide calm environment Do *not* incise or suck wound, apply ice, or use a tourniquet.	*Assessment/Noticing:* Look for: • Puncture wounds in skin. • Pain, swelling, redness, and/or bruising around bite(s). • Vesicles or hemorrhagic bullae that may form later. • Patient identification of minty, rubbery, or metallic taste. • Tingling or paresthesias on scalp, face, and lips. • Muscle twitching, weakness. • Nausea and vomiting. • Hypotension, seizures. • Clotting abnormalities or DIC. *Hospital Care:* • Obtain complete history of event (snake appearance, time of bite, prehospital interventions, and any past snakebites or antivenom therapy). • Give supplemental oxygen. • Insert two large-bore IV lines. • Infuse normal saline or Ringer's lactate. • Continuously monitor heart function and blood pressure. • Provide opioids to decrease pain. • Obtain coagulation panel, CBC, CK, type and crossmatch, urinalysis. • Obtain ECG. • Mark, measure, and record circumference of bitten extremity q15-30 minutes. • See Table 9-1 for envenomation severity. • Contact regional poison control for specific advice on antivenom dosing and medical management. • If indicated, administer Crotalidae, Polyvalent Immune Fab (CroFab) as ordered
Coral snakes	Bands of black, red, and yellow that encircle the snake's body Small maxillary fangs	Venom contains nerve and muscle toxins Blocks neurotransmission Toxic effects may be delayed up to 13 hours and then produce rapid clinical deterioration (Norris, 2015)	Definitively identify snake as a coral snake, if possible. Encircle affected extremity with an elastic bandage or roller gauze dressing (do not wrap so tightly that arterial flow is impeded); then splint. Leave on until the patient is treated at an acute care facility.	*Assessment/Noticing:* Look for: • Weakness, cranial nerve deficits (ptosis, diplopia, swallowing difficulty), altered level of consciousness, and respiratory paralysis (Norris, 2015). • Pain at the site, which may be described as mild and transient. • Difficult to find fang marks. *Hospital Care:* • Identify snake as a coral snake if possible. If the snake cannot be identified, treat as if venom were injected. • Be aware that toxic effects of venom may be delayed up to 13 hours and then produce rapid clinical deterioration (Norris, 2015). • Monitor for elevation in CK level from muscle breakdown and myoglobinuria. • Continually monitor cardiac function, blood pressure, and pulse oximetry. Be prepared to admit to a critical care unit. • Be prepared to provide aggressive airway management if respiratory insufficiency or severe neurologic impairment occurs. • Provide interventions to decrease risk for aspiration. • Coral snake antivenom is not manufactured in the United States. Supportive care is recommended (Norris, 2015). • Teach the patient that effects of a severe bite can persist for many days (Norris, 2015). • Contact regional poison control for specific advice on patient management.

TABLE 9-2   **Quick Reference for Bites and Stings—cont'd**

ORGANISM	CHARACTERISTICS	PATHOPHYSIOLOGY	FIRST AID/PRE-HOSPITAL CARE	INTERPROFESSIONAL COLLABORATIVE CARE
Brown recluse spiders	Medium-size, light brown, fiddle-shaped mark from eyes down their back (Fig. 9-4) Live in boxes, closets, basements, sheds, garages	Venom causes cellular damage and impaired tissue integrity	Apply cold compresses over site of bite. Do not apply heat because it increases enzyme activity and potentially worsens wound. Elevate affected extremity, provide local wound care, and rest.	*Assessment/Noticing:* Look for: • Central bite mark, which may appear as a bleb or vesicle with edema and erythema. • Description of bite as painless, stinging, or sharp. • Center of bite to become bluish-purple. • Central part of the wound to become dark and necrotic over the following 1-3 days (Fig. 9-5) for some patients. This is called the classic *red, white, and blue sign* associated with severe bites. • Systematic toxicity, which rarely occurs (rash, fever, chills, nausea, vomiting, malaise, joint pain). • Rare, severe systemic complications (loxoscelism), which may include hemolytic anemia, thrombocytopenia, DIC, and death. *Hospital Care:* • Hospitalization is rarely indicated. • Teach patient supportive care measures. • Topical antiseptic and sterile dressings can be applied to wound. • Antibiotics may be prescribed. • Administer tetanus prophylaxis as needed. • For extensive wounds, débridement and skin grafting may be needed.
Black widow spiders	Female shiny black with a red hourglass pattern on abdomen (hourglass pattern is faint in males) Inhabit cool, damp environments such as log piles, vegetation, and rocks; also live in barns, sheds, and garages	Venom is neurotoxic; produces a syndrome known as latrodectism in which the venom causes neurotransmitter release from nerve terminals	Apply ice pack to decrease action of neurotoxin. Monitor for systemic toxicity; support airway, breathing, and circulation as needed. Transport to acute care facility as soon as possible.	*Assessment/Noticing:* Look for: • Description of bite as nearly painless to sharply painful. • Tiny papule or small, red punctate mark. • Systemic complications, which usually develop within an hour of bite and involve neuromuscular system. • Concerns that may include severe abdominal pain, muscle rigidity and spasm, hypertension, nausea, and vomiting. This may be initially incorrectly diagnosed as an acute abdomen because of similarity in symptoms. *Hospital Care:* • Monitor older adults, especially those with cardiovascular disease, for complications as sequelae of hypertension. • Monitor vital signs, especially blood pressure and respiratory function. • Observe for seizures related to rapidly rising blood pressure. • Administer opioid pain medication and muscle relaxants (e.g., diazepam) as ordered. • Administer tetanus prophylaxis as needed. • Monitor for signs of pulmonary edema, uncontrollable hypertension, respiratory arrest, and/or shock. • Administer antivenom as ordered. Monitor for signs of anaphylaxis and serum sickness. • Contact regional poison control for specific advice on antivenom dosing and medical management.

Continued

TABLE 9-2   Quick Reference for Bites and Stings—cont'd

ORGANISM	CHARACTERISTICS	PATHOPHYSIOLOGY	FIRST AID/PRE-HOSPITAL CARE	INTERPROFESSIONAL COLLABORATIVE CARE
Scorpions	Found within the United States, although not typically in the Midwest or New England Bark scorpion lives in southwestern United States; its sting can be potentially fatal (Fig. 9-6)	Venom injected via stinging apparatus on tail; effects are neurotoxic	Transport to acute care facility as soon as possible.	*Assessment/Noticing:* Look for: • Symptoms arise immediately after the sting, reaching crisis level within 12 hours. • Gentle tapping at the site of sting usually causes increased pain. • Sting site may not be reddened. • Severe systemic symptoms include excessive salivation, hyperactivity, high fever, hypertension, GI disorders, tachycardiac, cardiac dysfunction, pulmonary edema, nervous system involvement, and (rarely) death. *Hospital Care:* • Monitor older adults, especially those with cardiovascular disease, for complications as sequelae of hypertension. • Monitor vital signs, especially blood pressure and respiratory function. • Observe for seizures related to rapidly rising blood pressure. • Provide basic wound care with antiseptic agent and apply ice pack to sting site. • Administer tetanus prophylaxis as needed. • Administer analgesic and sedative agents with caution. • Be very cautious if administering opioids, benzodiazepines, and barbiturates, as these can cause loss of airway reflexes and precipitate respiratory failure. • Contact regional poison control for specific information on pharmacologic agents for scorpion stings.
Bees and wasps	Found all over United States; "Africanized" or "killer" bees found in southwestern United States	Venom injected through stings; most can sting repeatedly when disturbed; only honeybees can sting just once	Quickly remove stinger with tweezers or by gently scraping or brushing it off with the edge of a knife blade, credit card, or needles (if present) (Auerbach, 2016b) and apply ice pack. Ensure that airway, breathing, and circulation are maintained. If patient has history of allergic reactions to stings or has wheezing, facial swelling, and respiratory distress, epinephrine must be given immediately. Allergic adult patients typically carry an epinephrine autoinjector (e.g., EpiPen®, Auvi-Q™).* (See Chapter 20 for further discussion of epinephrine administration for anaphylaxis management.) Follow with antihistamine.	*Assessment/Noticing:* Look for: • Wheal-and-flare skin reactions; swelling can be extensive and involve an entire limb or body area. • Urticaria (hives), pruritus (itching), and swelling of lips and tongue in patients who have allergy to the venom. • Monitor for anaphylaxis, a true medical emergency evidenced by respiratory distress with bronchospasm, laryngeal edema, hypotension, decreased mental status, and cardiac dysrhythmias. • Systemic effects develop based on venom load and patient sensitivity. These may include generalized edema, nausea, vomiting, diarrhea, destruction of red and white blood cells and platelets, damage to the blood vessel walls, acute kidney injury, renal failure, liver injury, cardiac complications, and multi-system organ failure. *Hospital Care:* • Administer oxygen. • Continuously monitor cardiac function and blood pressure. • Administer antihistamines, albuterol, and corticosteroids as ordered. • Be certain that advanced life support drugs and resuscitation equipment are readily available. • Observe patients who have sustained multiple stings for several hours. Be prepared to admit to critical care if toxic venom effects are noted. • See Table 9-2 for a quick reference regarding bites and stings.

CBC, Complete blood count; *CK,* creatine kinase; *DIC,* disseminated intravascular coagulation; *ECG,* electrocardiogram.

*In 2015 Sanofi U.S voluntarily recalled all AUVI-Q on the market, including the 0.15-mg and 0.3-mg strengths, in lot numbers 2081278 through 3037230, which expire October 2015 through December 2016. Patients may still have one of these in their possession; therefore educate patients about this recall. New approval for AUVI-Q was given in February 2017.

❓ **CLINICAL JUDGMENT CHALLENGE 9-1**
Safety QSEN

You are working as a nurse at a camp for adult leaders. The area of the camp is known for having rattlesnakes present. One of the leaders calls you on the phone and reports that a rattlesnake has bitten another leader.
1. Which initial teaching may have prevented exposure of the leaders to rattlesnakes?
2. What will you tell the leader who has called you by phone?
3. What is the priority of care of the individual who has been bitten?
4. Which interventions will you prioritize when the leader and the bitten patient reaches your location?

⚠️ **NURSING SAFETY PRIORITY** QSEN
Drug Alert

All patients who have sustained multiple stings (particularly more than 50) are observed in an emergency care setting for several hours to monitor for the development of toxic venom effects. A critical care admission may be needed.

⚠️ **NURSING SAFETY PRIORITY** QSEN
Action Alert

Teach anyone who develops an allergic reaction to bee or wasp stings to always carry a prescription epinephrine autoinjector and wear a medical alert tag or bracelet.

LIGHTNING INJURIES

❖ PATHOPHYSIOLOGY

Lightning is a year-round force of nature responsible for multiple injuries and deaths each year. It is caused by an electric charge generated within thunderclouds that may become cloud-to-ground lightning—the most dangerous form to people and structures. Young adult males account for the majority of lightning-related deaths. Most lightning-related injuries occur in the summer months during the afternoon and early evening because of increased thunderstorm activity and greater numbers of people spending time outside. Anyone without adequate shelter, including golfers, hikers, campers, beach-goers, and swimmers, is at risk.

Lightning has an enormous magnitude of energy and a different current flow than a typical high-voltage electric shock. The duration of contact is nearly instantaneous, resulting in a flashover phenomenon—an effect that may account for the relatively low overall mortality rate. Because water is a conductor of electricity and current takes the path of least resistance to the ground, any wetness on the body increases the flashover effect of a lightning strike. Lightning flashover produces an explosive force that can injure victims directly and cause them to fall or to be thrown. The clothing and shoes of victims may be damaged or blown off in the process.

Lightning produces injury by directly striking a victim, splashing off a nearby object, or traveling through the ground. Although few people die after a lightning strike, many survivors are left with permanent disabilities.

👤 **CHART 9-6   Patient and Family Education: Preparing for Self-Management**

Lightning Strike Prevention

- Observe weather forecasts when planning to be outside.
- Seek shelter when you hear thunder. Safe choices include going inside the nearest building or an enclosed vehicle. However, isolated sheds and the entrances to caves are dangerous. Do not stand under an isolated tall tree or structure (e.g., ski lift, flagpole, boat mast, power line) in an open area such as a field, ridge, or hilltop; lightning seeks the highest point. A stand of dense trees offers better protection.
- Leave the water immediately (including an indoor shower or bathtub) and move away from any open bodies of water.
- Avoid metal objects such as chairs or bleachers; put down tools, fishing rods, garden equipment, golf clubs, and umbrellas; stand clear of fences, exposed pipes, motorcycles, bicycles, tractors, and golf carts.
- If camping in a tent, stay away from the metal tent poles and wet walls.
- Once inside a building, stay away from open doors, windows, fireplaces, metal fixtures, and plumbing.
- Turn off electrical equipment, including computers, televisions, and stereos.
- Stay off a hard-wired telephone. Lightning can enter through the telephone line and produce head and neck trauma, including cataracts and tympanic membrane disruption. Death can result.
- If you are caught out in the open and cannot seek shelter, attempt to move to lower ground such as a ravine or valley; stay away from any tall trees or objects that could result in a lightning strike splashing over to you; place insulating material between you and the ground (e.g., sleeping pad, rain parka, life jacket). A lightning strike is imminent if your hair stands on end, you see blue halos around objects, and hear high-pitched or crackling noises. If you cannot move away from the area immediately, crouch on the balls of your feet and tuck your head down to minimize the target size; do not lie on the ground or have hand contact with the ground.

Data from Auerbach, P. S., Donner, H. J., & Weiss, E. A. (2013). *Field guide to wilderness medicine* (4th ed.). St. Louis: Mosby.

Health Promotion and Maintenance

Injuries caused by lightning strike are highly preventable. Teach people to stay indoors during an electrical storm. Chart 9-6 lists common prevention strategies. For more information the Wilderness Medical Society (http://wms.org) also offers evidence-based practice guidelines for the prevention and treatment of lightning injuries (Davis et al., 2014).

❖ INTERPROFESSIONAL COLLABORATIVE CARE
◆ Assessment: Noticing

Both the cardiopulmonary and the central nervous systems are profoundly affected by lightning injuries. *The most lethal initial effect of massive electrical current discharge on the cardiopulmonary system is cardiac arrest.* Because cardiac cells are autorhythmic, an effective cardiac rhythm may return spontaneously. However, prolonged respiratory arrest from impairment of the medullary respiratory center can produce hypoxia and subsequently a second cardiac arrest. Therefore, when attempting to manage multiple victims of a lightning strike, provide care to those who are in cardiopulmonary arrest first. Initiate resuscitation measures with immediate airway and ventilatory management, chest compressions, and other appropriate life support interventions.

People who survive the immediate lightning strike may be treated in a less emergent fashion. However, these victims can have serious myocardial injury, which may be manifested by electrocardiogram (ECG) and myocardial perfusion abnormalities such as angina and dysrhythmias. The initial appearance of mottled skin and decreased-to-absent peripheral pulses usually arises from arterial vasospasm and typically resolves spontaneously in several hours.

Central nervous system (CNS) injury is common in lightning strike victims. A classic finding is an immediate but temporary paralysis, known as *keraunoparalysis*, that affects the lower limbs to a greater extent than the upper limbs. This condition usually resolves within hours, but the patient must be evaluated for spinal injury. Other signs and symptoms and complications resulting from lightning strikes include cataracts, tympanic membrane rupture, cerebral hemorrhage, depression, and post-traumatic stress disorder. Lightning strikes also cause skin burns. Most burns are superficial and heal without incident. Patients may have full-thickness burns, charring, and contact burns from overlying metal objects. A characteristic skin manifestation of lightning is the appearance of tree-like branching or ferning marks on the skin called Lichtenberg figures or keraunographic markings. These skin manifestations are not considered burns and are thought to be caused by the coagulation of blood cells in the capillaries.

◆ *Interventions: Responding*

First Aid/Prehospital Care. Because of lightning's powerful impact to the body, patients are at great risk for multi-system trauma. The full extent of injury may not be known until thorough monitoring and diagnostic evaluation can be performed in the hospital. Initial care includes spinal stabilization with priority attention to maintenance of an adequate airway, effective breathing, and circulation through standard basic and advanced life support measures. Cardiopulmonary resuscitation (CPR) is performed immediately when a person is in cardiac arrest. If cardiopulmonary or CNS injury is present, skin burns are *not* an initial priority. However, if time and resources permit, a sterile dressing may be applied to cover the sites. *Victims of lightning strike are not electrically charged; the rescuer is in no danger from physical contact.* Nonetheless, the storm can present a continued threat to everyone in the vicinity who lacks adequate shelter. Contrary to popular belief, lightning can and does strike in the same place more than once.

Hospital Care. Once in the acute care hospital setting, the focus of care is advanced life support management, including cardiac monitoring to detect cardiac dysrhythmias and a 12-lead ECG. The patient may require mechanical ventilation until spontaneous breathing returns. Collaborate with the health care team to perform a thorough physical and diagnostic evaluation to identify obvious and occult (hidden) traumatic injuries because the patient may have suffered a fall or blast effect during the strike. A computed tomography (CT) scan of the head may be performed to identify intracranial hemorrhage. A creatine kinase (CK) measurement may be requested to detect skeletal muscle damage resulting from the lightning strike. In severe cases, rhabdomyolysis (circulation of by-products of skeletal muscle destruction) can lead to renal failure. Burn wounds are assessed and treated according to standard burn care protocols. Tetanus prophylaxis is necessary for burns or any break in skin integrity. Some institutions transfer these victims to a burn center for follow-up management.

COLD-RELATED INJURIES

Two common cold-related injuries are hypothermia and frostbite. Both types of injury can be prevented by implementing protection from the cold. Teach patients at risk ways to prevent these injuries through methods to maintain thermoregulation, which can range from alterations in COMFORT to major systemic complications.

Health Promotion and Maintenance

When participating in cold-weather activities, clothing choices are critical to the prevention of hypothermia and frostbite. Teach the importance of wearing synthetic clothing because it moves moisture away from the body and dries fast. Cotton clothing, especially as an undergarment, holds moisture, becomes wet, and contributes to the development of hypothermia. It should be strictly avoided in a cold outdoor environment; this rule applies to gloves and socks as well. Wet socks and gloves promote frostbite in the toes and fingers. Wearing too many pairs of socks can decrease circulation and lead to frostbite.

Clothing should be layered so it can be easily added or removed as the temperature changes. The inner layers, such as polyester fleece, provide warmth and insulation. The purpose of the outer layer is to block the wind and provide moisture protection. This layer is best made of a windproof, waterproof, breathable fabric. A hat is an essential clothing item that significantly decreases body heat loss through the head. Face protection with a facemask should be used on particularly cold days when wind chill poses a risk. Sunscreen (minimum sun protection factor [SPF] 30) and sunglasses are also important to protect skin and eyes from the sun's harmful rays.

Teach people to keep water, extra clothing, blankets, and food in their car when driving in winter in case the vehicle becomes stranded. Maintaining personal fitness and conditioning is also an important consideration to prevent hypothermia and frostbite. People should not diet or restrict food or fluid intake when participating in winter outdoor activities. Malnutrition and dehydration contribute to cold-related illnesses and injuries. Finally, it is important for people to know their physical limits and to come in out of the cold when these limits have been reached.

HYPOTHERMIA

❖ *PATHOPHYSIOLOGY*

Hypothermia is a core body temperature below 95°F (35°C). Common predisposing conditions that promote hypothermia include:

- Cold-water immersion
- Acute illness (e.g., sepsis)
- Traumatic injury
- Shock states
- Immobilization
- Cold weather (especially for the homeless and people working outdoors)
- Advanced age
- Selected medications (e.g., phenothiazines, barbiturates)
- Alcohol intoxication and substance abuse
- Malnutrition
- Hypothyroidism

• Inadequate clothing or shelter (e.g., the homeless population)

An environmental temperature below 82°F (28°C) can produce impaired thermoregulation and hypothermia in any susceptible person. *Therefore people, especially older adults, are actually at risk on a year-round basis in most areas of the world.* Wind chill is a significant factor: heat loss increases as wind speed rises. Wet conditions further increase heat loss through evaporation. Weather is the most common cause of hypothermia for outdoor sports enthusiasts and for those with inadequate clothing or shelter. It is also a problem for the older adult, the homeless, and the poor who cannot afford heating.

❖ INTERPROFESSIONAL COLLABORATIVE CARE

◆ Assessment: Noticing

Hypothermia is commonly divided into three categories by severity: *mild* (90° to 95°F [32° to 35°C]); *moderate* (82.4° to 90°F [28° to 32°C]); and *severe* (below 82.4°F [28°C]). Treatment decisions are based on the severity of hypothermia. Chart 9-7 summarizes by category the common key features for the patient who is hypothermic.

◆ Interventions: Responding

First Aid/Prehospital Care. For treatment of *mild hypothermia,* the person needs to be sheltered from the cold environment, have all wet clothing removed, and undergo passive or active external rewarming. Passive methods involve applying warm clothing or blankets. Active methods incorporate heating blankets, warm packs, and convective air heaters or warmers to speed rewarming. If a heating blanket is used, monitor the patient's skin at least every 15 to 30 minutes to reduce the risk for burn injury.

In the case of mild, uncomplicated hypothermia as the only health problem, having the victim drink warm high-carbohydrate liquids that do not contain alcohol or caffeine can aid in rewarming. Alcohol is a peripheral vasodilator; both alcohol and caffeine are diuretics. These effects can potentially worsen dehydration and hypothermia.

Hospital Care. General management principles apply to both *moderate* and *severe* hypothermia. Protect patients from further heat loss and handle them gently to prevent ventricular fibrillation. Positioning the patient in the supine position prevents orthostatic changes in blood pressure from cardiovascular instability. Follow standard resuscitation efforts with special attention to maintenance of airway, breathing, and circulation as recommended by the American Heart Association (2015):

• Administer drugs with caution and/or spaced at longer intervals because metabolism is unpredictable in hypothermic conditions.
• Remember that drugs can accumulate without obvious therapeutic effect while the patient is cold but may become active and potentially lead to drug toxicity as effective rewarming is under way.
• Consider withholding IV drugs, except vasopressors, until the core temperature is above 86°F (30°C).
• Initiate CPR for patients without spontaneous circulation.
• For a hypothermic patient in ventricular fibrillation or pulseless ventricular tachycardia, one defibrillation attempt is appropriate. Be aware that defibrillation attempts may be ineffective until the core temperature is above 86°F (30°C).

Treatment of *moderate* hypothermia may involve both active external and core (internal) rewarming methods. Applying external heat with heating blankets can promote core temperature "after-drop" by producing peripheral vasodilation. **After-drop** is the continued decrease in core body temperature after the victim is removed from the cold environment; it is caused by the return of cold blood from the periphery to the central circulation. Therefore the patient's trunk should be actively rewarmed before the extremities. Core rewarming methods for moderate hypothermia include administration of warm IV fluids; heated oxygen or inspired gas to prevent further heat loss via the respiratory tract; and heated peritoneal, pleural, gastric, or bladder lavage.

▶▶ CHART 9-7   Key Features

Hypothermia

Mild
• Shivering
• Dysarthria (slurred speech)
• Decreased muscle coordination
• Impaired cognition ("mental slowness")
• Diuresis (caused by shunting of blood to major organs)

Moderate
• Muscle weakness
• Increased loss of coordination
• Acute confusion
• Apathy
• Incoherence
• Possible stupor
• Decreased clotting (caused by impaired platelet aggregation and thrombocytopenia)

Severe
• Bradycardia
• Severe hypotension
• Decreased respiratory rate
• Cardiac dysrhythmias, including possible ventricular fibrillation or asystole
• Decreased neurologic reflexes
• Decreased pain responsiveness
• Acid-base imbalance

❗ NURSING SAFETY PRIORITY QSEN

Critical Rescue

Recognize that patients who are *severely* hypothermic are at high risk for cardiac arrest. Respond by avoiding active *external* rewarming with heating devices because it is dangerous and contraindicated in this population due to rapid vasodilation.

The treatment of choice for *severe* hypothermia is to use *extracorporeal* rewarming methods such as cardiopulmonary bypass or hemodialysis. Cardiopulmonary bypass is the fastest core rewarming technique. However, this device is not available in all hospitals. It also requires specialized personnel and resources to operate it properly. Monitor for early signs of complications that can occur after rewarming such as fluid, electrolyte, and metabolic abnormalities; acute respiratory distress syndrome (ARDS); acute renal failure; and pneumonia.

A long-standing principle in the treatment of patients with hypothermic cardiac arrest is that "no one is dead until he or she is warm and dead." There is a factual basis to this statement when considering the number of survivors who have suffered a prolonged hypothermic cardiac arrest. Prolonged resuscitation efforts may not be reasonable in cases in which survival appears highly unlikely such as in an anoxic event followed by a hypothermic cardiac arrest.

FROSTBITE

❖ PATHOPHYSIOLOGY

Another significant cold-related injury that may or may not be associated with hypothermia is frostbite. The main risk factor is inadequate insulation against cold weather (i.e., either the skin is exposed to the cold, or the person's clothing offers insufficient protection, leading to injury). Wet clothing in particular is a poor insulator and facilitates the development of frostbite. Fatigue, dehydration, and poor nutrition are other contributing factors. People who smoke, consume alcohol, or have impaired peripheral circulation have a higher incidence of frostbite. Any previous history of frostbite further increases a person's susceptibility.

❓ NCLEX EXAMINATION CHALLENGE 9-2
Health Promotion and Maintenance

The community nurse is educating a client about frostbite prevention. Which factors will the nurse teach that are risk factors for developing frostbite? **Select all that apply.**
A. Dehydration
B. Smoking history
C. Previous frostbite
D. Excessive fatigue
E. Active smoker
F. Wearing wool socks
G. History of diabetes

❖ INTERPROFESSIONAL COLLABORATIVE CARE
◆ Assessment: Noticing

Frostbite occurs when body tissue freezes and causes damage to TISSUE INTEGRITY. Like burns, frostbite injuries can be superficial, partial, or full thickness. By contrast, **frostnip** is a type of superficial cold injury that may produce pain, numbness, and pallor or a waxy appearance of the affected area but is easily relieved by applying warmth; it does not cause tissue damage (impaired TISSUE INTEGRITY). Frostnip typically develops on skin areas such as the face, nose, finger, or toes. Untreated, it is a precursor to more severe forms of frostbite.

First-degree frostbite, the least severe type of frostbite, involves **hyperemia** (increased blood flow) of the involved area and edema formation. In *second-degree frostbite*, large clear-to-milky fluid-filled blisters develop with partial-thickness skin necrosis (Fig. 9-7). *Third-degree frostbite* appears as small blisters that

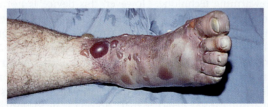

FIG. 9-7 Edema and blister formation 24 hours after frostbite injury occurring in an area covered by a tightly fitted boot. (From Auerbach, P. S. (2008). *Wilderness medicine* (5th ed.). Philadelphia: Mosby; courtesy Cameron Bangs, MD.)

contain dark fluid and an affected body part that is cool, numb, blue, or red and does not blanch. Full-thickness and subcutaneous tissue necrosis occurs and requires débridement. In *fourth-degree frostbite*, the most severe form, there are no blisters or edema; the part is numb, cold, and bloodless. The full-thickness necrosis extends into the muscle and bone. At this stage, gangrene develops, which may require amputation of the affected part. Of note, except for frostnip, other degrees of frostbite may all have the same general appearance while the body part is frozen; the differentiating features of each degree of frostbite only become apparent after the part is thawed. Gangrene may evolve over days to weeks after injury.

◆ Interventions: Responding

First Aid/Prehospital Care. Recognition of frostbite is essential to early, effective intervention and prevention of further damage to TISSUE INTEGRITY. Asking a partner to frequently observe for early signs of frostbite such as a white, waxy appearance to exposed skin, especially on the nose, cheeks, and ears is an effective strategy to identify the problem before it worsens. In people with dark skin, skin becomes paler, waxy, and somewhat gray. In this case the best remedy is to have the person seek shelter from the wind and cold and attend to the affected body part. Superficial frostbite is easily managed using body heat to warm the affected area. Teach patients to place their warm hands over the affected areas on their face or to place cold hands under the arms.

Hospital Care. Patients with more severe and deeper forms of frostbite need aggressive management. For all degrees of partial-thickness–to–full-thickness frostbite, rapid rewarming in a water bath at a temperature range of 104° to 108°F (40° to 42°C) is indicated to thaw the frozen part (Della-Giustina & Ingebretsen, 2013). Because patients experience severe pain during the rewarming process, this intervention is best accomplished in a medical facility; however, it may be done in another setting if no other options exist for prompt transport or rescue. Administer analgesics, especially IV opiates, and IV rehydration. Ibuprofen 400 mg to 800 mg PO should also be administered every 8 hours as it decreases thromboxane production in the inflammatory cascade and may reduce secondary tissue injury in frostbite (Auerbach, 2016b; Della-Giustina & Ingebretsen, 2013).

⚠ NURSING SAFETY PRIORITY [QSEN]
Critical Rescue

Recognize that dry heat or massage should not be used as part of the warming process for frostbitten areas because these actions can produce further damage to TISSUE INTEGRITY. Respond by using other interventions such as a rapid rewarming water bath of 104° to 108°F (40° to 42°C), to preserve tissue.

When the rewarming process is complete, handle the injured areas gently and elevate them above heart level if possible to decrease tissue edema. Sometimes splints are used to immobilize extremities during the healing process. Assess the person at least hourly for the development of compartment syndrome—a limb-threatening complication caused by severe neurovascular impairment. Observe for early manifestations, which include increasing alteration in levels of COMFORT (pain even after analgesics are given) and paresthesias (painful tingling and numbness). Compare the affected extremity with the unaffected one to assess for pallor. Assess for pulses and muscle weakness. Management of compartment syndrome is discussed in detail in Chapter 51.

Frostbite destroys tissue and produces a deep tetanus-prone wound; the patient should be immunized to prevent tetanus. Apply only loose, nonadherent sterile dressings to the damaged areas. Avoid compression of the injured tissues. Both topical and systemic antibiotics may be used. Once a patient's frozen part has thawed, do not allow it to refreeze, which worsens the injury.

In cases of severe, deep frostbite, débridement of necrotic tissue may be needed to evaluate tissue viability and provide wound management. Amputation may be indicated for patients with severe injuries or those who develop gangrene or severe compartment syndrome.

ALTITUDE-RELATED ILLNESSES

❖ PATHOPHYSIOLOGY

High-altitude illnesses, also known as **high-altitude disease (HAD)** or *altitude sickness,* cause pathophysiologic responses in the body as a result of exposure to low partial pressure of oxygen at high elevations. Although most consider high altitude to be an elevation over 5000 feet, millions of people worldwide who ascend to or live at altitudes above 2500 feet are at risk for acute and chronic mountain sickness.

As altitude increases, atmospheric (barometric) pressure decreases. Oxygen makes up 21% of the pressure. Therefore, as this pressure falls, the partial pressure of oxygen in the air decreases, resulting in less available oxygen to humans. The pathophysiologic consequence is hypoxia. Hypoxia is more pronounced as elevation increases. Elevations higher than 18,000 feet are extreme altitudes. Supplemental oxygen is necessary at these levels in nonacclimatized people to prevent altitude-related illnesses, including death, from occurring during abrupt ascent.

The cause of HAD is an interaction of environmental and genetic factors. Those who are obese or have chronic illnesses, especially cardiovascular problems, are more at risk than those who are thinner and healthier. Dehydration and CNS depressants such as alcohol also increase the risk. The age of the person does not seem to be a factor in altitude-related illnesses.

The process of adapting to high altitude is called *acclimatization.* **Acclimatization** involves physiologic changes that help the body adapt to less available oxygen in the atmosphere. As the carotid bodies sense a decline in PaO_2 at about 5000 feet, they increase the respiratory rate to improve oxygen delivery. This mechanism is called the *hypoxic-ventilatory response.* Increased respiratory rate causes **hypocapnia** (decreased carbon dioxide) and respiratory alkalosis, which limit further increases in respiratory rate. Rapid eye movement (REM) sleep is impaired. Hypoxia can occur from periods of apnea. Within 24 to 48 hours of being at high altitude, the kidneys excrete the excess bicarbonate, which helps the pH to return to normal and ventilatory rate to again increase.

Increased sympathetic nervous system activity increases heart rate, blood pressure, and cardiac output. Pulmonary artery pressure rises as an effect of generalized hypoxia-induced pulmonary vasoconstriction. Cerebral blood flow increases to

🧬 GENETIC/GENOMIC CONSIDERATIONS
Patient-Centered Care **QSEN**

Genetic differences among certain ethnic groups who live in high-altitude areas have been studied. For example, chronic mountain sickness is less common in Tibetans and Ethiopians than in Andeans (Ronen et al., 2014).

The pathogenesis of mountain sickness is associated with unidentified variations in hypoxia-related genes and the genes responsible for the human leukocyte antigen (HLA) system. Examples of genes with variants that may contribute to the development of HAD include:

- *EPO* (erythropoietin), which regulates red blood cell production
- *HIF1A* (hypoxia-inducible factor), which mediates the effects of hypoxia on body cells
- *EDN1* (endothelin), which causes vasoconstriction and thus increases blood pressure
- *NOS3* (endothelial nitric oxide synthase), which makes nitric acid in vascular tissue to maintain vessel tone and altitude adaptation

At this time, no clinical genetic testing to determine a person's risk for altitude sickness is available; however, further research is being conducted to identify specific gene variations that contribute to altitude-related illnesses.

maintain cerebral oxygen delivery. Hypoxia also induces red blood cell production by stimulating the release of erythropoietin. The result is an increase in red blood cells and hemoglobin concentration. Over time polycythemia can develop in people who remain in a high-altitude environment.

People who plan to climb to high altitudes are advised to ascend slowly, over the course of days or even weeks, depending on the degree of elevation. Ascending too rapidly is the primary cause of altitude-related illnesses. They are much more common in people who sleep at elevations above 8000 feet.

The three most common clinical conditions that are considered high-altitude illnesses are acute mountain sickness (AMS), high-altitude cerebral edema (HACE), and high-altitude pulmonary edema (HAPE). AMS may occur with HACE and/or HAPE; the underlying pathophysiology is hypoxia. Chronic mountain sickness can occur in people who live at high elevations. Although each syndrome has several unique manifestations, the basic assessment and management approach are the same.

❖ INTERPROFESSIONAL COLLABORATIVE CARE
◆ Assessment: Noticing

Assessment findings for the typical patient with AMS include reports of throbbing headache, anorexia, nausea, and vomiting. Feeling chilled, irritable, and apathetic is also associated with AMS. The syndrome produces effects similar to an alcohol-induced hangover. The patient may relate a feeling of extreme illness. Vital signs are variable: the patient can be tachycardic or bradycardic, have normal blood pressure, or have postural hypotension. He or she may experience dyspnea both on exertion and at rest. Exertional dyspnea is expected as a person adjusts to high altitude. However, dyspnea at rest is abnormal and may signal the onset of HAPE.

If AMS progresses to *high-altitude cerebral edema (HACE),* the extreme form of this disorder, the patient cannot perform ADLs and has extreme apathy. A key sign of HACE is the development of ataxia (defective muscular coordination). The patient also has a change in mental status with confusion and impaired judgment. Cranial nerve dysfunction and seizures may occur. If untreated, a further decline in the patient's level of consciousness results. Stupor, coma, and death can result from brain swelling and the subsequent damage caused by increased intracranial pressure over the course of 1 to 3 days.

High-altitude pulmonary edema (HAPE) often appears in conjunction with HACE but may occur during the progression of AMS within the first 2 to 4 days of a rapid ascent to high altitude, commonly on the second night. It is the most common cause of death associated with high altitude. Patients notice poor exercise tolerance and a prolonged recovery time after exertion. Fatigue, weakness, and other signs and symptoms of AMS are present. Important clinical indicators of HAPE include a persistent dry cough and cyanosis of the lips and nail beds. Tachycardia and tachypnea occur at rest. Crackles may be auscultated in one or both lungs. Pink, frothy sputum is a late sign of HAPE. A chest x-ray demonstrates pulmonary infiltrates and pulmonary edema. Arterial blood gas analysis shows respiratory alkalosis and hypoxemia (decreased oxygen). Pneumonia also may be present. Pulmonary artery pressure is usually very elevated because of pulmonary edema.

◆ **Interventions: Responding**

First Aid/Prehospital Care. The most important intervention to manage serious altitude-related illnesses is descent to a lower altitude. Patients must be monitored carefully for any evidence of symptom progression. With mild AMS, the victim should be allowed to rest and acclimate at the current altitude. The person is instructed not to ascend to a higher altitude, especially for sleep, until symptoms lessen. If symptoms persist or worsen, he or she should be moved to a lower altitude as soon as possible. Even a descent of about 1600 feet may improve the patient's condition and reverse altitude-related pathologic effects. Oxygen should also be administered if available to effectively treat symptoms of AMS.

Prevention and Treatment. The oral drug *acetazolamide* (Diamox, Apo-Acetazolamide ✦) is commonly used to both prevent and treat AMS. Acetazolamide is a carbonic anhydrase inhibitor. It acts by causing a bicarbonate diuresis, which rids the body of excess fluid and induces metabolic acidosis. The acidotic state increases respiratory rate and decreases the occurrence of periodic respiration during sleep at night. In this way it helps patients acclimate faster to a high altitude. For best results, the drug should be taken 24 hours before ascent and be continued for the first 2 days of the trip.

! NURSING SAFETY PRIORITY QSEN

Drug Alert

Because acetazolamide is a sulfa drug, ask about an allergy to sulfa before the patient takes the drug because it may cause hypersensitivity reactions in those who are sulfa sensitive.

Another drug that is indicated in the treatment of moderate-to-severe AMS is dexamethasone (Decadron). The mechanism of action of this drug is unclear for AMS treatment, but it reduces cerebral edema by acting as an anti-inflammatory in the CNS. It does not speed acclimatization like acetazolamide does, but it does relieve the symptoms of AMS. Symptoms may recur when the drug is stopped, an effect termed the *rebound phenomenon*.

For the treatment of HACE, early recognition of ataxia or a change in level of consciousness should prompt a rapid descent by rescuers or companions to a lower altitude. While undergoing descent, the patient can be given supplemental oxygen and dexamethasone. If mental status is severely impaired and the patient's airway is at risk, all drugs should be given parenterally. Ultimately the patient with HACE must be admitted to the hospital. Critical care management may be necessary.

Like HACE, early recognition of HAPE is essential to improve the patient's chance for survival. Phosphodiesterase inhibitors such as tadalafil (Cialis) and sildenafil (Viagra) may be used to prevent HAPE because of their pulmonary vasodilatory effects. When it occurs, HAPE is a serious condition that requires quick evacuation to a lower altitude, oxygen administration, and bedrest to save the patient's life. If descent must be delayed because of weather conditions or other factors, oxygen administration as soon as possible is essential. Keep the patient warm at all times. Drugs are not substitutes for descent and oxygen. However, the treatment of HAPE may include the calcium channel blocker *nifedipine* (Procardia, Adalat ✦, Apo-Nifed ✦) to decrease pulmonary vascular resistance. Hospital admission is required. In uncomplicated cases of HAPE recovery occurs quickly, but effects such as weakness and fatigue may persist for 2 weeks.

Chart 9-8 summarizes best practices for preventing, recognizing, and treating altitude-related illnesses.

? NCLEX EXAMINATION CHALLENGE 9-3

Physiological Integrity

The nurse is caring for a client who was brought to the emergency department after being found very ill on a mountain climb. Which assessment findings does the nurse recognize as symptoms of high-altitude pulmonary edema (HAPE)? **Select all that apply.**
A. Respiratory acidosis
B. Cyanosis of the lips
C. Tachycardia at rest
D. Bilateral crackles
E. Persistent dry cough

◎ CHART 9-8 Best Practice for Patient Safety & Quality Care QSEN

Preventing, Recognizing, and Treating Altitude-Related Illnesses

- Plan a slow ascent to allow for acclimatization.
- Learn to recognize signs and symptoms of altitude-related illnesses.
- Avoid overexertion and overexposure to cold; rest at present altitude before ascending further.
- Ensure adequate hydration and nutrition.
- Avoid alcohol and sleeping pills when at high altitude.
- For progressive or advanced acute mountain sickness (AMS), recognize symptoms and implement an immediate descent; provide oxygen at high concentration.
- To prevent the occurrence of AMS, discuss the use of acetazolamide (Diamox) and other agents as indicated with your health care provider.
- Protect skin and eyes from the harmful ultraviolet rays of the sun at high altitude. Wear sunscreen (at least SPF 30) and high-quality wraparound sunglasses or goggles.

SPF, Sun protection factor.

DROWNING

❖ PATHOPHYSIOLOGY

Drowning is a leading cause of accidental death in the United States. It occurs when a person suffers primary respiratory impairment from submersion or immersion in a liquid medium (usually water). Near-drowning was previously defined as recovery after submersion; however, this term is no longer used because language that describes drowning incidents has been standardized. Today the drowning process is considered a continuum with outcomes that range from survival to death.

Health Promotion and Maintenance

Prevention is the key to avoiding drowning incidents. When providing health teaching, include these points:

- Constantly observe people who cannot swim and are in or around water.
- Do not swim alone.
- Test the water depth before diving in head first; never dive into shallow water.
- Avoid alcoholic beverages when swimming and boating and while in proximity to water.
- Ensure that water rescue equipment such as life jackets, flotation devices, and rope is immediately available when around water.

❖ INTERPROFESSIONAL COLLABORATIVE CARE

◆ Assessment: Noticing

When water is aspirated into the lungs, the quantity and makeup of the water are key factors in the pathophysiology of the drowning event. Aspiration of both fresh water and salt water causes surfactant to wash out of the lungs. Surfactant reduces surface tension within the alveoli, increases lung compliance and alveolar radius, and decreases the work of breathing. Loss of surfactant destabilizes the alveoli and leads to increased airway resistance. Salt water—a hypertonic fluid—also creates an osmotic gradient that draws protein-rich fluid from the vascular space into the alveoli. In both cases, pulmonary edema results. Salt water and fresh water aspiration cause similar degrees of lung injury. Another concern is water quality; the victim's outcome may be negatively affected by contaminants in the water such as chemicals, algae, microbes, sand, and mud. These substances can worsen lung injury and cause a lung infection.

The duration and severity of hypoxia are the two most important factors that determine outcomes for victims of drowning. Very cold water seems to have a protective effect. Successful resuscitations have been reported even after prolonged arrest intervals. Hypothermia might offer some protection to the hypoxic brain by reducing cerebral metabolic rate. The diving reflex is a physiologic response to asphyxia, which produces bradycardia; a reduction in cardiac output; and vasoconstriction of vessels in the intestine, skeletal muscles, and kidneys. These physiologic effects are thought to reduce myocardial oxygen use and enhance blood flow to the heart and cerebral tissues. Survival may be linked to some combination of the effects of hypothermia and the diving reflex.

The cause of the drowning should also be determined if possible. The patient may have suffered a medical condition or injury that caused the drowning event such as a seizure, myocardial infarction, stroke, or spinal cord injury while in the water. Injuries sustained from diving into shallow water or body surfing, such as cervical spine trauma, can also increase the difficulty of rescue and resuscitation efforts.

◆ Interventions: Responding

First Aid/Emergency Care. Immediate emergency care focuses on a safe rescue of the victim. Potential rescuers must consider their own swimming abilities and limitations and any natural or human-made hazards before attempting to save the victim; failure to do so could place additional lives in jeopardy. *Once rescuers gain access to the victim, the priority is safe removal from the water.* Spine stabilization with a board or flotation device should be considered only for victims who are at high risk for spine trauma (e.g., history of diving, use of a water slide, signs of injury or alcohol intoxication), as opposed to all drowning victims. Time is of the essence; efforts directed toward a rapid rescue have the most potential benefit. Initiate airway clearance and ventilatory support measures, including delivering rescue breaths as soon as possible while the patient is still in the water. If hypothermia is a concern, handle the victim gently to prevent ventricular fibrillation.

! NURSING SAFETY PRIORITY QSEN

Critical Rescue

Recognize that you must not attempt to get the water out of the victim's lungs; respond by delivering abdominal or chest thrusts *only* if airway obstruction is suspected.

Hospital Care. Once the person is safely removed from the water, airway and cardiopulmonary support interventions begin, including oxygen administration, endotracheal intubation, CPR, and defibrillation, if necessary. In the clinical setting, gastric decompression with a nasogastric or orogastric tube is needed to prevent aspiration of gastric contents and improve ventilatory function. After a period of artificial ventilation by mask, the victim typically has a distended abdomen, which impairs movement of the diaphragm and decreases lung ventilation. Patients who experience drowning require complex care to support their major body systems. The full spectrum of critical care technology may be needed to manage the pathophysiologic complications of drowning, including pulmonary edema, infection, acute respiratory distress syndrome (ARDS), and CNS impairment. These complications are discussed elsewhere in this text.

? CLINICAL JUDGMENT CHALLENGE 9-2

Patient-Centered Care QSEN

The emergency department (ED) nurse is caring for a patient who is a drowning victim. The patient has cold, blue skin and significant abdominal swelling.

1. What further information will the nurse need to obtain from the paramedics who bring the client to the ED?
2. How does the nurse explain the major pathophysiologic event of drowning to the patient's significant other?
3. The paramedics state that the patient was submerged in saltwater from the ocean. How does that environment affect the patient?
4. What should the nurse know about a patient's potential cervical spine injury as it pertains to drowning?

GET READY FOR THE NCLEX® EXAMINATION!

▌ KEY POINTS

Review these Key Points for each NCLEX Examination Client Needs Category.

Safe and Effective Care Environment
- Collaborate with the interprofessional health care team to provide the most comprehensive care for patients with environment emergencies. **QSEN: Teamwork and Collaboration**

Health Promotion and Maintenance
- Teach people how to prevent heat-related illnesses as outlined in Chart 9-1, cold-related conditions, and bites and stings as described in Charts 9-4 and 9-5.
- Teach people that the best way to prevent lightning injury is to avoid places where lightning is likely to strike (see Chart 9-6).
- Teach people that hypothermia and frostbite can be prevented by selecting appropriate layered clothing; cotton should not be worn.

Physiological Integrity
- Remember that bites, stings, lightning injury, and cold injury can compromise TISSUE INTEGRITY. **QSEN: Safety**
- Recall that the priority for first aid for heat stroke after a patent airway is established is to cool the patient as quickly as possible (see Chart 9-3). **QSEN: Safety**
- Recall that the management of a patient who has a snakebite depends on the severity of envenomation (venom injection) (see Table 9-1).

- Remember that the priority for first aid/prehospital care when a patient has a poisonous snakebite is to decrease the venom circulation by administering antivenom drugs. **QSEN: Safety**
- Remember that cold applications, such as ice, should be used as first aid/prehospital care for poisonous spider bites.
- Understand that the effect of the bark scorpion venom is neurotoxic; monitor the patient for signs of respiratory failure that may require mechanical ventilation. **QSEN: Safety**
- Remember that epinephrine is the drug of choice for bee and wasp sting allergic reactions, followed by antihistamine drugs. **QSEN: Safety**
- Recall that lightning causes central nervous system, cardiovascular complications, and skin burns.
- Teach patients that in moderate-to-severe cases of hypothermia, coagulopathy (abnormal clotting) or cardiac failure can occur.
- Remember that the priority for care of a patient with a cold injury is warming; alcohol should be avoided.
- Review Chart 9-8, which outlines best practice strategies for preventing, recognizing, and treating altitude-related illnesses.
- Remember that drowning victims often require cardiopulmonary support, including CPR, and are at risk for pulmonary infection, ARDS, and central nervous system impairment.

SELECTED BIBLIOGRAPHY

Asterisk indicates a classic or definitive work on this subject.

*American Heart Association. (2015). *Advanced cardiovascular life support provider manual*. Dallas: Author.

Audet, G., Quinn, C., & Leon, L. (2015). Point-of-care cardiac troponin test accurately predicts heat stroke severity in rats. *American journal of physiology. Regulatory, integrative and comparative physiology*, *309*(10), R1264–R1272.

*Auerbach, P. S. (2016a). *Wilderness medicine* (6th ed.). Philadelphia: Mosby.

Auerbach, P. S. (2016b). *Medicine for the outdoors: The essential guide to first aid and medical emergencies* (6th ed.). Philadelphia: Elsevier.

*Auerbach, P. S., Donner, H. J., & Weiss, E. A. (2013). *Field guide to wilderness medicine* (4th ed.). St. Louis: Mosby.

Davis, C., Engeln, A., Johnson, E., McIntosh, S. E., Zafren, K., Islas, A. A., et al. (2014). Wilderness Medical Society practice guidelines for the prevention and treatment of lightning injuries: 2014 update. *Wilderness & environmental medicine*, *25*(4), S86–S95.

Della-Giustina, D., & Ingebretsen, R. (Eds.), (2013). *Advanced wilderness life support* (8th ed.). Utah: AdventureMed.

Norris, R. L. (2015). *Coral snake envenomation*, http://emedicine.medscape.com/article/771701-overview.

Ronen, R., Zhou, D., Bafna, V., & Haddad, C. (2014). The genetic basis of chronic mountain sickness. *Physiology*, *29*(6), 403–412. doi:10.1152/physiol.00008.2014.

CHAPTER 10

Principles of Emergency and Disaster Preparedness

Linda Laskowski-Jones

 http://evolve.elsevier.com/Iggy/

PRIORITY AND INTERRELATED CONCEPTS

The priority concepts for this chapter are:
- SAFETY
- TEAMWORK AND INTERPROFESSIONAL COLLABORATION
- COMMUNICATION

LEARNING OUTCOMES

Safe and Effective Care Environment

1. Apply triage principles to prioritize care delivery in a disaster situation.
2. Identify the roles of the nurse and interprofessional team in emergency preparedness and response.
3. Describe components of an emergency preparedness and response plan.
4. Develop a personal emergency preparedness plan.

Psychosocial Integrity

5. Describe the role of the nurse in supporting people in various stages of adaptation who are coping with life changes after disaster.

Physiological Integrity

6. Explain ways to maintain physical SAFETY when responding to disaster and mass casualty situations.

Defined as an event in which illness or injuries exceed resource capabilities of a health care facility or community because of destruction and devastation, a **disaster** can be either *internal* to a health care facility or *external* from situations that create casualties in the community. Both internal and external disasters can occur simultaneously, such as when Superstorm Sandy incapacitated several hospitals on the Atlantic Coast of New York and New Jersey in late October 2012 (Fig. 10-1).

TYPES OF DISASTERS

An event occurring inside a health care facility or campus that could endanger the SAFETY of patients or staff is considered to be an *internal* disaster. The event creates a need for evacuation or relocation. It often requires extra personnel and the activation of the facility's emergency preparedness and response plan (also called an *emergency management plan*). Examples of potential internal disasters include fire, explosion, loss of critical utilities (e.g., electricity, water, computer systems, and COMMUNICATION capabilities), and violence. Each health care organization develops policies and procedures for preventing these events through organized facility and security management plans. The most important outcome for any internal disaster is to maintain patient, staff, and visitor safety.

An event outside the health care facility or campus, somewhere in the community, which requires the activation of the facility's emergency management plan is considered an *external* disaster. The number of facility staff and resources may not be adequate for the incoming emergency department (ED) patients. External disasters can be either natural such as a hurricane, earthquake, or tornado, or technologic such as an act of terrorism with explosive devices or a malfunction of a nuclear reactor with radiation exposure. Recent external disasters include the 2015 Ebola virus crisis in a Dallas hospital, the 2013 Boston Marathon bombing, and the West Texas fertilizer plant explosion. St. John's Regional Medical Center in Joplin, Missouri, had an internal disaster compounding an external disaster in 2011 when it was directly hit by an EF-5 tornado that destroyed a large part of the town. Of the 142 dead, 6 people inside the hospital died (Letner, 2011).

Internal and external disasters can result in many casualties, including death. Multi-casualty and mass casualty (disaster) events are not the same. The main difference is based on the scope and scale of the incident, considering the number and severity of victims or casualties involved. Both require specific response plans to activate necessary resources. In general, a **multi-casualty event** can be managed by a hospital using local resources; a **mass casualty event** overwhelms local medical capabilities and may require the collaboration of multiple agencies and health care facilities to handle the crisis. State, regional, and/or national resources may be needed to support the areas affected by the event. Trauma centers have a special role in all

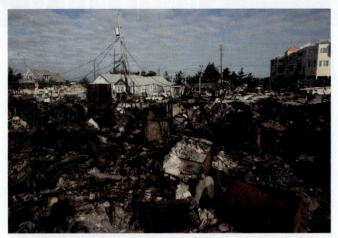

FIG. 10-1 The destruction after Superstorm Sandy ravaged the East Coast in 2012. (Copyright © The American National Red Cross 2012.)

CHART 10-1   Best Practice for Patient Safety & Quality Care QSEN

Nurse's Role in Responding to Health Care Facility Fires

- Remove any patient or staff from immediate danger of the fire or smoke.
- Discontinue oxygen for all patients who can breathe without it.
- For patients on life support, maintain their respiratory status manually until removed from the fire area.
- Direct ambulatory patients to walk to a safe location.
- If possible, ask ambulatory patients to help push wheelchair patients out of danger.
- Move bedridden patients from the fire area in bed, by stretcher, or in a wheelchair; if needed, have one or two staff members move patients on blankets or carry them.
- After everyone is out of danger, seek to contain the fire by closing doors and windows and using an ABC extinguisher (can put out any type of fire) if possible.
- Do not risk injury to yourself or staff members while moving patients or attempting to extinguish the fire.

emergency preparedness activities because they provide a critical level of expertise and specialized resources for complex injury management.

To maintain ongoing disaster preparedness, hospital personnel participate in emergency training and drills regularly. In the United States, The Joint Commission (2017) mandates that hospitals have an emergency preparedness plan that is tested through drills or actual participation in a real event at least twice a year. One of the drills or events must involve community-wide resources and an influx of actual or simulated patients to assess the ability of collaborative efforts and command structures. In addition, accredited health care organizations are required to take an "all-hazards approach" to disaster planning. Using this approach, preparedness activities must address *all credible threats* to the safety of the community that could result in a disaster situation. Disaster drills are ideally planned based on a risk assessment or vulnerability analysis that identifies the events most likely to occur in a particular community. For example, a flood is more likely in the Gulf of Mexico, and an avalanche is more likely in ski areas of the Rocky Mountains. Unfortunately, since the threat of gun violence is now a risk in all communities, "active-shooter" drills are commonplace in health care settings. It is essential that staff actively participate in these drills and take them seriously to enable their ability to act rapidly and maintain their ongoing competency. The importance of training has been emphasized in the wake of many disaster responses and has been credited with saving lives.

Hospitals are not the only health care agencies that are required to practice disaster drills. Nursing homes and other long-term care (LTC) facilities are also mandated to have annual drills to prepare for mass casualty events. Part of the response plan must include a method for evacuation of residents from the facility in a timely and safe manner.

An evacuation plan is also part of fire prevention and preparedness plans for health care facilities. The Life Safety Code® published by the National Fire Protection Association (2016) provides guidelines for building construction, design, maintenance, and evacuation. The Centers for Medicare and Medicaid Services (CMS) (2016) requires every health care facility to practice at least one fire drill or actual fire response once a year. Patient evacuation is not required if the event is a

drill. All facility personnel are mandated to have training on fire prevention and responsiveness each year. Chart 10-1 lists general guidelines for fire responsiveness and building evacuation to ensure safety.

IMPACT OF EXTERNAL DISASTERS

The events of September 11, 2001, substantially changed hospital and community disaster planning efforts. With the shocking terrorist attacks on the Twin Towers of the World Trade Center and the Pentagon, the loss of life in a field in Pennsylvania, and the actual and perceived threat of domestic terrorism, including the anthrax exposure that followed, hospital emergency preparedness concepts became integrated into the daily operations of emergency departments (EDs) by necessity. Weapons of mass destruction (WMDs) became a focus of public health risk.

The term "NBC" was coined to describe **n**uclear, **b**iologic, and **c**hemical threats. In response, emergency medical services (EMS) agencies and hospitals improved SAFETY by upgrading their decontamination facilities, equipment, and all levels of personal protective equipment to better protect staff. ED physician and nursing staff now routinely undergo hazardous materials (HAZMAT) training and learn how to recognize patterns of illness in patients who present for treatment that potentially indicate biologic terrorism agents such as anthrax or smallpox (Fig. 10-2). Protocols for the pharmacologic treatment of infectious disease agents and stockpiles of antibiotics and nerve agent antidotes are readily available.

The most immediate outcome of improving emergency preparedness after September 11, 2001, is that the ability to competently handle the more typical multi-casualty or mass casualty event such as a bus crash, tornado, chemical plant incident, or building collapse has been greatly improved in many communities. However, disaster situations can still exceed the scope of usual day-to-day crisis operations, pointing to the necessity of well-defined personal, facility, regional and national emergency preparedness plans, and ongoing drills. Research continues to call for nurses to be leaders in disaster preparedness and response (Veenema et al., 2016).

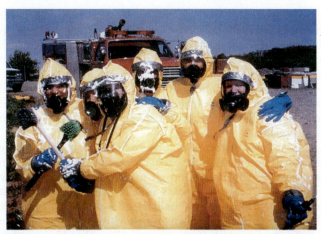

FIG. 10-2 Hazardous materials (HAZMAT) training to decontaminate people exposed to toxic agents in an outdoor decontamination area. (Courtesy Meg Blair, PhD, RN.)

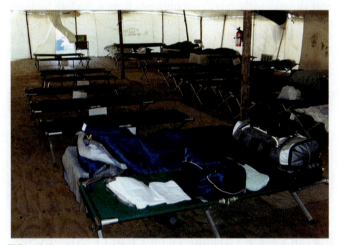

FIG. 10-3 Temporary shelter set up for homeless victims of Hurricane Katrina in New Orleans. (Courtesy Jeanne McConnell, MSN, RN.)

In 2005 Hurricane Katrina made landfall in Louisiana and other Gulf states as a category 4 storm and caused more than 1000 deaths and devastating environmental and property damage. Volunteers from all over the United States and local, regional, and federal agencies took part in the large-scale disaster evacuation, rescue, and relief effort that severely challenged available resources and established disaster plans. Critical systems failed and were eventually re-established through TEAMWORK AND INTERPROFESSIONAL COLLABORATION with multiple agencies to ensure that the most basic human needs were met (Fig. 10-3). Hurricane Katrina overwhelmed the existing emergency care system and caused the mobilization of a national mutual aid response on a level that had not been experienced in recent U.S. history.

Health care facilities must proactively address structural changes to provide SAFETY and protection from flooding and utilities failures. Although Superstorm Sandy, the event that made landfall in New York City in October 2012, was downgraded from a category 1 hurricane, the flooding that occurred destroyed critical hospital equipment, including emergency power generators, in the lower levels of several health care facilities, causing the loss of utilities and crippling operations. Hospitals that were severely impacted had to evacuate patients to other facilities, many of which were already overwhelmed by an influx of patients from the storm's damage in the community. Staff worked for several days in harsh conditions, carrying glow sticks and flashlights and wearing headlamps while evacuating critical patients via stairwells since elevators were nonfunctional.

Lessons learned from Hurricane Katrina, Superstorm Sandy, earthquakes in Japan and Haiti, tsunamis, and terrorist attacks, prompt improved facility design, staff preparation, and coordination of efforts that are beneficial for future disasters. These insights also can be applied to health care facility and community agency plans for pandemic infections, including influenza.

A **pandemic** (an infection or disease that occurs throughout the population of a country or the world) leads a vast number of people to seek medical care, even the "worried well." Although not yet ill, the "worried well" want evaluation, preventive treatment, or reassurance from a health care provider. The most recent global biologic threat is the Ebola virus disease outbreak that devastated West Africa in 2014 and 2015. The extremely high risk of contagion from blood and body fluids, and the deadly nature of the virus itself, prompted public health agencies and health facilities worldwide to initiate screening criteria for returning travelers from West Africa and facility-specific procedures to prevent exposure. These involved procuring effective personal protective equipment (PPE), teaching staff how to don and doff the PPE without self-contamination, and securing appropriate facilities and resources to isolate patients who are undergoing evaluation or treatment. Managing health care workers' fear of caring for these patients can pose ethical and leadership challenges that must be addressed through safety measures to protect staff, focused education, and utilization of evidence-based care standards (Casey, 2015).

Pandemic influenza outbreaks such as the 2009-2010 swine flu outbreak caused by the H1N1 virus raise significant concerns that the resource capabilities of the entire health care system could be overwhelmed and that community systems and critical supply chains could be severely damaged. Worker illness, absenteeism, and personal choices to remain quarantined to avoid being exposed to the illness negatively affect the number of health care staff available to care for patients. Because of the mass casualty nature of pandemic influenza, emergency preparedness planners must collaborate to incorporate strategies for handling an influx of ill patients into the system as part of ongoing disaster readiness. Quarantine of selected nursing units or the entire hospital could become necessary, prompting closure until the risk has passed.

Common to all mass casualty events, the goal of **emergency preparedness** is to effectively meet the extraordinary need for resources such as hospital beds, staff, drugs, PPE, supplies, and medical devices such as mechanical ventilators. The U.S. government stockpiles critical equipment and supplies in case they are needed for a pandemic influenza outbreak and organizes large-scale vaccination programs (see Chapter 23 for more information on emerging infections). Each state has its own specific emergency preparedness plan for pandemic influenza, including who would receive vaccines in a mass casualty event.

EMERGENCY PREPAREDNESS AND RESPONSE

Mass Casualty Triage

Bystanders will always be first on the scene of a disaster. Resources such as the Department of Homeland Security's

TABLE 10-1   Comparison of Triage Under Usual Versus Mass Casualty Conditions

TRIAGE UNDER USUAL CONDITIONS	TRIAGE UNDER MASS CASUALTY CONDITIONS
Emergent (immediate threat to life)	Emergent or class I (red tag) (immediate threat to life)
Urgent (major injuries that require immediate treatment)	Urgent or class II (yellow tag) (major injuries that require treatment)
Nonurgent (minor injuries that do not require immediate treatment)	Nonurgent or class III (green tag) (minor injuries that do not require immediate treatment)
Does not apply	Expectant or class IV (black tag) (expected and allowed to die)

(2016) "Stop the Bleed" can be helpful teaching tools so individuals know what to do before professional emergency services arrive. A key process in any multi-casualty or mass casualty response is effective **triage** to rapidly sort ill or injured patients into priority categories based on their acuity and survival potential.

Triage functions may be performed by EMS providers in the field such as:

- Emergency medical technicians (EMTs) and paramedics
- Nurse and physician field teams who are called from the hospital to a disaster scene to assist EMS providers
- Nurse and physician hospital teams to assess and reassess incoming patients

Triage concepts in a mass casualty incident differ from the "civilian triage" methods discussed in Chapter 8 that are practiced during usual emergency operations (Table 10-1). Although disaster triage practices can vary widely based on local EMS protocols, some concepts are fairly universal. Most mass casualty response teams in the field (at the disaster site) and in the hospital setting use a **disaster triage tag system** that categorizes triage priority by color and number:

- Emergent (class I) patients are identified with a red tag.
- Patients who can wait a short time for care (class II) are marked with a yellow tag.
- Nonurgent or "walking wounded" (class III) patients are given a green tag.
- Patients who are expected (and allowed) to die or are dead are issued a black tag (class IV).

! NURSING SAFETY PRIORITY **QSEN**

Action Alert

In mass casualty or disaster situations, implement a military form of triage with the overall desired outcome of doing the greatest good for the greatest number of people. This means that patients who are critically ill or injured and might otherwise receive attempted resuscitation during usual operations may be triaged into an "expectant" or "black-tagged" category and allowed to die or not be treated until others received care.

Typical examples of *black-tagged* patients are those with massive head trauma, extensive full-thickness body burns, and high cervical spinal cord injury requiring mechanical ventilation. The rationale for this very difficult decision is that limited resources must be dedicated to saving the most lives rather than expending valuable resources to save one life at the possible expense of many others.

In general, *red-tagged* patients have immediate threats to life such as airway obstruction or shock, and they require immediate attention. *Yellow-tagged* patients have major injuries such as open fractures with a distal pulse and large wounds that need treatment within 30 minutes to 2 hours. *Green-tagged* patients have minor injuries that can be managed in a delayed fashion, generally more than 2 hours. Examples of green-tagged injuries include closed fractures, sprains, strains, abrasions, and contusions.

Green-tagged patients are often referred to as the "walking wounded" because they may actually evacuate themselves from the mass casualty scene and go to the hospital in a private vehicle. Green-tagged patients usually make up the greatest number in most large-scale multi-casualty situations. Therefore they can overwhelm the system if provisions are not made to handle them as part of the disaster plan. Also, because they often come to the hospital on their own, the hospital may not be able to determine how many actual casualties will arrive. A related concern is that green-tagged patients who self-transport may unknowingly carry contaminants from a nuclear, biologic, or chemical incident into the hospital environment with potentially disastrous consequences. ED staff must anticipate these issues and collaborate to devise emergency response plans accordingly, including appropriate decontamination measures.

⊕ CULTURAL/SPIRITUAL CONSIDERATIONS

Patient-Centered Care **QSEN**

As a component of culturally competent care, disaster triage processes should also incorporate strategies to accommodate vulnerable patient populations such as the very young, the elderly, people with disabilities, the mentally ill, and those who require devices such as a mechanical ventilator or home oxygen (Danna & Bennett, 2013).

? NCLEX EXAMINATION CHALLENGE 10-1

Physiological Integrity

After a mass casualty event, the nurse is triaging clients in the field. Which client is correctly classified?
A. 38-year-old with an open femur fracture: black tag
B. 42-year-old with multiple abrasions and contusions: yellow tag
C. 54-year-old with third-degree burns over 90% of the body: green tag
D. 61-year-old who is having difficulty breathing and wheezing: red tag

Once patients are in the triage area of the hospital, they typically receive a special bracelet with a disaster number. Preprinted labels with this number can be applied to chart forms and personal belongings. Digital photos may be used as part of the identification process in some systems. The standard hospital registration process and identification band can be applied after the patient's identity is confirmed.

Automated tracking systems using infrared and radiofrequency technology (RFT) are available in some EDs to track a patient's triage priority on arrival, location, and process of care. The interactions the patient has with caregivers can also be tracked. This is an important SAFETY strategy if the patient is later found to have contaminants or a disease that could pose a risk to staff members who had close contact and require decontamination or prophylaxis (Laskowski-Jones, 2008). These systems are valuable components of the hospital's emergency preparedness infrastructure because they can rapidly portray the overall census and acuity of patients. They also enable ED leaders to determine how many casualties of a particular acuity level a hospital can safely accept from the incident scene.

Notification and Activation of Emergency Preparedness/ Management Plans

When the number of casualties exceeds the usual resource capabilities, a disaster situation exists. What may be considered a routine day in the ED of a large urban trauma center could be defined as a disaster for a small rural community hospital if the same number of patients arrived. Therefore each facility decides when criteria are met to declare a disaster. Flexibility is needed because resources may change by time of day and by day of the week. For example, hospitals typically have the fewest staff available after midnight on the weekend. An incident that occurs in this time frame may require activation of the emergency preparedness plan to bring extra resources into the hospital. The same incident during weekday business hours might be handled with on-site personnel alone without the need for activation of the plan.

Notification that a multi-casualty or mass casualty situation exists usually occurs by radio, cellular, or electronic COMMUNICATION between the ED and EMS providers at the scene. A state or regional emergency management agency may also notify the ED of the event. Each hospital has its own policy that specifies *who* has the authority to activate and *how* to activate the disaster or emergency preparedness plan. Group paging systems, telephone trees, and instant computer-based automated alert messages are the most common means of notifying essential personnel of a mass casualty incident or disaster.

A catastrophic event such as a major earthquake or tornado, or a terrorist incident involving weapons of mass destruction (WMDs), also requires the TEAMWORK AND INTERPROFESSIONAL COLLABORATION of volunteers from all members of the health care team in the region. The media may be contacted to facilitate COMMUNICATION by broadcasting messages to the health care community-at-large via television, radio, or social media (Woo et al, 2015). For such incidents, the National Guard, the American Red Cross, the public health department, various military units, a Medical Reserve Corps (MRC), or a Disaster Medical Assistance Team (DMAT) can be activated by state and federal government authorities.

- An MRC is made up of a group of volunteer medical and public health care professionals, including physicians and nurses. They offer their services to health care facilities or to the community in a supportive or supplemental capacity during times of need such as a disaster or pandemic disease outbreak. This group may help staff hospitals or community health settings that face personnel shortages and establish first aid stations or special-needs shelters. As a means to alleviate ED and hospital overcrowding, the MRC may also set up an acute care center (ACC) in the community for patients who need acute care (but not intensive care) for days to weeks.
- A DMAT is a medical relief team made up of civilian medical, paraprofessional, and support personnel that is deployed to a disaster area with enough medical equipment and supplies to sustain operations for 72 hours (U.S. Department of Health & Human Services, 2015). DMATs are part of the National Disaster Medical System (NDMS) in the United States. They provide relief services ranging from primary health care and triage to evacuation and staffing to assist health care facilities that have become overwhelmed with casualties. *Because licensed health care providers such as nurses act as federal employees when they are deployed, their professional licenses are recognized and valid in all states.* Additional examples of services provided by the NDMS include:

- Disaster Mortuary Operational Response Teams (DMORTs) to manage mass fatalities
- National Veterinary Response Teams (NVRTs) for emergency animal care; and
- International Medical Surgical Response Teams (IMSURTs) to establish fully functional field surgical facilities wherever they are needed in the world

Nurses can join these teams, complete the required training, and offer their expertise as part of a coordinated federal response team in times of critical need (U.S. Department of Health & Human Services, 2016).

Before going to the incident in the field, all members of the interprofessional team must have adequate training to prepare them to recognize the risks in an unstable environment (Laskowski-Jones, 2010; Yin et al., 2012). Such risks can include the potential for structural collapse, becoming the secondary target of a terrorist attack, interpersonal violence in unsecured locales, and working in an environment in which contagious diseases and natural hazards are possible (e.g., poisonous snake bites and mosquito-borne illnesses). Disaster workers must take measures such as obtaining prophylactic medications and vaccinations, having a personal evacuation plan, and ensuring access to necessary supplies and protective equipment so they do not become victims as well.

The National Disaster Life Support Foundation, Inc. (2014) offers Core, Basic, and Advanced Disaster Life Support training courses that include all essential aspects of disaster response and management. They include the core competencies of disaster management to all levels of health care professionals. In addition, the Federal Emergency Management Agency (FEMA) (2016) provides numerous online resources, including Community Emergency Response Team (CERT) training so people are better prepared for disasters and are able to respond more self-sufficiently to incidents and hazard situations in their own communities. These courses include mass casualty triage education.

Hospital Emergency Preparedness: Personnel Roles and Responsibilities

Nurses play a major role in the emergency preparedness or emergency management plan. Because multiple health system resources are necessary to effectively manage the disaster, the Hospital Incident Command System is typically established for organization and structure.

Hospital Incident Command System

The facility-level organizational model for disaster management is the Hospital Incident Command System (HICS), which is a part of the National Incident Management System (NIMS) implemented by the Department of Homeland Security and FEMA to standardize disaster operations. In this system, roles are formally structured under the hospital or long-term care facility incident commander with clear lines of authority and accountability for specific resources (FEMA, 2016). Officers are named to oversee essential emergency preparedness functions such as public information, safety and security, and medical command. Chiefs are appointed to manage logistics, planning, finance, and operations as appropriate to the type and scale of the event. In turn, chiefs delegate specific duties to other departmental officers and unit leaders. The idea is to achieve a manageable span of control over the personnel or resources allocated to achieve efficiency. FEMA offers free courses on the NIMS model and HICS structure through its website located at www.training.fema.gov/IS/.

Because mass casualty events typically involve large numbers of people and can create a chaotic work environment, many EMS agencies and health care facilities use brightly colored vests with large lettering to help identify key leadership positions. Specific job action sheets are distributed to all personnel with leadership roles in HICS that pre-define reporting relationships and list prioritized tasks and responsibilities. The HICS personnel also establish an emergency operations center (EOC) or command center in a designated location with accessible communication technology. They then use their collective expertise to manage the overall incident. All internal requests for additional personnel and resources and COMMUNICATION with field teams and external agencies should be coordinated through the EOC to maintain unity of command.

The roles and responsibilities of health care personnel in a mass casualty event or disaster are defined within the institution's emergency response or preparedness plan (Table 10-2). Each plan can be as individual as the particular facility's operations. However, virtually all plans identify certain key functions. For example, one of the primary roles to be established at the onset of an incident is that of a hospital incident commander who assumes overall leadership for implementing the institutional plan. This person is usually either a physician in the ED or a hospital administrator who has the authority to activate resources. This role can also be fulfilled by a nursing supervisor functioning as the on-site hospital administrator after usual business hours. The hospital incident commander's role is to take a global view of the entire situation and facilitate patient movement through the system, while bringing in personnel and supply resources to meet patient needs. For example, a hospital incident commander might dictate that all patients due to be discharged from an inpatient unit be moved to a lounge area immediately to free up hospital beds for mass casualty victims. He or she could also direct departments such as physical therapy or a surgical clinic to cancel their usual operations to convert the space into a minor treatment area. The incident commander assists in the organization of hospital-wide services to rapidly expand hospital capacity, recruit paid or volunteer staff, and ensure the availability of medical supplies.

Another typical role defined in hospital or other health care emergency preparedness plans is that of the medical command physician. He or she focuses on determining the number, acuity, and medical resource needs of victims arriving from the incident scene to the hospital and organizing the emergency health care team response to the injured or ill patients. Responsibilities include identifying the need for and calling in specialty-trained providers such as:

- Surgeons (trauma, neuro, orthopedic, plastic, and/or burn)
- Pulmonologists
- Infectious disease physicians
- Industrial hygienists
- Radiation safety personnel

In smaller hospitals with limited specialty resources, the medical command physician might also help determine which patients should be transported out of the facility to a higher level of care or to a specialty hospital (e.g., burn center).

Closely affiliated with the medical command physician is the triage officer. This person is generally a physician in a large hospital who is assisted by triage nurses. When physician resources are limited, an experienced nurse may assume this role. The triage officer rapidly evaluates each person who presents to the hospital, even those who come in with triage tags in place. Patient acuity is re-evaluated for appropriate disposition to the area within the ED or hospital best suited to meet the patient's needs.

Many other roles and responsibilities can be defined within the institutional emergency response plan and may include the supply officer, the COMMUNICATIONS officer, the infection control officer, and the community relations/public information officer, to name a few. The community relations or public information officer is an especially important role to delineate in advance. Mass casualty incidents tend to attract a large amount of media attention. This staff member can draw media away from the clinical areas so essential hospital operations are not hindered. He or she can also serve as the liaison between hospital administration and the media to release only appropriate and accurate information.

Role of Nursing in Health Care Facility Emergency Preparedness and Response

Nurses play key roles before, during, and after a disaster. The core components of the nursing process apply in the overall assessment of the emergency situation; the identification of needs, capabilities, and priorities; and planning, implementing, and evaluating the disaster response. Before an event, nurses contribute to developing internal and external emergency response plans, including defining specific nursing roles. Nurses take into account the security needs; COMMUNICATION methods; training; alternative treatment areas; staffing for high-demand or surge situations; and requirements for resources, equipment, and supplies. They then test the plans by actively participating in disaster drills and evaluating the outcomes.

During an actual disaster, the ED charge nurse, trauma program manager, and other ED nursing leadership personnel act in collaboration with the medical command physician and triage officer to organize nursing and ancillary services to meet patient needs. Telephone trees or automated group notification systems may be activated to call in ED nurses who are not

---

TABLE 10-2 Summary of Key Personnel Roles and Functions for Emergency Preparedness and Response Plan

PERSONNEL ROLE	PERSONNEL FUNCTION
Hospital incident commander	Physician or administrator who assumes overall leadership for implementing the emergency plan
Medical command physician	Physician who decides the number, acuity, and resource needs of patients
Triage officer	Physician or nurse who rapidly evaluates each patient to determine priorities for treatment
Community relations or public information officer	Person who serves as a liaison between the health care facility and the media

working or are not scheduled to work. ED areas are identified and prepared to stage, triage, resuscitate, and treat the disaster victims. Efforts are made to quickly discharge or admit other ED patients as appropriate to make room for the new arrivals. ED nurses apply principles of triage to prioritize care delivery as disaster victims enter the system and direct patients to the designated areas best suited to meet their needs. To maintain ongoing readiness, ED nurses require disaster response education that specifically addresses their roles in the ED environment and in overall hospital operations (Whetzel et al., 2013).

Nursing roles in a disaster extend to all areas within a health care facility. The level of involvement is determined by the scope and scale of the disaster. In any mass casualty event, nurses from medical-surgical nursing units may be asked, in collaboration with the health care provider, to recommend patients for discharge to free up inpatient beds for disaster victims. Patients who are the most medically stable may be discharged early, including those who:

- Were admitted for observation and are not bedridden
- Are having diagnostic evaluations and are not bedridden
- Are soon scheduled to be discharged or could be cared for at home with support from family or home health care services
- Have had no critical change in condition for the past 3 days
- Could be cared for in another health care facility such as rehabilitation or long-term care

? NCLEX EXAMINATION CHALLENGE 10-2

Safe and Effective Care Environment

A number of nurses are floated to the ED to care for clients affected by an earthquake. Which appropriate float nurse assignments will the ED charge nurse make? **Select all that apply.**
A. GI laboratory nurse assigned to clients undergoing sedation
B. Orthopedic nurse assigned to accompany clients to radiology
C. Nursing administrator assigned to monitor loved ones in the waiting room
D. Community health nurse assigned to care for clients with fractures
E. Medical-surgical nurse assigned to health care worker who is feeling overwhelmed

General staff nurses also may be recruited to collaborate in providing care for stable ED patients, thus allowing ED nurses to focus their efforts on aiding the mass casualty victims. Critical care unit nurses need to identify patients who can be transferred out of the unit to rapidly expand critical care bed capacity. In addition, they can supplement ED nurses in the resuscitation setting or assist in monitored care and transport to critical care units. Hospital and ED nurse leaders also typically direct the ancillary departments to deliver supplies, instrument trays, medications, food, and personnel to meet service demands.

Hospital staff of all levels may be required to alter their routine operations to accommodate a high volume of patients, including those with special needs such as decontamination, burn management, or quarantine. Inpatient unit nurses may be assigned a higher number of patients than usual. They may also be asked to provide care in nontraditional locations such as hallways or lounges to help rapidly decompress the ED so new arrivals can be readily managed.

Emergency plans dictate specific actions by all members of the interprofessional team such as who should be called when

the plan is activated, who should report, where to report, which supplies or equipment carts should be brought to a pre-designated location, and which type of paperwork or system should be implemented for patient identification in a large-scale event. Some staff may even have their roles changed completely. For example, administrative nurses may be reassigned to fulfill a clinical responsibility for a nursing unit. The key concept is that staff members are expected to remain flexible in a mass casualty situation and perform at their highest level to address the needs of both the health care system and the patients. The greatest good for the greatest number of people is still the organizing principle when considering roles and responsibilities in mass casualty events—not necessarily individual staff preferences. However, the SAFETY of all patients is vital.

Creativity and flexibility of nursing leaders and nursing staff are essential to provide the staffing coverage necessary for a large-scale or extended incident. The willingness of staff to show up for work is directly impacted by their concerns for their home and family in a disaster; inadequate staffing can jeopardize a facility's ability to provide care. A **personal emergency preparedness plan** developed by each nurse can help in such situations. It should outline the preplanned specific arrangements that are to be made for child care, pet care, and older adult care if the need arises, especially if the event prevents returning home for an extended period.

? NCLEX EXAMINATION CHALLENGE 10-3

Safe and Effective Care Environment

The experienced nurse is teaching a new nurse about hospital emergency plans and personal emergency preparedness. Which specific arrangements should the experienced nurse discuss? **Select all that apply.**
A. Assembly of a "go bag"
B. Plans for child and/or elder care
C. Neighbor who is willing to care for dog
D. Who will be called when the plan is activated
E. How long an emergency is expected to last
F. Where a nurse is expected to report if the emergency plan is activated
G. Names, addresses, and telephone numbers to be used if a crisis occurs

! NURSING SAFETY PRIORITY QSEN

Action Alert

Include emergency contact names, addresses, and telephone numbers to use in a crisis as part of a personal emergency preparedness plan. In addition, preassemble **personal readiness supplies** or a **"go bag"** (disaster supply kit) for the home and automobile with clothing and basic survival supplies, which allows for a rapid response for disaster staffing coverage (Table 10-3). "Go bags" are needed for all members of the family, including pets, in the event the disaster requires evacuation of the community or people to take shelter in their own homes.

When called to respond to work during a mass casualty event or pandemic infectious disease outbreak, some nurses may experience ethical and moral conflict among their own personal preparedness for disaster response, family obligations, and professional responsibilities (Bell et al., 2014; Nash, 2015). The American Nurses Association (ANA) Code of Ethics for Nurses with Interpretive Statements (2015) offers general

TABLE 10-3 Basic Supplies for Personal Preparedness (3-Day Supply)

- Backpack
- Clean, durable weather-appropriate clothing; sturdy footwear
- Potable water—at least 1 gallon per person per day for at least 3 days
- Food–nonperishable, no cooking required
- Headlamp or flashlight—battery powered; extra batteries and/or chemical light sticks (**Note:** a headlamp is superior because it allows hands-free operation)
- Pocket knife or multi-tool
- Personal identification (ID) with emergency contacts and phone numbers, allergies, and medical information; lists of credit card numbers and bank accounts (keep in watertight container)
- Towel and washcloth; towelettes, soap, hand sanitizer
- Paper, pens, and pencils; regional maps
- Cell phone and charger
- Sunglasses/protective and/or corrective eyewear
- Emergency blanket and/or sleeping bag and pillow
- Work gloves
- Personal first aid kit with over-the-counter (OTC) and prescription medications
- Rain gear
- Roll of duct tape and plastic sheeting
- Radio—battery powered or hand-crank generator
- Toiletries (toothbrush and toothpaste, comb, brush, razor, shaving cream, mirror, feminine supplies, deodorant; shampoo, lip balm, sunscreen, insect repellent, toilet paper)
- Plastic garbage bags and ties, resealable plastic bags
- Matches in a waterproof container
- Whistle
- Household liquid bleach for disinfection

 CHART 10-2 Best Practice for Patient Safety & Quality Care QSEN

Preventing Staff Acute Stress Disorder and Post-Traumatic Stress Disorder Following a Mass Casualty Event

- Use available counseling.
- Encourage and support co-workers.
- Monitor each other's stress level and performance.
- Take breaks when needed.
- Talk about feelings with staff and managers.
- Drink plenty of water and eat healthy snacks for energy.
- Keep in touch with family, friends, and significant others.
- Do not work more than 12 hours per day.

Adapted from Papp, E. (2005). Preparing for disasters: Helping yourself as you help others. *The American Journal of Nursing, 105*(5), 112.

guidance that can be helpful to nurses. Each person has to make a personal choice about whether to be involved in helping during the emergency or when to become involved.

EVENT RESOLUTION AND DEBRIEFING

When the last major casualties have been treated and no more are expected to arrive in numbers that could overwhelm the health care system, the incident commander considers "standing down" or deactivating the emergency response plan. Although the casualties may have left the ED, other areas in the hospital may still be under stress and need the support of the supplemental resources provided by emergency plan activation. Before terminating the response, it is essential to ensure that the needs of the other hospital departments have been met and all are in agreement to resume normal operations.

A vital consideration in event resolution is staff and supply availability to meet ongoing operational needs. If nursing staff and other personnel were called in from home during their off hours or if they worked well beyond their scheduled shifts to meet patient and departmental needs, provision for adequate rest periods should be made. Exhaustion poses a risk to patient safety and to the nurse when he or she must drive home. Sleeping quarters at the hospital might be necessary in this case, especially if the disaster event contributed to treacherous travel conditions.

Severe shortages of supplies also pose a threat to usual operations at the conclusion of a mass casualty incident. Taking inventory and restocking the ED are high-priority assignments. Teamwork and interprofessional collaboration between the ED and the central supply department are essential

to resolving stock availability problems. Instrument trays must be washed, packaged, and re-sterilized. Critical supplies that have been depleted from hospital stores must be reordered and delivered to the hospital quickly. Contracts with key vendors outlining emergency re-supply expectations and arrangements should be a part of the hospital's overall emergency preparedness plan.

Two general types of **debriefing**, or formal systematic review and analysis, occur after a mass casualty incident or disaster. The first type entails bringing in critical incident stress debriefing (CISD) teams to provide sessions for small groups of staff to promote effective coping strategies. The second type of debriefing involves an administrative review of staff and system performance during the event to determine whether opportunities for improvement in the emergency management plan exist.

Critical Incident Stress Debriefing

CISD is only one component of a much broader critical incident stress management (CISM) program. CISM programming addresses pre-crisis through post-crisis interventions for small-to-large groups, including communities. After working through the turmoil and the emotional impact of the incident and the aftermath, the staff may find it difficult to "get back to normal." Without intervention during *and* after the emergency, they may develop acute stress disorder (ASD), or post-traumatic stress disorder (PTSD). ASD, although similar to PTSD, focuses on dissociative symptoms such as numbing, reduced awareness, depersonalization, derealization, or amnesia, experienced within the first month after a traumatic event; it is also predictive of subsequent PTSD (Gibson, 2016). PTSD can lead to multiple characteristic psychological and physical effects, including flashbacks, avoidance, less interest in previously enjoyable events, detachment, rapid heart rate, and insomnia. People suffering from PTSD can have great difficulty relating in their usual way to family and friends. Ultimately, professional "burnout" can stem from the inability to cope with the stress effectively. A resource for CISM is the International Critical Incident Stress Foundation, Inc. (2016); their mission is "to provide leadership, education, training, consultation, and support services in comprehensive crisis intervention and disaster behavioral health services to the emergency response professions, other organizations, and communities worldwide". Chart 10-2 lists recommendations proposed by several national organizations to help prevent staff ASD and PTSD following an emergency situation.

A CISD team comprises two or three specially trained people who come together quickly when called to deal with the emotional needs of health care team members after a particularly devastating or disturbing incident. The team leader typically has background in a mental health/behavioral health field. The co-leader is ideally a peer of the group being debriefed. Thus, if nurses are debriefed, a nurse member of the CISD team is generally assigned to the session. CISD-trained physicians, police, firefighters, EMTs, and paramedics may also be used, depending on the needs of the group. The third member of the team is known as the "doorkeeper." This person is responsible for keeping inappropriate people out (e.g., media, spectators) and talking with anyone who leaves the session early in an effort to have him or her return or accept follow-up care. Staff involved in the incident need protected time to undergo stress debriefing, which generally lasts from 1 to 3 hours per session.

Typical "ground rules" for stress debriefing include strict confidentiality of information shared during the session and unconditional acceptance of the thoughts and feelings expressed by people within the group. The usual arrangement for the most effective group interaction is a circular configuration of chairs in a private setting. Food should be available so hunger is not a distraction. CISD group leaders encourage group discussion by asking a series of questions designed to get everyone involved to tell his or her own story about the incident and explain the personal impact. The group leaders enable participants to place the incident into perspective and dispel any feelings of blame or guilt. They also educate participants about self-care concepts and coping strategies to use immediately. People who require more than a CISD session may need referral for mental health/behavioral health counseling.

Administrative Review

The second type of debriefing is an administrative evaluation directed at analyzing the hospital or agency response to an event while it is still in the forefront of the minds of everyone who participated in it. The goal of this debriefing is to discern what went right and what went wrong during activation and implementation of the emergency preparedness plan so needed changes can be made. Typically, representatives from all groups who were involved in the incident come together soon after plan activation has been discontinued. They each are given an opportunity to hear and express both positive and negative comments related to their experiences with the event. In the days after the plan activation, written critique forms are also solicited to gain additional information after participants have had time to consider their overall impressions of the response and the impact it had on their respective departments or clinical areas.

Although drills are important, implementing the emergency preparedness plan during an actual mass casualty event is the most effective means of "reality testing" the plan's utility. Feedback provided by participants can be used to modify or revise the plan and create new processes in preparation for future events.

ROLE OF NURSING IN COMMUNITY EMERGENCY PREPAREDNESS AND RESPONSE

During a community disaster, nurses and other emergency personnel may be needed for triage, first aid/emergency care, and shelter assistance. The first action of first responders in a disaster is to remove people from danger, both the injured and uninjured. Firefighters and other disaster-trained emergency personnel typically manage this job; unless they have had specific search-and-rescue training, nurses are not usually involved in this process. In all cases developing and maintaining accurate *situational awareness* are critical for appropriate priority setting and SAFETY in a rapidly changing environment.

After removal from danger, victims are triaged by health care personnel as described earlier in this chapter. After triage, nurses often provide on-site first aid and emergency care. They may also be involved in teaching and supervising volunteers. The American Red Cross sets up shelters for people who have lost their homes or have been evacuated from their homes.

Nurses may also need to teach those living temporarily in shelters about procedures that will be needed for SAFETY when they return home. For example, clean drinking water may not be available for several days or longer. Community residents may need to boil their water before drinking. If electricity and gas are not available, an outdoor grill or camp stove can be used for this purpose. As alternative procedures, commercial water purification filters, sterilizing ultraviolet pens, or 10 to 20 drops of chlorine bleach added to a gallon of water will make the water safe to drink.

Human waste management creates another challenge if toilets do not flush. If not managed safely, enteric pathogens spread disease. A toilet bowl or bucket lined with a plastic bag can be used for human waste. To sanitize it and provide odor control, chlorine bleach can be added, and the bag tied and sealed. Portable toilet chemicals or chlorinated lime may be used as alternatives. To prevent a toxic gas reaction, remind residents not to mix any chemicals. Treated human waste bags can be buried in the ground. In an austere environment a pit can be dug in the ground as an improvised toilet. In all cases, emphasize the importance of handwashing with soap and water or using a hand sanitizer to prevent disease transmission.

PSYCHOSOCIAL RESPONSE OF SURVIVORS TO MASS CASUALTY EVENTS

One of the most important roles of the nurse during and after a community disaster is health assessment (also known as "noticing"), including psychosocial health. Experiencing a disaster can produce both immediate and long-lasting psychological and psychosocial effects in people personally affected by the event. Depending on the nature and magnitude of the incident, survivors experience the tragic loss of loved ones, pets, property, and valued possessions. They and their loved ones may have suffered injuries or illnesses brought about by the catastrophe. Lifestyles, roles, and routines are drastically altered, preventing people from achieving any sense of normalcy in the hours, days, and perhaps even weeks and months that follow a disaster. Coping abilities in survivors are severely stressed, leading to many individual responses, which can range from functional and adaptive behaviors to maladaptive coping.

Survivors have to confront feelings of vulnerability resulting from the devastating event, knowing that it could occur again. This may be a particularly relevant issue for people who live in areas prone to acts of terrorism or natural disasters. The decision, be it voluntary or involuntary, to abandon a family home or geographic region and then relocate to a "safe" area either temporarily or permanently results in a further sense of loss, grief, and disorientation. Some people may feel guilty about living through an event that caused so many others to die. The range of intense emotions can appear as physical illness and as psychological and social dysfunction.

When helping people in crisis after a mass casualty event, be calm and reassuring. Establish rapport through active listening and honest COMMUNICATION. Survivors benefit from talking about their experiences and putting them in chronological order, which provides clarity and helps them begin to problem solve. Offer resources whenever possible to help survivors gain a sense of personal control. Help survivors adapt to their new surroundings and routines through simple, concrete explanations. Convey caring behaviors, and provide a sense of safety and security to the best extent possible. If available, request that crisis counselors respond and assist in providing compassionate support to victims and their families.

A disaster may cause some survivors to develop acute stress disorder (ASD) or post-traumatic stress disorder (PTSD). People who are unable to sleep, are easily startled, have "flash-backs" to relive the disaster, or report "feeling numb" 2 weeks or more after a disaster or traumatic event are at risk for PTSD.

Nurses caring for survivors with these symptoms should perform further assessment. One tool that can be used to assess survivor response to a disaster is the Impact of Event Scale—Revised (IES-R). The IES-R is a 22-item self-administered questionnaire that includes several subscales such as avoidance. Before giving the tool, determine the patient's reading level because it is written at a 10th-grade reading level. The tool should not be used for patients with short-term memory loss. For this reason, many older survivors often are not adequately assessed for post-disaster PTSD. Assess all older survivors of a disaster for this complication when possible.

? CLINICAL JUDGMENT CHALLENGE 10-1
Patient-Centered Care QSEN

You are part of a DMAT team that has been dispatched to help a community after an EF-3 tornado touched down in a rural, underserved area. You have been notified that so far six people have been identified as killed, and over 100 have been identified as injured. The main street of the town has been demolished, and many people are without shelter.
1. How do you prepare to maintain your own personal health and safety while assisting others?
2. Which resources do you anticipate may be of highest need for this population?
3. Many residents are fearful about being transported to a facility several counties away, as most have lived in this town for their entire life. How would you respond?
4. After returning from the DMAT mission, you notice that a peer who served with you appears to feel disengaged with regular nursing employment and exhibits signs of depression. How will you support this nurse?

! NURSING SAFETY PRIORITY QSEN
Action Alert

A high score on any IES-R subscale indicates a need for further evaluation and counseling. Refer the patient to a social worker, psychiatric mental health nurse specialist, or qualified mental health counselor. A high score on all subscales requires referral to a psychiatrist, clinical psychologist, or psychiatric mental health nurse practitioner or clinical specialist to evaluate the possibility of current or past trauma, such as abuse or neglect.

GET READY FOR THE NCLEX® EXAMINATION!

KEY POINTS

Review these Key Points for each NCLEX Examination Client Needs Category.

Safe and Effective Care Environment
- Describe the hospital emergency preparedness and response team that all hospitals are required to have in case of mass casualty (disaster). **QSEN: Teamwork and Collaboration**
- Apply principles of triage by using the typical triage system for a mass casualty situation, which includes an additional category for patients allowed to die (black-tagged) (see Table 10-1). **Ethics**
- Describe the special roles that are assigned in a mass casualty incident as identified in Table 10-2.
- Understand how to assist in determining the need for initiating the emergency preparedness plan based on available resources and staffing. **QSEN: Teamwork and Collaboration**
- Develop a personal emergency preparedness plan (see Table 10-3).
- Compare key nursing and interprofessional team roles in emergency preparedness and in response plan and debriefing. **QSEN: Teamwork and Collaboration**
- Recall that nurses play a major role in triage, first aid and emergency care, and shelter assistance in external community disasters.

Psychosocial Integrity
- Assess survivors and families for their ability to adapt to the effects of disaster changes or traumatic events, including acute stress disorder (ASD) or post-traumatic stress disorder (PTSD). **QSEN: Patient-Centered Care**
- Provide emotional support to the person and/or family coping with life changes resulting from a disaster through active listening and appropriate referrals. **QSEN: Patient-Centered Care**
- Be honest with victims and their families. Avoid giving false reassurance. Offer orienting information and help them adapt to their changed or new surroundings. **Ethics**
- Provide support by taking precautions to prevent staff from developing ASD or PTSD as outlined in Chart 10-2.
- Recognize that older adults may not be properly assessed for ASD or PTSD. **Health Care Disparities**

Physiological Integrity
- Take precautions for meeting basic needs in a mass casualty situation; know your own limitations and develop situational awareness when responding. **QSEN: Safety**

SELECTED BIBLIOGRAPHY

Asterisk indicates a classic or definitive work on this subject.

American Nurses Association. (2015). *Code of Ethics for Nurses with Interpretive Statements*. http://www.nursingworld.org/MainMenu-Categories/EthicsStandards/CodeofEthicsforNurses/Code-of-Ethics-For-Nurses.html.

Bell, M. A., Dake, J. A., Price, J. H., Jordan, T. R., & Rega, P. (2014). A national survey of emergency nurses and avian influenza threat. *Journal of Emergency Nursing*, 40(3), 212–217.

Casey, D. (2015). A nurse's obligations to patients with Ebola. *Nursing 2015*, 45(11), 47–49.

Centers for Medicare and Medicaid Services (CMS). (2016). *Life safety code requirements*. www.cms.gov/Medicare/Provider-Enrollment-and-Certification/CertificationandComplianc/LSC.html.

Danna, D. & Bennett, M. J. (2013). Providing culturally competent care during disasters: Strategies for nurses. *Journal of Continuing Education in Nursing*, 44(4), 151–152.

Department of Homeland Security. (2016). *Stop the bleed*. https://www.dhs.gov/stopthebleed.

Federal Emergency Management Agency (FEMA) (2016). *Resources for National Disaster Recovery Framework*. www.fema.gov/resources.

Gibson, L. (2016). *Acute stress disorder*. http://www.ptsd.va.gov/professional/treatment/early/acute-stress-disorder.asp.

International Critical Incident Stress Foundation, Inc. (2016). *Mission statement*. http://www.icisf.org/about-us/mission-statement/.

*Laskowski-Jones, L. (2008). Change management at the hospital front door: Integrating automatic patient tracking in a high-volume emergency department and Level I trauma center. *Nurse Leader*, 6(2), 52–57.

*Laskowski-Jones, L. (2010). When disaster strikes: Ready, or not? (Editorial). *Nursing*, 40(4), 6.

*Letner, J. (2011). *A fist coming out of the sky: Six miles of terror*. The Joplin Globe. www.joplinglobe.com/local/x564433625/A-fist-coming-out-of-the-sky-Six-miles-of-terror.

Nash, T. (2015). Unveiling the truth about nurses' personal preparedness for disaster response: A pilot study. *Medsurg Nursing*, 24(6), 425–431.

National Disaster Life Support Foundation, Inc. (2014). *Types of training centers*. http://www.ndlsf.org/index.php/training-centers/types-of-training-centers.

National Fire Protection Association. (2016). *Codes and standards*. www.nfpa.org/codes and standards.aspx.

*Papp, E. (2005). Preparing for disasters: Helping yourself as you help others. *American Journal of Nursing*, 105(5), 112.

The Joint Commission. (2017). *Emergency management resources*. http://www.jointcommission.org/emergency_management.aspx.

U.S. Department of Health & Human Services. (2015). *Disaster Medical Assistance Team (DMAT)*. http://www.phe.gov/preparedness/responders/ndms/teams/pages/dmat.aspx.

U.S. Department of Health & Human Services. (2016). *National Disaster Medical System*. http://www.phe.gov/Preparedness/responders/ndms/Pages/default.aspx.

Veenema, T., Griffin, A., Gable, A., MacIntyre, L., Simons, N., Couig, M., et al. (2016). Nurses as leaders in disaster preparedness and response. A call to action. *Journal of Nursing Scholarship*, 48(2), 187–200.

Whetzel, E., Walker-Cillo, G., Chan, G. K., & Trivett, J. (2013). Emergency nurse perceptions of individual and facility emergency preparedness. *Journal of Emergency Nursing*, 39(1), 46–52.

Woo, J., Lee, G., Cho, J., Yang, J., Lim, Y., Kim, J., et al. (2015). Disaster medical responses to the disaster scene of long-distance on highway-field triage and disaster communication by social media for 106-vehicle chain collision in Yeong-Jong Grand Bridge. *Journal of Korean Society of Emergency Medicine*, 26(5), 449–457.

Yin, H., He, H., Arbon, P., Zhu, J., Tan, J., & Zhang, L. (2012). Optimal qualifications, staffing and scope of practice for first responder nurses in disaster. *Journal of Clinical Nursing*, 21(1–2), 264–271.

11 | CHAPTER

Assessment and Care of Patients With Problems of Fluid and Electrolyte Balance

M. Linda Workman

 http://evolve.elsevier.com/Iggy/

PRIORITY AND INTERRELATED CONCEPTS

The priority concept for this chapter is FLUID AND ELECTROLYTE BALANCE.

✳ The FLUID AND ELECTROLYTE BALANCE concept exemplar for this chapter is Dehydration, p. 167.

The interrelated concept for this chapter is PERFUSION.

LEARNING OUTCOMES

Safe and Effective Care Environment

1. Collaborate with the interprofessional team to perform a complete assessment of patients for FLUID AND ELECTROLYTE BALANCE.
2. Protect the patient with a problem of FLUID AND ELECTROLYTE BALANCE from injury and complications, especially those related to PERFUSION.
3. Teach the patient and caregiver(s) how home safety is affected by problems of FLUID AND ELECTROLYTE BALANCE.

Health Promotion and Maintenance

4. Teach all adults measures to take to prevent problems of FLUID AND ELECTROLYTE BALANCE.

Psychosocial Integrity

5. Implement nursing interventions to help the patient and family cope with the psychosocial impact of continuing risk for problems with FLUID AND ELECTROLYTE BALANCE.

Physiological Integrity

6. Apply knowledge of anatomy and physiology to perform an evidence-based assessment for the patient who has a problem with FLUID AND ELECTROLYTE BALANCE.
7. Interpret assessment findings for the patient experiencing a problem of FLUID AND ELECTROLYTE BALANCE.
8. Teach the patient and caregivers about diagnostic procedures and drug therapies associated with conditions affecting FLUID AND ELECTROLYTE BALANCE.

ANATOMY AND PHYSIOLOGY REVIEW

Optimal body function depends on maintaining FLUID AND ELECTROLYTE BALANCE in each body fluid space (compartment). Keeping this balance within normal ranges is part of homeostasis. Because the range of normal is so narrow, the body has many control actions (known as *homeostatic mechanisms*) to prevent dangerous changes (Walker, 2016).

Water (fluid) makes up about 55% to 60% of total weight for younger adults and 50% to 55% of total weight for older adults. This water is divided into two main compartments (spaces)—the fluid outside the cells (**extracellular fluid [ECF]**) and the fluid inside the cells (**intracellular fluid [ICF]**). The ECF space is about one third (about 15 L) of the total body water. The ECF includes **interstitial fluid** (fluid between cells, "third space"); blood, lymph, bone, and connective tissue water; and the transcellular fluids. Transcellular fluids include cerebrospinal fluid, synovial fluid, peritoneal fluid, and pleural fluid. ICF is about two thirds (about 25 L) of total body water. Fig. 11-1 shows normal total body water distribution.

Water delivers dissolved nutrients and electrolytes to all organs, tissues, and cells. In health the volume of water in the fluid compartments remains within the normal range, although the water moves constantly between compartments. Changes in either the amount of water or the amount of electrolytes in body fluids can reduce the function of all cells, tissues, and organs.

Body fluids are composed of water and particles dissolved or suspended in water. The solvent is the water portion of fluids. Solutes are the particles dissolved or suspended in the water. Solutes vary in type and amount from one fluid space to another. When solutes express an overall electrical charge, they are known as *electrolytes.*

Three processes control FLUID AND ELECTROLYTE BALANCE to keep the internal environment stable even when the external environment changes. These processes (filtration, diffusion, and osmosis) determine whether fluids and particles move across cell membranes.

FILTRATION

Physiologic Action

Filtration is the movement of fluid (water) through a cell or blood vessel membrane because of water pressure (hydrostatic pressure) differences on both sides of the membrane. This pressure is caused by water volume pressing against confining membranes.

Water molecules in a confined space constantly press outward against the membranes, creating hydrostatic pressure (also

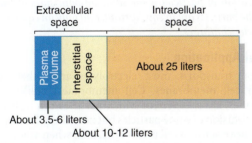

FIG. 11-1 Normal distribution of total body water in adults.

known as *water pressure*). This is a "water-pushing" pressure, because it forces water outward from a confined space through a membrane (Fig. 11-2).

The amount (volume) of water in any body fluid space determines the hydrostatic pressure of that space. Blood, which is "thicker" than water (more *viscous*), is confined within the blood vessels. Blood has hydrostatic pressure because of its weight and volume and also from the pressure in arteries generated by the pumping action of the heart.

The hydrostatic pressures of two fluid spaces can be compared whenever a porous (permeable) membrane separates the two spaces. If the hydrostatic pressure is the same in both fluid spaces, there is no pressure difference between the two spaces, and the hydrostatic pressure is at *equilibrium*. If the hydrostatic pressure is not the same in both spaces, disequilibrium exists. This means that the two spaces have a graded difference (*gradient*) for hydrostatic pressure: one space has a higher hydrostatic pressure than the other. *The human body constantly seeks equilibrium.* When a gradient exists, water movement (filtration) occurs until the hydrostatic pressure is the same in both spaces (see Fig. 11-2).

Water moves through the membrane (filters) from the space with higher hydrostatic pressure to the space with lower pressure. Filtration continues only as long as the hydrostatic pressure gradient exists. Equilibrium is reached when enough fluid leaves one space and enters the other space to make the hydrostatic pressure in both spaces equal. Then water molecules are evenly exchanged between the spaces, but no net movement of fluid occurs. Neither space gains or loses water molecules, and the hydrostatic pressure in both spaces is the same.

Clinical Application

Blood pressure is an example of a hydrostatic filtering force. It moves whole blood from the heart to capillaries where filtration can occur to exchange water, nutrients, and waste products between the blood and the tissues. The hydrostatic pressure difference between the capillary blood and the interstitial fluid (fluid in the tissue spaces) determines whether water leaves the blood vessels and enters the tissue spaces.

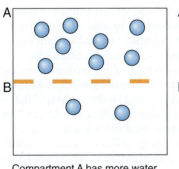

Compartment A has more water molecules and greater hydrostatic pressure than does compartment B.

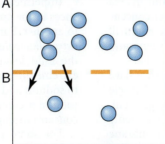

Water molecules move down the hydrostatic pressure gradient from compartment A through the permeable membrane into compartment B, which has a lower hydrostatic pressure.

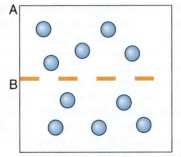

Enough water molecules have moved down the hydrostatic pressure gradient from compartment A into compartment B that both sides now have the same amount of water and the same amount of hydrostatic pressure. An equilibrium of hydrostatic pressure now exists between the two compartments, and no further *net* movement of water will occur.

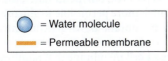

○ = Water molecule
▬ = Permeable membrane

FIG. 11-2 The process of filtration.

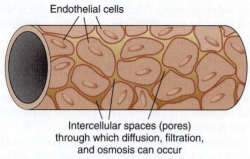

FIG. 11-3 The basic structure of a capillary.

Capillary membranes are only one cell layer thick, making a thin "wall" to hold blood in the capillaries. Large spaces (**pores**) in the capillary membrane help water filter freely when a hydrostatic pressure gradient is present (Fig. 11-3).

Edema (excess tissue fluid) forms with changes in hydrostatic pressure differences between the blood and the interstitial fluid such as in right-sided heart failure (McCance et al., 2014). In this condition the volume of blood in the right side of the heart increases because the right ventricle is too weak to pump blood well into lung blood vessels. As blood backs up into the venous and capillary systems, the capillary hydrostatic pressure rises until it is higher than the pressure in the interstitial space. Excess filtration from the capillaries into the interstitial tissue space then forms visible edema.

DIFFUSION

Physiologic Action

Diffusion is the movement of particles (solute) across a permeable membrane from an area of higher particle concentration to an area of lower particle concentration (*down a concentration gradient*). Particles in a fluid have random movement from the vibration of atoms in the nucleus. Random movement allows molecules to bump into each other in a confined fluid space. Each collision increases the speed of particle movement. The more particles (higher concentration) present in the confined fluid space, the greater the number of collisions.

As a result of the collisions, molecules in a solution spread out evenly through the available space. They move from an area of higher molecule concentrations to an area of lower concentrations until an equal concentration (amount) is present in all areas. Spaces with many particles have more collisions and faster particle movement than spaces with fewer particles.

A concentration gradient exists when two fluid spaces have different concentrations of the same type of particles. Particle collisions cause them to move down the concentration gradient. Any membrane that separates two spaces is struck repeatedly by particles. When the particle strikes a pore in the membrane that is large enough for it to pass through, diffusion occurs (Fig. 11-4). The chance of any single particle hitting the membrane and going through a pore is much greater on the side of the membrane with a higher solute particle concentration.

The speed of diffusion is related to the difference in amount of particles (concentration gradient) between the two sides of the membrane. The degree of difference is the *steepness* of the gradient: the larger the concentration difference between the two sides, the steeper the gradient. Diffusion is more rapid when the gradient is steeper (just as a ball rolls downhill faster when the hill is steep than when the hill is nearly flat). Particles

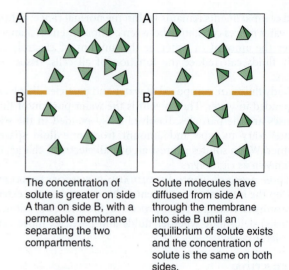

The concentration of solute is greater on side A than on side B, with a permeable membrane separating the two compartments.

Solute molecules have diffused from side A through the membrane into side B until an equilibrium of solute exists and the concentration of solute is the same on both sides.

FIG. 11-4 Diffusion of solute particles through a permeable membrane from an area of higher solute concentration to an area of lower solute concentration until an equilibrium is reached.

move from the fluid space with a higher concentration of solute particles to the fluid space with a lower concentration of solute particles.

Particle diffusion continues as long as a concentration gradient exists between the two sides of the membrane. *When the concentration of particles is the same on both sides of the membrane, the particles are in equilibrium, and only an equal exchange of particles continues.*

Clinical Application

Diffusion transports most electrolytes and other particles through cell membranes. Cell membranes, unlike capillary membranes, are *selective* for which particles can diffuse. They permit diffusion of some particles but not others. Some particles cannot move across a cell membrane, even when a steep "downhill" gradient exists, because the membrane is **impermeable** (closed) to that particle. For these particles the concentration gradient is maintained across the membrane.

Impermeability and special transport systems cause differences in the amounts of specific particles from one fluid space to another. For example, usually the fluid outside the cell (the *extracellular fluid [ECF]*) has ten times more sodium ions than the fluid inside the cell (the *intracellular fluid [ICF]*). This extreme difference is caused by cell membrane impermeability to sodium and by special "sodium pumps" that move any extra sodium present inside the cell out of the cell "uphill" against its concentration gradient and back into the ECF.

For some particles diffusion cannot occur without help, even down steep concentration gradients, because of selective membrane permeability. One example is glucose. Even though the amount of glucose may be much higher in the ECF than in the ICF (creating a steep gradient for glucose), glucose cannot cross some cell membranes without the help of insulin. Insulin binds to insulin receptors on cell membranes, which then makes the membranes much more permeable to glucose. Then glucose can cross the cell membrane down its concentration gradient into the cell.

Diffusion across a cell membrane that requires a membrane-altering system (e.g., insulin) is called **facilitated diffusion**. This type of movement is still a form of diffusion because it does not require extra energy.

OSMOSIS

Physiologic Action

Osmosis is the movement of *water only* through a selectively permeable *(semipermeable)* membrane. For osmosis to occur, a membrane must separate two fluid spaces, and one space must have particles that cannot move through the membrane. (The membrane is impermeable to this particle.) A concentration gradient of this particle must also exist. Because the membrane is impermeable to these particles, they cannot cross the membrane, but water molecules can.

For the fluid spaces to have equal concentrations of the particle, the water molecules move down their concentration gradient from the side with the higher concentration of water molecules (and a lower concentration of particles along with a greater hydrostatic pressure) to the side with the lower concentration of water molecules (and a higher concentration of particles along with a lower hydrostatic pressure). This movement continues until both spaces contain the same proportions of particles to water. Dilute fluid is less concentrated and has fewer particles and more water molecules than more concentrated fluid. Thus water moves by osmosis down its hydrostatic pressure gradient from the dilute fluid to the more concentrated fluid until a concentration equilibrium occurs (Fig. 11-5).

At this point the *concentrations* of particles in the fluid spaces on both sides of the membrane are equal, even though the total amounts of particles and volumes of water are different. *The concentration equilibrium occurs by the movement of water molecules rather than the movement of solute particles.*

Particle concentration in body fluid is the major factor that determines whether and how fast osmosis and diffusion occur (McLafferty et al., 2014). This concentration is expressed in milliequivalents per liter (mEq/L), millimoles per liter (mmol/L), and milliosmoles per liter (mOsm/L). Osmolarity is the number of milliosmoles in a *liter* of solution; osmolality is the number of milliosmoles in a *kilogram* of solution. Because 1 L of water weighs 1 kg, in human physiology osmolarity and osmolality are considered the same, although osmolarity is the actual concentration measured most often. The normal osmolarity value for plasma and other body fluids ranges from 270 to about 300 mOsm/L. The body functions best when the osmolarity of all body fluid spaces is close to 300 mOsm/L. When all fluids have this particle concentration, the fluids are isosmotic or isotonic (also called normotonic) to each other.

Fluids with osmolarities greater than 300 mOsm/L are hyperosmotic, or hypertonic, compared with isosmotic fluids. These fluids have a *greater* osmotic pressure than do isosmotic fluids and tend to pull water from the isosmotic fluid space into the hyperosmotic fluid space until an osmotic balance occurs. If a hyperosmotic (hypertonic) IV solution (e.g., 3% or 5% saline) were infused into a patient with normal extracellular fluid (ECF) osmolarity, the infusing fluid would make the adult's blood hyperosmotic. To balance this situation, the interstitial fluid would be pulled into the circulation in an attempt to dilute the blood osmolarity back to normal. In addition, fluid would also be drawn from the intracellular fluid (ICF) compartment. As a result, the interstitial and ICF volumes would shrink, and the plasma volume would expand.

Fluids with osmolarities of less than 270 mOsm/L are hypo-osmotic, or hypotonic, compared with isosmotic fluids.

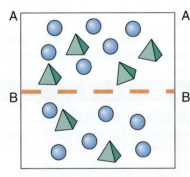 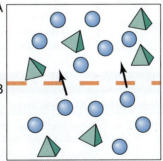 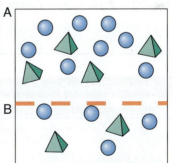

Side A has more solute molecules than does side B, even though the number of water molecules is the same on both sides. Thus side A has a greater osmotic (water pulling) pressure than does side B.

DISEQUILIBRIUM
Side A 1.5:1 ratio of water to solute
Side B   3:1 ratio of water to solute

Movement of water occurs by osmosis toward side A because it has greater osmotic pressure. The membrane is *not* permeable to the solute molecules, so the actual number of solute molecules on side A and side B does not change. *Only the water molecules move, because the membrane is not permeable to the solute molecules.*

Enough water molecules have moved from side B into side A that the actual concentration of solute is now the same on both sides, with a ratio of water to solute of 2:1. An equilibrium of osmotic pressure now exists between the two compartments, and no further *net* movement of water molecules or solute molecules will occur.

EQUILIBRIUM
Side A 2:1 ratio of water to solute
Side B 2:1 ratio of water to solute

○ = Water molecule
▬ = Permeable membrane
△ = Solute molecule

FIG. 11-5 The process of osmosis to generate a concentration equilibrium (but not a volume equilibrium) for a solute particle that cannot move through a cell membrane.

Hypo-osmolar fluids have a *lower* osmotic pressure than isosmotic fluids, and water is pulled from the hypo-osmotic fluid space into the isosmotic fluid spaces of the interstitial and ICF fluids. As a result, the interstitial and ICF fluid volumes would expand, and the plasma volume would shrink. An example of a hypotonic IV fluid is 0.45% saline.

Clinical Application

Osmosis and filtration act together at the capillary membrane to maintain both extracellular fluid (ECF) and intracellular fluid (ICF) volumes within their normal ranges. The thirst mechanism is an example of how osmosis helps maintain homeostasis. The feeling of thirst is caused by the activation of cells in the brain that respond to changes in ECF osmolarity. These cells, so very sensitive to changes in ECF osmolarity, are called *osmoreceptors*. When an adult loses body water but most of the particles remain, such as through excessive sweating, ECF volume is decreased, and its osmolarity is increased (is hypertonic). The cells in the thirst center shrink as water moves from the cells into the hypertonic ECF. The shrinking of these cells triggers an adult's awareness of thirst and increases the urge to drink. Drinking replaces the amount of water lost through sweating and dilutes the ECF osmolarity, restoring it to normal.

? NCLEX EXAMINATION CHALLENGE 11-1

Physiological Integrity

What **immediate** response does the nurse expect as a result of infusing 1 L of an isotonic intravenous solution into a client over a 3-hour time period if urine output remains at 100 mL per hour?
A. Extracellular fluid (ECF) osmolarity increases; body weight increases.
B. Extracellular fluid (ECF) osmolarity decreases; body weight decreases.
C. Extracellular fluid (ECF) osmolarity is unchanged; body weight increases.
D. Extracellular fluid (ECF) osmolarity is unchanged; body weight decreases.

FLUID BALANCE

BODY FLUIDS

Fluid balance is closely linked to and affected by electrolyte concentrations. Table 11-1 lists the normal ranges of the major serum electrolytes. Chart 11-1 lists the normal electrolyte values for people older than 60 years.

Age, gender, and amount of fat affect the amount and distribution of body fluids. An older adult has less total body water than a younger adult. Chart 11-2 shows age-related changes in fluid balance. An obese adult has less total water than a lean adult of the same weight because fat cells contain almost no water.

🧑 GENDER HEALTH CONSIDERATIONS

Patient-Centered Care QSEN

Women of any age have less total body water and a higher risk for dehydration than men of similar sizes and ages. This difference is because men tend to have more muscle mass than women and because women have more body fat. (Muscle cells contain mostly water, and fat cells have little water.)

Body fluids are constantly filtered and replaced as fluid balance is maintained through intake and output. The total amount of water in each fluid space is stable, but water in all spaces is exchanged continually while maintaining constant fluid volume.

Fluid intake is regulated through the thirst drive. Fluid enters the body as liquids and solid foods, which contain up to 85% water (Table 11-2). A rising blood osmolarity or a decreasing blood volume triggers the sensation of thirst (Arai et al., 2013). An adult takes in about 2300 mL of fluid daily from food and liquids.

Fluid loss occurs through several routes (see Table 11-2). The kidney is the most important and the most sensitive water loss route because it is regulated and adjustable. The volume

TABLE 11-1	Serum Electrolyte Concentrations and Significance of Abnormal Values		
ELECTROLYTE	**REFERENCE RANGE**	**CANADIAN UNITS**	**SIGNIFICANCE OF ABNORMAL VALUES**
Sodium (Na⁺)	136-145 mEq/L	136-145 mmol/L	*Elevated:* Hypernatremia; dehydration; kidney disease; hypercortisolism *Low:* Hyponatremia; fluid overload; liver disease; adrenal insufficiency
Potassium (K⁺)	3.5-5.0 mEq/L	3.5-5.0 mmol/L	*Elevated:* Hyperkalemia; dehydration; kidney disease; acidosis; adrenal insufficiency; crush injuries *Low:* Hypokalemia; fluid overload; diuretic therapy; alkalosis; insulin administration; hyperaldosteronism
Calcium (Ca²⁺)	9.0-10.5 mg/dL	2.25-2.75 mmol/L	*Elevated:* Hypercalcemia; hyperthyroidism; hyperparathyroidism *Low:* Hypocalcemia; vitamin D deficiency; hypothyroidism; hypoparathyroidism; kidney disease; excessive intake of phosphorus-containing foods and drinks
Chloride (Cl⁻)	98-106 mEq/L	98-106 mmol/L	*Elevated:* Hyperchloremia; metabolic acidosis; respiratory alkalosis; hypercortisolism *Low:* Hypochloremia; fluid overload; excessive vomiting or diarrhea; adrenal insufficiency; diuretic therapy
Magnesium (Mg²⁺)	1.8-2.6 mEq/L	0.74-1.07 mmol/L	*Elevated:* Hypermagnesemia; kidney disease; hypothyroidism; adrenal insufficiency *Low:* Hypomagnesemia; malnutrition; alcoholism; ketoacidosis

Data from Pagana, K., Pagana, T., & Pagana, T. (2017). *Mosby's diagnostic and laboratory test reference* (13th ed.). St. Louis: Mosby; and Pagana, K., Pagana, T., & Pike-MacDonald, S. (2013). *Mosby's Canadian manual of diagnostic and laboratory tests* (1st ed.). St. Louis: Mosby.

CHART 11-1   Nursing Focus on the Older Adult

Normal Plasma Electrolyte Values for People Older Than 60 Years

	REFERENCE RANGE		CANADIAN UNITS	
ELECTROLYTE	60-90 YEARS	>90 YEARS	60-90 YEARS	>90 YEARS
Calcium (Ca^{2+})	9.0-10.5 mg/dL	8.2-9.6 mg/dL	2.2-2.75 mmol/L	2.05-2.40 mmol/L
Chloride (Cl^-)	98-106 mEq/L	98-111 mEq/L	98-106 mmol/L	98-111 mmol/L
Magnesium (Mg^{2+})	1.8-2.6 mEq/L	1.8-2.6 mEq/L	0.74-1.07 mmol/L	0.74-1.07 mmol/L
Potassium (K^+)	3.5-5.0 mEq/L	3.5-5.0 mEq/L	3.5-5.0 mmol/L	3.5-5.0 mmol/L
Sodium (Na^+)	136-145 mEq/L	132-146 mEq/L	136-145 mmol/L	132-146 mmol/L

Data for adults >90 years from Tietz, N. W. (Ed.). (1995). *Clinical guide to laboratory tests* (3rd ed.). Philadelphia: Saunders.
Data for adults 60 to 90 years from Pagana, K., Pagana, T., & Pagana, T. (2017). *Mosby's diagnostic and laboratory test reference* (13th ed.). St. Louis: Mosby; and Pagana, K., Pagana, T., & Pike-MacDonald, S. (2013). *Mosby's Canadian manual of diagnostic and laboratory tests* (1st ed.). St. Louis: Mosby.

CHART 11-2   Nursing Focus on the Older Adult

Impact of Age-Related Changes on Fluid Balance

SYSTEM	CHANGE	RESULT
Skin	Loss of elasticity Decreased turgor Decreased oil production	Skin becomes an unreliable indicator of fluid status, especially the back of the hand Dry, easily damaged skin
Kidney	Decreased glomerular filtration Decreased concentrating capacity	Poor excretion of waste products Increased water loss, increasing the risk for dehydration
Muscular	Decreased muscle mass	Decreased total body water Greater risk for dehydration
Neurologic	Diminished thirst reflex	Decreased fluid intake, increasing the risk for dehydration
Endocrine	Adrenal atrophy	Poor regulation of sodium and potassium, increasing the risk for hyponatremia and hyperkalemia

Data from Touhy, T., & Jett, K. (2016). *Ebersole and Hess' toward health aging* (9th ed.). St. Louis: Mosby.

TABLE 11-2   Routes of Fluid Ingestion and Excretion

INTAKE	OUTPUT
Measurable	
Oral fluids	Urine
Parenteral fluids	Emesis
Enemas*	Feces
Irrigation fluids*	Drainage from body cavities
Not Measurable	
Solid foods	Perspiration
Metabolism	Vaporization through the lungs

*Measured by subtracting the amount returned from the amount instilled.

control it. In a healthy adult insensible water loss is about 500 to 1000 mL/day. This loss increases greatly during thyroid crisis, trauma, burns, states of extreme stress, and fever. Patients at risk for excess insensible water loss include those being mechanically ventilated, those with rapid respirations, and those undergoing continuous GI suctioning. Water loss through stool increases greatly with severe diarrhea or excessive fistula drainage. If not balanced by intake, insensible loss can lead to severe dehydration and electrolyte imbalances.

HORMONAL REGULATION OF FLUID BALANCE

Three hormones help control FLUID AND ELECTROLYTE BALANCE. These are aldosterone, antidiuretic hormone (ADH), and natriuretic peptide (NP).

Aldosterone is secreted by the adrenal cortex whenever sodium levels in the extracellular fluid (ECF) are low. Aldosterone prevents both water and sodium loss. When aldosterone is secreted, it acts on the kidney nephrons, triggering them to reabsorb sodium and water from the urine back into the blood. This action increases blood osmolarity and blood volume. Aldosterone also promotes kidney potassium excretion.

Antidiuretic hormone (ADH), or vasopressin, is released from the posterior pituitary gland in response to changes in blood osmolarity. The hypothalamus contains the osmoreceptors that are sensitive to changes in blood osmolarity. Increased blood

lost through urine elimination daily varies, depending on the amount of fluid taken in and the body's need to conserve fluids.

The minimum amount of urine per day needed to excrete toxic waste products is 400 to 600 mL. This minimum volume is called the obligatory urine output. If the 24-hour urine output falls below the obligatory output amount, wastes are retained and can cause lethal electrolyte imbalances, acidosis, and a toxic buildup of nitrogen.

The ability of the kidneys to make either concentrated or very dilute urine helps maintain fluid balance. The kidney works with various hormones to maintain fluid balance when extracellular fluid (ECF) concentrations, volumes, or pressures change.

Other normal water loss occurs through the skin, the lungs, and the intestinal tract. Water losses also can result from salivation, drainage from fistulas and drains, and GI suction. This loss is called insensible water loss because no mechanisms osmolarity, especially an increase in the level of plasma sodium, results in a slight shrinkage of these cells and triggers ADH release from the posterior pituitary gland. Because the action of ADH retains just water, it only indirectly regulates electrolyte retention or excretion.

ADH acts on kidney nephrons, making them more permeable to water. As a result, more water is *reabsorbed* by these tubules and returned to the blood, decreasing blood osmolarity by making it more dilute. When blood osmolarity decreases with low plasma sodium levels, the osmoreceptors swell slightly and inhibit ADH release. Less water is then reabsorbed, and more is excreted in the urine, bringing extracellular fluid (ECF) osmolarity up to normal.

Natriuretic peptides (NPs) are hormones secreted by special cells that line the atria of the heart (atrial natriuretic peptide [ANP]) and the ventricles of the heart. (The peptide secreted by the heart ventricular cells is known as brain natriuretic peptide [BNP].) These peptides are secreted in response to increased blood volume and blood pressure, which stretch the heart tissue. NP binds to receptors in the nephrons, creating effects that are opposite of aldosterone. Kidney reabsorption of sodium is inhibited at the same time that urine output is increased. The outcome is decreased circulating blood volume and decreased blood osmolarity.

SIGNIFICANCE OF FLUID BALANCE

The Renin-Angiotensin II Pathway

The most important body fluids to keep in balance for optimal function are the blood volume (plasma volume) and the fluid inside the cells (intracellular fluid). Maintaining blood volume at a sufficient level for blood pressure to remain high enough to ensure adequate PERFUSION is critical for life. A major regulator of fluid balance is the renin-angiotensin II pathway, also known as the renin-angiotensin system (RAS).

Because low blood volume and low blood pressure can rapidly lead to death, the body has many compensatory mechanisms that guard against low plasma volume. These involve specific responses to change how water and sodium are handled to maintain blood pressure.

Because the kidney is a major regulator of water and sodium balance to maintain blood pressure and perfusion to all tissues and organs, the kidneys monitor blood pressure, blood volume, blood oxygen levels, and blood osmolarity (related to sodium concentration). When the kidneys sense that any one of these parameters is getting low, they begin to secrete a substance called *renin* that sets into motion a group of hormonal and blood vessel responses to ensure that blood pressure is raised back up to normal. Fig. 11-6 summarizes these responses.

So the triggering event for renin secretion is any change in the blood indicating that PERFUSION is at risk. Low blood pressure is a triggering event because it reduces perfusion to tissues and organs. Anything that reduces blood volume (e.g., dehydration, hemorrhage) below a critical level *always* lowers blood pressure. Low blood oxygen levels also are triggering events because with too little oxygen in the blood it cannot supply the needed oxygen and the tissues and organs could die. A low blood sodium level also is a triggering event because sodium and water are closely linked. Where sodium goes, water follows.

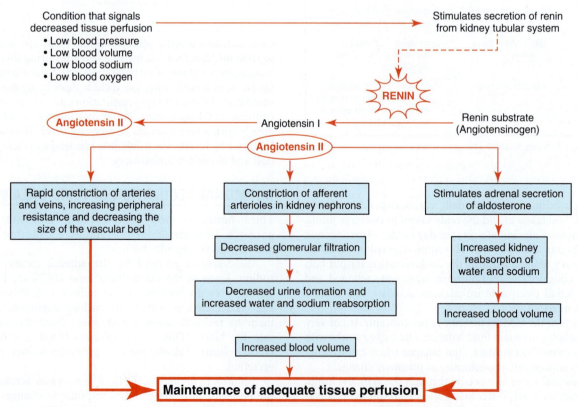

FIG. 11-6 The role of the renin-angiotensin II pathway in fluid and electrolyte balance and blood pressure regulation.

So anything that causes the blood to have too little sodium prevents water from staying in the blood. The result is low blood volume with low blood pressure and poor tissue perfusion.

Once the kidneys sense that PERFUSION is at risk, special cells in the kidney tubule begin to secrete renin into the blood. Renin then activates *angiotensinogen*. Activated angiotensinogen is *angiotensin I*, which is activated by the enzyme *angiotensin-converting enzyme* or *ACE* to its most active form, angiotensin II (McCance et al., 2014).

Angiotensin II starts several actions to increase blood volume and blood pressure. First it constricts arteries and veins throughout the body. This action increases peripheral resistance and reduces the size of the vascular bed, which raises blood pressure as a compensatory mechanism without adding more blood volume. Angiotensin II also constricts the size of the arterioles that feed the kidney nephrons. This action results in a lower glomerular filtration rate and a huge reduction of urine output. Decreasing urine output prevents further water loss so more is retained in the blood to help raise blood pressure. Angiotensin II also causes the adrenal glands to secrete the hormone aldosterone. Aldosterone is nicknamed the "water-and-sodium-saving hormone" because it causes the kidneys to reabsorb water and sodium, preventing them from being excreted into the urine. This response allows more water and sodium to be returned to the blood, increasing blood pressure, blood volume, and PERFUSION.

Clinical Application

The renin-angiotensin II pathway is stimulated whenever the patient is in shock. This is why urine output is used as an indicator of PERFUSION adequacy after surgery or any time the patient has undergone an invasive procedure and is at risk for hemorrhage.

This pathway also is related to management of *hypertension* (high blood pressure). Patients who have hypertension are often asked to limit their intake of sodium. The reason for this is that a high sodium intake raises the blood level of sodium, causing more water to be retained in the blood volume and raising blood pressure. Drug therapy for hypertension management may include diuretic drugs that increase the excretion of sodium so less is present in the blood, resulting in a lower blood volume. Another class of drugs often used to manage blood pressure is the "ACE inhibitors" (ACEIs). These drugs disrupt the renin-angiotensin II pathway by reducing the amount of angiotensin-converting enzyme (ACE) made so less angiotensin II is present. With less angiotensin II, there is less vasoconstriction and reduced peripheral resistance, less aldosterone production, and greater excretion of water and sodium in the urine. All of these responses lead to decreased blood volume and blood pressure. Another class of drugs used to manage hypertension is the angiotensin receptor blockers (ARBs). These drugs disrupt the renin-angiotensin II pathway by blocking the receptors that bind with angiotensin II so the tissues cannot respond to it and blood pressure is lowered. The most recent class of drugs to manage hypertension by changing the renin-angiotensin II pathway is the direct renin inhibitors. These drugs act early in the pathway and prevent the enzyme renin from changing angiotensinogen into angiotensin I. These drugs may be combined with an ARB to block the pathway in more than one place, leading to greater reduction in blood pressure. See Chapter 36 for more information about antihypertensive agents.

DISTURBANCES OF FLUID AND ELECTROLYTE BALANCE

 FLUID AND ELECTROLYTE BALANCE CONCEPT EXEMPLAR Dehydration

❖ *PATHOPHYSIOLOGY*

In **dehydration** fluid intake or retention is less than what is needed to meet the body's fluid needs, resulting in a deficit of fluid volume, especially plasma volume. It is a condition rather than a disease and can be caused by many factors (Table 11-3). Dehydration may be an *actual* decrease in total body water caused by either too little intake of fluid or too great a loss of fluid. It also can occur without an actual loss of total body water such as when water shifts from the plasma into the interstitial space. This condition is called *relative* dehydration.

CONSIDERATIONS FOR OLDER ADULTS
Patient-Centered Care (QSEN)

Older adults are at high risk for dehydration because they have less total body water than younger adults. In addition, many older adults have decreased thirst sensation and may have difficulty with walking or other motor skills needed for obtaining fluids. They also may take drugs such as diuretics, antihypertensives, and laxatives that increase fluid excretion. Assess the FLUID AND ELECTROLYTE BALANCE status of all older adults in any setting.

Dehydration may occur with just water (fluid) loss or with water and electrolyte loss (isotonic dehydration). *Isotonic dehydration is the most common type of fluid loss problem.* Fluid is lost only from the extracellular fluid (ECF) space, including both the plasma and the interstitial spaces. There is no shift of fluids between spaces, so the intracellular fluid (ICF) volume remains normal (Fig. 11-7). Circulating blood volume is decreased (**hypovolemia**) and leads to reduced perfusion. The body's defenses compensate during dehydration to maintain

TABLE 11-3 **Common Causes of Fluid Imbalances**	
Dehydration	**Fluid Overload**
• Hemorrhage	• Excessive fluid replacement
• Vomiting	• Kidney failure (late phase)
• Diarrhea	• Heart failure
• Profuse salivation	• Long-term corticosteroid therapy
• Fistulas	• Syndrome of inappropriate antidiuretic hormone (SIADH)
• Ileostomy	
• Profuse diaphoresis	• Psychiatric disorders with polydipsia
• Burns	
• Severe wounds	• Water intoxication
• Long-term NPO status	
• Diuretic therapy	
• GI suction	
• Hyperventilation	
• Diabetes insipidus	
• Difficulty swallowing	
• Impaired thirst	
• Unconsciousness	
• Fever	
• Impaired motor function	

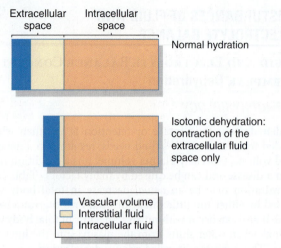

Extracellular space   Intracellular space

Normal hydration

Isotonic dehydration: contraction of the extracellular fluid space only

■ Vascular volume
□ Interstitial fluid
■ Intracellular fluid

FIG. 11-7 Changes in fluid compartment volumes with dehydration. (© 1992 by M. Linda Workman. All rights reserved.)

PERFUSION to vital organs in spite of hypovolemia. The main defense is increasing vasoconstriction and peripheral resistance to maintain blood pressure and circulation.

Health Promotion and Maintenance

Mild dehydration is very common among healthy adults and is corrected or prevented easily by matching fluid intake with fluid output. Teach all adults to drink more fluids, especially water, whenever they engage in heavy or prolonged physical activity or live in dry climates or at higher altitudes. Beverages with caffeine can increase fluid loss, as can drinks containing alcohol; thus these beverages should not be used to prevent or treat dehydration.

❖ INTERPROFESSIONAL COLLABORATIVE CARE

Dehydration can occur in any setting. Mild dehydration can be managed in the home or other residential setting. Severe dehydration may require temporary hospitalization, depending on the cause and the effects on PERFUSION.

◆ Assessment: Noticing

History. Ask specific questions about food and liquid intake. Also assess the types of fluids and foods ingested to determine amount and osmolarity. Many patients do not know that solid foods contain liquid. Other foods such as ice cream, gelatin, and ices are liquids at body temperature and are included when calculating fluid intake.

Collect specific information about exact intake and output volumes and obtain serial daily weight measurements. If possible, weigh the patient directly rather than asking what he or she weighs. Weight loss is an indication of dehydration. *Because 1 L of water weighs 2.2 lbs (1 kg), changes in daily weights are the best indicators of fluid losses or gains. A weight change of 1 lb corresponds to a fluid volume change of about 500 mL.*

Ask specific questions about prescribed and over-the-counter drugs and check the dosage, the length of time taken, and the patient's adherence to the drug regimen. Older adults may use diuretics or laxatives that can lead to impaired FLUID AND ELECTROLYTE BALANCE.

Ask about the presence of kidney or endocrine diseases. Assess the patient's level of consciousness and mental status because changes in mental status occur with fluid imbalance.

Ask the patient about changes in ring or shoe tightness. A sudden decrease in tightness may indicate dehydration.

Physical Assessment/Signs and Symptoms. Nearly all body systems are affected by dehydration to some degree. The most obvious changes occur in the cardiovascular and integumentary systems.

Cardiovascular changes are good indicators of hydration status because of the relationship between plasma fluid volume, blood pressure, and PERFUSION. Heart rate increases to help maintain blood pressure with less blood volume. Peripheral pulses are weak, difficult to find, and easily blocked. Blood pressure also decreases, as does pulse pressure, with a greater decrease in diastolic blood pressure. Hypotension is more severe with the patient in the standing position than in the sitting or lying position (**orthostatic** or **postural hypotension**). Measure blood pressure first with the patient lying down, then sitting, and finally standing. (These measures are also called *ortho checks* or *ortho changes*.) As the blood pressure decreases when changing position, perfusion to the brain decreases, causing light-headedness and dizziness. This problem increases the risk for falling, especially among older adults.

Neck veins are normally distended when a patient is in the supine position, and hand veins are distended when lower than the level of the heart. Neck veins normally flatten when the patient moves to a sitting position. With dehydration, neck and hand veins are flat, even when the neck and hands are not raised above the level of the heart.

Respiratory changes include an increased rate because the decreased blood volume reduces perfusion and gas exchange. The increased respiratory rate is a compensatory mechanism that attempts to maintain oxygen delivery when perfusion is decreased.

Skin changes can indicate dehydration. Assess the skin and mucous membranes for color, moisture, and turgor. Assess skin turgor by checking:
- How easily the skin over the back of the hand and arm can be gently pinched between the thumb and the forefinger to form a "tent"
- How soon the pinched skin resumes its normal position after release

In dehydration skin turgor is poor, with the tent remaining for minutes after pinching the skin. The skin is dry and scaly.

CONSIDERATIONS FOR OLDER ADULTS
Patient-Centered Care QSEN

Assess skin turgor in an older adult by pinching the skin over the sternum or on the forehead rather than on the back of the hand (Fig. 11-8). With aging the skin loses elasticity and tents on hands and arms even when the adult is well hydrated.

In dehydration oral mucous membranes may be dry and covered with a thick, sticky coating and may have cracks and fissures. The tongue surface may have deep furrows.

Neurologic changes with dehydration include changes in mental status and temperature with reduced PERFUSION in the brain. Changes in cognition are more common among older adults and may be the first indication of a fluid imbalance.

The patient with dehydration often has a low-grade fever, and fever can also cause dehydration. For every degree (Celsius)

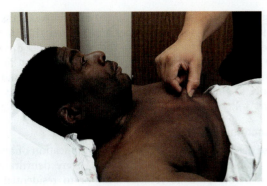

FIG. 11-8 Examining the skin turgor of an older patient.

increase in body temperature above normal, a minimum of an additional 500 mL of body fluid is lost.

Kidney changes in dehydration affect urine volume and concentration. Monitor urine output, comparing total output with total fluid intake and daily weights. The urine may be concentrated, with a specific gravity greater than 1.030, and have a dark amber color and a strong odor. *Urine output below 500 mL/day for a patient without kidney disease is cause for concern.* Use daily weights to assess fluid loss. Weight loss over a half pound per day is fluid loss.

Laboratory Assessment. No single laboratory test result confirms or rules out dehydration. Instead dehydration is determined by laboratory findings along with signs and symptoms (see Table 11-1). Usually laboratory findings with dehydration show elevated levels of hemoglobin, hematocrit, serum osmolarity, glucose, protein, blood urea nitrogen, and electrolytes because more water is lost and other substances remain, increasing blood concentration (hemoconcentration). Hemoconcentration is not present when dehydration is caused by hemorrhage because loss of all blood and plasma products occurs together.

？ NCLEX EXAMINATION CHALLENGE 11-2

Safe and Effective Care Environment

When evaluating the hydration status of a new 84-year-old nursing home client, the nurse observes tenting of the skin on the back of the client's hand. What is the nurse's **best** action?
A. Assess the skin turgor on the client's forehead.
B. Ask the client when he or she last had anything to drink.
C. Examine the client's dependent body areas, especially the ankles.
D. Document this observation in the client's record as the only action.

◆ Analysis: Interpreting

The priority problems for the patient who has dehydration are:
1. Dehydration due to excess fluid loss or inadequate fluid intake
2. Potential for injury due to blood pressure changes and muscle weakness

◆ Planning and Implementation: Responding

The focus of management for the patient with dehydration is to prevent further fluid loss, to increase fluid volumes to normal, and to prevent injury. Nursing priorities include fluid replacement, drug therapy, and patient safety.

◎ CHART 11-3 Best Practice for Patient Safety & Quality Care QSEN

The Patient With Dehydration

- When possible, provide oral fluids that meet the patient's dietary restrictions (e.g., sugar-free, low-sodium, thickened).
- Collaborate with other members of the interprofessional team to determine the amount of fluids needed during a 24-hour period.
- Ensure that fluids are offered and ingested on an even schedule at least every 2 hours throughout 24 hours.
- Teach unlicensed assistive personnel to actively participate in the hydration therapy and not to withhold fluids to prevent incontinence.
- Infuse prescribed IV fluids at a rate consistent with hydration needs and any known cardiac, pulmonary, or kidney problems.
- Monitor the patient's response to fluid therapy at least every 2 hours for indicators of adequate rehydration or the need for continuing therapy, especially:
  - Pulse quality
  - Urine output
  - Pulse pressure
  - Weight (every 8 hours)
- Monitor for and report indicators of fluid overload, including:
  - Bounding pulse
  - Difficulty breathing
  - Neck vein distention in the upright position
  - Presence of dependent edema
- Assess the IV line and the infusion site at least hourly for indications of infiltration, extravasation, or phlebitis (e.g., swelling around the site, pain, cordlike veins, reduced drip rate).
- Administer drugs prescribed to correct the underlying cause of the dehydration (e.g., antiemetics, antidiarrheals, antibiotics, antipyretics).

Restoring Fluid Balance

Planning: Expected Outcomes. The patient with dehydration is expected to have sufficient fluid volume for adequate perfusion. Indicators include that the patient has:
- Blood pressure at or near his or her normal range
- Daily urine output within 500 mL of total daily fluid intake (or at least 30 mL per hour)
- Moist mucous membranes
- Normal skin turgor

Interventions. Interventions for restoring fluid balance include fluid replacement and drug therapy.

Fluid Replacement. Replacement of fluids is key to correcting dehydration and preventing death from reduced PERFUSION. Best practices for nursing care of the patient with dehydration are listed in Chart 11-3. Mild-to-moderate dehydration is corrected with oral fluid replacement if the patient is alert enough to swallow and can tolerate oral fluids. Encourage fluid intake and measure the amount ingested.

Provide fluid the patient enjoys and time the intake schedule. Dividing the total amount of fluids needed by nursing shifts helps meet fluid needs more evenly over 24 hours with less danger of overload. Offer the conscious patient small volumes of fluids hourly.

Coordinate with unlicensed assistive personnel (UAP) to meet patients' specific fluid needs. Teach UAP to offer 60 to 120 mL of fluid every hour to patients who are dehydrated or who are at risk for dehydration. If incontinence is a concern, ensure that UAP understand that withholding fluids is not appropriate to prevent the problem. Instruct them to take the time to stay with patients while they drink the fluid and to note the exact amount ingested.

Use of oral rehydration solutions (ORSs) for rehydration therapy is an effective way to replace fluids. Specifically formulated solutions containing glucose and electrolytes are absorbed even when the patient is vomiting or has diarrhea. These are more often used in the home setting; in long-term care; and for patients who have poor veins, making IV therapy difficult. A variety of commercial ORSs are available over the counter.

When dehydration is severe or the patient cannot tolerate oral fluids, IV fluid replacement is needed. Calculation of how much fluid to replace is based on the patient's weight loss and symptoms. The rate of fluid replacement depends on the degree of dehydration and the patient's cardiac, pulmonary, or kidney status.

The type of fluid prescribed varies with the patient's cardiac status and blood osmolarity (Bridges, 2013; Pierce et al., 2016). Crystalloids are IV fluids that contain water, minerals (electrolytes), and sometimes other water-soluble substances such as glucose. These fluids rapidly disperse to all body fluid compartments and are most useful when dehydration includes both the intracellular and extracellular compartments. Colloids are IV fluids that contain larger non–water-soluble molecules that increase the osmotic pressure in the plasma volume. These fluids are most useful in helping to maintain plasma volume with a lower infused volume (Pierce et al., 2016). Table 11-4 lists types of common IV fluids. *The two most important areas to monitor during rehydration are pulse rate and quality and urine output.*

Drug Therapy. Drug therapy may correct some causes of the dehydration. Antidiarrheal drugs are prescribed when diarrhea causes dehydration. Antimicrobial therapy may be used in patients with bacterial diarrhea. Antiemetics may be used when vomiting causes dehydration. Antipyretics to reduce fever are helpful when fever makes dehydration worse.

Preventing Injury

Planning: Expected Outcomes. The patient with dehydration is expected to avoid injury. Indicators include that the patient:
- Asks for assistance when ambulating
- Does not fall

Interventions. Patient safety issues and strategies are priorities of care before and during other therapies for dehydration. Monitor vital signs, especially heart rate and blood pressure. The patient with dehydration is at risk for falls because of orthostatic hypotension, dysrhythmia, muscle weakness, and possible confusion. Assess his or her muscle strength, gait stability, and level of alertness. Instruct the patient to get up slowly from a lying or sitting position and to immediately sit down if he or she feels light-headed. Stress the importance of asking for assistance to ambulate. Implement other fall precautions listed in Chart 3-4.

Care Coordination and Transition Management

Because dehydration is a symptom or complication of another health problem or drug therapy, even severe dehydration is resolved before patients return home or to residential care. Education is the most important management strategy to prevent recurrence among adults who remain at some risk for recurrence such as patients who have diabetes insipidus or diabetes mellitus. See Chapter 62 for a detailed discussion of the care coordination needed for diabetes insipidus and Chapter 64 for care coordination for diabetes mellitus.

◆ *Evaluation: Reflecting*

Depending on the cause of dehydration, most patients return to an acceptable fluid balance with proper management. Indications that the patient's underlying cause of dehydration is well managed and that the imbalance is corrected include that the patient:
- Maintains a daily fluid intake of at least 1500 mL (or drinks at least 500 mL more than his or her daily urine output)
- Can state the indications of dehydration

❓ NCLEX EXAMINATION CHALLENGE 11-3
Safe and Effective Care Environment

For which clients is it **most** important for the nurse to check frequently for dehydration? **Select all that apply.**
A. 24-year-old athlete who is NPO for 4 hours awaiting an appendectomy
B. 42-year-old client who has diabetes insipidus
C. 56-year-old client recently diagnosed with syndrome of inappropriate antidiuretic hormone (SIADH)
D. 68-year-old client with poorly controlled type 2 diabetes mellitus
E. 72-year-old client taking 80 mg of furosemide orally every day
F. 74-year-old undergoing a bowel preparation with multiple enemas before colon surgery

TABLE 11-4 Characteristics of Common Intravenous Therapy Solutions

SOLUTION	OSMOLARITY (mOsm/L)	pH	CALORIES (Kcal) PER LITER	TONICITY
0.9% saline	308	5	0	Isotonic
0.45% saline	154	5	0	Hypotonic
5% dextrose in water (D$_5$W)	272	3.5-6.5	170	Isotonic*
10% dextrose in water (D$_{10}$W)	500	3.5-6.5	340	Hypertonic*
5% dextrose in 0.9% saline	560	3.5-6.5	170	Hypertonic*
5% dextrose in 0.45% saline	406	4	170	Hypertonic*
5% dextrose in 0.225% saline	321	4	170	Isotonic*
Ringer's lactate	273	6.5	9	Isotonic
5% dextrose in Ringer's lactate	525	4-6.5	179	Hypertonic*

Data from Trissel, L. (2013). *Handbook on injectable drugs* (17th ed.). Bethesda, MD: American Society of Hospital-System Pharmacists.
*Solution tonicity at the time of administration. Within a short time after administration, the dextrose is metabolized, and the tonicity of the infused solution decreases in proportion to the osmolarity or tonicity of the nondextrose components (electrolytes) within the water.

- Starts fluid replacement at the first indication of dehydration
- Correctly follows treatment plans for ongoing health problems that increase the risk for dehydration

FLUID OVERLOAD

❖ PATHOPHYSIOLOGY

Fluid overload, also called *overhydration*, is an excess of body fluid. It is a clinical indication of a problem in which fluid intake or retention is *greater* than the body's fluid needs. The most common type of fluid overload is hypervolemia (Fig. 11-9) because the problems result from excessive fluid in the extracellular fluid (ECF) space. Most problems caused by fluid overload are related to excessive fluid in the vascular space or to dilution of specific electrolytes and blood components. The conditions leading to fluid overload are related to excessive intake or inadequate excretion of fluids. See Table 11-3 for causes of fluid overload. Fig. 11-10 outlines the adaptive changes the body makes in response to mild or moderate fluid overload, especially increased urine output, and edema formation. When overload is severe or occurs in an adult with poor cardiac or kidney function,

it can lead to heart failure and pulmonary edema. Dilution of sodium and potassium can lead to seizures, coma, and death.

❖ INTERPROFESSIONAL COLLABORATIVE CARE

◆ Assessment: Noticing

Patients with fluid overload often have pitting edema (Fig. 11-11). Other symptoms are usually seen in the cardiovascular, respiratory, neuromuscular, integumentary, and GI systems (Chart 11-4).

Fluid overload is diagnosed based on assessment findings and the results of laboratory tests. Usually serum electrolyte values are normal; but decreased hemoglobin, hematocrit, and serum protein levels may result from excessive water in the vascular space (**hemodilution**).

◆ Interventions: Responding

The focus of priority nursing interventions is to ensure patient safety, restore normal fluid balance, provide supportive care until the imbalance is resolved, and prevent future fluid overload. Drug therapy, nutrition therapy, and monitoring are the basis of intervention.

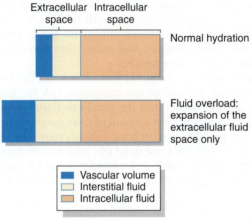

FIG. 11-9 Changes in fluid compartment volumes with fluid overload. (© 1992 by M. Linda Workman. All rights reserved.)

Extracellular space | Intracellular space — Normal hydration

Fluid overload: expansion of the extracellular fluid space only

■ Vascular volume
□ Interstitial fluid
■ Intracellular fluid

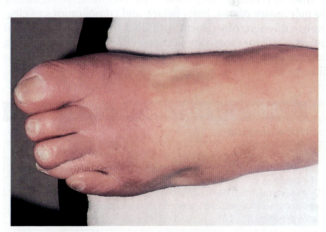

FIG. 11-11 Pitting edema of the left foot and ankle.

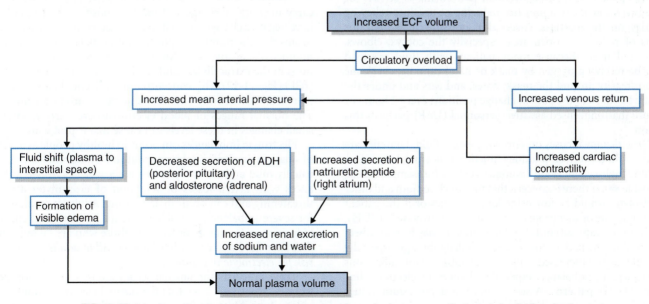

FIG. 11-10 Adaptive actions and mechanisms to prevent cardiac and pulmonary complications during fluid overload. (*ADH*, Antidiuretic hormone; *ECF*, extracellular fluid.)

CHART 11-4 Key Features

Fluid Overload

Cardiovascular Changes
- Increased pulse rate
- Bounding pulse quality
- Elevated blood pressure
- Decreased pulse pressure
- Elevated central venous pressure
- Distended neck and hand veins
- Engorged varicose veins
- Weight gain

Respiratory Changes
- Increased respiratory rate
- Shallow respirations
- Shortness of breath
- Moist crackles present on auscultation

Skin and Mucous Membrane Changes
- Pitting edema in dependent areas
- Skin pale and cool to touch

Neuromuscular Changes
- Altered level of consciousness
- Headache
- Visual disturbances
- Skeletal muscle weakness
- Paresthesias

Gastrointestinal Changes
- Increased motility
- Enlarged liver

Patient safety is the first priority. Interventions are implemented to prevent fluid overload from becoming worse, leading to pulmonary edema, heart failure, and complications of electrolyte dilution. Any patient with fluid overload, regardless of age, is at risk for these complications. Older adults or those with cardiac problems, kidney problems, pulmonary problems, or liver problems are at greater risk.

! NURSING SAFETY PRIORITY QSEN

Critical Rescue

Assess the patient with fluid overload at least every 2 hours to recognize pulmonary edema, which can occur very quickly and can lead to death. If indications of worsening fluid overload are present (bounding pulse, increasing neck vein distention, presence of crackles in lungs, increasing peripheral edema, reduced urine output), respond by notifying the health care provider.

The patient with fluid overload and edema is at risk for skin breakdown. Use a pressure-reducing or pressure-relieving overlay on the mattress. Assess skin pressure areas daily for signs of redness or open area, especially the coccyx, elbows, hips, and heels. Because many patients with fluid overload may be receiving oxygen by mask or nasal cannula, check the skin integrity around the mask, nares, and ears and under the elastic band. Help the patient change positions every 2 hours or ensure that unlicensed assistive personnel (UAP) perform this action.

Drug therapy focuses on removing excess fluid. Diuretics are used for fluid overload if kidney function is normal. Drugs may include high-ceiling (loop) diuretics such as furosemide (Lasix, Furoside ✦). If there is concern that too much sodium and other electrolytes would be lost using loop diuretics or if the patient has syndrome of inappropriate antidiuretic hormone (SIADH), conivaptan (Vaprisol) or tolvaptan (Samsca) may be prescribed.

Monitor the patient for response to drug therapy, especially weight loss and increased urine output. Observe for indications of electrolyte imbalance, especially changes in electrocardiogram (ECG) patterns. Assess sodium and potassium values every 8 hours or whenever they are drawn.

Nutrition therapy for the patient with *chronic* fluid overload may involve restrictions of both fluid and sodium intake. Often sodium restriction involves only "no added salt" to ordinary table foods when fluid overload is mild. For more severe fluid overload, the patient may be restricted to 2 g/day to 4 g/day of sodium. When sodium restriction is ongoing, teach the patient and family how to check food labels for sodium content and how to keep a daily record of sodium ingested. Explain to the patient and family the reason for any fluid restriction and the importance of adhering to the restriction.

Monitoring intake and output and weight provides information on therapy effectiveness. Teach UAP that these measurements need to be accurate, not just estimated, because treatment decisions are based on these findings. Schedule fluid offerings throughout the 24 hours. Teach UAP to check urine for color and character and to report these findings. If the patient is receiving IV therapy, infuse the exact amount prescribed.

Fluid retention may not be visible. Rapid weight gain is the best indicator of fluid retention and overload. Metabolism can account for only a half-pound (250 g) of weight gain in 1 day. Each pound (0.5 kg) of weight gained (after the first half pound) equates to about 500 mL of retained fluid. Weigh the patient at the same time every day (before breakfast), using the same scale. Have the patient wear the same type of clothing for each weigh-in. When in-bed weights are taken, lift tubing and equipment off the bed. Record the number of blankets and pillows on the bed at the initial weigh-in and ensure that ongoing weights always include the same number.

If the patient is discharged to home before the fluid overload has completely resolved or has continuing risk for fluid overload, teach him or her and the family to monitor weight at home. Teach them to keep a record of daily weights to show the health care provider at checkups. Patients may choose to use mobile "apps" to record and trend this information. Instruct the patient to call the health care provider for more than a 3-lb (1.5-kg) gain in a week or more than a 2-lb (1-kg) gain in 24 hours.

ELECTROLYTE BALANCE AND IMBALANCES

Electrolytes, or **ions**, are substances dissolved in body fluid that carry an electrical charge. **Cations** have positive charges; **anions** have negative charges. Body fluids are electrically neutral, which means that the number of positive ions is balanced by an equal number of negative ions. Most ions have different concentrations in the extracellular fluid (ECF) and the intracellular fluid (ICF) (Fig. 11-12). This concentration difference helps maintain membrane excitability and allows nerve impulse transmission. The normal ranges of blood electrolytes are narrow, so even small changes in these levels can cause major problems.

Electrolyte imbalances can occur in healthy people as a result of changes in fluid intake and output. These imbalances are usually mild and are easily corrected. Severe electrolyte imbalances with actual losses or retention of electrolytes are life threatening and can occur in any setting. Adults at greatest risk for severe imbalances are older patients, patients with chronic kidney or endocrine disorders, and those who are taking drugs that alter fluid and electrolyte balance. *All ill adults are at some risk for electrolyte imbalances.*

Table 11-1 lists the normal serum levels of the major electrolytes, and Chart 11-1 lists the normal electrolyte values for older adults. Most electrolytes enter the body in ingested food.

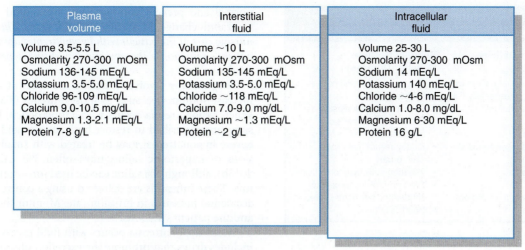

Plasma volume	Interstitial fluid	Intracellular fluid
Volume 3.5-5.5 L Osmolarity 270-300 mOsm Sodium 136-145 mEq/L Potassium 3.5-5.0 mEq/L Chloride 96-109 mEq/L Calcium 9.0-10.5 mg/dL Magnesium 1.3-2.1 mEq/L Protein 7-8 g/L	Volume ~10 L Osmolarity 270-300 mOsm Sodium 135-145 mEq/L Potassium 3.5-5.0 mEq/L Chloride ~118 mEq/L Calcium 7.0-9.0 mg/dL Magnesium ~1.3 mEq/L Protein ~2 g/L	Volume 25-30 L Osmolarity 270-300 mOsm Sodium 14 mEq/L Potassium 140 mEq/L Chloride ~4-6 mEq/L Calcium 1.0-8.0 mg/dL Magnesium 6-30 mEq/L Protein 16 g/L

FIG. 11-12 The electrolyte composition of various body fluids.

Electrolyte balance occurs when dietary intake of electrolytes matches kidney electrolyte excretion or reabsorption. For example, serum potassium level is maintained between 3.5 and 5.0 mEq/L (mmol/L). The high potassium level in foods such as meat and citrus fruit could increase the ECF potassium level and lead to major problems. In health, kidney excretion of potassium keeps pace with potassium intake and prevents major changes in the blood potassium level.

CONSIDERATIONS FOR OLDER ADULTS

Patient-Centered Care QSEN

> Older adults are at risk for electrolyte imbalances as a result of age-related organ changes. Always ask the older adult which drug(s) he or she takes because older adults are more likely to be taking drugs that affect fluid and electrolyte balance.

SODIUM

Sodium (Na$^+$) is the major *cation* (positively charged particle) in the extracellular fluid (ECF) and maintains ECF osmolarity. Sodium levels of the ECF are high (136 to 145 mEq/L [mmol/L]), and the intracellular fluid (ICF) sodium levels are low (about 14 mEq/L [mmol/L]). Keeping this difference in sodium levels is vital for muscle contraction, cardiac contraction, and nerve impulse transmission. Sodium levels and movement influence water balance because "where sodium goes, water follows." The ECF sodium level determines whether water is retained, excreted, or moved from one fluid space to another. Changes in plasma sodium levels seriously change fluid volume and the distribution of other electrolytes.

Sodium enters the body through the ingestion of many foods and fluids. Foods with the highest sodium levels are those that are processed or preserved such as smoked or pickled foods, snack foods, and many condiments. Foods lowest in sodium include fresh fish and poultry and most fresh vegetables and fruit.

Despite variation in daily sodium intake, blood sodium levels usually remain within the normal range. Serum sodium balance is regulated by the kidney under the influences of aldosterone, antidiuretic hormone (ADH), and natriuretic peptide (NP) (see the Hormonal Regulation of Fluid Balance section).

Low serum sodium levels inhibit the secretion of ADH and NP and trigger aldosterone secretion. Together these compensatory actions increase serum sodium levels by increasing kidney reabsorption of sodium and enhancing kidney loss of water.

High serum sodium levels inhibit aldosterone secretion and stimulate secretion of ADH and NP. Together these hormones increase kidney sodium excretion and water reabsorption.

HYPONATREMIA

❖ PATHOPHYSIOLOGY

Hyponatremia is an electrolyte imbalance in which the serum sodium (Na$^+$) level is below 136 mEq/L (mmol/L). Sodium imbalances often occur with a fluid imbalance because the same hormones regulate both sodium and water balance. The problems caused by hyponatremia occur from two changes—reduced excitable membrane depolarization and cellular swelling.

Excitable cell membrane depolarization depends on high extracellular fluid (ECF) levels of sodium being available to cross cell membranes and move into cells in response to a stimulus. Hyponatremia makes depolarization slower so excitable membranes are less excitable.

With hyponatremia the osmolarity of the ECF is lower than that of the intracellular fluid (ICF). As a result, water moves into the cell, causing swelling. Even a small amount of swelling can reduce cell function. Larger amounts of swelling can make the cell burst (*lysis*) and die.

Many conditions and drugs can lead to hyponatremia (Table 11-5). A common cause of low sodium levels is the prolonged use and overuse of diuretics, especially in older adults. When these drugs are used to manage fluid overload, sodium is lost along with water. Hyponatremia can result from the loss of total body sodium, the movement of sodium from the blood to other fluid spaces, or the dilution of serum sodium from excessive water in the plasma.

❖ INTERPROFESSIONAL COLLABORATIVE CARE

◆ Assessment: Noticing

The signs and symptoms of hyponatremia are caused by its effects on excitable cellular activity. The cells especially affected are those involved in cerebral, neuromuscular, and intestinal smooth muscle and cardiovascular functions.

TABLE 11-5 Common Causes of Hyponatremia

Actual Sodium Deficits	Relative Sodium Deficits (Dilution)
• Excessive diaphoresis	• Excessive ingestion of hypotonic fluids
• Diuretics (high-ceiling diuretics)	• Psychogenic polydipsia
• Wound drainage (especially GI)	• Freshwater submersion accident
• Decreased secretion of aldosterone	• Kidney failure (nephrotic syndrome)
• Hyperlipidemia	• Irrigation with hypotonic fluids
• Kidney disease (scarred distal convoluted tubule)	• Syndrome of inappropriate antidiuretic hormone secretion
• Nothing by mouth	• Heart failure
• Low-salt diet	
• Cerebral salt-wasting syndrome	
• Hyperglycemia	

Cerebral changes are the most obvious problems of hyponatremia. Behavioral changes result from cerebral edema and increased intracranial pressure. Closely observe and document the patient's behavior, level of consciousness, and cognition. A sudden onset of acute confusion or increased confusion is often seen in older adults who have low serum sodium levels (Reynolds, 2015). When sodium levels become very low, seizures, coma, and death may occur (Schreiber, 2013b).

Neuromuscular changes are seen as general muscle weakness. Assess the patient's neuromuscular status during each nursing shift for changes from baseline. Deep tendon reflexes diminish, and muscle weakness is worse in the legs and arms. Assess muscle strength and deep tendon reflex responses as described in Chapter 41.

! NURSING SAFETY PRIORITY QSEN
Action Alert

If muscle weakness is present, immediately check respiratory effectiveness because ventilation depends on adequate strength and function of respiratory muscles.

Intestinal changes include increased motility, causing nausea, diarrhea, and abdominal cramping. Assess the GI system by listening to bowel sounds and observing stools. Bowel sounds are hyperactive, and bowel movements are frequent and watery.

Cardiovascular changes are seen as changes in cardiac output. The cardiac responses to hyponatremia with **hypovolemia** (decreased plasma volume) include a rapid, weak, thready pulse. Peripheral pulses are difficult to palpate and are easily blocked. Blood pressure is decreased, and the patient may have severe orthostatic hypotension, leading to light-headedness or dizziness. The central venous pressure is low.

When hyponatremia occurs with **hypervolemia** (fluid overload), cardiac changes include a full or bounding pulse with normal or high blood pressure. Peripheral pulses are full and difficult to block; however, they may not be palpable if edema is present.

◆ Interventions: Responding

The cause of the low sodium level is determined to plan appropriate management. Interventions with drug therapy and nutrition therapy are used to restore serum sodium levels to normal and prevent complications from fluid overload or a too-rapid change in serum sodium level. *The priorities for nursing care of the patient with hyponatremia are monitoring the patient's response to therapy and preventing hypernatremia and fluid overload.*

Drug therapy involves reducing the doses of any drugs that increase sodium loss such as most diuretics (Kaufman, 2014). When hyponatremia occurs with a fluid deficit, IV saline infusions are prescribed to restore both sodium and fluid volume. Severe hyponatremia may be treated with small-volume infusions of hypertonic saline, most often 3% saline (Schreiber, 2013b), although 5% saline can be used for extreme hyponatremia. These infusions are delivered using a controller to prevent accidental increases in infusion rate. Monitor the infusion rate and the patient's response.

When hyponatremia occurs with fluid excess, drug therapy includes drugs that promote the excretion of water rather than sodium such as conivaptan (Vaprisol) or tolvaptan (Samsca) (Friedman & Cirulli, 2013). Drug therapy for hyponatremia caused by inappropriate secretion of antidiuretic hormone (ADH) may include lithium (Carbolith, Lithane ♣) and demeclocycline (Declomycin). Assess hourly for signs of excessive fluid loss, potassium loss, and increased sodium levels.

Nutrition therapy can help restore sodium balance in mild hyponatremia. Therapy involves increasing oral sodium intake and restricting oral fluid intake. Collaborate with the registered dietitian (RD) to teach the patient about which foods to increase in the diet. Fluid restriction may be needed long-term when fluid overload is the cause of the hyponatremia or when kidney fluid excretion is impaired. Nursing actions for patient safety, skin protection, monitoring, and patient and family teaching are the same as those for fluid overload.

? NCLEX EXAMINATION CHALLENGE 11-4
Safe and Effective Care Environment

A client is receiving 250 mL of a 3% sodium chloride solution intravenously for severe hyponatremia. Which signs or symptoms indicate to the nurse that this therapy is effective?
A. The client reports hand swelling.
B. Bowel sounds are present in all four abdominal quadrants.
C. Serum potassium level has decreased from 4.4 mEq/L (mmol/L) to 4.2 mEq/L (mmol/L).
D. Blood pressure has increased from 100/50 mm Hg to 112/70 mm Hg.

HYPERNATREMIA
❖ PATHOPHYSIOLOGY

Hypernatremia is a serum sodium level over 145 mEq/L (mmol/L). It can be caused by or can cause changes in fluid volume. Table 11-6 lists causes of hypernatremia.

As serum sodium level rises, a larger difference in sodium levels occurs between the extracellular fluid (ECF) and the intracellular fluid (ICF). More sodium is present to move rapidly across cell membranes during depolarization, making excitable tissues more easily excited. This condition is called **irritability**, and excitable tissues over-respond to stimuli. In addition, water moves from the cells into the ECF to dilute the hyperosmolar ECF. Thus, when serum sodium levels are high, severe cellular dehydration with cellular shrinkage occurs.

TABLE 11-6 Common Causes of Hypernatremia

Actual Sodium Excesses	Relative Sodium Excesses
• Hyperaldosteronism	• Nothing by mouth
• Kidney failure	• Increased rate of metabolism
• Corticosteroids	• Fever
• Cushing's syndrome or disease	• Hyperventilation
• Excessive oral sodium ingestion	• Infection
• Excessive administration of sodium-containing IV fluids	• Excessive diaphoresis
	• Watery diarrhea
	• Dehydration

Eventually the dehydrated excitable tissues may no longer be able to respond to stimuli.

❖ INTERPROFESSIONAL COLLABORATIVE CARE

◆ Assessment: Noticing

Symptoms of hypernatremia vary with the severity of sodium imbalance and whether a fluid imbalance is also present. Changes are first seen in excitable membrane activity, especially nerve, skeletal muscle, and cardiac function.

Nervous system changes start with altered cerebral function. Assess the patient's mental status for attention span and cognitive function. In hypernatremia with normal or decreased fluid volumes, the patient may have a short attention span and be agitated or confused. When hypernatremia occurs with fluid overload, the patient may be lethargic, stuporous, or comatose.

Skeletal muscle changes vary with the degree of sodium increases. Mild rises cause muscle twitching and irregular muscle contractions. As hypernatremia worsens, the muscles and nerves are less able to respond to a stimulus, and muscles become progressively weaker. Late, the deep tendon reflexes are reduced or absent. Muscle weakness occurs bilaterally and has no specific pattern. Observe for twitching in muscle groups. Assess muscle strength by having the patient perform handgrip and arm flexion against resistance as described in Chapters 41 and 49. Assess deep tendon reflexes by lightly tapping the patellar (knee) and Achilles (heel) tendons with a reflex hammer and measuring the movement.

Cardiovascular changes include decreased contractility because high sodium levels slow the movement of calcium into the heart cells. Measure blood pressure and the rate and quality of the apical and peripheral pulses. Pulse rate is increased in patients with hypernatremia and hypovolemia. Peripheral pulses are difficult to palpate and are easily blocked. Hypotension and severe orthostatic (postural) hypotension are present, and pulse pressure is reduced. Patients with hypernatremia and hypervolemia have slow-to-normal bounding pulses. Peripheral pulses are full and difficult to block. Neck veins are distended, even with the patient in the upright position. Blood pressure, especially diastolic blood pressure, is increased.

◆ Interventions: Responding

Drug and nutrition therapies are used to prevent further sodium increases and to decrease high serum sodium levels. *Nursing care priorities for the patient with hypernatremia include monitoring his or her response to therapy and ensuring patient safety by preventing hyponatremia and dehydration.*

Drug therapy is used to restore fluid balance when hypernatremia is caused by fluid loss. Isotonic saline (0.9%) and dextrose

5% in 0.45% sodium chloride are most often prescribed (Schreiber, 2013a). Although the dextrose 5% in 0.45% sodium chloride is hypertonic in the IV bag, once it is infused, the glucose is rapidly metabolized, and the fluid is really hypotonic. Hypernatremia caused by reduced kidney sodium excretion requires drug therapy with diuretics that promote sodium loss such as furosemide (Lasix, Furoside ✦) or bumetanide (Bumex, Burinex ✦). Assess the patient hourly for symptoms of excessive losses of fluid, sodium, or potassium.

Nutrition therapy to prevent or correct mild hypernatremia involves ensuring adequate water intake, especially among older adults. Dietary sodium restriction may be needed to prevent sodium excess when kidney problems are present. Collaborate with the dietitian to teach the patient how to determine the sodium content of foods, beverages, and drugs. Nursing actions for patient safety, skin protection, monitoring, and patient and family teaching are similar to those for fluid overload.

POTASSIUM

Potassium (K^+) is the major cation of the intracellular fluid (ICF). The normal plasma potassium level ranges from 3.5 to 5.0 mEq/L (mmol/L) (see Table 11-1). The normal ICF potassium level is about 140 mEq/L (mmol/L). Keeping this large difference in potassium concentration between the ICF and the extracellular fluid (ECF) is critical for excitable tissues to depolarize and generate action potentials.

Because potassium levels in the blood and interstitial fluid are so low, any change seriously affects physiologic activities. For example, a decrease in blood potassium of only 1 mEq/L (from 4 mEq/L [mmol/L] to 3 mEq/L) [mmol/L] is a 25% difference in total ECF potassium concentration.

Almost all foods contain potassium. It is highest in meat, fish, and many (but not all) vegetables and fruits. It is lowest in eggs, bread, and cereal grains. Typical potassium intake is about 2 to 20 g/day. Despite heavy potassium intake the healthy adult keeps plasma potassium levels within the narrow range of normal values.

The main controller of ECF potassium level is the sodium-potassium pump within the membranes of all body cells. This pump moves extra sodium ions from the ICF and moves extra potassium ions from the ECF back into the cell. In this way the serum potassium level remains low, and the cellular potassium remains high. At the same time, this action also helps the serum sodium level remain high and the cellular sodium level remain low.

About 80% of potassium is removed from the body by the kidney. Kidney excretion of potassium is enhanced by aldosterone.

HYPOKALEMIA

❖ PATHOPHYSIOLOGY

Because most potassium (K^+) is inside cells, minor changes in extracellular potassium levels cause major changes in cell membrane excitability. Hypokalemia is a serum potassium level below 3.5 mEq/L (mmol/L). *It can be life threatening because every body system is affected.*

Low serum potassium levels reduce the excitability of cells. As a result, the cell membranes of all excitable tissues such as nerve and muscle are less responsive to normal stimuli. Gradual potassium loss may have no symptoms until the loss is extreme.

TABLE 11-7	Common Causes of Hypokalemia
Actual Potassium Deficits	**Relative Potassium Deficits**
• Inappropriate or excessive use of drugs: • Diuretics • Digitalis-like drugs • Corticosteroids • Increased secretion of aldosterone • Cushing's syndrome • Diarrhea • Vomiting • Wound drainage (especially GI) • Prolonged nasogastric suction • Heat-induced excessive diaphoresis • Kidney disease impairing reabsorption of potassium • Nothing by mouth	• Alkalosis • Hyperinsulinism • Hyperalimentation • Total parenteral nutrition • Water intoxication • IV therapy with potassium-poor solutions

Rapid reduction of serum potassium levels causes dramatic changes in function. Table 11-7 lists causes of hypokalemia.

Actual potassium depletion occurs when potassium loss is excessive or when potassium intake is not adequate to match normal potassium loss. Relative hypokalemia occurs when total body potassium levels are normal but the potassium distribution between fluid spaces is abnormal or diluted by excess water.

❖ INTERPROFESSIONAL COLLABORATIVE CARE

◆ Assessment: Noticing

Age is important because urine concentrating ability decreases with aging, which increases potassium loss. Older adults are more likely to use drugs that lead to potassium loss.

Drugs, especially diuretics, corticosteroids, and beta-adrenergic agonists or antagonists, can increase potassium loss through the kidneys. Ask about prescription and over-the-counter drug use. In patients taking digoxin (Lanoxin, Novo-Digoxin ✦, Toloxin ✦), hypokalemia increases the sensitivity of the cardiac muscle to the drug and may result in digoxin toxicity, even when the digoxin level is within the therapeutic range. Ask whether the patient takes a potassium supplement such as potassium chloride (KCl) or eats foods that have high concentrations of potassium such as bananas, citrus juices, raisins, and meat. The patient may not be taking the supplement as prescribed because of its unpleasant taste.

Disease can lead to potassium loss. Ask about chronic disorders, recent illnesses, and medical or surgical interventions. A thorough nutrition history, including a typical day's food and beverage intake, helps identify patients at risk for hypokalemia.

Respiratory changes occur because of respiratory muscle weakness, resulting in shallow respirations. Assess the patient's breath sounds, ease of respiratory effort, color of nail beds and mucous membranes, and rate and depth of respiration.

❗ NURSING SAFETY PRIORITY QSEN

Action Alert

Assess respiratory status of a patient with hypokalemia at least every 2 hours because respiratory insufficiency is a major cause of death.

Musculoskeletal changes include skeletal muscle weakness. A stronger stimulus is needed to begin muscle contraction. Patients may be too weak to stand. Hand grasps are weak, and deep tendon reflexes are reduced (hyporeflexia). Severe hypokalemia causes flaccid paralysis. Assess for muscle weakness and the patient's ability to perform ADLs.

Cardiovascular changes are assessed by palpating the peripheral pulses. In hypokalemia the pulse is usually thready and weak. Palpation is difficult, and the pulse is easily blocked. Pulse rate ranges from very slow to very rapid, and an irregular heartbeat (dysrhythmia) may be present. Measure blood pressure with the patient in the lying, sitting, and standing positions, because orthostatic (postural) hypotension occurs with hypokalemia.

Neurologic changes from hypokalemia include altered mental status. The patient may have short-term irritability and anxiety followed by lethargy that progresses to acute confusion and coma as hypokalemia worsens.

Intestinal changes occur with hypokalemia because GI smooth muscle contractions are decreased, which leads to decreased peristalsis. Bowel sounds are hypoactive, and nausea, vomiting, constipation, and abdominal distention are common. Measure abdominal girth and auscultate for bowel sounds in all four abdominal quadrants. *Severe hypokalemia can cause the absence of peristalsis* (paralytic ileus).

Laboratory data confirm hypokalemia (serum potassium value below 3.5 mEq/L [mmol/L]). Hypokalemia causes ECG changes in the heart, including ST-segment depression, flat or inverted T waves, and increased U waves. *Dysrhythmias can lead to death, particularly in older adults who are taking digoxin.*

◆ Interventions: Responding

Interventions for hypokalemia focus on preventing potassium loss, increasing serum potassium levels, and ensuring patient safety. Drug and nutrition therapies help restore normal serum potassium levels. *The priorities for nursing care of the patient with hypokalemia are ensuring adequate gas exchange, patient safety for falls prevention, prevention of injury from potassium administration, and monitoring the patient's response to therapy.* Chart 11-5 highlights best practice activities when caring for a patient with hypokalemia.

Drug therapy for management and prevention of hypokalemia includes additional potassium and drugs to prevent potassium loss (Scotto et al., 2014). Most potassium supplements are potassium chloride, potassium gluconate, or potassium citrate. The amount and route of potassium replacement depend on the degree of loss.

Potassium is given intravenously for severe hypokalemia. The drug is available in different concentrations, and it carries a high-alert warning as a concentrated electrolyte solution. The Joint Commission's National Patient Safety Goals mandate that concentrated potassium be diluted and added to IV solutions only in the pharmacy by a registered pharmacist and that vials of concentrated potassium not be available in patient care areas. *Before infusing any IV solution containing potassium chloride (KCl), check and re-check the dilution of the drug in the IV solution container.*

Potassium is a severe tissue irritant and is never given by IM or subcutaneous injection. Tissues damaged by potassium can become necrotic, causing loss of function and requiring surgery. IV potassium solutions irritate veins and cause phlebitis. Check the prescription carefully to ensure that the patient receives the

◎ CHART 11-5 Best Practice for Patient Safety & Quality Care QSEN

The Patient With Hypokalemia

- Question the continued use of drugs that increase excretion of potassium (e.g., thiazide and loop diuretics).
- Give prescribed oral potassium supplement, well diluted and with a meal or just after a meal or snack to prevent nausea and vomiting.
- Prevent accidental overdose of IV potassium by checking and re-checking the concentration of potassium in the IV solution, ensuring that the maximum concentration is no greater than 1 mEq (mmol)/10 mL of solution.
- Establish an IV access in a large vein with a high volume of flow, avoiding the hand.
- Assess the IV access for placement and an adequate blood return before administering potassium-containing solutions.
- Use a controller for solution delivery, maintaining an infusion rate not faster than 5-10 mEq (mmol) of potassium per hour.
- Assess the IV site hourly.
- Stop the infusion immediately if the patient reports pain or burning or if any sign of infiltration occurs.
- If possible, monitor electrocardiography continuously.
- Monitor patient responses every 1-2 hours to determine therapy effectiveness and the potential for hyperkalemia.
- Indications of therapy effectiveness:
  - Respiratory rate is greater than 12 breaths/min.
  - Oxygen saturation is at least 95% (or has returned to the patient's normal baseline).
  - The patient can cough effectively.
  - Hand-grasp strength increases.
  - Deep tendon reflexes are present.
  - Bowel sounds are present and active.
  - Pulse is easily palpated and regular.
  - Systolic blood pressure when standing remains within 20 mm Hg of the systolic pressure obtained when the patient is sitting or lying down.
  - ST segment returns to the isoelectric line.
  - T waves increase in size and are positive.
  - U waves decrease or disappear.
  - Patient's cognition resembles his or her prehypokalemic state.
  - Serum potassium level is between 3.5 and 5.0 mEq/L (mmol/L).
- Indications of hyperkalemia:
  - Heart rate is less than 60 beats/min.
  - P waves are absent.
  - T waves are tall.
  - PR intervals are prolonged.
  - QRS complexes are wide.
  - Deep tendon reflexes are hyperactive.
  - Bowel sounds are hyperactive.
  - Numbness or tingling is present in the hands and feet and around the mouth.
  - The patient is anxious.
  - Serum potassium level is above 5.0 mEq/L (mmol/L).
- Keep patient on bedrest until hypokalemia resolves or provide assistance when out of bed to prevent falls.

⚠ NURSING SAFETY PRIORITY QSEN

Drug Alert

A dilution no greater than 1 mEq (mmol/L) of potassium to 10 mL of solution is recommended for IV administration. The maximum recommended infusion rate is 5 to 10 mEq/hr (mmol/hr); this rate is never to exceed 20 mEq/hr (mmol/hr) under any circumstances. In accordance with National Patient Safety Goals, potassium is not given by IV push to avoid causing cardiac arrest.

correct amount of potassium. Assess the IV site hourly and ask the patient whether he or she feels burning or pain at the site.

⚠ NURSING SAFETY PRIORITY QSEN

Action Alert

If infiltration of solution containing potassium occurs, stop the IV solution immediately, remove the venous access, and notify the health care provider or Rapid Response Team. Document these actions along with a complete description of the IV site.

Oral potassium preparations may be taken as liquids or solids. Potassium has a strong, unpleasant taste that is difficult to mask, although it can be mixed with many liquids. Because potassium chloride can cause nausea and vomiting, give the drug during or after a meal and advise patients using the drug at home not to take it on an empty stomach.

Diuretics that increase the kidney excretion of potassium can cause hypokalemia, especially high-ceiling (loop) diuretics (e.g., furosemide [Lasix, Furoside ✦] and bumetanide [Bumex, Burinex ✦]) and the thiazide diuretics. These drugs are avoided in patients with hypokalemia. A potassium-sparing diuretic may be prescribed to increase urine output without increasing potassium loss. Potassium-sparing diuretics include spironolactone (Aldactone, TEVA-spironolactone ✦), triamterene (Dyrenium, TEVA-triamterene ✦), and amiloride (Midamor, Novamilor ✦).

Nutrition therapy involves collaboration with a dietitian to teach the patient how to increase dietary potassium intake. Eating foods rich in potassium helps prevent further loss, but supplementation is needed to restore normal potassium levels.

Implement safety measures with a patient who has muscle weakness from hypokalemia, including the fall precautions listed in Chart 3-4. Be sure to have the patient wear a gait belt when ambulating with assistance.

Respiratory monitoring is performed at least hourly for severe hypokalemia. Also check oxygen saturation by pulse oximetry to determine breathing effectiveness. Assess respiratory muscle effectiveness by checking the patient's ability to cough. Examine the face, oral mucosa, and nail beds for pallor or cyanosis. Evaluate arterial blood gas values (when available) for decreased blood oxygen levels (**hypoxemia**) and increased arterial carbon dioxide levels (**hypercapnia**), which indicate inadequate gas exchange.

❓ CLINICAL JUDGMENT CHALLENGE 11-1

Safety; Patient-Centered Care QSEN

A patient with severe hypokalemia from an accidental overdose of furosemide is to receive IV potassium replacement through a peripheral inserted central catheter placed in the right upper arm. The ordered IV solution contains 120 mEq (mmol/L) of potassium chloride in 1000 mL of normal saline to be infused at a rate of 150 mL/hr.
1. Should this solution be infused using a pump or controller? Why or why not?
2. How many mEq of potassium per hour will the patient receive at this rate?
3. Is this rate permissible? Explain your rationale.
4. Which parameter changes would indicate to you that the patient is responding well to this therapy?
5. For which changes should you assess to determine whether the patient is becoming hyperkalemic?

HYPERKALEMIA

❖ PATHOPHYSIOLOGY

Hyperkalemia is a serum potassium level higher than 5.0 mEq/L (mmol/L). Even small increases above normal values can affect excitable tissues, especially the heart.

A high serum potassium increases cell excitability, causing excitable tissues to respond to less intense stimuli. The heart is very sensitive to serum potassium increases; and hyperkalemia interferes with electrical conduction, leading to heart block and ventricular fibrillation.

The problems that occur with hyperkalemia are related to how rapidly ECF potassium levels increase. Sudden potassium rises cause severe problems at serum levels between 6 and 7 mEq/L (mmol/L). When serum potassium rises slowly, problems may not occur until potassium levels reach 8 mEq/L (mmol/L) or higher.

Hyperkalemia is rare in people with normal kidney function (Hannibal, 2015). Most cases of hyperkalemia occur in hospitalized patients and in those undergoing medical treatment (Adis Medical Writers, 2015). Those at greatest risk are chronically ill patients, debilitated patients, and older adults (Table 11-8).

❖ INTERPROFESSIONAL COLLABORATIVE CARE

◆ Assessment: Noticing

Age is important because kidney function decreases with aging. Ask about kidney disease; diabetes mellitus; recent medical or surgical treatment; and urine output, including frequency and amount of voidings. Ask about drug use, particularly potassium-sparing diuretics and angiotensin-converting enzyme inhibitors (ACEIs) (Adis Medical Writers, 2015). Obtain a nutrition history to determine the intake of potassium-rich foods and the use of salt substitutes (which contain potassium).

Ask whether the patient has had palpitations, skipped heartbeats, or other cardiac irregularities; and muscle twitching leg weakness, or unusual tingling or numbness in the hands, feet, or face. Ask about recent changes in bowel habits, especially diarrhea.

Cardiovascular changes are the most severe problems from hyperkalemia and are the most common cause of death in patients with hyperkalemia. Cardiac symptoms include bradycardia; hypotension; and ECG changes of tall, peaked T waves, prolonged PR intervals, flat or absent P waves, and wide QRS

complexes. Ectopic beats may appear. Complete heart block, asystole, and ventricular fibrillation are life-threatening complications of severe hyperkalemia.

Neuromuscular changes with hyperkalemia have two phases. Skeletal muscles twitch in the early stages of hyperkalemia, and the patient may be aware of tingling and burning sensations followed by numbness in the hands and feet and around the mouth (paresthesia). As hyperkalemia worsens, muscle weakness occurs, followed by flaccid paralysis. The weakness moves up from the hands and feet and first affects the muscles of the arms and legs. Respiratory muscles are not affected until serum potassium levels reach lethal levels.

Intestinal changes include increased motility with diarrhea and hyperactive bowel sounds. Bowel movements are frequent and watery.

Laboratory data confirm hyperkalemia (potassium level over 5.0 mEq/L [mmol/L]). If it is caused by dehydration, levels of other electrolytes, hematocrit, and hemoglobin also are elevated. Hyperkalemia caused by kidney failure occurs with elevated serum creatinine and blood urea nitrogen, decreased blood pH, and normal or low hematocrit and hemoglobin levels.

◆ Interventions: Responding

Interventions for hyperkalemia focus on reducing the serum potassium level, preventing recurrences, and ensuring patient safety. Drug therapy is key. *The priorities for nursing care of the patient with hyperkalemia are assessing for cardiac complications, patient safety for falls prevention, monitoring the patient's response to therapy, and health teaching.*

Drug therapy can restore potassium balance by enhancing potassium excretion and promoting the movement of potassium from the extracellular fluid (ECF) into the cells. A newly approved drug to treat hyperkalemia is patiromer (Veltassa). This oral drug binds with potassium in the GI tract and decreases its absorption (Aschenbrenner, 2016).

Stop potassium-containing infusions and keep the IV access open. Withhold oral potassium supplements and provide a potassium-restricted diet.

Increasing potassium excretion helps reduce hyperkalemia if kidney function is normal. Potassium-excreting diuretics are prescribed. When kidney problems exist, more invasive interventions may be needed (see Chapter 68).

Movement of potassium from the extracellular fluid (ECF) to the intracellular fluid (ICF) can help reduce serum potassium levels temporarily. Potassium movement into the cells is enhanced by insulin. Insulin increases the activity of the sodium-potassium pumps, which move potassium from the ECF into the cell. IV fluids containing glucose and insulin are prescribed to help decrease serum potassium levels (usually 100 mL of 10% to 20% glucose with 10 to 20 units of regular insulin). These IV solutions are hypertonic and are infused through a central line or in a vein with a high blood flow to avoid local vein inflammation. Observe the patient for indications of hypokalemia and hypoglycemia during this therapy.

Cardiac monitoring allows for the early recognition of dysrhythmias and other symptoms of hyperkalemia on cardiac muscle. Compare recent ECG tracings with the tracings obtained when the patient's serum potassium level was close to normal.

Health teaching is key to the prevention of hyperkalemia and the early detection of complications. The teaching plan includes diet, drugs, and recognition of the indicators of hyperkalemia. Collaborate with the dietitian to teach the patient and family

TABLE 11-8	Common Causes of Hyperkalemia
Actual Potassium Excesses	**Relative Potassium Excesses**
• Overingestion of potassium-containing foods or medications: • Salt substitutes • Potassium chloride • Rapid infusion of potassium-containing IV solution • Bolus IV potassium injections • Transfusions of whole blood or packed cells • Adrenal insufficiency • Kidney failure • Potassium-sparing diuretics • Angiotensin-converting enzyme inhibitors (ACEIs)	• Tissue damage • Acidosis • Hyperuricemia • Uncontrolled diabetes mellitus

! NURSING SAFETY PRIORITY QSEN
Critical Rescue

Assess anyone who has or is at risk for hyperkalemia to recognize cardiac changes. If the patient's heart rate falls below 60 beats/min or if the T waves become spiked, both of which accompany hyperkalemia, respond by notifying the Rapid Response Team.

about which foods to avoid (those high in potassium). Foods that are low in potassium are listed in Chart 11-6. Instruct the patient and family to read the labels on drug and food packages to determine the potassium content. Warn them to avoid salt substitutes, which contain potassium.

? NCLEX EXAMINATION CHALLENGE 11-5
Health Promotion and Maintenance

Which food items selected by a client who must restrict potassium because of a continuing risk for hyperkalemia indicates to the nurse that more teaching is needed?
A. Strawberries, Cheerios, eggs
B. Cantaloupe, broccoli, sweet potatoes
C. Apple pie, black coffee with sugar, carrot sticks
D. Whole wheat toast with butter, canned pineapple chunks

CHART 11-6 Patient and Family Education: Preparing for Self-Management

Nutritional Management of Hyperkalemia

You Should Avoid
- Meats, especially organ meat and preserved meat
- Dairy products
- Dried fruit
- Fruits high in potassium:
  - Bananas
  - Cantaloupe
  - Kiwi
  - Oranges
- Vegetables high in potassium:
  - Avocados
  - Broccoli
  - Dried beans or peas
  - Lima beans
  - Mushrooms
  - Potatoes (white or sweet)
  - Seaweed
  - Soybeans
  - Spinach

You May Eat
- Eggs
- Breads
- Butter
- Cereals
- Sugar
- Fruits low in potassium (fresh, frozen, or canned):
  - Apples
  - Apricots
  - Berries
  - Cherries
  - Cranberries
  - Grapefruit
  - Peaches
  - Pineapple
- Vegetables low in potassium:
  - Alfalfa sprouts
  - Cabbage
  - Carrots
  - Cauliflower
  - Celery
  - Eggplant
  - Green beans
  - Lettuce
  - Onions
  - Peas
  - Peppers
  - Squash

Data from Pennington, J. A., & Spungen, J. S. (2010). *Bowes and Church's food values of portions commonly used* (19th ed.). Philadelphia: Lippincott Williams & Wilkins.

CALCIUM

Calcium (Ca^{2+}) is an ion having two positive charges *(divalent cation)* that exists in the body in a bound form and an ionized (unbound or free) form. Bound calcium is usually attached to serum proteins, especially albumin. Ionized calcium is present in the blood and other extracellular fluid (ECF) as free calcium. Free calcium is the active form and must be kept within a narrow range in the ECF (see Table 11-1). Calcium has a steep gradient between ECF and intracellular fluid (ICF) because the amount of calcium in the ICF is very low. This mineral is important for maintaining bone strength and density, activating enzymes, allowing skeletal and cardiac muscle contraction, controlling nerve impulse transmission, and allowing blood clotting.

Calcium enters the body by dietary intake and absorption through the intestinal tract. Absorption of dietary calcium requires the active form of vitamin D. Calcium is stored in the bones. When more calcium is needed, parathyroid hormone (PTH) is released from the parathyroid glands. PTH increases serum calcium levels by:
- Releasing free calcium from bone storage sites (bone *resorption* of calcium)
- Stimulating vitamin D activation to help increase intestinal *absorption* of dietary calcium
- Inhibiting kidney calcium excretion
- Stimulating kidney calcium *reabsorption*

When excess calcium is present in plasma, PTH secretion is inhibited, and the secretion of *thyrocalcitonin (TCT),* a hormone secreted by the thyroid gland, is increased. TCT causes the plasma calcium level to decrease by inhibiting bone resorption of calcium, inhibiting vitamin D–associated intestinal uptake of calcium, and increasing kidney excretion of calcium in the urine.

HYPOCALCEMIA
❖ PATHOPHYSIOLOGY

Hypocalcemia is a total serum calcium (Ca^{2+}) level below 9.0 mg/dL or 2.25 mmol/L. Because the normal blood level of calcium is so low, any change in calcium levels has major effects on function.

Calcium is an excitable membrane stabilizer, regulating depolarization and the generation of action potentials. It decreases sodium movement across excitable membranes, slowing the rate of depolarization. Low serum calcium levels increase sodium movement across excitable membranes, allowing depolarization to occur more easily and at inappropriate times.

Hypocalcemia is caused by many chronic and acute conditions, as well as medical or surgical treatments. Table 11-9 lists causes of hypocalcemia. Acute hypocalcemia results in the rapid onset of life-threatening symptoms. Chronic hypocalcemia occurs slowly over time, and excitable membrane symptoms may not be severe because the body has adjusted to the gradual reduction of serum calcium levels.

❖ INTERPROFESSIONAL COLLABORATIVE CARE
◆ Assessment: Noticing

Assess the nutrition history for the risk for hypocalcemia. Ask the patient about his or her intake of dairy products and whether he or she takes a calcium supplement regularly.

One indicator of hypocalcemia is a report of frequent, painful muscle spasms ("charley horses") in the calf or foot

TABLE 11-9	Common Causes of Hypocalcemia
Actual Calcium Deficits	**Relative Calcium Deficits**

• Inadequate oral intake of calcium
• Lactose intolerance
• Malabsorption syndromes:
  • Celiac sprue
  • Crohn's disease
• Inadequate intake of vitamin D
• End-stage kidney disease
• Diarrhea
• Steatorrhea
• Wound drainage (especially GI)
	• Hyperproteinemia
	• Alkalosis
	• Calcium chelators or binders
	• Citrate
	• Mithramycin
	• Penicillamine
	• Sodium cellulose phosphate (Calcibind)
	• Aredia
	• Acute pancreatitis
	• Hyperphosphatemia
	• Immobility
	• Removal or destruction of parathyroid glands

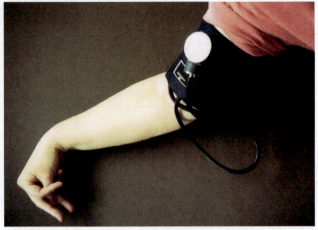

FIG. 11-13 Palmar flexion indicating a positive Trousseau's sign in hypocalcemia.

GENDER HEALTH CONSIDERATIONS

Patient-Centered Care QSEN

Postmenopausal women are at risk for chronic calcium loss. This problem is related to reduced weight-bearing activities and a decrease in estrogen levels. As they age, many women decrease weight-bearing activities such as running and walking, which allows osteoporosis to occur at a more rapid rate. In addition, the estrogen secretion that protects against osteoporosis diminishes. Teach older women to continue walking and other weight-bearing activities.

during rest or sleep. Ask about a history of recent orthopedic surgery or bone healing. Thyroid surgery, therapeutic irradiation of the upper middle chest and neck area, or a recent anterior neck injury increases the risk for hypocalcemia. Most symptoms of acute hypocalcemia are caused by overstimulation of the nerves and muscles.

Neuromuscular changes often occur first in the hands and feet. Paresthesias occur at first, with sensations of tingling and numbness. If hypocalcemia continues or worsens, muscle twitching or painful cramps and spasms occur. Tingling may also affect the lips, nose, and ears. These problems may signal the onset of neuromuscular overstimulation and tetany.

Assess for hypocalcemia by testing for Trousseau's and Chvostek's signs. To test for Trousseau's sign, place a blood pressure cuff around the arm, inflate the cuff to greater than the patient's systolic pressure, and keep the cuff inflated for 1 to 4 minutes. Under these hypoxic conditions, a positive Trousseau's sign occurs when the hand and fingers go into spasm in palmar flexion (Fig. 11-13). To test for Chvostek's sign, tap the face just below and in front of the ear to trigger facial twitching of one side of the mouth, nose, and cheek (Fig. 11-14).

Cardiovascular changes involve heart rate and ECG changes. The heart rate may be slower or slightly faster than normal, with a weak, thready pulse. Severe hypocalcemia causes severe hypotension and ECG changes of a prolonged ST interval and a prolonged QT interval (Moore et al., 2014).

Intestinal changes include increased peristaltic activity. Assess the abdomen for hyperactive bowel sounds. The patient may report painful abdominal cramping and diarrhea.

Skeletal changes are common with chronic hypocalcemia. Calcium leaves bone storage sites, causing a loss of bone density

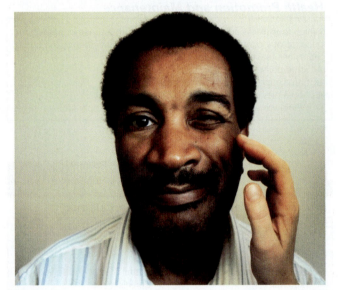

FIG. 11-14 Facial muscle response indicating a positive Chvostek's sign in hypocalcemia.

(osteoporosis). The bones are less dense, more brittle, and fragile and may break easily with slight trauma. Vertebrae become more compact and may bend forward, leading to an overall loss of height. See Chapter 50 for discussion of osteoporosis.

Ask about changes in height and any unexplained bone pain. Observe for spinal curvatures and any unusual bumps or protrusions in bones that may indicate old fractures.

◆ Interventions: Responding

Interventions focus on restoring normal calcium levels and preventing complications. These include drug therapy, nutrition therapy, reducing environmental stimuli, and preventing injury. Patient safety during restoration of serum calcium levels is a nursing care priority.

Drug therapy includes direct calcium replacement (oral and IV) and drugs that enhance the absorption of calcium such as vitamin D. When neuromuscular symptoms are troublesome, drugs that decrease nerve and muscle responses also may be used.

Nutrition therapy involves a calcium-rich diet for patients with mild hypocalcemia and for those who are at continuing risk for hypocalcemia. Collaborate with the dietitian to help the patient select calcium-rich foods.

Environmental management for safety is needed because the excitable membranes of the nervous system and the skeletal system are overstimulated in hypocalcemia. Reduce stimulation by keeping the room quiet, limiting visitors, adjusting the lighting, and using a soft voice.

Injury prevention strategies are needed because the patient with long-standing calcium loss may have brittle, fragile bones that fracture easily and cause little pain. When lifting or moving a patient with fragile bones, use a lift sheet rather than pulling the patient. Observe for normal range of joint motion and for any unusual surface bumps or depressions over bony areas that may indicate bone fracture.

HYPERCALCEMIA
❖ PATHOPHYSIOLOGY

Hypercalcemia is a total serum calcium level above 10.5 mg/dL or 2.62 mmol/L. Even small increases above normal have severe effects, and all systems are affected. Hypercalcemia causes excitable tissues to be less sensitive to normal stimuli, thus requiring a stronger stimulus to function. The excitable tissues affected most by hypercalcemia are the heart, skeletal muscles, nerves, and intestinal smooth muscles. Causes of hypercalcemia are listed in Table 11-10.

❖ INTERPROFESSIONAL COLLABORATIVE CARE
◆ Assessment: Noticing

The signs and symptoms of hypercalcemia are related to its severity and how quickly the imbalance occurred. The patient with a mild but rapidly occurring calcium excess often has more severe problems than the patient whose imbalance is severe but has developed slowly.

Cardiovascular changes are the most serious and life-threatening problems of hypercalcemia. Mild hypercalcemia at first causes increased heart rate and blood pressure. Severe or prolonged calcium imbalance depresses electrical conduction, slowing heart rate.

Measure pulse rate and blood pressure and observe for indications of poor PERFUSION such as cyanosis and pallor. Examine ECG tracings for dysrhythmias, especially a shortened QT interval.

Hypercalcemia allows blood clots to form more easily whenever blood flow is poor. Blood clotting is more likely in the lower legs, the pelvic region, areas where blood flow is blocked by internal or external constrictions, and areas where venous obstruction occurs.

Assess for slowed or impaired PERFUSION. Measure and record calf circumferences with a soft tape measure. Assess the feet for temperature, color, and capillary refill to determine PERFUSION to and from the area.

Neuromuscular changes include severe muscle weakness and decreased deep tendon reflexes without paresthesia. The patient may be confused and lethargic.

Intestinal changes are first reflected as decreased peristalsis. Constipation, anorexia, nausea, vomiting, abdominal distention, and pain are common. Bowel sounds are hypoactive or absent. Assess abdominal size by measuring abdominal girth with a soft tape measure in a line circling the abdomen at the umbilicus.

◆ Interventions: Responding

Interventions for hypercalcemia focus on reducing serum calcium levels through drug therapy; rehydration; and, depending on the cause and severity, dialysis. Cardiac monitoring is also important.

Drug therapy involves preventing increases in calcium and drugs to lower calcium levels. IV solutions containing calcium (e.g., Ringer's lactate) are stopped. Oral drugs containing calcium or vitamin D (e.g., calcium-based antacids) are discontinued.

Fluid volume replacement can help restore normal serum calcium levels. IV normal saline (0.9% sodium chloride) is usually given because sodium increases kidney excretion of calcium.

Thiazide diuretics are discontinued and replaced with diuretics that enhance the excretion of calcium such as furosemide (Lasix, Furoside ✦). Calcium chelators (calcium binders) help lower serum calcium levels. Such drugs include plicamycin (Mithracin) and penicillamine (Cuprimine).

Drugs to prevent hypercalcemia include agents that inhibit calcium resorption from bone such as phosphorus, calcitonin (Calcimar), bisphosphonates (etidronate [Didronel, Etidrocal ✦, NOVO-etidronatecal ✦]), and prostaglandin synthesis inhibitors (aspirin, NSAIDs).

Cardiac monitoring of patients with hypercalcemia is needed to identify dysrhythmias and decreased cardiac output. Compare recent ECG tracings with the patient's baseline tracings. Especially look for changes in the T waves and the QT interval and changes in rate and rhythm.

MAGNESIUM

Magnesium (Mg^{2+}) is a cation mostly stored in bones and cartilage. Little magnesium is present in the blood (see Table 11-1). The intracellular fluid (ICF) has more magnesium, and it has more functions inside the cells than in the blood. It is important for skeletal muscle contraction, carbohydrate metabolism, generation of energy stores, vitamin activation, blood coagulation, and cell growth.

HYPOMAGNESEMIA

Hypomagnesemia is a serum magnesium (Mg^{2+}) level below 1.8 mEq/L or 0.74 mmol/L. It is most often caused by decreased absorption of dietary magnesium or increased kidney magnesium excretion. Two major causes of hypomagnesemia are inadequate intake and the use of loop or thiazide diuretics. Table 11-11 lists additional causes of hypomagnesemia.

TABLE 11-10 Common Causes of Hypercalcemia	
Actual Calcium Excesses	**Relative Calcium Excesses**
• Excessive oral intake of calcium	• Hyperparathyroidism
• Excessive oral intake of vitamin D	• Malignancy
• Kidney failure	• Hyperthyroidism
• Use of thiazide diuretics	• Immobility
	• Use of glucocorticoids
	• Dehydration

TABLE 11-11 Common Causes of Magnesium Imbalance

Hypomagnesemia	Hypermagnesemia
• Malnutrition	• Increased magnesium intake:
• Starvation	• Magnesium-containing antacids and laxatives
• Diarrhea	• IV magnesium replacement
• Steatorrhea	• Decreased kidney excretion of magnesium resulting from kidney disease
• Celiac disease	
• Crohn's disease	
• Drugs (diuretics, aminoglycoside antibiotics, cisplatin, amphotericin B, cyclosporine)	
• Citrate (blood products)	
• Ethanol ingestion	

The effects of hypomagnesemia are caused by increased membrane excitability and the accompanying serum calcium and potassium imbalances. Excitable membranes, especially nerve cell membranes, may depolarize spontaneously.

Cardiovascular changes associated with hypomagnesemia are serious. Low magnesium levels increase the risk for hypertension, atherosclerosis, hypertrophic left ventricle, and a variety of dysrhythmias (McCance et al., 2014). The dysrhythmias include premature contractions, atrial fibrillation, ventricular fibrillation, and long QT intervals. One aspect of the conduction problems is that, when serum magnesium levels are low, intracellular potassium levels are also low. This changes the resting membrane potential in cardiac muscle cells, slowing normal conduction and triggering ectopic beats. Low magnesium levels also are associated with greater cardiac muscle cell damage after myocardial infarction.

Neuromuscular changes are caused by increased nerve impulse transmission. Normally magnesium inhibits nerve impulse transmission at synapse areas. Decreased levels increase impulse transmission from nerve to nerve or from nerve to skeletal muscle. The patient has hyperactive deep tendon reflexes, numbness and tingling, and painful muscle contractions. Positive Chvostek's and Trousseau's signs may be present because hypomagnesemia may occur with hypocalcemia (see the earlier discussion of these assessment signs of neuromuscular changes in the Hypocalcemia section). The patient may have tetany and seizures as hypomagnesemia worsens.

Intestinal changes are from decreased intestinal smooth muscle contraction. Reduced motility, anorexia, nausea, constipation, and abdominal distention are common. A paralytic ileus may occur when hypomagnesemia is severe.

Interventions for hypomagnesemia aim to correct the imbalance and manage the specific problem that caused it. In addition, because hypocalcemia often occurs with hypomagnesemia, interventions also aim to restore normal serum calcium levels.

Drugs that promote magnesium loss such as high-ceiling (loop) diuretics, osmotic diuretics, aminoglycoside antibiotics, and drugs containing phosphorus are discontinued. Magnesium is replaced intravenously with magnesium sulfate ($MgSO_4$) when hypomagnesemia is severe. Assess deep tendon reflexes at least hourly in the patient receiving IV magnesium to monitor effectiveness and prevent hypermagnesemia. If hypocalcemia is also present, drug therapy to increase serum calcium levels is prescribed.

HYPERMAGNESEMIA

Hypermagnesemia is a serum magnesium level above 2.6 mEq/L or 1.07 mmol/L. Table 11-11 lists the specific causes of hypermagnesemia.

Magnesium is a membrane stabilizer. Most symptoms of hypermagnesemia occur as a result of reduced membrane excitability. They usually are not apparent until serum magnesium levels exceed 4 mEq/L (1.6 mmol/L).

Cardiac changes include bradycardia, peripheral vasodilation, and hypotension. These problems become more severe as serum magnesium levels increase. ECG changes show a prolonged PR interval with a widened QRS complex. Bradycardia can be severe, and cardiac arrest is possible. Hypotension is also severe, with a diastolic pressure lower than normal. *Patients with severe hypermagnesemia are in grave danger of cardiac arrest.*

Central nervous system changes result from depressed nerve impulse transmission. Patients may be drowsy or lethargic. Coma may occur if the imbalance is prolonged or severe.

Neuromuscular changes include reduced or absent deep tendon reflexes. Voluntary skeletal muscle contractions become progressively weaker and finally stop.

Hypermagnesemia has no direct effect on the lungs; however, when the respiratory muscles are weak, respiratory insufficiency can lead to respiratory failure and death.

Interventions for hypermagnesemia focus on reducing the serum level and correcting the underlying problem that caused the imbalance. All oral and parenteral magnesium is discontinued. When kidney failure is not present, giving magnesium-free IV fluids can reduce serum magnesium levels. High-ceiling (loop) diuretics such as furosemide (Lasix, Furoside ✦) can further reduce serum magnesium levels. When cardiac problems are severe, giving calcium may reverse the cardiac effects of hypermagnesemia.

❓ CLINICAL JUDGMENT CHALLENGE 11-2

Patient-Centered Care; Evidence-Based Practice; Teamwork and Collaboration **QSEN**

A 73-year-old patient who is being managed for viral cardiomyopathy with heart failure is going home today after an acute exacerbation of his heart failure. He is has been taking furosemide 40 mg orally daily, rivaroxaban 20 mg orally daily, lisinopril 5 mg orally daily, and carvedilol 25 mg orally twice daily. He is now being prescribed to also take magnesium 500 mg orally once daily. He tells you that he understands why he is to continue to take the previously prescribed drugs but wants to know how the magnesium will help him. Your responsibility is to help him become a partner in his therapy to prevent worsening heart failure.

1. Is this patient at risk for dehydration or fluid overload? Explain this risk.
2. Which parameters will you teach him to self-monitor at home for indications of needing to see the health care provider? Provide a rationale for your selection.
3. Which electrolytes are most likely to be disturbed by his drug therapy. Explain your selections and the directions of the potential disturbances.
4. What will you tell him about the magnesium?
5. Which additional members of the interprofessional team would be most helpful in this patient's management and why?

GET READY FOR THE NCLEX® EXAMINATION!

KEY POINTS

Review these key points for each NCLEX Examination Client Needs Category.

Safe and Effective Care Environment
- Assess any patient with a problem of fluid and electrolyte balance for fall risk. **QSEN: Safety**
- Supervise the oral fluid therapy and intake and output measurement aspects of care delegated to unlicensed assistive personnel. **QSEN: Safety**
- Use a pump or controller to deliver IV fluids to patients with fluid overload. **QSEN: Safety**
- Do not give IV potassium at a rate greater than 20 mEq/hr (mmol/hr). **QSEN: Safety**
- Never give potassium supplements by the IM, subcutaneous, or IV push routes. **QSEN: Safety**
- Use a pump or controller when giving IV potassium-containing solutions. **QSEN: Safety**
- Assess the IV site hourly of an adult receiving IV solutions containing potassium and document its condition. **QSEN: Safety**
- Use a gait belt when assisting a patient with muscle weakness to walk or transfer. **QSEN: Safety**
- Use a lift sheet to move or reposition a patient with chronic hypocalcemia. **QSEN: Safety**

Health Promotion and Maintenance
- Encourage all patients to maintain an adequate fluid intake (minimum of 1.5 L per day) unless another condition requires fluid restriction. **QSEN: Evidence-Based Practice**
- Teach all adults to increase fluid intake when exercising, when in hot or dry environments, or during conditions that increase metabolism (e.g., fever). **QSEN: Patient-Centered Care**
- Instruct patients at risk for fluid imbalance to weigh themselves on the same scale daily, close to the same time each day, and with about the same amount of clothing on each time and to monitor these daily weights for changes or trends. **QSEN: Patient-Centered Care**
- Ensure access to adequate fluids for patients who cannot talk or who have limited mobility. **QSEN: Patient-Centered Care**
- Instruct caregivers of older adults who have cognitive impairments or mobility problems to schedule offerings of fluids at regular intervals throughout the day. **QSEN: Evidence-Based Practice**

- Teach patients how to determine electrolyte content of processed foods by reading labels. **QSEN: Patient-Centered Care**

Psychosocial Integrity
- Explain the purpose of fluid restriction to the patient and the family to ensure cooperation and prevent any misunderstandings. **QSEN: Patient-Centered Care**
- Assess patients who have a sudden change in cognition for a change in fluid and electrolyte balance. **QSEN: Patient-Centered Care**
- Determine the patient's food preferences and dislikes when planning an electrolyte-restricted diet. **QSEN: Patient-Centered Care**

Physiological Integrity
- Assess skin turgor on the forehead or sternum of older patients. **QSEN: Evidence-Based Practice**
- Use daily weights to determine fluid gains or losses. **QSEN: Evidence-Based Practice**
- Ask patients about the use of drugs such as diuretics, laxatives, salt substitutes, and antihypertensives that may alter fluid and electrolyte balance. **QSEN: Patient-Centered Care**
- Monitor the cardiac and pulmonary status at least every hour when patients with dehydration are receiving IV fluid replacement therapy. **QSEN: Patient-Centered Care**
- Collaborate with the registered dietitian to teach patients about diets that are restricted in potassium, sodium, or calcium. **QSEN: Teamwork and Collaboration**
- Immediately stop the infusion of potassium-containing solutions if infiltration is suspected. **QSEN: Evidence-Based Practice**
- Assess all patients with hyperkalemia for cardiac dysrhythmias and ECG abnormalities, especially tall T waves, conduction delays, and heart block. **QSEN: Evidence-Based Practice**
- Assess the respiratory status of all patients with hypokalemia. **QSEN: Evidence-Based Practice**
- Assess the bowel sounds; heart rate, rhythm and quality; and muscle strength to evaluate the patient's responses to therapy for an electrolyte imbalance. **QSEN: Evidence-Based Practice**

SELECTED BIBLIOGRAPHY

Adis Medical Writers. (2015). Minimize drug-induced hyperkalemia by increasing awareness and using preventative strategies. *Drugs & Therapy Perspectives, 31*(1), 28–33.

Arai, S., Stotts, N., & Puntillo, K. (2013). Thirst in critically ill patients. From physiology to sensation. *American Journal of Critical Care, 22*(4), 328–335.

Aschenbrenner, D. (2016). The FDA approves one new hyperkalemia drug, requires drug interaction study for another. *American Journal of Nursing, 116*(2), 23.

Bridges, E. (2013). Using functional hemodynamic indicators to guide fluid therapy. *The American Journal of Nursing, 113*(5), 42–50.

Crawford, A. (2014). Hyperkalemia: Recognition and management of a critical electrolyte disturbance. *Journal of Infusion Nursing, 37*(3), 167–175.

Friedman, B., & Cirulli, J. (2013). Hyponatremia in critical care patients: Frequency, outcome, characteristics, and treatment with the vasopressin V2-receptor antagonist tolvaptan. *Journal of Critical Care, 28*, 219.e1–219.e12.

Hannibal, G. (2015). Severe hyperkalemia with sine wave ECG pattern. *AACN Advanced Critical Care, 26*(2), 177–180.

Kaufman, G. (2014). Diuretics: How they work, cautions and contraindications. *Nursing & Residential Care, 16*(2), 83–86.

Maday, K. (2013). Understanding electrolytes: Important diagnostic clues to patient status. *Journal of the American Association of Physician Assistants, 26*(1), 26–31.

McCance, K., Huether, S., Brashers, V., & Rote, N. (2014). *Pathophysiology: The biologic basis for disease in adults and children* (7th ed.). St. Louis: Mosby.

McLafferty, E., Johnstone, C., Hendry, C., & Farley, A. (2014). Fluid and electrolyte balance. *Nursing Standard, 28*(29), 42–49.

Moore, S., Winkelman, C., & Daum, B. (2014). Influence of calcium abnormalities on the ECG. *AACN Advanced Critical Care, 25*(3), 297–304.

Moritz, M. (2013). Case studies in fluid and electrolyte therapy. *Journal of Infusion Nursing, 36*(4), 270–277.

Pagana, K., Pagana, T., & Pagana, T. (2017). *Mosby's diagnostic and laboratory test reference* (13th ed.). St. Louis: Mosby.

Pagana, K., Pagana, T., & Pike-MacDonald, S. (2013). *Mosby's Canadian manual of diagnostic and laboratory tests* (1st ed.). St. Louis: Mosby.

Parli, S., Ruf, K., & Magnuson, B. (2014). Pathophysiology, treatment, and prevention of fluid and electrolyte abnormalities during refeeding syndrome. *Journal of Infusion Nursing, 37*(3), 197–202.

Pierce, J., Shen, Q., & Thimmesch, A. (2016). The ongoing controversy: Crystalloids versus colloids. *Journal of Infusion Nursing, 39*(1), 40–44.

Reynolds, I. G. (2015). Recognizing acute hyponatremia. *American Nurse Today, 10*(7), 26.

Ruiz, C. (2015). Tracing angioedema to its source. *American Nurse Today, 10*(11), 24.

Schreiber, M. (2013a). Understanding hypernatremia. *Nursing2013 Critical Care, 8*(3), 8–10.

Schreiber, M. (2013b). Understanding hyponatremia. *Nursing2013 Critical Care, 8*(2), 8–10.

Scotto, C., Fridline, M., Menhart, C., & Klions, H. (2014). Preventing hypokalemia in critically ill patients. *American Journal of Critical Care, 23*(2), 145–149.

Touhy, T., & Jett, K. (2016). *Ebersole and Hess' toward health aging* (9th ed.). St. Louis: Mosby.

Trissel, L. (2013). *Handbook on injectable drugs* (17th ed.). Bethesda, MD: American Society of Hospital-System Pharmacists.

United States Food and Drug Administration (USFDA). (2015). *FDA approves new drug to treat hyperkalemia.* http://www.fda.gov/NewsEvents/Newsroom/PressAnnouncements/ucm468546.htm.

Walker, M. (2016). Fluid and electrolyte imbalances: Interpretation and assessment. *Journal of Infusion Nursing, 39*(6), 382–386.

Wunderlich, R. (2013). Principles in the selection of intravenous solutions replacement: Sodium and water balance. *Journal of Infusion Nursing, 36*(2), 126–130.

CHAPTER 12

Assessment and Care of Patients With Problems of Acid-Base Balance

M. Linda Workman

 http://evolve.elsevier.com/Iggy/

PRIORITY AND INTERRELATED CONCEPTS

The priority concept for this chapter is ACID-BASE BALANCE.

✳ The ACID-BASE BALANCE concept exemplar for this chapter is Acidosis, p. 190.

LEARNING OUTCOMES

Safe and Effective Care Environment

1. Collaborate with the interprofessional team to perform a complete assessment of patients for ACID-BASE BALANCE.

Health Promotion and Maintenance

2. Explain how physiologic aging changes the effectiveness of mechanisms to maintain ACID-BASE BALANCE and increases the risk for imbalance.
3. Teach all adults measures to take to prevent disturbances of ACID-BASE BALANCE.

Psychosocial Integrity

4. Implement patient-centered nursing interventions to help the patient and family cope with the psychosocial

impact of continuing risk for disturbances of ACID-BASE BALANCE.

Physiological Integrity

5. Apply knowledge of anatomy, physiology, and pathophysiology to perform an evidence-based assessment for the patient with a disturbance of ACID-BASE BALANCE.
6. Interpret assessment findings for the patient experiencing a disturbance of ACID-BASE BALANCE.
7. Teach the patient and caregivers about diagnostic procedures associated with conditions affecting ACID-BASE BALANCE.

As defined in Chapter 2, ACID-BASE BALANCE is the maintenance of arterial blood pH between 7.35 and 7.45 through regulation of hydrogen ion (H^+) production and elimination. The pH is an indirect measure of the free hydrogen ion level in the blood and other body fluids. Maintaining the pH within the narrow normal range is critical for life and body function. Even small changes in the free hydrogen ion level (pH) of body fluids can cause major problems in function. Thus the level of free hydrogen ions, formed from acids, must be rigidly controlled.

The normal free hydrogen ion level of blood and other body fluids is quite low (less than 0.0001 mEq/L [mmol/L]), and its concentration is calculated in negative logarithm units. The value of pH is *inversely* related (negatively related) to the level of free hydrogen ions. Thus the *lower* the pH value of a fluid, the *higher* the level of free hydrogen ions in that fluid. The pH of a solution may range from 1 (as acidic as possible) to 14 (as alkaline as possible), with 7 being neutral. *A change of 1 pH unit actually represents a tenfold change in free hydrogen ion level* (McCance et al., 2014). Therefore any pH unit change (e.g., a

change from 7.4 to 7.3) represents a large increase in the free hydrogen ion level.

Maintaining ACID-BASE BALANCE is important because changes from normal pH interfere with many functions. These include:

- Changing the shape and reducing the function of hormones and enzymes
- Changing the distribution of other electrolytes, causing fluid and electrolyte imbalances
- Changing excitable membranes, making the heart, nerves, muscles, and GI tract either less or more active than normal
- Decreasing the effectiveness of many drugs

MAINTAINING ACID-BASE BALANCE

Most body fluids have a pH value between 7.35 and 7.45 even though they contain acidic substances and basic substances. This value is slightly alkaline rather than strictly neutral (7.0 is neutral). Normal body fluid pH remains at this near-neutral value when the acids and bases are nearly balanced, limiting the total number of free or unbalanced hydrogen ions. ACID-BASE BALANCE occurs by matching the rate of hydrogen ion production (which is a continuous normal process) with hydrogen ion loss.

ACID-BASE CHEMISTRY

Acids

Acids are substances that release hydrogen ions when dissolved in water (H_2O) or body fluids, *increasing* the amount of free hydrogen ions in that solution. The strength of an acid is measured by how easily it releases a hydrogen ion in solution. A strong acid such as hydrochloric acid (HCl) separates completely in water and releases *all* of its hydrogen ions, as shown in Fig. 12-1.

$$HCl + H_2O \leftrightarrow H^+ + Cl^- + H_2O$$

Hydrochloric Water Hydrogen Chloride Water
acid   ion   ion

FIG. 12-1 Release of hydrogen ions by a strong acid (hydrochloric acid) in which the strong acid completely dissociates in water.

A weak acid releases only *some*, not all, of its hydrogen ions. In the following example each molecule of acetic acid (CH_3COOH), a weak acid, contains a total of four hydrogen molecules. When acetic acid combines with water, as shown in Fig. 12-2, it releases only *one* of its four hydrogen molecules, keeping the other three hydrogen molecules bound to the molecule (CH_3COO^-).

$$CH_3COOH + H_2O \leftrightarrow H^+ + CH_3COO^- + H_2O$$

Acetic acid   Water Hydrogen Acetic acid   Water
(not ionized)   ion   (ionized)

FIG. 12-2 Release of hydrogen ions by a weak acid (acetic acid) in which the weak acid only partially dissociates in water and most of its hydrogen ions remain bound.

Bases

A base binds free hydrogen ions in solution and *lowers* the amount of free hydrogen ions in solution. Strong bases bind hydrogen ions easily. Examples are sodium hydroxide (NaOH) and ammonia (NH_3).

Weak bases bind hydrogen ions less readily. An example of a weak base is bicarbonate (HCO_3^-). Although a weak base, the many bicarbonate ions in the body are critical in preventing major changes in body fluid pH.

Buffers

Buffers are critical in keeping body fluid pH at normal levels because they can react either as an acid (releasing a hydrogen ion) or as a base (binding a hydrogen ion). How a buffer reacts depends on the existing pH of that fluid. Buffers always try to bring the fluid as close as possible to the normal body fluid pH of 7.35 to 7.45. If the fluid is basic (with few free hydrogen ions), the buffer *releases hydrogen ions* into the fluid (Fig. 12-3). If the fluid is acidic (with many free hydrogen ions), the buffer *binds some of the excess hydrogen ions*. In this way buffers act like hydrogen ion "sponges," soaking up hydrogen ions when too many are present and squeezing out hydrogen ions when too few are present. This flexibility allows buffers to keep body fluid pH in the normal range.

Liquids with a pH of 7.0 are neutral by having a free hydrogen ion level in which the amount and strength of acids and bases are equal. Fig. 12-4 shows the concept of neutral pH in which the combined *strength* and *amount* of all acids are equal to the combined *strength* and *amount* of all bases in a given solution. With human acid-base homeostasis, the relative amounts and

AAABBB   AAAABBB   AAABB
AAABBB   AAAABBB   AAABB
AAABBB   AAAABBB   AAABB

Neutral or acid-   Acidic (acid excess)   Acidic (base deficit)
base balance   (actual acidosis)   (relative acidosis)

FIG. 12-4 Concept of acidic versus normal pH. (A = acid; B = base.)

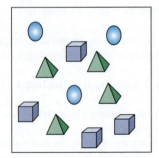

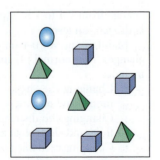

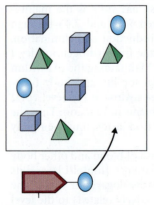

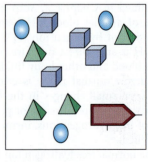

Fluid pH 7.38 (normal). The number and strength of acid components are equal to the number and strength of base components. Hydrogen ion concentration is limited and constant.

Fluid pH 7.51 (alkaline). The number and strength of base components are greater than the number and strength of acid components. Hydrogen ion concentration is below normal.

Buffer is added to the alkaline fluid.

The buffer acts as an acid, releasing a hydrogen ion.

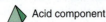 Acid component   Base component   Hydrogen ion   Buffer

FIG. 12-3 Action of buffer in solution. (© 1992 by M. Linda Workman. All rights reserved.)

strengths of acids and bases are nearly equal, and normally hydrogen ion production is balanced with hydrogen ion loss so the overall free hydrogen ion levels remain constant.

Liquids with a pH ranging from 1.0 to 6.99 have more or stronger (or both) acids compared with bases. These liquids are *acidic* (see Fig. 12-4), with more free hydrogen ions released than bound, increasing the amount of free hydrogen ions in the liquid.

Liquids with a pH ranging from 7.01 to 14.0 have more or stronger (or both) bases compared with acids. These liquids are *basic,* in which more hydrogen ions are being bound than released, decreasing the amount of free hydrogen ions (Fig. 12-5).

AAABBB   **AAABBBB**   **AABBB**
AAABBB   **AAABBBB**   **AABBB**
AAABBB   **AAABBBB**   **AABBB**

Neutral   Alkaline (base excess)   Alkaline (acid deficit)

FIG. 12-5 Concept of alkaline versus normal pH. (A = acid; B = base.)

BODY FLUID CHEMISTRY

Bicarbonate Ions

Body fluids contain different types of acids and bases. The most common base in human body fluid is bicarbonate (HCO_3^-); the most common acid is carbonic acid (H_2CO_3). In health the body keeps these substances at a constant ratio of 1 molecule of carbonic acid to 20 free bicarbonate ions (1:20) (Fig. 12-6). To maintain this ratio, both carbonic acid and bicarbonate must be carefully controlled. This constant ratio is related to balancing the production and elimination of carbon dioxide (CO_2) and hydrogen ions (H^+).

Relationship Between Carbon Dioxide and Hydrogen Ions

A key process in understanding ACID-BASE BALANCE is the carbonic anhydrase equation. This equation, driven by the enzyme carbonic anhydrase, shows how hydrogen ion levels and carbon dioxide levels are directly related to one another so an increase in one causes an equal increase in the other (Fig. 12-7).

$$CO_2 + H_2O \leftrightarrow H_2CO_3 \leftrightarrow HCO_3^- + H^+$$

FIG. 12-7 The carbonic anhydrase equation showing that the concentration of carbon dioxide is directly related to the concentration of hydrogen ions.

Carbon dioxide is a gas that forms carbonic acid when combined with water, making carbon dioxide a part of carbonic acid. Carbonic acid is not stable, and the body needs to keep a 1:20 ratio of carbonic acid to bicarbonate. When carbonic acid is formed from water and carbon dioxide, it begins to separate into free hydrogen ions and bicarbonate ions. *Therefore the carbon dioxide content of a fluid is directly related to the amount of hydrogen ions in that fluid. Whenever conditions cause carbon dioxide to increase, more free hydrogen ions are created. Likewise, whenever free hydrogen ion production increases, more carbon dioxide is produced.*

When excess carbon dioxide is produced, the equation shifts to the *right,* causing an *increase* in hydrogen ions (and a *decrease* in pH), as shown in Fig. 12-8. When very little carbon dioxide is produced, no free hydrogen ions are created by this equation.

$$CO_2 + H_2O \rightarrow H_2CO_3 \rightarrow HCO_3^- + H^+$$

FIG. 12-8 Increased carbon dioxide levels force the equation to the right and increase the concentration of hydrogen ions proportionately.

When excess hydrogen ions are present, the carbonic anhydrase equation shifts to the *left,* causing the creation of more carbon dioxide, as shown in Fig. 12-9. When the amount of free hydrogen ions in body fluids is low, no extra carbon dioxide is produced.

$$CO_2 + H_2O \leftarrow H_2CO_3 \leftarrow HCO_3^- + H^+$$

FIG. 12-9 Increased hydrogen ion levels force the equation to the left and increase the concentration of carbon dioxide levels proportionately.

How is the relationship between free hydrogen ions and carbon dioxide helpful? Carbon dioxide is a gas that can be eliminated during exhalation, and this action is important for ACID-BASE BALANCE. When any condition causes the hydrogen ion concentration of body fluids to increase, extra CO_2 is produced in the same proportion. This extra CO_2 is eliminated during exhalation, helping to bring the hydrogen ion concentration down to normal. Whenever the CO_2 level changes, the pH changes to the same degree, in the opposite direction. Thus, when the CO_2 level of a liquid increases, the pH drops, indicating more free hydrogen ions (more acidic). Likewise, when the CO_2 level of a liquid decreases, the pH rises, indicating fewer free hydrogen ions (more alkaline).

An increase in bicarbonate causes the amount of hydrogen ions to decrease and the pH to increase, becoming more alkaline (basic). Likewise, a decrease in bicarbonate causes the free hydrogen ion level to increase and the pH to decrease, becoming more acidic.

Because the kidneys control bicarbonate levels and the lungs control CO_2 levels, pH is also the result of how well the kidneys

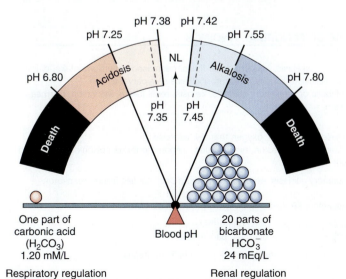

FIG. 12-6 Normal ratio of carbonic acid to bicarbonate is 1:20. (From McCance, K., Huether, S., Brashers, V., & Rote, N. [2014]. *Pathophysiology: The biologic basis for disease in adults and children* [7th ed.]. St. Louis: Mosby.)

are functioning to retain or eliminate bicarbonate divided by how well the lungs are functioning to eliminate carbon dioxide (Fig. 12-10). A problem in either organ system can lead to disturbed ACID-BASE BALANCE.

$$pH = \frac{\text{(Slow but powerful response)}}{\text{Lung function = Carbon dioxide levels}} \frac{\text{Kidney function = Bicarbonate levels}}{\text{(Rapid but limited response)}}$$

FIG. 12-10 Contribution of pH balance by kidney and lung function.

Sources of Acids and Bicarbonate

When acids are present in body fluids, free hydrogen ions are released and must be controlled for ACID-BASE BALANCE. Acids and hydrogen ions are produced continuously through normal body physiologic work and metabolism.

Normal metabolism of carbohydrate, protein, and fat creates natural waste products. Carbohydrate metabolism forms carbon dioxide (CO_2). Carbon dioxide is exhaled by the lungs during breathing. One factor that determines blood pH is how much CO_2 is produced by body cells during metabolism versus how rapidly that CO_2 is removed by breathing. Protein breakdown forms sulfuric acid. Fat breakdown forms fatty acids and ketoacids.

Incomplete breakdown of glucose, which occurs whenever cells metabolize under anaerobic (no oxygen) conditions, forms lactic acid. Anaerobic conditions occur with hypoxia, sepsis, and shock. Incomplete breakdown of fatty acids, occurring when large amounts of fatty acids are being metabolized, forms ketoacids.

Cell destruction allows cell contents to be released, including the structures that contain acids. These released acids in the extracellular fluid (ECF) increase free hydrogen ion levels.

Bicarbonate, a weak base, is the main buffer of the ECF. It comes from the GI absorption of ingested bicarbonate, pancreatic production of bicarbonate, movement of cellular bicarbonate into the ECF, kidney reabsorption of filtered bicarbonate, and the breakdown of carbonic acid. Once bicarbonate is in the ECF, it is kept at a level 20 times greater than that of carbonic acid.

ACID-BASE REGULATORY ACTIONS AND MECHANISMS

As long as body cells are healthy, they continuously produce acids, carbon dioxide, and free hydrogen ions. Despite this production, hydrogen ion, bicarbonate, oxygen, and carbon dioxide levels are kept within normal limits when ACID-BASE BALANCE controlling actions are normal. Chart 12-1 lists the normal values in arterial and venous blood. This homeostasis depends on:

- Hydrogen ion production being consistent and not excessive
- CO_2 loss from the body through breathing keeping pace with all forms of hydrogen ion production

To keep the free hydrogen ion level (pH) of the ECF within the narrow normal range, the body has chemical, respiratory, and kidney actions (mechanisms) for acid-base balance (Table 12-1).

Chemical Acid-Base Control Actions

Buffers are the first line of defense against changes in free hydrogen ion levels. These buffers are always present in body fluids and act fast to reduce or raise the amount of free hydrogen ions to normal. By acting as hydrogen ion "sponges," buffers can bind hydrogen ions when too many are present or release hydrogen ions when not enough are present.

Buffers are composed of chemicals or proteins. The two most common chemical buffers are bicarbonate (which is active in

---

CHART 12-1   Laboratory Profile

Acid-Base Assessment

TEST	NORMAL RANGE FOR ADULTS		SIGNIFICANCE OF ABNORMAL FINDINGS
	ARTERIAL	**VENOUS**	
pH			
Adult <90 yr	7.35-7.45	7.31-7.41	Increased: Metabolic alkalosis, loss of gastric fluids, decreased potassium intake, diuretic therapy, fever, salicylate toxicity, respiratory alkalosis, hyperventilation
>90 yr	7.25-7.45	7.31-7.41	Decreased: Metabolic or respiratory acidosis, ketosis, renal failure, starvation, diarrhea, hyperthyroidism
PaO$_2$			
Adult <90 yr	80-100 mm Hg		Increased: Increased ventilation, oxygen therapy, exercise
>90 yr	70-90 mm Hg		Decreased: Respiratory depression, high altitude, carbon monoxide poisoning, decreased cardiac output
PaCO$_2$	35-45 mm Hg	40-50 mm Hg	Increased: Respiratory acidosis, emphysema, pneumonia, cardiac failure, respiratory depression
			Decreased: Respiratory alkalosis, excessive ventilation, diarrhea
Bicarbonate	21-28 mEq/L	24-29 mEq/L	Increased: Metabolic alkalosis, bicarbonate therapy
	(21-28 mmol/L)	(24-29 mmol/L)	Decreased: Metabolic acidosis, diarrhea, pancreatitis
Lactate	3-7 mg/dL	5-20 mg/dL	Increased: Hypoxia, exercise, insulin infusion, alcoholism, pregnancy
	0.3-0.8 mmol/L	0.6-2.2 mmol/L	Decreased: Fluid overload

PaCO$_2$, Partial pressure of arterial carbon dioxide; *PaO$_2$,* partial pressure of arterial oxygen.
Data from Pagana, K., Pagana, T., & Pagana, T. (2017). *Mosby's diagnostic and laboratory test reference* (13th ed.). St. Louis: Mosby; and Pagana, K., Pagana, T., & Pike-MacDonald, S. (2013). *Mosby's Canadian manual of diagnostic and laboratory tests* (1st ed.). St. Louis: Mosby.

TABLE 12-1   Acid-Base Regulatory Mechanisms

MECHANISM TYPE	KEY CHARACTERISTICS
Chemical	
Protein buffers (albumin, globulins, hemoglobin)	Very rapid response
Chemical buffers (bicarbonate, phosphate)	Provide immediate response to changing conditions
	Can handle relatively small fluctuations in hydrogen ion production during normal metabolic and health conditions
Respiratory	
Increased hydrogen ions or increased carbon dioxide:	Primarily assist buffering systems when the fluctuation of hydrogen ion concentration is acute
Triggers the brain to increase the rate and depth of breathing, causing more carbon dioxide to be lost and decreasing the hydrogen ion concentration	
Decreased hydrogen ions or decreased carbon dioxide:	
Inhibits brain stimulation, leading to decreased rate and depth of breathing, causing carbon dioxide to be retained and increasing the hydrogen ion concentration	
Kidney	
Actions to decrease pH:	The most powerful regulator of acid-base balance
Increased kidney excretion of bicarbonate	Respond to large or chronic fluctuations in hydrogen ion production or elimination
Increased kidney reabsorption of hydrogen ions	Slowest response (hours to days)
Actions to increase pH:	Longest duration
Decreased kidney excretion of bicarbonate	
Decreased kidney reabsorption of hydrogen ions	

both the extracellular fluid [ECF] and intracellular fluid [ICF]) and phosphate (which is active in the ICF). Protein buffers are the most common buffers. Extracellular protein buffers are albumin and globulins. A major intracellular protein buffer is hemoglobin (McCance et al., 2014). When the amount of free hydrogen ions in the blood increases, some of the excess hydrogen ions cross the membranes of red blood cells and bind to the large numbers of hemoglobin molecules in each red blood cell. Binding of hydrogen ions to hemoglobin results in fewer hydrogen ions remaining in the blood, bringing blood pH back up toward normal.

Respiratory Acid-Base Control Actions

When chemical buffers alone cannot prevent changes in blood pH, the respiratory system is the second line of defense against changes. Breathing controls the amount of free hydrogen ions by controlling the amount of carbon dioxide (CO_2) in arterial blood. Because CO_2 is converted into hydrogen ions with the carbonic anhydrase reaction, the CO_2 level is *directly* related to the hydrogen ion level. Breathing rids the body of any excess CO_2.

The CO_2 level in venous blood increases with metabolism. This CO_2 moves into lung capillary blood. Because the amount (pressure) of CO_2 is far higher in lung capillary blood than it is in the air in the alveoli, CO_2 diffuses freely from the blood into the alveolar air. Once in the alveoli, CO_2 is exhaled during breathing and is lost from the body. Because the amount of CO_2 in room air is nearly zero, CO_2 can continue to be exhaled even when breathing is impaired.

Respiratory regulation of ACID-BASE BALANCE is under the control of the central nervous system (Fig. 12-11). Special receptors in the respiratory areas of the brain are sensitive to changes in the amount of CO_2 in brain tissues. As the amount of CO_2 begins to rise above normal in brain blood and tissues, these central receptors trigger the neurons to increase the rate and depth of breathing (**hyperventilation**). As a result, more

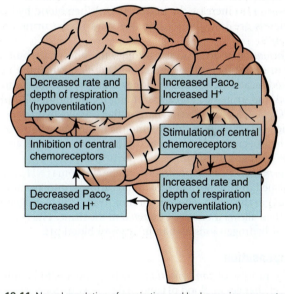

FIG. 12-11 Neural regulation of respiration and hydrogen ion concentration. (*H⁺*, Hydrogen ion, *PacO₂*, partial pressure of arterial carbon dioxide.)

CO_2 is exhaled ("blown off") from the lungs, and the CO_2 level in the ECF decreases. When the arterial CO_2 level returns back down to normal, the rate and depth of breathing return to levels that are normal for the patient.

If the amount of ECF free hydrogen ions is too low, the CO_2 level also is too low. Central receptors sense these low CO_2 levels and stop or slow the neuron activity in the respiratory centers of the brain, decreasing the rate and depth of breathing (**hypoventilation**). As a result, less CO_2 is lost through the lungs, and more CO_2 is retained in arterial blood. This retention of already-formed CO_2, together with the normal production of CO_2 from metabolism, results in a rapid return of the arterial

CO_2 levels (and hydrogen ion levels) back up to normal. When these levels are normal, the rate and depth of breathing also return to normal levels.

The respiratory system's response in ACID-BASE BALANCE is rapid. Changes in the rate and depth of breathing occur within minutes after changes in the hydrogen ion level or CO_2 level of the ECF occur.

Kidney Acid-Base Control Actions

The kidneys are the third line of defense against wide changes in body fluid pH. Kidney actions are stronger for regulating ACID-BASE BALANCE but take 24 to 48 hours to completely respond. When blood pH changes are persistent, kidney actions to increase excretion and reabsorption rates of acids or bases (depending on which way pH changes) start. These actions are kidney movement of bicarbonate, formation of acids, and formation of ammonium.

Kidney movement of bicarbonate is the first kidney pH control action. It occurs in the kidney tubules in two ways: (1) kidney movement of bicarbonate produced elsewhere in the body, and (2) kidney movement of bicarbonate produced in the kidneys. Much of the bicarbonate made in other body areas is excreted in the urine. When blood hydrogen ion levels are high, this bicarbonate is reabsorbed from the kidneys back into circulation, where it can help buffer excess hydrogen ions. The kidney tubules also can make additional bicarbonate and reabsorb it to increase the buffer effect. When blood hydrogen ion levels are low, the bicarbonate stays in the urine and is excreted.

Formation of acids occurs through the phosphate-buffering system inside the cells of the kidney tubules. When the newly created bicarbonate made in kidney cells is reabsorbed into the blood, the urine has an excess of anions, including phosphate (HPO_4^{2-}). This negatively charged fluid draws hydrogen ions (which have a positive charge) into the urine. Once in the urine, the hydrogen ion binds to phosphate ions, forming an acid (H_2PO_4) that is then excreted in the urine.

Formation of ammonium converts the ammonia (NH_3), which is formed during normal protein breakdown, into ammonium (NH_4^+) in the urine. The ammonium "traps" the hydrogen ions and then allows them to be excreted in the urine. The result is a loss of hydrogen ions and an increase in blood pH.

Compensation

In the process of *compensation*, the body adapts to attempt to correct changes in blood pH and maintain ACID-BASE BALANCE. A pH below 6.9 or above 7.8 is usually fatal. The normal pH range for human extracellular fluid (ECF) is 7.35 to 7.45. Both the kidneys and the lungs can compensate for acid-base imbalances, but they are not equal in their final responses. The respiratory system is much more sensitive to acid-base changes and can begin compensation efforts within seconds to minutes after a change in pH. However, these efforts are limited and can be overwhelmed easily. The kidney compensatory actions are much more powerful and result in rapid changes in ECF composition. However, these more powerful actions are not fully triggered unless the acid-base imbalance continues for several hours to several days.

Respiratory compensation occurs through the lungs, usually to correct for acid-base imbalances from metabolic problems. For example, when prolonged running causes buildup of lactic acid, hydrogen ion levels in the ECF increase, causing the pH

to drop. To bring the pH back to normal, breathing is triggered in response to increased carbon dioxide levels. Both the rate and depth of respiration increase. These respiratory efforts cause the blood to lose carbon dioxide with each exhalation, so ECF levels of carbon dioxide and free hydrogen ions gradually decrease. When the lungs can *fully compensate*, the pH returns to normal (Blevins, 2014).

Kidney compensation results when a healthy kidney works to correct for changes in blood pH that occur when the respiratory system either is overwhelmed or is not healthy. For example, in an adult with chronic obstructive pulmonary disease (COPD), the respiratory system cannot exchange gases adequately. Carbon dioxide is retained continuously, hydrogen ion levels increase, and the blood pH falls (becomes more acidic). The kidneys oppose this by excreting more hydrogen ions and increasing the movement of bicarbonate back into the blood. Then blood pH remains either within or closer to the normal range. When adaptive actions are completely effective, acid-base problems are *fully compensated*; and the pH of the blood returns to normal, even though the levels of oxygen and bicarbonate may be abnormal (Blevins, 2014).

However, sometimes the respiratory problem causing the acid-base imbalance is so severe that kidney actions can only *partially compensate* and the pH is not quite normal. Partial compensation prevents the acid-base imbalance from becoming severe (Blevins, 2014; Larkin & Zimmanck, 2015).

❓ NCLEX EXAMINATION CHALLENGE 12-1
Physiological Integrity

How are blood hydrogen ion levels and blood carbon dioxide levels related?
A. These two blood values are negatively related to the extent that, as carbon dioxide levels rise, the concentration of hydrogen ions decreases.
B. Carbon dioxide is attached to and becomes part of hydrogen ions in the blood so the loss of one always leads to the loss of the other.
C. There is no relation between blood hydrogen ion level and carbon dioxide, making the concentration of each substance independent of the other.
D. Blood hydrogen ion levels and blood carbon dioxide levels are directly related so, when the level of one increases, the level of the other increases to the same degree.

ACID-BASE IMBALANCES

Acid-base imbalances are problems of ACID-BASE BALANCE resulting from changes in the blood hydrogen ion level or pH. These changes are caused by problems with the acid-base regulatory actions or exposure to dangerous conditions. Imbalances in which blood pH is below normal reflect acidosis, and imbalances in which blood pH is above normal reflect alkalosis. Acid-base imbalances impair the function of many organs and can be life threatening.

✦ ACID-BASE BALANCE CONCEPT EXEMPLAR
Acidosis
❖ *PATHOPHYSIOLOGY*

In acidosis the ACID-BASE BALANCE of the blood and other extracellular fluid (ECF) is upset by an excess of hydrogen ions (H^+). This is seen as an arterial blood pH below 7.35. The amount of acids present is greater than normal compared with the amount or strength of bases.

Acidosis is not a disease; it is a condition caused by a disorder or pathologic process. It can be caused by metabolic problems, respiratory problems, or both. Patients at greatest risk for acute acidosis are those with problems that impair breathing. Older adults with chronic health problems are at greater risk for developing acidosis (Chart 12-2) (McCance et al., 2014).

Acidosis can result from an actual or relative increase in the amount or strength of acids. An *actual acid excess* results in acidosis by either overproducing acids (and release of hydrogen ions) or undereliminating normally produced acids (retention of hydrogen ions). Either way, more hydrogen ions are present than should be. Problems that increase acid production include diabetic ketoacidosis and seizures. Problems that decrease acid elimination include respiratory impairment and kidney impairment.

In *relative* acidosis the amount of acids does not increase. Instead the amount or strength of the bases decreases (to create a *base deficit*), which makes the fluid relatively more acidic than basic. A relative acidosis *(base deficit)* is caused by either overeliminating or underproducing bicarbonate ions (HCO_3^-) (see Fig. 12-4). Problems that underproduce bases include pancreatitis and dehydration. A condition that overeliminates bases is diarrhea.

Regardless of its cause, acidosis causes major changes in body function. The main problems occur because hydrogen ions are positively charged ions. An increase in hydrogen ions creates imbalances of other positively charged electrolytes, especially potassium. The changes in potassium levels because of excess hydrogen ions are described in the Laboratory Assessment section for acidosis. These electrolyte imbalances then disrupt the functions of nerves, cardiac muscle, and skeletal muscle. Symptoms of acidosis first appear in the musculoskeletal, cardiac, respiratory, and central nervous systems. Even slight increases in blood hydrogen ion levels reduce the activity of many hormones and enzymes, leading to death.

Acidosis can be caused by metabolic problems, respiratory problems, or combined metabolic and respiratory problems. Specific causes of acidosis are listed in Table 12-2.

Metabolic Acidosis

Four processes can result in metabolic acidosis: overproduction of hydrogen ions, underelimination of hydrogen ions, underproduction of bicarbonate ions, and overelimination of bicarbonate ions.

Overproduction of hydrogen ions can occur with excessive breakdown of fatty acids, anaerobic glucose breakdown *(lactic acidosis),* and excessive intake of acids. Excessive breakdown of fatty acids occurs with diabetic ketoacidosis or starvation. When insufficient glucose is available for fuel, the body breaks down fats (lipids). The products of excessive fatty acid breakdown are strong acids *(ketoacids),* which release large amounts of hydrogen ions.

Lactic acidosis occurs when cells use glucose without adequate oxygen *(anaerobic metabolism);* glucose then is incompletely broken down and forms lactic acid. This acid releases hydrogen ions, causing acidosis. Lactic acidosis occurs whenever

---

CHART 12-2 **Nursing Focus on the Older Adult**

The Older Patient Experiencing Acid-Base Imbalance

When Obtaining a Patient's History

- Assess risk factors for acid-base imbalance, including drugs, chronic health problems (especially kidney disease, pulmonary disease), and acute health problems.
- Ask the patient to list all prescribed and over-the-counter drugs (especially diuretics and antacids). If the patient is unable to provide this information, ask the family to bring the drugs in from home.
- Ask the patient to recall which liquids were taken in the past 24 hours and whether urination amounts have changed.

When Assessing the Patient

- Compare the patient's mental status with what the family, significant other, or health record states is the patient's baseline.
- Observe the rate and depth of respiration.
- Determine whether the patient can complete a sentence without stopping for breath.
- Examine the color of nail beds and mucous membranes.
- Obtain a urine specimen and observe for color and character. Test for specific gravity and pH.
- Examine skin turgor for dehydration. Attempt to pinch the skin to form a tent over the sternum and on the forehead. If a tent forms, record how long it remains.
- Measure the rate and quality of the pulse.
- Monitor clinical responses and laboratory values while the acid-base imbalance is being corrected.
- Administer IV therapy by pump or controller.

Modified from Touhy, T., & Jett, K. (2016). *Ebersole & Hess' Toward healthy aging: Human needs & nursing response.* St. Louis: Elsevier.

TABLE 12-2 **Common Causes of Acidosis**

PATHOLOGY	CONDITION
Metabolic Acidosis	
Overproduction of hydrogen ions	Excessive oxidation of fatty acids: Diabetic ketoacidosis Starvation Hypermetabolism: Heavy exercise Seizure activity Fever Hypoxia, ischemia Excessive ingestion of acids: Ethanol or methanol intoxication Salicylate intoxication
Underelimination of hydrogen ions	Kidney failure
Underproduction of bicarbonate	Kidney failure Pancreatitis Liver failure Dehydration
Overelimination of bicarbonate	Diarrhea
Respiratory Acidosis	
Underelimination of hydrogen ions	Respiratory depression: Anesthetics Drugs (especially opioids) Electrolyte imbalance Inadequate chest expansion: Muscle weakness Airway obstruction Alveolar-capillary block

the body has too little oxygen to meet metabolic oxygen demands (e.g., heavy exercise, seizure activity, reduced oxygen).

Excessive intake of acids floods the body with hydrogen ions. Agents that cause acidosis when ingested in excess include ethyl alcohol, methyl alcohol, and acetylsalicylic acid (aspirin).

Underelimination of hydrogen ions leads to acidosis when hydrogen ions are produced at the normal rate but are not removed at the same rate they are produced. Most hydrogen ion loss occurs through the lungs and the kidneys. Kidney failure causes acidosis when the kidney tubules cannot secrete hydrogen ions into the urine and they are retained. Severe lung problems also can result in retention of CO_2 with a corresponding retention of hydrogen ions.

Underproduction of bicarbonate ions (base deficit) leads to acidosis when hydrogen ion production and removal are normal but too few bicarbonate ions are present to balance the hydrogen ions. Because bicarbonate is made in the kidneys and pancreas, kidney failure and impaired liver or pancreatic function can cause a base-deficit acidosis.

Overelimination of bicarbonate ions (base deficit) leads to acidosis when hydrogen ion production and removal are normal but too many bicarbonate ions have been lost. One cause of base deficit acidosis is diarrhea.

Respiratory Acidosis

Respiratory acidosis results when respiratory function is impaired and the exchange of oxygen (O_2) and carbon dioxide (CO_2) is reduced. This problem causes CO_2 retention, which leads to the same increase in hydrogen ion levels and acidosis (McCance et al., 2014). (See the carbonic anhydrase equation in Fig. 12-7.)

Unlike metabolic acidosis, respiratory acidosis results from only one cause—retention of CO_2, causing increased production of free hydrogen ions. Table 12-2 lists the four types of respiratory problems and their possible causes.

Respiratory depression results from depressed function of the brainstem neurons that trigger breathing movements. This lowered rate and depth of breathing leads to poor gas exchange and retention of carbon dioxide. Common causes include anesthetic agents, opioids, and poisons. Physical respiratory depression occurs when respiratory neurons are damaged or destroyed by trauma or when problems in the brain increase the intracranial pressure. Problems causing cerebral edema and respiratory depression include brain tumors, cerebral aneurysm, stroke, and fluid overload.

Inadequate chest expansion reduces gas exchange and leads to acidosis. Chest expansion can be restricted by skeletal trauma or deformities, respiratory muscle weakness, or external constriction. Respiratory muscle weakness, caused by electrolyte imbalances, fatigue, muscular dystrophy, muscle damage, or muscle breakdown, reduces chest movement. External conditions such as casts, tight scar tissue around the chest, obesity, and the internal condition of ascites can restrict chest movement.

Airway obstruction prevents air movement into and out from the lungs *(ventilation)* and leads to poor gas exchange, CO_2 retention, and acidosis. External obstruction can be caused by clothing, neck edema, and local lymph node enlargement. Internal obstruction can be caused by aspiration of foreign objects, bronchoconstriction, mucus, and edema.

Reduced alveolar-capillary diffusion causes poor gas exchange and leads to CO_2 retention and acidosis. Disorders that reduce diffusion include pneumonia, pneumonitis, tuberculosis,

emphysema, acute respiratory distress syndrome, chest trauma, pulmonary emboli, pulmonary edema, and drowning.

In addition to pathologic conditions, improper mechanical ventilation can cause respiratory acidosis. If either the tidal volume or the number of ventilations per minute is set too low, the patient can develop respiratory acidosis because the ventilations are not sufficient to rid the body of excess CO_2 (Lian, 2013).

Combined Metabolic and Respiratory Acidosis

Metabolic and respiratory acidosis can occur at the same time. Uncorrected acute respiratory acidosis always leads to poor oxygenation and lactic acidosis (McCance et al., 2014). For example, an adult who has diabetic ketoacidosis and chronic obstructive pulmonary disease has a combined metabolic and respiratory acidosis. Combined acidosis is more severe than either metabolic acidosis or respiratory acidosis alone.

❖ INTERPROFESSIONAL COLLABORATIVE CARE

Episodes of acidosis that are severe enough to require intervention are usually managed in an acute care setting. Patients are discharged from the hospital when ACID-BASE BALANCE is restored. For patients who are at continuing risk for acidosis, especially respiratory acidosis, management interventions must be continued in the home or other residential setting.

◆ Assessment: Noticing

History. Collect data about risk factors related to the development of acidosis. Information about age, nutrition, and current symptoms is especially important.

Older adults are more at risk for problems leading to acid-base imbalance, including cardiac, kidney, or pulmonary impairment (Touhy & Jett, 2016). They also may be taking drugs that disrupt ACID-BASE BALANCE, especially diuretics and aspirin. Ask about specific risk factors such as any type of breathing problem, kidney failure, diabetes mellitus, diarrhea, pancreatitis, and fever.

Obtain a detailed nutrition history to determine total caloric intake and the proportions of carbohydrates, fats, and proteins ingested. Ask whether the patient has fasted or followed a strict diet within the past week.

Ask about headaches, behavior changes, increased drowsiness, reduced alertness, reduced attention span, lethargy, anorexia, abdominal distention, nausea or vomiting, muscle weakness, or increased fatigue. Ask the patient to relate activities of the previous 24 hours to identify activity intolerance, behavior changes, and fatigue. Because the central nervous system is often depressed in acidosis, you may need to obtain this information from the patient's family.

Physical Assessment/Signs and Symptoms. Symptoms of acidosis are similar whether the cause is metabolic or respiratory (Chart 12-3). Acidosis reduces the ability of excitable membranes to respond appropriately, especially in cardiovascular tissue, neurons, skeletal muscle, and GI smooth muscle.

Cardiovascular changes are first seen with mild acidosis and are more severe as the condition worsens. Early changes include increased heart rate and cardiac output. With worsening acidosis or with acidosis and hyperkalemia (elevated blood potassium levels), heart rate decreases, T waves become tall and peaked, and QRS complexes are widened. Peripheral pulses may be hard to find and are easily blocked. Hypotension occurs with vasodilation.

Central nervous system (CNS) changes include depression of CNS function. Problems may range from lethargy to confusion, especially in older patients. As acidosis worsens, the patient may become unresponsive.

Neuromuscular changes include reduced muscle tone and deep tendon reflexes as a result of the accompanying hyperkalemia.

 NURSING SAFETY PRIORITY **QSEN**

Critical Rescue

Assess the cardiovascular system **first** in any patient at risk for acidosis because acidosis can lead to cardiac arrest from the accompanying hyperkalemia. If cardiac changes are present, respond by reporting these changes immediately to the health care provider.

⟫ **CHART 12-3   Key Features**

Acidosis

Cardiovascular Signs and Symptoms
- Delayed electrical conduction:
  - Ranges from bradycardia to heart block
  - Tall T waves
  - Widened QRS complex
  - Prolonged PR interval
- Hypotension
- Thready peripheral pulses

Central Nervous System Signs and Symptoms
- Depressed activity (lethargy, confusion, stupor, coma)

Neuromuscular Signs and Symptoms
- Hyporeflexia
- Skeletal muscle weakness
- Flaccid paralysis

Respiratory Signs and Symptoms
- Kussmaul respirations (in metabolic acidosis with respiratory compensation)
- Variable respirations (generally ineffective in respiratory acidosis)

Integumentary Signs and Symptoms
- Warm, flushed, dry skin in metabolic acidosis
- Pale-to-cyanotic and dry skin in respiratory acidosis

Assess arm muscle strength by having the patient squeeze your hand. Assess leg muscle strength by having the patient push both feet against a flat surface (such as a box or a board) while you apply resistance to the opposite side of the surface. Muscle weakness is bilateral and can progress to paralysis.

Respiratory changes may cause the acidosis and can be caused by the acidosis (Larkin & Zimmanck, 2015). Assess the patient's rate, depth, and ease of breathing. Use pulse oximetry to determine how well oxygen is delivered to the peripheral tissues.

If acidosis is metabolic in origin, the rate and depth of breathing increase as the hydrogen ion level rises. Breaths are deep and rapid and not under voluntary control, a pattern called Kussmaul respiration.

If acidosis is caused by respiratory problems, breathing efforts are reduced. Respirations are usually shallow and rapid. Muscle weakness makes this problem worse.

Skin changes occur with metabolic or respiratory acidosis. With metabolic acidosis breathing is unimpaired, the rate is increased, and CO_2 is lost. This causes vasodilation and makes the skin and mucous membranes warm, dry, and pink. With respiratory acidosis breathing is ineffective, and skin and mucous membranes are pale to cyanotic.

Psychosocial Assessment. Cognitive changes may be the first signs of acidosis. Assess the patient's mental status for awareness of time, place, and person (see Chapter 41). Determine whether the patient is able to perform simple cognitive tasks such as counting backward by threes. Behavior changes may accompany acidosis. Observe and document the patient's behavior by description (objectively) rather than by interpretation (subjectively). Ask family members if the patient's behavior is typical for him or her and establish a baseline for comparison with later assessment findings.

Laboratory Assessment. Arterial blood pH is the laboratory value used to confirm acidosis. Acidosis is present when arterial blood pH is less than 7.35. However, this test alone does not indicate what is causing the acidosis. Symptoms of metabolic acidosis and respiratory acidosis are similar, but their treatments are different. *Therefore it is critical to obtain and interpret other laboratory data such as arterial blood gas (ABG) values and blood levels of electrolytes* (Chart 12-4).

Metabolic acidosis is reflected by several changes in ABG values. The pH is low (<7.35) because buffering and respiratory compensation are not adequate to keep the amount of free

---

◢ **CHART 12-4   Laboratory Profile**

Acid-Base Imbalances (Uncompensated)

	LABORATORY VALUE CHANGES						
IMBALANCE	**pH**	**HCO₃⁻**	**PaO₂**	**PaCO₂**	**K⁺**	**Ca²⁺**	**Cl⁻**
Metabolic acidosis	↓	↓	Ø	Ø and ↓	↑	Ø	Ø and ↑
Respiratory acidosis	↓	Ø or ↑↓	↓	↑	↑	Ø	↑↓
Combined acidosis	↓	↓↑	↓	↑	↑	Ø	↑
Metabolic alkalosis	↑	↑	Ø	Ø and ↑	↓	↓	↓
Respiratory alkalosis	↑	Ø or ↑↓	Ø	↓↓	↓	↓	↑
Combined alkalosis	↑	↑	Ø	↓	↓	↓	↓

↑, Above normal; ↓, below normal; ↑↓, value can increase or decrease depending on other factors; Ø, normal; *Ca²⁺*, calcium ions; *Cl⁻*, chloride ions; *PaCO₂*, partial pressure of arterial carbon dioxide; *PaO₂*, partial pressure of arterial oxygen; *HCO₃⁻*, bicarbonate ions; *K⁺*, potassium ions.

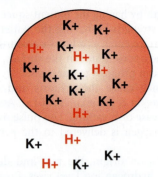

Under normal conditions, the intracellular potassium content is much greater than that of the extracellular fluid. The concentration of hydrogen ions is low in both compartments.

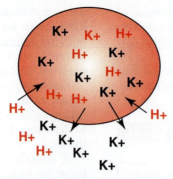

In acidosis, the extracellular hydrogen ion content increases and the hydrogen ions move into the intracellular fluid. To keep the intracellular fluid electrically neutral, an equal number of potassium ions leave the cell, creating a relative hyperkalemia.

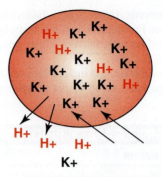

In alkalosis, more hydrogen ions are present in the intracellular fluid than in the extracellular fluid. Hydrogen ions move from the intracellular fluid into the extracellular fluid. To keep the intracellular fluid electrically neutral, potassium ions move from the extracellular fluid into the intracellular fluid, creating a relative hypokalemia.

FIG. 12-12 Movement of potassium (K^+) in response to changes in the extracellular fluid hydrogen ion (H^+) concentration.

hydrogen ions at a normal level. The bicarbonate level is low (<21 mEq/L [mmol/L]). It is low because (1) bicarbonate has been lost, causing a base-deficit acidosis; (2) bicarbonate production is inadequate, causing a base-deficit acidosis; or (3) bicarbonate may be bound to other substances. The partial pressure of arterial oxygen (PaO_2) is normal because gas exchange is not impaired. The partial pressure of arterial carbon dioxide ($PacO_2$) is normal or even slightly decreased because gas exchange is adequate and carbon dioxide retention is not a factor.

The serum potassium level is often high in acidosis as the body attempts to maintain electroneutrality during buffering. Fig. 12-12 shows the movement of potassium ions as serum pH changes. As the blood hydrogen ion level rises, some of the excess hydrogen ions enter red blood cells for intracellular buffering. The movement of hydrogen ions into the cells creates an excess of positive ions inside the cells. To balance these extra positive charges, an equal number of potassium ions (that also have a positive charge) move from the cells into the blood. This increases the blood potassium level, causing hyperkalemia (Gooch, 2015).

Respiratory acidosis is reflected by several changes in ABG values. The pH is low (<7.35) because of the increased amount of free hydrogen ions in the blood. Buffering and kidney compensation are not adequate to keep the amount of free hydrogen ions at a normal level. If the kidneys partially compensate for this acidosis, pH is low but not as abnormal as could be expected with the degree of CO_2 retention.

The partial pressure of arterial oxygen (PaO_2) is low, and the partial pressure of arterial carbon dioxide ($PacO_2$) is high because the pulmonary problem impairs gas exchange, causing poor oxygenation and CO_2 retention. *(The hallmarks of respiratory acidosis are a decreasing PaO_2 coupled with a rising $PacO_2$.)* Because carbon dioxide diffuses more easily across the alveolar membrane than oxygen, a decreased PaO_2 usually occurs before an increased $PacO_2$.

The serum bicarbonate level is variable. A patient with rapid onset of respiratory acidosis often has a normal bicarbonate level because kidney compensation has not started. When the

acidosis persists for 24 hours or longer, kidney compensation increases the levels of bicarbonate. Chronic respiratory acidosis is indicated by an elevated bicarbonate level and increased $PacO_2$.

Serum potassium levels are elevated in acute respiratory acidosis. They are normal or low in chronic respiratory acidosis when kidney compensation is present.

💡 NCLEX EXAMINATION CHALLENGE 12-2
Physiological Integrity

Which blood laboratory values does the nurse need to evaluate to determine whether the client's acidosis has a respiratory origin or a metabolic origin? **Select all that apply.**
A. Calcium
B. HCO_3^-
C. Lactic acid (lactate)
D. $PaCO_2$
E. PaO_2
F. pH
G. Potassium

◆ *Analysis: Interpreting*

Patients experiencing acidosis have problems associated with the decreased function of excitable membranes. For metabolic acidosis these problems include hypotension and decreased perfusion, impaired memory and cognition, and increased risk for falls. For patients who have respiratory acidosis in addition to the general problems, life-threatening problems are related to the cause of the respiratory impairment. The priority collaborative problem for the patient experiencing respiratory acidosis is:

1. Decreased gas exchange due to underlying pulmonary disease

◆ *Planning and Implementation: Responding*

Interventions for acidosis focus on correcting the underlying problem and monitoring for changes. Remember that acidosis is not a disease. It is a symptom of another health problem. To ensure appropriate interventions, first identify the specific type of acidosis present.

Metabolic Acidosis. Interventions for metabolic acidosis include hydration and drugs or treatments to control the problem causing the acidosis. For example, if the acidosis is a result of diabetic ketoacidosis, insulin is given to correct the hyperglycemia and halt the production of ketone bodies. Rehydration and antidiarrheal drugs are given if the acidosis is a result of prolonged diarrhea. *Bicarbonate is administered only if serum bicarbonate levels are low and the pH is less than 7.2 (Ellis, 2015).*

Nursing priorities include continuously monitoring the patient for indications either that he or she is responding to the treatment or the acidosis is becoming worse. The cardiovascular and skeletal muscle systems are sensitive to acidosis and are the most important systems to monitor. Interpreting ABG results is an important part of monitoring.

Respiratory Acidosis

Improving Gas Exchange

Planning: Expected Outcomes. The patient being managed for respiratory acidosis is expected to have a reduction in acidosis signs and symptoms. Indications include:

- Arterial pH approaching 7.35
- PaO_2 levels above 90 mm Hg
- $PaCO_2$ levels below 45 mm Hg or at least 15 mm Hg below the patient's admission level

Interventions. Interventions for the patient who has a condition that causes him or her to remain at continued risk include drug therapy, oxygen therapy, pulmonary hygiene (positioning and breathing techniques), and ventilatory support. These interventions are the same as those used for a patient who has chronic obstructive pulmonary disease (COPD), which is the most common health problem associated with continuing risk for respiratory acidosis. A brief overview of these interventions is provided here. For in-depth discussion of these interventions, see Chapter 30 under the Gas Exchange Exemplar: Chronic Obstructive Pulmonary Disease.

Drug therapy is focused on improving ventilation and gas exchange rather than directly on altering pH. Drug categories useful for respiratory acidosis include bronchodilators, anti-inflammatories, and mucolytics.

Oxygen therapy helps promote gas exchange for patients with respiratory acidosis. Carefully monitor oxygen saturation levels to ensure that the lowest flow of oxygen that prevents hypoxemia is used to avoid oxygen-induced tissue damage.

Ventilation support with mechanical ventilation may be needed for patients who cannot keep their oxygen saturation at 90% or who have respiratory muscle fatigue. Chapter 32 discusses the nursing care needs of patients who are being mechanically ventilated.

Preventing complications is a nursing priority when caring for a patient with respiratory acidosis. Monitoring breathing status hourly and intervening when changes occur are critical in preventing complications. Listen to breath sounds and assess how easily air moves into and out of the lungs. Check for any muscle retractions, the use of accessory muscles (especially the neck muscles [sternocleidomastoids]), and whether breathing produces a grunt or wheeze that can be heard without a stethoscope. Assess nail beds and oral membranes for cyanosis (a late finding).

Care Coordination and Transition Management

Because respiratory acidosis is a symptom or complication of another health problem, most often COPD, care during the acute phase occurs in a hospital setting. Ongoing management for continuing risk is the same as for COPD. See Chapter 30 for a detailed discussion of the care coordination needed for this problem.

◆ Evaluation: Reflecting

Depending on the cause of the respiratory acidosis and the patient's continuing risk, some patients may not return to full ACID-BASE BALANCE, even with meticulous care. Indications that the patient's underlying disease process is well managed and that the imbalance is reduced include the expected outcomes that he or she:

- Maintains adequate gas exchange
- Has an arterial pH above 7.2 and closer to 7.35
- Has a PaO_2 level above 90 mm Hg or at least 10 mm Hg higher than his or her admission level
- Has a $PaCO_2$ levels below 45 mm Hg or at least 15 mm Hg below his or her admission level

---

? CLINICAL JUDGMENT CHALLENGE 12-1

Patient-Centered Care; Safety; Evidence-Based Practice **QSEN**

A patient who comes to the emergency department for a sports injury suddenly goes into cardiac arrest and has neither a pulse nor any respiratory effort. He is successfully resuscitated within 5 minutes of the initial arrest.

1. Which specific type of impairment of acid-base balance would this situation cause? Provide a rationale for your choice.
2. Should you prepare to administer intravenous sodium bicarbonate? Why or why not?
3. Should oxygen be applied to this patient in the initial post-resuscitation period? Why or why not?

ALKALOSIS

❖ PATHOPHYSIOLOGY

In patients with alkalosis, the ACID-BASE BALANCE of the blood is disturbed and has an excess of bases, especially bicarbonate (HCO_3^-). The amount or strength of the bases is greater than normal compared with the amount of the acids. Alkalosis is a *decrease* in the free hydrogen ion level of the blood and is reflected by an arterial blood pH *above* 7.45. Like acidosis, alkalosis is not a disease but rather is an indication of a problem. It can be caused by metabolic problems, respiratory problems, or both (Table 12-3).

Alkalosis can result from an actual or relative increase in the amount or strength (or both) of bases. In an actual base excess, alkalosis occurs when base (usually bicarbonate) is either overproduced or undereliminated.

In *relative* alkalosis the actual amount or strength of bases does not increase; but the amount of the acids decreases, creating an *acid deficit*. A relative base-excess alkalosis (actual acid deficit) results from an overelimination or underproduction of acids (Fig. 12-13).

The problems of alkalosis are serious and can be life threatening. Management focuses on correcting the cause

TABLE 12-3	Common Causes of Alkalosis
PATHOLOGY	**CONDITION**
Metabolic Alkalosis	
Increase of base components	Oral ingestion of bases: Antacids Parenteral base administration: Blood transfusion Sodium bicarbonate Total parenteral nutrition
Decrease of acid components	Prolonged vomiting Nasogastric suctioning Hypercortisolism Hyperaldosteronism Thiazide diuretics
Respiratory Alkalosis	
Excessive loss of carbon dioxide	Hyperventilation, fear, anxiety Mechanical ventilation Salicylate toxicity High altitudes Shock Early-stage acute pulmonary problems

AAABBB AAABBBB AABBB
AAABBB AAABBBB AABBB
AAABBB AAABBBB AABBB

Acid-base balance   Actual alkalosis (base excess)   Relative alkalosis (acid deficit)

FIG. 12-13 Concepts of actual and relative alkalosis. (A = acid; B = base.)

after identifying whether the alkalosis origin is respiratory or metabolic.

Whether metabolic, respiratory, or both, alkalosis affects specific functions. The pathologic effects are caused by the electrolyte imbalances that occur in response to decreased blood cation (positively charged particles) levels. Most problems of alkalosis are related to increased stimulation of the nervous, neuromuscular, and cardiac systems.

Metabolic alkalosis is an acid-base imbalance caused by either an increase of bases (base excess) or a decrease of acids (acid deficit). Base excesses are caused by excessive intake of bicarbonates, carbonates, acetates, and citrates. Excessive use of bicarbonate-containing antacids can cause a metabolic alkalosis. Other base excesses can occur during medical treatments such as citrate excesses during massive blood transfusions and IV sodium bicarbonate given to correct acidosis. The hallmark of a base excess acidosis is an ABG result with an elevated pH and an elevated bicarbonate level, along with normal oxygen and carbon dioxide levels.

Acid deficits can be caused by disease processes or medical treatment. Disorders causing acid deficits include prolonged vomiting, excess cortisol, and hyperaldosteronism. Treatments that promote acid loss causing metabolic alkalosis include thiazide diuretics and prolonged gastric suctioning.

Respiratory alkalosis is usually caused by an excessive loss of CO_2 through hyperventilation (rapid respirations). Patients may hyperventilate in response to anxiety, fear, or improper settings on mechanical ventilators. Hyperventilation can also result from direct stimulation of central respiratory centers because of fever, central nervous system lesions, and salicylates.

CHART 12-5 **Key Features**

Alkalosis

Central Nervous System Signs and Symptoms
- Increased activity
- Anxiety, irritability, tetany, seizures
- Positive Chvostek's sign
- Positive Trousseau's sign
- Paresthesias

Neuromuscular Signs and Symptoms
- Hyperreflexia
- Muscle cramping and twitching
- Skeletal muscle weakness

Cardiovascular Signs and Symptoms
- Increased heart rate
- Normal or low blood pressure
- Increased digitalis toxicity

Respiratory Signs and Symptoms
- Increased rate and depth of ventilation in respiratory alkalosis
- Decreased respiratory effort associated with skeletal muscle weakness in metabolic alkalosis

The hallmark of respiratory alkalosis is an ABG result with an elevated pH coupled with a low carbon dioxide level. Usually the oxygen and bicarbonate levels are normal.

❖ **INTERPROFESSIONAL COLLABORATIVE CARE**

◆ **Assessment: Noticing**

Symptoms of problems with ACID-BASE BALANCE regulation are the same for metabolic and respiratory alkalosis. Many symptoms are the result of the low calcium levels (**hypocalcemia**) and low potassium levels (**hypokalemia**) that usually occur with alkalosis (see Fig. 12-12). These problems change the function of the nervous, neuromuscular, cardiac, and respiratory systems (Chart 12-5).

Central nervous system (CNS) changes are caused by over-excitement of the nervous systems. Patients have dizziness, agitation, confusion, and hyperreflexia, which may progress to seizures. Tingling or numbness may occur around the mouth and in the toes. Other indicators of alkalosis with hypocalcemia are positive Chvostek's and Trousseau's signs (see Chapter 11).

Neuromuscular changes are related to the hypocalcemia and hypokalemia that occur with alkalosis. Nervous system activity increases, causing muscle cramps, twitches, and "charley horses." Deep tendon reflexes are hyperactive. **Tetany** (continuous contractions) of muscle groups also may be present. Tetany is painful and indicates a rapidly worsening condition.

Skeletal muscles may contract as a result of nerve stimulation, but they become weaker because of the hypokalemia. Handgrip strength decreases, and the patient may be unable to stand or walk. Respiratory efforts become less effective as the respiratory muscles weaken.

Cardiovascular changes occur because alkalosis increases myocardial irritability, especially when accompanied by hypokalemia. Heart rate increases, and the pulse is thready. When decreased blood volume is also present, the patient may have severe hypotension. The hypokalemia increases heart sensitivity to digoxin, which increases the risk for digoxin toxicity.

Respiratory changes, especially increases in the rate of breathing, are the main causes of respiratory alkalosis. Although the volume of air inhaled and exhaled with each breath is nearly normal, the total volume of air inhaled and exhaled each minute rises with the increased respiratory rate. The increased minute volume may be caused by anxiety or physiologic changes.

Arterial blood pH greater than 7.45 confirms alkalosis, but this test alone does not identify its cause. Because the symptoms of metabolic alkalosis and respiratory alkalosis are similar, it is critical to obtain additional laboratory data, especially arterial blood gas (ABG) values and specific serum electrolyte levels (see Chart 12-4) (Blevins, 2014).

❓ NCLEX EXAMINATION CHALLENGE 12-3

Health Promotion and Maintenance

A client asks why the provider has recommended that he breathe into a paper bag for several minutes when his anxiety disorder causes him to hyperventilate. What is the nurse's **best** response?

A. "Even your exhaled breath still has some oxygen in it, and rebreathing this air ensures that you won't pass out from lack of oxygen."

B. "When you breathe fast, you can lose too much carbon dioxide, and rebreathing this air keeps you from becoming dizzy and falling."

C. "Rapid breathing can lead to dehydration from excessive fluid loss, and rebreathing this air helps you retain fluid in the form of vapor moisture."

D. "Breathing into the bag for several minutes helps you become distracted from whatever is making you anxious and allows you to calm down."

◆ *Interventions: Responding*

Interventions are planned to prevent further losses of hydrogen, potassium, calcium, and chloride ions; to restore fluid balance; to monitor changes; and to provide for *patient safety*. Treatments that may have caused alkalosis (e.g., prolonged gastric suctioning, excessive infusion of certain IV solutions, drugs that promote hydrogen ion excretion) are modified or stopped. Drug therapy is prescribed to resolve the causes of alkalosis and to restore normal fluid, electrolyte, and ACID-BASE BALANCE. For example, the patient with metabolic alkalosis caused by diuretic therapy receives fluid and electrolyte replacement, and the diuretic therapy is adjusted or stopped. Antiemetic drugs are prescribed for vomiting. Monitor the patient's progress and adjust fluid and electrolyte therapy. Monitor electrolytes daily until they return to near normal.

During correction of alkalosis, a nursing care priority is prevention of injury from falls. The patient with alkalosis has hypotension and muscle weakness, which increase the risk for falls, especially among older adults. Implement the general falls prevention nursing interventions and the high-risk falls prevention nursing interventions outlined in Chart 2-4.

GET READY FOR THE NCLEX® EXAMINATION!

▌ KEY POINTS

Review these Key Points for each NCLEX Examination Client Needs Category.

Safe and Effective Care Environment

- Assess the cardiovascular system first in any patient at risk for acidosis because acidosis can lead to cardiac arrest from the accompanying hyperkalemia. **QSEN: Safety**
- Assess the airway of any patient who has acute respiratory acidosis. **QSEN: Safety**
- Assess heart rate and rhythm at least every 2 hours for any patient with an acid-base imbalance. **QSEN: Safety**
- Monitor the neurologic status at least every 2 hours in patients being treated for a problem with ACID-BASE BALANCE. **QSEN: Safety**
- Assess the ACID-BASE BALANCE of any patient with new-onset muscle weakness. **QSEN: Safety**
- Use fall precautions for any patient with a problem in ACID-BASE BALANCE. **QSEN: Safety**

Health Promotion and Maintenance

- Teach patients to take drugs as prescribed, especially diuretics, antihypertensives, and cardiac drugs. **QSEN: Patient-Centered Care**
- Instruct patients at continuing risk for respiratory acidosis to stop smoking. **QSEN: Patient-Centered Care**

Psychosocial Integrity

- Assess the gas exchange status of any patient with acute confusion. **QSEN: Patient-Centered Care**

- Perform a mental status assessment in any patient with or at risk for problems of ACID-BASE BALANCE. **QSEN: Patient-Centered Care**
- Assist patients who have anxiety-induced respiratory alkalosis to identify causes of anxiety. **QSEN: Patient-Centered Care**

Physiological Integrity

- Be aware of how the following principles, processes, and mechanisms influence the regulation of ACID-BASE BALANCE:
  - The normal pH of the body's extracellular fluids (including blood) is 7.35 to 7.45.
  - The more hydrogen ions present, the more acidic the fluid; the fewer hydrogen ions present, the more alkaline the fluid.
  - pH values below 7.35 indicate acidosis; pH values above 7.45 indicate alkalosis.
  - Anything that increases the CO_2 level in the blood increases the hydrogen ion content and lowers the pH.
  - Acids are normally formed in the body as a result of metabolism.
  - Chemical blood buffers are the immediate way that acid-base imbalances are corrected.
  - The lungs control the amount of CO_2 that is retained or exhaled.
  - The kidneys regulate the amount of hydrogen and bicarbonate ions that are retained or excreted by the body.

- If a lung problem causes retention of carbon dioxide, the healthy kidney compensates by increasing the amount of bicarbonate that is produced and retained.
- Acidosis reduces the excitability of cardiovascular muscle, neurons, skeletal muscle, and GI smooth muscle.
- Alkalosis increases the sensitivity of excitable tissues, allowing them to over-respond to normal stimuli and respond even without stimulation.

- Check the serum potassium level for any patient who has acidosis. **QSEN: Evidence-Based Practice**
- Monitor arterial blood gas (ABG) values to evaluate the effectiveness of therapy for acid-base imbalances. **QSEN: Patient-Centered Care**

SELECTED BIBLIOGRAPHY

Barnette, L., & Kautz, D. (2013). Creative ways to teach arterial blood gas interpretation. *Dimensions of Critical Care Nursing, 32*(2), 84–87.

Blevins, S. (2014). Making ABGs simple. *Medsurg Nursing, 23*(3), 185–186.

Ellis, M. (2015). Use of bicarbonate in patients with metabolic acidosis. *Critical Care Nurse, 35*(5), 73–75.

Gooch, M. (2015). Identifying acid-base and electrolyte imbalances. *The Nurse Practitioner, 40*(8), 37–42.

Jarvis, C. (2016). *Physical examination & health assessment* (7th ed.). St. Louis: Elsevier Saunders.

Larkin, B. G., & Zimmanck, R. J. (2015). Interpreting arterial blood gases successfully. *AORN Journal, 102*(10), 344–354.

Lian, J. X. (2013). Using ABGs to optimize mechanical ventilation. *Nursing, 43*(6), 46–52.

McCance, K., Huether, S., Brashers, V., & Rote, N. (2014). *Pathophysiology: The biologic basis for disease in adults and children* (7th ed.). St. Louis: Mosby.

Pagana, K., Pagana, T., & Pagana, T. (2017). *Mosby's diagnostic and laboratory test reference* (13th ed.). St. Louis: Mosby.

Pagana, K., Pagana, T., & Pike-MacDonald, S. (2013). *Mosby's Canadian manual of diagnostic and laboratory tests* (1st ed.). St. Louis: Mosby.

Touhy, T., & Jett, K. (2016). *Ebersole & Hess' Toward healthy aging: Human needs & nursing response*. St. Louis: Elsevier.

CHAPTER 13

Concepts of Infusion Therapy

Jeanette Spain Adams

 http://evolve.elsevier.com/Iggy/

PRIORITY AND INTERRELATED CONCEPTS

The priority concept for this chapter is FLUID AND ELECTROLYTE BALANCE.

The interrelated concept for this chapter is TISSUE INTEGRITY.

LEARNING OUTCOMES

Safe and Effective Care Environment

1. Prevent infusion administration errors by following best practices that ensure patient and staff safety.
2. Describe the benefits and limitations of selected safety-enhancing technologies used for infusion therapy.
3. Identify the evidence-based guidelines for prevention of intravenous (IV) catheter-related bloodstream infection (CRBSI).

Health Promotion and Maintenance

4. Describe the special needs and care for older adults receiving infusion therapy, including careful monitoring of FLUID AND ELECTROLYTE BALANCE.
5. Teach the patient and family about the type and care related to the patient's infusion therapy.

Physiological Integrity

6. Explain how to check the accuracy of prescriptions for infusion fluids and drug therapy to promote patient safety.

7. Identify the appropriate veins for peripheral IV catheter insertion.
8. Differentiate types of vascular access devices (VADs) used for peripheral and central IV therapy.
9. Outline evidence-based practice for inserting peripheral VADs.
10. Assess the patient's infusion site frequently for local complications, including impaired TISSUE INTEGRITY.
11. Prioritize nursing interventions for maintaining an infusion system.
12. Use clinical judgment to assess, prevent, document, and manage systemic complications related to infusion therapy and VADs.
13. Describe nursing care associated with intra-arterial, intraperitoneal, subcutaneous, intraosseous, and intraspinal infusion therapy.

Infusion therapy is the delivery of medications in solution and fluids by parenteral (piercing of skin or mucous membranes) route through a wide variety of catheter types and locations using multiple procedures. Intravenous (IV) therapy is the most common route for infusion therapy. It delivers solutions directly into the veins of the vascular system. This chapter focuses on access for and administration of all types of infusion therapy.

OVERVIEW

Infusion therapy is delivered in all health care settings, including hospitals, home care, ambulatory care clinics, primary health care providers' offices, and long-term care facilities. The most common reasons for using infusion therapy are to:

- Maintain FLUID BALANCE or correct fluid imbalance
- Maintain ELECTROLYTE or acid-base BALANCE or correct electrolyte or acid-base imbalance
- Administer medications
- Replace blood or blood products

IV therapy is the most common invasive therapy administered to hospitalized patients. Advances in medicine and technology have made it possible for people with chronic diseases such as diabetes mellitus, chronic kidney disease, and malabsorption syndromes to live long and productive lives. These patients often depend on long-term infusion therapy of some kind. They often have very poor vascular integrity; therefore accessing their peripheral veins takes a high level of skill.

Having a specialized team of infusion nurses to initiate and maintain infusion therapy has been recommended as best practice by the Centers for Disease Control and Prevention (CDC) to reduce complications of infusion therapy. These teams have demonstrated value in cost savings, patient satisfaction, and patient outcomes.

Infusion nurses may perform any or all of these activities:

- Develop evidence-based policies and procedures.
- Insert and maintain various types of peripheral, midline, and central venous catheters and subcutaneous and intraosseous accesses.
- Monitor patient outcomes of infusion therapy.
- Educate staff, patients, and families regarding infusion therapy.
- Consult on product selection and purchasing decisions.
- Provide therapies such as blood withdrawal, therapeutic phlebotomy, hypodermoclysis, intraosseous infusions, and administration of medications.

The registered nurse (RN) generalist is taught to insert peripheral IV lines; most institutions have a process for demonstrating competency for this skill. Depending on the state's nurse practice act, licensed practical/vocational nurses (LPNs/LVNs) and technicians may be trained and verified competent to perform the skill of peripheral IV insertion and assist with infusions. *The RN is ultimately accountable for all aspects of infusion therapy and delegation of associated tasks (Infusion Nurses Society [INS], 2016; Weinstein & Hagle, 2014).*

The Infusion Nurses Society (INS) publishes guidelines and standards of practice for policy and procedure development in all health care settings. These standards establish the criteria for all nurses delivering infusion therapy. The Infusion Nurses Certification Corporation (INCC) offers a written certification examination. Nurses who successfully complete this examination have mastered an advanced body of knowledge in this specialty and may use the initials *CRNI*, which stand for *certified registered nurse infusion.*

Types of Infusion Therapy Fluids

Many types of parenteral fluids are used for infusion therapy. These fluids are IV solutions, including parenteral nutrition, blood and blood components, biologics, and pharmacological therapy.

Intravenous Solutions

More than 200 IV fluids (solutions) are available that meet the requirements established by the United States Pharmacopeia (USP). Each solution is classified by its tonicity (concentration) and pH. Tonicity is typically categorized by comparison with normal blood plasma as osmolarity (mOsm/L). As discussed in Chapter 11, normal serum osmolarity for adults is between 270 and 300 mOsm/L. Parenteral solutions within that normal range are **isotonic**; fluids greater than 300 mOsm/L are **hypertonic**; and fluids less than 270 mOsm/L are **hypotonic**.

When an *isotonic* **infusate** (solution that is infused into the body) is used, water does not move into or out of the body's cells. Therefore patients, especially older adults, receiving isotonic solutions are at risk for fluid overload (see Chapter 11). *Hypertonic* solutions are used to correct altered FLUID AND ELECTROLYTE BALANCE and acid-base imbalances by moving water out of the body's cells and into the bloodstream. Electrolytes and other particles also move across cell membranes across a concentration gradient (from higher concentration to lower concentration). Parenteral nutrition solutions are hypertonic (see Chapter 60). Instead of moving water out of cells, *hypotonic*

infusates move water into cells to expand them. Patients receiving either hypertonic or hypotonic fluids are at risk for phlebitis and infiltration. **Phlebitis** is the inflammation of a vein caused by mechanical, chemical, or bacterial irritation. **Infiltration** occurs when IV solution leaks into the tissues around the vein.

The pH of IV solutions is a measure of acidity or alkalinity and usually ranges from 3.5 to 6.2. Extremes of both osmolarity and pH can cause vein damage, leading to phlebitis and **thrombosis** (blood clot in the vein). Thus fluids and medications with a pH value less than 5.0 and more than 9.0 and with an osmolarity more than 600 mOsm/L are best infused in the central circulation where greater blood flow provides adequate hemodilution (McClelland, 2014). For example, total parenteral nutrition (TPN) solutions have an osmolarity greater than 1400 mOsm/L. TPN should not be infused in peripheral circulation because it can damage blood cells and the endothelial lining of the veins and decrease perfusion.

> ⚠️ **NURSING SAFETY PRIORITY** [QSEN]
>
> **Drug Alert**
>
> Drugs such as amiodarone (Cordarone), vancomycin (Vancocin), and ciprofloxacin (Cipro IV) are venous irritants that have a pH less than 5.0. Phlebitis occurs when patients require long-term infusion of these drugs in peripheral circulation. Drugs with vasoconstrictive action (e.g., dopamine or chemotherapeutic agents [e.g., vinblastine]) are **vesicants** (chemicals that damage body tissue on direct contact) that can cause extravasation. **Extravasation** results in severe TISSUE INTEGRITY impairment as manifested by blistering, tissue sloughing, or necrosis from infiltration into the surrounding tissues. (See the Complications of Intravenous Therapy section for further explanation and Chapter 22 for more detail.) Monitor the IV insertion site carefully for early manifestations of infiltration, including swelling, coolness, or redness. If any of these symptoms are present, discontinue the drug immediately and notify the infusion therapy team, if available. If an infusion specialist is not available, notify the primary health care provider and remove the IV catheter.

Blood and Blood Components

Blood transfusion is given by using packed red blood cells, created by removing a large part of the plasma from whole blood. Other available blood components include platelets, fresh frozen plasma, albumin, and several specific clotting factors. Each component has detailed requirements for blood-type compatibility and infusion techniques. **For patient safety, The Joint Commission's (TJC) 2015 National Patient Safety Goals (NPSGs) require agencies to ensure that blood components are properly ordered, handled and dispensed, and administered, and that patients are appropriately monitored. Positive patient identification using two patient identifiers and requiring two qualified health care professionals is essential before any blood or blood component is administered. Automated bar coding can be used for positive patient identification in ambulatory care, acute care, and critical access hospitals, and office-based surgery-accredited programs.**

Most organizations use the International Society of Blood Transfusion (ISBT) universal bar-coding system to ensure the right blood for the right patient (Fig. 13-1). The ISBT system includes four components that must be present on the blood label both in bar code and in eye-readable format. These four components are (1) a unique facility identifier, (2) the lot number relating to the donor, (3) the product code, and (4) the ABO group and Rh type of the donor. Chapter 40 describes blood and blood product administration in more detail.

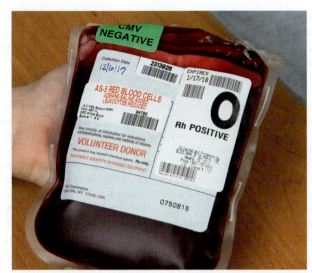

FIG. 13-1 Unit of blood showing the International Society of Blood Transfusion (ISBT) universal bar code for blood transfusions. (From Perry, A., Potter, P., & Ostendorf, W. [2017]. *Clinical nursing skills & techniques* [9th ed.]. St. Louis: Mosby.)

Drug Therapy

IV drugs provide a rapid therapeutic effect but can lead to immediate serious reactions, called **adverse drug events (ADEs).** Hundreds of drugs are available for infusion by a variety of techniques. As with all drug administration, nurses must be knowledgeable about drug indications, proper dosage, contraindications, and precautions. IV administration also requires knowledge of appropriate dilution, rate of infusion, pH and osmolarity, compatibility with other IV medications, appropriate infusion site (peripheral versus central circulation), potential for vesicant/irritant effects, and specific aspects of patient monitoring because of its immediate effect. *Regardless of familiarity with the drug, never assume that IV administration is the same as giving that drug by other routes.* New information is continuously being published, and new drugs are rapidly being introduced.

Medication safety is extremely important in all health care settings today. **The Joint Commission's 2014 NPSGs include as a major goal improving the safety of high-alert drugs. Examples of this type of drug are concentrated electrolyte solutions (e.g., potassium chloride), which require restricted access, prominent warnings about the concentration, and storage in a secured location.**

Procedures must be established to prevent errors resulting from look-alike, sound-alike drugs such as Celebrex IV (celecoxib) and Cerebyx (fosphenytoin). Other strategies to reduce errors include limiting available concentrations of drugs and dispensing all drugs, including catheter flush solutions, in single-dose containers. Smart pumps with drug libraries (see Infusion Systems section), in combination with computer provider (physician, nurse practitioner, physician assistant) order entry (CPOE) and bar-code medication administration (BCMA) systems, use recent technology to help reduce adverse drug events (ADEs). **Electronic medication administration records (MARs) and multiple checks by pharmacists, as required by The Joint Commission's NPSGs, also help reduce errors.**

Prescribing Infusion Therapy

A prescription for infusion therapy written by an authorized primary health care provider (physician, nurse practitioner, or physician assistant) is necessary before IV therapy begins. To be complete, the prescription for infusion fluids should include:

- Specific type of fluid
- Rate of administration written in milliliters per hour (mL/hr) or the total amount of fluid and the total number of hours for infusion (e.g., 125 mL/hr or 1000 mL/8 hrs)
- Drugs and the specific dose to be added to the solution such as electrolytes or vitamins
- A drug prescription should include:
  - Drug name, preferably by generic name
  - Specific dose and route
  - Frequency of administration
  - Time of administration
  - Length of time for infusion
  - Purpose (required in some health care agencies, especially nursing homes)

Some continuously infused drugs such as those for pain management are prescribed as milligrams per hour. The type and volume of dilution for infusion medications may be included in the prescription or calculated by the infusion pharmacist.

! NURSING SAFETY PRIORITY QSEN
Action Alert

Determine that the IV prescription is appropriate for the patient and clarify any questions with the primary health care provider before administration. Be sure to check for the accuracy and completeness of the treatment prescription. An example of an incomplete one is "5% dextrose in water to keep the vein open" (TKO or KVO). This statement does not specify the rate of infusion and is not considered complete.

Vascular Access Devices

An infusion catheter, also known as a **vascular access device (VAD),** is a plastic tube placed in a blood vessel to deliver fluids and medications. This catheter should not be confused with the ventricular assist device, also called a VAD. In this chapter VAD refers to vascular access devices. The specific type and purpose of the therapy determine whether the infusion can be given safely through peripheral veins or if the large central veins of the chest are needed. Advances in catheter materials and insertion techniques have radically expanded the types of VADs currently used. This discussion includes the description of each type of catheter used for peripheral and central IV therapy. Seven major types are described:

- Short peripheral catheters
- Midline catheters
- Peripherally inserted central catheters (PICCs)
- Nontunneled percutaneous central venous catheters (CVCs)
- Tunneled catheters
- Implanted ports
- Hemodialysis catheters

Assess the patient's needs for vascular access and choose the device that has the best chance of infusing the prescribed therapy for the required length of time. Depending on the patient and type of VAD to be inserted, a topical anesthetic agent or intradermal lidocaine HCl 1% may be helpful to decrease patient discomfort. Obtain a primary health care provider's prescription and check for patient allergies before administering any anesthetic.

? NCLEX EXAMINATION CHALLENGE 13-1

Safe and Effective Care Environment

A client receiving gentamycin intravenously reports that the peripheral IV insertion site has become painful and reddened. What action will the nurse take **first**?

A. Report the client's problem to the primary health care provider.

B. Document findings and actions in the electronic health record.

C. Change the IV insertion site to a new location.

D. Stop the infusion of the drug immediately.

PERIPHERAL INTRAVENOUS THERAPY

Short infusion catheters are the most commonly used vascular access devices (VADs) for peripheral IV therapy. They are usually placed in the veins of the arm. Another catheter used for peripheral IV therapy is a midline catheter.

Short Peripheral Catheters

Short peripheral catheters are composed of a plastic cannula built around a sharp stylet extending slightly beyond the cannula (Fig. 13-2). The stylet (sharp) allows for the venipuncture, and the cannula is advanced into the vein. Once the cannula is advanced into the vein, the stylet is withdrawn. These catheters are designed with a safety mechanism to cover the sharp end of the stylet after it is removed from the patient. The stylet is a hollow-bore, blood-filled needle that carries a high risk for exposure to bloodborne pathogens if needlestick injury occurs. A federal law enacted in 2000 amended the Bloodborne Pathogen Standards from the Occupational Safety and Health Administration (OSHA) requiring the use of catheters with an engineered safety mechanism to prevent needlesticks.

Insertion and Placement Methods

Short peripheral catheters are most often inserted into superficial veins of the forearm using sterile technique. In emergent situations these catheters can also be used in the external jugular vein of the neck. *Avoid the use of veins in the lower extremities of adults, if possible, because of an increased risk for deep vein thrombosis and infiltration.*

Short catheters range in length from ¾ inch to 1¼ inch, with gauge sizes from 26 gauge (the smallest) to 14 gauge (large bore). Choose the smallest-gauge catheter capable of delivering the prescribed therapy with consideration of all the contributing factors, including expected duration, vascular characteristics, and comorbidities (INS, 2016). Current design improves the fluid flow through the catheter while using a smaller gauge and thereby decreases the possibility of vein irritation from a large catheter. For example, a thin-walled 24-gauge Insyte catheter

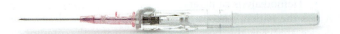

FIG. 13-2 BD Insyte Autoguard IV catheter. With the push of a button, the needle instantly retracts, reducing the risk for accidental needlestick injuries. (Courtesy and © Becton, Dickinson and Company.)

has about the same flow-rate ability as a 22-gauge non–thin-walled Angiocath. Larger gauge sizes allow for faster flow rates but also cause phlebitis more often. Table 13-1 lists each gauge size and its common uses.

The current recommendations for dwell (stay-in) time of short peripheral catheters do not include a specific time frame. The recommendations from both the CDC and the INS are that the catheter should be removed and/or rotated to a different site based on clinical indications (e.g., signs of phlebitis [warmth, tenderness, erythema or palpable venous cord], infection, or malfunction) (INS, 2016). This process requires conscientious and frequent assessment of the site. INS (2016) recommends assessment at least every 4 hours—every 1 to 2 hours for vulnerable patients and every 4 hours for continuous infusions for outpatient and home care patients; otherwise site assessment should be done once a day. If the patient's therapy is expected to be longer than 6 days, a midline catheter or PICC should be chosen (Wojnar, 2013). When selecting the site for insertion of a peripheral catheter, consider the patient's age, history, and diagnosis; the type and duration of the prescribed therapy; and, whenever possible, the patient's preference. Chart 13-1 lists the major criteria for the placement of peripheral VADs.

Vascular visualization technology (e.g., near infrared and ultrasound devices) are now available as tools to assist in IV line placement. Several different types of portable *vein transilluminators* are available such as VeinViewer, Veinlite LED, and AccuVein AV 300 (Fig. 13-3). Although they may have different mechanisms of action (some use infrared light and some use laser), these devices penetrate only up to about 10 mm and are limited to finding *superficial* veins.

Ultrasound-guided peripheral IV insertion can allow insertion into *deeper* veins (Arbique et al., 2014). This technology has been shown to be very valuable in assisting with cannulation

TABLE 13-1	Choosing the Gauge Size for Peripheral Catheters	
CATHETER GAUGE	**INDICATIONS**	**APPROXIMATE FLOW RATES**
24-26 gauge Smallest, shortest (¾ -inch length)	Not ideal for viscous infusions Expect blood transfusion to take longer Preferred for infants and small children	24 mL/min (1440 mL/hr)
22 gauge	Adequate for most therapies; blood can infuse without damage	38 mL/min (2280 mL/hr)
20 gauge (1-1¼ -inch length)	Adequate for all therapies Most providers of anesthesia prefer not to use a smaller size than this for surgery cases	65 mL/min (3900 mL/hr)
18 gauge	Preferred size for surgery Vein needs to be large enough to accommodate the catheter	110 mL/min (6600 mL/hr)
14-16 gauge	For trauma and surgical patients requiring rapid fluid resuscitation Needs to be in a vein that can accommodate it	Over 200 mL/min (12,000 mL/hr)

◎ **CHART 13-1** **Best Practice for Patient Safety & Quality Care** QSEN

Placement of Short Peripheral Venous Catheters

- Verify that the prescription for infusion therapy is complete and appropriate for infusion through a short peripheral catheter.
- For adults choose a site for placement in the upper extremity. DO NOT USE THE WRIST.
- Choose the patient's nondominant arm when possible.
- Choose a distal site and make all subsequent venipunctures proximal to previous sites.
- Do not use the arm on the side of a mastectomy, lymph node dissection, arteriovenous shunt or fistula, or paralysis.
- Avoid choosing a site in an area of joint flexion.
- Avoid choosing a site in a vein that feels hard or cordlike.
- Avoid choosing a site close to areas of cellulitis, dermatitis, or complications from previous catheter sites.
- Choose a vein of appropriate length and width to fit the size of the catheter required for infusion.
- Limit unsuccessful attempts to two per clinician and no more than four total (INS, 2016).

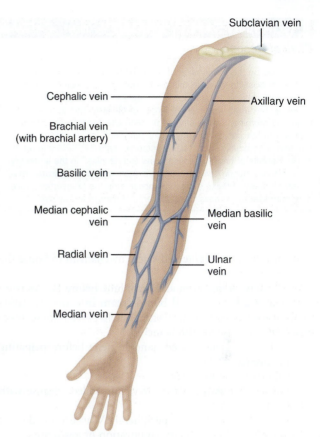

FIG. 13-4 Common IV sites in the inner arm.

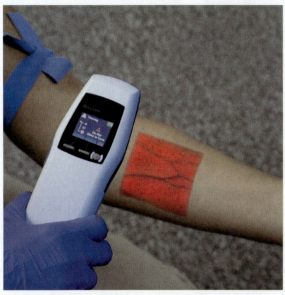

FIG. 13-3 The AccuVein AV300 is a vein illumination device that helps health care professionals locate veins for blood draw, IV infusion, and blood donation by projecting a pattern of light on the patient's skin to reveal the position of underlying veins on the skin's surface. The device uses red and infrared light, which the hemoglobin in blood absorbs to detect the position of the vein. (Courtesy AccuVein, LLC.)

of peripheral veins that the nurse cannot access with sight and touch. However, there are risks the nurse must be aware of when using ultrasound guidance. This technology should be used only by nurses who have been trained and whose competencies are maintained. Arteries and nerves lie parallel to deep veins, and training is needed to learn to identify these structures and avoid damaging them. In addition, when deeper veins are accessed, infiltration may go undetected until a significant amount of fluid has collected in the tissues. This complication can be particularly devastating if the solution is an irritant or vesicant.

For patients who need IV access but are at risk for fluid overload or do not need extra IV fluids, the peripheral vascular access device (VAD) can be converted into an intermittent IV lock, also called a *saline lock.* This device allows administration of specific drugs given IV push (e.g., furosemide [Lasix, Furoside]) or on an intermittent basis using a medication administration set. IV antibiotics are frequently given this way. In some cases the saline lock is placed in case there is a need for emergency drug administration via IV push. The intermittent device is flushed with saline before and after drug administration to ensure patency and prevent occlusion with a blood clot.

Site Selection and Skin Preparation

The most appropriate veins for peripheral catheter placement include the dorsal venous network (i.e., basilic, cephalic, and median veins and their branches) (Fig. 13-4). *However, cannulation of veins on the hand is not appropriate for older patients with a loss of skin turgor and poor vein condition and for active patients receiving infusion therapy in an ambulatory care clinic or home care. Use of veins on the dorsal surface of the hands should be reserved as a last resort for short-term infusion of nonvesicant and nonirritant solutions in young patients.*

Mastectomy, axillary lymph node dissection, lymphedema, paralysis of the upper extremity, and the presence of dialysis grafts or fistulas alter the normal pattern of blood flow through the arm. Using veins in the extremity affected by these conditions requires a primary health care provider's request and order. Short peripheral catheters are not recommended for obtaining routine blood samples.

Winged needles ("butterfly needles") are easy to insert but are associated with a high frequency of infiltration. They are most commonly used for injecting single-dose drugs or drawing blood samples. Like a short peripheral catheter, winged needles

! NURSING SAFETY PRIORITY **QSEN**

Critical Rescue

Avoid veins on the palmar side of the wrist because the median nerve is located close to veins in this area, making the venipuncture more painful and difficult to stabilize. The cephalic vein begins above the thumb and extends up the entire length of the arm. This vein is usually large and prominent, appearing as a prime site for catheter insertion. Damage to the nerve from any injury can result in permanent loss of function or complex regional pain syndrome, type 2 (CRPS) (Kim et al., 2014). Reports of tingling, feeling "pins and needles" in the extremity, or numbness during the venipuncture procedure can indicate nerve puncture. If any of these symptoms occur, stop the IV insertion procedure immediately, remove the catheter, and choose a new site.

should also have an engineered safety mechanism to house the needle when removed.

Aseptic skin preparation and technique before IV insertion are crucial. **Catheter-related bloodstream infection (CRBSI)** can occur from a peripheral IV site. To help prevent these infections, CDC recommendations include:

- Perform evidence-based hand hygiene before palpating the insertion site.
- Clip hair—do not shave.
- Ensure that skin is clean. If visibly soiled, cleanse with soap and water.
- Wear clean gloves for peripheral IV insertion; do not touch the access site after application of antiseptics.
- Prepare clean skin with a skin antiseptic (chlorhexidine 2% with 70% alcohol, 70% isopropyl alcohol, or povidone-iodine) with a back-and-forth motion for 30 seconds and allow the solution to dry before peripheral venous catheter insertion.
- Do not retouch the proposed insertion site. If retouching occurs, prepare the skin antiseptic again and allow to dry.

Midline Catheters

Midline catheters can be anywhere from 3 to 8 inches long, 3 to 5 Fr, and double or single lumen. They are inserted through the veins of the upper arm. The median antecubital vein is used most often if insertion is done without the aid of ultrasound guidance. With ultrasound guidance deeper veins can be accessed, and the insertion site can be farther above the antecubital fossa. The basilic vein is preferred over the cephalic vein because of its larger diameter and straighter path. It also allows greater hemodilution of the fluids and medications being infused. The catheter tip is located in the upper arm, with the tip residing no further into the venous network than the axillary vein (Fig. 13-5).

Midline catheters have been found to reduce the number of repeated IV cannulations, which reduces patient discomfort, increases patient satisfaction, and contributes to organizational efficiency (Owen, 2014). A midline catheter can be used when skin integrity or limited peripheral veins make it difficult to maintain a short peripheral catheter. Indications for these catheters include fluids for hydration and drug therapy that are given longer than 6 days and up to 4 weeks such as antibiotics, heparin, steroids, and bronchodilators. There are currently no recommendations for the optimal dwell time. In a 2014 study the average dwell time for midlines was identified as 6.9 days (Dumont et al., 2014). Because of the extended dwell time,

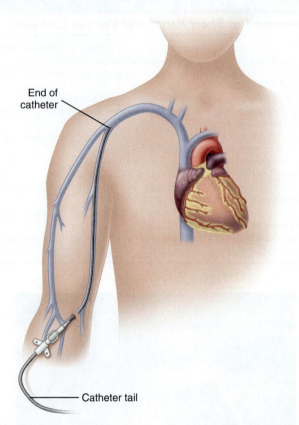

End of catheter

Catheter tail

FIG. 13-5 Midline catheter; the tip of this catheter resides in a peripheral vein.

strict sterile technique is used for insertion and dressing changes for a midline catheter. Additional education and skill assessment are required for the nurse to be qualified to insert midline catheters.

Midline catheters are considered to dwell in the peripheral circulation; the recommendations for infusates (fluids or drugs) are the same as for short peripheral IV lines. Fluids and medications infused through a midline catheter should have a pH between 5 and 9 and a final osmolarity of less than 600 mOsm/L (McClelland, 2014). The pH and osmolarity outside these parameters increase the risk for complications such as phlebitis and thrombosis. Midline catheters should not be used for infusion of **vesicant medications**—drugs that cause severe tissue damage if they escape into the subcutaneous tissue (**extravasation**). There is concern that at a midline tip location, larger amounts of the drug may extravasate before the problem is detected.

All parenteral nutrition formulas, including those with low concentrations of dextrose and solutions that have an osmolarity greater than 600 mOsm/L, should not be infused through a midline. Do not draw blood from these catheters routinely. Midline catheters should not be placed in extremities affected by mastectomy with lymphedema, paralysis, or dialysis grafts and fistulas. When using a double-lumen midline catheter, do not administer incompatible drugs simultaneously through both lumens because the blood flow rate in the axillary vein is not high enough to ensure adequate hemodilution and prevention of drug interaction in the vein. Currently new midlines with power-injectable technology are available for use with computed tomography.

? NCLEX EXAMINATION CHALLENGE 13-2
Physiological Integrity

The primary health care provider prescribes 1 L 5% D/0.45% NS to be infused over 8 hours. The nurse sets the rate at ___ mL/hr of IV solution.

CENTRAL INTRAVENOUS THERAPY

In **central IV therapy** the vascular access device (VAD) is placed in the central circulation, specifically within the superior vena cava (SVC) near its junction with the right atrium, also called the *caval-atrial junction (CAJ)*. Blood flow in the SVC is about 2 L/min compared with about 200 mL/min in the axillary vein. Most central vascular access devices require confirmation of tip location at the CAJ by chest x-ray before solutions are infused. However, newer technologies use either a magnet tip locator or identification of the CAJ by electrocardiogram rather than by x-ray. Both the Sherlock 3CG by Bard and the VasoNova/Teleflex systems have received Food and Drug Administration (FDA) approval as alternatives to chest x-ray or fluoroscopy to verify PICC tip location.

A number of types of central vascular access devices (CVADs) are available, depending on the purpose, duration, and insertion site availability. Several recent improvements in catheter materials allow antimicrobial and heparin coatings to reduce infection risk and improve the longevity of the catheter. Not all central-line catheters are approved for power injection used in radiologic tests. The catheter can rupture if it is not designed to handle the injection pressure necessary for some tests such as pulmonary CT angiography or CT angiography of the aorta (5 mL/sec and 300 per square inch [psi]). Even with power-injectable designed catheters, dislodgment may occur (Boon & Babu, 2013). Be sure to confirm if the PICC is power injectable or not.

Peripherally Inserted Central Catheters

A **peripherally inserted central catheter (PICC)** is a long catheter inserted through a vein of the antecubital fossa (inner aspect of the bend of the arm) or the middle of the upper arm. Nurses who insert these CVADs require special training and competency confirmation.

In adults the PICC length ranges from 18 to 29 inches (45 to 74 cm), with the tip residing in the superior vena cava (SVC) ideally at the caval-atrial junction (CAJ) (Fig. 13-6). Placement of the catheter tip in veins distal to the SVC is avoided. This inappropriate tip location, often called a *mid-clavicular catheter,* is associated with much higher rates of thrombosis than when the tip is located in the SVC at the CAJ. Mid-clavicular tip locations are used only when anatomic or pathophysiologic changes prohibit placing the catheter into the SVC.

PICCs should be inserted early in the course of therapy before veins of the extremity have been damaged from multiple venipunctures and infusions. Insertion methods using guide-wires and ultrasound systems greatly improve insertion success. The basilic vein is the preferred site for insertion; the cephalic

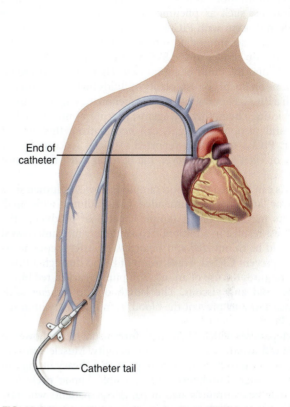

FIG. 13-6 Peripherally inserted central catheter (PICC) is placed peripherally in a vein of the upper arm with the tip resting in the superior vena cava.

vein can be used if necessary. Two brachial veins are not recommended because they are more difficult to access; they are deeper in the arm and run close to the brachial artery. *Sterile technique is used for insertion to reduce the risk for CRBSI. Before the catheter can be used for infusion, a chest x-ray indicating that the tip resides in the lower SVC is required when the catheter is not placed under fluoroscopy or with the use of the electrocardiogram tip-locator technique.*

PICCs are available in single-, dual-, or triple-lumen configurations and with both the Groshong valve and the pressure-activated safety valve (PASV). PICCs are also available as "Power PICCs" and can be used for contrast injection at a maximum of 5 mL/sec and a maximum pressure of 300 psi. They can also be connected to transducers and used to monitor central venous pressure.

The most common complications from PICCs include phlebitis, thrombophlebitis, deep vein thrombosis (DVT), and CRBSIs. When infections occur from a central line, they are also referred to as **central line-associated bloodstream infection, or CLABSI.** Thrombophlebitis and DVT can be very serious, threaten the integrity of the vein, and decrease perfusion. The smallest possible French size should be used to decrease the rate of upper-extremity DVT, a potentially life-threatening event.

CRBSI has been noted to be less common in PICCs than in other central venous catheters (CVCs) because of the insertion site in the upper extremity. The cooler, drier skin of the upper arm has fewer types and numbers of microorganisms, leading to lower rates of infection. Accidental arterial puncture or excessive bleeding can occur on insertion and is controlled by direct pressure. Infiltration and extravasation are rare. Insertion complications such as pneumothorax associated with other CVCs do not occur with PICCs.

PICCs can accommodate infusion of all types of therapy because the tip resides in the SVC where the rapid blood flow quickly dilutes the fluids being infused. Therefore there are no limitations on the pH or osmolality of fluids that can be infused through a PICC. For example, patients requiring lengthy courses of antibiotics, chemotherapy agents, parenteral nutrition formulas, and vasopressor agents can benefit from this type of catheter. PICCs have been reported to dwell successfully for months or even years; however, the optimal dwell time is not known.

PICCs can be used for blood sampling; however, lumen sizes of 4 Fr or larger are recommended. Using lumens with small diameters may not yield a sample capable of producing the needed test results. In addition, frequent entry into any central line should be minimized and treated with strict aseptic technique to prevent CRBSI. Transfusion of blood through a PICC usually requires the use of an infusion pump. Packed red blood cells are cold and viscous. The length of the catheter adds resistance and may prevent the blood from infusing within the 4-hour limit.

Teach patients with a PICC to perform usual ADLs; however, they should avoid excessive physical activity. Muscle contractions in the arm from physical activity such as heavy lifting can lead to catheter dislodgment and possible lumen occlusion. PICCs may be contraindicated in paraplegic patients who rely on their arms for mobility and in patients using crutches that provide support in the axilla.

PICC insertion is commonly performed in the patient's hospital room, an ambulatory care treatment facility, or the imaging department. Regardless of where they are inserted, the same precautions must be taken as with any other central line insertion using the **catheter-related bloodstream infection (CRBSI) prevention bundle**. Major components of this prevention bundle include:

- Hand hygiene
- Measuring upper arm circumference as a baseline before insertion (INS, 2016)
- Maximal barrier precautions on insertion
- Chlorhexidine skin antisepsis
- Optimal catheter site selection and post-placement care with avoidance of the femoral vein for central venous access in adult patients
- Daily review of line necessity with prompt removal of unnecessary lines

Other helpful interventions include use of a checklist for sterility during the procedure, a line cart with all equipment, and a stop sign on the door of the room to stop unnecessary traffic through the room during the procedure. The checklist should be completed by another professional health care member who can stop the inserter when any breaks in technique are observed (INS, 2016).

Nontunneled Percutaneous Central Venous Catheters

Nontunneled percutaneous central venous catheters (CVCs) are inserted by a physician, physician assistant, or nurse practitioner through the subclavian vein in the upper chest or the internal jugular veins in the neck using sterile technique.

NURSING SAFETY PRIORITY (QSEN)

Action Alert

The INS recommendation for flushing PICC lines not actively used is 5 mL of heparin (10 units/mL) in a 10-mL syringe at least daily when using a nonvalved catheter and at least weekly with a valved catheter. Use 10 mL of sterile saline to flush before and after medication administration; 20 mL of sterile saline is flushed after drawing blood. *Always use 10-mL barrel syringes to flush any central line because the pressure exerted by a smaller barrel poses a risk for rupturing the catheter.*

Occasionally the patient's condition may require insertion of the CVC in a femoral vein, but the rate of infection is very high. If the femoral site must be used, it is removed as soon as possible.

CVCs are usually 7 to 10 inches (18 to 25 cm) long and have one to as many as five lumens (Fig. 13-7). These catheters are also available with antimicrobial coatings such as chlorhexidine and silver sulfadiazine. The tip resides in the superior vena cava (SVC) and is confirmed by a chest x-ray. Nontunneled percutaneous CVCs are most commonly used for emergent or trauma situations, critical care, and surgery. There is no recommendation for optimal dwell time. However, these catheters are commonly used for short-term situations and are *not* the catheter of choice for home care or ambulatory clinic settings.

Insertion of these central catheters requires the patient to be placed in the Trendelenburg position, usually with a rolled

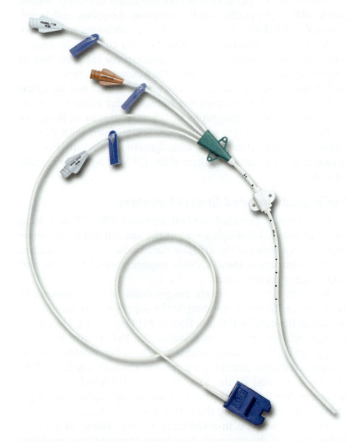

FIG. 13-7 Edwards Lifesciences PreSep central venous catheter (CVC); often placed in the subclavian or internal jugular vein with the tip of the catheter resting in the superior vena cava. (Courtesy Edwards Lifesciences, Irvine, CA.)

towel between the shoulder blades. This position may be difficult or contraindicated for patients with respiratory conditions, spinal curvatures, and increased intracranial pressure, especially for older adults. Trauma, surgery, or radiation in the neck or chest prohibits the use of these devices as well. Insertion with ultrasound guidance has been demonstrated to improve the safety of insertion in the internal jugular site (Bowen et al., 2014). The presence of a tracheotomy increases the risk for cross-contamination of the insertion site. The warmer, moister skin of the neck and upper chest has more types and higher numbers of microorganisms, resulting in more CRBSIs with this type of catheter.

Tunneled Central Venous Catheters

Tunneled central venous catheters are VADs that have part of the catheter lying in a subcutaneous tunnel, separating the points where the catheter enters the vein from where it exits the skin. This separation is intended to prevent the organisms on the skin from reaching the bloodstream (Fig. 13-8). Today these catheters are usually inserted by physicians in the radiology suite rather than placed surgically. The catheter has a cuff made of a rough material that is positioned inside the subcutaneous tunnel. These cuffs commonly contain antibiotics, which also reduce the risk for infection. The tissue granulates into the cuff, providing a mechanical barrier to microorganisms and anchoring the catheter in place.

The design of tunneled CVCs requires surgical techniques for insertion and removal. Single, dual, and triple lumens are available. These catheters were originally named for the physicians who designed them, including Broviac, Hickman, and Leonard catheters.

Tunneled catheters are used primarily when the need for infusion therapy is frequent and long term. Patients needing parenteral nutrition for months, years, or the remainder of their lives commonly choose a tunneled catheter. Tunneled catheters

are also chosen when several weeks or months of infusion therapy are needed and a PICC is not a good choice. For example, paraplegic patients needing 6 to 8 weeks of antibiotics are not good candidates for a PICC because of the excessive use of the upper extremities for mobility. Some oncology patients may prefer a tunneled catheter instead of an implanted port because they cannot tolerate the needlesticks required for accessing those devices.

Implanted Ports

Implanted ports are very different from other central vascular access devices (CVADs). This type of device is chosen for patients who are expected to require IV therapy for more than a year (Zhou et al., 2014). Implanted ports typically are inserted by a physician in the radiology department or a surgeon in the operating suite. Implanted ports consist of a portal body, a dense septum over a reservoir, and a catheter. They can be single or double lumen and come in various sizes. A subcutaneous pocket is surgically created to house the port body. The catheter is inserted into the vein and attached to the portal body. The septum is made of self-sealing silicone and is located in the center of the port body over the reservoir; the catheter extends from the side of the port body. The incision is closed, and no part of the catheter is visible externally; therefore this device has the least impact on body image (Fig. 13-9).

Some implanted ports are power injectable and can be used for obtaining contrast-enhanced computed tomography (CECT). These devices can withstand 5 mL/sec at up to 300 psi pressure. The BARD PowerPort can be identified by palpation of three bumps on the top of the septum and a triangular-shaped port. Be careful not to press firmly on the bumps because it can be painful to the patient. Be sure to use a power-injection–rated noncoring needle with this type of port when it is used for this purpose. These needles come with labeling identifying that they are power-injection rated (Fig. 13-10).

Venous ports may be placed on the upper chest or the upper extremity. The venous catheter may enter either the subclavian

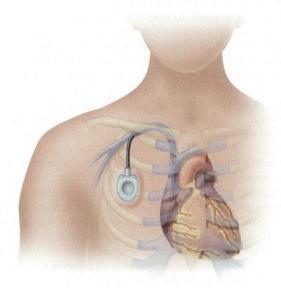

FIG. 13-8 Tunneled catheter. Part of this catheter lies in a subcutaneous tunnel, separating the point where the catheter enters the vein from where it exits the skin.

FIG. 13-9 Positioning of an implanted port.

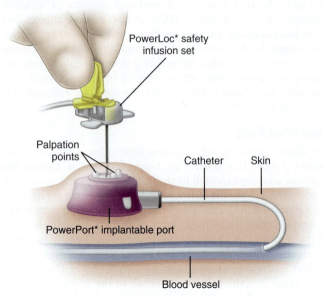

FIG. 13-10 A noncoring needle for accessing an implanted power port.

or internal jugular vein. Although an implanted port is most commonly used in the venous system, the catheter may be placed in arteries, the epidural space, or the peritoneal cavity, with the port pocket located over a bony prominence.

Implanted ports are accessed by using a noncoring needle (a common brand name is *Huber*) that is specially designed with a deflected tip. This design slices through the dense septum without coring out a small piece of it, thus preserving the integrity of the septum. Port bodies placed in the chest have a larger septum and usually tolerate about 2000 punctures. Port bodies placed in the upper extremity are smaller and are rated to tolerate about 750 punctures.

Port access should be done only by formally trained health care professionals using a mask and aseptic technique. Implanted ports are used most often for patients receiving chemotherapy. These patients are immune compromised, making them highly susceptible to infection. Before puncture, palpate the port to locate the septum. Carefully palpate to feel the shape and depth of the port body to ensure puncture of the septum, not the attached catheter. Some have attached extension sets and wings to stabilize the needle. One important feature is an engineered safety mechanism to contain the needle when it is removed from the septum. Because the dense septum holds tightly to the needle, there can be a rebound when it is pulled from the septum, which can result in needlestick injury to the nurse.

Implanted ports need to be flushed after each use and at least once a month between courses of therapy. This procedure is done to prevent clot formation in the internal chamber of the port and is often referred to as "locking" or "de-accessing." The INS recommendation for locking or de-accessing a port is the use of a 10-mL syringe with either heparin 10 units per milliliter or preservative-free 0.9% normal saline (INS, 2016). When the port is not accessed, there is no external catheter requiring a dressing. Puncture of the skin over the port is required to gain access to the port body, causing pain for some patients. Topical anesthetic creams can be used to make the access procedure more tolerable.

! NURSING SAFETY PRIORITY QSEN

Drug Alert

Before giving a drug through an implanted port, always check for blood return. INS (2016) defines blood return "as the color and consistency of whole blood upon aspiration" (p.S147). If there is no blood return, withhold the drug until patency and adequate noncoring needle placement of the port are established. Serious extravasations of vesicant drugs can occur because a fibrin sheath (flap or tail) may occur at the tip of the catheter, clot it, and cause retrograde subcutaneous leakage.

Hemodialysis Catheters

Hemodialysis catheters have very large lumens to accommodate the hemodialysis procedure or a pheresis procedure that harvests specific blood cells. They may be tunneled for long-term needs or nontunneled for short-term needs. A hemodialysis catheter is critical to the management of renal failure and must function well. CRBSIs and vein thrombosis are common problems; therefore this catheter should not be used for administration of other fluids or drugs except in an emergency.

The concentration of heparin used to lock hemodialysis catheters ranges from 1000 to 10,000 units/mL. Researchers have demonstrated that using 1000 units/mL reduces the incidence of postinsertion bleeding but may be associated with an increased need for recombinant tissue plasminogen activator (tPA) to maintain patency. A flush of 1000 units heparin/mL or a solution of 4% sodium citrate in the amount of the dwell volume of each lumen has been recommended. Heparin is most often used because sodium citrate has not been as commercially available in the preparation needed. To prevent systemic anticoagulation and subsequent bleeding, be sure to aspirate the heparin from the lumens before use.

INFUSION SYSTEMS

Nurses administering infusion therapies need to understand how infusion systems work. This knowledge ensures that the patient can benefit from a particular system's advantages while minimizing any potential complications.

Containers

Infusion containers are made of glass or plastic. *Glass* bottles were the original fluid container to be mass produced. They are easily sterilized, and it is easy to read the amount of fluid remaining in the bottle. Also, glass is inert and thus cannot interact with some drugs such as plastic can. However, glass bottles are heavy and cannot be used easily in many situations such as patient transport during emergencies. These containers require an air vent for fluids to flow freely from them. The most common method is to use an administration set with a special filtered vent. Some bottles may have a straw tube open to the room air through the rubber stopper in the bottle and extending to above the level of the fluid. Bottles with a venting straw do not have a barrier to prevent contaminants in the air from entering the fluid.

Plastic containers are considered *closed systems* because they do not rely on outside air to allow the fluid to infuse. Instead atmospheric pressure pushes against the flexible sides of the

container, allowing the fluid to flow by gravity. For this reason plastic containers do not require vented administration sets. These containers are lightweight, resistant to breaking, easier to store, and easy to use in emergency conditions. Therefore they are used more frequently than glass containers.

All plastic containers were commonly made of polyvinyl chloride (PVC). To increase flexibility and strength, PVC required the addition of a plasticizer such as di-2-ethylhexyl-phthalate or DEHP. Concern has been growing in the past few years over the exposure of patients to this chemical because it can leach from the plastic fluid container or tubing and infuse into the patient with the IV fluid or medication. The FDA has determined that there is little to no risk posed to most patients by exposure to the amount of DEHP released from IV bags with infusion of crystalloids or drugs. However, there is concern about the buildup of chemical exposure from many sources over a lifetime and specifically the potential effects of DEHP on the development of the male reproductive system (Meer et al., 2014). Therefore many hospitals are using PVC-free and DEHP-free IV bags, especially for high-risk groups.

One disadvantage of removing DEHP from the plastic bags is that the bags are less pliable and more prone to rupture. Some institutions do not allow these bags to be sent through a pneumatic tube system because the pressure exerted has caused the bags to rupture during transport.

A problem with plastic containers is that they are not compatible with insulin, nitroglycerin, lorazepam (Ativan), fat emulsions, and lipid-based drugs. Nitroglycerin and insulin adhere to the walls of the PVC container, making it impossible to know exactly how much medication the patient is receiving. Another concern with plastic bags is the accuracy of reading the amount of fluid remaining in the container and the residual volume in some sets. As much as 20% of a medication in an attached 100-mL bag may not be infused, which in a 24-hour period may result in a patient missing a whole dose of medication (Lee, 2015).

! NURSING SAFETY PRIORITY QSEN

Action Alert

Regardless of the type of fluid container being used, check it for cracks or pinholes before use. Always observe the fluid for **turbidity** (cloudiness) or any unusual color that could indicate contamination.

Administration Sets

The administration set is the connection between the catheter and the fluid container. Numerous sets are available in many different configurations. The type and purpose of the infusion determine the type of administration set needed. Some sets are *generic,* meaning that they are appropriate for most infusions. Other sets are used for specific types of infusions such as blood transfusion. Still others are *dedicated,* meaning that they must be used with a specific manufacturer's infusion controlling device. Information that describes their proper use is provided on the packaging of administration sets.

Secondary Administration Sets

A primary continuous administration set is used to infuse the primary IV fluid by either a gravity infusion or an electronic infusion pump. A short **secondary administration set**, also known as a **piggyback set**, is attached to the primary set at a Y–injection site and is used to deliver intermittent medications (Fig. 13-11). Directions and diagrams for use typically are on the packaging. Once attached, these sets should remain connected as an infusion system. Primary and secondary continuous infusion administration sets used to infuse fluids other than parenteral nutrition and lipids can be used for up to 96 hours unless the closed system has been compromised (INS, 2016).

FIG. 13-11 Secondary IV administration set attached to the primary set at a Y-injection site. (Courtesy Rick Brady, Riva, Maryland. In Lilley, L., Collins, S., & Snyder, J. [2014]. *Pharmacology and the nursing process* [7th ed.]. St. Louis: Mosby.)

Intermittent Administration Sets

When no primary continuous fluid is being infused, use an intermittent administration set to infuse multiple doses of medications through a catheter that has been capped with a needleless connection device. Remove the medication bag from the previous dose and attach the new one. Remove the sterile cap covering the distal end of the set and attach the set to the catheter. Because both ends of the set are being manipulated with each dose, the INS standards of practice state that this set should be changed every 24 hours. When the administration set is used for infusion of parenteral nutrition or lipid solution, change it every 24 hours. Change blood tubing within 4 hours.

Administration sets are sterile in the fluid pathway and under the sterile caps on each end of the set. The set is not packaged as a completely sterile product and cannot be added to a sterile field. Careful attention is required to maintain the sterility of the spike and the connection end of the tubing to prevent introduction of microorganisms into the catheter and bloodstream.

Add-on Devices

Several other types of add-on devices include short extension sets, injection caps, and filters. Extension sets may be packaged

as a sterile product for adding to a sterile field; however, always check the product label for this information.

Administration sets have two ways to connect to the catheter hub: a slip lock or a Luer-Lok. The *slip lock* is a male end that slips into the female catheter hub. A *Luer-Lok* connection has the same male end with a threaded collar that requires twisting onto the corresponding threads of the catheter hub. All connections, including *extension sets*, should have a Luer-Lok design to ensure that the set remains firmly connected. Loose connections lead to fluid leakage and increase the risk for contamination and subsequent bloodstream infection. When using a central venous catheter, a Luer-Lok connection is critical to reduce the risk for air embolism. Tape is not considered an adequate mechanism for securing set connections.

Luer-Lok devices may be purposefully or accidentally disconnected. Patients or visitors may disconnect the system to allow the patient to get out of bed or the chair, or the device may become accidentally disconnected when the patient turns or moves. In either case be sure to reconnect the device by following the proper sequence to reassemble the IV system components. Fatalities have resulted when nurses have accidently reconnected IV tubing to a tracheostomy or other inappropriate port.

Filters may be part of the administration set or separate add-on pieces. Their purpose is to remove particulate matter, microorganisms, and air from the infusion system. Filter sizes depend on the pore size, with common sizes being 1.2 microns used to filter lipid-containing parenteral nutrition and 0.2 microns intended to remove all particles and bacteria. Filters should be placed as close to the catheter hub as possible.

Particulate matter in the IV fluid, a primary reason to use filters, comprises undissolved, unintended substances and may include rubber pieces, glass particles, cotton fibers, drug particles, paper, and metal fibers. These particles become trapped in the small circulation of the lungs. A red blood cell is about 5 microns in diameter and is the largest size that can pass through the pulmonary capillary bed; IV fluids may contain particles larger than 5 microns. For patients receiving infusion therapy for long periods, a significant number of particles could block the blood flow through the pulmonary circulation. Microcirculation in the spleen, kidneys, and liver could also be affected. Particulate matter has also been implicated in the development of phlebitis in peripheral veins.

Other concerns with using filters include the possibility for their rupture, their use with certain drugs that bind to the filter surface, using the incorrect size of filter for drugs with large molecules, and choosing a filter that will not tolerate the pressure exerted by infusion pumps. Rupture is most commonly associated with the exertion of high pressure exceeding the limit tolerated by the specific filter. Some drugs cannot be filtered because they are retained inside the filter because of their chemical nature or molecule size. For these reasons medication filtration during the process of admixing is commonly used today as an alternative to final filtration at the bedside. Drugs of a very small quantity should be administered below the filter.

Filters used on blood administration sets have much larger pore size and are not interchangeable with filters used for fluids and medications. A standard blood filter ranges from 170 to 260 microns and removes microclots and other debris caused by blood collection and storage. Microaggregate filters have a pore size of 20, 40, or 80 microns and are used to remove degenerating platelets, white blood cells, and fibrin strands. Leukocyte-removal filters are used to remove white blood cells that cause febrile and allergic blood transfusion reactions.

Needleless Connection Devices

In July 1992, the Occupational Safety and Health Administration (OSHA) published guidelines entitled *Occupational Exposure to Bloodborne Pathogens, Final Rule*. This document requires health care organizations to initiate engineering controls "that isolate or remove the bloodborne pathogen hazard from the workplace." This standard was amended in 2001 with the passage of the Needlestick Safety and Prevention Act. This regulation requires the use of devices engineered with safety mechanisms and mandates that staff who perform these tasks be directly involved with selecting products. It also requires each employer to maintain a sharps injury log with details of each incident. Many products are designed to minimize health care workers' exposure to contaminated needles. Luer-Lok–activated devices are the most common design for needleless systems today.

Although these devices have reduced the incidence of accidental needlesticks for health care professionals, it is imperative that the connector be disinfected with alcohol or chlorhexidine/alcohol before and after each use with a *vigorous scrub* for 5 to 60 seconds (INS, 2016). This method is known as "scrub the hub." Blood and bacteria can be trapped in the crevices, and meticulous disinfecting is required with each use.

Various designs are available for connectors that provide positive or negative displacement of fluid when the needleless syringe is removed. Needleless positive-pressure valve (PPV) connectors were developed to prevent backflow of blood into the IV catheter, thereby decreasing chances of thrombus formation and CRBSI. Several newer connectors are silver-impregnated to reduce bacterial growth (Fig. 13-12). Be sure to check which type of connector valve is used in your facility because the flushing technique differs depending on type.

Conclusive studies are needed to determine the best design for needleless systems. Until then, implement these interventions to reduce infection risk:

- Clean all needleless system connections vigorously with antimicrobial for 60 seconds (usually 70% alcohol or alcohol and 2% chlorhexidine swabs) before connecting infusion sets or syringes, paying special attention to the small ridges in the Luer-Lok device. Newer caps that are impregnated with alcohol or chlorhexidine may be used to keep the port aseptic; however, these will

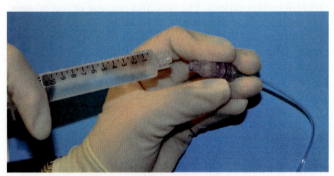

FIG. 13-12 Example of a needleless connector.

increase costs, and research is needed to demonstrate the benefit.

- Do not tape connections between tubing sets.
- Use evidence-based hand hygiene guidelines from the CDC and OSHA.

Rate-Controlling Infusion Devices

The ability to regulate the rate and volume of infusions is critical to the safe and accurate administration of medications and fluids to patients. Nurses have a choice of numerous devices that can be electronically or mechanically regulated.

Electronic infusion devices (IV pumps) are used universally in acute care institutions. They are also used in long-term care settings and at home. In addition, "smart pumps" provide the latest infusion computer technology to promote patient safety and save nursing time. *Remember that the use of pumps does not decrease your responsibility to carefully monitor the patient's infusion site and the infusion rate.*

In inpatient settings IV pumps are pole mounted. As their name implies, these electronic devices with battery backup pump drugs or fluids under pressure. They accurately measure the volume of fluid being infused by using one of three mechanisms:

- A syringe-type mechanism that fills and empties
- A wavelike, peristaltic action that pushes fluid along the tubing
- A series of microchambers that fill and empty

Regardless of the pumping mechanism, these devices require dedicated cassette tubing designed to match the pump.

Syringe pumps use an electronic or battery-powered piston to push the plunger continuously at a selected milliliter-per-hour rate. The use of syringe pumps is limited to small-volume continuous or intermittent infusions and depends on the syringe size. Antibiotics and patient-controlled analgesia are frequently delivered with syringe pumps. Patients requiring fluid restrictions can also benefit from using a syringe pump because smaller yet accurate volumes can be used to dilute medications.

Ambulatory pumps are generally used for home care patients and allow them to return to their usual activities while receiving infusion therapy. These pumps have a wide range of sizes, with some requiring a backpack, but they usually weigh less than 6 lb. They are typically used to accurately deliver continuous infusions such as parenteral nutrition, pain medication, and many programmable drug schedules. Frequent battery recharging or replacement is usually necessary.

Electronic infusion devices can be programmed in many different ways and require a thorough knowledge of the specific brand being used. Infusion rate and the volume to be infused are usually entered in single milliliter increments, but some can be programmed as fractions of a milliliter. Some pumps allow the rate to be programmed to taper or ramp up and down at the beginning and ending of the infusion. Secondary syringe infusion, secondary infusion rate, remote site programming, adjustable infusion pressure, and integration into the nurse call system also are possible.

Electronic infusion devices have a variety of alarms such as air-in-line, upstream and downstream occlusion, infusion complete, and low-battery or power warnings. All devices must have some mechanism to prevent free flow of the infusing fluid or medication. When the cassette or tubing is removed from the pump, this mechanism automatically stops fluid flow until it is properly replaced in the pump. This safety measure prevents accidental rapid infusion of large amounts of fluid or medication, which could lead to serious clinical problems.

In the past few years, smart pumps (infusion pumps with dosage calculation software) have been promoted to reduce adverse drug events (ADEs). Incorrect programming of pumps without this feature is one of the most common types of drug errors, especially in hospitals. Multiple libraries of drug information are stored in the pump manufacturer's medical management system. This software allows the facility to preprogram dosing limits, especially for high-alert drugs. Examples of smart pumps are the B. Braun Outlook 400ES and the Baxter Sigma Spectrum infusion system.

The newest development in smart pumps is a wireless network connection. Drug libraries can be updated via a wireless connection, thus eliminating the necessity of manually updating each pump. In addition to preventing drug errors, smart-pump systems record potential errors that would have occurred without these safety mechanisms (Waterson, 2013).

Dose-track technology is intended to transmit the infusion data to the institution's pharmacy so the correct patient receives the correct medication. Dose-guard technology alerts the nurse if institution-defined dose limits are exceeded. These newer technologies provide safeguards for patients to keep them safe. However, the "smarter" the pump, the more extensive the programming steps, and the more alarms to which the nurse must respond. In addition, technology and wireless connections can fail. The challenge for nurses is to maintain the skill of manual dose calculation and rate control, acknowledge and validate all alarms, and guard against becoming desensitized to alarms.

Mechanically regulated devices can be used to deliver intermittent medications such as antibiotics or continuous pain medications in community-based health or home care settings. In acute care settings devices called "infusers" may be found in surgical services. They are powered by positive pressure from the collapsing balloon or roller returning to its coiled position.

The systems include elastomeric balloons, spring-coiled syringes and containers, and a multi-chambered fluid container placed in a mechanical roller (Accufuser or ON-Q PainBuster) (Fig. 13-13). These small portable devices do not require power sources such as batteries or electricity. They deliver a preset infusion rate, and fluid volume is determined by the size of the fluid container; however, most hold only 50 to 100 mL.

NURSING CARE FOR PATIENTS RECEIVING INTRAVENOUS THERAPY

Educating the Patient

The current trend in health care demands that we partner with our patients to provide the best patient-centered care. In 2010 The Joint Commission added the requirement that all patients who have central lines placed in the hospital must have education on prevention of catheter-related bloodstream infection (CRBSI). Before catheter insertion, educate the patient and family about:

- The type of catheter to be used
- Hand hygiene and aseptic technique for care of the catheter
- The therapy required
- Alternatives to the catheter and therapy

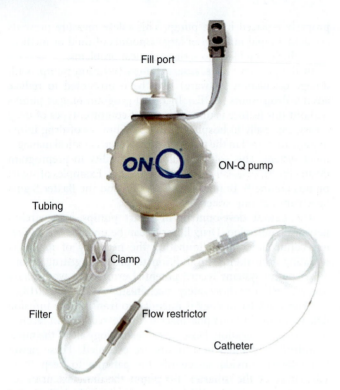

FIG. 13-13 ON-Q PainBuster pump (mechanical infuser). (Courtesy Kimberly-Clark Corporation.)

- Activity limitations
- Any signs or symptoms of complications that should be reported to a health care professional

Provide written information before placement of a long-term catheter and continue to assess the patient's knowledge level and provide more information or answers as needed. Most manufacturers of PICCs, tunneled catheters, and implanted ports provide patient information booklets. However, specific information about the chosen procedures and supplies may be required. Conversation and pictures are helpful for patients who are literacy challenged (have a low reading level ability.) Patients who do not speak or read English will need a translator.

Performing the Nursing Assessment

All central VADs require documentation of tip location at the CAJ by electrocardiogram technology, fluoroscopy, or chest x-ray. The initial verbal and subsequent written report should contain specific information about the catheter tip location in relation to anatomic structures. The nurse's knowledge of accurate tip location is required before beginning infusion through the catheter. Repeating the x-ray during catheter use may be necessary if the patient reports unusual pain or sensation.

Nursing assessment for all infusion systems should be systematic. Begin with the insertion site and work upward, following the tubing. Know the type of catheter your patient has in place. Be sure to find out the length of catheter, the insertion site, and tip location to perform a complete assessment. Assess the insertion site by looking for redness, swelling, hardness, or drainage. Also assess the skin underneath the dressing especially for signs of medical adhesive–related skin injury (MARSI) (INS,

2016). Lightly palpate the area over the dressing. When a midline catheter or PICC is used, assess the entire extremity and upper chest for signs of phlebitis and thrombosis. When a tunneled catheter is used, assess the exit site, the entire length of the tunnel, and the point where the catheter enters the vein. For a well-healed catheter, it may not be possible to detect the vein entrance site. On newly inserted catheters there could be a small puncture site with a suture or other securement device. For implanted ports, assess the incision and surgically created subcutaneous pocket.

Assess the integrity of the dressing, making sure that it is clean, dry, and adherent to the skin on all sides. Check all connections on the administration set and ensure that they are secure. Be sure that they are not taped. Check the rate of infusion for all fluids by either counting drops or checking the infusion pump. Assess the amount of fluid that has infused from the container. Is it accurate, or is it infusing too fast or too slow? Adjust the rate to the prescribed flow rate. Check all labels on containers for the patient's name and fluid or medication. *Be sure that the correct solution is being infused!*

! NURSING SAFETY PRIORITY QSEN
Action Alert

Remind unlicensed assistive personnel (UAP) to avoid taking blood pressures in an extremity with any type of catheter in place. If a short peripheral catheter is being used for continuous infusion, the compression while taking the blood pressure can increase venous pressure, causing fluid to overflow from the puncture site and infiltration. When a midline catheter or PICC is being used, compression from the blood pressure cuff could increase vein irritation and lead to phlebitis.

Draw blood samples in the extremity opposite from all catheters. Blood should not be drawn from a venipuncture site proximal to (above) an infusing peripheral catheter because the infusing fluid could alter the results of the test to be performed. Venipuncture at or near the insertion site of a midline catheter or PICC could damage the catheter, add to areas of venous inflammation, and decrease perfusion.

Securing and Dressing the Catheter

Adequate catheter securement is vital to prevent many complications. Tape, sutures, and specially designed securement devices can be used for this purpose. For a short peripheral catheter, tape strips are most common; however, the tape should be *clean.* Tape strips from a peripheral IV start kit are preferred. Strips of tape should not be taken from rolls of tape moved between patient's rooms, from other procedures, or from uniform pockets. Precutting tape and placing it on the patient's bedrails, your uniform or scrubs, or other object should also be avoided to prevent transmission of microorganisms.

Newer *securement devices* are designed for all catheter types and provide an evidence-based method to prevent VAD movement (INS, 2016). Recent studies have shown that these devices such as the StatLock IV stabilization device prevent peripheral and central catheters from becoming dislodged (Fig. 13-14) (see the Evidence-Based Practice box). In addition, they prevent complications such as phlebitis and infiltration. To prevent skin tears, remove the adhesive on a StatLock with 70% alcohol.

PICCs and nontunneled percutaneous central catheters may be sutured in place; however, this creates additional breaks in the skin that could become infected. If these sutures are loose or broken, notify the primary health care provider to replace

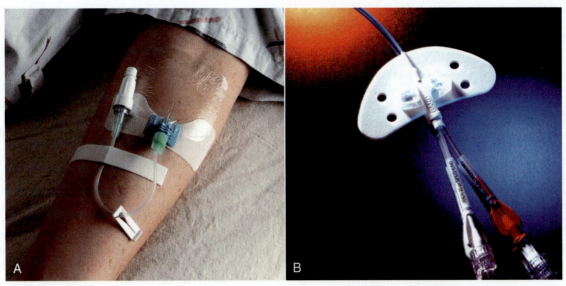

FIG. 13-14 The StatLock provides a standardized method to prevent catheter movement. (Courtesy Venetec International, San Diego, CA.)

EVIDENCE-BASED PRACTICE QSEN

What Is the Best Method for Securing a Patient's Central Venous Access Device?

Ullman, A.J., Cooke, M., & Rickard, C.M. (2015). Examining the role of securement and dressing products to prevent central venous access device failure: A narrative review. *Journal of the Association for Vascular Access, 20*(2), 99–110.

Central venous catheters require stabilization to ensure an extended lifeline. Dislodgment is one of the major complications associated with failure of the access device. The researchers undertook a narrative methodology to explore the fundamental principles of securement and dressing products to prevent central venous access device failure. The researchers use a narrative review that included articles that reported the underpinning of central catheter securement and dressing to prevent dislodgment failure, which totaled 21 studies out of the 213 studies retrieved.

Findings included characteristics focused on providing a microbial barrier for contamination and colonization, reducing external and internal motion, and the effect of dressing disruption. The researchers concluded that patients with central venous access devices are a heterogenous group and there is not one securement device that fits everyone. Individualized assessment is required to select the appropriate securement. Future studies are needed to determine the most effective securement that is cost-effective for all populations.

Level of Evidence: 1

This study used a narrative research review and analysis methodology to determine best practices for use of IV securement devices.

Commentary: Implications for Practice and Research

This research validated the effectiveness of IV catheter securement and stabilization devices for all patients receiving central infusion therapy. Clinicians need to recognize the priority of using an appropriate securement and dressing for the patient. Institutions need to recognize the long-term savings of using a securement and dressing to prevent catheter failure for improved patient outcomes. Future clinical research and innovative solutions need to be ongoing.

them. IV catheter sutures are being replaced with securement devices and Dermabond glue in some facilities, which can decrease infection and avoid the need to remove sutures after infusion therapy is discontinued.

Tunneled catheters usually have sutures placed near the skin exit site, which are removed after the tunnel has healed. The incision over an implanted port pocket will have sutures until it has healed. After it is healed and when it is not accessed, no dressing is required. When an implanted port is accessed, the sterile occlusive dressing should cover the entire needle and site.

Sterile dressings used over the insertion site protect the skin and puncture site. For a short *peripheral* catheter, the transparent membrane dressings do not require routine changes. Short peripheral lines do not usually dwell longer than a few days; and, as long as the dressing is dry, clean, and intact, it does not have to be changed. Any VAD dressing should be changed when it is loose or soiled.

For central lines and midline catheters, tape and sterile gauze or a transparent membrane dressing may be used. Change tape and gauze dressings every 48 hours; change transparent membrane dressings such as Tegaderm, every 5 to 7 days (INS, 2016). The initial dressing on a midline catheter or PICC is usually tape and gauze, changed within 24 hours after insertion because some bleeding is likely. Transparent membrane dressings can be used for subsequent dressing. For patients who develop erythema (redness) from Tegaderm, the IV3000 dressing from Smith and Nephew may be used. Document when you change the sterile dressing and your IV site assessments in the appropriate electronic health record according to agency policy.

When changing the dressing, remove it by pulling laterally from side to side. It can also be removed by holding the external catheter and pulling it off toward the insertion site. *Never pull it off by pulling away from the insertion site because this could dislodge the catheter!*

After removing the dressing from a midline catheter or any central venous catheter, note the external catheter length. Compare this length with the original length at insertion. If the

! NURSING SAFETY PRIORITY (QSEN)

Action Alert

> Site protection may be needed for short peripheral catheters or for port access needles. Plastic shields can be placed over the site to prevent accidental bumping or pressure from clothing. Make sure that you can easily assess the site frequently. Never place a restraint or opaque dressing over a peripheral IV site, especially when infusing an irritant or vesicant.

length has changed, the catheter tip location has also changed and may no longer be in a vein appropriate for infusion. Follow agency policy or notify the primary health care provider about the length change. A chest x-ray may be needed, and careful assessment of the type of therapy and remaining length of therapy will likely be required.

Protect the external catheter, dressing, and all attached tubing from water because it is a source of contamination. *Remind unlicensed assistive personnel (UAP) to cover the extremity where the IV line is located when giving the patient a bath.* A plastic bag or wrap can be taped over the extremity to keep the dressing and site dry.

? CLINICAL JUDGMENT CHALLENGE 13-1

Evidence-Based Practice; Safety (QSEN)

> A new graduate nurse is being oriented to your medical-surgical nursing unit. Today he is assigned to care for three patients. One patient is an older adult with an infiltrated peripheral IV line in her forearm. The second patient has a PICC line for antibiotic therapy, and the third patient has an arterial implanted port for chemotherapy. As his preceptor, you are responsible for teaching him how to assess patients with these devices and prevent and/or monitor for complications. Your unit has several memory checklists for IV care that you plan to review with him.
> 1. Which best clinical practices will you teach the new nurse about how to care for patients who have a PICC line?
> 2. For which life-threatening complication is the patient with the implanted port most at risk?
> 3. You observe the new nurse as he prepares to restart the IV line for the older-adult patient. He chooses a vein in the dorsum of the hand. What is your best response about his IV site selection?
> 4. What is the value of memory checklists to ensure consistency among nurses caring for patients receiving IV therapy?

Changing Administration Sets and Needleless Connectors

Plan the change of administration sets and fluid containers to occur at the same time, if possible, to minimize the number of times the system is opened. For short peripheral catheters, the administration set and catheter should also be changed at the same time to avoid excessive manipulation of the catheter. Document these changes per agency policy.

Needleless connector devices can be changed when the administration set is changed. If it is being used for intermittent infusions, the device should be changed at least once per week. Fluid leakage from the device indicates that the integrity has been compromised, and it should be changed immediately.

Precautions to prevent *air emboli* are required when changing the set or connectors attached to any catheter; however, central venous catheters require special attention. Most catheters

have a pinch clamp that can be closed during this procedure. Techniques used to increase the intrathoracic pressure and prevent air embolism during IV set change include:

- Placing the patient in a flat or Trendelenburg position to ensure that the catheter exit site is at or below the level of the heart
- Asking the patient to perform a Valsalva maneuver by holding his or her breath and bearing down
- Timing the IV set change to the expiratory cycle when the patient is spontaneously breathing
- Timing the IV set change to the inspiratory cycle when the patient is receiving positive-pressure mechanical ventilation

Controlling Infusion Pressure

Fluid flow through the infusion system requires that the pressure on the external side be greater than the pressure at the catheter tip. Fluid flow can be slowed or obstructed by many causes. Inside the catheter lumen, resistance is created by the catheter length and diameter or by deposits of fibrin, thrombus, or drug precipitate. Near the catheter tip, resistance to flow comes from the catheter tip impinging on the vein wall, thrombus, or venous spasm.

All catheter manufacturers have warnings about the use of excessive pressure. Gravity and infusion pumps do not exert pressure too high for the catheter to handle; however, excessive pressure from syringes can lead to catheter damage. For this reason use 10-mL syringes for central venous catheters. Although these larger syringes generate less pressure, it is still possible to reach excessive pressure levels if great force is applied against a syringe attached to a catheter that is partially occluded.

Flushing the Catheter

Catheter flushing prevents contact between incompatible drugs and maintains patency of the lumens. Normal saline alone or normal saline followed by heparinized saline may be used. When using valved catheters and certain positive fluid-displacement needleless devices, normal saline alone is acceptable because these devices have mechanisms that prevent the backflow of blood into the catheter lumen.

! NURSING SAFETY PRIORITY (QSEN)

Critical Rescue

> Assess catheter patency carefully before each use. Use sterile technique to flush with normal saline while applying slow, gentle pressure to the syringe plunger. If you feel any resistance, stop the procedure immediately! If you continue, catheter rupture or forcing a blood clot into circulation could result. During the flushing procedure always aspirate for a brisk blood return from the catheter lumen.
> If the catheter will not yield a blood return, further diagnostic studies may be needed to determine the cause of the problems. Thrombolytic agents such as alteplase (Cathflo Activase) may be used to dissolve blood clots in venous catheters.

For short peripheral catheters, usually 3 mL normal saline is adequate to flush the catheter. For all other catheters 5 to 10 mL of preservative-free normal saline is needed. Bacteriostatic normal saline is limited to no more than 30 mL in a 24-hour period in adults. By using 10 mL before and after each dose of medication, it is easy to exceed this limitation. Check your agency's policy and procedure about specific flushing amounts.

Flush catheters immediately after each use. Delay in disconnecting the intermittent administration set and flushing the catheter could cause lumen occlusion from blood that backflows into the lumen when the infusion pressure is lower than venous pressure.

All fluids used to flush catheters should be obtained from single-dose containers or prefilled syringes. Vials used for multiple doses contribute to medication errors and increase the risk for contamination.

Obtaining Blood Samples From Central Venous Catheters

Short peripheral catheters should not be used routinely for obtaining blood samples. This additional manipulation could lead to vein irritation that requires removal of the catheter. Central venous catheters and midlines can be used for obtaining blood samples after a careful assessment of the risks versus the benefits. If your patient has no peripheral venipuncture sites or is fearful of needles, using the central venous catheter may be appropriate. The risks associated with obtaining blood samples from a central venous catheter are numerous. This procedure requires additional hub manipulation, which is a major cause of CRBSI. Consider the laboratory tests needed and the types of fluids that have recently been infused. For example, heparin interferes with coagulation studies, and electrolytes in the fluid may alter the results of serum electrolytes. Drawing blood from catheters for blood culture should not be done within an hour of completion of antimicrobial infusions.

If blood sampling from a central venous catheter is the best alternative, vigorous cleaning of the connections with 70% alcohol is necessary. Use methods that do not require exposed needles. Vacuum tubes attached via a "vacutainer" to the catheter hub eliminate the need to transfer the blood from a syringe into the tubes. For small-diameter catheters, the vacuum in the tube may cause the catheter to temporarily collapse, preventing the backflow of blood into the tube. In this situation small syringes should be used because they create less pressure on aspiration, the opposite of what small syringes do on injection. Transfer of the blood from the syringe to the vacuum tube requires the use of a "vacutainer needle holder." This device keeps the needle housed in a plastic case and covered, preventing needlestick injuries (Fig. 13-15). After blood draw from any catheter, a flush of 10 to 20 mL sterile normal saline is necessary to ensure a patent line. Be sure to clear the line and cap of blood to prevent a breeding ground for infection.

Removing the Vascular Access Device

To remove a short peripheral IV line, lift opposite sides of the transparent dressing and pull laterally to remove the dressing from the site while stabilizing the catheter. Slowly withdraw the catheter from the skin and immediately cover the puncture site with dry gauze. Hold pressure on the site until hemostasis is achieved. Assess the catheter tip to make sure that it is intact and completely removed. Document the time of catheter removal and the appearance of the IV site.

Removal of midline catheters and PICCs must be performed with the same slow, gentle techniques used to insert the catheter. Veins can develop venospasms when rapid or forceful techniques are used. After explaining to the patient that this procedure will

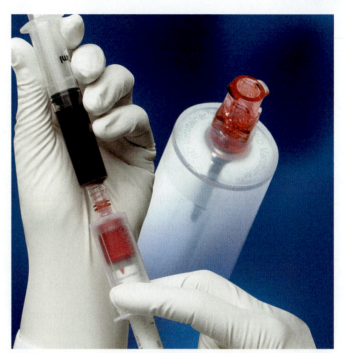

FIG. 13-15 Vacutainer needle holder prevents needlestick injuries when drawing blood. (Courtesy and © Becton, Dickinson and Company.)

not be painful, remove the dressing and withdraw the catheter in short segments by pulling from the insertion site. *If you feel resistance, always stop and never apply force to the catheter. Extreme traction or force could cause the catheter to break and embolize (travel) to the heart or pulmonary circulation.*

Simple distraction techniques and deep breathing may be sufficient to relax the patient and remove the catheter. If these fail, replace the dressing and apply heat; allow time for the vein wall to relax. Keeping the extremity warm and dry and asking the patient to drink warm liquids could facilitate removal. Use of medications to relax the vein wall may be required if the catheter cannot be removed after several hours. Imaging studies may also be needed to determine whether the cause is a thrombosis instead of venospasm.

Nontunneled percutaneous central catheters are removed by clipping any sutures and withdrawing the catheter in short segments. Venospasm does not commonly occur when removing these catheters because the vein diameter is large.

To prevent venous air embolism when removing any central venous catheter (including PICCs), position the patient in a flat supine or Trendelenburg position according to agency policy. To ensure that the intrathoracic pressure is higher than atmospheric pressure, have the patient hold his or her breath or perform a Valsalva maneuver during removal. If the patient is mechanically ventilated, time the removal to the delivery of an inhalation by the ventilator. Be sure to keep the catheter clamped during this procedure. When a central venous catheter is removed, a tract between the skin and vein may create a conduit that could allow air to be pulled into the vein.

After removal, measure the catheter length and compare it with the length documented on insertion. *If the entire catheter length was not removed, contact the primary health care provider immediately!* Removal of tunneled catheters and implanted ports is usually performed by nurse practitioners or physicians.

Documenting Intravenous Therapy

Intravenous therapy is risk prone. Nurses can protect themselves from malpractice claims with conscientious assessment, intervention, and documentation. Be sure that you document after insertion of a vascular access device (VAD) and throughout the course of the therapy. When inserting a venous catheter, remember to document the:

- Date and time of the VAD insertion
- Name of the nurse (you) who inserted the VAD
- Vein that was used for insertion
- Type of VAD used
- Number of insertion attempts and locations of attempts before successful insertion
- Response of the patient to the VAD insertion process
- Type of dressing applied
- Type of securement device, if used
- Special barrier precautions used, if any
- Patient and family education provided related to IV therapy

During the course of the patient's infusion therapy, be sure to continue documenting in the electronic health record your assessments and any interventions needed as a result of complications. Follow your agency's policies and procedures for additional requirements.

COMPLICATIONS OF INTRAVENOUS THERAPY

Complications from IV therapy can be minor and limited or life threatening. Serious life-altering or life-threatening complications are dramatically increasing in frequency and severity and present a tremendous financial burden to the U.S. health care system. Catheter-related bloodstream infection (CRBSI) is one of the most serious problems, often resulting in patient death. They are more common in patients with central VADs but can also occur with peripheral catheters.

Catheter-Related Bloodstream Infection

The Institute for Healthcare Improvement identified CRBSI as one of several preventable hospital-acquired infections (HAIs). As part of their previous *100,000 Lives Campaign*, a number of evidence-based interventions were combined into the CRBSI prevention bundle. As a nurse your accountability is to ensure that these interventions are followed (Table 13-2).

Other Complications of Intravenous Therapy

Local complications of IV therapy occur at or near the catheter. A priority for care for patients with IV therapy is to prevent, assess, and detect these complications. In some cases nurses also manage these problems. Definitions, causes, signs and symptoms, treatment, and prevention of local complications are summarized in Table 13-3. *Systemic complications* of IV therapy involve the entire vascular system or multiple systems. Information on common systemic complications can be found in Table 13-4. For central venous catheters (CVCs), complications can occur during the insertion procedure or during the dwell time (Table 13-5). Tables 13-6 and 13-7 are the INS criteria for grading phlebitis and infiltrations. Document all assessments and complications in the patient's electronic health record. Notify the infusion therapy team and/or primary health care provider per agency policy when complications occur.

TABLE 13-2   The Catheter-Related Bloodstream Infection (CRBSI) Prevention Bundle

- Use a *checklist* during insertion to make sure that everything is done correctly. Tell anyone who violates the correct steps to stop the procedure immediately.
- *Hand hygiene* before inserting a central line must be thorough (i.e., no quick scrub). Anyone who touches the central line must also perform thorough hand hygiene.
- *Maximal barrier precautions* during line insertion require that the patient be draped from head to toe with a sterile barrier.
- The primary health care provider who inserts the VAD wears sterile *gloves, gown, and mask*. Anyone in the room during the procedure must also wear a mask.
- *Traffic in and out of the room must be minimized.* Many institutions use a "stop" sign on the door of the room to prevent people from coming in and going out during the procedure and a special "central line cart" to ensure that they have everything they need in the room.
- *Chlorhexidine is used for skin disinfection* because it has best outcomes for preventing infection.
- *Use preferred sites.* PICC in the upper arm and subclavian veins are the first choice. The next preference is the internal jugular vein, and the least preferred is the femoral vein.
- *Post-placement care* requires meticulous dressing changes and care of all parts of the IV system such as keeping ports and stopcocks clean; hanging bags using sterile technique; vigorously scrubbing catheter hub with alcohol when used.
- *Review daily the need* for the patient's VAD. The incidence of CRBSI increases each day the device is in place. As soon as it is determined that the patient no longer needs the IV line, it should be removed.

PICC, Peripherally inserted central catheter; *VAD,* vascular access device.

INTRAVENOUS THERAPY AND CARE OF THE OLDER ADULT

The aging process causes numerous changes in all body functions, and yet aging occurs differently in each person. Nutrition, environment, genetics, social factors, and education are just a few of the factors that influence the older adult's needs. Because all body functions are affected, IV therapy can be affected by these changes.

Skin Care

Aging skin becomes thinner and loses subcutaneous fat, decreasing the skin's ability for thermal regulation. Fewer nerve endings mean the decreased ability to feel pain. Older patients *may* not perceive acute pain from traumatic venipuncture requiring excessive probing or multiple attempts. However, this action increases the risk for fluid leakage and subsequent infiltration or extravasation injury. Inserting and removing a catheter and dressing could tear the skin layers.

Skin antisepsis is extremely important because of the decreased immunity seen as part of the aging process. Lipids are normally found in skin as a protective agent, and alcohol easily dissolves lipids. Although greater numbers of organisms may be killed, the skin can also become excessively dry and cracked. Current recommendations call for using friction when cleaning the skin to penetrate the layers of the epidermis. However, excessive friction may damage fragile skin and cause impaired TISSUE INTEGRITY. Chlorhexidine is the preferred

Text continued on p. 222

TABLE 13-3   Local Complications of Intravenous Therapy

COMPLICATION	CAUSE	SIGNS AND SYMPTOMS	INTERVENTIONS	PREVENTION
Infiltration				
Leakage of a nonvesicant IV solution or medication into the extravascular tissue	Peripheral catheter has punctured opposite vein wall Obstruction of blood flow causing backflow through original entrance site Inflammatory process causing fluid leakage at the capillary level Fibrin sheath fully encasing a central venous catheter, leading to retrograde flow and leakage from venipuncture site Damaged septum of implanted port Dislodged port access needle	IV rate slows Increasing edema around site Patient report of skin tightness; blanching or coolness of skin; burning, tenderness, or general discomfort at the insertion site; fluid leaking from puncture site; absence of a blood return (though this may not be reliable with a short peripheral catheter)	Stop infusion and remove short peripheral catheter immediately after identification of problem. Apply sterile dressing if weeping from tissue occurs. Elevate extremity. Warm or cold compresses may be used according to the solution infiltrated and organizational policy. Warm compresses increase circulation to the area and speed healing. Cool compresses may be used to relieve discomfort and reduce swelling. Insert a new catheter in the opposite extremity. For all central venous catheters, obtain a study to determine the cause of the problem. For implanted port, remove and insert a new port access needle. Rate the infiltration using the INS Infiltration Scale and document (Table 13-7).	Catheter stabilization—use smallest catheter appropriate; avoid area of flexion or use armboard. Avoid placing restraints at IV site. Make successive venipunctures proximal to the previous site. Monitor site frequently; educate patient about activities and signs and symptoms. Central venous catheters—obtain a brisk blood return before using the catheter for infusion. Frequently assess proper positioning of port access needle. Stabilize it well and protect from clothing.
Extravasation				
Leakage of a vesicant IV solution or medication into the extravascular tissue Can occur with both peripheral and central catheters	Same as for infiltration	Same as for infiltration Blistering and tissue sloughing may not appear for a few days and resolves over 1-4 wks with infiltration of some chemotherapeutic agents such as anthracycline and alkylating agents	Stop infusion and disconnect administration set. Aspirate drug from short peripheral catheter or port access needle. Leave short peripheral catheter or port access needle in place to deliver antidote, if indicated by established policy. If possible, aspirate residual drug from the exit site of a central venous catheter. Administer antidote according to established policy. Apply cold compresses for all drugs EXCEPT vinca alkaloids and epipodophyllotoxins. Photograph site. Monitor at 24 hrs, 1 wk, 2 wks, and as needed. Surgical interventions may be required. Provide written instructions to patient and family.	Same as for infiltration. Know the vesicant potential before giving any IV medication. Prevention is key.

Continued

TABLE 13-3	**Local Complications of Intravenous Therapy—cont'd**			
COMPLICATION	**CAUSE**	**SIGNS AND SYMPTOMS**	**INTERVENTIONS**	**PREVENTION**
Phlebitis				
Inflammation of the vein Post-infusion phlebitis presents within 48-96 hrs after the catheter has been removed	Mechanical cause from insertion technique, catheter size, and lack of catheter securement Chemical cause from extremes of pH and/or osmolarity of the fluid or medication Bacterial cause from a break in aseptic technique, poor securement, and extended dwell time	Patient may report pain at the IV site; nurse may observe that vein appears red and inflamed along the length; vein may become hard and cordlike (Table 13-6)	Remove short peripheral catheter at the first sign of phlebitis; use warm compresses to relieve pain. Monitor frequently. Document using Phlebitis Scale. Insert a new catheter using the opposite extremity. Mechanical phlebitis occurring in the first week after PICC insertion may be treated without catheter removal. Apply continuous heat; rest and elevate the extremity. Significant improvement is seen in 24 hrs, and complete resolution is seen within 72 hrs. Remove catheter if treatment is unsuccessful.	Choose the smallest-gauge catheter for the required therapy. Avoid sites of joint flexion or stabilize with an armboard. Avoid infusing fluids or medications with a pH below 5.0 or above 9.0 through a peripheral vein. Avoid infusing fluids or medications with a final osmolarity above 500 mOsm/L through a peripheral vein. Rotate sites every 72-96 hrs according to established policy. Adequately secure the catheter. Use aseptic technique. For PICCs, teach patient to avoid excessive physical activity with the extremity.
Thrombosis				
Blood clot inside the vein	Anything that damages the endothelial lining of the intima can initiate clot formation Traumatic venipuncture Multiple venipuncture attempts Use of catheters too large for the chosen vein Hypercoagulable state and venous stasis	Slowed or stopped infusion rate Swollen extremity Tenderness and redness Engorged peripheral veins of the ipsilateral chest and extremity	Stop infusion and remove short peripheral catheter immediately. Apply cold compresses to decrease blood flow and stabilize the clot. Elevate extremity. Surgical intervention may be required. For central venous catheters, notify the physician and obtain requests for a diagnostic study. Low-dose thrombolytic agents can be used to lyse the clot.	Use evidence-based venipuncture technique. Make only two attempts to perform venipuncture. Choose the smallest-gauge catheter in the largest vein possible. Secure catheter adequately. Use armboards if short peripheral catheters are placed in areas of joint flexion. Ensure adequate hydration to avoid changes in blood composition and flexion of the extremity. Prophylactic low-dose warfarin (Coumadin, Warfilone ♦) may be prescribed for patients with a central venous catheter.
Thrombophlebitis				
Presence of a blood clot and vein inflammation	Same as for phlebitis and thrombosis	Same as for phlebitis and thrombosis	Same as for phlebitis and thrombosis. Apply cold compresses initially, followed by warm.	Same as for phlebitis and thrombosis.
Ecchymosis and Hematoma				
Ecchymosis results from infiltration of blood into the surrounding tissue Hematoma results from uncontrolled bleeding	Unskilled or multiple IV insertion attempts Patients with coagulopathy or fragile veins (e.g., older adults and patients on steroids) Accidental laceration of a large vein or artery	Swelling Bruising Pain or tenderness	When removing device, apply light pressure; excessive pressure could cause other fragile veins in the area to rupture. For hematoma, apply direct pressure until bleeding has stopped. Elevate extremity, apply ice for first 24 hours and then warm compress for comfort.	Avoid veins that cannot be easily seen or palpated. Use extra caution in patients with coagulopathies. Use evidence-based venipuncture technique.

TABLE 13-3 Local Complications of Intravenous Therapy—cont'd

COMPLICATION	CAUSE	SIGNS AND SYMPTOMS	INTERVENTIONS	PREVENTION
Site Infection				
Invasion of microorganisms at the insertion site in the absence of simultaneous bloodstream infection	Break in aseptic technique during insertion or the handling of sterile equipment	Site appears red, swollen, and warm; patient may report tenderness at the site; may observe purulent or malodorous exudates	Clean exit site with alcohol, expressing drainage if present. For short peripheral catheter, midline catheter, or PICC, remove using sterile technique and avoid contact between skin and catheter.	Use strict aseptic technique when inserting, maintaining, or removing catheters. Practice evidence-based hand hygiene.
Infection localized at the insertion site, the port pocket, or subcutaneous tunnel	Lack of proper hand hygiene and skin antisepsis		Send catheter tip for culture, if requested. Clean site with alcohol and cover with dry, sterile dressing; physician to evaluate for septic phlebitis and need for antimicrobial therapy or surgical intervention.	Ensure that dressing remains clean, dry, and adherent to skin at all times.
Venous Spasm				
Sudden contraction of the vein	Normal response to irritation or injury of the vein wall	Cramping or pain at or above the insertion site	Temporarily slow infusion rate. Apply warm compress. Do not immediately remove short peripheral catheter.	Allow time for vein diameter to return to normal after tourniquet removal and before advancing catheter.
		Numbness in the area Slowing of the infusion rate Inability to withdraw midline catheter or PICC	If occurring during midline catheter or PICC removal, do not apply tension or attempt forceful removal. Reapply a dressing, apply heat, encourage patient to drink warm liquids, and keep extremity covered and dry. 12-24 hrs may be required before catheter can be removed.	Infuse fluids at room temperature if possible. For a midline catheter or PICC, gently withdraw the catheter in short segments.
Nerve Damage				
Inadvertent piercing or complete transection of a nerve	Venipuncture near known nerve locations Unanticipated nerve locations	Reports of tingling or feeling "pins and needles" at or below the insertion site Numbness at or near the insertion site	Immediately stop the insertion procedure if the patient reports extreme pain. Remove the catheter if reports of discomfort do not improve when the catheter is secured.	Avoid using the cephalic vein near the wrist. Avoid using veins on the palm side of the wrist. Adequately secure the catheter, but avoid tape that is too tight. Support areas of joint flexion with an armboard.

INS, Infusion Nurses Society; *PICC,* peripherally inserted central catheter.

TABLE 13-4 Systemic Complications of Intravenous Therapy

COMPLICATION	CAUSE	SIGNS AND SYMPTOMS	INTERVENTIONS	PREVENTION
Circulatory Overload				
Disruption of fluid homeostasis with excess fluid in the circulatory system	Infusion of fluids at a rate greater than the patient's system can accommodate	Patient may report shortness of breath and cough; patient's blood pressure is elevated, and there is puffiness around the eyes and edema in dependent areas; patient's neck veins may be engorged, and nurse may hear moist breath sounds.	Slow the IV rate and notify physician; raise patient to an upright position; monitor vital signs and administer oxygen as prescribed; administer diuretics as prescribed.	Monitor intake and output carefully and notify physician as soon as an imbalance is noticed between the patient's intake and output.

Continued

TABLE 13-4 | **Systemic Complications of Intravenous Therapy—cont'd**

COMPLICATION	CAUSE	SIGNS AND SYMPTOMS	INTERVENTIONS	PREVENTION
Speed Shock Systemic reaction to the rapid infusion of a substance unfamiliar to the patient's circulatory system	Rapid infusion of drugs or bolus infusion, which causes the drug to reach toxic levels quickly	Patient may report light-headedness or dizziness and chest tightness; nurse may note that patient has a flushed face and an irregular pulse; without intervention, patient may lose consciousness and go into shock and cardiac arrest.	Immediately discontinue the drug infusion and hang isotonic solution to keep the vein open; monitor vital signs carefully and notify physician for further treatments.	Be aware of the appropriate infusion rate of medications and adhere to them; use of infusion control devices helps to prevent speed shock.
Catheter Embolism A shaving or piece of catheter breaks off and floats freely in the vessel	Anything that damages the catheter—during insertion, dressing change, excessive force with flushing, or medication administration	Depending on where the catheter embolizes, this could be life threatening. Cardiopulmonary arrest could occur.	Emergently notify the physician. Remove the catheter and apply a tourniquet high on the limb of the catheter site; inspect catheter to determine how much may have embolized; an x-ray is taken to determine the presence of any catheter piece; surgical intervention may be necessary.	When inserting over-the-needle catheters, never reinsert the needle into the catheter; avoid pulling a through-the-needle catheter back through the needle during insertion. Avoid scissors near the catheter with dressing changes.

TABLE 13-5 | **Complications During the Dwell of Central Venous Catheters**

COMPLICATION	POSSIBLE CAUSES	SIGNS AND SYMPTOMS	TREATMENT	PREVENTION
Catheter Migration Movement of a properly placed catheter tip to another vein No change in the external catheter length	Changes in intrathoracic pressure caused by coughing, vomiting, sneezing, heavy lifting, and congestive heart failure	For migration to the jugular vein—reports of hearing a running stream or gurgling sound on the side of catheter insertion For migration to the azygos vein—back pain between the shoulder blades Neurologic complications if medications are infused	Stop all infusions and flush catheter. Notify physician. Obtain a chest x-ray, if required, to assess tip location. Spontaneous repositioning back to the SVC is possible. Repositioning by radiology may be required.	Place catheter tip properly in the lower third of the SVC near the junction with the right atrium. Instruct patient to perform usual ADLs but to avoid excessive physical activity.
Catheter Dislodgment Movement of catheter into or out of the insertion site	Inadequate catheter securement Excessive physical activity with a PICC	External catheter length has changed, also changing the internal tip location No other signs or symptoms may be noticed immediately	Stop all infusions and flush catheter. NEVER re-advance the catheter into the insertion site. Determine the amount of external catheter length and compare with the length documented on insertion. Notify the physician or nurse inserting the catheter for further assessment.	Use proper catheter securement device. Instruct patient to perform normal ADLs but to avoid excessive physical activity.
Catheter Rupture Catheter is broken, damaged, or separated from hub or port body	Forcefully flushing a catheter with any size syringe against resistance Using scissors to remove a dressing Catheter compression of a subclavian-inserted catheter between the clavicle and first rib (also known as *pinch-off syndrome*)	Fluid leaking from insertion site Pain or swelling during infusion Reflux of blood into the catheter extension Inability to aspirate blood from catheter	Repair the damaged segment; depends on the availability of a repair kit designed for the specific brand of catheter being used; repair may be considered a temporary measure instead of a permanent treatment. Remove catheter.	NEVER use excessive force when flushing a catheter, regardless of syringe size. On injection, small syringes generate more pressure than larger syringes. Use of a 10-mL syringe is generally recommended for flushing procedures. Insert catheter through jugular or upper-extremity sites instead of subclavian site.

TABLE 13-5   Complications During the Dwell of Central Venous Catheters—cont'd

COMPLICATION	POSSIBLE CAUSES	SIGNS AND SYMPTOMS	TREATMENT	PREVENTION
Lumen Occlusion				
Catheter lumen is partially or totally blocked	Drug or mineral precipitate (calcium, diazepam, and phenytoin are common) Lipid sludge from long-term infusion of fat emulsion Blood clots and fibrin sheath caused by blood reflux into lumen Allowing administration sets to remain connected for extended periods after medication has infused	Infusion stops or pump alarm sounds Inability or difficulty administering fluids Inability or difficulty drawing blood Increased resistance to flushing of the catheter	Assess history of catheter use. A suddenly developing problem may indicate contact between incompatible medications. A problem that develops over an extended period may indicate a gradual clot formation. For drug precipitate, determine the pH of the precipitated drug. Use hydrochloric acid for acidic drug. Use sodium bicarbonate for alkaline drugs. For blood clot use thrombolytic enzymes such as alteplase.	Always flush with normal saline between, before, and after each medication given through the catheter. Use positive-pressure flushing techniques when a negative fluid-displacement needleless connector is being used. Use a positive fluid-displacement needleless connector. Flush catheters immediately when medication infusion is complete.
Catheter-Related Bloodstream Infection (CRBSI)				
Pathogenic organisms invade the patient's circulation The CDC has specific criteria to classify these infections	Lack of sterile field during insertion Inadequate skin antiseptic agents and application techniques Manipulation of the catheter hub leading to intraluminal contamination Inadequate hand hygiene Long dwell time	Early symptoms include fever, chills, headache, and general malaise	Change the entire infusion system from solution to IV device; notify physician, obtain cultures, and administer antibiotics as prescribed. If the infusate is the suspected cause, send a specimen to the laboratory for evaluation.	Maintain sterile technique. Use the recommended CRBSI prevention bundle.

CDC, Centers for Disease Control and Prevention; *PICC,* peripherally inserted central catheter; *SVC,* superior vena cava.

TABLE 13-6   Phlebitis Scale From INS Standards of Practice

GRADE	CLINICAL CRITERIA
0	No symptoms
1	Erythema with or without pain
2	Pain at access site with erythema and/or edema
3	Pain at access site with erythema and/or edema Streak formation Palpable cord
4	Pain at access site with erythema and/or edema Streak formation Palpable venous cord more than 1 inch long Purulent drainage

Data from Infusion Nurses Society (INS). (2016). Infusion therapy standards of practice. *Journal of Infusion Nursing, 39*(1S), S96.

TABLE 13-7   Infiltration Scale From INS Standards of Practice

GRADE	CLINICAL CRITERIA
0	No symptoms
1	Skin blanched Edema <1 inch in any direction Cool to touch With or without pain
2	Skin blanched Edema 1-6 inches in any direction Cool to touch With or without pain
3	Skin blanched, translucent Gross edema >6 inches in any direction Cool to touch Mild-to-moderate pain Possible numbness
4	Skin blanched, translucent Skin tight, leaking Skin discolored, bruised, swollen Gross edema >6 inches in any direction Deep pitting tissue edema Circulatory impairment Moderate-to-severe pain Infiltration of any amount of blood product, irritant, or vesicant

Data from Infusion Nurses Society (INS). (2016). Infusion therapy standards of practice. *Journal of Infusion Nursing, 39*(1S), S96.

agent, and the product currently available contains alcohol. Check for allergies to iodine before using iodine or iodophors. Iodophors such as povidone-iodine require contact with the skin for a minimum of 2 minutes to be effective. All antiseptic solutions must be thoroughly dry before applying the dressing or tape.

Skin should never be shaved before venipuncture, but excessive amounts of hair should be clipped. Shaving causes micro-abrasions that can lead to infection. The skin of an older adult may be more delicate and therefore more easily nicked while shaving.

Skin and TISSUE INTEGRITY can easily be compromised by the application of tape or dressings. Use of skin protectant solutions puts a protective barrier between the skin and dressing and improves the adherence of the dressing to the skin. Removal of tape and dressings may require adhesive remover solutions, or an alcohol pad may accomplish the same purpose. Securement devices such as the StatLock require the use of a skin protectant (e.g., Skin-Prep) before applying the device. The protectant prevents skin tearing when the device is removed.

Vein and Catheter Selection

Vein and catheter selection are of highest importance in older adults. Choose insertion sites carefully after considering the patient's skin integrity, vein condition, and functional ability. The general principle of starting with the most distal sites usually indicates use of hand veins. *However, avoid fragile skin and small, tortuous veins on the back of the hand (dorsum); select the initial IV site higher on the arm.*

Venous distention must be accomplished with a flat tourniquet; however, the veins may require longer to adequately distend. Allowing a tourniquet to remain in place for extended periods causes an overfilling of the vein and can result in a hematoma when the vein is punctured. On extremely fragile skin the tourniquet application can lead to ecchymotic areas or skin tears. Protect the skin by placing a washcloth or the patient's gown between the skin and tourniquet. A tourniquet may not be required in veins that are already distended; however, carefully palpate these veins to determine their condition. Avoid hard, cordlike veins. Blood pressure cuffs can also be used for venous distention. Inflate the cuff and release until the pressure is slightly less than diastolic pressure. Other methods to distend veins include:

- Tapping lightly, but avoiding forceful slapping
- Asking the patient to open and close the fist so the muscles can force blood into the veins, making sure that the hand is relaxed when the venipuncture is attempted
- Placing the extremity lower than the heart
- Applying warm compresses or a heating pad (be careful not to make it too hot) to the entire extremity for 10 to 20 minutes and removing just before making the venipuncture

As with all patients, venipuncture technique requires adequate skin and vein stabilization during the puncture and complete catheter advancement. Veins of an older adult are more likely to roll away from the needle. Low angles of 10 to 15 degrees between the skin and catheter will improve your success with venipuncture.

As soon as the catheter enters the vein, it may be necessary to release the tourniquet. Release of venous pressure from the puncture can lead to ecchymosis. Allowing the tourniquet to remain in place during the complete catheter advancement could increase this problem.

! NURSING SAFETY PRIORITY QSEN
Action Alert

Catheter securement may mean that administration sets are placed out of easy reach of a confused patient. Use flexible netting over the extremity to help prevent the patient from pulling at the dressing or tubing, while allowing easy access to the site. A device such as the I.V. House UltraDressing shown in Fig. 13-16 can also protect the site. Do not use rolled bandages to cover the extremity because they prevent insertion site assessment. Complications may progress to an advanced state before they are noticed.

Choosing a midline catheter or PICC may be best in older patients with poor skin turgor; limited venous sites; or veins that are fragile, tortuous, or hard. These catheters are placed in the upper extremity where venous distention techniques can be used. Inserting nontunneled percutaneous central catheters in older adults can be much more challenging. Venous distention for insertion requires the Trendelenburg position and a well-hydrated patient. Fluid volume deficit prevents adequate distention of the subclavian or jugular veins. Patients with conditions such as chronic obstructive pulmonary disease and kyphosis cannot tolerate the Trendelenburg position. Tunneled catheters and implanted ports may be appropriate after considering the surgical techniques required to insert these catheters.

Cardiac and Renal Changes

Because of changes in cardiac and renal status in older adults, the accuracy of infusion volume and flow rate measurements is

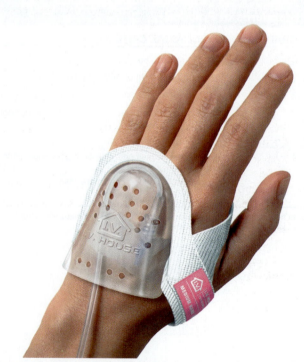

FIG. 13-16 I.V. House UltraDressing IV site protector, a safety device used for IV site protection, guards the integrity of the older adult's skin while helping secure the site. (Courtesy I.V. House, Hazelwood, MO.)

very important in the older adult. The primary health care provider's prescription for infusion therapy should be assessed for appropriateness for the patient's condition. Older adults are very prone to fluid overload and resulting heart failure. Electronic controlling devices may be required to ensure the necessary accuracy. Signs and symptoms of fluid overload are described in Chapter 11.

When fluid restrictions are required, medications could be diluted in small quantities and delivered using a syringe pump or a manual IV push. Consult with a pharmacist to determine the smallest amount of diluent required. This alternative may allow the patient to have more fluid to drink. Serum sodium levels should be considered when normal saline is routinely used for dilution in patients with hypertension or cardiac problems.

CLINICAL JUDGMENT CHALLENGE 13-2

Patient-Centered Care; Teamwork and Collaboration; Informatics QSEN

A 79-year-old obese woman with diabetes is transferred from the hospital to the skilled nursing facility (SNF) where you work as a charge nurse. The resident is being managed with IV cefoxitin 2 g IV piggyback (IVPB) every 8 hours for osteomyelitis resulting from an infected diabetic foot ulcer. On review of her admission orders, you note that she has a newly inserted intermittent saline lock in her right forearm and is prescribed to receive the antibiotic for 4 more weeks.

1. The SNF policy for administration of drugs prescribed every 8 hours is a 6 PM–2 AM–10 AM schedule. Would you schedule her antibiotic at these times? Why or why not?
2. Two days later as you are planning to end your shift, the resident reports that her IV site seems red and swollen. Which action will you take at this time? What will you document on the resident's electronic health record?
3. Is a peripheral vascular access device (VAD) the best choice for this resident? Why or why not? With whom will you or the oncoming nurse collaborate to make this decision? What does the evidence say about the type of VAD that would be best to meet this resident's needs? Where would you go to find the answer to this clinical question?
4. Using the SBAR technique, what will you report to the oncoming nurse about the resident's IV complications?

An increasing number of patients with chronic illness require repeated and frequent IV therapies. Many of these patients are vein depleted and need vein preservation. Subcutaneous and intraosseous routes have demonstrated effectiveness in emergency resuscitation. These procedures may also be beneficial for routine infusion of isotonic, nonirritant, nonvesicant solutions in patients with chronic illness and vein depletion (Benson, 2015).

Specific therapies requiring infusion into arteries and peritoneal, epidural, and intrathecal space are also available. These therapies are most commonly used to administer chemotherapy, lytic therapy, or pain medication.

SUBCUTANEOUS INFUSION THERAPY

Subcutaneous infusion therapy has been used for a variety of drug infusions. Most commonly it is used for administration of pain medications and insulin therapy. It is beneficial for palliative care patients who cannot tolerate oral medications, when IM injections are too painful, or when vascular access is not available or is too difficult to obtain.

Hypodermoclysis or "clysis" involves the slow infusion of isotonic fluids into the patient's subcutaneous tissue. Although common in the early twentieth to mid-twentieth century, this method had not been widely used again until the 1990s. The growth of geriatric and palliative health care has helped spur the use of this method of infusion therapy for selected patients and the emergent biologics.

Hypodermoclysis can be used for short-term fluid volume replacement. The patient must have sufficient sites of intact skin without infection, inflammation, bruising, scarring, or edema. The most common sites are the front and sides of the thighs and hips, the upper abdomen, and the area under the clavicle. Unlike IV therapy, the upper extremities should not be used because fluid is absorbed more readily from sites with larger stores of adipose tissue. Hypodermoclysis is not appropriate for emergency resuscitations and should not be used if the fluid replacement needs (Smith, 2014).

Hyaluronidase may be prescribed by the primary health care provider and is mixed with each liter of infusion fluid. This substance is an enzyme that improves the absorption of the infusion from the subcutaneous tissue.

A small-gauge (25 to 27) winged infusion or "butterfly" needle, a small-gauge short peripheral catheter, or an infusion set specially designed for subcutaneous infusion can be chosen. The subcutaneous infusion sets have a small needle extending at a right angle from a flat disk that helps stabilize the needle.

When choosing the infusion site, consider the patient's level of activity. The area under the clavicle or the abdomen prevents difficulty with ambulation. Clip excess hair in the area and clean the chosen site with the antiseptic solution, preferably 2% chlorhexidine gluconate in 70% isopropyl alcohol to prevent infection (Smith, 2014). Prime the infusion tubing and the attached subcutaneous infusion set or winged needle. Gently pinch an area of about 2 inches (5 cm) and insert the needle using sterile technique. After securing the needle, cover the site with a transparent dressing. Flow rates for hydration fluids begin at 30 mL/hr. After 1 hour the rate can be increased if the patient has experienced no discomfort. The maximum rate is usually 2 mL/min or 120 mL/hr. Assess the site every 4 hours while in a hospital setting and at least twice daily while at home. Redness, warmth, leakage, bruising, swelling, and reports of pain indicate tissue irritation and possible impaired tissue integrity. If these symptoms occur, remove the infusion needle. Rotate the site at least once a week. More frequent rotation may be needed, depending on TISSUE INTEGRITY (INS, 2016).

Other complications include pooling of the fluid at the insertion site and an uneven fluid drip rate. Both of these problems may be resolved by restarting the infusion in another location. An infusion pump may also be used. Small ambulatory infusion pumps can be used to allow for greater mobility.

INTRAOSSEOUS INFUSION THERAPY

Intraosseous (IO) therapy allows access to the rich vascular network in the red marrow of bones. Although IO has previously been regarded as a pediatric procedure, it is now considered acceptable for use in adults. Victims of trauma, burns, cardiac arrest, diabetic ketoacidosis, and other life-threatening conditions benefit from this therapy because often clinicians cannot access these patients' vascular systems for traditional IV therapy (Benson, 2015). IO catheters may be established in the prehospital setting when IV access cannot be readily obtained in an emergency.

Absorption rates of large-volume parenteral (LVP) infusions and drugs administered via the IO route are similar to those achieved with peripheral or central venous administration. The IO route should be used only during the immediate period of resuscitation and should not be used longer than 24 hours (Benson, 2015). After establishing access, efforts should continue to obtain IV access as well.

There are few contraindications for IO infusion. The only absolute contraindication is fracture in the bone to be used as a site. Conditions such as severe osteoporosis, osteogenesis imperfecta, or other conditions that increase the risk for fracture with insertion of the IO needle and skin infection over the site may also be contraindications for some patients. Repeated attempts to access the same site should be avoided (Anson et al., 2015).

Any needle could be used to provide therapy and access the medullary space (marrow). However, 15- or 16-gauge needles specifically designed for IO therapy are preferred. New technology using a battery-powered drill has improved the ease of IO insertion. A number of sites can be used, including the proximal tibia (tibial tuberosity), distal femur, medial malleolus (inner ankle), proximal humerus, and iliac crest. The proximal tibia is the most common site accessed for IO therapy (Fig. 13-17).

If IV access cannot be obtained within the first few minutes of resuscitation procedures, IO therapy may be attempted. The leg is restrained, and the site is cleaned with an antiseptic agent such as chlorhexidine. After successful insertion the needle must be secured to prevent movement out of the bone. The same doses of fluids and medications can be infused by IO therapy as IV. An infusion pump may be used for rapid flow rates.

During the procedure most patients rate the pain as a 2 or 3 on a scale of 0 to 10. Lidocaine 1% is used to anesthetize the skin, the subcutaneous tissue, and the periosteum to promote comfort. Pain is also reported during the initial infusion. This may be reduced by injecting 0.5 mg/kg of preservative-free lidocaine through the IO port before initiating the infusion (Phillips & Gorski, 2014).

Improper needle placement with infiltration into the surrounding tissue is the most common complication of IO therapy. An accumulation of fluid under the skin at either the insertion site or on the other side of the limb indicates that the needle either is not far enough in to penetrate the bone marrow or is too far into the limb and has protruded through the other side of the shaft. Needle obstruction occurs when the puncture has been accomplished but flushing has been delayed. This delay may cause the needle to become clotted with bone marrow.

Osteomyelitis is an unusual but serious complication of IO therapy. You can help prevent this with meticulous aseptic technique, hand hygiene, and removal of the catheter as soon as it is no longer needed.

Compartment syndrome is a condition in which increased tissue pressure in a confined anatomic space causes decreased perfusion (peripheral blood flow to the area). The decreased circulation to the area leads to hypoxia and pain in the area. Although the complication is rare in IO therapy, the nurse should monitor the site carefully and alert the primary health care provider promptly if the patient exhibits any signs of decreased circulation to the limb such as coolness, swelling,

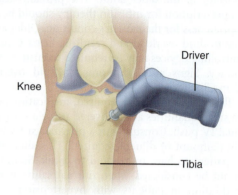

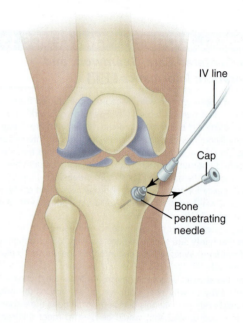

FIG. 13-17 Proximal tibial intraosseous (IO) access.

mottling, or discoloration. Without improvement in perfusion to the limb, the patient could ultimately require amputation of the limb. Nursing assessment and interventions for compartment syndrome are discussed in detail in Chapter 51.

INTRA-ARTERIAL INFUSION THERAPY

Catheters are placed into arteries to obtain repeated arterial blood samples, to monitor various hemodynamic pressures continuously, and to infuse chemotherapy agents or fibrinolytics (intra-arterial infusion therapy). Catheters placed in the radial, brachial, or femoral arteries are used for obtaining blood samples and arterial pressure monitoring. Arterial waveforms and pressures are converted to digital values displayed on attached monitors. Between the catheter and the monitor is a special administration set capable of handling high infusion pressure, a pressurized fluid container, a continuous flush attachment, a three-way stopcock, and a transducer. The transducer is positioned at the level of the patient's atrium and secured to an IV pole to enable correct arterial pressure measurements.

The pulmonary artery is used to monitor pressures in the heart and lungs. This artery is cannulated via the large central venous system and through the right side of the heart. Hemodynamic monitoring and how to interpret these values are described in Chapter 38.

Chemotherapy agents administered arterially allow infusion of a high concentration of drug directly to the tumor site before it is diluted in blood or metabolized by the liver or kidneys. Drug infusion through the same blood supply feeding the tumor optimizes cell destruction at the tumor site while minimizing systemic side effects. The most common arterial sites include the hepatic and celiac arteries for liver tumors, although the carotid artery for tumors of the head, neck, or brain and pelvic arteries for cervical tumors have been used. Arterial catheter insertion can be performed through the skin via a surgical procedure or by an interventional radiologist. Implanted ports are commonly used for extended therapies. For short-term therapy, an external catheter may be used for 3 to 7 days, although the risks for complications increase during dwell time.

! NURSING SAFETY PRIORITY (QSEN)

Critical Rescue

Carefully secure all junctions on the administration sets with Luer-Lok devices. Life-threatening hemorrhage can occur if an accidental disconnection occurs! When an infusion pump is used, be sure that it has a pressure high enough to overcome arterial pressure. Closely monitor the arterial insertion site and affected extremity. Assess the extremity for warmth, sensation, capillary refill, and pulse.

When the carotid artery is involved, perform neurologic assessments. When a femoral catheter is used, apply antiembolic stockings or other measures to prevent deep vein thrombosis. Complications from arterial catheters are similar to those from venous catheters, including infection, bleeding from the insertion site, hemorrhage from a catheter disconnection, catheter migration, infiltration, and catheter lumen or arterial occlusion. Specialized training is required to manage patients with arterial catheters.

INTRAPERITONEAL INFUSION THERAPY

Intraperitoneal (IP) infusion therapy is the administration of chemotherapy agents into the peritoneal cavity. IP therapy is used to treat intra-abdominal malignancies such as ovarian and GI tumors that have moved into the peritoneum after surgery.

Catheters used for IP therapy may be an implanted port for long-term treatment or an external catheter for temporary use. These catheters, including those attached to an implanted port, have large internal lumens with multiple side-holes along the catheter length to allow for delivery of large quantities of fluid. Administration of IP therapy includes three phases: the instillation phase; the dwell phase, usually 1 to 4 hours; and the drain phase. Because this treatment involves the delivery of biohazardous agents, additional competency is required to handle the infusion properly.

The patient should be in the semi-Fowler's position for the infusion. He or she may experience nausea and vomiting caused by increasing pressure on the internal organs from the infusing fluid. Pressure on the diaphragm may cause respiratory distress.

Reducing the flow rate and treatment with antiemetic drugs may be needed. Severe pain may indicate that the catheter has migrated, and an abdominal x-ray is needed to determine its location.

During the dwell and drainage phases, the patient may need assistance in frequently moving from side to side to distribute the fluid evenly around the abdominal cavity. After the fluid has drained, the catheter is flushed with normal saline, although heparinized saline may be used in implanted ports. Catheter lumen occlusion is caused by the formation of fibrous sheaths or fibrin clots or plugs inside the catheter or around the tip.

Exit site infection, indicated by redness, tenderness, and warmth of the tissue around the catheter, can occur. Microbial peritonitis and inflammation of the peritoneal membranes from the invasion of microorganisms are other complications. If peritonitis occurs, the patient may experience a fever and report abdominal pain. Abdominal rigidity and rebound tenderness may be present. This condition is preventable by using strict aseptic technique in the handling of all equipment and infusion supplies. Management includes antimicrobial therapy administered either IV or intraperitoneally.

INTRASPINAL INFUSION THERAPY

The spinal column is covered by three layers: the dura mater, or outermost covering; the arachnoid, or middle layer; and the pia mater, which is closest to the spinal cord. Two spaces used for infusion are the epidural space between the dura mater and vertebrae and the subarachnoid space. The epidural space consists of fat, connective tissue, and blood vessels that protect the spinal cord. Medications infused into the epidural space must diffuse through the dura mater, and there is the possibility that some drug will be absorbed systemically. Intrathecal medications are infused into the subarachnoid space and directly into the cerebral spinal fluid, allowing reduced doses (Prager et al., 2014). Care of patients with these therapies requires competency training and validation.

Postoperative and chronic pain is the primary indication for epidural infusion (see Chapter 4). Opioids administered epidurally slowly diffuse across the dura mater to the dorsal horn of the spinal cord. They lock onto receptors and block pain impulses from ascending to the brain. The patient receives pain relief from the level of the injection caudally (toward the toes). Local anesthetics administered epidurally work on the sensory nerve roots in the epidural space to block pain impulses. The primary health care provider administers the first dose of medication; then, depending on state law, the type of medication, and facility policies, nurses trained in epidural therapy may administer subsequent doses.

Intrathecal infusion of chemotherapy has been used for treating central nervous system (CNS) cancers. The belief was that lower total body doses delivered directly to the tumor would help prevent side effects. Intrathecal infusion has also been used to manage chronic pain and treat spasticity of neurologic diseases such as cerebral palsy, multiple sclerosis, reflex sympathetic dystrophy, and traumatic and anoxic acquired brain injuries (Shamsoddini et al., 2014).

A temporary catheter used for epidural therapy can be a percutaneous catheter that is secured at the site and extends up the back toward the shoulder. These catheters are used for postoperative pain management and usually dwell for only several hours or a few days. Infection and subsequent meningitis and catheter migration are the possible complications.

Epidural catheters used for longer periods include a tunneled catheter and implanted port. Tunneled catheters are tunneled toward the abdomen and have a subcutaneous cuff to act as a barrier to infection. The external catheter exits the skin on the abdomen so it can be reached easily for use by the patient or caregiver. An epidural implanted port is the same design as an IV implanted port and is accessed with the same noncoring needle. The catheter extends from the lumbar puncture site to the port pocket and is located over a bony prominence on the abdomen through a subcutaneous tunnel. Surgically implanted pumps can also be used to deliver epidural and intrathecal infusion.

Using sterile technique, an intraspinal catheter usually is inserted in the lumbar region. The external part of a temporary epidural catheter is laid along the back toward the head and usually extends over the shoulder. The entire catheter length is taped for added security. Dressings are usually not routinely changed because they are used only for short periods. If bleeding or fluid leakage requires dressing removal, use extreme care to prevent dislodging the catheter.

For a tunneled catheter or implanted port, the entire subcutaneous tunnel and port pocket should be assessed frequently. Measurement of an external catheter segment could help identify catheter migration.

An in-line filter is used on all intraspinal infusions to block the infusion of particulate matter. Medications commonly contain preservatives such as alcohol, phenols, or sulfites; however, these are toxic to the CNS. All medications used for intraspinal infusion must be free of preservatives. Alcohol and products containing alcohol should not be applied to the insertion site because the solution could track along the catheter and cause nerve damage. Povidone-iodine solutions are preferred for skin antisepsis before insertion and during catheter dwell, including tunneled catheter exit sites and implanted port pockets.

Complications from epidural and intrathecal infusion can be caused by the type of medication being infused or can be related to the catheter. It is important to know the specific location of the intraspinal catheter because the doses of medications are quite different. When used for pain management, doses are usually 10 times greater for epidural than for intrathecal infusion. Assess the patient for response to the drugs being given, level of alertness, respiratory status, and itching.

Catheter-related complications include infection, bleeding, leakage of cerebrospinal fluid (CSF), occlusion of the catheter lumen, and catheter migration. It is important to be aware of coagulopathy and timing of anticoagulant therapy when epidural catheters are inserted. An epidural hematoma can cause neurologic damage if not corrected promptly. Infection in the patient receiving either epidural or intrathecal therapy could be the result of a lack of asepsis when handling the medication or during the administration. Evidence of local infection such as redness or swelling at the catheter exit site may be present. The patient may also exhibit neurologic and systemic signs of infection (e.g., meningitis) such as headache, stiff neck, or temperature higher than 101° F (38.3° C). Report any neurologic change to the primary health care provider immediately!

GET READY FOR THE NCLEX® EXAMINATION!

KEY POINTS

Review these Key Points for each NCLEX Examination Client Needs Category.

Safe and Effective Care Environment

- Check infusion administration prescriptions for accuracy and completeness before implementing them. **QSEN: Safety**
- Prevent infusion administration errors by using smart pumps and other emerging technology-based safety infusion systems; these devices do not replace careful monitoring and assessment of the patient receiving infusion therapy. **QSEN: Informatics**
- Devices engineered with safety mechanisms are required by the Occupational Safety and Health Administration (OSHA) to prevent staff injuries from needles, thus preventing blood-borne pathogen hazards. **QSEN: Safety**
- Use the evidence-based catheter-related bloodstream infection (CRBSI) prevention bundle during insertion and care of patients who have central lines, including using a checklist during insertion, hand hygiene, maximal barrier precautions, and chlorhexidine for skin disinfection (see Table 13-2). **QSEN: Evidence-Based Practice**

Health Promotion and Maintenance

- Older adults present special challenges when infusion therapy is used; physiologic changes of TISSUE INTEGRITY and cardiac/renal systems must be considered.

- Use small IV catheters for older adults and insert using a 10- to 15-degree angle to prevent rolling of the vein. **QSEN: Patient-Centered Care**
- Teach patients and their families about the patient's infusion therapy, including purpose, type, and safety precautions.

Physiological Integrity

- Infusion therapy is the delivery of parenteral medications and fluids through a wide variety of catheters and locations.
- Infusion therapy is used for establishing FLUID AND ELECTROLYTE BALANCE, achieving optimum nutrition, maintaining hemostasis, and treating or preventing illnesses with medications.
- Vascular access devices (VADs) are catheters that are used to deliver fluids and electrolytes and medications into the intravascular space.
- Common types of VADs include short peripheral catheters, midline catheters, peripherally inserted central catheters (PICCs), nontunneled percutaneous and tunneled central catheters, implanted ports, and hemodialysis catheters.
- Use best practice for placement of short peripheral VADs, including avoiding the small veins of the hands (see Chart 13-1). **QSEN: Evidence-Based Practice**
- Document care for the patient receiving IV therapy, including the type of VAD inserted. **QSEN: Informatics**

- The type of VAD that is used depends on the reason for infusion therapy, the patient's condition, and the length of therapy. **Clinical Judgment**
- Choose the appropriate peripheral catheter gauge size of the VAD, depending on its purpose (see Table 13-1).
- PICCs, tunneled central catheters, and implanted ports are commonly used for long-term infusion therapy.
- Infusion controllers and pumps are electronic devices used to regulate the flow of infusion fluids and medications, but be sure to monitor the infusion rate.
- Nursing care for patients receiving all types of infusion therapy includes using sterile technique when starting the therapy and when changing components of the infusion system, changing and securing the site dressing, and assessing the site for local complications (see Table 13-3). **QSEN: Evidence-Based Practice**
- Assess and document the presence of phlebitis using the INS Phlebitis Scale (see Table 13-6). **QSEN: Evidence-Based Practice**
- Use normal saline to flush IV catheters on a periodic basis per agency policy.
- Assess, prevent, and manage systemic complications related to IV therapy as outlined in Table 13-4. **Clinical Judgment**

- Assess, prevent, and manage complications during the course of central IV therapy as listed in Table 13-5. **Clinical Judgment**
- Subcutaneous therapy of fluids (hypodermoclysis) involves a slow infusion for a short time; the thighs, hips, and abdomen are commonly used.
- Intraosseous infusion therapy allows fluids and medications to be absorbed by the rich vascular network of the bones; it is used for both children and adults, particularly in emergency situations.
- Arterial therapy is used primarily for the administration of chemotherapy agents directly into a tumor site; the liver is the most common arterial site for this purpose.
- Intraperitoneal therapy is used for chemotherapy agent administration into the peritoneal cavity, especially for ovarian and gastrointestinal tumors that have metastasized into the peritoneum.
- Epidural and intrathecal administration of medications are the common uses for intraspinal infusion. Epidural infusions are usually for pain management; intrathecal infusions are usually chemotherapy agents used for cancers that cross the blood-brain barrier into the central nervous system.

SELECTED BIBLIOGRAPHY

Anson, J. A., Sinz, E. H., & Swick, J. T. (2015). The versatility of intraosseous vascular access in perioperative medicine: A case series. *Journal of Clinical Anesthesia, 27*(1), 63–67.

Arbique, D., Bordelon, M., Dragoo, R., & Huckaby, S. (2014). Ultrasound-guided access for peripheral intravenous therapy. *Med-Surg Matters, 23*(3), 1–15.

Benson, G. (2015). Intraosseous access to the circulatory system: An under-appreciated option for rapid access. *Journal of Perioperative Practice, 25*(7/8), 140–143.

Boon, K. L., & Babu, S. B. (2013). Dislodgement of a power-injectable peripherally inserted central catheter after power injection: A case report. *Journal of the Association for Vascular Access, 18*(1), 27–29.

Bowen, M. E., Mone, M. C., Nelson, E. W., & Scaife, C. L. (2014). Image-guided placement of long-term central venous catheters reduces complications and cost. *American Journal of Surgery, 208*(6), 937–941.

Dumont, C., Getz, O., & Miller, S. (2014). Evaluation of midline vascular access: A descriptive study. *Nursing, 44*(10), 60–66.

Infusion Nurses Society. (2016). Infusion therapy standards of practice. *Journal of Infusion Nursing, 39*(1S), S96.

Kim, H. J., Park, S. H., & Shin, H. Y. (2014). Brachial plexus injury as a complication after nerve block or vessel puncture. *The Korean Journal of Pain, 27*(3), 210–218.

Lee, P. (2015). IV administration: Making a decision. *British Journal of Healthcare Management, July*(Suppl.), 10–15.

McClelland, M. (2014). IV therapies for patients with fluid and electrolyte imbalances. *Med-Surg Matters, 23*(5), 4–8.

Meer, P. F., Reesink, H. W., Panzer, S., Wong, J., Ismay, S., Keller, A., et al. (2014). Should DEHP be eliminated in blood bags? *Vox Sanguinis, 106*(2), 176–195.

O'Grady, N., Alexander, M., Burns, L. A., Dellinger, E. P., Garland, J., Heard, S. O., et al. (2011). *Guidelines for the prevention of intravascular catheter-related infections.* Atlanta: Centers for Disease Control and Prevention.

Owen, K. (2014). The use of 8 cm midlines in community IV therapy. *British Journal of Nursing, 23*, S18–S20.

Phillips, L. D., & Gorski, L. (2014). *Manual of I.V. therapeutics: Evidence-based practice for infusion therapy* (6th ed.). Philadelphia: F.A. Davis.

Prager, J., Deer, T., Levy, R., Bruel, B., Buchser, E., Caraway, D., et al. (2014). Best practices for intrathecal drug delivery for pain. *Neuromodulation, 17*(4), 354–372.

Shamsoddini, A., Amirsalari, S., Hollisaz, M. T., & Rahimnia, A. (2014). Management of spasticity in children with cerebral palsy. *Iranian Journal of Pediatrics, 24*(4), 345–351.

Smith, L. S. (2014). Clinical queries. Hypodermoclysis with older adults. *Nursing, 44*(12), 66.

The Joint Commission. (2015). *National Patient Safety Goals: NPSG.01.03.01 eliminate transfusion errors related to patient misidentification.* www.jointcommmission.org/hap_2015_npsg/.

Waterson, J. (2013). Making smart pumps smarter, making IV therapy safer. *British Journal of Nursing, 22*(S14), 22–27.

Weinstein, S., & Hagle, M. (2014). *Plumer's principles and practice of infusion therapy.* Philadelphia: Lippincott Williams & Wilkins.

Wojnar, D. (2013). Peripherally inserted central catheter: Compliance with evidence-based indications for insertion in an inpatient setting. *Journal of Infusion Nursing, 36*(4), 291–296.

14 | CHAPTER

Care of Preoperative Patients

Cynthia L. Danko and Rebecca M. Patton

e http://evolve.elsevier.com/Iggy/

PRIORITY AND INTERRELATED CONCEPTS

The priority concept for this chapter is SAFETY.

The interrelated concepts for this chapter are:
• TEAMWORK AND INTERPROFESSIONAL COLLABORATION
• ETHICS

LEARNING OUTCOMES

Safe and Effective Care Environment

1. Collaborate with the interprofessional team to coordinate high-quality care for patients in the preoperative setting.
2. Differentiate SAFETY implications associated with the various types and purposes of surgery.
3. Examine risk factors associated with potential threats to patient and personnel SAFETY.
4. Ensure SAFETY by protecting patients from injury, wrong-site surgery, and health care–associated infection during the preoperative period.

Health Promotion and Maintenance

5. Teach patients about preoperative preparations and postsurgical interventions to prevent complications.

Psychosocial Integrity

6. Implement nursing interventions to decrease the psychosocial impact of the preoperative experience.
7. Using principles of ETHICS, respond with advocacy to patient concerns and needs.

Physiological Integrity

8. Apply knowledge of anatomy and physiology to perform a complete preoperative assessment.
9. Implement evidence-based nursing interventions to reduce the risk for preoperative complications.
10. Interpret clinical and laboratory data to assess the patient's response to drugs, anesthesia, and surgery.

Advances in surgical techniques, anesthesia, pharmacology, medical devices, and supportive interventions have greatly benefitted patients undergoing surgery. New interventions and advances in anesthetic agents and techniques have made surgery safer than ever before. Outpatient ambulatory care facilities, known as *ambulatory surgical centers (ASCs)*, are being used for many surgical procedures outside acute care hospitals and account for about two thirds of surgical procedures performed in the United States (American Hospital Association, 2015). Additional factors that have had a positive impact on perioperative care include Population Health Management, Triple Aims, and Value Based Purchasing (Douglas et al., 2016; Hohenberger & Delahanty, 2015; Zhao et al., 2015).

These positive changes affect the role of the perioperative nurse and have an impact on how patient teaching is performed and perioperative care is provided. Each of these initiatives

focuses on health care costs, value-added elements of care and SAFETY, and quality outcomes. However, all changes keep the patient as the central focus of interprofessional care during the surgical experience (Fig. 14-1).

Cost reduction is a driving force for the management of the surgical patient. Shortened stays and ambulatory surgeries are common. Patient histories may be conducted by telephone or online before surgery rather than in person. Some patients may be observed only after surgery and not admitted as an inpatient. In response to the ongoing health care delivery changes and the use of multiple settings, nurses have modified their interventions, remaining focused on patient care before (**preoperative**), during (**intraoperative**), and after (**postoperative**) surgery. Together these time periods are known as the **perioperative** experience.

Patient SAFETY throughout the perioperative period is the number-one priority and requires TEAMWORK AND

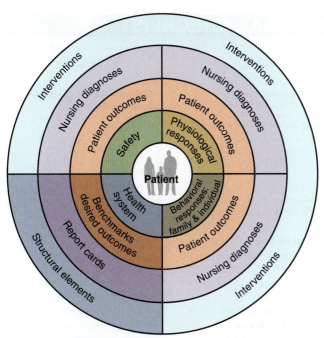

FIG. 14-1 Perioperative patient-focused model. (Redrawn from Rothrock, J. C., & Smith, D. A. [2000]. Selecting the perioperative patient focused model. *AORN Journal, 71*[5], 1030-1037. doi:10.1016/s0001-2092(06)61552-4.)

INTERPROFESSIONAL COLLABORATION. Fig. 14-2 shows an overview of a surgical safety checklist as recommended by the World Health Organization (WHO), The Joint Commission, and the Association of periOperative Registered Nurses (AORN). Quality measures such as wrong-site surgery, patient falls, hospital-acquired pressure injuries, and vascular catheter-associated infections must now be reported to the Centers for Medicare and Medicaid Services (CMS). These data are used for tracking patient outcomes and ensuring patient-centered care and accountability on the part of health care facilities.

Because surgery is invasive and involves exposure to various anesthetic agents and drugs, positioning, and other environmental hazards, complications are common. Some complications are predictable and are considered preventable or "never events." As a result, The Joint Commission (TJC) partnered with other groups and agencies in 2006 and developed a plan for the reduction and eventual elimination of preventable surgical complications known as the Surgical Care Improvement Project (SCIP). Implementation of a set of core compliance measures resulted in a change in the process of managing surgical care. Extensive data about the core measures were collected and publically reported to demonstrate compliance with the process change. Research has demonstrated the effectiveness of the SCIP measures on lowering surgical site infections (SSIs) (Guido et al., 2014). In 2015, data on most measures were no longer collected because the actions associated with this initiative evolved into standard practice for most perioperative departments. Although the SCIP initiative has changed practice in many perioperative settings, additional research is needed to explore the overall impact and the complexity of SSI risks.

The current SCIP foci remain on infection prevention, prevention of serious cardiac events, prevention of venous thromboembolism (VTE) (also known as deep vein thrombosis [DVT]), and maintaining normothermia. Table 14-1 provides

an overview of these core measures as currently addressed in the perioperative environment. The preoperative areas of responsibility for these core measures and their prevention strategies are highlighted in the appropriate areas of this chapter. In addition, some core measures also are discussed in patient care chapters most associated with the complication.

OVERVIEW

The preoperative period begins when the patient is scheduled for surgery and ends at the time of transfer to the surgical suite. As a perioperative nurse, you will function primarily as an advocate. The perioperative nurse collaborates with the other team members to plan and implement an individualized care plan for the surgical patient. The surgical environment demands the use of knowledge, judgment, and skills based on the principles of nursing science. Perioperative nursing places special emphasis on SAFETY, advocacy, and patient education, although ensuring a "culture of safety" is the responsibility of all health care team members.

The Association of periOperative Registered Nurses (AORN) is the specialty organization that provides ETHICS and practice standards and recommended practices for safe care for patients undergoing operative and other invasive procedures. AORN has developed a perioperative-specific vocabulary known as the Perioperative Nursing Data Set (PNDS) that describes nursing interventions and outcomes in the perioperative environment. PNDS is integral to evidence-based practice. The Perioperative Patient Focused Model illuminates the relationship among the patient, the family, and the care provided by the perioperative nurse (see Fig. 14-1). The model is the fundamental basis of the PNDS (AORN, 2011). The graphic represents the patient and the family and the extension of the nursing domains. When available in the electronic health record, PNDS can help the perioperative nurse recognize the link between interventions and outcomes (Behairy, 2015).

The patient's readiness for surgery is critical to the outcome. Preoperative care focuses on preparing the patient for the surgery and ensuring patient SAFETY. This care includes assessing patient knowledge and educational needs. Implement interventions needed before surgery to reduce anxiety and complications and promote patient compliance after surgery. In addition, during the nursing assessment before surgery, validate, clarify, and reinforce information the patient has received from the surgical team. Problems identified may warrant further patient assessment or intervention before the procedure. **As required by The Joint Commission's National Patient SAFETY Goals (NPSGs), communication and collaboration with the surgical team are essential so correct actions are taken to achieve the desired outcome.**

Categories and Purposes of Surgery

Surgical procedures are categorized by the purpose, body location, extent, and degree of urgency. Table 14-2 explains the categories and gives examples of surgical procedures.

Surgical Settings

The term **inpatient** refers to a patient who is admitted to a hospital. The patient may be admitted the day before or, more often, the day of surgery (often termed same-day admission [SDA]), or he or she may already be an inpatient when surgery is needed. The terms **outpatient** and **ambulatory** refer to a

COMPREHENSIVE SURGICAL CHECKLIST

Blue = World Health Organization (WHO)   Green = The Joint Commission - Universal Protocol 2016 National Patient Safety Goals   Teal = Joint Commission and WHO

PREPROCEDURE CHECK-IN	SIGN-IN	TIME-OUT	SIGN-OUT
In Preoperative Ready Area	Before Induction of Anesthesia	Before Skin Incision	Before the Patient Leaves the Operating Room
Patient or patient representative actively confirms with registered nurse (RN):	RN and anesthesia professional confirm:	Initiated by designated team member: All other activities to be suspended (except in case of life-threatening emergency)	RN confirms:
Identity ☐ Yes Procedure and procedure site ☐ Yes Consent(s) ☐ Yes Site marked ☐ Yes ☐ N/A by the person performing the procedure **RN confirms presence of:** History and physical ☐ Yes Preanesthesia assessment ☐ Yes Nursing assessment ☐ Yes Diagnostic and radiologic test results ☐ Yes ☐ N/A Blood products ☐ Yes ☐ N/A Any special equipment, devices, implants ☐ Yes ☐ N/A	Confirmation of the following: identity, procedure, procedure site, and consent(s) ☐ Yes Site marked ☐ Yes ☐ N/A by person performing the procedure Patient allergies ☐ Yes ☐ N/A Pulse oximeter on patient ☐ Yes Difficult airway or aspiration risk ☐ No ☐ Yes (preparation confirmed) Risk of blood loss (> 500 mL) ☐ Yes ☐ N/A # of units available _____ Anesthesia safety check completed ☐ Yes **Briefing:** All members of the team have discussed care plan and addressed concerns ☐ Yes	Introduction of team members ☐ Yes **All:** Confirmation of the following: identity, procedure, incision site, consent(s) ☐ Yes Site is marked and visible ☐ Yes ☐ N/A Fire Risk Assessment and Discussion ☐ Yes (prevention methods implemented) ☐ N/A Relevant images properly labeled and displayed ☐ Yes ☐ N/A Any equipment concerns ☐ Yes ☐ N/A **Anticipated Critical Events** **Surgeon:** States the following: ☐ Critical or nonroutine steps ☐ Case duration ☐ Anticipated blood loss **Anesthesia professional:** Antibiotic prophylaxis within 1 hour before incision ☐ Yes ☐ N/A Additional concerns ☐ Yes ☐ N/A **Scrub person and RN circulator:** Sterilization indicators confirmed ☐ Yes Additional concerns ☐ Yes ☐ N/A **RN:** Documented completion of time out ☐ Yes	Name of operative procedure: _____ Completion of sponge, sharp, and instrument counts ☐ Yes ☐ N/A Specimens identified and labeled ☐ Yes ☐ N/A Equipment problems to be addressed ☐ Yes ☐ N/A Discussion of Wound Classification ☐ Yes **To all team members:** What are the key concerns for recovery and management of this patient? _____ _____ _____ _____ **Debriefing with all team members:** Opportunity for discussion of – team performance – key events – any permanent changes in the preference card June 2016

Include in Preprocedure check-in as per institutional custom:
Beta blocker medication given
☐ Yes ☐ N/A
Venous thromboembolism prophylaxis ordered
☐ Yes ☐ N/A
Normothermia measures
☐ Yes ☐ N/A

The Joint Commission does not stipulate which team member initiates any section of the checklist except for site marking. The Joint Commission also does not stipulate where these activities occur. See the Universal Protocol for details on the Joint Commission requirements.

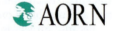

FIG. 14-2 Comprehensive surgical checklist. (Created in collaboration with AORN Perioperative Nursing Specialist Robin Chard, PhD, RN, CNOR, AORN; President Charlotte Guglielmi, RN, BSN, MA, CNOR; contributors to the WHO Surgical Safety Checklist, including Atul Gawande, MD, MPH; and representatives from The Joint Commission.)

patient who goes to the surgical area the day of the surgery and returns home on the same day (i.e., *same-day surgery [SDS]*). Hospital-based ambulatory surgical centers, freestanding surgical centers, physicians' offices, and ambulatory care centers are common. Regardless of the surgical setting, patient SAFETY, teamwork and interprofessional collaboration, and use of professional ETHICS remain priorities.

The advantages of outpatient surgery centers include cost-effective care, service-oriented processes, and a high degree of patient satisfaction. The complexity of procedures being performed in outpatient surgery centers (e.g., laparoscopic cholecystectomy, total knee replacements) places more responsibility on the patient and family, especially for care after surgery. Often a case manager is needed to coordinate post-discharge care for the patient to ensure follow-up treatments and avoid postprocedure hospital admission.

❖ INTERPROFESSIONAL COLLABORATIVE CARE
◆ Assessment: Noticing

The surgical patient assessment begins in the preoperative phase and continues throughout the perioperative experience.

Using a patient-centered approach focuses the assessment on the patient's physical, psychosocial, and spiritual needs. The assessment process is key to identifying potential patient problems, planning care, and forecasting potential outcomes.

History. Data collection about the patient before surgery begins in various settings (e.g., the surgeon's office, the preadmission or admission office, the inpatient unit, the telephone, the Internet). Completing an assessment and gathering data should take place in a private setting to ensure that the patient's confidentiality is protected. Privacy increases the patient's comfort with the interview process and may help reduce the stress associated with the surgery and anesthesia.

Essential data elements include:
- Age
- Use of tobacco, alcohol, or illicit substances, including marijuana
- Current drugs (prescribed and over-the-counter)
- Use of complementary or alternative practices such as herbal therapies, folk remedies, or acupuncture
- Medical history
- Prior surgical procedures and how these were tolerated

TABLE 14-1 Surgical Care Improvement Project (SCIP) Core Measure Overview

CORE MEASURE IDENTIFICATION	MEASUREMENT NAME/DESCRIPTION
SCIP Infection-1 (SCIP Inf-1)	*Prophylactic Antibiotic Received Within One Hour Prior to Surgical Incision* The purpose is to use short-duration antibiotics to establish bactericidal blood and tissue levels by the time the surgical incision is made.
SCIP Infection-2 (SCIP Inf-2)*	*Prophylactic Antibiotic Selection for Surgical Patients* The purpose is to ensure that prophylactic antibiotics are used for patients who are at increased risk for surgical site infections. The guidelines for risk and for the exact antibiotic to be used are specific to each type of surgical procedure and follow evidence-based published recommendations.
SCIP Infection-3 (SCIP Inf-3)*	*Prophylactic Antibiotics Discontinued Within 24 Hours After Surgery End Time* The purpose is to ensure that prophylactic antibiotic therapy provides benefit without risk. Prolonged prophylactic antibiotic therapy has not been shown to increase benefit and is known to increase the risk for *C. difficile* infection and the development of microorganisms that are resistant to antimicrobial drugs.
SCIP Infection-4 (SCIP Inf-4)†	*Cardiac Surgery Patients With Controlled 6 AM Postoperative Blood Glucose* (Applies to cardiac surgery patients only) The purpose is to avoid hyperglycemia (which is defined as blood glucose levels above 200 mg/dL and is associated with increased complications and mortality) in cardiac surgery patients, especially patients undergoing coronary artery bypass graft surgery and patients with diabetes who are having cardiac surgery.
SCIP Infection-6 (SCIP Inf-6)*	*Surgery Patients With Appropriate Hair Removal* The purpose is to avoid hair-removal procedures, specifically shaving, that cause skin abrasions and increase the risk for surgical site infections. If hair must be removed from the surgical site, removal is performed with electric clippers or chemical depilatories.
SCIP Infection-9 (SCIP Inf-9)	*Urinary Catheter Removed on Postoperative Day 1 (POD 1) or Postoperative Day 2 (POD 2) With Day of Surgery Being Day Zero* The purpose is to avoid urinary catheter–associated urinary tract infections, which increase with longer-duration indwelling catheters. It is unacceptable to have an indwelling urinary catheter in place longer than 48 hours after surgery unless there is a documented specific and medically validated reason for it.
SCIP Infection-10 (SCIP Inf-10)	*Surgery Patients With Perioperative Temperature Management* The purpose is to prevent prolonged hypothermia, which is associated with impaired wound healing, serious cardiac complications, altered drug metabolism, coagulation problems, and a higher incidence of surgical site infections. Temperature must be measured within 15 minutes from the end of anesthesia administration. Intentional hypothermia must be documented.
SCIP CARD-2*	*Surgery Patients on Beta-Blocker Therapy Prior to Arrival Who Received a Beta-Blocker During the Perioperative Period* The purpose is to ensure that patients with specific medical conditions receive beta-blocker therapy before surgery and continue the therapy in the immediate postoperative period. This evidence-based action has resulted in a significant reduction in coronary events, cardiovascular mortality, and overall mortality.
SCIP Venous thromboembolism-1 (SCIP VTE-1)*	*Surgery Patients With Recommended Venous Thromboembolism Prophylaxis Ordered* The purpose is to reduce the complications from postoperative venous thromboembolism (VTE). Surgery is a major risk factor responsible for VTE formation and subsequent pulmonary embolism. Although VTE prophylaxis is effective, it is underused. Specific preoperative and postoperative VTE prophylaxis strategies are recommended on the basis of patient risk, type and duration of surgery, and extent of expected postoperative immobilization.
SCIP Venous thromboembolism-2 (SCIP VTE-2)*	*Surgery Patients Who Received Appropriate Venous Thromboembolism Prophylaxis Within 24 Hours Prior to Surgery to 24 Hours After Surgery* The purpose is to reduce the complications from postoperative venous thromboembolism (VTE), particularly among patients undergoing the types of surgeries in which the risk is highest.

Data from The Joint Commission. (2014). *National Patient Safety Goals.* www.jointcommission.org/surgical_care_improvement_project/.
C. difficile, Clostridium difficile.
*Retired in 2015 by CMS and JC. Initiatives have evolved into standard practice; therefore data measurement and submission to CMS no longer required.
†Retired in 2016 by CMS and JC. Initiatives have evolved into standard practice; therefore data measurement and submission to CMS no longer required.

- Prior experience with anesthesia, pain control, and management of nausea or vomiting
- Autologous or directed blood donations
- Allergies, including sensitivity to latex products
- General health
- Family history
- Type of surgery planned
- Knowledge about and understanding of events during the perioperative period
- Adequacy of the patient's support system

When taking a history, assess the patient for problems that increase the risk for complications during and after surgery. Some of these problems are listed in Table 14-3. The American Society of Anesthesiologists (ASA) created the **ASA Physical Status Classification system** to assess the fitness of patients before surgery (American Society of Anesthesiologists, 2014). See Table 14-4 for definitions of the ASA system. Each surgical patient is assigned a classification by the anesthesia provider to indicate overall physical health or sickness before surgery. The ASA Classification has been associated with

TABLE 14-2   Selected Categories of Surgical Procedures

CATEGORY	DESCRIPTION	CONDITION OR SURGICAL PROCEDURE
Reasons for Surgery		
Diagnostic	Performed to determine the origin and cause of a disorder or the cell type for cancer	Breast biopsy Exploratory laparotomy Arthroscopy
Curative	Performed to resolve a health problem by repairing or removing the cause	Cholecystectomy Appendectomy Hysterectomy
Transplant	Replacing malfunctioning structures	Kidney transplant Heart transplant Liver transplant
Restorative	Performed to improve a patient's functional ability	Total knee replacement Finger reimplantation
Palliative	Performed to relieve symptoms of a disease process but does not cure	Colostomy Nerve root resection Tumor debulking Ileostomy
Cosmetic	Performed primarily to alter or enhance personal appearance	Liposuction Revision of scars Rhinoplasty Blepharoplasty
Urgency of Surgery		
Elective	Planned for correction of a nonacute problem	Cataract removal Hernia repair Hemorrhoidectomy Total joint replacement
Urgent	Requires prompt intervention; may be life threatening if treatment is delayed more than 24-48 hrs	Intestinal obstruction Bladder obstruction Kidney or ureteral stones Bone fracture Eye injury Acute cholecystitis
Emergent	Requires immediate intervention because of life-threatening consequences	Gunshot or stab wound Severe bleeding Abdominal aortic aneurysm Compound fracture Appendectomy
Surgical Approach		
Simple	Only the most overtly affected areas involved in the surgery	Simple/partial mastectomy
Minimally invasive surgery (MIS)	Surgery performed in a body cavity or body area through one or more endoscopes; can correct problems, remove organs, take tissue for biopsy, re-route blood vessels and drainage systems; is a fast-growing and ever-changing type of surgery	Arthroscopy Tubal ligation Hysterectomy Lung lobectomy Coronary artery bypass Cholecystectomy
Radical	Extensive surgery beyond the area obviously involved; is directed at finding a root cause	Radical prostatectomy Radical hysterectomy

patient's risks before surgery and provides a baseline for intraoperative care.

Older patients are at increased risk for complications from both anesthesia and surgery (Deiner et al., 2014). The normal aging process decreases immune system functioning and delays wound healing. The frequency of chronic illness increases in older patients. Gas exchange is more profoundly affected by general anesthetic agents and opioid analgesics. Age-related changes in kidney and liver function may delay the elimination of anesthetic and analgesic agents, increasing the risk for

adverse reactions. See Chart 14-1 for other changes in older adults that may alter the operative response or risk.

Drugs and substance use may affect patient responses to surgery. Tobacco use increases the risk for pulmonary complications because of changes to the lungs, blood vessels, and chest cavity. Alcohol and illicit substance use can alter the patient's responses to anesthesia and pain medication. Withdrawal of alcohol before surgery may lead to delirium tremens. Prescription and over-the-counter drugs may also affect how the patient reacts to the operative experience. Adverse effects can occur with the use of

TABLE 14-3 Selected Factors That Increase the Risk for Surgical Complications

Age
- Older than 65 years

Medications
- Antihypertensives
- Tricyclic antidepressants
- Anticoagulants
- Nonsteroidal anti-inflammatory drugs (NSAIDs)
- Immunosuppressives

Medical History
- Decreased immunity
- Diabetes
- Pulmonary disease
- Cardiac disease
- Hemodynamic instability
- Multi-system disease
- Coagulation defect or disorder
- Anemia
- Dehydration
- Infection
- Hypertension
- Hypotension
- Any chronic disease

Prior Surgical Experiences
- Less-than-optimal emotional reaction
- Anesthesia reactions or complications
- Postoperative complications

Health History
- Malnutrition or obesity
- Drug, tobacco, alcohol, or illicit substance use or abuse
- Altered coping ability
- Herbal use

Family History
- Malignant hyperthermia
- Cancer
- Bleeding disorder
- Anesthesia reactions or complications

Type of Surgical Procedure Planned
- Neck, oral, or facial procedures (airway complications)
- Chest or high abdominal procedures (pulmonary complications)
- Abdominal surgery (paralytic ileus, venous thromboembolism)

some herbs. Thus a thorough assessment and documentation of past and current use of herbs or botanicals is essential.

Medical history is important to obtain because many chronic illnesses increase surgical risks and need to be considered when planning care. For example, a patient with systemic lupus erythematosus may need additional drugs to offset the stress of the surgery. A patient with immunity issues such as rheumatoid arthritis may need special considerations during the positioning process because of decreased movement and mobility. Any infection present requires intervention before surgery, which may include cancellation of the procedure.

Ask the patient specifically about cardiac problems because complications from anesthesia occur more often in patients with cardiac problems (Devereaux & Sessler, 2015). A patient with a history of rheumatic heart disease may be prescribed antibiotics before surgery. Cardiac problems that increase surgical risks include coronary artery disease, angina, myocardial infarction (MI) within 6 months before surgery, heart failure, hypertension, and dysrhythmias. These problems impair the patient's ability to withstand hemodynamic changes and alter the response to anesthesia. The risk for an MI during surgery is higher in patients who have heart problems. Patients with cardiac disease who are prescribed beta-blocking drugs should continue the therapy before surgery and in the immediate postoperative period (Wong & Irwin, 2016).

Pulmonary complications during or after surgery are more likely to occur in older patients, those with chronic respiratory problems, and smokers because of smoking- or age-related lung changes. Increased chest rigidity and loss of lung elasticity reduce anesthetic excretion. Smoking increases the blood level of carboxyhemoglobin (carbon monoxide on oxygen-binding sites of the hemoglobin molecule), which decreases oxygen delivery to organs. Action of cilia in pulmonary mucous

TABLE 14-4 ASA PHYSICAL STATUS CLASSIFICATION SYSTEM

ASA PS CLASSIFICATION	DEFINITION	EXAMPLES, INCLUDING, BUT NOT LIMITED TO:
ASA I	Normal healthy patient	Healthy, nonsmoking, no or minimal alcohol use
ASA II	Patient with mild systemic disease	Mild diseases only without substantive functional limitations; examples include (but not limited to): current smoker, social alcohol drinker, pregnancy, obesity (30 < BMI < 40), well-controlled DM/HTN, mild lung disease
ASA III	Patient with severe systemic disease	Substantive functional limitations; one or more moderate-to-severe diseases; examples include (but not limited to): poorly controlled DM or HTN; COPD; morbid obesity (BMI ≥40); active hepatitis; alcohol dependence or abuse; implanted pacemaker; moderate reduction of ejection fraction; ESRD undergoing regularly scheduled dialysis; premature infant PCA <60 weeks; history (>3 months) of MI, CVA, TIA, or CAD/stents
ASA IV	Patient with severe systemic disease that is a constant threat to life	Examples include (but not limited to): recent (<3 months) MI, CVA, TIA, or CAD/stents, ongoing cardiac ischemia or severe valve dysfunction, severe reduction of ejection fraction, sepsis, DIC, ARD or ESRD not undergoing regularly scheduled dialysis
ASA V	Moribund patient who is not expected to survive without the operation	Examples include (but not limited to): ruptured abdominal/thoracic aneurysm, massive trauma, intracranial bleed with mass effect, ischemic bowel in the face of significant cardiac pathology or multiple organ/system dysfunction
ASA VI	Declared brain-dead patient whose organs are being removed for donor purposes	

ARD, Acute renal dysfunction; *BMI*, body mass index; *CAD*, coronary artery disease; *COPD*, chronic obstructive pulmonary disease; *CVA*, cerebrovascular accident; *DIC*, disseminated intravascular coagulopathy; *DM*, diabetes mellitus; *ESRD*, end-stage renal disease; *HTN*, hypertension; *MI*, myocardial infarction; *PCA*, post-conceptual age; *TIA*, transient ischemic attack.

NOTE: The addition of "E" denotes Emergency surgery. (An emergency is defined as existing when delay in treatment of the patient would lead to a significant increase in the threat to life or body part.) Adopted in 2014 by the American Society of Anesthesiologists (ASA).

CHART 14-1 Nursing Focus on the Older Adult

Age-Related Changes as Surgical Risk Factors

PHYSIOLOGIC CHANGE	NURSING INTERVENTIONS	RATIONALES
Cardiovascular System		
Decreased cardiac output Increased blood pressure	Determine normal activity levels and note when the patient tires.	Knowing limits helps prevent fatigue.
Decreased peripheral circulation	Monitor vital signs, peripheral pulses, and capillary refill.	Having baseline data helps detect deviations.
Respiratory System		
Reduced vital capacity Loss of lung elasticity	Teach coughing and deep-breathing exercises.	Pulmonary exercises help prevent pulmonary complications.
Decreased oxygenation of blood	Monitor respirations and breathing effort.	Having baseline data helps detect deviations.
Renal/Urinary System		
Decreased blood flow to kidneys Reduced ability to excrete waste Decline in glomerular filtration rate	Monitor intake and output. Assess overall hydration. Monitor electrolyte status.	Ongoing assessment helps detect fluid and electrolyte imbalances and decreased renal function.
Nocturia common	Assist frequently with toileting needs, especially at night.	Frequent toileting helps prevent incontinence and falls.
Neurologic System		
Sensory deficits Slower reaction time Cognitive impairment	Orient the patient to the surroundings. Allow extra time for teaching the patient. Keep patient informed of activities before implementation	An individualized preoperative teaching plan is developed based on the patient's orientation and any neurologic deficits.
Decreased ability to adjust to changes in the surroundings	Provide for the patient's safety.	Safety measures help prevent falls and injury.
Musculoskeletal System		
Increased incidence of deformities related to osteoporosis or arthritis	Assess the patient's mobility. Teach turning and positioning. Encourage ambulation.	Interventions help prevent complications of immobility.
	Place on falls precautions, if indicated.	Safety measures help prevent injury.
Skin		
Dry with less subcutaneous fat makes the skin at greater risk for damage; slower skin healing increases risk for infection	Assess the patient's skin before surgery for lesions, bruises, and areas of decreased circulation.	Having baseline data helps detect changes and evaluate interventions.
	Pad bony prominences.	Padding can protect at-risk areas.
	Use pressure-avoiding or pressure-reducing overlays.	Overlays can prevent pressure injury formation by redistributing body weight.
	Avoid applying tape to skin.	Tape removal damages thin skin.
	Teach the patient to change position at least every 2 hours. Use safe patient-handling devices to avoid shearing during patient movement.	Changing position frequently helps prevent reduced blood flow to an area and changes external pressure patterns.

membranes decreases, which leads to retained secretions and predisposes the patient to infection (pneumonia) and atelectasis (collapse of alveoli). Atelectasis reduces gas exchange and causes intolerance of anesthesia. It is also a common problem after general anesthesia.

Chronic lung problems such as asthma, emphysema, and chronic bronchitis also reduce the elasticity of the lungs, which reduces gas exchange. As a result, patients with these problems have reduced tissue oxygenation.

Previous surgical procedures and anesthesia affect the patient's readiness for surgery. Previous experiences, especially with complications, may increase anxiety about the scheduled surgery. Assess the patient's past experiences with anesthesia and all allergies. These data provide information about tolerance of and possible fears about the use of anesthesia. The

family medical history and problems with anesthetics may indicate possible reactions to anesthesia such as malignant hyperthermia (see Chapter 15). This information will be critical for the anesthesia team's plan of care.

An allergy to certain substances alerts you to a possible reaction to anesthetic agents or to substances that are used before or during surgery. For example, povidone-iodine (e.g., Betadine) used for skin cleansing contains the same allergens found in shellfish. Patients who are allergic to shellfish may have an adverse reaction to povidone-iodine. The patient with an allergy to avocados, bananas, strawberries, and other fruits may also have a latex sensitivity or allergy. Patients who have an egg, peanut, or soy allergy may be at risk for a reaction to propofol (Diprivan), which is an anesthetic agent often used in the induction and maintenance of anesthesia, although literature suggests that there is less risk for anaphylaxis to the components of propofol (egg, soy, legumes, peanuts) than previously documented (Mehta & Chehade, 2014). Carefully assess all patients for food allergies during the preoperative phase. Document in the electronic health record and communicate any allergies to all members of the perioperative team.

Blood donation for surgery can be made by the patient (autologous donations) a few weeks before the scheduled surgery date. If blood is needed during or after surgery, an autologous blood transfusion can be given. This practice eliminates transfusion reactions and reduces the risk for acquiring bloodborne disease. Specific patient criteria, which may vary by surgical type and patient's health status, must be met to qualify for autologous transfusion.

A special tag is placed on the blood bag when an autologous blood donation has been made. **The blood donor center gives the patient a matching tag that he or she wears or brings to the surgical area before surgery as required by The Joint Commission's National Patient Safety Goals (NPSGs).** This procedure helps ensure that patients receive only their own donated blood.

Patients may wish to have family and friends donate blood exclusively for their use, if needed. This practice (called *directed blood donation*) is possible only if the blood types are compatible and the donor's blood is acceptable. Directed donation is not practiced in all blood donation centers. When directed blood donations are used, a special tag is attached to the blood bag. This tag notes the names of the patient and the donor and bears the patient's signature.

Ask whether autologous or directed blood donations have been made and document this information in the electronic health record. It is important to know the specific blood collection center where the donation was made and whether the blood has arrived before the patient goes into surgery. The hospital receives and stores the blood units until they are used or are no longer needed. Unused blood is returned to the collection center.

Increased use of "bloodless surgery" and minimally invasive surgery (MIS) provides alternatives for patients with religious or medical restrictions to blood transfusions. (Part of professional ETHICS requires interprofessional team members to honor patient requests based on religious views.) These programs reduce the need for transfusion during and after surgery. Some techniques used are limiting blood samples (the number of samples and the volume of blood drawn per sample) before surgery and stimulating the patient's own red blood cell production with epoetin alpha (e.g., Epogen, Procrit). Supplemental iron, folic acid, vitamin B_{12}, and vitamin C may be prescribed to help red blood cell formation. Newer equipment and surgical techniques cause less blood loss. Such advances include intraoperative cell salvage machines commonly known as *cell savers,* which suction, wash, and filter blood so it can be given back to the patient's body instead of being discarded. One advantage to this is that the patient receives his or her own blood instead of donor blood, so there is no risk of contracting outside diseases. Because the blood is recirculated, there is no limit to the amount of blood that can be given back to the patient. The cell salvage is a cost-effective and safe option for autologous transfusion. Cell salvage is also a viable alternative for patients with religious objections to receiving blood transfusions (Kudela et al., 2015). It is important to assess, monitor, teach, and advocate for the patient during the bloodless surgery process.

Discharge planning is started before surgery. Assess the patient's home environment, self-care capabilities, and support systems and anticipate postoperative needs before surgery. *All patients, regardless of how minor the procedure or how often they have had surgery, should have discharge planning.* Older patients and dependent adults may need transportation referrals to and from the physician's office or the surgical setting. A home care nurse may be needed to monitor recovery and provide instructions. Patients with few support systems may need follow-up care at home. Some patients need a planned direct admission to a rehabilitation facility or center for physical therapy after surgery, especially joint-replacement surgery. Shortened hospital stays require adequate discharge planning to achieve the desired outcomes after surgery.

? NCLEX EXAMINATION CHALLENGE 14-1

Safe and Effective Care Environment

A client was originally scheduled for surgery at noon. The surgeon is delayed, and the surgery has been rescheduled for 3:00 PM. How will the nurse plan to administer the preoperative prophylactic antibiotic?

A. Give at noon as originally prescribed.
B. Cancel orders; preoperative prophylactic antibiotics are given optionally.
C. Adjust the administration time to be given within 1 hour before surgery.
D. Hold the preoperative antibiotic so it can be administered immediately following surgery.

Physical Assessment/Signs and Symptoms. The preoperative patient may be any age, with a health status that varies from well to debilitated. Perform a complete assessment before surgery to obtain baseline data. Use this information to identify current health problems, potential complications related to anesthesia, and risk for complications that may occur after surgery.

Begin the assessment by obtaining a complete set of vital signs. You may need to obtain vital signs several times at different time intervals for accurate baseline values. Previous vital signs from another admission (if available) are helpful to compare with current vital signs. Abnormal vital signs may require postponement of surgery until the problem is treated and the patient's condition is stable. Also assess for anxiety, which could increase blood pressure, pulse, and respiratory rate. Document these findings as part of the overall assessment.

Throughout the assessment focus on problem areas identified from the patient's history and on all body systems affected by the surgical procedure. The older adult (Chart 14-2; see also Chapter 3) or chronically ill patient is at increased risk for complications during and after surgery. The number of serious diseases (morbidity) and death (mortality) during or after surgery is higher in older and chronically ill patients (Deiner et al., 2014; Oresanya et al., 2014).

Report any abnormal assessment findings to the surgeon and to anesthesia personnel, as required by The Joint Commission's NPSGs. In this way, you are a proactive patient advocate exercising professional legal and ETHICAL responsibility and demonstrating critical thinking skills. Often established protocols or care maps identify which interventions are to be performed before surgery.

CHART 14-2   Nursing Focus on the Older Adult

Specific Considerations When Planning Care for the Older Preoperative Patient

- Greater incidence of chronic illness (e.g., hypertension, diabetes, cardiac)
- Greater incidence of malnutrition and dehydration
- More allergies
- Increased abnormal laboratory values (anemia, low albumin level)
- Increased incidence of impaired self-care abilities
- Inadequate support systems
- Decreased ability to withstand the stress of surgery and anesthesia
- Increased risk for cardiopulmonary complications after surgery
- Risk for a change in mental status when admitted (e.g., related to unfamiliar surroundings, change in routine, drugs)
- Increased risk for a fall and resultant injury
- Mobility changes

Cardiovascular status is critical to assess because cardiac problems are associated with many surgery-related deaths. Check the patient for hypertension, which is common, is often undiagnosed, and can affect the response to surgery. Cardiac assessment includes listening to heart sounds for rate, regularity, and abnormalities. Ask whether the patient has ever had a venous thromboembolism (VTE). Examine the patient's hands and feet for temperature, color, peripheral pulses, capillary refill, and edema. Report any problems (e.g., absent peripheral pulses, pitting edema, cardiac symptoms, chest pain, shortness of breath, and dyspnea) to the surgeon for further assessment and evaluation. (Cardiac assessment is discussed in Chapter 33.)

Respiratory status considers age, smoking history (including exposure to secondhand smoke), and any chronic illness. Obese patients may have undiagnosed respiratory problems such as obstructive sleep apnea (OSA), which can lead to complications from anesthesia (Ramly et al., 2015; Shah et al., 2016). Observe the patient's posture; respiratory rate, rhythm, and depth; overall respiratory effort; and lung expansion. Document any clubbing of the fingertips (swelling at the base of the nail beds caused by a chronic lack of oxygen) or cyanosis. Auscultate the lungs to assess for any abnormal breath sounds (crackles, wheezes, rubs). (More information on respiratory assessment is found in Chapter 27.)

Kidney function affects the excretion of drugs and waste products, including anesthetic and analgesic agents. If kidney function is reduced, fluid and electrolyte balance can be altered, especially in older patients. Ask about problems such as urinary frequency, **dysuria** (painful urination), **nocturia** (awakening during nighttime sleep because of a need to void), difficulty starting urine flow, and **oliguria** (scant amount of urine). Ask the patient about the appearance and odor of the urine. Assess the patient's usual fluid intake and degree of continence. If the patient has kidney or urinary problems, consult with the surgeon about further workup. (Kidney/urinary assessment is discussed further in Chapter 65.)

Kidney impairment with a reduced glomerular filtration rate decreases the excretion of drugs and anesthetic agents. As a result, drug responses may be prolonged. Scopolamine (Buscopan ✦), morphine, other opioids, benzodiazepines, and barbiturates often cause confusion, disorientation, apprehension,

and restlessness when given to patients with decreased kidney function.

Neurologic status includes the patient's overall mental status, level of consciousness, orientation, and ability to follow commands. This information is needed before planning preoperative teaching and care after surgery. A problem in any of these areas affects the type of care needed during the surgical experience. Determine the patient's baseline neurologic status to be able to identify changes that may occur later. Also assess for any motor or sensory deficits. (See Chapter 41 for complete nervous system assessment.) **The Joint Commission's NPSGs require that you ensure patient SAFETY by assessing the patient's risk for falling, especially older patients.** Evaluate factors such as mental status, muscle strength, steadiness of gait, and sense of independence to determine the patient's risk. Document the patient's ability to ambulate and the steadiness of gait as baseline data.

The usual neurologic status of a mentally impaired patient may be difficult to assess. Psychiatric issues may be overlooked in the perioperative environment; but an assessment of coping skills, a mental health history, and recent behavioral changes is the minimum standard of care for patients at risk or patients with previously diagnosed mental illness. The patient who has been independent and oriented at home may become disoriented in the hospital setting. Family members can often provide information about what the patient was like at home.

Musculoskeletal status problems may interfere with positioning during and after surgery. For example, patients with arthritis may be able to assume surgical positions but have discomfort after surgery from prolonged joint immobilization. Other anatomic features such as the shape and length of the neck and the shape of the chest cavity may interfere with respiratory and cardiac function or require special positioning during surgery.

! NURSING SAFETY PRIORITY **QSEN**
Action Alert

Ask about a history of joint replacement and document the exact location of any prostheses. Communicate this information to operating room personnel to ensure that electrocautery pads, which could cause an electrical burn, are not placed on or near the area of the prosthesis. Other areas to avoid when placing electrocautery pads include on or near bony prominences, pacemakers, scar tissue, hair, tattoos, weight-bearing surfaces, pressure points, and metal piercings.

Nutrition status, especially malnutrition and obesity, can increase surgical risk. Surgery increases metabolic rate and depletes potassium and vitamins C and B, all of which are needed for wound healing and blood clotting. In poorly nourished patients decreased serum protein levels may slow recovery. Negative nitrogen balance may result from depleted protein stores. This problem increases the risk for skin breakdown, delayed wound healing, possible dehiscence or evisceration (see Chapter 16), dehydration, and sepsis.

Some older patients may have poor nutrition because of chronic illness, diuretic or laxative use, poor dietary planning or habits, anorexia, lack of motivation, or financial limitations (Touhy & Jett, 2015). Indications of poor fluid or nutrition status include:

- Brittle nails
- Muscle wasting

- Dry or flaky skin, decreased skin turgor, and hair changes (e.g., dull, sparse, dry)
- Orthostatic (postural) hypotension
- Decreased serum protein levels and abnormal serum electrolyte values

The obese patient is often malnourished because of an imbalanced diet. Obesity increases the risk for poor wound healing because of excessive *adipose* (fatty) tissue. Fatty tissue has few blood vessels, little collagen, and decreased nutrients, all of which are needed for wound healing. Obesity stresses the heart and reduces the lung volumes, which can affect the surgery and recovery. Obese patients may need larger drug doses and may retain them longer after surgery.

Skin assessment is an important component of the preoperative assessment. Assess skin color, turgor, and temperature; signs of breakdown; open sores; or areas that may be exposed to excessive pressure during the surgical procedure. Be attentive to body piercing, body modifications, and tattoos. Document these findings and communicate this information to members of the interprofessional perioperative team so precautions can be taken to prevent injury during surgery. Keeping patients safe and free from skin injury caused by pressure injuries, surgical burns, or bruises is the responsibility of all members of the team. Many insurers no longer reimburse hospitals for care provided to patients who develop skin breakdown or pressure injuries during the perioperative period.

Psychosocial Assessment. Most patients have some degree of anxiety or fear before surgery. The extent of these reactions varies according to the type of surgery, the perceived effects of the surgery and its potential outcome, and the patient's personality. Surgery may be seen as a threat to life, body image, self-esteem, self-concept, or lifestyle. Patients may fear death, pain, helplessness, a change in role or work status, a diagnosis of life-threatening conditions, possible disabling or crippling effects, or the unknown.

Anxiety or fear affects the patient's ability to learn, cope, and cooperate with teaching and operative procedures. Anxiety may also influence the amount and type of anesthetic needed and may slow recovery. In some cases, severe preoperative anxiety can increase the degree of pain after surgery. Be aware of potential anxiety when interviewing the patient and planning teaching.

Perform a psychosocial assessment to determine the patient's level of anxiety, coping ability, and support systems. Provide information and support to the patient and family as needed. Identify coping mechanisms used by the patient under similar situations or in the past when confronted with a stressful situation. Ask open-ended questions about the patient's feelings about the entire surgical experience. Factors that influence coping include age, previous surgical or sick-role experiences, and physical discomfort. Indications of anxiety include anger, crying, restlessness, profuse sweating, increased pulse rate, palpitations, sleeplessness, diarrhea, and urinary frequency.

Laboratory Assessment. Laboratory tests before surgery provide baseline data about the patient's health and help predict potential complications. The patient scheduled for surgery in an ambulatory surgical center or admitted to the hospital on the morning of or day before surgery may have preadmission testing (PAT) performed from 24 hours to 28 days before the scheduled surgery. These test results are usually valid unless there has been a change in the patient's condition that warrants repeated testing or the patient is taking drugs that can alter laboratory values (e.g., warfarin [Coumadin], aspirin, diuretics). Some facilities have time limits for tests, especially pregnancy testing or any other test results that would require altering the surgical plan.

The choice of laboratory testing before surgery varies among facilities and depends on the patient's age, medical history, and type of anesthesia planned (Rothrock, 2014). The most common tests include:

- Urinalysis
- Blood type and screen
- Complete blood count or hemoglobin level and hematocrit
- Clotting studies (prothrombin time [PT], international normalized ratio [INR], activated partial thromboplastin time [aPTT], platelet count)
- Electrolyte levels
- Serum creatinine and blood urea nitrogen levels
- Depending on a female patient's age and the nature of the planned procedure, a pregnancy test may also be needed

Urinalysis is performed to assess for abnormal substances in the urine such as protein, glucose, blood, and bacteria. If kidney disease is suspected or if the patient is older, the physician may request other tests to determine the type and degree of disease present.

Report electrolyte imbalances or other abnormal laboratory results to the anesthesia team and the surgeon before surgery begins. **Hypokalemia** (decreased serum potassium level) increases the risk for toxicity if the patient is taking digoxin, slows recovery from anesthesia, and increases cardiac irritability. **Hyperkalemia** (increased serum potassium level) increases the risk for dysrhythmias, especially with the use of anesthesia.

> **! NURSING SAFETY PRIORITY** **QSEN**
>
> ***Critical Rescue***
>
> Review laboratory findings to recognize any potassium imbalance. If either hypokalemia or hyperkalemia is present, respond by communicating this information to the surgical team so the imbalance can be corrected before surgery.

Other studies may be needed, depending on the patient's medical history. For example, baseline arterial blood gas (ABG) values are assessed before surgery for patients with chronic pulmonary problems. Laboratory values and their significance are found in Chapters 11, 12, 39, and 65.

Imaging Assessment. A chest x-ray may be requested before surgery. Healthy adults are often not required to have a chest x-ray. A chest x-ray determines the size and shape of the heart, lungs, and major vessels and provides evidence of the presence of pneumonia or tuberculosis. It also provides baseline data in case of complications. Abnormal x-ray findings alert the surgeon to potential cardiac or pulmonary complications. Heart failure, cardiomyopathy, pneumonia, or infiltrates may cause cancellation or delay of elective surgery. For emergency surgery, x-ray results help the anesthesia provider select anesthesia type.

Other imaging studies are based on patient need, medical history, and the nature of the surgical procedure. For example, a patient with back pain may have computed tomography (CT) scans or magnetic resonance imaging (MRI) examinations before spinal surgery to identify the exact location of the problem.

CHART 14-3   Focused Assessment

The Preoperative Patient

As part of the cardiopulmonary assessment, take and record vital signs; report:
- Hypotension or hypertension
- Heart rate less than 60 or more than 120 beats/min
- Irregular heart rate
- Chest pain
- Shortness of breath or dyspnea
- Tachypnea
- Pulse oximetry reading of less than 94%

Assess for and report any signs or symptoms of infection, including:
- Fever
- Purulent sputum
- Dysuria or cloudy, foul-smelling urine
- Any red, swollen, draining IV or wound site
- Increased white blood cell count

Assess for and report signs or symptoms that could contraindicate surgery, including:
- Increased prothrombin time (PT), international normalized ratio (INR), or activated partial thromboplastin time (aPTT)
- Hypokalemia or hyperkalemia
- Patient report of possible pregnancy or positive pregnancy test

Assess for and report other clinical conditions that may need further evaluation before proceeding with the surgical plans, including:
- Change in mental status
- Vomiting
- Rash
- Recent administration of an anticoagulant drug

Assess and determine functionality of any implantable cardiovascular devices:
- Pacemaker
- Implantable cardioverter defibrillators (ICDs)

Evaluate patient and family past medical history that may need further evaluation:
- History of ischemic heart disease and interventions
- History of cerebrovascular disease and interventions

NCLEX EXAMINATION CHALLENGE 14-2

Safe and Effective Care Environment

Which assessment data finding for a client scheduled for total knee replacement surgery is **most** important for the nurse to communicate to the surgeon and the anesthesia provider before the procedure? **Select all that apply.**
A. The oxygen saturation is 97%.
B. The serum potassium level is 3.0 mEq/L (3.0 mmol/L).
C. The client took a total of 1300 mg of aspirin yesterday.
D. The client requests to talk with a registered dietitian about weight loss.
E. The client took a regularly scheduled antihypertensive drug with a sip of water 2 hours ago.
F. After receiving the preoperative medications, the client tells the nurse that he lied on the assessment form and that he really is a current smoker.

Other Diagnostic Assessment. An electrocardiogram (ECG) may be required for patients older than a specific age who are to have general anesthesia. The age varies among facilities but is often 40 to 45 years. An ECG may also be required for patients with a history of cardiac disease or those at risk for cardiac complications. It provides baseline information on new or existing cardiac problems such as an old myocardial infarction (MI). A patient with a known cardiac problem may need a cardiology consultation before surgery.

Drugs for problem prevention such as nitroglycerin, beta-blockers, and antibiotics may be needed throughout the perioperative period to reduce or prevent stress on the heart. Abnormal or potentially life-threatening ECG results may cause the cancellation of surgery until the patient's cardiac status is stable.

A focused assessment of the preoperative patient is shown in Chart 14-3.

◆ Analysis: Interpreting

The priority collaborative problems for preoperative patients are:
1. Need for health teaching due to unfamiliarity with surgical procedures and preparation
2. Anxiety due to new or unknown experience, possibility of pain, and possible surgical outcomes

◆ Planning and Implementation: Responding

The role of the perioperative nurse in the preoperative setting is to advocate for the patient and coordinate all aspects of care before the patient transfer to the operating room. The preoperative nurse participates in the assessment of risk for the surgical patient and collaborates with other members of the perioperative team to safely transition the patient to the intraoperative phase of care (Malley et al., 2015) (see the Evidence-Based Practice box).

Providing Information

Planning: Expected Outcomes. The patient needs to know what to expect during and after surgery, as well as how to participate in his or her recovery as indicated by consistently demonstrating these behaviors:
- Explaining in his or her own words the purpose and expected results of the planned surgery
- Asking questions when a term or procedure is not known
- Adhering to the NPO requirements
- Stating an understanding of preoperative preparations (e.g., skin preparation, bowel preparation)
- Demonstrating correct use of exercises and techniques to be used after surgery for the prevention of complications (e.g., splinting the incision, using an incentive spirometer, performing leg exercises, ambulating as early as permitted)

Interventions. Because the surgical experience is foreign to many people, focus on teaching the patient and family members. Teaching may begin in the surgeon's office for planned or elective surgery. Pamphlets, written instructions, approved websites, and video recordings or DVDs may be given or sent to the patient. More teaching may occur when the patient has preadmission testing. Some facilities hold classes before surgery for groups of patients or show videos for those who are having the same or similar surgical procedures. A tour of the operating suite and the postanesthesia care unit (PACU) may be included.

Explore the patient's level of knowledge and understanding. Increased access to information via the Internet may be helpful but is also a concern. Some Internet information may not be accurate or may not apply to a specific patient's plan of care.

The Joint Commission's NPSGs require that you provide information about informed consent, dietary restrictions, specific preparation for surgery (bowel and skin preparations), exercises after surgery, and plans for pain management to promote patients' participation and help achieve the

EVIDENCE-BASED PRACTICE (QSEN)

Preoperative Assessment—Does It Assist With Transitions in Care in the Perioperative Environment?

Malley, A., Kenner, C., Kim, T., & Blakeney, B. (2015). The role of the nurse and the preoperative assessment in patient transitions. *AORN Journal, 102*(2), 181.e1-181.e9.

Perioperative care occurs in a complex environment that involves numerous members of the interdisciplinary team, multiple transitions of care, various communication pathways, and extensive use of technology. The nursing preoperative assessment is designed to highlight patient vulnerabilities that significantly increase the risk for perioperative surgical and anesthesia complications.

Information obtained during the preoperative phase is used to evaluate the patient's status and plan for interventions that effectively meet care needs and minimize poor outcomes. During this assessment, the nurse serves as a patient advocate by accurately communicating the plan of care to interdisciplinary team members during transitions in care levels.

Research identifies communication as a critical element in maintaining patient safety in the perioperative environment. Lack of communication contributes to adverse events and unexpected negative outcomes. Using Dr. Afaf Meleis' transitions theory as a framework, the complexities of the transitions inherent in the perioperative environment were studied in this research.

Level of Evidence: 3

The study is a qualitative descriptive design used to identify: (1) nursing's contributions to transitions in care as the patient moved between care settings in the perioperative environment, and (2) the role of the preoperative assessment in the transitions. Focus groups were conducted with 24 nurses in a 975-bed medical center. Five open-ended questions were presented to the participants. Time was allotted for the nurses to provide detailed information about the use of the nursing preoperative assessment and the gaps in information incurred as patients moved between care settings. As recurring patterns emerged, four themes were identified:

1. Understanding patient vulnerabilities
2. Multidimensional communication
3. Managing patients' expectations
4. Nursing's role in compensating for gaps

Because the study was conducted in a single academic health care setting with a small number of participants, findings may not be transferable to all other health care settings.

Commentary: Implications for Practice and Research

Nurses contribute to transitions in care by integrating and reconciling data from diverse sources. Identifying "red flags" that emerge during transitions in care were critical. The preoperative assessment, which established an accurate patient baseline, was viewed as helpful in identifying the red flags for both preoperative and postoperative nurses. Additional research is needed to discern how nurses and other members of the interdisciplinary team can identify and address patient vulnerabilities in the perioperative environment.

---

expected outcome. A sample educational checklist is shown in Table 14-5. Because education occurs in a variety of settings, coordination of patient teaching efforts is challenging. When you care for the patient just before surgery (same-day, ambulatory surgery [outpatient] unit, inpatient hospital unit), assess the patient's and family members' knowledge and provide additional information as needed. If the patient is receiving sedation or general anesthesia, stress the importance of having another adult drive the patient home after the procedure. Document information in the electronic health record about who was involved in teaching, what specifically was taught, and which education materials were given to the patient and family.

Ensuring Informed Consent. Surgery of any type involves invasion of the body and requires informed consent from the patient or legal guardian (Fig. 14-3). **The Joint Commission's NPSGs state that patients deserve to be informed and involved in decisions affecting their health care.** Consent implies that the patient has sufficient information to understand:

- The nature of and reason for surgery
- Who will be performing the surgery and whether others will be present during the procedure (e.g., students, vendors)
- All available options and the benefits and risks associated with each option
- The risks associated with the surgical procedure and its potential outcomes
- The risks associated with the use of anesthesia
- The risks, benefits, and alternatives to the use of blood or blood products during the procedure

Informed consent is one way to help ensure patient SAFETY and reflects professional ETHICS. It helps protect the patient from any unwanted procedures and protects the surgeon and the facility from lawsuit claims related to unauthorized surgery or

TABLE 14-5 **Preoperative Teaching Checklist**
Consider these items when planning individualized preoperative teaching for patients and families:
• Fears and anxieties
• Surgical procedure
• Preoperative routines (e.g., NPO, blood samples, showering)
• Invasive procedures (e.g., lines, catheters)
• Coughing, turning, deep breathing
• Incentive spirometer
• How to use
• How to tell when used correctly
• Lower extremity exercises
• Stockings and pneumatic compression devices
• Early ambulation
• Splinting
• Pain management

uninformed patients. Written record of informed consent is documented on a "consent form" but can also be documented in the surgeon's notes. The consent form documents the patient's consent and signature for the procedure(s) listed.

As a competent adult, it is the patient's right to refuse treatment for any reason, even when refusal might lead to death. For example, in the case of Jehovah's Witnesses, some patients will not accept blood transfusions because of their religious convictions.

It is the surgeon's responsibility to provide a complete explanation of the planned surgical procedure and to have the consent form signed before sedation is given and before surgery is performed. The perioperative nurse *is not responsible for providing detailed information about the surgical procedure. The nurse's role is to clarify facts that have been presented by the*

GENERAL REQUEST AND CONSENT

FOR OFFICE USE ONLY:
Patient Name: _____
Date of Birth: _____
Date of Procedure: _____

I _____ request and give consent to _____
(Type or print patient name)   (Type or print Doctor or Practitioner Name(s))

to perform the following procedure(s) _____
(Please list site and side if appropriate)

_____

The benefits, risks, complications, and alternatives to the above procedure(s) have been explained to me.

I understand that the procedure(s) will be performed at Christiana Care by and under supervision of my doctor or practitioner. My doctor or practitioner may use the services of other doctors or practitioners, or members of the resident staff as he or she deems necessary or advisable.

I authorize my doctor or practitioner and his or her associates and assistants to perform such additional procedures, which in their judgment are necessary and appropriate to carry out my diagnosis or treatment.

I authorize the hospital to retain, preserve and use for scientific, teaching or transplant purposes, or to make other dispositions of, at their convenience, any specimens, tissues, or parts taken from my body during the course of this operation.

I consent to observers in the operating room in accordance with hospital policy. I consent to photography or video taping of my surgical procedure for educational purposes, provided my identity remains anonymous and confidential.

I agree to being given blood or blood products as deemed advisable during the course of my procedure. The risks, benefits, and alternatives to receiving blood or blood products have been explained to me.

I consent to the administration of sedation or analgesia during my procedure. The risks, benefits, and alternatives to receiving sedation or analgesia have been explained to me.

If anesthesia is required, I consent to the administration of anesthesia by members of the Department of Anesthesiology. I also consent to the use of non-invasive and invasive monitoring techniques as deemed necessary. I understand that anesthesia involves risks that are in addition to those resulting from the operation itself including, but not limited to, dental injury, hoarseness, vocal cord injury, infection, nerve injury, corneal abrasion, seizures, heart attack, stroke and even death.

Please initial one of the following statements (females only):

_____ To the best of my knowledge I am not pregnant.   _____ I believe I am pregnant.

I certify that I have read and understand the above consent statements. In addition, I have been offered the opportunity to ask my doctor or practitioner any questions I have regarding the procedure(s) to be performed and they have been answered to my satisfaction. I acknowledge that I have been given no guarantee or assurance as to the results that may be obtained from the procedure(s).

_____   _____   _____   _____
Signature of Patient or Decision Maker   Date and Time   Doctor or Practitioner Signature   Date and Time

_____   _____
Relationship to Patient if Decision Maker   Doctor ID # or Print Name

_____   _____   _____
Witness Signature   Date and Time   Practitioner Print Name/Title

_____
Witness Print Name

Telephone
Consent: _____
Name of person obtained from/Relationship to Patient

_____   _____   _____   _____
Witness's (es') Signature(s)   Date and Time   Witness's (es') Signature(s)   Date and Time

_____   _____
Witness's (es') Print Name(s)   Witness's (es') Print Name(s)

FIG. 14-3 Surgical consent form. (Courtesy Christiana Care Health Services, Newark, DE.)

surgeon and dispel myths that the patient or family may have about the surgical experience. The nurse must verify that the consent form is signed, and he or she may serve as a witness to the signature, not to the fact that the patient is informed (Rock & Hoebeke, 2014).

> ⚠ **NURSING SAFETY PRIORITY** QSEN
> *Action Alert*
>
> If you believe that the patient has not been adequately informed, that he or she has questions about his or her procedure, or there is a discrepancy related to surgical site, it is your professional and ETHICAL duty to contact the surgeon and request that he or she see the patient for further clarification. Document this action in the electronic health record.

Patients who cannot write may sign with an X, which must be witnessed by two people. In an emergency, telephone or telegram authorization is acceptable and should be followed up with written consent as soon as possible. The number of witnesses (usually two) and the type of documentation vary according to the facility policy. For a life-threatening situation in which every effort has been made to contact the individual with medical power of attorney, consent is desired but not essential. In place of written or oral consent, written consultation by at least two physicians who are not associated with the case may be requested by the surgeon. This formal consultation legally supports the decision for surgery until the appropriate individual can sign a consent form. If the patient is not capable of giving consent and has no family, the court can appoint a legal guardian to represent the patient's best interests.

A blind patient may sign his or her own consent form, which usually needs to be witnessed by two people. Patients who do not speak the general language of the facility or who are hearing impaired may require a qualified translator and a second witness. Many facilities have consent forms written in more than one language and also have health care professionals who are proficient with American Sign Language. Qualified translators may be health care professionals or other types of hospital employee. Family members should not serve as translators because the health care team may not be able to validate that the medical information is being translated accurately. Translators are part of the interprofessional care team and are required to keep patient information confidential.

Some surgical procedures such as sterilization and experimental procedures may require a special permit in addition to the standard consent. National and local governing bodies and the individual facility determine which procedures require a separate permit. Separate consents for anesthesia and blood products may be required.

Surgical procedures that are site specific, such as left, right, or bilateral, require patient identification before surgery. **As required by The Joint Commission's NPSGs, to ensure that the correct site is selected and the wrong site is avoided, the site is marked by a licensed independent practitioner and, whenever possible, involves the patient.** The surgeon is accountable and should be present during the procedure. The nurse is an important part of this SAFETY measure. Before starting the operative procedure, facilities use a "time-out" procedure to verify the correct site, patient, and procedure. The perioperative nurse is in a position of ensuring that these SAFETY measures

are implemented immediately before the procedure is started (AORN, 2015). The "time-out" involves the participation of all members of the procedure team, including the surgeon, anesthesia provider, circulating nurse, scrub person, and any other active participants.

> ⚠ **NURSING SAFETY PRIORITY** QSEN
> *Action Alert*
>
> At a minimum the patient's identity, correct side and site, correct patient position, and agreement on the proposed procedure must be verified by all members of the surgical team before the incision.

Patient Self-Determination. Patients receiving medical care have the right to have or to initiate advance directives such as a living will or durable power of attorney, as mandated by the Patient Self-Determination Act. Advance directives provide legal instructions to the primary health care providers about the patient's wishes and are to be followed. *Surgery does not provide an exception to a patient's advance directives or living will* (AORN, 2016a). Chapter 7 discusses advance directives in more detail.

Implementing Dietary Restrictions. Regardless of the type of surgery and anesthesia planned, the patient is restricted to NPO status before surgery. **NPO** means no eating, drinking (including water), or smoking (nicotine stimulates gastric secretions). The exact amount of time a patient must be NPO before surgery is controversial. Patients, especially older adults, who fast for 8 or more hours may have imbalances of fluids, electrolytes, and blood glucose levels. The American Society of Anesthesiologists (ASA) recommends a reduced NPO time—6 or more hours for easily digested solid food and 2 hours for clear liquids (Gebremedhn & Nagaratnam, 2014). A major problem is that these guidelines for duration of fasting have not been implemented universally.

NPO status ensures that the stomach contains a limited volume of gastric secretions, which decreases the risk for aspiration. Outpatients and patients who are scheduled for admission to the hospital on the same day that surgery is performed must receive written and oral instructions about when to begin NPO status.

> ⚠ **NURSING SAFETY PRIORITY** QSEN
> *Action Alert*
>
> Emphasize the importance of adhering to the prescribed NPO restriction. Failure to adhere can result in postponing or canceling surgery and an increased risk for aspiration during or after surgery.

Administering Regularly Scheduled Drugs. On the day of surgery, the patient's usual drug schedule may need to be altered. Consult the medical health care provider and the anesthesia provider for instructions about drugs such as those taken for diabetes, cardiac disease, or glaucoma and regularly scheduled anticonvulsants, antihypertensives, anticoagulants, antidepressants, and corticosteroids. The surgeon may prescribe some drugs, including over-the-counter drugs such as aspirin, other NSAIDs, and herbal supplements, to be stopped until after surgery. Other drugs may be given IV to maintain the drug level in the blood. *Drugs for cardiac disease, respiratory disease, seizures, and hypertension are commonly allowed with a sip of water before surgery.* Some antihypertensive or antidepressant drugs are withheld on the day of surgery to reduce adverse effects on blood pressure during surgery. Even when beta blockers are not part of a patient's usual medications, they may be prescribed for some patients who are at risk for cardiac problems. Check with the primary health care provider, surgeon, or anesthesia provider to determine whether a specific patient requires perioperative therapy with beta-blocking drugs.

The patient who takes insulin for diabetes may be given a reduced dose of intermediate- or long-acting insulin based on the blood glucose level, or regular (fast-acting) insulin in divided doses on the day of surgery. As an alternative, an IV infusion of 5% dextrose in water may be given with the insulin to prevent low blood sugar during surgery. Because of the many treatment approaches to diabetes, clarify drug and IV prescriptions with the primary health care provider. (See Chapter 64 for more information about diabetes.)

Intestinal Preparation. Bowel or intestinal preparations are performed to prevent injury to the colon and reduce the number of intestinal bacteria. Bowel evacuation is needed for major abdominal, pelvic, perineal, or perianal surgery. In addition, colonoscopy procedures, routinely performed in outpatient ambulatory care facilities, require the patient to follow a strict preoperative protocol for bowel evacuation. The surgeon's preference and the type of surgical procedure determine the type of bowel preparation. An enema ordered to be given until return flow is clear is a stressful procedure, especially for the older patient. Repeated enemas can cause electrolyte imbalance, fluid volume imbalances, vagal stimulation, and postural (orthostatic) hypotension. Enemas cause severe anal discomfort in patients with hemorrhoids. Some physicians prescribe potent laxatives instead of enemas, especially for older patients. Bowel preparations can exhaust the patient, and SAFETY precautions must be taken to prevent falls.

Skin Preparation. The skin is the body's first line of defense against infection. A break in this barrier increases the risk for infection, especially for older patients. Skin preparation before surgery is the first step to reduce the risk for surgical site infection (AORN, 2016b).

One or two days before the scheduled surgery, the surgeon may ask the patient to shower using an antiseptic solution. Instruct the patient to be especially careful to clean well around the proposed surgical site. If the patient is hospitalized before surgery, showering and cleaning are repeated the night before surgery or in the morning before transfer to the surgical suite. This cleaning reduces contamination of the surgical field and the number of organisms at the site. Remove any soil or debris from the surgical site and surrounding areas.

Factors that predispose to wound contamination and surgical site infection (SSI) include bacteria found in hair follicles, disruption of the normal protective mechanisms of the skin, and nicks in the skin. Shaving of hair creates the potential for infection. **Hair clipping with electrical clippers and depilatories are to be used for hair removal as required by The Joint Commission's NPSGs (Markatos et al., 2015).**

The Centers for Disease Control and Prevention (CDC) recommends that, if shaving is necessary, the hair should be removed using disposable sterile supplies and aseptic principles *immediately* before the start of the surgical procedure. If needed, shaving is performed in the treatment room, the holding area of the operating suite, or the operating room (OR). Fig. 14-4 shows areas of hair removal for various surgical procedures.

Preparing the Patient for Tubes, Drains, and Vascular Access. Prepare the patient for possible placement of tubes, drains, and vascular access devices. Preparation reduces the patient's anxiety and fear and the family's negative reaction. Be careful not to scare the patient while providing information about the purpose of each tube.

Tubes of all sorts are common after surgery. A nasogastric (NG) tube may be inserted before abdominal surgery to decompress or empty the stomach and the upper bowel. Usually the tube is placed after the induction of anesthesia, when insertion is less disturbing to the patient and is easier to perform. The patient may need an indwelling urinary (Foley) catheter before, during, or after surgery to keep the bladder empty and monitor kidney function.

Drains are often placed during surgery to help remove fluid from the surgical site. Some drains are under the dressing; others are visible and require emptying. Drains come in various shapes and sizes (see Chapter 16). Inform the patient that drains are often used routinely and that generally they are not painful but may cause some discomfort. Discuss the reasons drains should not be kinked or pulled.

Vascular access is placed for patients receiving a general anesthetic and for most patients receiving other types of anesthetics. Access is needed to give drugs and fluids before, during, and after surgery. Patients who are dehydrated or are at risk for dehydration may receive fluids before surgery.

CONSIDERATIONS FOR OLDER ADULTS
Patient-Centered Care QSEN

Older adult patients are at greater risk for dehydration because their fluid reserves are lower than those of young or middle-age adults. Hemodynamic monitoring of older adult patients and patients with cardiac disease receiving IV fluids is essential. (See Chapter 13 for more information on IV therapy.)

The IV access is usually placed in the arm using a large-bore, short catheter (e.g., 18-gauge, 1-inch catheter) or in the back of the hand using a smaller-bore (20-gauge) catheter. A larger vein provides the least resistance to fluid or blood infusion, especially in an emergency when rapid infusion may be needed. Depending on the patient's needs and the facility policies, the IV access can be placed before surgery when the patient is in the hospital room, in the holding or admission area of the surgical suite, or in the OR.

Postoperative Procedures and Exercises. Teach the patient and family members about exercises and procedures (e.g., checking dressings, obtaining vital signs frequently) to be performed after surgery. Family members can be helpful in reminding patients to perform the exercises. Teaching before surgery reduces apprehension and fear, increases cooperation and participation in care after surgery, and decreases respiratory and vascular complications. When the fear or anxiety level is high, explore the patient's feelings before beginning to teach the procedures.

Discussion, demonstration with return demonstration, and practice by the patient aid in the ability to perform various breathing (Chart 14-4) and leg (Chart 14-5) exercises after surgery. Stress the need to begin exercises early in the recovery phase and to continue them, with 5 to 10 repetitions each, every 1 to 2 hours after surgery for at least the first 48 hours. Explain that the patient may need to be awakened for these activities.

Procedures and Exercises to Prevent Respiratory Complications. *Breathing exercises* include deep, or diaphragmatic, breathing

Head surgery

Unilateral chest surgery

Thoracoabdominal surgery

Abdominal surgery

Forearm, elbow or hand surgery

Gynecologic surgery

Genitourinary surgery

Hip surgery

Thigh and leg surgery

Foot/lower leg surgery

Ankle, foot or toe surgery

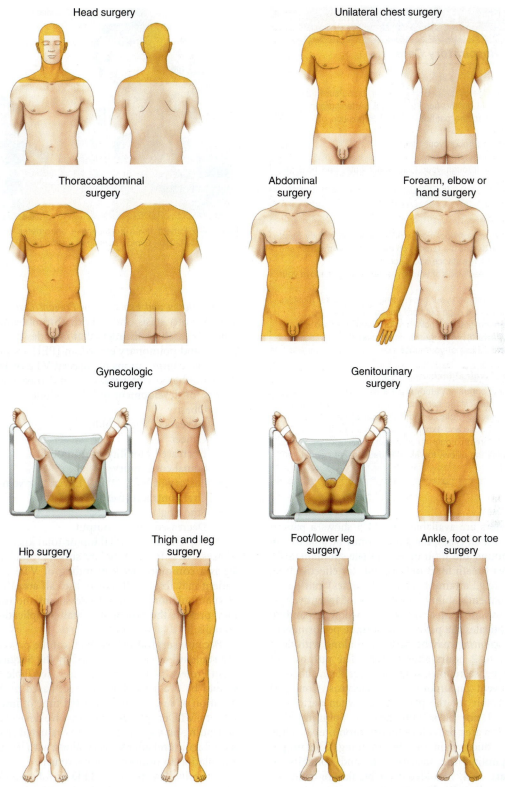

FIG. 14-4 Skin preparation of common surgical sites. Shaded areas indicate preparation sites.

to enlarge the chest cavity and expand the lungs. After demonstrating and explaining the technique, urge the patient to practice deep breathing.

For patients with chronic lung disease or limited chest expansion, as seen in older patients because of the aging process, expansion breathing exercises are useful. For the patient having chest surgery, expansion breathing exercises strengthen accessory muscles and are started before surgery. Expansion breathing after surgery during chest physiotherapy (percussion, vibration, postural drainage) may help loosen secretions and maintain an adequate air exchange.

Incentive spirometry is another way to encourage the patient to take deep breaths. Its purposes are to promote complete lung expansion and prevent pulmonary problems. Various types of

CHART 14-4 Patient and Family Education: Preparing for Self-Management

Perioperative Respiratory Care

Deep (Diaphragmatic) Breathing

1. Sit upright on the edge of the bed or in a chair, being sure that your feet are placed firmly on the floor or a stool. (After surgery, deep breathing is done with the patient in Fowler's position or in semi-Fowler's position.)
2. Take a gentle breath through your mouth.
3. Breathe out gently and completely.
4. Take a deep breath through your nose and mouth, and hold this breath to the count of five.
5. Exhale through your nose and mouth.

Expansion Breathing

1. Find a comfortable upright position, with your knees slightly bent. (Bending the knees decreases tension on the abdominal muscles and decreases respiratory resistance and discomfort.)
2. Place your hands on each side of your lower rib cage, just above your waist.
3. Take a deep breath through your nose, using your shoulder muscles to expand your lower rib cage outward during inhalation.
4. Exhale, concentrating first on moving your chest, then on moving your lower ribs inward, while gently squeezing the rib cage and forcing air out of the base of your lungs.

Splinting of the Surgical Incision

1. Unless coughing is contraindicated, place a pillow, towel, or folded blanket over your surgical incision and hold the item firmly in place.
2. Take three slow, deep breaths to stimulate your cough reflex.
3. Inhale through your nose and exhale through your mouth.
4. On your third deep breath, cough to clear secretions from your lungs while firmly holding the pillow, towel, or folded blanket against your incision.

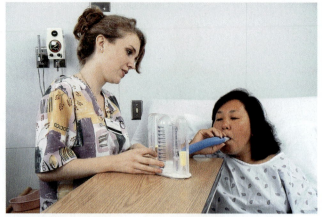

FIG. 14-5 Patient using an incentive spirometer. (From Perry, A. G., & Potter, P. A. (2010). *Clinical nursing skills and techniques* (7th ed.). St. Louis: Mosby.)

incentive spirometers are available; Fig. 14-5 shows a patient using one type. With all types, the patient must be able to seal the lips tightly around the mouthpiece, inhale spontaneously, and hold his or her breath for 3 to 5 seconds for effective lung expansion. Goals (e.g., attaining specific volumes) can be set according to the patient's ability and the type of incentive spirometer. Seeing a ball move up a column or a bellows expanding reinforces and motivates the patient to continue performance.

Coughing and splinting may be performed along with deep breathing every 1 to 2 hours after surgery. The purposes of coughing are to expel secretions, keep the lungs clear, allow full aeration, and prevent pneumonia and atelectasis. Coughing may be uncomfortable for the patient; but, when performed correctly, it should not harm the incision. Splinting (i.e., holding) the incision area provides support, promotes a feeling of security, and reduces pain during coughing. The proper technique for splinting the incision site and coughing is described in Chart 14-4. A folded bath blanket or pillow is helpful to use as a splint. Cardiac surgery patients may receive their own heart-shaped pillow for splint use.

The use of routine coughing exercises after surgery is controversial. Some surgeons believe that coughing may harm the surgical wound and that it would be better to use other, safer measures for lung hygiene, such as deep-breathing and incentive spirometer exercises. When routine coughing exercises should be avoided for a specific patient such as after a hernia repair or craniotomy, the surgeon usually writes a "do not cough" order.

Procedures and Exercises to Prevent Cardiovascular Complications. Venous stasis and venous thromboembolism (VTE) (a group of vascular disorders that includes deep vein thrombosis [DVT] and pulmonary embolism [PE]) are potential but often avoidable complications of surgery. VTE or DVT can lead to a PE if the blood clot breaks off and travels to the lungs. Risk factors for development of VTE include:

- Obesity
- 40 years of age or older
- Cancer
- Decreased mobility or immobility
- Spinal cord injury
- History of VTE, DVT, PE, varicose veins, or edema
- Oral contraceptives use
- Smoking
- Decreased cardiac output
- Hip fracture or total hip or total knee surgery

Always assess for VTE before surgery. Sudden swelling in one leg is a common physical finding of VTE caused by DVT. A patient may feel a dull ache in the calf area that becomes worse with ambulation. A careful assessment and timely intervention may prevent the potentially fatal complication of pulmonary embolism.

Because surgical-related VTE can be prevented, prophylaxis is a standard of care established by the Surgical Care Improvement Project (SCIP) core measures (see Table 14-1). All patients should be evaluated for VTE risk based on history, type and duration of surgery, and expected time of immobilization after surgery. VTE prophylaxis may involve devices and drug therapy, depending on a specific patient's evaluated risk. Devices may be used during and after surgery, along with leg exercises and early ambulation to promote venous return.

Antiembolism stockings (TED or Jobst stockings) and elastic (Ace) wraps provide graduated compression of the legs, starting at the end of the foot and ankle. Measure the patient's leg length and circumference before ordering the stocking size. Elastic wraps are used when the legs are too large or too small for the stockings. Help the patient apply the stockings or wraps and ensure that they are neither too loose (are ineffective) nor too tight (inhibit blood flow). They need to be worn properly and should be removed two to three times per day for 30 minutes for skin inspection and skin care.

👤 **CHART 14-5** **Patient and Family Education: Preparing for Self-Management**

Postoperative Leg Exercises

Exercise No. 1

1. Lie in bed with the head of your bed elevated to about 45 degrees.
2. Beginning with your right leg, bend your knee, raise your foot off the bed, and hold this position for a few seconds.
3. Extend your leg by straightening your knee and lower the leg to the bed.
4. Repeat this sequence four more times with your right leg; then perform this same exercise five times with your left leg.

Exercise No. 2

1. Beginning with your right leg, point your toes toward the bottom of the bed.
2. With the same leg, point your toes up toward your face.
3. Repeat this exercise several times with your right leg; then perform this same exercise with your left leg.

Exercise No. 3

1. Beginning with your right leg, make circles with your ankle, first to the left and then to the right.
2. Repeat this exercise several times with your right leg; then perform this same exercise with your left leg.

Exercise No. 4

1. Beginning with your right leg, bend your knee and *push* the ball of your foot into the bed or floor until you feel your calf and thigh muscles contracting.
2. Repeat this exercise several times with your right leg; then perform this same exercise with your left leg.

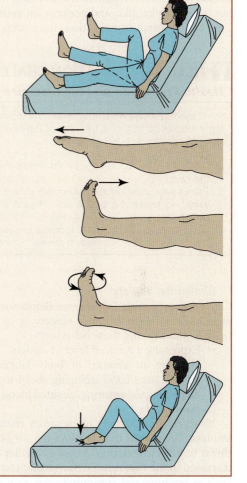

Pneumatic compression devices enhance venous blood flow by providing intermittent periods of compression on the legs. Measure the patient's legs and order the correct size. Place the boots on the patient's legs and set and check the compression pressures (usually 35 to 55 mm Hg). *Unless these devices are applied properly, there is no benefit (Elpern et al., 2013).* Fig. 14-6 shows various types of sequential compression devices. Antiembolism stockings may be worn in addition to the boots and may reduce some of the uncomfortable sensations of the boots (e.g., itching, sweating, and heat).

Leg exercises also promote venous return. Teach the leg exercises outlined in Chart 14-5 and urge the patient to practice them before surgery. The exercises are important, even when other devices are used.

Mobility soon after surgery (early ambulation) has many cardiovascular and other benefits. It stimulates intestinal motility, enhances lung expansion, mobilizes secretions, promotes venous return, prevents joint rigidity, and relieves pressure. For most types of surgery, teach the patient to turn at least every 2 hours after surgery while confined to bed. Teach patients how to use the bed side rails safely for turning and how to protect the surgical wound by splinting when turning. Assure patients that assistance and pain medication will be given as needed to reduce any anxiety and pain they may have with this activity.

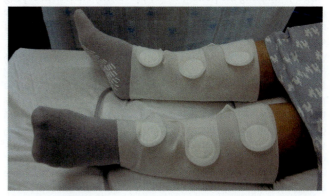

FIG. 14-6 External pneumatic compression device used to promote venous return and prevent deep vein thrombosis (DVT). (From Angelo, R., Ryu, R., & Esch, J. (2010). *AANA advanced arthroscopy: The shoulder.* Philadelphia: Saunders.)

For certain surgical procedures, such as some brain, spinal, and orthopedic procedures, the surgeon may prescribe turning restrictions. Ask the surgeon about other interventions to prevent complications of immobility in patients with turning restrictions. During preoperative teaching, inform the patient of anticipated turning restrictions.

Most patients are allowed and encouraged to get out of bed the day of or the day after surgery. Assist the patient into a chair or with ambulation after the surgery, the next day, or when the surgeon specifies. If a patient must remain in bed, help him or her turn, deep breathe, and perform leg exercises at least every 2 hours to prevent complications from immobility.

❓ NCLEX EXAMINATION CHALLENGE 14-3
Health Promotion and Maintenance

What client teaching will the nurse provide regarding postoperative leg exercises to minimize the risk for development of deep vein thrombosis after surgery?
A. Only perform each exercise one time to prevent overuse.
B. Begin exercises by sitting at a 90-degree angle on the side of the bed.
C. Point toes of one foot toward bottom of bed; then point toes of same leg toward his or her face. Repeat several times; then switch legs.
D. Bend knee, and push heel of foot into the bed until the calf and thigh muscles contract. Repeat several times; then switch legs.

Minimizing Anxiety
Planning: Expected Outcomes. Before surgery, the patient is expected to have manageable anxiety as indicated by consistently demonstrating these behaviors:
- Expressing a reduced level of anxiety
- Showing an absence of body language indicators of anxiety (e.g., hand wringing, facial tension, restlessness, dilated pupils, sweating, elevated blood pressure, elevated pulse rate)

Interventions. Anxiety often causes restlessness and sleeplessness. The patient may perceive the surgical experience as a threat to life and function. Assess his or her level of anxiety as discussed in the Psychosocial Assessment section. Interventions such as teaching and communicating with the patient before surgery, enabling the patient to use previously successful coping mechanisms, and giving antianxiety drugs may help reduce the anxiety. Incorporate available support systems into the plan of care.

Preoperative teaching involves first assessing the patient's knowledge about the surgical experience (see the Providing Information section) and then providing factual information to promote his or her understanding. Allow ample time for questions. Respond to the questions accurately and refer unanswered questions to the proper professional. During the discussion, continually assess the patient's responses and anxiety level. Be careful not to provide information that might increase anxiety. The informed, educated patient is better able to anticipate events and maintain self-control and is thus less anxious.

Encouraging communication by having the patient state feelings, fears, and concerns can help reduce anxiety. Use an honest and open approach so the patient can express feelings freely without fear of ridicule or judgment. Keep the patient informed by clarifying information, answering questions, and allaying fears about the surgery.

Promoting rest is helpful because the stress and anxiety of impending surgery often interfere with the patient's ability to sleep and rest the night before surgery. The period before surgery is physically and emotionally stressful. To help the patient relax, determine what he or she usually does to relax and fall asleep. If the patient is able, urge him or her to continue these methods of relaxation. A back rub is relaxing and can be performed by a nurse, unlicensed assistive personnel (UAP), or family member. The surgeon may prescribe a sedative or hypnotic drug to help the patient rest for surgery.

Distraction may be used as an intervention for anxiety, especially in the 24 hours immediately before surgery. Listening to music may decrease anxiety, as may watching television, reading, or visiting with family members.

Teaching family members helps reduce anxiety by increasing the likelihood of support and involvement in the patient's care. Assess the readiness and desire of the family to take an active part in the patient's care. A positive sign of family interest is that of members asking questions about the surgical experience. After family readiness is determined, keep family members informed and encourage their involvement in all aspects of education. Emphasize the important role of the family before surgery, but guide discussions and practice sessions so the patient is the focus of the discussion. Family members can encourage and help the patient practice exercises to be performed after surgery.

Inform the family of the time for surgery, if known, and of any schedule changes. If the patient is an outpatient, provide clear directions to the patient and family regarding any specific night-before procedures, what time and where to report, and what to bring with them. Encourage the family to stay with the patient before surgery for support.

Most families are anxious about the surgery planned for their loved one. To reduce their anxiety, explain the routines expected before, during, and after surgery. Tell the family that, after the patient leaves the hospital room or admission area, there is usually a 30- to 60-minute preparation period in the operating area (holding room, treatment area) before the surgery actually begins. After surgery, the patient is taken to the postanesthesia care unit (PACU) usually for 1 to 2 hours before returning to the hospital room or discharge area. The length of stay in the PACU depends on the type of surgery, the type of anesthesia, any complications, and the patient's responses. Tell the family about the best place to wait for the patient or surgeon according to the facility policy and the surgeon's preference. Many hospitals and surgical centers have surgical waiting areas so families can wait in comfortable surroundings and be easily located when the procedure is completed. Often families are provided with a beeper to let them know when to report to a specific area to receive updates about the patient's status, meet with the surgeon, or see the patient.

Preoperative Electronic Health Record Review. Review the patient's electronic health record to ensure that all documentation, preoperative procedures, and orders are completed. Check the surgical informed consent form and, if indicated, any other special consent forms to see that they are signed and dated and that they contain the witnesses' signatures. Confirm that the scheduled procedure, including the identification of left versus right when necessary, is what is listed on the consent form. Even though it might be obvious, inform the patient that the site for surgery will be marked before the procedure begins. **If possible, encourage the patient to assist with the marking, as suggested by The Joint Commission's NPSGs. Document allergies according to facility policy.** Accurate measuring and recording of height and weight are important for proper dosage of the anesthetic agents. Ensure that the results of all laboratory, radiographic, and diagnostic tests are on the electronic health record. Document any abnormal results, and report them to the surgeon and the anesthesia provider. If the patient is an autologous blood donor or has had directed blood donations made, those special slips must be included in the electronic health record. Record a current set of vital signs (within 1 to 2 hours of the scheduled surgery time), and document any significant physical or psychosocial observations.

Report special needs, concerns, and instructions (including advance directives) to the surgical team, as required by The Joint Commission's NPSGs. For example, advise the surgical team if the patient is a member of Jehovah's Witnesses and does not accept blood products or if the patient is hard of hearing and does not have his or her hearing aid. This information helps the surgical team provide continuity of care while the patient is in the surgical area.

Preoperative Patient Preparation. Facilities usually require the patient to remove most clothing and wear a hospital gown into the OR; however, underpants may be worn in above-the-waist surgery; and socks may be worn, except in foot or leg surgery. If prescribed by the surgeon, apply antiembolism stockings or pneumatic compression devices before surgery. In some ambulatory settings, such as for cataract surgery, no or minimal clothing is removed.

Patients are advised to leave all valuables at home. If he or she has valuables, including jewelry, money, or clothes, they are given to a family member or locked in a safe place, according to the facility policy. If rings cannot be removed, assess the risk for swelling. If swelling makes it necessary, rings may be cut off to avoid further injury. It is preferable that all pierced jewelry be removed before surgery. Religious emblems may be pinned or fastened securely to the patient's gown. Care must be provided to avoid loss or theft of these items. Some facilities have paper emblems from a religious leader.

The patient wears an identification band that clearly gives the first and last name, hospital number, surgeon, and birthdate. An additional bracelet, usually red, identifies any allergies. A bracelet indicating that a blood sample for type and screen has been drawn may be worn, depending on the facility policy.

If dentures are to be removed, including partial dental plates, place them in a labeled denture cup. Denture removal is a SAFETY measure to prevent aspiration and obstruction of the airway. If a patient has any capped teeth, document this finding on the checklist.

All prosthetic devices, such as artificial eyes and limbs, are removed and given to a family member or safely stored, as are contact lenses, glasses, wigs, and toupees. Check and remove hairpins and clips, which can conduct electrical current used during surgery and cause scalp burns.

Some facilities allow hearing aids in the surgical suite to help communication before and after surgery. Some facilities allow dentures, wigs, and glasses to be worn into the operating suite to prevent embarrassment to the patient. These items are removed when absolutely necessary. If the patient is sent to surgery with any assistive devices (e.g., hearing aid, glasses), communicate this to the perioperative nurse to prevent accidental loss of or damage to the device. In the electronic health record, document all valuables going into the operating room with the patient.

The removal of fingernail polish or artificial nails is controversial. Polish and artificial nails have been thought to affect the accuracy of pulse oximetry readings. Recent studies have indicated that pulse oximetry readings taken on fingers are affected by brown or blue polish but not by red or lighter color polish. In addition, pulse oximetry does not have to be measured on fingers only. Some facilities still require that at least one artificial nail must be removed to monitor oxygen saturation by pulse oximetry.

After the patient is prepared for surgery and just before transport into the operating suite, ask the patient to empty the bladder. This action prevents incontinence or overdistention and is a starting point for intake and output measurement.

Preoperative Drugs. Preoperative drugs may be prescribed, regardless of the type of planned anesthesia. Various drugs reduce anxiety, promote relaxation, prevent laryngospasm, reduce vagal-induced bradycardia, inhibit oral and gastric secretions, and decrease the amount of anesthetic needed for the induction and maintenance of anesthesia. Drug selection is based on the patient's age, physical and psychological condition, medical history, and height and weight; other drugs the patient takes routinely; test results; and the type and extent of the planned surgical procedure. If more than one response is required, combination therapy may be prescribed.

Drug types for preoperative purposes may include sedatives (e.g., hydroxyzine [Atarax, Vistaril]); hypnotics (e.g., lorazepam [Ativan]); anxiolytics (e.g., midazolam [Versed]); opioid analgesics (e.g., morphine, hydromorphone); and an anticholinergic agent (e.g., atropine). Other specific-purpose drugs also may be added. For example, if rapid emptying of the stomach is needed, metoclopramide (Reglan) may be prescribed. When procedures are long or stress ulcers are likely, an H_2 histamine blocker (e.g., cimetidine [Tagamet]; ranitidine [Zantac]) is used.

Preoperative drugs may be given when the patient is "on call" to the surgical suite. **After positively identifying the patient as required by The Joint Commission's NPSGs, (using the armband and asking the patient to state his or her name and birthdate) and making sure that the operative permit is signed, give the correct drugs in the correct doses.** Then raise the side rails, place the call light within easy reach of the patient, and remind him or her not to try to get out of bed. Place the bed in a low position. Tell the patient that he or she may become drowsy and have a dry mouth as a result of the drugs.

A more common practice is for the preoperative drugs to be given *after* the patient is transferred to the preoperative area. This practice permits the surgical team and anesthesia personnel to make more accurate assessments and have last-minute discussions with a patient not yet affected by drugs. In addition, after the patient is in the preoperative area, drugs can be given by the IV route. Monitoring equipment such as continuous pulse oximetry and ECG is more readily available in this area. The oral or IM route is used less often because of variable absorption rates. **The surgeon may prescribe a prophylactic antibiotic to be given right before or during surgery to reduce the risk for a surgical site infection, as suggested by The Joint Commission's NPSGs. When needed, the antibiotic is given within 60 minutes before the incision is made, as mandated by the Surgical Care Improvement Project (SCIP) core measures, SCIP Inf-1** (see Table 14-1).

Patient Transfer to the Surgical Suite. In the immediate preoperative period, review and update the patient's electronic health record, reinforce teaching, ensure that the patient is correctly dressed for surgery, and give prescribed preoperative drugs. Use an electronic or hard-copy preoperative checklist for a smooth, efficient transfer to the surgical suite (Fig. 14-7). The patient, along with the signed consent form, the completed

PREOPERATIVE CHECKLIST

PATIENT INFORMATION

Date and Time of Arrival to Presurgical Holding Area:_____

INITIAL APPROPRIATELY

1. Hospital identification band intact and legible including patient name, date of birth, medical record number ____ Yes ____ No	
A. If yes, which arm? _____	
B. If no, make and apply arm band	
C. Is the extremity involved in the surgery? ____ Yes ____ No	
D. If yes, change to another extremity ____ Yes ____ No	

	IN PLACE	REMOVED
2. Glasses, contact lenses		
3. Hearing aid(s)		
4. Jewelry, piercings, religious medals, ring taped to finger		
5. Dentures (full, partial)		
6. Other prostheses (list)		
7. Hairpiece, wig, pins/combs		
8. Makeup, nail polish		
9. Clothing		

	YES	NO
10. Antiembolic stockings, compression devices		
11. Patient voided		
12. Advance directives on MR		
13. IV started by:		
14. Permission for surgeon to speak to family		
15. Family has pager #		
16. Informed consent signed, witnessed, on chart		

INITIAL APPROPRIATE COLUMN

	YES	NO
17. Site of site-specific surgery verified by patient and surgeon		
18. History and physical on chart		
19. Pregnancy test date within the past 10 days for females age 11–55 (unless documented hysterectomy)		
20. Type and screen verified with blood bank		
21. Test results (circle those on chart) CBC H&H UA EPI PT/PTT METAPNL ECG CXR		
22. OR notified of latex allergy		
23. ID plate on chart		
24. NPO with appropriate meds		

LIST KNOWN ALLERGIES

PRE-OP MEDS & DOSAGES	**TIME**

VITAL SIGNS		**TIME**
BP	Pulse	
Resp	O$_2$ sat	
Temp Ht	Wt	
MISCELLANEOUS		**YES/NO**
Risk for falls		
Communication barrier		

COMMENTS _____

_____

_____

RN _____ **PHONE/PAGER**_____ **DATE**_____ **TIME**_____

FIG. 14-7 Preoperative checklist.

preoperative checklist, and the patient identification card, is transported to the surgical suite.

Most patients in the hospital setting are transferred to the surgical suite on a stretcher with the side rails up. In special circumstances (e.g., patients requiring traction, those having some types of orthopedic surgery, those who should be moved as little as possible), the patient is transferred in the hospital bed. Other factors that influence the decision to transfer in a bed are the patient's age, size, and physical condition. In ambulatory settings, patients either walk or are transferred to the surgical suite on a stretcher or in a wheelchair.

◆ Evaluation: Reflecting

Evaluate the care of the preoperative patient based on the identified patient problems. The expected outcomes include that the patient:
- States understanding of the informed consent and preoperative procedures
- Demonstrates postoperative exercises and techniques for prevention of complications
- Verbalizes reduced anxiety

⚐ CLINICAL JUDGMENT CHALLENGE 14-1

Patient-Centered Care (QSEN)

You are caring for a patient who is scheduled for surgery, which must be performed under general anesthesia, to alleviate pain and stabilize the spinal column. During the preoperative assessment in which the patient's husband is present, you ask the patient if she has had anything to eat or drink since midnight. The patient states, "I have not eaten anything since midnight. I only drank a can of soda this morning before I came to the hospital." The patient's husband immediately responds, "This won't keep her from having surgery, will it? I better not have to take off from work another day for this nonsense."
1. What are the possible implications of the patient's consumption of soda before surgery?
2. What is your response to the patient's disclosure that she has consumed a can of soda on the morning of the scheduled surgery?
3. How would you address the husband's response?
4. Would you tell the surgeon about the patient's consumption of soda? Why or why not?
5. What teaching will you provide at this time?

GET READY FOR THE NCLEX® EXAMINATION!

KEY POINTS

Review these Key Points for each NCLEX Examination Client Needs Category.

Safe and Effective Care Environment
- Determine the purpose and expected outcomes of surgery for each patient.
- Assess each patient's risk factors for threats to SAFETY.
- Ensure that proper patient identification occurs (ID bands).
- Use at least two appropriate identifiers (e.g., patient identification number, patient name and/or birthdate as stated by the patient) when providing instruction, administering drugs, marking surgical sites, and performing any procedure. *Do not use room number or bed number to identify the patient.* **QSEN: Safety**
- Validate that the informed consent has been properly executed (signed by the patient, surgeon, and witness as necessary). Confirm that presurgical checklist is complete and accurate.
- Communicate to the perioperative team any physical or laboratory change that may alter the patient's response to drugs, anesthesia, or surgery. **QSEN: Safety**
- Ask the patient to explain in his or her own words which surgical procedure is being done and why.
- If the patient's explanation of the scheduled surgery is not consistent with the documentation, notify the surgeon and request that he or she speak to the patient. **QSEN: Safety**
- Validate correct patient, correct procedure, correct operative site (left, right, spinal level). **QSEN: Safety**
- Confirm that the operative permit or any other legal documents are signed before preoperative drug administration. **Ethics**
- After the patient has received preoperative drugs, keep the side rails up and the bed in the low position. **QSEN: Safety**
- Communicate during hand-off to the operating room personnel all care that has been provided and what care may still be needed.

Health Promotion and Maintenance
- Teach patients about preoperative preparations and specific postoperative interventions to prevent complications (incision splinting, deep-breathing exercises, range-of-motion exercises—as described in Charts 14-4 and 14-5). **QSEN: Patient-Centered Care**

Psychosocial Integrity
- Assess the patient's and family members' knowledge about the scheduled surgical procedure to identify learning needs. **QSEN: Patient-Centered Care**
- Encourage the patient to express his or her feelings regarding the surgical procedure or its possible outcome(s).
- Explain and provide written information for all diagnostic procedures, restrictions, and follow-up care to the patient and his or her family. **Ethics**
- Communicate to the perioperative team any concerns, fears, or preferences the patient has. **Ethics**
- Implement appropriate interventions to reduce patient anxiety.

Physiological Integrity
- Perform a complete and accurate preoperative assessment.
- Ensure that dentures and any other personal items are removed from the patient before he or she is transferred to the surgical suite.
- Apply prescribed antiembolic stockings, sequential compression boots, or other devices to reduce or prevent vascular complications. **QSEN: Evidence-Based Practice**
- Communicate to the perioperative team any physical or laboratory change(s) that may alter the patient's response to drugs, anesthesia, or surgery. **QSEN: Safety**

SELECTED BIBLIOGRAPHY

American Hospital Association (2015). Utilization and volume. In *Trends affecting hospitals and health systems.* http://www.aha.org/research/reports/tw/chartbook/index.shtml.

American Society of Anesthesiologists (2014). *ASA physical status classification system.* https://www.asahq.org/resources/clinical-information/asa-physical-status-classification-system.

Association of periOperative Registered Nurses (AORN) (2011). *Perioperative nursing data set: The perioperative nursing vocabulary* (3rd ed.). Denver: Author.

Association of periOperative Registered Nurses (AORN) (2015). *Correct site surgery tool kit.* https://www.aorn.org/guidelines/clinical-resources/tool-kits/correct-site-surgery-tool-kit.

Association of periOperative Registered Nurses (AORN) (2016a). *Guideline for transfer of patient care information. 2016 guidelines for perioperative practice.* Denver: Author.

Association of periOperative Registered Nurses (AORN) (2016b). *Guideline for preoperative patient skin antisepsis. 2016 guidelines for perioperative practice.* Denver: Author.

Behairy, A. (2015). Nursing students' opinions towards nursing diagnoses. *International Journal of Nursing Didactics, 5*(11), 1–6. doi:10.15520/ijnd.2015.vol5.iss11.112.01-06.

Deiner, S., Westlake, B., & Dutton, R. P. (2014). Patterns of surgical care and complications in the elderly. *Journal of the American Geriatrics Society, 62*(5), 829–835. http://doi.org/10.1111/jgs.12794.

Devereaux, P. J., & Sessler, D. I. (2015). Cardiac complications in patients undergoing major noncardiac surgery. *New England Journal of Medicine, 373,* 2258–2269. doi:10.1056/NEJMra1502824.

Douglas, C., Aroh, D., Colella, J., & Quadri, M. (2016). Value-based care model: Building essentials for value-based purchasing, The Hackensack UMC. *Nursing Administration Quarterly, 40*(1), 51–59. doi:10.1097/NAQ.0000000000000136.

Elpern, E., Killeen, K., Patel, G., & Senecal, G. (2013). The application of intermittent pneumatic compression devices for thromboprophylaxis. *The American Journal of Nursing, 113*(4), 30–36.

Gebremedhn, E. G., & Nagaratnam, V. B. (2014). Audit on preoperative fasting of elective surgical patients in an African academic medical center. *World Journal of Surgery, 38*(9), 2200–2204. http://doi.org/10.1007/s00268-014-2582-3.

Guido, C., Weinberg, D., Wong, H., & Kahn, L. L. (2014). The effect of surgical care improvement project (SCIP) compliance on surgical site infections (SSI). *Medical Care, 52*(2 Suppl. 1), S66–S73.

Hohenberger, H., & Delahanty, K. (2015). Patient-centered care—enhanced recovery after surgery and population health management. *AORN Journal, 102*(6), 578–583.

Kudela, M., Dzvincuk, P., Marek, R., Huml, K., Hejtmanek, P., & Pilka, R. (2015). The gynecological surgery of Jehovah's Witnesses. *Gynecology & Obstetrics (Sunnyvale), 5*(6), 297. doi:10.4172/2161-0932.1000297.

Malley, A., Kenner, C., Kim, T., & Blakeney, B. (2015). The role of the nurse and the preoperative assessment in patient transitions. *AORN Journal, 102*(2), 181.e1–181.e9. http://doi.org/10.1016/j.aorn.2015.06.004.

Markatos, K., Kaseta, M., & Nikolaou, V. S. (2015). Perioperative skin preparation and draping in modern total joint arthroplasty: Current evidence. *Surgical Infections, 16*(3), 221–225. doi:10.1089/sur.2014.097.

Mehta, H., & Chehade, M. (2014). Safety of propofol use in patients with food allergies. *Journal of Allergy and Clinical Immunology, 133* (2 Suppl.), AB152.

Munday, G. S., Deveaux, P., Roberts, H., Fry, D. F., & Polk, H. C. (2014). Impact of implementation of the Surgical Care Improvement Project and future strategies for improving quality in surgery. *The American Journal of Surgery, 208*(5), 835–840.

Oresanya, L. B., Lyons, W. L., & Finlayson, E. (2014). Preoperative assessment of the older patient: A narrative review. *The Journal of the American Medical Association, 311*(20), 2110–2120. doi:10.1001/jama.2014.4573.

Ramly, E., Kaafarani, H. M. A., & Velmanhos, G. C. (2015). The effect of aging on pulmonary function: Implications for monitoring and support of the surgical and trauma patient. *Surgical Clinic of North America, 95,* 53–69. doi.org/10.1016/j.suc.2014.09.009.

Rock, M., & Hoebeke, R. (2014). Informed consent: Whose duty to inform? *Medsurg Nursing, 23*(3), 189–191, 194.

Rothrock, J. (2014). *Alexander's care of the patient in surgery* (15th ed.). St. Louis: Elsevier.

Shah, U., Wong, J., Wong, D. T., & Chung, F. (2016). Preoxygenation and intraoperative ventilation strategies in obese patients: A comprehensive review. *Current Opinion in Anesthesiology, 29*(1), 109–118. doi:10.1097/ACO.0000000000000267.

Touhy, T., & Jett, K. (2015). *Ebersole & Hess' Toward Healthy Aging* (9th ed.). St. Louis: Elsevier.

Wong, S. S. C., & Irwin, M. G. (2016). Peri-operative cardiac protection for non-cardiac surgery. *Anesthesia, 71,* 29–39. doi:10.1111/anae.13305.

Zhao, M., Haley, D. R., Spaulding, A., & Balogh, H. A. (2015). Value-based purchasing, efficiency, and hospital performance. *Health Care Manager, 34*(1), 4–13. doi:10.1097/HCM.0000000000000048.

CHAPTER 15

Care of Intraoperative Patients

Cynthia L. Danko and Rebecca M. Patton

http://evolve.elsevier.com/Iggy/

PRIORITY AND INTERRELATED CONCEPTS

The priority concept for this chapter is SAFETY.

The interrelated concepts for this chapter are:
- GAS EXCHANGE
- TISSUE INTEGRITY
- TEAMWORK AND INTERPROFESSIONAL COLLABORATION

LEARNING OUTCOMES

Safe and Effective Care Environment

1. Collaborate with the interprofessional team to coordinate high-quality care for patients in the intraoperative setting.
2. Maintain SAFETY by using appropriate patient identifiers when administering drugs, ensuring informed consent, and verifying surgical sites during the intraoperative period.
3. Ensure SAFETY by protecting patients from injury, poor thermoregulation, and health care–associated infection during the intraoperative period.

Psychosocial Integrity

4. Implement nursing interventions to minimize stressors for the patient and family regarding the intraoperative experience.

5. Using ethical principles, respond with advocacy to patient and family concerns and needs during the intraoperative period.

Physiological Integrity

6. Apply knowledge of anatomy, physiology, and principles of aging to prioritize care and prevent patient harm resulting from skin breakdown and positioning injury during the intraoperative period.
7. Implement nursing interventions to minimize risk for potential intraoperative emergencies such as malignant hyperthermia, allergic reactions, and cardiac events.

As one of the most complex and demanding environments in the health care setting, the challenges of managing patient care during a surgical procedure in the operating room (OR) requires expertise and TEAMWORK AND INTERPROFESSIONAL COLLABORATION within the perioperative team. Perioperative nursing as a specialty, in the inpatient or ambulatory setting, provides care for patients undergoing operative or other invasive procedures and has a distinct clinical focus. Nursing care during this period affects the patient's physical needs, spiritual needs, comfort, SAFETY, dignity, and psychological status. Patient-centered care is the key to optimal outcomes in the OR. Recognizing the patient as the source of control and including the family in the plan of care plan ensure compassionate and coordinated care based on the preferences, values, and needs of the patient (QSEN, 2016). Specific procedures and policies may differ among hospital and OR settings but should all reflect the standards and recommended practices as established by the

Association of periOperative Registered Nurses (AORN) (2016a). Perioperative nurses practice within a specific, patient-focused model that incorporates professional practice with attainable, measurable outcomes.

The patient undergoing surgery may recognize the experience as a time of great anxiety, fear, and vulnerability. Few other episodes of care put patients in such a defenseless condition as a surgical procedure. Continual communication with the patient provides a level of comfort and control in a situation that seems out of his or her control. Patient engagement and positive patient experiences have been linked to clinical SAFETY and effectiveness (Doyle et al., 2013).

OVERVIEW

The *intraoperative period* begins when the patient enters the surgical suite and ends at the time of transfer to the postanesthesia recovery area, same-day surgery unit, or intensive care unit. The priorities for perioperative nurses are SAFETY and patient advocacy by preventing, reducing, avoiding, and managing the risk factors in the perioperative environment. In the OR the patient is at risk for infection, impaired skin TISSUE INTEGRITY, increased anxiety, inadequate thermoregulation and altered body temperature, and injury related to positioning and other intraoperative interventions. The surgical phase is filled with unfamiliar experiences and uncertain outcomes.

Members of the Surgical Team

The surgical team consists of a multidisciplinary interprofessional cohort of caregivers representing several clinical specialties. Each team member has specific duties in the OR and uses his or her expertise to enhance the care and SAFETY of the perioperative patient. The number of assistants, circulating nurses, and scrub nurses depends on the complexity and length of the surgical procedure. For minor procedures only a circulating nurse and scrub person may be needed in addition to the surgeon. More complex procedures may require additional nursing staff to either circulate or scrub. See Table 15-1, which identifies perioperative team member responsibilities and duties.

The Surgical Suite—Patient and Team Safety

Protecting the patient when he or she is unable to protect himself or herself during surgery is the priority for all members of the surgical team. Patient SAFETY and safety of personnel in the OR are addressed through various means.

Construction and design of the OR suite centers on preventing infection by reducing contaminants through controlled air exchanges in the room, maintaining recommended temperature and humidity levels, and limiting the traffic and activities in the OR by means of sliding door closures and designated traffic patterns.

Electrical and fire SAFETY is an integral part of the design process. Multiple outlets on separate circuits are required to avoid overloads that prevent short circuits and the potential loss of power. The nurse ensures safety through the use of electrical equipment that meets specific standards. All equipment used during surgery must be functional and in proper working condition as determined by the safety procedure of that facility.

Electrosurgical devices are a primary energy source in the OR. Proper placement of grounding pads; inspection of the electrosurgical device; and avoiding patient contact with metal components of the OR table, other electrical equipment, or pooling preparation solutions help to prevent surgical burns and injury.

All OR personnel strive to prevent fire and complications from the use of electrical devices or hazardous substances. Ignition sources, oxidizers, and fuels (commonly referred to as the *fire triangle;* Fig. 15-1A) are present in the OR and increase the risk for fires (Seifert et al., 2015). Such events are rare but can occur during any procedure. Completing a fire risk assessment for each patient is critical to determine the likelihood for a fire occurrence. Eliminating any elements of the fire triangle avoids or minimizes the risk for injury (see Fig. 15-1B). Managing room temperature (between 68° and 73°F [20° to 23°C]) and humidity (30% to 60%) at recommended levels is optimal for fire SAFETY (AORN, 2015a). The entire surgical team must remain knowledgeable of emergency measures to take in the event of a fire.

Patient SAFETY *devices* and nursing interventions are used to manage risk during surgical procedures. Safety straps are required for the patient, and the OR bed is locked in place. Blankets or warming units are used to prevent hypothermia from inadequate thermoregulation, and interventions (e.g., positioning devices, gel pads, frames) are used to prevent skin breakdown and injury during the positioning process.

The OR setting presents multiple occupational hazards that can put the surgical team at risk for injury, resulting in lost work time and potential long-term disability. Working conditions in the OR that could lead to injury include lifting and transferring patients; carrying heavy instrument sets; moving equipment; and exposure to sharps, bloodborne pathogens, anesthetic gases, radiation, and chemicals. Slips, trips, and falls related to clutter in the room; cords on the floor; or wet surfaces can also lead to unsafe conditions in the work environment.

The use of patient-transfer and personal protective equipment (gowns, non-powdered gloves, masks, and eye protection), ongoing monitoring of the environment for trace anesthetic gases, and monitoring of radiation badges worn by personnel (for exposure levels to radiation) and lead shielding are basic safety precautions that are used in the OR to manage personnel safety and minimize known risk factors. Constant awareness of the environment and adherence to practice standards will reduce staff injuries. Observing safety precautions and using safe patient-handling devices to move patients are effective for both patients and staff.

Surgical Suite Layout

The surgical suite is located out of the mainstream of the hospital and adjacent to the postanesthetic care unit (PACU) and support services (e.g., blood bank, pathology, and laboratory departments). Traffic flow is restricted to reduce contamination from outside the suite. Within the suite, clean and contaminated areas are separate. The surgical area is divided into three zones—unrestricted, semi-restricted, and restricted—to ensure proper movement of patients and personnel.

Surgical departments contain areas related to patient care, surgery, surgical support, and staff areas. Patient care areas include an admission or holding area, the ORs, and the PACU. Support areas include instrument storage, cabinets for sterile supplies, separate utility rooms for clean and soiled equipment, and a clean linen room. Staff areas include locker rooms and staff lounges.

The OR is equipped with tables and equipment based on the needs of each patient and the complexity of the procedure. A communication system links the OR with the main desk of the surgical suite, including monitors for in-room cameras and an intercom with separate systems for routine and emergency calls.

OR design continues to evolve as technology advances. The use of computers, video, and digital imaging has transformed ORs into high-tech care settings. Many ORs have voice-activated command systems to operate some equipment and robotic technology that can transmit surgical images to remote sites.

Minimally Invasive and Robotic Surgery

Minimally invasive surgery (MIS) is a common practice and now is the preferred technique for many types of surgery, including cholecystectomy, cardiac surgery, splenectomy, and spinal surgery. It is even being used for cancer surgeries such as the removal of a

TABLE 15-1 Perioperative Team Members—Responsibilities and Duties

TEAM MEMBER	RESPONSIBILITIES	DUTIES/INTERVENTIONS
Surgeon	Manages the surgical procedure and makes surgical judgments about the patient's care	Initiates, participates, and completes the essential components of the surgical procedure
Surgical assistant • Another surgeon • Physician • Physician Assistant/Surgical Assistant • Resident • Intern • Advanced practice nurse • Certified registered nurse first assistant	Under the direction of the surgeon (and within the legal scope of practice for each role/state), the assistant performs specific task during the surgical procedure	The assistant may hold retractors, suction the wound, cut tissue, suture and dress wounds
Anesthesiologist (MD)	Administers anesthetic agents and continually monitors patient status	Plans medications for anesthesia, analgesia, and blocks Monitors major bodily functions (such as breathing, heart rate and rhythm, body temperature, blood pressure, and blood oxygen levels) during surgery Addresses any problems that might arise during surgery
Certified registered nurse anesthetist (CRNA)	Administers anesthetic agents under the supervision of physician (either anesthesiologist or surgeon)	Provides fluids and blood products as needed; medications for anesthesia, analgesia, and blocks; monitors patient during surgery by assessing: • Level of anesthesia (using a peripheral nerve stimulator) • Cardiopulmonary function (electrocardiographic [ECG] monitoring) • Capnography (monitors ventilation for nonintubated patients) • Vital signs • Intake and output
Circulator—registered nurse	Uses clinical decision-making skills to develop a plan of care and coordinates care delivery to patients and their family members; coordinates, oversees, and implements nursing care interventions to support the patient during the surgical procedure	Sets up the operating room, gathers supplies, anticipates equipment needed, and inspects all equipment for safety and functionality; prepares positioning devices and ensures that the physical environment is clean and at the proper temperature for the patient's arrival Throughout the surgery the circulating nurse: • Protects the patient's privacy • Ensures the patient's safety • Monitors traffic in the room • Assess urinary output and blood loss • Communicates finding to surgeon and anesthesiologist • Monitors sterile field and provides sterile supplies and medications to the sterile field • Anticipates the patient's and surgical team's needs • Communicates patient's status to family member(s) per protocol • Documents care, events, interventions, and findings
Scrub person—registered nurse or certified surgical technologist (CST)	Provides patient care at the surgical field, assisting the surgeon and assistants; maintains the integrity, safety, and efficiency of the sterile field during the procedure	Sets up the sterile field, hands up sterile instrumentation/equipment With the circulating nurse, maintains accurate count of sponges, sharps, and instruments and monitors the amount of irrigation fluid and medication used
Specialty team members (e.g., cardiac, orthopedic, ophthalmology)	Provide patient care in surgical specialty areas; assess, maintain, and recommend equipment, instruments, and supplies used in that specialty	May circulate or scrub on procedures in a specific surgical specialty; participate in scheduling process for surgical cases and organize personnel in the clinical specialty area
Laser nurse	Coordinates activities and equipment for surgical cases using laser technology	Functions as coordinator for laser cases, monitors laser function, maintains safety, and completes documentation required for a laser log
Perfusionist	Specialized health care professional who uses the heart-lung machine during cardiac surgery and other surgeries that require cardiopulmonary bypass to manage the patient's physiological status.	Sets up heart-lung machine and continually monitors and manages the patient's blood flow, fluids, and electrolyte levels just before, during, and on completion of the cardiac bypass procedure

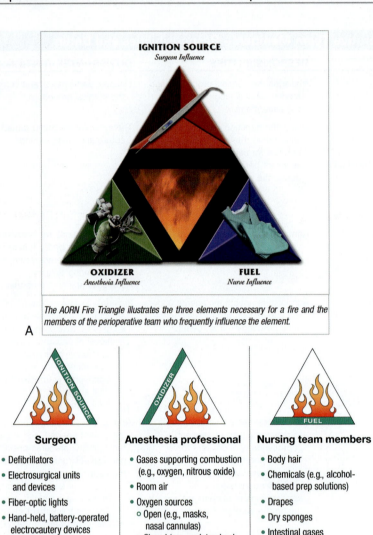

FIG. 15-1 A, Fire Triangle from Association of periOperative Nurses. (AORN). **B,** Role of team members in managing components of the fire triangle. (**A** reprinted with permission from *Guidelines for Perioperative Practice.* Copyright © 2017, AORN, Inc, 2170 S. Parker Road, Suite 400, Denver, CO 80231. All rights reserved. **B** from Seifert, P. C., Peterson, E., Graham, K. [2015]. Crisis management of fire in the OR. *AORN Journal*, Feb; 101[2]:250-63. DOI: 10.1016/j.aorn.2014.11.002.)

lung lobe (lobectomy) or even the entire lung (pneumonectomy) and colectomy. Benefits of MIS include reduced surgery time for some surgeries, smaller incisions, reduced blood loss, faster recovery time, and less pain after surgery.

During MIS one or more small incisions are made in the surgical area, and an **endoscope** (a tube that allows viewing and manipulation of internal body areas) is placed through the opening (Fig. 15-2). These instruments may be rigid, semi-rigid, or flexible and usually have self-contained light sources. Endoscopes have different functions and configurations for different surgical purposes. For example, laparoscopes are used for abdominal surgery, arthroscopes are used for joint surgery, and ureteroscopes are used for urinary tract surgery.

In addition to being used for examination and obtaining specimens for biopsy, endoscopes can be used for organ removal, reconstruction, blood vessel grafting, and many other procedures. Cutting, suturing, stapling, cautery, and laser surgery can all be performed through or with endoscopes. An important

part of MIS for abdominal surgery, pelvic surgery, and surgery in some other body cavity areas is injecting gas or air into the cavity before the surgery to separate organs and improve visualization. This injection is known as **insufflation** and may contribute to complications and patient discomfort. This factor is considered when deciding whether to perform a procedure by traditional surgery or endoscopy.

Patient preparation for endoscopic surgery is similar to the preparation for the same procedure when performed by open surgical methods. An endoscopic surgical procedure has a chance for becoming an open surgical procedure, depending on which patient- or procedure-related variables are discovered or develop during the surgery.

Robotic technology takes MIS to a new level and is changing how surgery is performed and how the OR is organized. Many gynecologic, urologic, and cardiovascular procedures are being performed by using robotics. The robotic system consists of a console, surgical arm cart, and video cart (Fig. 15-3). The

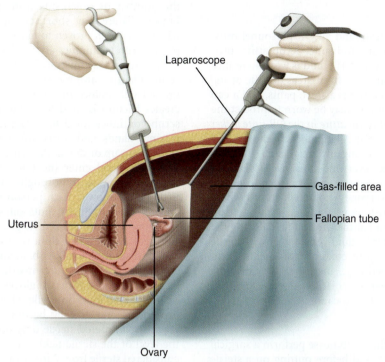

FIG. 15-2 How an operative laparoscope is used.

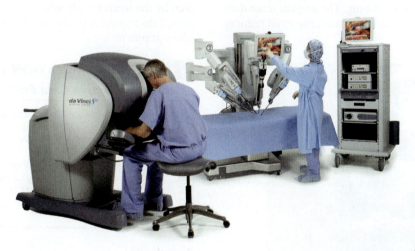

FIG. 15-3 Operating room layout for robotic surgery with da Vinci Robotic Surgery System. (©2016 Intuitive Surgical, Inc.)

surgeon first inserts the required instruments and positions the articulating arms; he or she then breaks scrub and performs the surgery while sitting at the console. A three-dimensional (3-D) view of the patient's anatomy allows precise control and dexterity. This new technology requires additional education for the perioperative nurse.

Mechanical trauma and thermal injury are two types of injury that a patient can incur during MIS and robotic surgery (The Joint Commission, 2014). Both MIS and robotic surgery are limited by the cost of special equipment, OR settings, and the lengthy training and practice periods for the surgeon to become proficient in even one procedure using these methods.

Health and Hygiene of the Surgical Team

People are a source of contamination in the surgical setting from the bacteria on skin, on hair, and in the airways. To avoid transmitting these organisms to the patient, policies and procedures for special health standards and dress must be followed. All members of the surgical team and support personnel in the surgical suite must be free of communicable diseases. No one who has an open wound, cold, or any infection should participate in surgery.

Good personal hygiene and frequent handwashing help prevent and control infection. Jewelry carries many organisms and should be minimal. All personnel must wash their hands before and after contact with patients and performing procedures. Hands of surgical personnel may be cultured on a regular basis to assess for potential health care–associated infections and to identify sources of pathogens. Further interventions or cultures are needed if quality reports indicate a problem. Adhering to proper surgical attire policies and the surgical scrub protocols also helps prevent contaminations.

Surgical Attire

All members of the surgical team and all OR personnel must wear scrub attire while in the surgical suite. Scrub attire, provided by the hospital, is clean, not sterile, and is worn to reduce contamination and risk for infection from areas outside of the surgical setting. Basic surgical attire is a shirt, pants, and a cap or hood (Fig. 15-4). Shoe coverings may be worn to protect the shoes. *Staff change into clean surgical attire in the OR suite locker rooms, not at home* (AORN, 2016b). All members of the surgical team must cover their hair, including any facial hair.

In addition to basic attire, everyone must wear personal protective equipment (mask, eyewear, non-powdered gloves, head covering, and gown). Everyone who enters an OR where a sterile field is present must wear a mask. Surgical team members who are scrubbed and at the surgical field during the surgery must also wear a sterile fluid-resistant gown, sterile non-powdered gloves, and eye protectors or face shields. Team members who are *not* scrubbed (e.g., anesthesia provider, circulating nurse) may wear cover scrub jackets that are snapped or buttoned closed and eyewear, as warranted.

Surgical Scrub

The surgeon, assistants, and the scrub nurse perform a surgical scrub after putting on a mask and before putting on a sterile gown and non-powdered gloves (Fig. 15-5). Rings, watches, and bracelets are removed before scrubbing. *The surgical scrub does not make the skin sterile.* Correctly performed, the scrub reduces the number of organisms from the hands, arms, and nails. Fingernails are kept short, clean, and healthy. Artificial nails, which have been proven to harbor organisms even after appropriate scrub techniques are used, should not be worn.

A surgical antimicrobial solution is used for the surgical scrub. Plain or antimicrobial soap is used for washing hands immediately before the surgical scrub. Vigorous rubbing that creates friction is used from the fingertips to the elbow. The scrub continues for 3 to 5 minutes, followed by a rinse. For rinsing, hands and arms are positioned so water runs off, rather than up or down, the arms (AORN, 2016c). After scrubbing, personnel enter the OR with their hands held higher than the elbows and thoroughly dry their hands and forearms with a sterile towel. Each person is then assisted into a sterile gown *("gowning")* and puts on sterile non-powdered gloves *("gloving")*. Alcohol-based surgical scrub products will reduce transient and resident flora on the hands as effectively as the standard surgical scrub with an antimicrobial agent when used according to manufacturer instructions (Shen et al., 2015).

Gowns, non-powdered gloves, and materials used at the operative field must be sterile. These items are changed between procedures and as they become contaminated. The surgical gown is considered sterile only on the front from the chest to the level of the sterile field. The entire sleeves of the gown are considered sterile from 2 inches above the elbow to the cuff. The back of the gown is not considered sterile because it cannot be seen by the wearer. Only when they are properly scrubbed and attired do members of the surgical team handle sterile drapes and equipment.

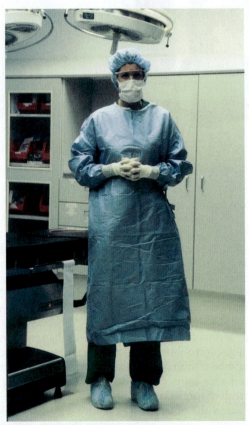

FIG. 15-4 Typical attire for all scrubbed personnel. Note complete hair covering, eye shields, mask, and the sterile gloves over the sleeves of the sterile gown. Note that, when not in use, the hands are typically folded in front of the body, never below the waist.

❓ NCLEX EXAMINATION CHALLENGE 15-1

Safe and Effective Care Environment

A scrub person is discussing artificial nail use with the nurse. The scrub person states, "I do not use artificial nails; I'm wearing gel polish to strengthen my nails." What is the appropriate nursing response?
A. "I understand. That is my nail treatment of choice also."
B. "Hand hygiene is enhanced by covering natural nails."
C. "Wear double gloves to prevent puncture or contamination."
D. "Gel polish is a type of artificial nail that alters skin flora and impedes hand hygiene."

Anesthesia

Anesthesia reduces or temporarily eliminates sensory perception. Anesthesia administration has evolved into a precise science. Anesthesia providers include an anesthesiologist, a certified registered nurse anesthetist (CRNA) working under the direction of an anesthesiologist or another physician, or an anesthesiologist assistant (AA)—(working under the direction of an anesthesiologist).

Anesthesia is an induced state of partial or total loss of sensory perception, with or without loss of consciousness. The purposes of anesthesia are to block nerve impulse transmission, suppress reflexes, promote muscle relaxation and, in some cases, achieve a controlled level of unconsciousness. Anesthesia providers document medications given, vital signs, and other interventions during the procedure in a separate section of the electronic health record.

Usually the anesthesia provider selects the type of anesthesia to be used after consulting with the patient and surgeon and after considering specific patient risk factors. The nurse and the

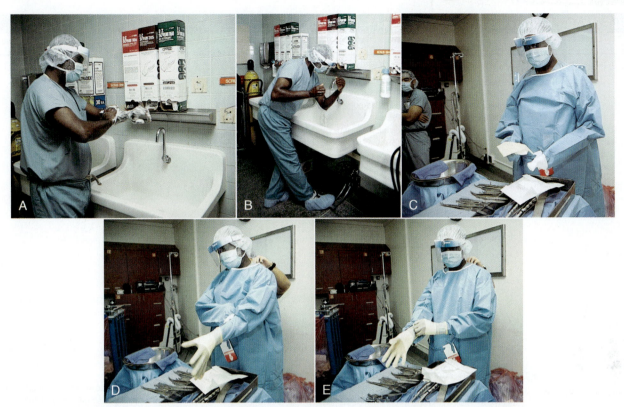

FIG. 15-5 The scrubbing, gowning, and gloving process. **A,** The surgical scrub. **B,** Rinsing. Note the water falling off the hands and arms. Also note the foot-operated handle that controls the water flow. (After scrubbing and rinsing, the scrub nurse dries his hands and arms with a sterile towel inside the operating room and then is assisted into a sterile gown.) **C,** The scrub nurse prepares sterile non-powdered gloves. Note that the scrub nurse's hands are *inside* the sleeve of the gown and that he is touching the sterile gloves only with the sterile sleeve. **D,** The scrub nurse puts on his first sterile glove while the sterile gown is being tied in the back. Note again that his hand never emerges from under the sterile sleeve. **E,** The scrub nurse puts on his second sterile glove.

anesthesia provider collaborate to assess and address the patient's preferences and fears about the anesthesia intervention. Patient health problems are factors in the selection and dose of anesthetic. Selection is also influenced by:

1. Type and duration of the procedure
2. Area of the body having surgery
3. SAFETY issues to prevent injury, such as airway management
4. Status of procedure (elective, emergent)
5. Pain management options after surgery
6. How long it has been since the patient ate, had any liquids, or had any drugs
7. Patient position needed for the surgical procedure
8. Requirement of the patient to be alert enough to follow instructions during surgery
9. Patient's previous responses and reactions to anesthesia

The physical status of a patient is ranked according to a classification system developed by the American Society of Anesthesiologists (ASA). The anesthesiologist assesses the patient and assigns him or her to one of six categories based on current health and the presence of diseases and disorders. The categories rank patients in a range from a totally healthy patient (ASA1 ranking) to a patient who is brain dead (ASA6 ranking) (American Society of Anesthesiologists, 2014) (see Chapter 14, Table 14-4). This system is used to estimate potential risks during surgery and patient outcomes.

Anesthesia care begins with selecting and administering preoperative drugs (see Chapter 14). The nurse must know the actions of the drugs used, contraindications, and their effects during and after surgery. Anesthetic agents affect many systems and have the potential to negatively impact other health conditions. For example, most anesthetics are metabolized by the liver and excreted by the kidneys. Liver or kidney impairment increases anesthetic effects and the risk for toxicity. In addition, interactions may occur between the anesthetics and other drugs the patient has received.

Anesthesia can be induced in many ways (Table 15-2). The most common forms of anesthesia used in North America include general, regional, and local anesthesia. Less commonly used forms include hypnosis, cryothermia (use of cold), and acupuncture.

General Anesthesia

General anesthesia is a reversible loss of consciousness induced by inhibiting neuronal impulses in areas of the central nervous system (CNS). This state can be achieved with a single agent or a combination of agents. General anesthesia depresses the CNS, resulting in **analgesia** (pain relief or pain suppression), **amnesia** (memory loss of the surgery), and unconsciousness. General anesthesia is used most often in surgery of the head, neck, upper torso, and abdomen. For certain procedures, muscle relaxation is also required. This is achieved with paralytic agents.

TABLE 15-2	Features of Various Types of Anesthesia
TYPE	**FEATURES**
General: inhalation	Most controllable method
	Suppresses central nervous system activity and results in unconsciousness
	Medications administered either as inhalation agents, intravenous, or combination of the two
	Inhalation agents either inhaled through a breathing mask or endotracheal tube
	Intravenous medications given
	Induction and reversal accomplished with pulmonary ventilation
	Must be used in combination with other anesthetic agents for painful or prolonged procedures
	Limited muscle relaxant effects
	Postoperative nausea and shivering common
General: intravenous	Rapid and pleasant induction
	Low incidence of postoperative nausea and vomiting
	Must be metabolized and excreted from the body for complete reversal
	Contraindicated in presence of liver or kidney disease
	Increased cardiac and respiratory depression
Balanced	Minimal disturbance to physiologic function
	Can be used with older and high-risk patients
	Drug interactions can occur
Regional or local: spinal, epidural, nerve block	Local anesthetic agent injected around major nerves or the spinal cord to block sensation and pain from limited part of the body
	Allows participation and cooperation by the patient
	Gag and cough reflexes stay intact
	Less disruption of physical and emotional body functions
	No way to control agent after administration
	Increased nervous system stimulation (overdose)
	Not practical for extensive procedures because of the amount of drug that would be required to maintain anesthesia
	Often used for lower abdominal, pelvic, rectal, or lower-extremity surgery; involves injecting a single dose of the anesthetic agent directly into the spinal cord in the lower back, causing numbness in the lower body

Stages of General Anesthesia. Induction of general anesthesia involves four stages. Table 15-3 lists the expected patient responses and nursing care for each stage. The speed of **emergence** (recovery from the anesthesia) depends on the anesthetic agent, the duration of anesthesia administration, and whether a reversal agent is used. Gagging, vomiting, and restlessness may occur during emergence, although not all patients have these responses. Suction equipment must be available at all times. During recovery, shivering, rigidity, and slight cyanosis may occur. These responses are caused by a temporary change in the body's thermoregulation. The nurse provides warm blankets, radiant heat, and oxygen to decrease the effects of emergence.

Administration of General Anesthesia. General anesthesia agents are administered by inhalation and IV injection. A combination of types of agents (balanced anesthesia) is used to provide hypnosis, amnesia, analgesia, muscle relaxation, and reduced reflexes with minimal disturbance of physiologic function. This method provides safe and controlled anesthetic delivery, especially for older and high-risk patients. An example of balanced anesthesia is the use of thiopental or propofol for induction, morphine or fentanyl for analgesia, and pancuronium or rocuronium for muscle relaxation. Agent selection is based on the individual patient risks (age, comorbidities, airway issues, anesthesia history, and current drugs) and the specific surgical procedure (type and duration of procedure).

Other drugs such as hypnotics, opioid analgesics, and neuromuscular blocking agents may be used as part of the anesthesia plan. Hypnotics and opioid analgesics can be used for sedation before surgery, for IV moderate sedation for short procedures, and as an adjunct to general anesthesia during surgery. The neuromuscular blocking agents are used to relax the jaw and vocal cords immediately after induction so the endotracheal tube can be placed. These drugs also may be used during surgery to provide continued muscle relaxation.

Complications of General Anesthesia. Complications can range from minor harm (e.g., sore throat) to death. Improvement in anesthesia care and surgical techniques has resulted in a decline in anesthesia-related deaths, even among higher-risk patients. Although the anesthesia provider has the main responsibility for monitoring patient responses during surgery, the circulating nurse also remains alert for changes in the patient's condition.

Malignant hyperthermia (MH), an inherited muscle disorder, is an acute, life-threatening complication of certain drugs used for general anesthesia. It is characterized by many problems, including inadequate thermoregulation. The reaction begins in skeletal muscles exposed to the drugs, causing increased calcium levels in muscle cells and increased muscle metabolism. Serum calcium and potassium levels are increased, as is the metabolic rate, leading to acidosis, cardiac dysrhythmias, and a high body temperature.

MH may start immediately after anesthesia induction, several hours into the procedure, or even after anesthesia is completed. Symptoms, caused by increased muscle calcium and increased metabolism, include tachycardia, dysrhythmias, muscle rigidity of the jaw and upper chest, hypotension, tachypnea, skin mottling, cyanosis, and **myoglobinuria** (muscle proteins in the urine). The most sensitive indication is an unexpected rise in the end-tidal carbon dioxide level with a decrease in oxygen saturation and tachycardia. Extremely elevated temperature, as high as 111.2°F (44°C), is a late sign of MH. Survival depends on early diagnosis and the immediate

TABLE 15-3 The Four Stages of General Anesthesia and Related Nursing Interventions

DESCRIPTION	NURSING INTERVENTIONS	RATIONALES
Stage 1 (Analgesia and Sedation, Relaxation)		
Begins with induction and ends with loss of consciousness.	Close operating room doors, dim the lights, and control traffic in the operating room.	Avoiding external stimuli in the environment promotes relaxation.
Patient feels drowsy and dizzy, has a reduced sensation to pain, and is amnesic.	Position patient securely with safety belts.	Using safety measures in stage 1 prepares for stage 2.
Hearing is exaggerated.	Keep discussions about the patient to a minimum.	Being sensitive to the patient maintains his or her dignity.
Stage 2 (Excitement, Delirium)		
Begins with loss of consciousness and ends with relaxation, regular breathing, and loss of the eyelid reflex.	Avoid auditory and physical stimuli.	Sensory stimuli can contribute to the patient's response.
Patient may have irregular breathing, increased muscle tone, and involuntary movement of the extremities.	Protect the extremities.	Safety measures help prevent injury.
Laryngospasm or vomiting may occur.	Assist the anesthesiologist or CRNA with suctioning as needed.	Adequate suctioning of vomitus can prevent aspiration.
Patient is susceptible to external stimuli.	Stay with patient.	Staying with the patient is emotionally supportive.
Stage 3 (Operative Anesthesia, Surgical Anesthesia)		
Begins with generalized muscle relaxation and ends with loss of reflexes and depression of vital functions.	Assist the anesthesiologist or CRNA with intubation.	Providing assistance helps promote smooth intubation and prevent injury.
The jaw is relaxed, and breathing is quiet and regular. The patient cannot hear. Sensations (i.e., to pain) are lost.	Place patient into operative position. Prepare (scrub) the patient's skin over the operative site as directed.	Performing procedures as soon as possible promotes time management to minimize total anesthesia time for the patient.
Stage 4 (Danger)		
Begins with depression of vital functions and ends with respiratory failure, cardiac arrest, and possible death. Respiratory muscles are paralyzed; apnea occurs. Pupils are fixed and dilated.	Prepare for and assist in treatment of cardiac and/or pulmonary arrest. Document occurrence in the patient's chart.	Teamwork and preparedness help decrease injuries and complications and promote the possibility of a desired outcome for the patient.

CRNA, Certified registered nurse anesthetist.

actions of the entire surgical team. Dantrolene sodium, a skeletal muscle relaxant, is the drug of choice along with other interventions (Rosenberg et al., 2015).

? NCLEX EXAMINATION CHALLENGE 15-2
Safe and Effective Care Environment

Which emergency care does the nurse recognize that will be implemented for a client with malignant hyperthermia? **Select all that apply.**
A. Removal of endotracheal tube
B. Cessation (stopping) of surgery when possible
C. Insertion of Foley catheter to monitor urine output
D. Transfer of patient to intensive care unit when stabilized
E. Assessment of arterial blood gases (ABGs) for respiratory alkalosis
F. Use of active cooling techniques such as a cooling blanket and ice packs around the axillae and groin

! NURSING SAFETY PRIORITY QSEN
Critical Rescue

Recognize that you must monitor patients for the cluster of elevated end-tidal carbon dioxide level, decreased oxygen saturation, and tachycardia to identify symptoms of malignant hyperthermia. If these changes begin, respond by alerting the surgeon and anesthesia provider immediately.

When the patient has a known history for MH, treatment with dantrolene can begin before, during, and after surgery to prevent it. Chart 15-1 lists best practices for care of the patient with MH. AORN recommends that all ORs have a dedicated MH cart containing drugs for management (normal saline, dantrolene, sodium bicarbonate, insulin, 50% dextrose, lidocaine, calcium chloride), a protocol card listing interventions, and the MH hotline number. Additional nursing care and anesthesia support are needed during this perioperative emergency.

🧬 GENETIC/GENOMIC CONSIDERATIONS
Patient-Centered Care QSEN

Malignant hyperthermia (MH) is a genetic disorder with an autosomal-dominant pattern of inheritance. The patient with a genetic predisposition for MH is at risk when exposed to halothane, enflurane, isoflurane, desflurane, sevoflurane, and succinylcholine. The problem is most common in young adult males (despite the autosomal-dominant pattern of inheritance) because of gender differences in muscle mass. The muscle biopsy tested with the caffeine halothane contracture test (CHCT) is still considered the most commonly used MH test (Rosenberg et al., 2015). There is also a genetic test that is performed on blood to assess whether a mutation in the *RYR1* gene is present. Usually the cost of the genetic test is not covered by insurance. Always ask the patient about any previous problems or difficulties with anesthesia.

CHART 15-1 Best Practice for Patient Safety & Quality Care QSEN

Emergency Care of the Patient With Malignant Hyperthermia

- Stop all volatile inhalation anesthetic agents and succinylcholine.
- If an endotracheal tube (ET) is not already in place, intubate immediately.
- Ventilate the patient with 100% oxygen at the highest possible flow rate to flush anesthetics and lower end-tidal carbon dioxide.
- Administer dantrolene sodium (Dantrium) IV at a dose of 2 to 3 mg/kg. Repeat as needed.
- If possible, terminate surgery. If termination is not possible, maintain general anesthesia with IV anesthetic agents that do not trigger malignant hyperthermia (MH) (IV sedatives, narcotics, amnestics and nondepolarizing neuromuscular blockers).
- Assess arterial blood gases (ABGs) and serum chemistries for metabolic acidosis and hyperkalemia.
- If metabolic acidosis is evident by ABG analysis, administer sodium bicarbonate IV.
- If hyperkalemia is present, administer 10 units of regular insulin in 50 mL of 50% dextrose IV.
- Use active cooling techniques:
  - Administer iced saline (0.9% NaCl) IV at a rate of 15 mL/kg every 15 minutes as needed.
  - Apply a cooling blanket over the torso.
  - Pack bags of ice around the patient's axillae, groin, neck, and head.
  - Lavage the stomach, bladder, rectum, and open body cavities with sterile iced normal saline.
- Insert a nasogastric tube and a rectal tube.
- Monitor core body temperature to assess effectiveness of interventions and avoid hypothermia.
- Monitor cardiac rhythm by electrocardiography (ECG) to assess for dysrhythmias.
- Insert a Foley catheter to monitor urine output.
- Treat any dysrhythmias that do not resolve on correction of hyperthermia and hyperkalemia with antidysrhythmic agents. Avoid *calcium channel blockers*.
- Administer intravenous fluids at a rate and volume sufficient to maintain urine output above 2 mL/kg/hr.
- Monitor urine for presence of blood or myoglobin.
- If urine output falls below 2 mL/kg/hr, consider using osmotic or loop diuretics, depending on the patient's cardiac and kidney status.
- Contact the Malignant Hyperthermia Association of the United States (MHAUS) hotline for more information regarding treatment: (800) 644-9737.
- Transfer the patient to the intensive care unit (ICU) when stable.
- Continue to monitor the patient's temperature, ECG, ABGs, electrolytes, creatine kinase, coagulation studies, and serum and urine myoglobin levels until they have remained normal for 24 hours.
- Instruct the patient and family about testing for MH risk.
- Refer the patient and family to the Malignant Hyperthermia Association of the United States at (800) 986-4287 or www.mhaus.org.
- Report the incident to the North American Malignant Hyperthermia Registry at the Malignant Hyperthermia Association of the United States: (800) 644-9737.

Data from Malignant Hyperthermia Association of the United States. (2016). *Managing an MH crisis.* http://www.mhaus.org/healthcare-professionals/managing-a-crisis.

Overdose of anesthetic can occur if the patient's metabolism and drug elimination are slower than expected, such as with patients who are older or who have liver or kidney problems. Drugs (e.g., antihypertensives, diuretics, and herbal supplements) can alter metabolism, and interactions can occur between the anesthetic and the patient's regular drugs. Accurate information about the patient's height, weight, and medical history, especially liver and kidney function, is vital in determining the anesthetic type and dosage.

Unrecognized hypoventilation is an anesthesia-induced complication. Failure of adequate GAS EXCHANGE can lead to cardiac arrest, permanent brain damage, and death. Monitoring standards include the use of capnography (an end-tidal carbon dioxide monitor) to confirm carbon dioxide levels in the patient's expired gas (Spiegel, 2013) and a breathing system–disconnect monitor to detect any break in the breathing circuit equipment.

Intubation complications can include many problems (e.g., broken teeth and caps, swollen lip, vocal cord trauma). Difficult intubation may be caused by anatomic issues or disease presence (e.g., small oral cavity, tight jaw joint, tumor). Improper neck extension during intubation may cause injury. The surgeon should be in the OR during the intubation process in case of complications. In difficult airway situations, a tracheotomy may be needed if the endotracheal tube (ET) is unable to be placed. Intubation causes tracheal irritation and edema. A common complaint after surgery is a sore throat.

Local or Regional Anesthesia

Local or regional anesthesia briefly disrupts sensory nerve impulse transmission, providing a reversible regional loss of sensation in a predetermined area of the body to reduce pain and facilitate the surgical procedure (Gmyrek & Elston, 2015). Motor function may or may not be affected. The patient remains conscious and can follow instructions. The gag and cough reflexes remain intact, and the risk for aspiration is low. This type of anesthesia may be supplemented with sedatives, opioid analgesics, or hypnotics to reduce anxiety and increase comfort. The OR nurse provides the patient with information, directions, and emotional support before, during, and after the procedure.

Local Anesthesia. Local anesthesia is delivered topically (applied to the skin or mucous membranes of the area to be anesthetized) and by local infiltration (injected directly *into* the tissue around an incision, wound, or lesion). The term *local anesthesia* may mean *any* form of anesthesia that is not general or monitored anesthesia.

Regional Anesthesia. Regional anesthesia is a type of local anesthesia that blocks multiple peripheral nerves and reduces sensation in a specific body region. It can be used for a variety of conditions and procedures. Anesthesia and surgeon preference along with patient input can determine the use of regional anesthetics. Regional anesthesia is often used when pain management after surgery is desired such as after a total knee replacement. If the patient has eaten and the surgery is an emergency, it may be possible to perform surgery with the patient under regional anesthesia to decrease the risk for aspiration. Regional anesthesia includes field block, nerve block, spinal, and epidural (Table 15-4). Figs. 15-6 and 15-7 show common sites of nerve blocks, spinal anesthesia, and epidural anesthesia.

The nurse's role in providing regional anesthesia includes:
- Assisting the anesthesia provider
- Positioning the patient comfortably and safely
- Offering information and reassurance
- Staying with the patient and providing emotional support
- Observing for breaks in sterile technique
- Recognizing and responding to signs and symptoms of possible reactions to the anesthetics

Complications of Local or Regional Anesthesia. Complications of local or regional anesthesia are related to patient sensitivity to the anesthetic agent (anaphylaxis), incorrect delivery technique, systemic absorption, and overdose. Complications seen early after administration of a local anesthetic agent include edema and inflammation. Abscess formation, tissue necrosis, and/or gangrene may occur later. Abscesses result from contamination during injection of the agent. Necrosis and gangrene may occur as a result of prolonged blood vessel constriction in the injected area.

Systemic toxicity of a local agent may result in adverse reactions in the central nervous and cardiovascular systems (Gmyrek & Elston, 2015). The nurse continually assesses for restlessness; excitement; incoherent speech; headache; blurred vision; metallic taste; nausea; tremors; seizures; and increased pulse, respiration, and blood pressure. Interventions include establishing an open airway, giving oxygen, and notifying the surgeon. Usually a fast-acting barbiturate is needed for treatment. If the toxic reaction is untreated, unconsciousness, hypotension, apnea, cardiac arrest, and death may result.

Cardiac arrest may occur as a rare complication of spinal anesthesia. Epinephrine is given to prevent cardiac arrest in patients who develop sudden, unexplained bradycardia.

Moderate Sedation

Moderate sedation (conscious sedation) is the IV delivery of sedative, hypnotic, and opioid drugs to reduce sensory perception but allow the patient to maintain a patent airway. The amnesia action is short, and the patient has a rapid return to normal function and activities. Etomidate (Amidate), diazepam (Valium, Vivol ♣, Novo-Dipam ♣), midazolam (Versed), fentanyl (Sublimaze), alfentanil (Alfenta), propofol (Diprivan), and morphine sulfate are the most commonly used drugs. Moderate sedation is used to reduce the level of consciousness during minor surgical procedures, endoscopy, cardiac catheterization, closed fracture reduction, and cardioversion.

Selection of patients for moderate sedation is based on specific criteria. The physician determines whether the patient is a candidate. In most states, a registered nurse may administer moderate sedation under physician supervision and within the state-defined scope of nursing practice. Additional credentialing is required, which may include advanced training in IV drug delivery, airway management, and advanced cardiac life support (ACLS).

The nurse monitors the patient during and after the procedure for response to the procedure and the drugs. The airway, level of consciousness, oxygen saturation, capnography (measure of carbon dioxide level), electrocardiogram (ECG) status, and vital signs are monitored every 15 to 30 minutes until the patient is awake and oriented and vital signs have returned to baseline levels (AORN, 2016d).

The nurse performs evaluation of consciousness during and after moderate sedation. A variety of sedation scales are available to use based on patient and procedural situations. The Ramsay Sedation Scale (RSS) was developed for ICU patients and is one of the scoring systems most widely used during moderate sedation (Lazear, 2014). Additional scales are listed in Table 15-5. Each scale has specific patient responses or behaviors to a continuum of environmental stimulation indicating degree of arousal from sedation or readiness for discharge.

TABLE 15-4	**Types of Regional Anesthesia**
ANESTHESIA TYPE	**DEFINITION AND COMMON USE**
Field block	Series of injections *around* the operative field
	Most commonly used for chest procedures, hernia repair, dental surgery, and some plastic surgeries
Nerve block	Injection of the local anesthetic agent *into* or *around* one nerve or group of nerves in the involved area
	Most commonly used for limb surgery or to relieve chronic pain
Spinal anesthesia	Injection of an anesthetic agent into the cerebrospinal fluid in the subarachnoid space
	Most commonly used for lower abdominal, pelvic, hip, and knee surgery
Epidural anesthesia	Injection of an agent into the epidural space (see Fig. 15-7)
	Most commonly used for anorectal, vaginal, perineal, hip, and lower-extremity surgeries

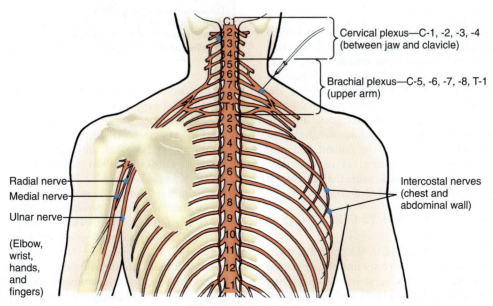

FIG. 15-6 Nerve block sites.

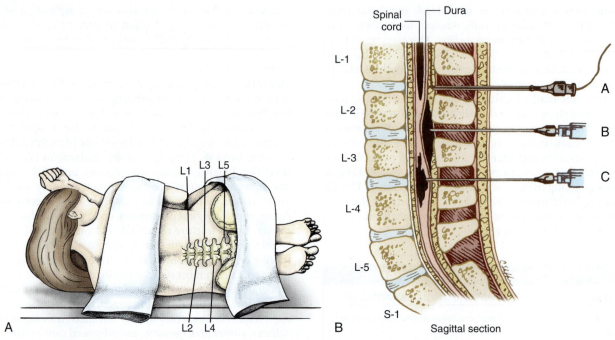

FIG. 15-7 Administration of spinal and epidural anesthesia. (**B** from Rothrock, J. [2014]. *Alexander's care of the patient in surgery* [15th ed.]. St. Louis: Elsevier.)

TABLE 15-5   Scales Used to Evaluate Patient Responses to Moderate Sedation

Interprocedural Scales (Used During Procedure to Assess Level of Sedation)

- Modified Observer's Assessment of Alertness/Sedation Scale
- Ramsay Sedation Scale (RSS)
- Sedation-Agitation Score
- Richmond Agitation-Sedation Scale (RASS)
- Motor Activity Assessment Scale

Postprocedure Scales (Used After Procedure to Determine Readiness for Discharge)

- Postanesthesia Discharge Scoring System (PADSS)
- Modified Postanesthesia Discharge Scoring System (MPADSS)
- Modified Aldrete Score

The patient receiving IV moderate sedation can be discharged to home with a responsible adult if capnography indicates GAS EXCHANGE is adequate and arousal from sedation is at a preprocedural level. If the patient returns to the general medical-surgical nursing unit, the unit nurses continue monitoring. The patient is expected to be sleepy but arousable for several hours after the procedure. Oral intake is not permitted until 30 minutes after the patient received the last dose of sedation or according to the physician's orders. If the patient had oral endoscopy, return of the gag reflex is required before oral intake. When fluids are permitted, the nurse makes sure that the patient is awake and positioned upright to avoid aspiration.

❖ INTERPROFESSIONAL COLLABORATIVE CARE
◆ Assessment: Noticing

History. On arrival in the surgical suite, the patient is taken to the preoperative holding area or directly into the operating suite. The preoperative holding area nurse or the circulating nurse greets the patient on arrival. **As indicated in The Joint**

Commission's National Patient Safety Goals (NPSGs), *correct identification of the patient is the responsibility of every member of the health care team.* Check the patient's identification bracelet and ask, "What is your name and birthdate?" This practice prevents errors by drowsy or confused patients. For example, avoid asking a patient, "Are you Mr. Gates?" He may respond inappropriately if he is anxious or sedated. The nurse always validates patient identification for safety using two unique identifiers. The electronic health record and identification bracelet should be consistent with the information the patient shares with the perioperative staff.

> **! NURSING SAFETY PRIORITY** **QSEN**
>
> ***Action Alert***
>
> The Joint Commission's NPSGs require that you verify the patient's identity with two types of identifiers (name, date of birth, electronic health record number, telephone number, or other person-specific identifier). Ask the patient to tell you his or her name.

After completing the identification process, the nurse validates that the surgical consent form has been signed and witnessed. The nurse asks, "What kind of operation are you having today?" to ascertain that the patient's perception of the procedure, the surgical consent, the surgeon's order, and the operative schedule are the same. *When the procedure involves a specific site, validating the side on which a procedure is to be performed (e.g., for amputation, cataract removal, hernia repair) is the responsibility of each health care professional before and at the time of surgery. The Joint Commission now recommends that the patient and the licensed independent practitioner who is ultimately accountable for the procedure and will be present during the procedure (usually the surgeon performing the surgery) mark the surgical site (The Joint Commission [TJC], 2017).* Before proceeding, each health care professional thoroughly investigates *any* discrepancy and notifies the surgeon and anesthesia provider. The Joint Commission (TJC) has developed a Universal Protocol for Preventing Wrong Site, Wrong Procedure, Wrong Person Surgery; and the Association of periOperative Registered Nurses has developed recommendations based on this protocol (AORN, 2015b). The nurse asks the patient about any allergies and determines whether autologous blood was donated. A special allergy bracelet on the patient's wrist and the medical record must be verified with what has been communicated.

> ### ⚠ NURSING SAFETY PRIORITY QSEN
> #### *Critical Rescue*
>
> Assess the patient's knowledge of his or her scheduled surgical procedure and site. If you recognize that the patient's description of the surgical site is different from that listed on the informed consent, respond by contacting the surgeon to validate the procedure with the patient and to mark the correct site.

The nurse checks the patient's attire to ensure adherence with facility policy. Dentures and dental prostheses, jewelry (including body piercing), eyeglasses, contact lenses, hearing aids, wigs, and other prostheses are removed. Denture removal before anesthesia is controversial because, although the denture plate may come loose and obstruct the airway, the anesthesia provider may request that dentures be left in place to ensure a snug fit of the bag-mask. In some facilities, patients may wear eyeglasses and hearing aids until after anesthesia induction.

Electronic Health Record Review. The circulating nurse and anesthesia provider review the patient's electronic health record in the perioperative holding area or the operating room (OR). This record provides information to identify patient needs during surgery and allows the nurse to assess and plan specific care during and after surgery. It is the main source of information on the type and location of the planned surgery. The nurse checks the medical record to ensure that required data are present before surgery is started.

Advance Directives and Do-Not-Resuscitate Orders. Ethical dilemmas may occur during or after surgery. As a patient advocate, the nurse may have to intervene on behalf of the patient's rights and wishes. The nurse must be familiar with the advance directives and do-not-resuscitate (DNR) orders for each patient. It may be difficult for some health care providers in the surgical setting to care for a patient who has an existing DNR order. Some agencies suspend DNR orders while a patient is undergoing a surgical procedure. The position statement of the Association of periOperative Registered Nurses states that automatically suspending a DNR or allow-natural-death order during surgery undermines a patient's right to self-determination (AORN, 2014).

Allergies and Previous Reactions to Anesthesia or Transfusions. The nurse asks about allergies and previous reactions to anesthesia and blood transfusions. Allergies to iodine products or shellfish indicate a risk for a reaction to the agents used to clean the surgical area. Latex allergies are assessed with all patients because anaphylaxis can occur with latex contact during surgery. Latex-free equipment and supplies are used when there is a latex allergy. The nurse documents the allergy in the medical record and communicates the allergy information to the entire surgical team.

> ### ? CLINICAL JUDGMENT CHALLENGE 15-1
> #### *Patient-Centered Care; Teamwork and Collaboration; Ethics* QSEN
>
> You are caring for a 70-year-old patient who was alert and oriented to person, place, and time during the preoperative assessment. At that time, the patient confirmed that she has a current do-not-resuscitate (DNR) order in place and stated that she is "ready to die" if surgery to remove a malignant tumor "does not go well." During the surgery, complications arise, and members of the interprofessional health care team prepare to administer life-saving measures.
> 1. How do you serve as the patient's advocate at this time?
> 2. What information do you communicate to the interprofessional health care team?
> 3. Should the DNR order be suspended during surgery, especially if it appears that the patient can be saved?
> 4. What information will you share with the family when they ask why you did not save their loved one?

> ### ⚠ NURSING SAFETY PRIORITY QSEN
> #### *Action Alert*
>
> Advance directives are to be honored in the surgical environment regardless of the situation.

The patient's previous experience with anesthesia helps the surgical team anticipate needs and plan interventions. For example, if a patient is restless or agitated as a reaction to anesthesia, the nurse must plan patient SAFETY interventions (including padding for the side rails and protective restraints). The use of blood products during surgery will be influenced by the patient's history, religious beliefs, preferences, and past transfusion reactions.

> ### ? NCLEX EXAMINATION CHALLENGE 15-3
> #### *Safe and Effective Care Environment*
>
> The nurse is performing an assessment on a client who has arrived in the preoperative holding area. Which client statement requires **immediate** nursing intervention?
> A. "I'm a little bit anxious about my surgery."
> B. "When I eat shrimp, my tongue swells, and I have difficulty breathing."
> C. "This left knee replacement will help me walk much more comfortably again."
> D. "Before I get discharged home, I want to have my eyeglasses and hearing aids returned."

Autologous Blood Transfusion. Autologous blood transfusion (reinfusing the patient's own blood) may be used for surgery. Chapters 14 and 40 discuss autologous transfusion in more detail. Chart 15-2 outlines best practices for autologous blood transfusion using blood salvage techniques during surgery.

Laboratory and Diagnostic Test Results. The OR nurse reviews the most recent laboratory findings and test results to inform the surgical team about the patient's health and alert them for potential problems. These results are usually obtained within 24 to 48 hours before surgery for hospitalized patients and within 4 weeks for ambulatory surgery patients. The nurse reports all abnormal findings or results to the surgeon and

CHART 15-2   Best Practice for Patient Safety & Quality Care QSEN

Intraoperative Autologous Blood Salvage and Transfusion

- Be aware of the cell-processing method to be used.
- Make sure that collection containers are labeled for the patient.
- Assist with sterile setup as necessary.
- Assist with processing and reinfusing procedures as needed.
- Document the transfusion process.
- Monitor the patient's vital signs during the transfusion procedure.

anesthesia provider. Laboratory values greater or less than the normal range are potentially life threatening during surgery (see Chapter 14). For example, if the hemoglobin level is less than 10 g/dL, oxygen transport and GAS EXCHANGE are reduced, affecting the amount and type of anesthesia used.

Medical History and Physical Examination Findings. The nurse performs a final assessment to identify risk factors related to patient SAFETY, starting with the patient's age and general physical condition. Older patients and those who are thin or overweight are at greater risk for injury during the positioning process. Assessing mental status is important because confused patients and those who are unable to either follow instructions or communicate may not be able to tell you when a problem exists. Patients who have impaired sensory perception of any type are at increased risk for injury. Specific drugs, such as long-term steroid use (which increases capillary fragility and thins the skin) or immunosuppressives (which inhibit the immune system and may delay healing), and limitations of range or motion, require modification during positioning and may increase risk for injury for some patients.

The OR nurse ensures that the medical history and physical examination findings, including usual pulse and blood pressure, are recorded. This information provides baseline data to assess the patient's reaction to the surgery and anesthesia. Drugs taken before surgery may affect the patient's reaction to surgery and wound healing. For example, aspirin and other NSAIDs can increase clotting time and the risk for hemorrhage.

NCLEX EXAMINATION CHALLENGE 15-4

Safe and Effective Care Environment

The nurse is caring for four clients who will undergo surgery today. Which client does the nurse recognize as at **highest** risk for surgical complication?
A. 52-year old who takes aspirin daily
B. 58-year old who has well-controlled type II diabetes
C. 64-year old who has just received presurgical prophylactic antibiotics
D. 69-year old who will be discharged after surgery to an extended-care facility

Knowing the patient's medical history and age allows the nurse to plan interventions for the care and SAFETY of high-risk patients. The nurse carefully monitors older patients (Chart 15-3) and those with cardiac disease for potential fluid overload.

After completing the electronic health record review, the nurse may insert an IV catheter and administer preoperative medications as ordered. Providing patient-centered care by

CHART 15-3   Nursing Focus on the Older Adult

Intraoperative Nursing Interventions

- Allow patients to retain eyeglasses, dentures, and hearing aids until anesthesia has begun.
- Use a small pillow under the patient's head if his or her head and neck are normally bent slightly forward.
- Lift patients into position to prevent shearing forces on fragile skin.
- Position arthritic and artificial joints carefully to prevent postoperative pain and discomfort from strain on those joints.
- Pad bony prominences to prevent pressure sores.
- Provide extra padding for patients with decreased peripheral circulation.
- Use warming devices to prevent hypothermia.
- Cover the patient's head and feet.
- Warm IV and irrigation fluids as indicated by agency policy and manufacturer recommendations.
- Follow strict aseptic technique.
- Carefully monitor intake and output, including blood loss.

Data from Oster, K., & Oster, C. (2015). Special needs population: Care of the geriatric patient population in the perioperative setting. A*ORN Journal, 101*(4), 443-456.

involving the patient in the plan and addressing identified needs will optimize care and may improve the overall surgical experience. Emotional support, ongoing explanation of procedures, and including family as appropriate will help decrease patient's anxiety in the preoperative period. After the preoperative routine is completed, the patient is moved to the OR.

NURSING SAFETY PRIORITY QSEN

Action Alert

Once the patient has been moved into the OR, do not leave him or her alone. Apply a safety belt across the mid-thigh area of the patient to protect him or her from falls/injury.

◆ *Analysis: Interpreting*

The priority collaborative problems for patients during surgery are:
1. Potential for injury due to improper perioperative positioning
2. Potential for infection due to invasive procedures
3. Decreased GAS EXCHANGE due to anesthesia, pain, reduced respiratory effort

◆ *Planning and Implementation: Responding*

Preventing Injury

Planning: Expected Outcomes. The patient is expected to be free of injury as indicated by:
- Adequate capillary refill and peripheral pulses in all extremities
- Sensory perception and motor function after surgery at the same level as before surgery
- Absence of injury to the skin (redness, open skin areas, bruising, burns)
- Absence of retained surgical items

Interventions. Interventions are needed to prevent injury from positioning based on patient risk factors, anesthesia method, and type and duration of the surgical procedure. Proper positioning is critical. Pressure injuries and nerve injuries can occur if attention is not paid to all areas of the body that are in contact with the OR table. The circulating nurse pads the operating bed with foam and/or silicone gel pads and coordinates the patient's transfer to the operating table. The skin is assessed, especially of older patients, for bruising or injury, and extra padding is placed as indicated (Spruce & VanWicklin, 2015).

The patient is usually in a supine position after transfer to the operating bed. Anesthesia may be initiated with the patient supine, and the patient then may be repositioned for surgery (Fig. 15-8). Before or just after anesthesia induction and before positioning begins, a time-out is conducted to prevent wrong-site, wrong-side, wrong-procedure or wrong-person surgery. A time-out is a critical pause in the progression of care to confirm the patient's identity, the procedure and the site, and other pertinent information. The time-out is initiated by a member of the surgical team and is documented in the electronic health record (Fig. 15-9) by the circulating nurse. Once the time-out has been completed, patient care activities such as positioning, skin preparation, and draping of the surgical site may begin.

The circulating nurse coordinates positioning of the patient for surgery and modifies the position according to the patient's risk factors and special needs. The OR nurse ensures that there is an adequate number of personnel to assist in positioning the patient.

Factors influencing the positioning process include:
- The surgical site (procedure being performed)
- The age, weight, and size of the patient
- The anesthetic delivery technique
- Pain on movement (conscious patient)
- The surgeon's preference

- Any pulmonary, skeletal, or muscular limitations such as arthritis, joint replacements, emphysema, or implanted devices

Chart 15-4 lists best practices to prevent complications related to intraoperative positioning, and thus prolonged immobility, during surgery.

The dorsal recumbent (supine), prone, lithotomy, and lateral positions are most often used for surgery. Fig. 15-8 shows many surgical positions and the use of protective padding. When general anesthesia is used, the surgical team positions the patient slowly to prevent hypotension from blood vessel dilation. Proper positioning is ensured by assessing for:
- Optimal exposure of the operative site and IV line
- Adequate access to the patient for the anesthesia provider
- Interference with circulation and breathing
- Anatomic alignment
- Protection of skeletal and neuromuscular structures
- Patient comfort, SAFETY, and dignity

Care is modified to reduce the potential injury from specific positions. For example, patients in the lithotomy position may develop leg swelling, pain in the legs or back, reduced foot pulses, or reduced sensory perception from compression of the peroneal nerve. Following the nursing process addresses the key aspects of properly positioning a patient in the OR. Assess the patient risk factors before surgery; plan for the availability of personnel, equipment, and positioning devices based on patient specific need; implement the positioning plan once the patient is in the OR; and evaluate the final position before prepping and draping to ensure safe intraoperative care and minimize the risk of a positioning injury.

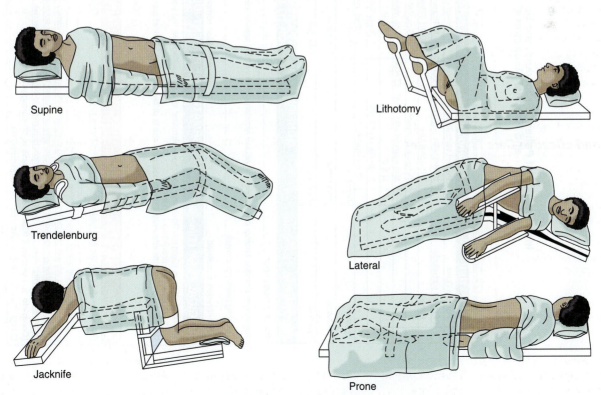

Supine

Trendelenburg

Jacknife

Lithotomy

Lateral

Prone

FIG. 15-8 Common surgical positions.

Identification of Patient, Procedure, and Surgical Side/Sites, and Fire Risk Assessment

Procedure: _____

Date of Procedure: _____

Preoperative verification process to be completed by assigned personnel in designated areas. Mark appropriate blocks.

PEP	Sending Unit	Prep & Holding/Admission Area	Surgical Site Marking Verification
Posting Card	Patient verbalizes	Patient verbalizes	Side 1
Patient verbalizes	ID Bracelet (e.g., Name & DOB)	ID Bracelet (e.g., Name & DOB)	* Not applicable (N/A) meets exemption criteria (see instructions on side 2).
Other	OR Schedule	OR Schedule	* After 2 methods of verification (patient verbalized, consent, H & P, other), the patient (in presence of RN) will write "yes" with a permanent marker on or as near to surgical site:
	Surgical Consent	Surgical Consent	☐ N/A ☐ RIGHT ☐ LEFT
	Site marked with "yes" ☐ N/A	Site marked with "yes" ☐ N/A	
	H & P	H & P	Signature _____ Print Name _____ Date / Time
	X-ray Report / X-ray	X-ray Report / X-ray	Side/Sites Marked by:
	Other studies	Other studies	

Signature: _____   Signature: _____

Print Name: _____   Print Name: _____

Date/Time: _____   Date/Time: _____

COMMENTS

Signature _____ Date/Time

ANESTHESIA (Time-out)   CONFIRMATION OF PATIENT IDENTIFICATION, PROCEDURE & SURGICAL SITE PRIOR TO THE START OF ANESTHESIA BLOCK

The anesthesiologist _____ (Provider Name(s)) and the identification assistant (perianesthesia nurse, operating room RN, another anesthesia provider, another physician or physician assistant) have verbally agreed that _____ (Patient Name) will have the following block performed: _____

Re-verification completed _____ Identification Assistant

Re-verification completed _____

SURGICAL TEAM (Time-out)   CONFIRMATION OF PATIENT IDENTIFICATION, PROCEDURE, SURGICAL SITE, AND AS APPLICABLE, IMPLANT WITH START OF PROCEDURE

The surgical team (Surgeon/Resident, Anesthesia Provider, and Circulating RN) has verbally agreed that _____ (Patient Name) will have the above procedure performed.

Document procedure/site only if the procedure/site is different or left blank at top of form.

Circulating RN: _____

Signature / Print Name _____ Date / Time

SURGICAL TEAM   SURGICAL SITE FIRE RISK ASSESSMENT SCORE

Alcohol based prep solution had sufficient time for fumes to dissipate.   ☐ YES ☐ NO ☐ N/A

Verified by: _____

(Circle appropriate option)	Y	N
• Surgical site or incision above the xiphoid	1	0
• Open oxygen source (Patient receiving supplemental oxygen via any variety of face mask or nasal cannula)	1	0
• Available ignition source (i.e., electrosurgery unit, laser, fiberoptic light source)	1	0

(Circulating RN Signature) _____

Print Name: _____

Total Score _____

Scoring 3 = High risk; 2 = Low risk w/potential to convert to high risk; 1 = Low risk

(Complete this section if Risk Score increases to "3" during procedure)

☐ High Risk Fire Protocol Initiated   Signature/Title: _____   ☐ High Risk Fire Protocol initiated   Time: _____

FIG. 15-9 Identification of patient, procedures, and surgical side/sites and fire risk assessment. (Courtesy Christiana Care Health Services, Newark, DE.)

CHART 15-4 Best Practice for Patient Safety & Quality Care QSEN

Prevention of Complications Related to Intraoperative Positioning

Prevention of Brachial Plexus Complications (Paralysis, Loss of Sensation in Arm and Shoulder)
- Pad the elbow if tucked at the side.
- Avoid excessive abduction (less than 90 degrees).
- Secure the arm firmly on a padded armboard, positioned at shoulder level, and extended less than 90 degrees.

Prevention of Radial Nerve Complications (Wrist Drop)
- Support the wrist with padding.
- Be careful not to overtighten wrist straps.

Prevention of Medial or Ulnar Nerve Complications (Hand Weakness, Claw Hand)
- Place the safety strap above or below the nerve locations (do not overtighten).
- Place the arm of supine patient with palm up.

Prevention of Peroneal Nerve Complications (Foot Drop)
- Pad knees and ankles.
- Maintain minimal external rotation of the hips.
- Support the lower extremities.
- Be careful not to overtighten leg straps.

Prevention of Tibial Nerve Complications (Loss of Sensation on the Plantar Surface of the Foot)
- Place the safety strap above the ankle.
- Do not place equipment on lower extremities.
- Urge operating room (OR) personnel to avoid leaning on the patient's lower extremities.

Prevention of Joint Complications (Stiffness, Pain, Inflammation, Limited Motion)
- Place a pillow or foam padding under bony prominences.
- Maintain the patient's extremities in good anatomic alignment.
- Slightly flex joints and support with pillows, trochanter rolls, or pads.

Data from Association of periOperative Registered Nurses. (2016). Recommended practices for positioning the patient in the perioperative practice setting. In *Perioperative standards and recommended practices* Denver, p. 649-688; and Rothrock, J. (2014). *Alexander's Care of the patient in surgery* (15th ed.). St. Louis: Elsevier.

Before the incision occurs, during the procedure, and upon closing the surgical wound, surgical counts are done to acknowledge and verify that all surgical items (sponges, instruments, and sharps) are present and accounted for. Retained surgical items (RSIs) pose immediate and long-term risks for patients. RSIs can cause pain, infection, and the need for additional surgery to remove the item. Any discrepancies in the surgical counting process must be investigated and resolved before the patient leaves the OR. All team members must participate in resolving any count-related events.

Preventing Infection
Planning: Expected Outcomes. The patient is expected to have an uninfected surgical wound or wounds. Indicators include:
- Aseptic technique is maintained throughout the surgical procedure.
- Wound edges are closed and not excessively red or swollen.
- Wound is free from purulent drainage.
- White blood cell counts remain at expected levels after surgery.
- Patient is afebrile.

Interventions. Surgical wound infections interfere with recovery, delay wound healing, contribute to rising health care costs, and are a source of nosocomial infections. The Centers for Disease Control and Prevention (CDC) defines surgical site infections as occurring 30 days after surgery (CDC, 2016). **Aseptic technique must be strictly practiced by all OR personnel to ensure that the patient is free from infection, as required by The Joint Commission's NPSGs.**

Assess the risk for infection by identifying patients with health problems such as diabetes mellitus, reduced immunity, obesity, and kidney disease. Interventions that minimize risk for infection include performing prescribed skin preparation, protecting against cross-contamination, keeping traffic to a minimum, and administering prescribed antimicrobial prophylaxis. Surgery increases risk for wound complications such as infection, incisional dehiscence, and loss of body fluids. Sterile surgical technique and the use of protective drapes, skin closures, and dressings reduce complications and promote wound healing. When a wound is already infected or is at high risk for infection, antibiotics may be used directly in the wound before wound closure.

Skin and tissue closures include sutures, staples, special tape, and tissue adhesive (surgical "glue"). Fig. 15-10 shows commonly used wound closures. They are used to:
- Hold wound edges in place until wound healing is complete
- Occlude blood vessels, preventing poor clotting and hemorrhage
- Prevent wound contamination and infection

Sutures are absorbable or nonabsorbable. *Absorbable sutures* dissolve over time by body enzymes. *Nonabsorbable sutures* become encapsulated in the tissue during the healing process and remain in the tissue unless they are removed. Body enzymes do not affect nonabsorbable sutures. Retention (stay) sutures (see Fig. 15-10) may be used in addition to standard sutures for patients at high risk for impaired wound healing (obese patients, patients with diabetes, and those taking steroids).

After the incision is closed, the surgeon may inject a local anesthetic or instill an antibiotic into the wound. A gauze or spray dressing may be applied to protect the incision from contamination. A variety of dressings are used to absorb drainage, protect the wound, and support the incision. A pressure dressing may be applied to prevent poor clotting and bleeding. One or more drains (see Chapter 16) may be inserted to remove secretions and fluids around the surgical area. These secretions, if not drained, slow healing and promote bacterial growth, which could result in wound infection.

At the end of the surgical procedure, the surgical team safely transfers the patient from the operating bed to a stretcher or bed. The circulating nurse and anesthesia provider go with the patient to the postanesthesia care unit (PACU) and communicate the hand-off report to the PACU nurse (see Chapter 16).

Preventing Hypoventilation
Planning: Expected Outcomes. The patient is expected to be free of respiratory complications related to impaired GAS EXCHANGE and hypoventilation as indicated by:
- Maintenance of SaO_2, PaO_2, and blood pH within normal limits

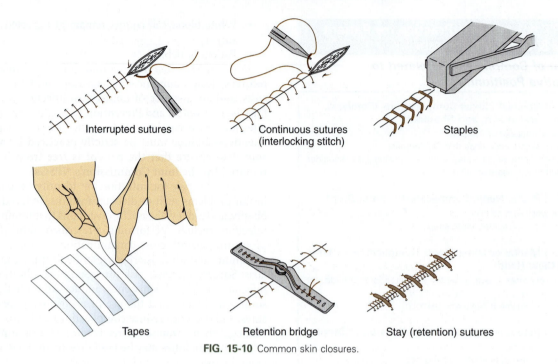

FIG. 15-10 Common skin closures.

- Vital signs within normal limits
- Return to presurgical level of cognitive function

Interventions. The purpose of interventions is to prevent respiratory and circulatory complications resulting from the effect of anesthesia on breathing and GAS EXCHANGE. The nurse, surgeon, and anesthesia provider monitor the patient throughout the procedure according to evidence-based practice standards. These standards, adopted by both the American Society of Anesthesiologists and the American Association of Nurse Anesthetists, include continuous monitoring of breathing, circulation, and cardiac rhythms; blood pressure and heart rate recordings every 5 minutes; and the constant presence of an anesthesia provider during the case.

◆ *Evaluation: Reflecting*

The nurse evaluates the care of the patient during surgery based on the identified priority patient problems. The expected outcomes include:

- Safe anesthesia care provided without complications
- Remains injury free related to surgical positioning or equipment (no skin tears, bruises, redness, or other injury over pressure points)
- Remains free of skin or tissue contamination and infection during surgery
- Maintains normal thermoregulation and body temperature

GET READY FOR THE NCLEX® EXAMINATION!

KEY POINTS

Review these Key Points for each NCLEX Examination Client Needs Category.

Safe and Effective Care Environment
Review preoperative checklist and informed consent forms, including any allergies.

- Highlight any known allergies. **QSEN: Safety**
- Ensure that all personnel entering the OR are wearing proper OR attire for their role.
- Observe for and inform OR personnel of any break in sterile field or sterile technique. **QSEN: Safety**
- Use appropriate patient identifiers when administering drugs or marking surgical sites. **QSEN: Safety**
- Report to the surgeon any discrepancy between the type and location of surgery the patient says is going to be performed and what the informed consent form indicates. **QSEN: Safety**
- Apply grounding pads as needed. **QSEN: Safety**

- Complete any needed skin preparation.
- Perform an accurate "sharps," sponge, and instrument count with the scrub nurse or surgical technologist. **QSEN: Safety**
- Complete a "time-out" with the entire surgical team before incision. **QSEN: Safety**

Psychosocial Integrity
- Communicate patient preferences or fears about anesthesia to the anesthesia provider. **QSEN: Patient-Centered Care**
- Respect the patient's privacy and dignity by minimizing body exposure. **Ethics**
- Stay with the patient during induction of anesthesia. **Ethics**
- Communicate information about the patient's status to waiting family members.
- Ensure that the patient's wishes, as expressed in the advance directives statement, are honored in the surgical setting. **Ethics**

Physiological Integrity

- Apply padding to the OR bed to maintain the patient's skin integrity. **QSEN: Evidence-Based Practice**
- Position the patient comfortably and safely.
- Maintain awareness of signs and symptoms of malignant hyperthermia. **QSEN: Safety**
- Monitor the patient's airway, level of consciousness, oxygen saturation, ECG, and vital signs during and immediately after moderate sedation. **QSEN: Safety**

- Assess the patient for tachycardia, increased end-tidal carbon dioxide level, and increased body temperature as indicators of malignant hyperthermia. **QSEN: Safety**
- Assess all skin areas and document findings before transferring the patient to the postanesthesia care unit.
- Communicate clearly and accurately information about patient's surgical experience when handing off the patient to the postanesthesia care nurse. **QSEN: Teamwork and Collaboration**

SELECTED BIBLIOGRAPHY

American Society of Anesthesiologists. (2014). *ASA physical status classification system.* https://www.asahq.org/resources/clinical-information/asa-physical-status-classification-system.

Association of periOperative Registered Nurses (AORN). (2014). *AORN position statement on perioperative care of patients with do-not-resuscitate or allow-natural-death orders.* https://www.aorn.org/guidelines/clinical-resources/position-statements.

Association of periOperative Registered Nurses (AORN). (2015a). *Fire Safety Tool Kit.* http://www.aorn.org/guidelines/clinical-resources/tool-kits/fire-safety-tool-kit.

Association of periOperative Registered Nurses (AORN). (2015b). *Correct Site Surgery Tool Kit.* https://www.aorn.org/guidelines/clinical-resources/tool-kits/correct-site-surgery-tool-kit.

Association of periOperative Registered Nurses (AORN). (2016a). *Guidelines for Perioperative Practice.* 2016 Edition. Denver, CO.

Association of periOperative Registered Nurses (AORN). (2016b). *Guideline for surgical attire. Guidelines for Perioperative Practice.* 2016 Edition. Denver, CO.

Association of periOperative Registered Nurses (AORN). (2016c). *Guideline for hand hygiene in the perioperative setting. Guidelines for Perioperative Practice.* Denver, CO.

Association of periOperative Registered Nurses (AORN). (2016d). *Guideline for care of the patient receiving moderate sedation/analgesia. Guidelines for Perioperative Practice.* Denver, CO.

Centers for Disease Control and Prevention (2016). *National health statistics report: Surgical site infection (SSI) event.* http://www.cdc.gov/nhsn/PDFs/pscManual/9pscSSIcurrent.pdf.

Doyle, C., Lennox, L., & Bell, D. (2013). A systematic review of evidence on the links between patient experience and clinical safety and effectiveness. *BMJ Open, 2013*(3), e001570. doi:10.1136/bmjopen-2012-001570.

Gmyrek, R., & Elston, D. (2015). *Local and regional anesthesia. Medscape reference drugs, diseases, & procedures.* http://emedicine.medscape.com/article/1831870-overview.

Lazear, S. (2014). *Moderate sedation/analgesia. NetCE Continuing Education.* http://www.netce.com/coursecontent.php?courseid=1072#chap.6.

Malignant Hyperthemia Association of the United States. (2016). *Managing an MH crisis.* http://www.mhaus.org/healthcare-professionals/managing-a-crisis.

Oster, K., & Oster, C. (2015). Special needs population: Care of the geriatric patient population in the perioperative setting. *AORN Journal, 101*(4), 443–456, quiz 457–459. doi:10.1016/j.aorn.2014.10.022.

Quality & Safety Education for Nurses (QSEN). (2016). *Pre-Licensure KSAs.* http://qsen.org/competencies/pre-licensure-ksas/.

Rosenberg, H., Pollock, N., Schiemann, A., Bulger, T., & Stowell, K. (2015). Malignant hyperthermia: A review. *Orphanet Journal of Rare Diseases, 10*(93), doi:10.1186/s13023-015-0310-1.

Rothrock, J. (2014). *Alexander's care of the patient in surgery* (15th ed.). St. Louis: Elsevier.

Seifert, P., Peterson, E., & Graham, K. (2015). Crisis management of fire in the OR. *AORN Journal, 101*(2), 250–263. doi:10.1016/j.aorn.2014.11.002.

Shen, N., et al. (2015). Comparative antimicrobial efficacy of alcohol-based hand rub and conventional surgical scrub in a medical center. *Journal of Microbiology, Immunology, and Infection, 48*(3), 322–328.

Spiegel, J. (2013). *End-tidal carbon dioxide: The most vital of vital signs. Anesthesiology News Special Edition:* October, 21-27.

Spruce, L., & VanWicklin, S. (2015). Back to basics: Positioning the patient. *AORN Journal, 100*(3), 298–305, doi. http://dx.doi.org/10.1016/j.aorn.2014.06.004.

The Joint Committee. (2014). *Potential risks of robotic surgery.* http://www.jointcommission.org/assets/1/23/Quick_Safety_Issue_Three_June_2014.pdf.

The Joint Commission (2017). *National Patient Safety Goals Effective January 2017.* https://www.jointcommission.org/assets/1/6/NPSG_Chapter_HAP_Jan2017.pdf.

Care of Postoperative Patients

Rebecca M. Patton and Cynthia Danko

http://evolve.elsevier.com/Iggy/

PRIORITY AND INTERRELATED CONCEPTS

The priority concepts for this chapter are:
- GAS EXCHANGE
- COMFORT
- SAFETY
- TISSUE INTEGRITY

LEARNING OUTCOMES

Safe and Effective Care Environment

1. Collaborate with the interprofessional team to coordinate high-quality care for patients in the postoperative period.
2. Ensure SAFETY by protecting patients from injury, infection, and complications of surgery during the postoperative period.

Health Promotion and Maintenance

3. Provide postoperative education for patients and family members after surgery.
4. Coordinate with the interprofessional health care team to obtain postsurgical supplies and assistive devices.

Psychosocial Integrity

5. Implement nursing interventions to minimize stressors for the patient and family regarding the postoperative experience.

Physiological Integrity

6. Perform ongoing, complete assessments of the patient throughout the postoperative period.
7. Implement appropriate pain relief strategies to improve COMFORT for the postoperative patient.
8. Apply knowledge of anatomy, physiology, and pathophysiology to prevent patient harm such as shock, respiratory depression, and impaired wound healing.
9. Prioritize nursing interventions for the patient during the postoperative period.
10. Collaborate with members of the interprofessional health care team when performing emergency procedures for surgical wound dehiscence or wound evisceration.

Ongoing evaluation and stabilization of patients after surgery takes place in a postanesthesia care unit (PACU or recovery room). Here nurses anticipate, prevent, and manage complications after surgery. The PACU, usually a large and open room that provides direct observation of all patients and easy access to supplies and emergency equipment, is usually located close to the surgical suite for ease of access and patient transfer. The patient area may be divided into individual cubicles, and privacy is managed using ceiling mounted curtains or floor screens that are fully closed during bedside procedures. Each cubicle has equipment to monitor and care for the patient such as oxygen, suction equipment, cardiac monitors, pulse oximetry, airway equipment, and emergency drugs.

OVERVIEW

The postoperative period starts with completion of the surgical procedure and transfer of the patient to a specialized area for monitoring such as the PACU or an ICU. This period may extend beyond discharge from the hospital until activity restrictions have been lifted. The period of postanesthesia care is divided into three phases that are based on the level of care needed, not the physical place of care. Not every patient needs to transition through all three phases.

Phase I care occurs immediately after surgery, most often in a PACU. For patients who have very complicated procedures or many serious health problems, phase I care may occur in an ICU. The length of time the patient remains at a phase I level of care depends on his or her health status, the surgical procedure, anesthesia type, and rate of progression to regain alertness and hemodynamic stability. It can range from less than 1 hour to days. This level requires ongoing monitoring of the airway, vital signs, and evidence of recovery that varies from every 5 to 15 minutes initially. The time between assessments gradually increases as the patient progresses toward recovery.

Phase II care focuses on preparing the patient for care in an extended-care environment such as a medical-surgical unit, step-down unit, skilled nursing facility, or home. This phase can occur in a PACU, on a medical-surgical unit, or in the same-day surgery (SDS) unit (ambulatory care unit) and may last only 15 to 30 minutes, although 1 to 2 hours is more typical. Patients are discharged from this phase when presurgery level of consciousness has returned, oxygen saturation is at baseline, and vital signs are stable. Some patients achieve this level of recovery in phase I and can be discharged directly to home. Others may require further observation.

Phase III care, known as the *extended-care environment*, most often occurs on a hospital unit or in the home. For patients who have continuing care needs that cannot be met at home, discharge may be from the hospital unit to an extended-care facility. Although vital signs continue to be monitored in this type of environment, the frequency ranges from several times daily to just once daily.

Ambulatory surgery units provide same-day procedural care. Patients recover in a PACU environment that advances them quickly from a phase I to a phase III level, preparing them for discharge to home. Discharge criteria must be met before the patient is discharged from the facility. If the patient experiences ongoing issues related to unstable vital signs, poor GAS EXCHANGE, excessive nausea and vomiting, or unmanageable alterations in COMFORT, admission to an acute care setting or extended-care facility may be necessary.

The actual time spent away from home after surgery varies according to age, physical health, self-care ability, support systems, type and length of the surgical procedure, anesthesia, any complications, home environmental conditions, and community resources. Preoperative assessment determines factors that may have an impact in the recovery process. Communication and planning for management of identified issues to the interprofessional postoperative care team aids in minimizing complications after surgery (Malley et al., 2015).

After the surgery is completed, the circulating nurse and the anesthesia provider accompany the patient to the PACU. For patients in critical condition, transfer may be directly from the operating room (OR) to the ICU. On arrival the anesthesia provider and the circulating nurse give the PACU nurse a verbal "hand-off" report to communicate the patient's condition and care needs.

==A hand-off report that meets the Joint Commission's National Patient Safety Goals requires effective communication between health care professionals.== It is at least a two-way verbal interaction between the health care professional giving the report and the nurse receiving it. The language used to give the report is clear and concise in interpretation. The nurse receiving the report focuses on the report and is not distracted by the environment, other responsibilities, or other caregivers. Standardizing the information reported helps prevent omission of critical patient-centered information and helps avoid

> ### CHART 16-1 Best Practice for Patient Safety & Quality Care QSEN
>
> #### Postoperative Hand-off Report
>
> - Type and extent of the surgical procedure
> - Type of anesthesia and length of time the patient was under anesthesia
> - Allergies (especially to latex or drugs)
> - Any health problems or pathophysiologic conditions
> - Any relevant events/complications during anesthesia or surgery such as a traumatic intubation
> - If intraoperative complications, how were they managed and patient responses (e.g., laboratory values, excessive blood loss, injuries)
> - Status of vital signs, including temperature and oxygen saturation
> - Intake and output, including current IV fluid administration and estimated blood loss
> - Type and amount of IV fluids or blood products
> - Medications administered and when last dose of pain medication given
> - When the next dose of medications is due, especially antibiotics, cardiac drugs
> - Primary language, any sensory impairments, any communication difficulties
> - Special requests that were verbalized by the patient before surgery, including communications with family
> - Preoperative and intraoperative respiratory function and dysfunction
> - Location and type of incisions, dressings, catheters, tubes, drains, or packing
> - Prosthetic devices
> - Joint or limb immobility while in the operating room, especially in the older patient
> - Other intraoperative positioning that may be relevant in the postoperative phase

irrelevant details (AORN, 2016). The receiving nurse takes the time to restate (report back) the information to verify what was said and to make certain that he or she has the same understanding as the reporting person. The receiving nurse takes the time to ask questions, and the reporting professional must respond to the questions until a common understanding is established. Chart 16-1 gives an example of critical information to include in a standard hand-off report.

The PACU nurse is skilled in the care of patients with multiple medical and surgical problems immediately after a surgical procedure. This area requires in-depth knowledge of anatomy and physiology, anesthetic agents, pharmacology, pain management, airway management, surgical procedures, and advanced cardiac life support (ACLS). The PACU nurse is skilled in assessment and can make knowledgeable, critical decisions if emergencies or complications occur. The patient is monitored continuously, and the anesthesia provider and surgeon are consulted as needed.

❖ INTERPROFESSIONAL COLLABORATIVE CARE

◆ Assessment: Noticing

History. Using the surgical team's report, the nurse creates an individualized plan of care. After receiving the report and assessing the patient, the nurse reviews the preoperative assessment and the electronic health record for information about the patient's history, physical condition, and emotional status. If the patient remains as an inpatient, the surgical and anesthesia information is incorporated into the postoperative plan of care. Table 16-1 identifies potential complications of surgery.

TABLE 16-1 Potential System Complications of Surgery

Respiratory System Complications
- Atelectasis
- Laryngeal edema
- Pneumonia
- Pulmonary edema
- Pulmonary embolism (PE)
- Ventilator dependence

Cardiovascular Complications
- Anaphylaxis
- Anemia
- Disseminated intravascular coagulation (DIC)
- Dysrhythmias
- Heart failure
- Hypertension
- Hypotension
- Hypovolemic shock
- Sepsis
- Venous thromboembolism (VTE), especially deep vein thrombosis (DVT)

Neurologic Complications
- Cerebral infarction
- Cognitive decline
- Visual loss

Neuromuscular Complications
- Hyperthermia
- Hypothermia
- Joint contractures
- Nerve damage and paralysis

GI Complications
- GI ulcers and bleeding
- Paralytic ileus

Kidney/Urinary Complications
- Acute kidney injury (AKI)
- Acute urinary retention
- Electrolyte imbalances
- Stone formation
- Urinary tract infection

Skin Complications
- Pressure injuries
- Skin rashes or contact allergies
- Wound infection
- Wound dehiscence
- Wound evisceration

Physical Assessment/Signs and Symptoms. Once the patient is assessed, the data are documented in the electronic health record or on a PACU flow chart record (Fig. 16-1). Assessment data include level of consciousness, temperature, pulse, respiration, oxygen saturation, and blood pressure. Examine the surgical area for bleeding. Monitor vital signs per facility policy, per surgeon orders, or as the patient's condition warrants. On discharge from the PACU, vital signs are measured as prescribed or as often as the patient's condition indicates.

! NURSING SAFETY PRIORITY QSEN

Action Alert

Respiratory assessment is the most critical assessment to perform after surgery for any patient who has undergone general anesthesia or moderate sedation or has received sedative or opioid drugs.

The health care team determines the patient's readiness for discharge from the PACU by the presence of a recovery score rating of 9 to 10 on the recovery scale (see Fig. 16-1) (see Chapter 15 for additional scoring algorithms). Other criteria for discharge (e.g., stable vital signs; normal body temperature; no overt bleeding; return of gag, cough, and swallow reflexes; the ability to take liquids; and adequate urine output) may be facility specific. After determining that all criteria have been met, the patient is discharged by the anesthesia provider to the hospital unit or to home. If an anesthesia provider has not been involved, which may be the case with local anesthesia or moderate sedation, the surgeon or nurse discharges the patient once the discharge criteria have been met.

CHART 16-2 Focused Assessment

The Patient on Arrival at the Medical-Surgical Unit After Discharge From the Postanesthesia Care Unit

Airway
- Is it patent?
- Is the neck in proper alignment?

Breathing
- What is the quality and pattern of the breathing?
- What is the respiratory rate and depth?
- Is the patient using accessory muscles to breathe?
- Is the patient receiving oxygen? At which setting and method of delivery?
- What is the pulse oximetry reading?

Cardiovascular Status
- Are these values within the patient's baseline range?
- Are peripheral pulses palpable?
- What is the rate and rhythm of the heartbeat?
- Are these values significantly different from when the patient was in the postanesthesia care unit (PACU)?

Mental Status
- Is the patient awake, able to be aroused, oriented, and aware?
- Does the patient respond to verbal stimuli?

Surgical Incision Site
- How is it dressed?
- Review the amount of drainage on the dressing immediately.
- Is there any bleeding or drainage under the patient?
- Are any drains present?
- Are the drains set properly (e.g., compressed if they should be compressed, not kinked, patient not lying on them)?
- How much drainage is present in the drainage container?

Temperature
- Is the value significantly different from baseline and when the patient was in the PACU?

Intravenous Fluids
- Which type of solution is infusing and with which additives?
- How much solution was remaining on arrival?
- How much solution was infused in the transport time from PACU?
- At what rate is the infusion supposed to be set? Is it?

Other Tubes
- Is there a nasogastric or intestinal tube?
- What is the color, consistency, and amount of drainage?
- Is suction applied to the tube if ordered? Is the suction setting correct?
- Is there a Foley catheter?
- Is the Foley draining properly?
- What is the color, clarity, and volume of urine output?

Assessment continues from the PACU to the intensive care or medical-surgical nursing unit. When the patient is discharged from the PACU to home, assessment and any needed nursing care are continued by home care nurses or by the patient or family members after home-going instructions are completed. When the patient is transferred to an inpatient unit, a comprehensive initial assessment is completed on arrival (Chart 16-2).

During the postoperative period, all patients remain at risk for pneumonia, shock, cardiac arrest, respiratory arrest, clotting and

FORREST GENERAL HOSPITAL
POST ANESTHESIA CARE UNIT RECORD

POST ANESTHESIA RECOVERY SCORE		MINUTES				
		in	30	60	90	out
Activity						
Able to move 4 extremities voluntarily or on command	= 2					
Able to move 2 extremities voluntarily or on command	= 1					
Able to move 0 extremities voluntarily or on command	= 0					
Respiration						
Able to deep breathe and cough freely	= 2					
Dyspnea or limited breathing	= 1					
Apneic	= 0					
Circulation						
BP ± 20 of Preanesthetic level	= 2					
BP ± 20-50 of Preanesthetic level	= 1					
BP ± 50 of Preanesthetic level	= 0					
Consciousness						
Fully Awake	= 2					
Arousable on calling	= 1					
Not Responding	= 0					
O₂ Saturation						
Able to maintain O₂ Sat > 92% on room air	= 2					
Needs O₂ to maintain O₂ Sat > 90%	= 1					
O₂ Sat < 90% even with O₂	= 0					
TOTAL						

Pre-op B.P. _____
Allergy

Airway: On Adm.
Jawthrust _____
Chin Hold _____
Endotracheal _____
Oral Airway _____
Mask Oxygen _____
Nasal Oxygen _____
Trach _____
T-Tube _____
Nasal Airway _____
Ventilator Settings _____

Addressograph

Time In _____ Time Out _____
Accompanied by _____
Type of anesthesia _____
Surgical Procedure:

PULSE - RESPIRATION - BLOOD PRESSURE
15 30 45   15 30 45   15 30 45   15 30 45
240 220 200 180 160 140 120 100 80 60 40 20

O₂ Sat.
Pain score
PAP

CODES

⊥ A-line
T B.P.

V Manual or
∧ NBP

Pulse •
Resp. ○

Siderails: Yes / No

Restraints: Yes / No

IV Type _____
Total IV in OR _____ cc
Blood in OR _____ units
Urinary Output in OR _____ cc
Est. Blood Loss _____ cc

Foley Cath. _____
Suprapubic _____
Ureteral _____
Levine _____

DRAINS

RN Signature _____

RN Signature _____

MEDICATIONS AND TREATMENTS

	AMT.	ROUTE	TIME
Demerol			
Morphine			
Phenergan			
Droperidol			
Zofran			
Toradol			

FIG. 16-1 Example of a postanesthesia care unit record. (Courtesy Forrest General Hospital, Hattiesburg, MS.)

venous thromboembolism (VTE), and GI bleeding. These serious complications can be prevented, or the consequences reduced with collaborative care. Nursing observations and interventions are part of critical rescue management for patient SAFETY and quality care.

Respiratory System. When the patient is admitted to the PACU, immediately assess for a patent airway and adequate GAS EXCHANGE. Although some patients may be awake and able to speak, talking is not a reliable indicator of adequate GAS EXCHANGE. An artificial airway such as an endotracheal tube (ET), a nasal trumpet, or an oral airway may be in place. If the patient is receiving oxygen, document the type of delivery device and the concentration or liter flow of the oxygen. Continuously monitor pulse oximetry for oxygen saturation (SpO₂). The SpO₂ should be above 95% (or at the patient's presurgery baseline).

> ⚠ **NURSING SAFETY PRIORITY** (QSEN)
>
> ### *Critical Rescue*
>
> If you recognize that your patient's oxygen saturation drops below 95% (or below his or her presurgery baseline), immediately respond by notifying the surgeon or anesthesia provider. If the patient's condition continues to deteriorate or he or she becomes symptomatic, an emergency response is imperative.

Assess the rate, pattern, and depth of breathing to determine adequacy of GAS EXCHANGE. A respiratory rate of less than 10 breaths per minute may indicate anesthetic- or opioid analgesic–induced respiratory depression. Rapid, shallow respirations may signal shock, cardiac problems, increased metabolic rate, or pain.

Auscultate over all lung fields to assess breath sounds. Also check symmetry of breath sounds and chest wall movement. For example, if the patient has an ET tube, it could move down into the right bronchus and prevent left lung expansion. In this case lung sounds on the left are absent or decreased, and only the right chest wall rises and falls with breathing.

Continue to inspect the chest wall for accessory muscle use, sternal retraction, and diaphragmatic breathing. These symptoms may indicate an excessive anesthetic effect, airway obstruction, or paralysis, which could result in hypoxia. Listen for snoring and **stridor** (a high-pitched crowing sound). Snoring and stridor occur with airway obstruction resulting from tracheal or laryngeal spasm or edema, mucus in the airway, or blockage of the airway from edema or tongue relaxation. When neuromuscular blocking agents are retained, the patient has muscle weakness, which could affect the diaphragm and impair GAS EXCHANGE. Indicators of muscle weakness include the inability to maintain a head lift, weak hand grasps, and an abdominal breathing pattern.

If the patient returns to an inpatient unit, an initial assessment is completed on arrival (see Chart 16-2), and he or she is then continually assessed for respiratory depression or hypoxemia. Listen to the lungs to check for effective expansion and abnormal breath sounds. Check the lungs at least every 4 hours during the first 24 hours after surgery and then every 8 hours or more often, as indicated. Older patients, smokers, and patients with a history of lung disease are at greater risk for respiratory complications after surgery and need more frequent assessment (Ramly et al., 2015). Obese patients are also at high risk for respiratory complications.

Cardiovascular System. *Vital signs* and heart sounds are assessed on admission to the PACU and then at least every 15 minutes until the patient's condition is stable. Automated blood pressure cuffs and cardiac monitoring assist in continuous assessment.

Assess vital signs after surgery for trends and compare them with those taken before surgery. Report blood pressure changes that are 25% higher or lower than values obtained before surgery (or a 15- to 20-point difference, systolic or diastolic) to the anesthesia provider or the surgeon. Decreased blood pressure, pulse pressure, and abnormal heart sounds indicate possible cardiac depression, fluid volume deficit, shock, hemorrhage, or the effects of drugs (see Chapters 11 and 37). Bradycardia could indicate an anesthesia effect or hypothermia. Older patients are at risk for hypothermia because of age-related changes in the hypothalamus (the temperature regulation center), low levels of body fat, or prolonged exposure to the cool environment of the OR suite (Touhy & Jett, 2015). An increased pulse rate could indicate hemorrhage, shock, or pain.

Cardiac monitoring is maintained until the patient is discharged from the PACU. For patients at risk for dysrhythmias, monitoring may continue either on telemetry units or on general medical-surgical units. In assessing the vital signs of a patient who is not being monitored continuously, compare the rate, rhythm, and quality of the apical pulse with the rate, rhythm, and quality of a peripheral pulse such as the radial pulse. A **pulse deficit** (a difference between the apical and peripheral pulses) could indicate a dysrhythmia.

Peripheral vascular assessment needs to be performed because anesthesia and positioning during surgery (e.g., the lithotomy position for genitourinary procedures) may impair the peripheral circulation and contribute to clotting and venous thromboembolism (VTE), especially deep vein thrombosis (DVT). Compare distal pulses on both feet for pulse quality, observe the color and temperature of extremities, evaluate sensation and motion, and determine the speed of capillary refill. Palpable pedal pulses indicate adequate circulation and perfusion of the legs.

Prophylactic interventions initiated before surgery for prevention of clot formations and VTE should be continued during the postoperative period as prescribed (Piazza et al., 2015). These interventions vary in type (e.g., drug therapy with anticoagulants or antiplatelet drugs, sequential compression devices, antiembolic stockings or elastic wraps, early ambulation), depending on the patient's specific risk factors. Any preventive strategies started before surgery are usually needed for at least the first 24 hours after surgery. It is important to daily reassess the patient's risk for clotting, VTE, and the effectiveness of all preventive strategies implemented. Assess the feet and legs for redness, pain, warmth, and swelling, which may occur with DVT. Foot and leg assessment may be performed once during a nursing shift or once daily, depending on the patient's risk for complications and the facility policy. (See Chapters 14 and 36 for more information on prevention of inappropriate clotting and VTE.)

Neurologic System. *Cerebral functioning* and the level of consciousness or awareness must be assessed in *all* patients who have received general anesthesia (Table 16-2) or any type of sedation. Observe for lethargy, restlessness, or irritability and

---

TABLE 16-2   Immediate Postoperative Neurologic Assessment: Return to Preoperative Level

Order of Return to Consciousness After General Anesthesia

1. Muscular irritability
2. Restlessness and delirium
3. Recognition of pain
4. Ability to reason and control behavior

Order of Return of Motor and Sensory Functioning After Local or Regional Anesthesia

1. Sense of touch
2. Sense of pain
3. Sense of warmth
4. Sense of cold
5. Ability to move

test coherence and orientation. Determine awareness by observing responses to calling the patient's name, touching the patient, and giving simple commands such as "Open your eyes" and "Take a deep breath." Eye opening in response to a command indicates wakefulness or arousability but not necessarily awareness. Assess the degree of orientation to person, place, and time by asking the conscious patient to answer questions such as, "What is your name?" (person), "Where are you?" (place), and "What day is it?" (time).

ⓘ CLINICAL JUDGMENT CHALLENGE 16-1
Safety (QSEN)

You are caring for a 57-year-old patient who came from the OR to the postanesthesia recovery unit 30 minutes ago after surgery for a hernia repair. He responds when you say his name, but he is mildly confused about where he is and why he is here. He continuously attempts to remove the oxygen cannula from his nose and says it itches, but allows you to gently replace it several times. Vital signs taken 15 minutes ago were BP 130/90, pulse 88, respirations 20. Vital signs now show BP 120/80, pulse 86, respirations 18.

1. Are any of the changes in vital signs a cause for concern? If so, which ones?
2. Should you be assessing for postsurgical bleeding? Why or why not? If so, where would you assess for this bleeding?
3. Should you remove oxygen from the patient? Why or why not?
4. Should you notify the surgeon or anesthesia provider? Why or why not?

👤 CONSIDERATIONS FOR OLDER ADULTS
Patient-Centered Care (QSEN)

For an older adult a rapid return to his or her level of orientation before surgery may not be realistic. Preoperative drugs and anesthetics may delay the older patient's return of orientation. Inform family members that most episodes of postoperative confusion or delirium resolve within a day or two (Rajesh, 2015).

Compare the patient's baseline neurologic status (obtained before surgery) with the findings after surgery. Patients who had altered cerebral functioning before surgery because of another condition usually continue to have the same alteration after surgery. After the patient is alert (and all other criteria have been met), he or she is discharged from the PACU. On the medical-surgical nursing unit, assess the level of consciousness every 4 to 8 hours or as indicated by the patient's condition and facility policy.

Motor and sensory function after general anesthesia are altered and must be assessed. General anesthesia depresses all voluntary motor function. Regional anesthesia alters the motor and sensory function of only part of the body. (See Chapter 15 for more information on anesthesia.)

Motor and sensory function after spinal and epidural anesthesia are profoundly affected. Assess the level of sensation loss remaining by lightly pricking the patient's skin with a needle or pin and having the patient indicate when the sensation feels sharp rather than dull (just pressure). Evaluate motor function by asking the patient to move each extremity. The patient who had epidural or spinal anesthesia remains in the PACU until sensory function (feeling) and voluntary motor movement of the legs have returned (see Table 16-2). It is critical to assess the strength of each limb and compare the results on both sides. Test for the return of sympathetic nervous system tone by gradually elevating the patient's head and monitoring for hypotension. Begin this evaluation after the patient's sensation has returned to at least the spinal dermatome level of T10 (see Chapter 41).

Specific assessment findings for complications of spinal and epidural anesthesia are listed in Chart 16-3. After the patient is transferred to the nursing unit, continue neurologic assessment as indicated.

◎ CHART 16-3 **Best Practice for Patient Safety & Quality Care** (QSEN)
Recognizing Serious Complications of Spinal and Epidural Anesthesia

Respiratory Depression (Can Occur if the Anesthetic Agent Moves Higher in the Epidural or Subarachnoid Space)
- What is the quality and pattern of the breathing?
- What is the respiratory rate and depth?
- Is the patient receiving oxygen? At which setting and method of delivery? What is the pulse oximetry result?
- Notify the anesthesia provider if pulse oximetry drops or if the patient is unable to increase the depth of respiration.

Hypotension (Can Occur When Regional Anesthesia Causes Widespread Vasodilation)
- What is the patient's blood pressure?
- Is the blood pressure now lower than in the preoperative or operative period?
- Has the pulse pressure widened?
- Notify the anesthesia provider if systolic blood pressure remains more than 10 mm Hg below the patient's baseline or if other manifestations of shock are present.
- Notify the anesthesia provider if hypotension is accompanied by other manifestations of autonomic nervous system blockade (bradycardia, nausea, vomiting).

Epidural Hematoma
- Assess for delayed or regressing return of sensory and motor function.
- If return is delayed or is taking longer than usual, alert the anesthesia provider.
- Determine whether sensory or motor deficits are improving, remaining the same, or worsening.
- If motor deficits are worsening or decreasing after brief improvement, notify the anesthesia provider immediately.
- Assess for return of deep tendon reflexes of extremities on both sides.
- Compare reflexes from one side of the body with the other.
- If reflexes regress, notify the anesthesia provider immediately.
- Assess pain level in the back.
- If the patient feels pressure or increasing back pain while coughing or straining, notify the anesthesia provider immediately.

Infection (Meningitis)
- Assess for mental status changes.
- Assess for increasing temperature.
- Assess for ability to turn the neck.
- Notify the anesthesia provider immediately for temperature elevations above 101° F (38.3° C), inability to move the neck, acute confusion.

Postdural Puncture Headache
- Assess for report of headache in the occipital region, especially when the patient is permitted to sit upright.

? NCLEX EXAMINATION CHALLENGE 16-1

Physiological Integrity

Which assessment is **most** important for the nurse to perform for the client admitted to the postanesthesia care unit (PACU) after surgery under general anesthesia?
A. Determining the client's level of consciousness
B. Checking for pain on dorsi and plantar flexion of the foot
C. Assessing the response to pin-prick stimulation from feet to mid-chest level
D. Comparing blood pressure taken in the right arm to blood pressure taken in the left arm

Fluid, Electrolyte, and Acid-Base Balance. NPO status before surgery, the loss of fluid during the procedure, and the type and amount of blood or fluid given affect the patient's fluid and electrolyte balance after surgery. Fluid volume deficit or fluid volume overload may occur after surgery. Sodium, potassium, chloride, and calcium imbalances may also result, as may changes in other electrolyte levels. Fluid and electrolyte imbalances occur more often in older or debilitated patients and in those with health problems such as diabetes mellitus, Crohn's disease, or heart failure.

Intake and output measurement is recorded in the operative record and is reported by the circulating nurse and anesthesia provider to the PACU nurse. Intake or output, including IV fluid intake, vomitus, urine, wound drainage, and nasogastric (NG) tube drainage are all recorded. The total intake and output from both the OR and the PACU must be accurate to assess fluid balance correctly within a 24-hour period.

Hydration status is assessed in the PACU and the medical-surgical unit. To determine hydration status, inspect the color and moisture of mucous membranes; the turgor, texture, and "tenting" of the skin (test over the sternum or forehead of an older patient); the amount of drainage on dressings; and the presence of axillary sweat. Measure and compare total output (e.g., NG tube drainage, urine output, wound drainage) with total intake to identify a possible fluid imbalance. Consider insensible fluid loss such as sweat when reviewing total output. Continue to assess intake and output as long as the patient is at risk for fluid imbalances. All patients receiving IV fluids or those who have a catheter, drains, or an NG tube are on an intake and output monitoring protocol. In addition, patients who have heart disease or kidney disease are monitored closely for fluid and electrolyte imbalances.

IV fluids are closely monitored to promote fluid and electrolyte balance. Isotonic solutions such as lactated Ringer's (LR), 0.9% sodium chloride (normal saline), and 5% dextrose with lactated Ringer's (D_5/LR) are used for IV fluid replacement in the PACU. After the patient returns to the medical-surgical unit, the type and rate of IV infusions are based on need.

Acid-base balance is affected by the patient's respiratory status; metabolic changes during surgery; and losses of acids or bases in drainage. For example, NG tube drainage or vomitus causes a loss of hydrochloric acid and leads to metabolic alkalosis. Monitor arterial blood gas (ABG) values and other laboratory values to identify potential consequences of an acid-base imbalance. (See Chapter 12 for more detailed information on acid-base imbalances.)

Kidney/Urinary System. Control of urination may return immediately after surgery or may not return for hours after general or regional anesthesia. The effects of preoperative drugs (especially atropine), anesthetic agents, or manipulation during surgery can cause urine retention. Assess for urine retention by inspection, palpation, and percussion of the lower abdomen for bladder distention or by the use of a bladder scanner (see Chapter 65). Assessment may be difficult to perform after lower abdominal surgery. Urine retention or incontinence may occur early after surgery and requires intervention such as intermittent (straight) catheterization or an indwelling catheter to empty the bladder.

When the patient has an indwelling urinary (Foley) catheter, assess the urine for color, clarity, and amount. If the patient is voiding, assess the frequency, amount per void, and any symptoms. Urine output should be close to the total intake for a 24-hour period. Consider sweat, vomitus, or diarrhea stools as sources of fluid output. Report a urine output of less than 30 mL/hr (240 mL per 8-hour nursing shift) to the surgeon. Decreased urine output may indicate hypovolemia or renal complications. (See Chapter 65 for kidney/urinary assessment.)

Gastrointestinal System. *Postoperative nausea and vomiting (PONV)* are among the most common reactions after surgery. Many patients who receive general anesthesia have some form of GI upset within the first 24 hours after surgery; however, some patients are more at risk than others (Smith & Ruth-Sahd, 2016). Patients with a history of motion sickness are more likely to develop nausea and vomiting after surgery. Obese patients may be at risk because many anesthetics are retained by fat cells and remain in the body longer. Abdominal surgery and the use of opioid analgesics reduce intestinal peristalsis after surgery. These problems increase the risk for prolonged nausea and vomiting after surgery. Preventive drug therapy, often started in the preoperative period, is effective in reducing the incidence. Drugs often used are a serotonin antagonist such as ondansetron (Zofran), a sedating H_1 histamine antagonist such as dimenhydrinate (Dramamine), and an anticholinergic agent such as scopolamine.

PONV can stress and irritate abdominal and GI wounds, increase intracranial pressure in patients who had head and neck surgery, elevate intraocular pressure in patients who had eye surgery, and increase the risk for aspiration. Assess the patient continuously for PONV. Often patients have nausea as the head of the bed is raised early after surgery. Help reduce this distressing symptom by having the patient in a side-lying position before raising the head slowly.

Intestinal peristalsis return may be delayed because of prolonged anesthesia time, the amount of bowel handling during surgery, and opioid analgesic use. In the PACU and later on the medical-surgical unit, assess for the return of peristalsis. *Patients who are recovering from abdominal surgery often have decreased or no peristalsis for at least 24 hours.* This problem may persist for several days for those who have GI surgery.

Listen for bowel sounds in all four abdominal quadrants and at the umbilicus. If NG suction is being used, turn off the suction before listening to prevent mistaking the sound of the suction for bowel sounds. *The presence of active bowel sounds usually indicates return of peristalsis; however, the absence of bowel sounds does not confirm a lack of peristalsis. The best indicator of intestinal activity is the passage of flatus or stool* (Rothrock, 2014). Abdominal cramping along with distention denotes trapped, nonmoving gas—not peristalsis.

Decreased peristalsis occurs in patients who have a paralytic ileus. The abdominal wall is distended with no visible intestinal movement. Assess for signs and symptoms of paralytic ileus (distended abdomen, abdominal discomfort, vomiting, no passage of flatus or stool). In some patients bowel sounds can be heard even when a true paralytic ileus is present. The passage of flatus or stool is the best indicator of resolution of a paralytic ileus.

A nasogastric (NG) tube may be inserted during surgery to decompress and drain the stomach, promote GI rest, and allow the lower GI tract to heal. It may also be used to monitor any gastric bleeding and prevent intestinal obstruction. Usually low suction is applied to promote drainage. Suction is either continuous or intermittent.

Record the color, consistency, and amount of the NG drainage every 8 hours. In some instances an occult blood test (Gastroccult) may be performed. Normal NG drainage fluid is greenish yellow. Red or pink drainage fluid indicates active bleeding, and brown liquid or drainage with a "coffee-ground" appearance indicates old bleeding. The NG tube should be secured to prevent any chance of displacement.

Assess the patient for complications related to NG tube use such as fluid and electrolyte imbalances, aspiration, and nares discomfort. To prevent aspiration, check the tube placement every 4 to 8 hours and before instilling any liquid, including drugs, into the tube. (See Chapter 55 for information on tube placement and care.) Electrolyte imbalances can result from NG drainage and tube irrigation with water instead of saline. Imbalances include fluid volume deficit, hypokalemia and hyponatremia (see Chapter 11), hypochloremia, and metabolic alkalosis (see Chapter 12).

! NURSING SAFETY PRIORITY (QSEN)
Action Alert

After gastric surgery do not move or irrigate the NG tube unless ordered.

Constipation may occur after surgery as a result of anesthesia, analgesia (especially opioids), decreased activity, and decreased oral intake. Assess the abdomen by inspection, auscultation, palpation, and percussion and record the elimination pattern to determine whether intervention is needed. *Auscultate before palpation or percussion because these two maneuvers are thought to affect peristalsis.* Increased dietary fiber intake, the use of mild laxatives or bulk-forming agents, or the use of enemas may be needed. Encourage ambulation as early as possible after surgery to promote peristalsis (Economou, 2015).

? NCLEX EXAMINATION CHALLENGE 16-2
Safe and Effective Care Environment

The PACU nurse caring for a client with a nasogastric (NG) tube notes that 300 mL of bright red blood has collected. What is the appropriate nursing action?
A. Document as a normal finding.
B. Immediately remove the NG tube.
C. Place the client in Trendelenburg position.
D. Call the client's surgeon to report the drainage.

Skin Assessment. The clean surgical wound regains TISSUE INTEGRITY (heals) at skin level in about 2 weeks in the absence of trauma, infection, connective tissue disease, malnutrition, or the use of some drugs such as steroids. Patients who are older, are obese, smoke, or have diabetes or whose immunity is reduced have delayed wound healing. Complete tissue integrity (healing) of all layers within the surgical wound may take 6 months to 2 years. The physical health and age of the patient, size and location of the wound, and stress on the wound all affect healing time. Head and facial wounds heal more quickly than abdominal and leg wounds because there is less stress on these locations and better blood flow to the head and neck area.

Normal Wound Healing. During the first few days of normal wound healing, the incised tissue regains blood supply and begins to bind together. Fibrin and a thin layer of epithelial cells seal the incision. After 1 to 4 days, epithelial cells continue growing in the fibrin, and strands of collagen begin to fill in the wound gaps. *This process continues for 2 to 3 weeks. At that time* TISSUE INTEGRITY *appears regained; however, healing is not complete for up to 2 years, until the scar is strengthened.* (See Chapters 24 and 25 for discussion of wound healing and wound infection.)

When the patient is an inpatient, the surgeon usually removes the original dressing on the first or second day after surgery. Assess the TISSUE INTEGRITY of the incision on a regular basis, at least every 8 hours, for redness, increased warmth, swelling, tenderness or COMFORT alterations, and the type and amount of drainage. Some drainage (e.g., changing from **sanguineous** (bloody) to serosanguineous to **serous** (serum-like, or yellow) is normal during the first few days. Serosanguineous drainage continuing beyond the fifth day after surgery or increasing in amount instead of decreasing is a sign of possible dehiscence (discussed in the next paragraph), and the surgeon should be notified. Crusting on the incision line is normal, as is a pink color to the line itself, which is caused by inflammation from the surgical procedure. Slight swelling under the sutures or staples is also normal. Redness or swelling of or around the incision line, excessive tenderness or pain on palpation, and purulent or odorous drainage indicate surgical site infection (SSI) and must be reported to the surgeon.

Impaired Wound Healing. Impaired healing and a breakdown of the surgical wound with loss of TISSUE INTEGRITY may be caused by infection, distention, stress at the surgical site, and other health problems (comorbidities) that cause delayed wound healing (e.g., diabetes, renal disease, immune deficiency). Wound **dehiscence** is a partial or complete separation of the outer wound layers, sometimes described as a *splitting open of the wound.* **Evisceration** is the total separation of all wound layers and protrusion of internal organs through the open wound (Fig. 16-2). *Evisceration is a surgical emergency; the surgeon is contacted immediately, and the patient returned to the OR.* Both dehiscence and evisceration occur most often between the fifth and tenth days after surgery. Wound separation occurs more often in obese patients and those with diabetes, immune deficiency, or malnutrition or in those who are using steroids. Dehiscence or evisceration may follow forceful coughing, vomiting, or straining and not splinting the surgical site during movement. The patient may state, "Something popped" or "I feel as if I just split open."

Dressings and Drains. Assess all dressings, including casts and elastic (Ace) bandages, for bleeding or other drainage on admission to the PACU and then hourly thereafter. When the patient

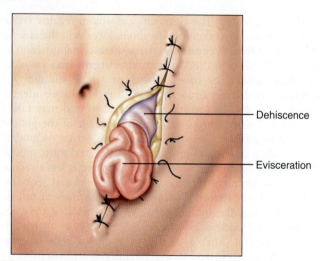

Dehiscence

Evisceration

FIG. 16-2 Complications of surgical wound healing. (From Harkreader, H., Hogan, M. A., & Thobaben, M. (2007). *Fundamentals of nursing: Caring and clinical judgment.* (3rd ed.). Philadelphia: Saunders.)

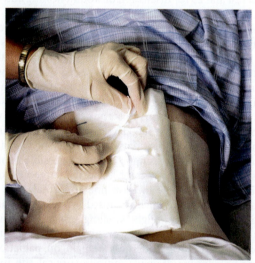

FIG. 16-3 Patient with a dressing held in place with Montgomery straps. (From Harkreader, H., Hogan, M. A., & Thobaben, M. (2007). *Fundamentals of nursing: Caring and clinical judgment.* (3rd ed.). Philadelphia: Saunders.)

is on the nursing unit, assess the dressing each time vital signs are taken (at least every 8 hours). During dressing inspection check for drainage and record its amount, color, consistency, and odor. If drainage is present on a dressing or cast, monitor its progression by outlining it with a pencil and indicating the date and time. Large amounts of sanguineous drainage may indicate poor clotting and possible internal bleeding. Check the area underneath the patient also, because drainage or blood may leak from the side of the dressing and not appear on the dressing itself.

Dressings vary with the surgical procedure and the surgeon's preference. Common dressings for large incisions consist of gauze or nonadherent pads covered with a larger absorbent pad held in place by tape, a tubular stretchy net, or Montgomery straps (Fig. 16-3). Some incisions may be covered with a transparent plastic surgical dressing (e.g., OpSite) or a spray in the OR. This type of dressing stays intact for 3 to 6 days, allows direct observation of the wound, prevents contamination, and eliminates the need for dressing changes. Ensure that the

dressing does not restrict circulation or sensation. This problem is most likely to occur when dressings are tight or completely encircle an arm or a leg. Chest dressings that are too tight or that encircle the chest can restrict breathing.

The surgeon inserts a drain into or close to the wound if more than a minimal amount of drainage is expected. A Penrose drain (a single-lumen, soft, open, latex tube) is a gravity-type drain under the dressing. Drainage on the dressing is expected with open-tube drains. Closed-suction drains such as Hemovac, VacuDrain, and Jackson-Pratt drains include a reservoir that collects drainage. Drainage on the dressing around the drain is not usually present. Assess closed drainage systems for maintenance of suction. Specialty drains such as a T-tube may be placed for specific drainage purposes. For example, a T-tube drains bile after a cholecystectomy. Chronic wounds or wounds that heal by delayed primary intention are typically drained with a negative-pressure wound device. Negative-pressure wound therapy has been shown to improve healing of closed surgical incisions and reduce SSI (Hudson et al., 2015). Fig. 16-4 shows commonly used drains.

Comfort Alterations/Pain Assessment. The patient almost always has pain or alterations in COMFORT after surgery. Pain is a subjective experience and must be assessed based on individual conditions (see the Evidence-Based Practice box). Pain after surgery is related to the surgical wound, tissue manipulation, drains, positioning during surgery, presence of an ET, and the patient's experience with pain (Ward, 2014). Assess the patient's discomfort and need for medication by considering the type, extent, and length of the surgical procedure. Assess for physical and emotional signs of acute pain such as increased pulse and blood pressure, increased respiratory rate, profuse sweating, restlessness, confusion (in the older adult), wincing, moaning, and crying. When possible, ask the patient to rate the pain before and after drugs are given (e.g., on a scale of 0 to 10, with 0 being no pain and 10 being extreme pain). Plan the patient's activities around the timing of analgesia to improve mobility. Observe for a return of baseline physical and emotional behaviors. (See Chapter 4 for further discussion of pain assessment.)

Pain assessment is continuous during PACU care. Pain remains poorly assessed in the older adult; and specific care should be taken to determine the level of pain in older patients, especially in patients who are cognitively impaired. Challenges in assessing pain in the older patient include poor communication (cognitive deficits), comorbidities, stoic character, and a reluctance to report alterations in COMFORT (Schofield, 2014). Drug dosages may need to be adjusted for the older patient to account for age-related changes (frailty, comorbidities, reduced physiological reserve (Schofield, 2014). After the patient is transferred from the PACU, the medical-surgical nurse continues to assess his or her COMFORT level. Pain can increase after surgery, when the patient is more awake and more active and the anesthetic agents and drugs given during surgery have been excreted.

Psychosocial Assessment. Consider the psychological, social, cultural, and spiritual issues of the patient as postoperative care is provided. This assessment may be difficult to perform in the PACU when the patient is drowsy or confused and may be deferred until he or she is more alert. The patient's age and medical history; the surgical procedure; and the impact of surgery on recovery, body image, roles, and lifestyle are all considerations to take into account.

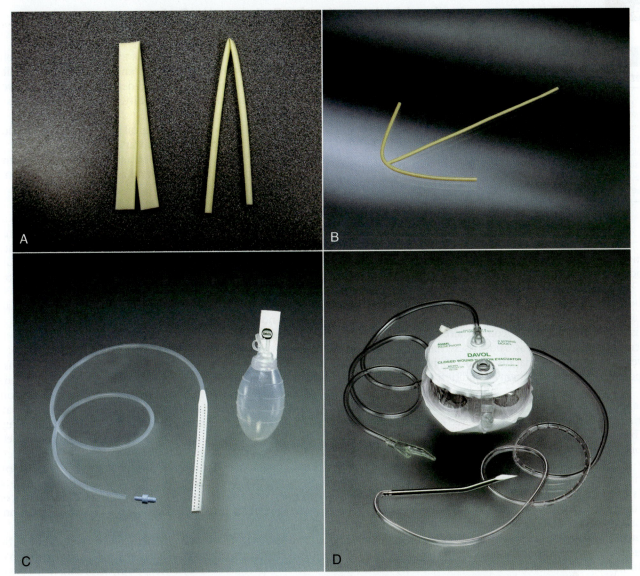

FIG. 16-4 Types of surgical drains. Gravity drains such as the Penrose **(A)** and the T-tube **(B)** drain directly through a tube from the surgical area. In closed-wound drainage systems such as the Jackson-Pratt **(C)** and Hemovac **(D)**, drainage collects in a collecting vessel by means of compression and reexpansion of the system. (**A** from Sirois, M. (2011). *Principles and practice of veterinary technology.* (3rd ed.). St. Louis: Mosby; **B** courtesy 2014 C. R. Bard, Inc. Covington, GA. Used with permission; **C** and **D** courtesy C.R. Bard, Inc., Covington, GA.)

EVIDENCE-BASED PRACTICE QSEN

Opioid Usage in Older Adults

Clarke, H., et al. (2014). Rates and risk factors for prolonged opioid use after major surgery: Population based cohort study. *BMJ, 348*, g1251. doi: http://dx.doi.org/10.1136/bmj.g1251.

Acute pain management in the postoperative older adult can be challenging. Subjectivity in the pain experience, physiologic differences in patients, and ongoing pharmacodynamic changes associated with aging create critical clinical challenges when intervening to manage postoperative pain. Inadequate management can contribute to persistent postsurgical pain for the older adult who already has chronic pain from degenerative bone, joint, and spine diseases.

Over 200 million patients worldwide experience a major surgical procedure annually. Patients typically experience some level of pain that requires management with drugs, often opioids, which are the key analgesic drugs most commonly prescribed. It can be challenging to effectively treat postoperative pain while managing patient concerns about long-term opioid use, potential misuse, and addiction.

Level of Evidence: 3

This population-based retrospective cohort study reviewed rates and associated risk factors of prolonged postoperative opioid use in older-adult patients who had never used opioids before surgery. Patients were older than 66 years and had major elective surgery, including cardiac, intrathoracic, intra-abdominal, and pelvic procedures in Ontario, Canada. Of the 39,140 patients included in the study, 49.2% (n=19,256) were discharged from hospital with an opioid prescription. After more than 90 postoperative days, 3.1% (n=1,229) continued to receive opioids. The analysis identified specific patient and surgical characteristics associated with prolonged opioid usage: of a lower income demographic, with specific comorbidities, use of specific preoperative drugs, having undergone a thoracic surgical procedure, and younger age (closer to 66).

Commentary: Implications for Practice and Research:

The study findings validate that opioids can be used appropriately to treat postoperative pain. Nurses must recognize patient and surgical characteristics and conditions that increase the risk for prolonged opioid usage. Appropriate initial and ongoing pain assessments are important to identify which patients may require interventions to prevent progression to prolonged postoperative opioid use.

CONSIDERATIONS FOR OLDER ADULTS

Patient-Centered Care QSEN

Pain remains poorly assessed in the older adult, and specific care should be taken to determine the level of pain in older patients, especially those who are cognitively impaired. Challenges in assessing pain in the older patient include poor communication (cognitive deficits), comorbidities, stoic character, and a reluctant to report pain (Schofield, 2014). Drug dosages may need to be adjusted for the older patient to account for age-related changes (e.g., frailty, comorbidities, reduced physiological reserve) (Schofield, 2014).

Indications of anxiety include restlessness; increased pulse, blood pressure, and respiratory rate; and crying. The patient may be anxious and ask questions about the results or findings of the surgical procedure. Reassure the patient that he or she is safe and that the surgeon will speak with him or her after he or she is fully awake. If the surgeon has already spoken with the patient, reinforce what was said. Assess the family members as well for any psychosocial discomfort or need for additional support related to the patient's condition and postoperative care.

Laboratory Assessment. Laboratory tests are performed after surgery to evaluate the patient's recovery responses. Tests are based on the surgical procedure, the patient's medical history, and clinical signs and symptoms after surgery. Common tests include analysis of electrolytes and a complete blood count. Changes in electrolyte, hematocrit, and hemoglobin levels often occur during the first 24 to 48 hours after surgery because of blood and fluid loss and the body's reaction to the surgical process. Fluid loss with minimal blood loss may cause elevated laboratory values. Such test results appear increased but actually are concentrated normal values.

An indication of infection is an increase in the band cells (immature neutrophils) in the white blood cell differential count, known as a "left-shift" or "bandemia." The source of infection may be the respiratory system, urinary tract, surgical wound, or IV site. Obtain specimens for culture and sensitivity testing and review the culture reports at 24, 48, and 72 hours. Notify the surgeon of positive culture results. (See Chapters 17 and 23 for information on infection.)

Arterial blood gas (ABG) tests may be needed for patients who have respiratory or cardiac disease, those undergoing mechanical ventilation after surgery, and those who had chest surgery. Review ABG results and notify the surgeon of any acid-base imbalance or hypoxemia that indicates poor GAS EXCHANGE. (For more discussion on arterial blood gases and acidosis, see Chapter 12.)

Urine and kidney laboratory tests also may be obtained (e.g., urinalysis, urine electrolyte levels, and serum creatinine levels). Other laboratory tests depend on the diagnosis, type of surgical procedure, and other health problems. For example, a serum amylase level may be ordered for a patient who had pancreatic surgery, and a blood glucose level may be ordered for a patient with diabetes.

◆ Analysis: Interpreting

The priority collaborative problems for patients in the immediate postoperative period are:

1. Potential for decreased GAS EXCHANGE due to the effects of anesthesia, pain, opioid analgesics, and immobility
2. Potential for infection and delayed healing due to wound location, decreased mobility, drains and drainage, and tubes
3. Acute pain due to the surgical incision, positioning during surgery, and endotracheal tube (ET) irritation
4. Potential for decreased peristalsis due to surgical manipulation, opioid use, and fluid and electrolyte imbalances

◆ Planning and Implementation: Responding

Improving Gas Exchange

Planning: Expected Outcomes. The patient is expected to attain and maintain optimal lung expansion and breathing patterns after surgery as indicated by:

- Partial pressure of arterial oxygen (Pao_2) within normal range
- Partial pressure of arterial carbon dioxide ($Paco_2$) within normal range
- Oxygen saturation values within normal range

Interventions

Airway Maintenance. After assessing respiratory status, an airway may need to be inserted if the patient does not demonstrate adequate GAS EXCHANGE. An oral airway pulls the tongue forward and holds it down to prevent obstruction. If the patient had oral surgery or has clenched teeth, a large tongue, or upper airway obstruction, insert a nasal airway (nasal trumpet) to keep the airway open. A manual resuscitation bag and emergency equipment for intubation or tracheostomy should remain readily available in the PACU area. For patients whose only airway is a tracheostomy or laryngectomy stoma, alert other staff members by posting signs in the room and notes on the chart.

Monitoring. Monitor the patient's oxygen saturation (Spo_2) for adequacy of GAS EXCHANGE with pulse oximetry with each set of vital signs or at least every hour, according to the patient's condition. Patients who normally have a low Pao_2 such as those with lung disease or older adults are at higher risk for hypoxemia. An older adult is often prescribed low-dose oxygen therapy for the first 12 to 24 hours after surgery to reduce confusion from anesthesia and sedation. Patients who received moderate sedation with a benzodiazepine such as midazolam (Versed) or lorazepam (Ativan, Nu-Loraz ✦) may be overly sedated or have respiratory depression sufficient to need reversal with flumazenil (Romazicon) (Chart 16-4). Hypothermia after surgery causes shivering, which increases oxygen demand and can induce hypoxemia. Many rewarming methods can be used, although prevention is more important. The highest incidence of impaired GAS EXCHANGE after surgery occurs on the second postoperative day.

Positioning. *In the PACU immediately position the patient in a semi-Fowler's position unless contraindicated. If the patient cannot have the head of the bed raised, either place him or her in a side-lying position or turn the head to the side to prevent aspiration.*

Oxygen Therapy. Impaired GAS EXCHANGE is prevented and managed with oxygen therapy. Apply oxygen by face tent, nasal cannula, or mask to eliminate inhaled anesthetic agents, increase oxygen levels, raise the level of consciousness, and reduce confusion. After the patient is fully reactive and stable, raise the head of the bed to support respiratory function.

CHART 16-4 Best Practice for Patient Safety & Quality Care QSEN

Emergency Care of the Patient Experiencing a Benzodiazepine Overdose

- Secure the airway and IV access before starting benzodiazepine antagonist therapy.
- Prepare to administer flumazenil* (Romazicon) in a dose of 0.2 mg to 1 mg IV (recommended for IV only).
- Repeat drug every 2 to 3 minutes up to 3 mg, as needed, depending on the patient's response.
- Give oxygen if hypoxia is present or if respirations are below 10 breaths/min.
- Have suction equipment available because flumazenil can trigger vomiting and a drowsy patient is at risk for aspiration.
- Continuously monitor vital signs and level of consciousness for reversal of overdose.
- Do not leave the patient until he or she is fully responsive.
- Continue to monitor the patient's vital signs and level of consciousness every 10 to 15 minutes for the first 2 hours because flumazenil is eliminated from the body more quickly than is the benzodiazepine.
- Determine the need for additional flumazenil therapy 1 to 2 hours after the patient initially becomes fully responsive.
- Observe the patient for tremors or convulsions because flumazenil can lower the seizure threshold in patients who have seizure disorders.
- Assess the IV site every shift because flumazenil can cause thrombophlebitis at the injection site.
- Observe the patient for side effects of flumazenil, including skin rash, hot flushes, dizziness, headache, sweating, dry mouth, and blurred vision. The incidence of these side effects increases with higher total doses of flumazenil.

*There are other benzodiazepine antagonists; however, flumazenil is used most often to manage adult complete or partial reversal of the sedative effects of benzodiazepine in cases in which general anesthesia was induced and or maintained with benzodiazepines, sedation was produced with benzodiazepines for diagnostic procedures, or in management of benzodiazepine overdose.

CHART 16-5 Nursing Focus on the Older Adult

Best Practice in Postoperative Skin Care

Improve perfusion to the wound to promote wound healing:
- Keep the patient adequately hydrated to maintain cardiac output.
- Keep the airway patent and provide adequate oxygenation.
- Keep the patient's oxygen saturation on pulse oximetry at greater than 93%.
- Use strict aseptic technique (e.g., IV or other catheters, indwelling urethral catheter, wound).
- Promote adequate sleep and rest periods throughout the day.
- If necessary, administer drugs to combat pain and sleeplessness.
- Provide rest periods throughout the day.
- Control the patient's room temperature.
- Place the patient on a safety program to prevent falls if indicated.
- Maintain the patient's psychosocial health.
- Maintain personal hygiene.
- Protect fragile skin.
- Minimize the use of tape on the skin.
- Use hypoallergenic tape or Montgomery straps.
- Change dressings as soon as they become wet.
- Lift the patient during transfer or repositioning.

For some patients oxygen therapy may continue through the second day after surgery. When hypoxemia occurs despite preventive care, interventions such as respiratory treatments and mechanical ventilation may be used to manage the cause of the hypoxemia.

Breathing Exercises. After the patient regains the gag and cough reflexes and meets criteria for extubation (if intubated), remove the airway or ET tube. Usual extubation criteria include the ability to raise and hold the head up and evidence of thoracic breathing. Help the patient splint the incision, cough, and deep breathe to promote GAS EXCHANGE and eliminate anesthetic agents. Chart 14-4 in Chapter 14 reviews breathing exercises and splinting of the surgical area. As soon as the patient is awake enough to follow commands, urge coughing, using the incentive spirometer, and breathing deeply hourly while awake throughout the postoperative period. The patient who is unable to remove mucus or sputum requires oral or nasal suctioning. Perform mouth care after removing secretions.

Movement. Assist the patient out of bed and to ambulate as soon as possible to help remove secretions and promote ventilation. Even when the patient has had extensive surgery, the expectation may be to get out of bed the day of or the first day after surgery. If this is not possible, help him or her turn

at least every 2 hours (side to side) and ensure that breathing exercises and leg exercises are performed (see Charts 14-4 and 14-5 in Chapter 14). Early ambulation reduces the risk for pulmonary complications, especially after abdominal, pelvic, or spinal surgery. It increases circulation to extremities and reduces the risk for clotting and venous thromboembolism (VTE), especially deep vein thrombosis (DVT). The patient may resist getting up, but you must stress the importance of activity to prevent complications. When indicated, offer the patient pain medication 30 to 45 minutes in advance of scheduled activities to allow for maximum effect of the analgesic agent.

Preventing Wound Infection and Delayed Healing

Planning: Expected Outcomes. The patient is expected to have incision healing without wound complications as indicated by:
- Wound edges remaining together
- No purulent drainage, induration, or redness in, from, or around the incision

Interventions. Nursing assessment of the surgical area is critical (see the Skin Assessment section). Although most wound complications do not require additional surgical intervention, emergency surgical procedures may be needed.

Nonsurgical Management. Wound care includes reinforcing the dressing, changing the dressing, and assessing the wound for healing and infection; caring for drains, including emptying drainage containers/reservoirs; measuring drainage; and documenting drainage features. Emphasize the importance of early deep-breathing exercises to prevent forceful coughing. Urge the patient to bend the hips when in the supine position to reduce tension on a chest or abdominal wound. Remind him or her to always splint the chest or abdominal incision when coughing. Promote wound healing and protection of the skin, especially for the older patient. Chart 16-5 lists best practices for skin care of the older patient after surgery.

Dressings. The surgeon usually performs the first dressing change to assess the wound, remove any packing, and advance (pull partially out) or remove drains. Before the first dressing change, reinforce the dressing (add more dressing material to the existing dressing) if it becomes wet from drainage. Document the added material and the color, type, amount, and odor of drainage fluid and time of observation. Assess the surgical site at least every shift and report any unexpected findings to the surgeon.

After removal of the dressing, the surgeon may leave the suture or staple line open to the air, which allows easy assessment of the wound and early detection of poor wound edge adherence, drainage, swelling, or redness. Some surgeons believe that air-drying promotes healing. However, a draining wound is always covered with a dressing.

Dressing changes are prescribed by the surgeon; however, the facility or unit may have standards or policies that dictate specific protocols for dressing changes and incision care. An unchanged wet or damp dressing is a source of infection. Change dressings using aseptic technique until the sutures or staples are removed.

Dressings vary with the surgical procedure and the surgeon's preference. Common dressings for large incisions consist of gauze or nonadherent pads covered with a larger absorbent pad held in place by tape, a tubular stretchy net, or Montgomery straps (see Fig. 16-3). Some incisions may be covered with a transparent plastic surgical dressing (e.g., OpSite) or a spray in the OR. This type of dressing stays intact for 3 to 6 days, allows direct observation of the wound, prevents contamination, and eliminates the need for dressing changes.

Wound or suture line care consists of changing gauze dressings at least once during a nursing shift or daily and may include cleaning the area with sterile saline or another prescribed solution. Some suture lines are left open to air without any dressing to cover the incision. The hospital policy, the unit's standards, and the surgeon's preference determine which solution, if any, is used to clean the wound and how often dressings are changed. For large dressing changes or drain removal, offer the patient a prescribed analgesic before the procedure. Always assess the skin for redness, rash, or blisters in areas where tape has been used. Tape can cause a skin reaction after surgery even among patients who are not known to be tape sensitive.

Skin sutures or staples are usually removed 5 to 10 days after surgery, although this varies up to 30 days, depending on the type of surgery and the patient's health. After sutures or staples are removed, the incision may then be secured with Steri-Strips, which stay in place until they fall off on their own. The surgeon or the nurse removes the sutures or staples, depending on agency policy. Clean the incision with the prescribed solution before removing sutures or staples. Before removing sutures examine the condition and healing stage of the wound. First remove every other suture or staple and re-assess the wound for integrity. If wound healing is progressing normally, the rest of the sutures or staples may then be removed. If the wound does not appear to be healing well or if any signs or symptoms of infection are present, notify the surgeon before removing any sutures.

Drains. Drains (see Fig. 16-4) may be placed in the wound or through a separate small incision (known as a *stab* wound) close to the incision during surgery. Drains provide an exit route for air, blood, and bile. Drains also help prevent deep infection and abscess formation during healing.

The Penrose drain is placed into the external aspect of the incision and drains directly onto the dressing and skin around the incision. Change a damp or soiled dressing and carefully clean under and around the Penrose drain. Then place absorbent pads under and around the exposed drain to prevent skin irritation, wound contamination, and infection. Whether sutured in place or not, the drain can be dislodged or pulled out accidentally during a dressing change. It is also possible for the drain to slip back through the wound into the patient. Usually this complication is prevented when the drain is first placed in the OR. The surgeon pins a sterile safety pin through the drain at an angle perpendicular to the drain and the wound, which prevents the drain from slipping. As the wound heals, the surgeon or nurse shortens (advances) the drain by pulling it out a short distance and trimming off the excess external part so only 2 to 3 inches of drain protrudes through the incision. The safety pin must be repositioned each time the drain is advanced. The drain remains in place until drainage stops.

Jackson-Pratt and Hemovac drains are two self-contained drainage systems that drain wounds directly through a tube via gravity and vacuum. These drains are sutured in place with a suture that seals the area when the drain is removed. Use sterile technique to empty the reservoir. Record the amount and color of drainage during every nursing shift or more often if prescribed. After emptying and compressing the reservoir to restore suction, secure the drain to the patient's gown (never to the sheet or mattress) to prevent pulling and stress on the surgical wound.

Drug Therapy. Wound infection is a major complication after surgery. It usually results from contamination during surgery, preoperative infection, debilitation, or immunosuppression. In accordance with the Surgical Care Improvement Project (SCIP) core measures for prevention of surgical site infection, a patient at risk for wound infection may have received antibiotic therapy with drugs that are effective against organisms common to the specific surgical site both before and during surgery. The need for these antibiotics is re-evaluated at 24 hours after surgery. If signs or symptoms of infection are not present, the antibiotic is discontinued at that time (SCIP Infection-3, see Table 14-1). If signs or symptoms of wound infection are present, they are documented to justify continuation of antibiotic therapy.

Wounds that become infected and open are treated with dressing changes and systemic antibiotic therapy. Depending on the surgeon's prescription, irrigate the wound (e.g., with sterile saline, hydrogen peroxide, povidone-iodine, or acetic acid), loosely pack it with solution-soaked gauze (e.g., neomycin, gentamicin, iodoform, povidone-iodine, saline, or acetic acid), and cover it with dry, sterile dressings. These wet-to-damp dressing changes, done two to three times daily, promote healing from within the wound and débridement (removal of the infected or dead tissue) as the wound heals. Negative-pressure wound-care systems, such as Wound VAC may be prescribed to help close the wound. Chapter 25 discusses these systems.

Surgical Management. Poorly healing, infected, or complicated wounds may require surgical intervention.

Management of Dehiscence. If dehiscence (wound opening) occurs, apply a sterile nonadherent (e.g., Telfa) or saline dressing to the wound and notify the surgeon. Instruct the patient to bend the knees and avoid coughing. A wound that becomes infected dehisces by itself, or it may be opened by the surgeon through an incision and drainage (I&D) procedure. In either case the wound is left open and is treated as described previously.

Management of Evisceration. An **evisceration** *(a wound opening with protrusion of internal organs) is a surgical emergency.* Chart 16-6 lists best practices for emergency care of the patient with surgical wound evisceration. Provide support by explaining what happened and reassuring the patient that the emergency will be handled competently.

! NURSING SAFETY PRIORITY **QSEN**

Critical Rescue

Monitor surgical incisions at least every 8 hours to recognize an impending evisceration. When a surgical wound evisceration occurs, respond by attending to the patient while another nurse immediately notifies the surgeon.

◎ CHART 16-6 Best Practice for Patient Safety & Quality Care **QSEN**

Emergency Care of the Patient With Surgical Wound Evisceration

1. Contact surgeon immediately or Rapid Response Team to bring any needed supplies into the patient's room.
2. Provide reassurance and support to ease the patient's anxiety. If possible, stay with the patient and instruct him or her to remain in bed.
3. Using sterile technique, unfold a sterile towel to create a sterile field.
4. Open an irrigation set and place the basin and syringe on the sterile field.
5. Open several large abdominal dressings and place them on the sterile field.
6. Put on the sterile gloves and place one or two of the large abdominal dressings into the basin to saturate them with warm saline solution.
7. Place the moistened dressings over the exposed viscera. Then place a sterile, waterproof drape over the dressings to prevent the sheets from getting wet.
8. If saline is not immediately available, cover the wound with gauze and moisten with sterile saline when available.
9. Do not attempt to reinsert the protruding organ or viscera.
10. Assess for manifestations of shock and document vital signs.
11. Place the patient in a supine position with the hips and knees bent.
12. Raise the head of the bed 15 to 20 degrees.
13. Continue assessing the patient, including vital signs assessment every 5 to 10 minutes until the surgeon arrives.
14. Keep dressings continuously moist by adding warmed sterile saline to the dressing as often as necessary. Do not let the dressing become dry.
15. When the surgeon arrives, report finding and interventions.
16. Document the incident, the activity in which the patient was engaged at the time of the incident, assessment, and interventions taken.
17. If necessary, prepare the patient for emergency surgery; start an IV infusion as ordered.
18. Don't allow the patient to have anything by mouth to decrease the risk of aspiration if surgery is planned.

Special Consideration: Best treatment is prevention. If a postoperative patient is at risk for poor healing, encourage adequate supply of protein, vitamins, and calories. Monitor dietary intake, identify deficiencies, and discuss with the surgeon and the dietitian.

The surgeon may prescribe a nasogastric (NG) tube to decompress the stomach and relieve internal pressure or to remove the stomach's contents if the patient has been eating and general anesthesia is needed. Prepare the patient for surgery (see Chapter 14) to close the wound. Regional or local anesthesia may be used, depending on the location and type of wound. Nausea and vomiting, which stress the already fragile incision, are reduced when regional or local anesthesia is used. To increase the incision's integrity, stay or retention sutures of wire or nylon are used along with standard sutures or staples (see Fig. 15-10).

Prevention. Patients also are at risk for developing pressure injuries from positioning during surgery, contact with damp surgical linens, and unpadded surfaces. Pressure injuries acquired during the surgical period prolong stays and increase the risk for complications. Early intervention of pressure injuries can prevent progression and complications.

Examine the patient's skin for areas of redness or open areas. Document and report any abnormalities. Use padding and positioning to relieve pressure. Treat any open areas according to facility guidelines and the surgeon's prescription. Ensure that information about the patient's skin condition in the PACU is communicated to the medical-surgical nurse. For patients at high risk, collaborate with a certified Wound, Ostomy, and Continence Registered Nurse (WOCRN) to plan preventive or interventional skin care.

Managing Pain

Planning: Expected Outcomes. The postoperative patient is expected to attain or maintain optimal COMFORT levels. Indicators include:

- Patient report that pain is controlled
- Absence of physiologic indicators of acute pain (increased heart rate and blood pressure)
- Absence of behavioral indicators of pain (e.g., facial grimacing, teeth clenching, guarding, rubbing the painful area)
- Willingness to ambulate and participate in self-care

Interventions. Pain management after surgery includes drug therapy and other methods of management such as positioning, massage, relaxation techniques, and diversion. Often the patient has better pain relief from a combination of approaches. Assess the patient's comfort level and the effectiveness of the therapies. See Chapter 4 for discussion of pain assessment and management. The patient who has optimal pain control is better able to cooperate with the therapies and exercises to prevent complications and promote rehabilitation.

Drug Therapy. *The use of opioids or other analgesics for pain management may mask or increase the severity of symptoms of an anesthesia reaction. Therefore give these drugs with caution, especially in the PACU when the patient's condition is not stable.* In the PACU pain drugs are usually given IV in small doses. After receiving any drug for pain, the patient remains in the PACU for a defined period (often 45 to 60 minutes). Assess for hypotension, respiratory depression, and other side effects. Within 5 to 10 minutes after an IV pain drug is given, assess the effectiveness of the drug (i.e., on a rating scale) in relieving pain and document the patient's response.

Opioid analgesics are given during the first 24 to 48 hours after surgery to control acute pain. Around-the-clock scheduling or the use of patient-controlled analgesia (PCA) systems is more effective and allows consistent blood levels more than does "on demand" scheduling. Common drugs include morphine (Statex ✦), hydromorphone (Dilaudid; Hydromorph

Contin ❧; Jurnista ❧), ketorolac (Toradol), codeine, butorphanol (Stadol), and oxycodone with aspirin (Percodan) or oxycodone with acetaminophen (Percocet).

⚠ NURSING SAFETY PRIORITY QSEN
Drug Alert

> The usual dosage for hydromorphone is much smaller (about one-fifth to one-tenth) that of morphine.

Assess the type, location, and intensity of the pain before and after giving pain medication. Monitor the patient's vital signs for hypotension and hypoventilation after giving opioid drugs. Chart 16-7 lists more information about analgesics used after surgery.

Patient-controlled analgesia (PCA) by IV infusion or internal pump (the catheter is sutured into or near the surgical area) and epidural analgesia are often used for better pain control. In PCA the patient adjusts the dosage of the analgesic based on the pain level and response to the drug. This method allows more consistent pain relief and more control by the patient. The maximum dose per hour is "locked in" to the pump so the patient cannot accidentally overdose. Common drugs used in PCA include morphine and hydromorphone.

Epidural analgesia can be given intermittently by the anesthesia provider or by continuous infusion through an epidural catheter left in place after epidural anesthesia. Common

🧓 CONSIDERATIONS FOR OLDER ADULTS
Patient-Centered Care QSEN

> Special care is needed when using PCA with older adults to prevent undertreating pain. Assess the patient's level of understanding of the delivery system and his or her comfort with the self-medication process. Reassure the patient that the system prevents accidental overdose.

drugs given by epidural catheter include the opioids fentanyl (Sublimaze), preservative-free morphine (Duramorph), and bupivacaine (Marcaine).

Take care not to overmedicate or undermedicate, especially with older patients. In assessing for overmedication, monitor vital signs, especially blood pressure and respiratory rate, and level of consciousness. Complications from the use of opioid analgesics include respiratory depression, hypotension, nausea, vomiting, and constipation. An opioid antagonist such as naloxone (Narcan) may be needed to reverse the acute effects of opioid depression. Because of the short effect of the opioid antagonist, monitor the patient's blood pressure and respirations every 15 to 30 minutes until the full effect of the opioid analgesic has passed. More doses of the antagonist may need to be given during this time because it is eliminated from the body more quickly than is the opioid. (See Chart 16-8 for more information on using opioid antagonists to reverse opioid overdose.) In addition, the patient may experience breakthrough pain after the opioid antagonist is given; therefore other interventions to achieve COMFORT are needed.

💊 CHART 16-7 Common Examples of Drug Therapy
Management of Postoperative Pain

DRUG	NURSING IMPLICATIONS
Opioids	
Morphine sulfate (Epimorph, Statex), and Hydromorphone hydrochloride (Dilaudid)	Monitor respiratory rate and blood pressure because respiratory depression can be severe and require medical intervention. Monitor GI motility and urine output because constipation and urinary retention can occur.
Codeine sulfate, codeine phosphate (Paveral)	Monitor respiratory status because respiratory depression can occur. Monitor GI motility because constipation when taking this drug is common and interventions may be indicated.
Butorphanol tartrate (Stadol)	Monitor neurologic status and for changes in level of consciousness because this medication can cause increased intracranial pressure. Monitor for respiratory depression.
Oxycodone hydrochloride and aspirin (Percodan, Endodan, Oxycodan)	Monitor for GI tolerance and function because the aspirin component of this drug can irritate the stomach. Constipation and GI bleeding can occur. Monitor coagulation studies (PT, aPTT) because the aspirin component of this drug may influence bleeding times and other coagulation study results.
Oxycodone hydrochloride and acetaminophen (Percocet, Endocet, Oxycocet)	Monitor blood pressure and respiratory status because hypotension and respiratory depression can occur. Monitor GI motility because constipation when taking this drug is common and interventions may be indicated.
NSAIDs	
Ketorolac tromethamine (Toradol)	Monitor for GI tolerance. GI bleeding, ulceration, and perforation can occur while taking this drug. Monitor for kidney effects, especially in older adult, because decreased urine output, increased serum creatinine, hematuria, and proteinuria can occur.
Ibuprofen (Motrin, Amersol, Novoprofen)	Monitor upper GI tolerance of medication; this drug can be given with food or milk to decrease irritation of the stomach. Monitor coagulation studies (PT, aPTT) and assess for signs of bleeding or delayed clotting so early detection can lead to avoidance of complications.

aPTT, Activated partial thromboplastin time; *PT,* prothrombin time.

CHART 16-8   Best Practice for Patient Safety & Quality Care QSEN

Emergency Care of the Patient Experiencing an Opioid Overdose

- Prepare to administer naloxone hydrochloride (Narcan)* in an initial dose of 0.4 mg-2 mg IV.
- If the desired degree of improvement in respiratory functions is not obtained, it may be repeated at 2- to 3-minute intervals up to 10 mg as needed, depending on the patient's response.
- Naloxone may be administered IV, IM, subcutaneously or intranasal spray. IV is most rapid onset and is recommended in emergency situations.
- Maintain an open airway.
- Give oxygen if hypoxia is present or if respirations are below 10 breaths/min.
- Have suction equipment available because naloxone can trigger vomiting and a drowsy patient is at risk for aspiration.
- Continuously monitor vital signs and level of consciousness for opioid reversal every 10-15 minutes for the first hour. Naloxone is eliminated from the body more quickly than is the opioid; and it may induce side effects, including blood pressure changes, tachycardia, and dysrhythmias.
- Do not leave the patient until he or she is fully responsive.
- Assess the patient for pain because reversal of the opioid also reverses the analgesic effects.
- Determine the need for additional antagonist therapy 1 hour after the patient initially becomes fully responsive.

*There are other opioid antagonists; however, naloxone hydrochloride is most often indicated for complete or partial reversal of opioid depression induced by natural and synthetic opioids. It is also indicated for suspected or known adult and opioid overdose in the postoperative period.

Assess for undermedication by asking the patient about degree of pain relief and observing for nonverbal cues of discomfort (e.g., restlessness, increased confusion, "picking" at bedcovers). Offer prescribed drug(s) after checking for hypotension and respiratory depression.

As recovery progresses, reduce the doses and frequency of drugs for pain control. Drugs are changed from injectable or PCA to oral as soon as the patient can tolerate oral agents. Nonopioid analgesics such as acetaminophen (Tylenol, Atasol ✦) and NSAIDs such as ibuprofen (Motrin, Novo-Profen ✦) and ketorolac (Toradol) are used alone or with an opioid analgesic. Antianxiety drugs may be given with an opioid analgesic to decrease pain-related anxiety, reduce muscle tension, and control nausea.

NURSING SAFETY PRIORITY QSEN

Drug Alert

Do not confuse Toradol (an NSAID used for short-term, acute-to-moderate pain) with Tramadol (an opioid drug used for central analgesia).

Complementary and Integrative Health. Other COMFORT measures that may lower the amount of pain drugs needed are provided in conjunction with drug therapy for pain control. Measures such as positioning, massage, relaxation, and diversion reduce anxiety and allow the patient to relax and rest.

In positioning the patient, consider the position during surgery, the location of the surgical incision and drains, and problems such as arthritis and chronic lung disease. Assist the patient to a position of comfort. Support the extremities with

CHART 16-9   Best Practice for Patient Safety & Quality Care QSEN

Nonpharmacologic Interventions to Reduce Postoperative Pain and Promote Comfort

- Find a general position of comfort for the patient.
- Use ice to reduce and prevent swelling as indicated.
- Cushion and elevate painful areas; avoid tension or pressure on these areas.
- Control or remove noxious stimuli.
- Provide adequate rest to increase pain tolerance.
- Encourage the patient's participation in diversional activities.
- Instruct the patient in relaxation techniques; use audio recordings or CDs and breathing exercises.
- Provide opportunities for meditation.
- Help the patient stimulate sensory nerve endings near the painful areas to inhibit ascending pain impulses.
- Help the patient stimulate the area contralateral (opposite) to the painful area.

NURSING SAFETY PRIORITY QSEN

Action Alert

Unless pillow support is ordered, do not place pillows under the knees and do not raise the knee gatch because this position could restrict circulation and increase the risk for venous thromboembolism.

pillows. Turn or help the patient turn at least every 2 hours while he or she is bedridden to prevent complications of immobility.

Based on orders for ambulation and assessment of the patient's tolerance, encourage the patient to increase activity progressively to prevent complications. When the patient first gets out of bed, assistance will be required to move him or her to the side of the bed and into a chair. Teach the patient to splint the surgical wound for support and comfort during the transfer.

Use gentle massage on stiff joints or a sore back to decrease discomfort. Assist the patient to a side-lying position and apply lotion with smooth, gentle strokes to increase blood flow to the area and promote relaxation. *Do not massage the calves because of the risk for loosening a clot and causing a life-threatening pulmonary embolus.*

Relaxation and diversion are also used to control acute episodes of pain during dressing changes and injections. (See Chapter 4 for how to instruct and guide the patient through these pain control methods.) Music and noise reduction may help decrease awareness of discomfort. Chart 16-9 lists other interventions that may help reduce pain and promote comfort.

Promoting Peristalsis. Decreased intestinal peristalsis with the possible development of a postoperative ileus (POI) can occur as a result of drug therapy, anesthesia/analgesia, operative manipulation, and increased sympathetic nervous system excitation from stress after any surgery but is most common after open abdominal procedures. Thus all postoperative patients are at some risk for POI. This complication is unpleasant for the patient, increases lengths of stay (Katrancha et al., 2014), and can lead to other avoidable complications such as wound dehiscence, nausea, vomiting, and deconditioning.

Planning: Expected Outcomes. The patient is expected to have return of intestinal peristalsis after surgery as indicated by:

- Presence of active bowel sounds in all four abdominal quadrants

- Passage of flatus and/or stool
- No abdominal distention or rigidity

Interventions. Nursing intervention to promote peristalsis include monitoring, ensuring adequate hydration, promotion of mobility, managing pain with nonopioid interventions, and when appropriate, pharmacologic management.

Monitoring with accurate assessment of the abdomen is key to determining recovery of intestinal peristalsis and recognizing possible POI early. Assess the abdomen for the presence and quality of bowel sounds, degree of distention, and firmness whenever vital signs are taken. First observe for distention and document whether this has increased or decreased since the last observation. Auscultate for bowel sounds in all four abdominal quadrants for up to 1 minute in each quadrant. Gently palpate the abdomen to determine degree of softness or whether any rigidity is present. Although the presence of bowel sounds, especially lower in the tract, does not indicate full peristalsis, the absence of sound does correlate with hypomotility. Ask the patient whether he or she has passed any flatus or stool. Although passage of either indicates some intestinal motility, it does not rule out POI.

Ensuring adequate hydration helps promote peristalsis because dehydration, fluid loss, and crystalloid excess can potentially decrease intestinal motility, leading to POI. Monitor IV fluid volume compared with urine output. Fluid volumes infused should be sufficient (for the adult without known kidney or cardiac problems) to maintain adequate urine output that is dilute in appearance.

Increased mobility, especially early ambulation, assists in return of peristalsis. Help the patient ambulate at least once per shift and increase the distance and time spent ambulating with each intervention. Document both the time and distance of each ambulation so progression can be continued by other caregivers.

Nonopioid pain management strategies can help reduce the amount of opioids needed to manage pain adequately. Opioids bind to GI receptors and contribute to decreased peristalsis and POI development. Work with the interprofessional team to use alternative pain control measures in addition to opioids in the postoperative period. See Chapter 4 for more discussion of nonopioid and nonpharmacologic pain management strategies.

Gum chewing in the early postoperative period has been suggested to promote intestinal peristalsis. Chewing gum stimulates digestive secretions, including gastric hormones that trigger increased motility without adding bulk to the GI system. A variety of nursing studies report this strategy to be acceptable to patients, low-cost, and successful in returning intestinal peristalsis after abdominal surgery (Katrancha et al., 2014).

Drug therapy can be useful both in preventing reduced peristalsis and promoting increased intestinal peristalsis. The opioid analgesics used for pain control work by binding to mu opioid receptors in the brain. Similar mu receptors in the GI system also are bound by opioids, which results in decreased peristalsis. Drugs known as peripherally acting mu opioid receptor antagonists (PAM-OR antagonists) can be given to prevent opioids from binding to mu receptors in the GI tract without interfering with the effectiveness of opioid pain relief. Thus the action of these drugs facilitates return to peristalsis after surgery. Two drugs approved for this purpose are alvimopan (Entereg) and methylnaltrexone (Relistor).

Other drugs that have been tried to promote peristalsis by directly stimulating GI motility are prokinetic agents. A common drug in this class is metoclopramide (Reglan, Maxeran). Because there is no evidence supporting its effectiveness in preventing POI, it is used less often today.

❓ NCLEX EXAMINATION CHALLENGE 16-3
Psychosocial Integrity

The nurse is caring for an older-adult client who reports being "afraid to get hooked" on opioid pain medication after surgery. What is the appropriate nursing response? **Select all that apply.**
A. "Why do you think you're going to get hooked?"
B. "Don't worry, I won't give you any opioid medications."
C. "Have you had concerns with drug dependence in the past?"
D. "Tell me what makes you most fearful about taking opioid medication."
E. "There are ways we can keep you from becoming dependent on these drugs."
F. "Older adults are much less likely to rely on pain medications than younger people."

Care Coordination and Transition Management

Many patients are discharged after a brief hospital stay or directly from the PACU (phase III level) to home. Because of the shortened length of hospital stays and the increase in ambulatory surgery, discharge planning, teaching, and referrals begin before surgery and continue after surgery.

Home Care Management. If the patient is discharged directly to home, assess information about the home environment for SAFETY and the availability of caregivers. Use the data obtained on admission before surgery to determine the patient's needs. For example, if the patient is unable or not allowed to climb stairs and lives in a two-story house with only one bathroom, advise him or her to rent a bedside commode. Other assistive devices may be needed such as a shower chair, walker, or recliner, based on assessment of the patient's living arrangements. Collaborate with the social worker or discharge planner to identify needs related to care after surgery, including meal preparation, dressing changes, drain management, drug administration, physical therapy, and personal hygiene. A referral to a home care nursing or physical therapy agency may be indicated.

The patient is usually concerned about complications, pain, changes in the usual activity level, or payment of the hospital bill. The more extensive the surgical procedure is, the more fearful the patient may be of assuming self-care. Support the patient and family members as they make discharge plans. The patient with visible scars after surgery may need more emotional support from and acceptance by his or her family. The patient may be angry about the surgical outcome or about role changes. He or she may be concerned about financial matters and work. The surgical outcome may not have met the patient's expectations, and further interventions may be needed to assist in the process of resolving his or her feelings. Ensure that referrals are made for additional counseling as indicated.

Self-Management Education. The teaching plan for the patient and family after surgery includes:
- Pain management
- Drug therapy with reconciliation of postoperative drugs
- SAFETY (e.g., understanding who to contact in case of complications, progressive increase in activity, needed assistive devices)

NCLEX EXAMINATION CHALLENGE 16-4

Health Promotion and Maintenance

Which client statement regarding appropriate pain control requires nursing intervention?
A. "I'll listen to music when I feel pain."
B. "Before exercise or physical therapy, I'll be sure I've taken my medication."
C. "If the prescribed dose of medication doesn't help my pain, I'll take an extra dose."
D. "I plan to keep a pain diary so I can see trends about when my pain worsens."

- Prevention of infection with care and assessment of the surgical wound
- Management of drains or catheters
- Nutrition therapy
- Follow-up with the surgeon

If dressing changes and drain or catheter care are needed, instruct the patient and family members on the importance of proper handwashing to prevent infection. Explain and demonstrate wound care to the patient and family, who then perform a return demonstration. During teaching sessions evaluate learning and promote adherence after discharge. At the same time, teach about the symptoms of complications such as wound infection. Also instruct the patient and family about what to do if complications occur.

Perform a drug reconciliation with the patient before discharge. Ensure that drugs for other health problems are resumed, as needed. Also ensure that drugs specific for the surgical procedure (and its complications) are available to the patient and that he or she understands how they are to be used, any side effects, and when they are to be discontinued. Teach the patient about drugs for pain, especially the proper dosage and frequency. Instruct the patient to notify the surgeon if pain is not controlled or if it suddenly increases. If antibiotics or other drugs are prescribed, stress the importance of completing the entire prescription.

A diet high in protein, calories, and vitamin C promotes wound healing. Supplemental vitamin C, iron, zinc, and other vitamins are often prescribed after surgery to aid in wound healing and red blood cell formation. Instruct the patient who needs dietary restrictions about the importance of following the prescribed diet while recovering from surgery. Encourage the older adult or weakened patient to continue using dietary supplements, if prescribed, between meals until the wound is completely healed and the energy levels are restored.

Surgery stresses the body, and time and rest are needed for healing. Teach the patient to increase activity level slowly, rest often, and avoid straining the wound or the surrounding area. The surgeon decides when the patient may climb stairs, return to work, drive, and resume other usual ADLs (e.g., housekeeping, gardening, and sexual activity). The surgeon will determine the amount of weight that the patient can lift safely after surgery (i.e., in pounds or kilograms). Instruct the patient in the use of proper lifting techniques and remind him or her about weights of frequently used items such as grocery bags, handbags, and common household items. A patient whose work involves a moderate amount of physical labor may return to work about 6 weeks after abdominal surgery. Stress the importance of adherence to prevent complications or disability.

Health Care Resources. A referral for a home care nurse may be needed for follow-up. This nurse provides nursing assessments, dressing supplies, education in self-care, and referrals for other services as needed. Such referrals may include Meals on Wheels, support groups, and homemaker services for housekeeping or food shopping.

! NURSING SAFETY PRIORITY QSEN

Action Alert

Always ensure that the patient and family receive written discharge instructions (including medication education sheets) to follow at home. Always ensure that the patient and family understand the instructions by having them explain them in their own words.

◆ Evaluation: Reflecting

Evaluate the care of the patient after surgery based on the identified priority patient problems. The expected outcomes include that the patient:

- Attains and maintains adequate lung expansion and respiratory function
- Has appropriate wound healing without complications
- Has acceptable pain management
- Has return of peristalsis

GET READY FOR NCLEX® EXAMINATION

KEY POINTS

Review the following key points for each NCLEX Examination Client Needs Category.

Safe and Effective Care Environment

- Examine individual patient factors for potential risks to SAFETY, especially risk for surgical site infection, hypoventilation, hypotension, venous thromboembolism, or injury during initial ambulation after surgery. **QSEN: Safety**
- Use aseptic technique during all dressing changes. **QSEN: Safety**

- Use established criteria to determine when a patient is ready to leave the postanesthesia care unit (PACU) for discharge to home or a medical-surgical nursing unit.
- Keep suction equipment, oxygen, and artificial breathing equipment near each patient bedside in the PACU. **QSEN: Safety**

Health Promotion and Maintenance

- Reinforce to the patient and family after surgery the specific interventions to use to prevent complications (e.g., hand hygiene, incision splinting, deep-breathing exercises, range-of-motion exercises—as described in Charts 14-4 and 14-5). **QSEN: Evidence-Based Practice**

- Encourage early ambulation.
- Stress the importance of following activity restrictions prescribed by the surgeon.
- Teach the patient and family about any drugs to be continued after discharge from the facility. **QSEN: Patient-Centered Care**
- Instruct the patient and family about the clinical signs and symptoms of complications and when to seek assistance. **QSEN: Patient-Centered Care**

Psychosocial Integrity

- Keep family members informed of the patient's progress during the time that he or she is in the postanesthesia recovery area. **Ethics**

- Reassure patients and family members that taking pain medication when needed, even opioids, does not make them drug abusers. **QSEN: Patient-Centered Care**

Physiological Integrity

- Begin every assessment of the patient after surgery by checking the airway and breathing effectiveness. **QSEN: Safety**
- Assess the incision site each shift (on the medical-surgical nursing unit).
- Offer alternative therapies for relaxation, pain reduction, and distraction such as massage, music therapy, and guided imagery.
- In the event of wound dehiscence or evisceration, have the patient lie flat (supine) with knees bent to reduce intra-abdominal pressure; apply sterile, nonadherent dressing materials to the wound; and follow the steps outlined in Chart 16-6. **QSEN: Evidence-Based Practice**

SELECTED BIBLIOGRAPHY

American Society of PeriAnesthesia Nurses. (2015). *2015-2017 Perianesthesia Nursing Standards, Practice Recommendations and Interpretive Statements.*

Association of periOperative Registered Nurses (AORN). (2016). *Guidelines for perioperative practice.* 2016 Edition. Denver, CO: AORN.

Economou, D. C. (2015). Bowel management: Constipation, diarrhea, obstruction, and ascites. In B. Ferrell, N. Coyle, & J. A. Paice (Eds.), *Oxford textbook of palliative nursing* (p. 221). New York: Oxford University Press. http://0-lib.myilibrary.com.lispac.lsbu.ac.uk?id=688359.

Hudson, D. A., Adams, K. G., Van Huyssteen, A., Martin, R., & Huddleston, E. M. (2015). Simplified negative-pressure wound therapy: Clinical evaluation of an ultraportable, no-canister system. *International Wound Journal, 12,* 195–201. doi:10.1111/iwj.12080.

Katrancha, E. D., & George, N. M. (2014). Postoperative ileus. *Medsurg Nursing, 23*(6), 387–390, 413.

Lemanski, C. (2015). Cochrane nursing care review: Pulse oximetry for perioperative monitoring. *Journal of Perianesthesia Nursing, 31*(1), 86–88.

Malley, A., Kenner, C., Kim, T., & Blakeney, B. (2015). The role of the nurse and the preoperative assessment in patient transitions. *AORN Journal, 102*(2), 181.e1–181.e9. doi:10.1016/j.aorn.2015.06.004.

Piazza, G., Hohlfelder, B., & Goldhaber, S. (2015). Prevention of venous thromboembolism: An evidence-based approach to thromboprophylaxis. In *Handbook for venous thromboembolism* (pp. 123–134). Chapter 13. Switzerland: Springer International Publishing. doi:10.1007/978-3-319-20843-5_13p.

Rajesh, M. C. (2015). Postoperative cognitive dysfunction (POCD) in geriatric population. *BMH Medical Journal, 2*(4), 110–112.

Ramly, E., Haytham, M. A., Kaafarani, H. M., & Velmahos, G. C. (2015). The effect of aging on pulmonary function implications for monitoring and support of the surgical and trauma patient. *Surgical Clinics of North America, 95*(2), 53–69.

Rothrock, J. (2014). *Alexander's care of the patient in surgery* (15th ed.). St. Louis: Elsevier.

Schofield, P. A. (2014). The assessment and management of perioperative pain in older adults. *Anaesthesia, 69*(Suppl. 1), 54–60.

Smith, C., & Ruth-Sahd, L. (2016). Reducing the incidence of postoperative nausea and vomiting begins with risk screening: An evaluation of the evidence. *Journal of Perianesthesia Nursing, 31*(2), 158–171.

Touhy, T., & Jett, K. (2015). *Ebersole & Hess' toward healthy aging* (9th ed.). St. Louis: Elsevier.

Ward, C. (2014). Procedure-specific postoperative pain management. *Medsurg Nursing, 23*(2), 107–110.

CHAPTER **17**

Principles of Inflammation and Immunity

M. Linda Workman

 http://evolve.elsevier.com/Iggy/

PRIORITY AND INTERRELATED CONCEPTS

The priority concept for this chapter is IMMUNITY.

LEARNING OUTCOMES

Health Promotion and Maintenance

1. Explain how physiologic aging affects IMMUNITY and the associated care of older adults.

Physiological Integrity

2. Interpret laboratory findings to assess the patient's risk for an IMMUNITY problem.
3. Explain how drug therapy alters IMMUNITY to interfere with transplant rejection.

OVERVIEW

As described in Chapter 2, IMMUNITY is protection from illness or disease that is maintained by the body's physiologic defense mechanisms. This protection requires the interaction of immunity and inflammation working together to control infection and other problems caused by harmful microorganisms or altered cells. Components of immunity include intact skin and mucous membranes and many different white blood cells (WBCs) and their products. In addition to protection, immunity plays a role in repair of damaged tissues.

Infectious diseases are common, but most adults are healthy more often than they are ill. IMMUNITY with inflammation is critical to maintaining health and preventing disease. When all the different parts and functions of immunity are working well, the adult is immunocompetent and has maximum protection against infection.

IMMUNITY is reduced by many diseases, injuries, and medical therapies. *Whether immunity is reduced temporarily or permanently, this reduction always endangers the patient's health.* Chapter 19 discusses reduced and inadequate immunity. Other problems occur when immunity is excessive or if some of its processes occur at inappropriate times. Chapters 18 and 20

discuss issues related to excess or inappropriate immunity responses such as hypersensitivity and autoimmune disease.

IMMUNITY uses many cells and their functions to fight against the effects of injury or invasion. Adults interact with many other large and small living organisms (bacteria, viruses, molds, spores, pollens, protozoa, and cells from other people or animals). As long as organisms do not enter the body, they pose no health threat. Body defenses to prevent organisms from entering include intact skin and mucous membranes, the microbiome, and natural chemicals that inhibit bacterial growth. These defenses are not perfect, and invasion can occur. However, most invasions do not result in disease or illness because of proper immunity.

IMMUNITY and the immune system stimulate processes that neutralize, eliminate, or destroy invading organisms. To protect without causing harm, immune system cells exert actions only against non-self proteins and cells. Immune system cells can distinguish between the body's own healthy self cells and non-self proteins and cells.

Self Versus Non-Self

Non-self proteins and cells include infected body cells, cancer cells, cells from other people, and invading organisms.

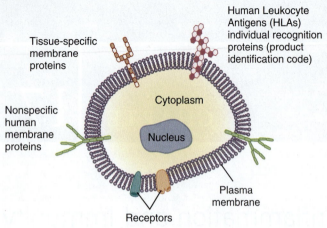

FIG. 17-1 Proteins on human cell plasma membranes.

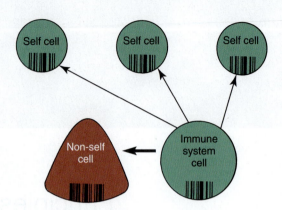

FIG. 17-2 Determination by immune system cell of self versus non-self cells.

Recognizing self versus non-self is called **self-tolerance**. This action prevents IMMUNITY from harming healthy body cells. Self-tolerance is possible because of the different proteins present on cell membranes.

Cells are surrounded by plasma membranes with different proteins on or through the surface (Fig. 17-1). For example, many different protein types are present on the liver cell membranes. Each of these protein types differs from that of all other protein types. Some protein types are specific markers for human tissues and are found only on human cells. In addition, each person's cells have unique surface proteins that are specific to that person known as **human leukocyte antigens (HLAs)**. These HLAs serve as a "universal product code" for that person and are identical only to the HLAs of an identical sibling. One adult's HLAs are recognized as "foreign," or non-self, by the immune system of another adult. Because the cell-surface proteins are non-self to another adult's immune system, they are **antigens**, which are proteins capable of stimulating an IMMUNITY response.

Human leukocyte antigens are on the surfaces of most body cells—not just leukocytes. They are a normal part of the person and determine the *tissue type* of a person, which is coded for by the specific genes he or she inherits from both parents. Other names for these HLAs are *human histocompatibility antigens* and *class I antigens.*

The HLAs are key for recognition and self-tolerance. The immune system cells constantly come into contact with other body cells and with any invader that enters the body. At each encounter the immune system cells compare the surface protein HLAs to determine whether the encountered cell belongs in the body (Fig. 17-2). If the encountered cell's HLAs match the HLAs of the immune system cell, the encountered cell is "self" and is not attacked. If the encountered cell's HLAs do not perfectly match the HLAs of the immune system cell, the encountered cell is non-self, or foreign. The immune system cell then takes action to neutralize, destroy, or eliminate this foreign invader.

A key element for recognition of non-self by cells involved in general immunity and those involved in specific immunity is the presence of **toll-like receptors (TLRs)** on these cells. Toll receptors were first discovered in fruit flies as a way that this insect recognizes and rids itself of pathogenic (disease-causing)

microorganisms. TLRs, which closely resemble the toll receptors, are known to be present on immune system cells of humans and other animals, as well as on defensive cells of insects and plants (Abbas et al., 2015). Their protective purpose is to interact with the surface of any invading organism and allow recognition that it is non-self so actions are taken to rid the body of this invader. TLRs also help immune system cells recognize damaged or unhealthy self cells.

IMMUNITY changes during an adult's life as a result of nutrition status, environmental conditions, drugs, disease, and age. Immunity is most efficient in adults who are in their 20s and 30s and slowly declines with increasing age (Touhy & Jett, 2016). Older adults have decreased immune function, increasing their risk for many health problems (Chart 17-1).

Organization of the Immune System

The immune system is present throughout the body. Most immune system cells come from the bone marrow. Some cells mature in the bone marrow; others leave the bone marrow and mature in different body sites. When mature, many immune system cells are released into the blood, where they circulate to most body areas and have specific effects.

The bone marrow is the source of all blood cells, including most immune system cells. The bone marrow produces immature, undifferentiated cells called **stem cells**. Stem cells are **pluripotent**, meaning that each cell has more than one potential outcome. When the stem cell is first generated in the bone marrow, it is undifferentiated, not yet committed to maturing into a specific blood cell type. This stem cell is flexible (pluripotent) and could become any one of many mature blood cells. Fig. 17-3 shows the possible outcomes for maturation of stem cells. The type of mature cell that the stem cell becomes depends on which pathway it follows.

The maturational pathway of any stem cell depends on body needs and the presence of specific growth factors that direct the cell to a pathway. For example, erythropoietin is a growth factor for red blood cells (**erythrocytes [RBCs]**). When immature stem cells are exposed to erythropoietin, they commit to the erythrocyte pathway and eventually become mature RBCs.

White blood cells (**leukocytes [WBCs]**) are the immune system cells that use a variety of actions to provide IMMUNITY. Table 17-1 lists the functions of different immune system cells.

CHART 17-1   Nursing Focus on the Older Adult

Changes in Immune Function Related to Aging

IMMUNE COMPONENT	FUNCTIONAL CHANGE	NURSING IMPLICATIONS
Inflammation	Reduced neutrophil function.	Neutrophil counts may be normal, but activity is reduced, increasing the risk for infection.
	Leukocytosis does not occur during acute infection.	Patients may have an infection but not show expected changes in white blood cell counts.
	Older adults may not have a fever during inflammatory or infectious episodes.	Not only is there potential loss of protection through inflammation, but also minor infections may be overlooked until the patient becomes severely infected or septic.
Antibody-mediated immunity	The total number of colony-forming B-lymphocytes and the ability of these cells to mature into antibody-secreting cells are diminished.	Older adults are less able to make new antibodies in response to the presence of new antigens. Thus they should receive immunizations such as "flu shots," the pneumococcal vaccination, and the shingles vaccination.
	There is a decline in natural antibodies, decreased response to antigens, and reduction in the amount of time the antibody response is maintained.	Older adults may not have sufficient antibodies present to provide protection when they are re-exposed to microorganisms against which they have already generated antibodies. Thus older patients need to avoid people with viral infections and receive "booster" shots for old vaccinations and immunizations, especially tetanus and pertussis (whooping cough).
Cell-mediated immunity	The number of circulating T-lymphocytes decreases.	Skin tests for tuberculosis may be falsely negative. Older patients are more at risk for bacterial and fungal infections, especially on the skin and mucous membranes, in the respiratory tract, and in the genitourinary tract.

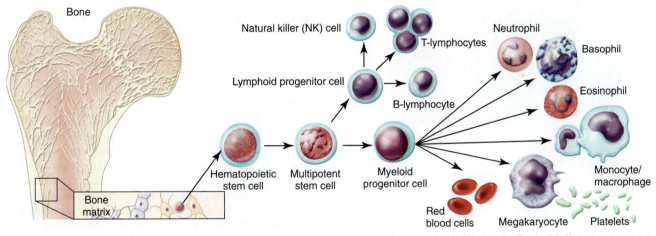

FIG. 17-3 Stem cell differentiation and maturation. (Modified from Goldman, L., & Schafer, A. (Eds.). (2012). *Goldman's Cecil medicine* (24th ed.). Philadelphia: Saunders.)

The leukocytes provide protection through these defensive actions:
- Recognition of self versus non-self
- Destruction of foreign invaders, cellular debris, and unhealthy or abnormal self cells
- Production of antibodies directed against invaders
- Complement activation
- Production of cytokines that stimulate increased formation of leukocytes in bone marrow and increase specific leukocyte activity

The three processes needed for human protection through IMMUNITY are (1) inflammation, (2) antibody-mediated immunity (AMI), and (3) cell-mediated immunity (CMI). Each process uses different defensive actions, and each influences or requires assistance from the other two processes (Fig. 17-4). *Therefore full immunity (immunocompetence) requires the function and interaction of all three processes.*

GENERAL IMMUNITY: INFLAMMATION

General immunity is nonspecific and is also called *innate-native immunity* or *natural immunity*. With inflammation, general immunity provides immediate protection against the effects of tissue injury and invading foreign proteins. Innate-native immunity is any natural protective feature of a human. It is a barrier to prevent organisms from entering the body and can

TABLE 17-1	Immune Functions of Specific Leukocytes	
VARIABLE	**LEUKOCYTE**	**FUNCTION**
Inflammation	Neutrophil	Nonspecific ingestion and phagocytosis of microorganisms and foreign protein
	Macrophage	Nonspecific recognition of foreign proteins and microorganisms; ingestion and phagocytosis Assists with antibody-mediated immunity and cell-mediated immunity
	Monocyte	Destruction of bacteria and cellular debris; matures into macrophage
	Eosinophil	Releases vasoactive amines during allergic reactions to limit these reactions
	Basophil	Releases histamine and heparin in areas of tissue damage
Antibody-mediated immunity	B-lymphocyte	Becomes sensitized to foreign cells and proteins with the assistance of macrophages and helper/inducer T-cells
	Plasma cell	Secretes immunoglobulins in response to the presence of a specific antigen
	Memory cell	Remains sensitized to a specific antigen and can secrete increased amounts of immunoglobulins specific to the antigen on re-exposure
Cell-mediated immunity	Helper/inducer T-cell	Enhances immune activity of all parts of general and specific immunity through secretion of various factors, cytokines, and lymphokines
	Cytotoxic/cytolytic T-cell	Selectively attacks and destroys non-self cells, including virally infected cells, grafts, and transplanted organs
	Natural killer cell	Nonselectively attacks non-self cells, especially body cells that have undergone mutation and become malignant; also attacks grafts and transplanted organs

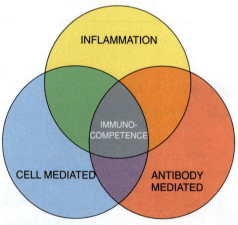

FIG. 17-4 The three divisions of immunity: inflammation, antibody-mediated immunity, and cell-mediated immunity. Optimal function of all three divisions is necessary for complete immunity.

attack organisms that have already entered the body. This type of IMMUNITY cannot be transferred from one adult to another and is not an adaptive response.

The inflammatory responses, the skin, mucosa, antimicrobial chemicals on the skin, complement, and natural killer cells compose general immunity. Inflammation is critical for health. General immunity and inflammation differ from specific immunity in two ways:

- Inflammatory protection is immediate but short term. It does not provide true immunity on repeated exposure to the same organisms.
- Inflammation is a *nonspecific* body defense to invasion or injury and can be started quickly by almost any event, regardless of where it occurs or what causes it.

So inflammation triggered by a scald burn to the hand is the same as inflammation triggered by bacteria in the middle ear. How widespread the symptoms of inflammation are depends on the intensity, severity, and duration of exposure to the

initiating event. For example, a splinter in the finger triggers inflammation only at the splinter site, whereas a burn injuring 50% of the skin leads to an inflammatory response involving the entire body.

Inflammation starts tissue actions that cause visible and uncomfortable symptoms that are important in ridding the body of harmful organisms. However, if the inflammatory response is excessive, tissue damage may result. Inflammation also helps start both antibody-mediated and cell-mediated actions to activate full IMMUNITY.

Infection

Inflammation occurs in response to tissue injury as well as to infection by organisms. *Infection is usually accompanied by inflammation; however, inflammation can occur without infection.* Inflammation without infection includes joint sprains, myocardial infarction, and blister formation. Inflammation caused by noninfectious invasion includes allergic rhinitis, contact dermatitis, and other allergic reactions. Inflammations from infection include otitis media, appendicitis, and viral hepatitis, among many others. *Inflammation does not always mean that an infection is present.*

Cell Types Involved in Inflammation

The leukocytes (white blood cells [WBCs]) involved in inflammation are neutrophils, macrophages, eosinophils, and basophils. An additional cell type important in inflammation is the tissue mast cell. Neutrophils and macrophages destroy and eliminate foreign invaders. Basophils, eosinophils, and mast cells release chemicals that act on blood vessels to cause tissue-level responses that help neutrophil and macrophage actions.

Neutrophils

Mature neutrophils make up between 55% and 70% of the normal total WBC count. Neutrophils come from the stem cells and complete the maturation process in the bone marrow (Fig. 17-5). They are also called *granulocytes* because of the

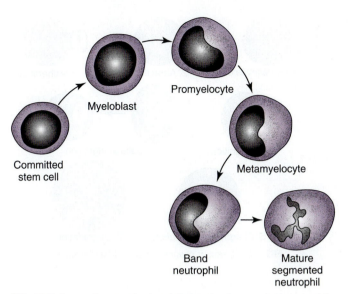

FIG. 17-5 Stem cell maturation into fully functional segmented neutrophils.

TABLE 17-2 **Values of a White Blood Cell Differential for Peripheral Blood Representing a Normal Count**

WBC TYPE	%	/MM³	×10⁹/L
Total WBC	**100**	**10,000**	**5-10**
Segs	50-62	5000-6200	5-6.2
Bands	5	500	0.5
Monos	2-8	100-700	0.1-0.7
Lymphs	20-40	1000-4000	1.0-4.0
Eosins	1-4	50-500	0.0-0.3
Basos	0.5-1.0	15-50	0.02-0.05

WBC, White blood cell.

large number of granules present inside each cell. Other names for neutrophils are based on their appearance and maturity. Mature neutrophils are also called *segmented neutrophils* ("segs") or *polymorphonuclear cells* ("polys," PMNs) because of their segmented nucleus. Less mature neutrophils are called *band neutrophils* ("bands" or "stabs") because of their nuclear shape.

Usually growth of a stem cell into a mature neutrophil requires 12 to 14 days. This time can be shortened by the presence of specific growth factors (cytokines) such as granulocyte-macrophage colony-stimulating factor (GM-CSF) and granulocyte colony-stimulating factor (G-CSF). The purpose and action of cytokines are described in the Cytokines section. In the healthy adult with full IMMUNITY, more than 100 billion fresh, mature neutrophils are released from the bone marrow into the circulation daily. This huge production is needed because the life span of each neutrophil is short—about 12 to 18 hours.

Neutrophil function provides protection after invaders, especially bacteria, enter the body. This powerful army of small cells destroys invaders by phagocytosis and enzymatic digestion, although each cell is small and can take part in only one episode of phagocytosis.

Mature neutrophils are the only stage of this cell capable of phagocytosis. Because this cell type causes continuous, instant, nonspecific protection against organisms, the percentage and actual number of mature circulating neutrophils are used to measure a patient's risk for infection: the higher the numbers, the greater the resistance to infection. This measurement is the absolute neutrophil count (ANC).

The differential of a normal WBC cell count shows the number and percent of the different types of circulating leukocytes (Table 17-2). Most circulating neutrophils are segmented neutrophils; only a small percentage are band neutrophils or less mature forms. Problems such as sepsis cause the circulating neutrophils to change from being mostly segmented neutrophils to being less mature forms. This situation is a left shift or *bandemia* because the segmented neutrophil (at the far right of the neutrophil pathway in Fig. 17-5) is no longer the most numerous type in circulation. Instead more of the circulating cells are bands—the less mature cell type found farther left on the neutrophil pathway.

A left shift indicates that the patient's bone marrow cannot produce enough mature neutrophils to keep pace with the continuing infection and is releasing immature neutrophils into the blood. These immature cells are of minimal benefit because they are not capable of phagocytosis.

Macrophages

Macrophages come from the committed myeloid stem cells in the bone marrow and form the mononuclear-phagocyte system. The stem cells first form monocytes, which are released into the blood at this stage. Until they mature, monocytes have limited activity. Most monocytes move from the blood into body tissues, where they mature into macrophages. Some macrophages become "fixed" in position within the tissues, whereas others can move within and between tissues. Macrophages in various tissues have slightly different appearances and names. The liver, spleen, and intestinal tract contain large numbers of these cells.

Macrophage function helps stimulate immediate inflammatory responses and also stimulates the longer-lasting immune responses of antibody-mediated IMMUNITY (AMI) and cell-mediated immunity (CMI). Macrophage functions include phagocytosis, repair, antigen presenting/processing, and secretion of cytokines for immune system control.

The inflammatory function of macrophages is phagocytosis. Macrophages can easily distinguish between self and non-self, and their large size makes them very effective at trapping invading cells. They have long life spans, and each cell can take part in many phagocytic events.

Basophils

Basophils come from myeloid stem cells and make up only about 1% of the total circulating WBC count. These cells cause the signs and symptoms of inflammation.

Basophil function acts on blood vessels with basophil chemicals (vasoactive amines), which include heparin, histamine, serotonin, kinins, and leukotrienes. Basophils have sites that bind the stem part of immunoglobulin E (IgE) molecules, which binds to and is activated by allergens. When allergens bind to the IgE on the basophil, the basophil membrane opens and releases the vasoactive amines into the blood, where most of them act on smooth muscle and blood vessel walls. Heparin inhibits blood and protein clotting. Histamine dilates arterioles and constricts small veins, slowing blood flow and decreasing venous return. This effect causes blood to collect in capillaries and arterioles. Kinins dilate arterioles and increase capillary permeability, causing blood plasma to leak into the interstitial space (*vascular leak syndrome*). Basophils stimulate both general inflammation and the inflammation of allergic reactions.

Eosinophils

Eosinophils come from the myeloid line and contain many vasoactive chemicals. Only 1% to 2% of the total WBC count normally is composed of eosinophils.

Eosinophil function is most active against infestations of parasitic larvae and also limits inflammatory reactions. Some eosinophil granules contain enzymes that degrade the vasoactive chemicals released by other leukocytes. This is why the number of circulating eosinophils increases during an allergic response.

Tissue Mast Cells

Tissue mast cells look like and have functions very similar to basophils and eosinophils. Although mast cells do originate in the bone marrow, they come from a different parent cell than leukocytes and do not circulate as mature cells (Abbas et al., 2015). Instead they differentiate and mature in tissues, especially those near blood vessels, lung tissue, skin, and mucous membranes. Mast cells have binding sites for the stems of IgE molecules and are involved in allergic reactions. They also respond to the inflammatory products released by T-lymphocytes. Tissue mast cells maintain and prolong inflammation and allergic reactions.

Complement

The complement system is a part of innate immunity. It is composed of a system of 20 different types of inactive plasma proteins that, when activated, act as enzymes and attract agents to enhance (or "complement") cell actions of innate immunity. When stimulated, each type of complement protein is activated, joins other activated complement proteins, surrounds an antigen, and "fixes" or sticks to the antigen. This action makes immune cell attachment to antigens more efficient. Complement fixation occurs quickly as a cascade.

Phagocytosis

A key process of inflammation is **phagocytosis**, the engulfing and destruction of invaders, which also rids the body of debris after tissue injury. Neutrophils and macrophages are most efficient at phagocytosis. Phagocytosis involves the seven steps shown in Fig. 17-6.

- *Exposure and invasion* occur as the first step in response to injury or invasion. Leukocytes that engage in phagocytosis and stimulate inflammation are present in the blood and extracellular fluids. Phagocytosis starts with invasion by organisms or foreign proteins.
- *Attraction* is the second step and brings the WBC into direct contact with the target (antigen, invader, or foreign protein). Damaged tissues secrete chemotaxins that attract neutrophils and macrophages and release debris that binds to the surface of invading proteins.
- *Adherence* binds the phagocytic cell to the surface of the target. *Opsonins* are substances that increase contact of the cell with its target by coating the target cell (antigen or organism). During inflammation coating the target

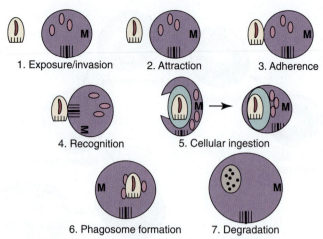

FIG. 17-6 Steps of phagocytosis. *M*, Macrophage.

makes it easier for phagocytic cells to stick to it. Substances that are opsonins are dead neutrophils, antibodies, and activated (fixated) complement components.
- *Recognition* occurs when the phagocytic cell sticks to the target cell and "recognizes" it as non-self. The phagocytic cells examine the universal product codes (human leukocyte antigens [HLAs]) of whatever they encounter. Recognition of non-self is made easier by opsonins on the target cell surface. Phagocytic cells start phagocytosis only when the target cell is recognized as non-self or debris.
- *Cellular ingestion* occurs when the target cell is brought inside the phagocytic cell by phagocytosis (engulfment).
- *Phagosome formation* occurs when the phagocyte's granules break and release enzymes that attack the ingested target.
- *Degradation* is the final step. The enzymes in the phagosome digest the engulfed target.

Sequence of Inflammation

Inflammation (inflammatory responses) occurs in a predictable three-stage sequence. The sequence is the same, regardless of the triggering event. Responses at the tissue level cause the **five cardinal symptoms of inflammation**: warmth, redness, swelling, pain, and decreased function. The timing of the stages may overlap.

Stage I is a vascular response that starts changes in blood vessels. Injured tissues and the leukocytes and tissue mast cells in this area secrete histamine, serotonin, and kinins that constrict the small veins and dilate the arterioles. These changes cause redness and warmth of the tissues. This increased blood flow increases delivery of nutrients to injured tissues.

Blood flow to the area increases (**hyperemia**), and edema forms at the site of injury or invasion. Capillary leak also occurs, allowing blood plasma to leak into the tissues. This response causes swelling and pain. Edema protects the area from further injury by creating a cushion of fluid. The duration of these responses depends on the severity of the initiating event, but usually they subside within 24 to 72 hours.

The macrophage is the major cell involved in stage I of inflammation. The action is rapid because macrophages are already in place at the site of injury or invasion. This action is limited because the number of macrophages is so small. To enhance the response, tissue macrophages secrete several cytokines. One is colony-stimulating factor (CSF), which triggers the bone marrow to shorten the time needed to produce white blood cells (WBCs) from 14 days to a matter of hours. Some cytokines cause neutrophils from the bone marrow to move to the site of injury or invasion, which leads to the next stage of inflammation.

Stage II is the cellular exudate part of the response. In this stage neutrophilia (an increased number of circulating neutrophils) occurs. Exudate in the form of pus occurs, containing dead WBCs, necrotic tissue, and fluids that escape from damaged cells.

Neutrophils, basophils, and tissue mast cells are active in this stage. Under the influence of cytokines, the neutrophil count can increase hugely within 12 hours after inflammation starts. Neutrophils attack and destroy organisms and remove dead tissue through phagocytosis. Basophils and tissue mast cells continue or sustain the initial responses

In acute inflammation the healthy adult produces enough mature neutrophils to keep pace with invasion and prevent the organisms from growing. At the same time the WBCs and inflamed tissues secrete cytokines, which allow tissue macrophages to increase and trigger bone marrow production of monocytes.

During this phase the arachidonic acid cascade starts to increase inflammation. This action begins by the conversion of fatty acids in plasma membranes into arachidonic acid (AA). The enzyme *cyclooxygenase* (COX) converts AA into chemicals that are further processed into the substances (mediators) that promote continued inflammation. Mediators include histamine, leukotrienes, prostaglandins, serotonin, and kinins. Anti-inflammatory drugs stop this cascade by preventing cyclooxygenase from converting AA into inflammatory mediators.

When an infection stimulating inflammation lasts longer than just a few days, the bone marrow begins to release immature neutrophils, reducing the number of circulating mature neutrophils. This problem limits helpful effects of inflammation and increases the risk for sepsis.

Stage III features tissue repair and replacement. Although this stage is completed last, it begins at the time of injury and is critical to the final function of the inflamed area.

WBCs involved in inflammation start the replacement of lost tissues or repair of damaged tissues by inducing the remaining healthy cells to divide. In tissues that cannot divide, WBCs trigger new blood vessel growth and scar tissue formation. Because scar tissue does not act like the tissue it replaces, function is lost wherever scar tissue forms. For example, when heart muscles are destroyed by a myocardial infarction (heart attack), scar tissue forms in the area to prevent a hole from forming in the heart wall as the ischemic cells die. The scar tissue serves only as a patch; it does not contract or act in any way like heart muscle. So if 20% of the left ventricle is replaced with scar tissue, the effectiveness of left ventricular contraction is reduced by 20%.

Inflammation alone cannot provide long-lasting IMMUNITY. Lymphocytes are the cells needed for long-lasting antibody-mediated immunity (AMI) and cell-mediated immunity (CMI).

SPECIFIC IMMUNITY

Specific IMMUNITY is an *adaptive* protection that results in long-term resistance to the effects of invading microorganisms. This means that the responses are not automatic, which is why

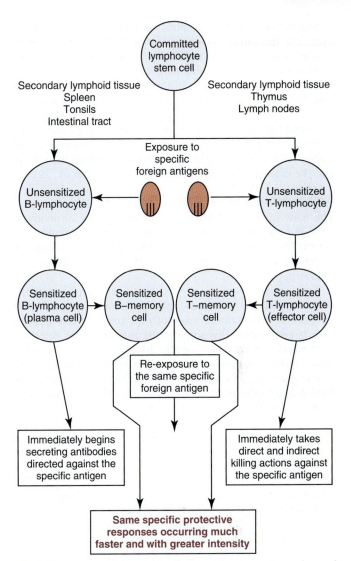

FIG. 17-7 B-lymphocyte and T-lymphocyte differentiation, maturation, and function.

specific immunity is also known as *acquired immunity*. The body has to learn to generate specific immune responses when it is infected by or exposed to specific organisms. Lymphocytes develop actions and products that provide true immunity. These cells develop specific actions in response to specific invasion (Fig. 17-7). The two divisions of specific immunity are antibody-mediated immunity and cell-mediated immunity. As indicated by Fig. 17-4, activation of both types of specific immunity require interactions with actions and cells of innate immunity.

Antibody-Mediated Immunity

Antibody-mediated immunity (AMI), also known as *humoral immunity*, uses antigen-antibody interactions to neutralize, eliminate, or destroy foreign proteins. Antibodies are produced by sensitized B-lymphocytes (B-cells).

B-cells become sensitized to a specific foreign protein (antigen) and produce antibodies directed specifically against that protein. The antibody, rather than the B-cell, then causes actions to neutralize, eliminate, or destroy that antigen. B-cells have the most direct role in AMI.

Macrophages and T-lymphocytes (discussed in the Cell-Mediated Immunity section) work with B-cells to generate antigen-antibody interactions. *For optimal AMI the entire immune system must function adequately.*

B-cells start as stem cells in the bone marrow, the primary lymphoid tissue, that commit to the lymphocyte pathway (see Fig. 17-3) and are then restricted in development. The lymphocyte stem cells released into the blood then migrate into many secondary lymphoid tissues to mature. The secondary lymphoid tissues for B-cells are the spleen, parts of lymph nodes, tonsils, and the mucosa of the intestinal tract (McCance et al., 2014).

Antigen-Antibody Interactions

The body learns to make enough of any specific antibody to provide long-lasting IMMUNITY against specific organisms or toxins. The seven steps for specific antibody production against a specific antigen are shown in Fig. 17-8 and described in the following paragraphs.

Exposure or invasion is needed for the antigen to enter the adult to generate an antibody, although not all exposures result in antibody production. Invasion by the antigen must occur in such large numbers that some of the antigen evades detection by the body's natural nonspecific defenses or overwhelms the ability of the inflammatory response to get rid of the invader.

For example, an adult who has never been exposed to the viral disease *influenza A* now baby-sits for three children who develop influenza symptoms within the next 10 hours. These children, in the presymptomatic stage, shed many millions of live influenza A virus particles by droplets from the upper respiratory tract. They expose the baby-sitter by drinking out of the baby-sitter's cup, kissing him or her on the lips, and sneezing and coughing into his or her face. During the 5 hours spent with the children, the baby-sitter is heavily invaded by the influenza A virus and will become sick with this disease within 2 to 4 days. While the virus is growing and the disease is developing, the baby-sitter's white blood cells (WBCs) are taking part in antibody-antigen actions to prevent him or her from having influenza A more than once.

Antigen recognition is the recognition of the antigen by unsensitized B-cells. This action requires the help of macrophages and helper/inducer T-cells.

Recognition is started by the macrophages of innate immunity. After the antigen surface has been altered by opsonization (see discussion of "adherence" in the Phagocytosis section), macrophages recognize the invading antigen as non-self and attach to the antigen. This attachment allows macrophages to "present" the attached antigen to the helper/inducer T-cell. Then the helper/inducer T-cell and the macrophages together process the antigen to expose the antigen's recognition sites (universal product code). After processing the antigen, the helper/inducer T-cells bring the antigen into contact with the B-cell so the B-cell can recognize the antigen as non-self.

1. Invasion of the body by new antigens in sufficient numbers to stimulate an immune response.

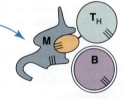

2. Interaction of macrophage (M) and helper/inducer T-cell (T$_H$) in the processing and presenting of the antigen to the unsensitized "virgin" B-lymphocyte (B).

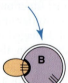

3. Sensitization of the virgin B-lymphocyte to the new antigen.

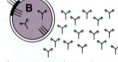

7. On re-exposure to the same antigen, the sensitized lymphocytes and their progeny produce large quantities of the antibody specific to the antigen. In addition, new "virgin" B-lymphocytes become sensitized to the antigen and also begin antibody production.

4. Antibody production by the B-lymphocyte. These antibodies are directed specifically against the initiating antigen. The antibodies are released from the B-lymphocyte and float freely in the blood and some other fluids.

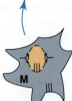

6. Antibody binding causes cellular events and attracts other leukocytes to the complex. The interaction of other leukocytes along with the cellular events results in the neutralization, destruction, or elimination of the antigen.

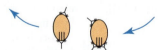

5. Antibodies bind to the antigen, forming an immune complex.

FIG. 17-8 Sequence of the seven steps required to stimulate antibody-mediated immunity.

Sensitization occurs when the B-cell recognizes the antigen as non-self and is now "sensitized" to this antigen. A single unsensitized B-cell can become sensitized only once. *So each B-cell can be sensitized to only one type of antigen.*

Sensitizing allows this B-cell to respond to any substance that carries the same antigens (codes) as the original antigen. The sensitized B-cell always remains sensitized to that specific antigen. In addition, all cells produced by that sensitized B-cell also are already pre-sensitized to that same specific antigen.

Immediately after it is sensitized, the B-cell divides and forms two types of B-lymphocytes, each one remaining sensitized to that specific antigen (see Fig. 17-7). One new cell becomes a plasma cell, which starts immediately to produce antibodies against the sensitizing antigen. The other new cell becomes a memory cell. The memory cell is a sensitized B-cell but does not produce antibodies until the next exposure to the same antigen (see discussion of sustained immunity [memory] later as an antigen-antibody interaction).

Antibody production and release allow the antibodies to search out specific antigens. Antibodies are produced by plasma cells; each plasma cell can make as many as 300 molecules of antibody per second. A plasma cell produces antibodies specific only to the antigen that originally sensitized the parent B-cell. For example, in the case of the baby-sitter who was invaded by the influenza A virus, the plasma cells from those B-cells sensitized to the influenza A virus can make only anti-influenza A antibodies. The antibody class (e.g., immunoglobulin G [IgG] or immunoglobulin M [IgM]) that the plasma cell produces may vary, but the antibody can be forever directed only against the influenza A virus.

Antibody molecules from plasma cells are released into the blood and body fluids (body "humors") as free antibodies that are separate from the B-cells. So this type of IMMUNITY may be called humoral immunity. *Circulating antibodies can be transferred from one adult to another and provide the receiving adult with immediate short-term immunity.*

Antibody-antigen binding is needed for anti-antigen actions. Antibodies are Y-shaped molecules (Fig. 17-9). The tips of the short arms of the Y recognize the specific antigen and bind to it. Because each antibody molecule has two tips (Fab fragments, or arms), each antibody can bind either to two separate antigens or to two areas of the same antigen.

The stem of the Y is the "Fc fragment." This area can bind to Fc receptor sites on white blood cells (WBCs). The WBC then not only has its own means of attacking antigens but also has the added power of having surface antibodies that can stick to antigens (see Fig. 17-9).

The binding of antibody to antigen may not be lethal to the antigen. Instead antibody-antigen binding starts other actions that neutralize, eliminate, or destroy the antigen.

Antibody-binding actions are triggered when an antibody binds to an antigen. The resulting actions of agglutination, lysis, complement fixation, precipitation, and inactivation can then neutralize, eliminate, or destroy the bound antigen.

Agglutination is a clumping action occurring when the antibodies link antigens together, forming large and small immune complexes (Fig. 17-10). The irregular shape of the antigen-antibody complex (see Fig. 17-10) increases the actions of macrophages and neutrophils.

Lysis is cell membrane destruction, and it occurs when antibodies bind to membrane-bound antigens of some invaders. Antibody binding makes holes in the invader's membrane, weakening the invader, especially bacteria and viruses. This response usually requires that complement be activated and "fixed" to the immune complex.

Complement activation and fixation are actions triggered by the IgG and IgM classes of antibodies that can remove or destroy antigen. (See discussion of complement in the General Immunity and Inflammation section for an explanation of how complement assists in immunity.) Binding of either IgG or IgM to an antigen provides a binding site for the first component of complement. Once the first complement molecule is activated, other proteins of the complement system are activated in a cascade.

Precipitation is similar to agglutination but has a larger response. With precipitation, antibody molecules bind so much antigen that large antigen-antibody complexes are formed. These complexes cannot stay in suspension in the blood. Instead they form a large precipitate, which then can be acted on and removed by neutrophils and macrophages.

Inactivation (neutralization) makes an antigen harmless without destroying it. Usually only a small area of the antigen, the *active site,* causes the harmful effects. When an antibody binds to an antigen's active site, covering it, the antigen is made harmless without destroying it.

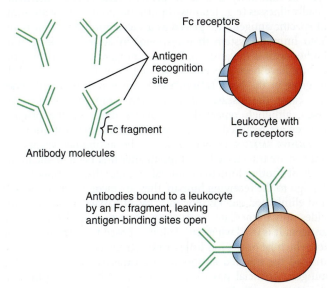

FIG. 17-9 Antibody structure and the Fc receptors on leukocytes.

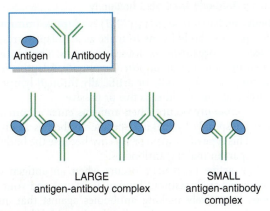

FIG. 17-10 Formation of large and small antigen-antibody complexes (immune complexes).

Sustained immunity (memory) provides us with long-lasting, true IMMUNITY to a specific antigen. This immunity results from memory B-cells made during lymphocyte sensitization. These memory cells remain sensitized to the specific antigen to which they were originally exposed. On re-exposure to the same antigen, the memory cells rapidly respond by dividing and forming new sensitized blast cells and plasma cells. The blast cells continue to divide, producing many more sensitized plasma cells. These new sensitized plasma cells rapidly make large amounts of the antibody specific for the sensitizing antigen.

Having memory cells respond on re-exposure to the same antigen that originally sensitized the B-cell allows a rapid and large immune response *(anamnestic response)* to the antigen. When so much antibody is made, the invading organisms may be removed completely, and illness does not result. This process prevents adults from becoming ill with any infectious disease more than once, even though they are exposed many times to the causative organism. Without immunologic memory, adults would be susceptible to diseases at every exposure to the organisms, and no long-term IMMUNITY would be generated (Abbas et al., 2015).

Antibody Classification

All antibodies are immunoglobulins, also called *gamma globulins*. A globulin is a protein that is globular rather than straight. Because antibodies are globular proteins, they are "globulins." The term **immunoglobulin** is used because they are globular proteins that provide IMMUNITY. Antibodies also are called **gamma globulins** because all free antibodies in the plasma separate out in the gamma fraction of plasma proteins during electrophoresis. The five antibody types are classified by differences in size, location, amount, and function (Table 17-3).

On first exposure to an antigen, the newly sensitized B-cell produces the IgM antibody type against the antigen. IgM is special because it forms itself into a five-member group with ten antigen binding sites. So even though antibody production is slow on first exposure, IgM is very efficient at antigen binding. This process ensures that the initial illness (e.g., influenza A) lasts only 5 to 10 days. On re-exposure to the same antigen, the already sensitized B-cell makes large amounts of the IgG type of antibody against that antigen. Although IgG does not form groups of five, the enormous amounts produced make IgG antibodies efficient at clearing the antigen and protecting the patient from becoming ill with the disease again.

Acquiring Antibody-Mediated Immunity

Antibody-mediated IMMUNITY (AMI) is **adaptive immunity** in which a person's body learns to make as an adaptive response to invasion by organisms or foreign proteins. Thus antibody-mediated immunity is an *acquired immunity*. Adaptive immunity occurs either naturally or artificially through lymphocyte responses and can be either active or passive.

Active immunity occurs when antigens enter a human and he or she responds by making specific antibodies against the antigen. This type of IMMUNITY is *active* because the body takes an active part in making antibodies.

Natural active IMMUNITY occurs when an antigen enters your body naturally without human assistance and your body responds by actively making antibodies against that antigen (e.g., influenza A virus). Usually the invasion that triggers antibody production also causes the disease. However, processes

TABLE 17-3	Antibody Classification
ANTIBODY	**FUNCTION**
IgA	"Secretory" antibody that is present in high concentrations in the secretions of mucous membranes and the intestinal mucosa Very low circulating levels Most responsible for preventing infection in the upper and lower respiratory tracts, the GI tract, and the genitourinary tract
IgD	Present in low blood concentrations in conjunction with IgM
IgE	Variable concentration in blood Associated with antibody-mediated hypersensitivity reactions Binds to mast cells and causes their degranulation when an allergen (antigen) binds to IgE antigen recognition sites
IgG	Composes at least 75% of circulating antibody population Is heavily expressed on second and subsequent exposures to antigens to provide sustained, long-term immunity against invading microorganisms Activates classic complement pathway and enhances neutrophil and macrophage actions
IgM	First antibody formed by a newly sensitized B-lymphocyte plasma cell Composes about 10% to 15% of circulating antibody population Especially effective at the antibody actions of agglutination and precipitation because of having 10 potential binding sites per molecule Activates complement pathway

occurring in your body at the same time as infection create immunity to that antigen so illness does not occur again after a second exposure to the same antigen. *Natural active immunity is the most effective and the longest lasting.*

Artificial active IMMUNITY is the protection developed by vaccination or immunization (Hogue & Meador, 2016). This type of immunity is used to prevent serious and potentially deadly illnesses (e.g., tetanus, diphtheria, polio). Small amounts of specific antigens are placed as a vaccination into your body. Your immune system then responds by actively making antibodies against the antigen. Because antigens used for this procedure have been specially processed to make them less likely to grow in the body (**attenuated**), this exposure usually does not cause the disease. Artificial active immunity lasts many years, although repeated but smaller doses of the original antigen are required as a "booster" to retain the protection.

Passive IMMUNITY occurs when the antibodies against an antigen are transferred to a human after first being made in the body of another human or animal. Because these antibodies are foreign to the receiving human, they are recognized as non-self and eliminated quickly. For this reason passive immunity provides only immediate, short-term protection against a specific antigen. It is used when an adult is exposed to a serious disease for which he or she has little or no actively acquired immunity. Instead the injected antibodies are expected to inactivate the antigen. Artificial passive immunity may be used to prevent disease or death for patients exposed to rabies, tetanus, and poisonous snake bites.

Natural passive IMMUNITY occurs when antibodies are passed from the mother to the fetus via the placenta or to the infant through colostrum and breast milk.

AMI works with inflammation to protect against infection. It provides effective long-lasting IMMUNITY only when its actions are combined with those of cell-mediated immunity.

? NCLEX EXAMINATION CHALLENGE 17-1
Physiological Integrity

Which white blood cell types are involved in the development of antibody-mediated immunity? **Select all that apply.**
A. Basophils
B. B-lymphocytes
C. Cytotoxic/cytolytic T-cells
D. Helper/inducer T-cells
E. Macrophages
F. Natural killer cells
G. Neutrophils

Cell-Mediated Immunity

Cell-mediated IMMUNITY (CMI), or cellular immunity, involves many white blood cell (WBC) actions and interactions. CMI also is adaptive or acquired true immunity that is provided by lymphocyte stem cells that mature in the secondary lymphoid tissues of the thymus and pericortical areas of lymph nodes (see Fig. 17-7). Certain CMI responses influence and regulate the activities of antibody-mediated immunity (AMI) and innate immunity (inflammation) by producing and releasing cytokines. For total or full immunity, CMI must function optimally.

Cell Types Involved in Cell-Mediated Immunity

The WBCs with the most important known roles in CMI include several specific T-lymphocytes (T-cells) along with a special population of cells known as *natural killer (NK) cells*. T-cells have a variety of subsets, each of which has a specific function.

Different T-cell subsets can be identified by the presence of "marker proteins" (antigens) on the cell membrane's surface. More than 200 different T-cell proteins have been identified on the cell membrane, and some of these are commonly used clinically to identify specific cells (Abbas et al., 2015). Most T-cells have more than one antigen on their cell membrane. For example, all mature T-cells contain T1, T3, T10, and T11 proteins.

The names that identify specific T-cell subsets include the specific membrane antigen and the overall actions of the cells in a subset. The three T-lymphocyte subsets that are critically important for the development and continuation of CMI are helper/inducer T-cells, suppressor T-cells, and cytotoxic/cytolytic T-cells. The natural killer cell (NK cell) also contributes to CMI.

Helper/inducer T-cells have the T4 protein on their membranes. These cells are usually called *T4+ cells* or T_H *cells*. The most correct name for helper/inducer T-cells is *CD4+* (cluster of differentiation 4).

Helper/inducer T-cells easily recognize self cells versus non-self cells. When they recognize non-self (antigen), helper/inducer T-cells secrete cytokines that can enhance the activity of other WBCs and increase overall immune function. These cytokines increase bone marrow production of stem cells and speed up their maturation. Thus helper/inducer T-cells act as organizers in "calling to arms" various squads of WBCs involved in inflammatory, antibody, and cellular protective actions.

Suppressor T-cells have the T8-lymphocyte antigen on membrane surfaces. These cells are commonly called *T8+ cells, CD8+ cells,* or T_S-*cells*. Suppressor T-cells help regulate CMI.

Suppressor T-cells prevent hypersensitivity (IMMUNITY *overreactions*) on exposure to non-self cells or proteins. This action prevents the formation of antibodies directed against normal, healthy self cells, which is the basis for many autoimmune diseases. The suppressor T-cells secrete cytokines that have an overall *inhibitory* action on most cells of the immune system.

Suppressor T-cells have the opposite action of helper/inducer T-cells. For optimal CMI, then, a balance between helper/inducer T-cell activity and suppressor T-cell activity must be maintained. This balance occurs when the helper/inducer T-cells outnumber the suppressor T-cells by a ratio of 2:1. When this ratio increases, indicating that helper/inducer T-cells vastly outnumber the suppressor cells, overreactions can occur, some of which are both tissue damaging and unpleasant. When the helper/suppressor ratio decreases, indicating fewer-than-normal helper/inducer T-cells, IMMUNITY is suppressed, and the person's risk for infections increases.

Cytotoxic/cytolytic T-cells are also called T_C-*cells*. Because they have the T8 protein present on their surfaces, they are a subset of suppressor cells. Cytotoxic/cytolytic T-cells destroy cells that contain a processed antigen's human leukocyte antigens (HLAs). This activity is most effective against self cells infected by parasites such as viruses or protozoa.

Parasite-infected self cells have both self HLA proteins (universal product code) and the parasite's antigens on the cell surface. This allows immune system cells to recognize the infected self cell as abnormal; and the cytotoxic/cytolytic T-cell can bind to it, punch a hole, and deliver a "lethal hit" of enzymes to the infected cell, causing it to lyse and die.

Natural killer (NK) cells are also known as *CD16+ cells* and are very important in providing CMI. These cells have direct cytotoxic effects on some non-self cells without first being sensitized. They conduct "seek and destroy" missions in the body to eliminate non-self cells. The NK cells are most effective in destroying unhealthy or abnormal self cells such as cancer cells and virally infected body cells (Kannan et al., 2014).

Cytokines

Cell-mediated IMMUNITY (CMI) regulates the immune system by producing cytokines. Cytokines are small protein hormones produced by the many WBCs (and some other tissues). Cytokines made by the macrophages, neutrophils, eosinophils, and monocytes are called monokines. Those produced by T-cells are called lymphokines. In addition, many other body cell types can produce and respond to cytokines.

Cytokines work like hormones: one cell produces a cytokine, which in turn exerts its effects on other cells of the immune system and on other body cells. The cells responding to the cytokine may be located close to or remote from the cytokine-secreting cell. Thus cytokines act like "messengers" that tell specific cells how and when to respond. The cells that change their activity when a cytokine is present are "responder" cells. For a responder cell to respond to the presence of a cytokine, the responder cell must have a specific receptor to which the cytokine can bind. Once the cytokine binds to its receptor, the responder cell changes its activity.

TABLE 17-4 Activity of Selected Cytokines

CYTOKINE	ACTIONS
Pro-inflammatory Cytokines	
Interleukin-1 (IL-1)	Induces fever
	Stimulates production of prostaglandins
	Increases growth of CD4+ T-cells
Interleukin-2 (IL-2)	Increases growth and differentiation of T-lymphocytes
	Enhances natural killer cell activity against cancer cells
Interleukin-6 (IL-6)	Stimulates liver to produce fibrinogen and protein C
	Increases rate of bone marrow production of stem cells
	Increases numbers of sensitized B-lymphocytes
Tumor necrosis factor (TNF)	Induces fever
	Major cytokine involved in rheumatoid arthritis damage
	Major cytokine involved in the acute inflammatory response to infectious bacteria and starts many of the systemic complications of severe infection or sepsis
	Participates in graft rejection
	Induces cell death
	Stimulates delayed hypersensitivity reactions and allergy
Growth Factors	
Granulocyte colony-stimulating factor (G-CSF)	Increases numbers and maturity of neutrophils
Granulocyte-macrophage colony-stimulating factor (GM-CSF)	Increases growth and maturation of myeloid stem cells
Erythropoietin	Increases growth and differentiation of erythrocytes
Thrombopoietin	Increases growth and differentiation of platelets

Cytokines control many inflammatory and immune responses and are controlled by interactions with other systems. Cytokines include the interleukins (ILs), interferons (INFs), colony-stimulating factors, tumor necrosis factor (TNFs), and transforming growth factors (TGFs). The interleukins are the largest group of cytokines, with interleukin-33 (IL-33) being the most recently defined (Abbas et al., 2015). Some cytokines have families and other classifications. Some cytokines are "pro-inflammatory" and increase the actions of natural immunity (inflammation). These currently include TNF-α, IL-1, IL-10, IL-12, and interferons (α [alpha], β [beta], and γ [gamma]). Other cytokines have a major influence on AMI and CMI activities. These include IL-2, IL-4, IL-5, IL-10, TGF-β, and INF-γ. Although there are many cytokines, not all functions are known or clinically useful at this time. Table 17-4 lists the cytokines that have current clinical importance. Chapters discussing specific diseases (e.g., lymphoma, rheumatoid arthritis) caused by or treated with certain cytokines have more information about the role of specific cytokines in the disease and its treatment.

Protection Provided by Cell-Mediated Immunity

Cell-mediated IMMUNITY (CMI) helps protect the body through the ability to differentiate self from non-self. The non-self cells most easily recognized by CMI are cancer cells and self cells infected by organisms that live within host cells, especially viruses. CMI watches for and rids the body of self cells that might potentially harm the body. *CMI is important in preventing the development of cancer and metastasis after exposure to carcinogens.*

❓ NCLEX EXAMINATION CHALLENGE 17-2

Health Promotion and Maintenance

A client has a white blood cell change in which the number of suppressor T-cells is way below normal and asks the nurse which type of health problem(s) could be expected as a result of this deficiency. What is the nurse's **best** response?
A. "You will need to receive booster vaccinations more often because your ability to make antibodies is reduced."
B. "Try to avoid crowds and people who are ill because you are now more susceptible to bacterial and viral infections."
C. "You will be more prone to allergic reactions when exposed to allergens or drugs."
D. "Your risk for cancer development is increased."

AGE-RELATED CHANGES IN IMMUNITY

Many IMMUNITY changes occur in older adults that reduce protection and increase risk for infection and the development of autoimmune diseases. These changes occur in both general immunity and in specific immunity. Review Chart 17-1 for nursing implications related to reduced immunity in the older adult.

Normal flora (microbiome) of skin, mucous membranes, and the GI tract change; and overgrowth of more pathogenic organisms occurs (Touhy & Jett, 2016). The number of neutrophils and macrophages are reduced, as are their functions. As a result, some of the normal responses to infection and injury are reduced. The older adult may not have a fever or any temperature elevation even with severe infection. The usual response of an increased white blood cell (WBC) count is delayed or absent. The number of toll-like receptors (TLRs) decreases (McCance et al., 2014). These changes result in less recognition of pathogens and an increase in the risk for infections of all types. In addition, because some of the usual responses are absent, identification and management of infection may be delayed until sepsis is present.

Changes in specific immune function include lower T-cell function (although lymphocyte numbers do not decrease). B-lymphocytes take longer to become sensitized and begin to make antibodies to new antigen exposures. Memory cells are much slower to respond to re-exposure of antigens. For these reasons repeat vaccinations to boost specific immunities developed in childhood are needed for older adults. With the loss of recognition of self, the amount of circulating autoantibodies increases, increasing the risk for autoimmune diseases in older adults (McCance et al., 2014).

TRANSPLANT REJECTION

Transplant rejection is caused by general and specific immunity functions of a host directed against tissues and organs transplanted from other people. Host natural killer (NK) cells and cytotoxic/cytolytic T-cells are the major cells responsible for the destructive attacks on transplanted organs *(grafts)* leading to host rejection of these helpful tissues. Because the solid organ

CLINICAL JUDGMENT CHALLENGE 17-1
Safety; Patient-Centered Care QSEN

When reviewing the vaccination record of a 74-year-old patient who has a chronic pulmonary disease, you note that, although he gets a flu shot every year and received the pneumonia vaccination 3 years ago, he has not received the pertussis (whooping cough) booster since he was 10 years old. When you recommend that he receive one now, he asks why.
1. Which type of immunity was provided by his previous pertussis vaccinations? Explain your choice.
2. What would another pertussis vaccination do for him now?
3. How will you answer his question? Provide a rationale for your response.

transplanted into the recipient (host) is seldom a perfectly identical match of human leukocyte antigens (HLAs) (unless the organ is obtained from an identical sibling) between the donated organ and the recipient host, the patient's immune system cells recognize a newly transplanted organ as non-self. Without intervention, the recipient's immune system starts immunologic actions that destroy these non-self cells, leading to rejection of the transplanted organ. Rejection is a complex series of responses that change over time and involve different components of IMMUNITY. Rejection can be hyperacute, acute, or chronic.

Hyperacute Rejection

Hyperacute rejection begins immediately on transplantation and is a result of antigen-antibody complexes that form in the blood vessels of the transplanted organ (Abbas et al., 2015). The recipient's blood has pre-existing antibodies to the antigens (including blood group antigens) present in the donated organ. The antigen-antibody complexes adhere to the lining of blood vessels and activate complement, which triggers small blood clots to form throughout the new organ. Widespread clotting occludes blood vessels and leads to ischemic necrosis, inflammation with phagocytosis of the necrotic blood vessels, and release of enzymes into the new organ. The enzymes cause massive cellular destruction within the transplanted organ.

Hyperacute rejection occurs mostly in transplanted kidneys but is less common now with better HLA matching. Symptoms of rejection are apparent within minutes of attachment of the donated organ to the recipient's blood supply. The process usually cannot be stopped once it has started, and the rejected organ is removed as soon as hyperacute rejection is diagnosed.

Acute Rejection

Acute rejection first occurs within 1 week to 3 months after transplantation and sporadically after that as a result of two mechanisms. The first mechanism is antibody mediated and results in vasculitis within the transplanted organ. This reaction differs from hyperacute rejection in that blood vessel necrosis (not occlusion) leads to organ destruction.

The second mechanism is cellular. The recipient's cytotoxic/cytolytic T-cells and NK cells enter the transplanted organ through the blood, penetrate the organ cells, start an inflammatory response, and cause lysis of the organ cells.

Diagnosis of acute rejection is made by laboratory tests that show impaired function of the donated organ and by biopsy of the donated organ. Symptoms of acute rejection vary with each patient and with the specific organ transplanted. For example, when acute rejection occurs in a transplanted kidney, the patient usually has some tenderness in the kidney area and may have other general symptoms of inflammation.

An episode of acute rejection after solid organ transplantation does not automatically mean that the patient will lose the new organ. Drug management of the recipient's immune responses at this time may limit the damage to the organ and allow the graft to be maintained.

Chronic Rejection

The origin of *chronic rejection* is related to chronic inflammation and scarring. The smooth muscles of arteries overgrow and occlude these vessels (Abbas et al., 2015). The organ tissues are replaced with fibrotic, scarlike tissue, and function is reduced in proportion to the amount of scarring. This type of reaction is long-standing and occurs continuously as a response to chronic ischemia caused by blood vessel injury. The results of chronic rejection are unique to different transplanted organs. For example, in transplanted lungs chronic rejection thickens small airways. In transplanted livers chronic rejection destroys bile ducts. In transplanted hearts this process is called *accelerated graft atherosclerosis (AGA)* and is the major cause of death in patients who have survived 1 or more years after heart transplantation.

Although good control over the recipient's immune function can delay this type of rejection, the process probably occurs to some degree with all transplanted solid organs obtained from donors who are not identical siblings of the recipients. Because the fibrotic changes are permanent, there is no cure for chronic graft rejection. When the fibrosis increases to the extent that the transplanted organ can no longer function, the only recourse is retransplantation.

Management of Transplant Rejection

Rejection of transplanted solid organs involves all three components of IMMUNITY, although cell-mediated immune (CMI) responses contribute the most to the rejection process. Approved drugs used to manage transplant rejection are listed in Chart 17-2.

Maintenance therapy is the continuous immunosuppression used after a solid organ transplant. The drugs used for routine therapy after solid organ transplantation are combinations of a calcineurin inhibitor, a corticosteroid, and an antiproliferative agent (Allison, 2016). Corticosteroids cause a general immunosuppression, which leave the patient at greater risk for infection. Although corticosteroids remain a part of therapy, the dosages are lower than in the past. Calcineurin inhibitors and antiproliferative agents are part of "selective immunosuppressant" therapy (Allison, 2016; Burchum & Rosenthal, 2016). These drugs more specifically target immunity components that are responsible for rejection. Which drugs are used depends on the transplant type and other patient-specific conditions. These are all oral agents and must be taken for the life of the transplanted organ. All are immunosuppressive to some degree, and the dosage is adjusted to the immune response of each patient. Treatment with these agents increases the risk for bacterial and fungal infections and for cancer development.

Rescue therapy is used to treat acute rejection episodes. The drug categories for this purpose are the monoclonal and polyclonal antibodies (see Chart 17-2). The drugs used for maintenance are often also used during rejection episodes at much higher dosages than for maintenance (Allison, 2016; Burchum & Rosenthal, 2016).

CHART 17-2 Common Examples of Drug Therapy

Drugs to Prevent Transplant Rejection

DRUG/CLASS	ROUTE	SIDE EFFECTS
Corticosteroids—Broadly inhibit cytokine production in most leukocytes, resulting in generalized immunosuppression		
Prednisone (Deltasone)	Oral	Hypertension Hyperlipidemia Osteoporosis Weight gain Cushingoid appearance Opportunistic infection Glaucoma GI ulcer formation Hyperglycemia
Prednisolone (Millipred, Orapred, Veripred)	Oral	Same as for prednisone
Calcineurin Inhibitors—The inhibition of calcineurin stops the production and secretion of IL-2, which then prevents the activation of lymphocytes involved in transplant rejection		
Cyclosporine (Sandimmune, Neoral, Gengraf)	Oral	Nephrotoxic Hypertension Tremor Coronary artery disease Hirsutism Gingival hyperplasia Opportunistic infections Malignancies Hyperuricemia Hepatoxicity
Tacrolimus (Astagraf XL, HECORIA, Prograf)	Oral	Nephrotoxic Hypertension Hyperkalemia Hypomagnesemia Hyperglycemia Opportunistic infections Malignancies
Antiproliferatives—The main action of all antiproliferatives is to inhibit something essential to DNA synthesis, which prevents cell division in activated lymphocytes. Some have additional immune suppressive actions		
Azathioprine (Azasan, Imuran)	Oral	Bone marrow suppression Thrombocytopenia Anemia Pancreatitis Hepatotoxicity Malignancies

DRUG/CLASS	ROUTE	SIDE EFFECTS
Mycophenolate (CellCept, Myfortic)	Oral	Leucopenia Thrombocytopenia Nausea Opportunistic infection Malignancies
Sirolimus (Rapamune)	Oral	Leucopenia Thrombocytopenia Hypercholesterolemia Hypertriglyceridemia
Everolimus (Afinitor, Zortress)	Oral	Acne GI upsets Hepatoxicity Cushingoid appearance Gingival hyperplasia Hyperglycemia Hyperlipidemia Hypertension Leucopenia
Monoclonal Antibodies—Specifically target the activation sites of T-lymphocytes, increasing their elimination from circulation		
Muromonab-CD3 (Orthoclone OKT3)	IV	Systemic inflammatory responses Aseptic meningitis Opportunistic infections Malignancies Hypersensitivity reactions
Basiliximab (Simulect)	IV	GI disturbances
Daclizumab (Zenapax)	IV	GI disturbances
Polyclonal Antibodies—Antibodies derived from other animals (horses, rabbits, rats) that bind to and eliminate most T-lymphocytes, thus stopping a transplant rejection episode		
Antithymocyte globulin— equine (Atgam)	IV	Leukopenia Serum sickness Thrombocytopenia Pruritus Fever Arthralgias Opportunistic infections Malignancies
Antithymocyte globulin— rabbit (RATG, Thymoglobulin)	IV	Same as for antithymocyte globulin—equine

GET READY FOR THE NCLEX® EXAMINATION!

KEY POINTS

Review the following key points for each NCLEX Examination Client Needs Category.

Health Promotion and Maintenance

- Remind adults, especially older adults, that vaccinations providing artificial active IMMUNITY require periodic "boosting" for best long-term effects.
- Remember that older adults may not have typical symptoms of infection or responses to tests as a result of reduced IMMUNITY.

Physiological Integrity

- Use the differential of the WBC count to determine the patient's risk for infection, the presence or absence of infection, the presence or absence of an allergic reaction, and whether an infection is bacterial or viral.
- Remind patients who receive transplanted organs (unless from an identical sibling) about the need to take immunosuppressive drugs daily to prevent transplant rejection.
- Teach patients who take immunosuppressive drugs long term that they have an increased risk for infection and cancer development.

SELECTED BIBLIOGRAPHY

Abbas, A., Lichtman, A., & Pillai, S. (2015). *Cellular and molecular immunology* (8th ed.). Philadelphia: Saunders.

Allison, T. (2016). Immunosuppressive therapy in transplantation. *Nursing Clinics of North America, 51*(1), 107–120.

Burchum, J., & Rosenthal, L. (2016). *Lehne's pharmacology for nursing care* (9th ed.). St. Louis: Elsevier.

Hogue, M., & Meador, A. (2016). Vaccines and immunization practice. *Nursing Clinics of North America, 51*(1), 121–136.

Kannan, R., Madden, K., & Andrews, S. (2014). Primer on immune oncology and immune response. *Clinical Journal of Oncology Nursing, 18*(3), 311–317.

McCance, K., Huether, S., Brashers, V., & Rote, N. (2014). *Pathophysiology: The biologic basis for disease in adults and children* (7th ed.). St. Louis: Mosby.

Pagana, K., Pagana, T., & Pagana, T. (2017). *Mosby's diagnostic and laboratory test reference* (13th ed.). St. Louis: Mosby.

Pagana, K., Pagana, T., & Pike-MacDonald, S. (2013). *Mosby's Canadian manual of diagnostic and laboratory tests* (1st ed.). St. Louis: Elsevier.

Rittle, C., & Francis, R. (2016). The critical role of nurses in promoting immunization for adults. *American Nurse Today, 11*(9), 42.

Touhy, T., & Jett, K. (2016). *Ebersole and Hess' toward health aging* (9th ed.). St. Louis: Mosby.

Care of Patients With Arthritis and Other Connective Tissue Diseases

Roberta Goff and Kathy Vanderbeck

ⓔ http://evolve.elsevier.com/Iggy/

PRIORITY AND INTERRELATED CONCEPTS

The priority concepts for this chapter are:
- Mobility
- Immunity

✳ The Mobility concept exemplar for this chapter is Osteoarthritis, p. 305.

✳ The Immunity concept exemplar for this chapter is Rheumatoid Arthritis, p. 318.

The interrelated concepts for this chapter are:
- Comfort
- Clotting

LEARNING OUTCOMES

Safe and Effective Care Environment

1. Collaborate with members of the interprofessional team to ensure quality care for patients with arthritis and other connective tissue diseases (CTDs).
2. Use clinical judgment to prioritize evidence-based interventions for patients with osteoarthritis (OA) and rheumatoid arthritis (RA) to promote Mobility.
3. Prioritize nursing interventions to help prevent and monitor for postoperative complications of total joint arthroplasty, including impaired Clotting, joint dislocation, and infection.

Health Promotion and Maintenance

4. Identify community resources to help patients achieve or maintain ADL independence and Mobility.
5. Teach patients evidence-based strategies for how to prevent osteoarthritis.
6. Teach patients how to prevent Lyme disease and detect it early if it occurs.

Psychosocial Integrity

7. Assess the patient's and family's response to arthritis or other CTD, their support systems, and available resources.

8. Assess the patient's and family's sources of stress and coping mechanisms when living with arthritis or other CTD.

Physiological Integrity

9. Interpret laboratory findings for patients with RA and other CTDs that affect Immunity.
10. Assess presence and extent of pain and suffering in patients with arthritis.
11. Teach patients and their families about the postoperative care required after a total joint arthroplasty, including promotion of Comfort.
12. Describe the nursing implications associated with drug therapy for patients with RA and other CTDs.
13. Select nursing interventions for patients who have systemic sclerosis.
14. Apply knowledge of pathophysiology to plan patient-centered collaborative care of patients with gout.
15. Outline current treatment strategies for patients with fibromyalgia syndrome and psoriatic arthritis.

Connective tissue disease (CTD) is the major focus of *rheumatology*, the study of rheumatic disease. A **rheumatic disease** is any disease or condition involving the musculoskeletal system. In this text CTDs are discussed separately from other musculoskeletal conditions because most CTDs are classified as autoimmune disorders. In autoimmune disease, antibodies attack healthy normal cells and tissues. For reasons that are unclear, the immune system does not recognize body cells as self and therefore triggers an immune response. The usual *protective* nature of the immune system does not function properly in patients with autoimmune CTDs.

Most common CTDs are characterized by chronic pain and progressive joint deterioration, which results in decreased functional ability and impaired Mobility. Some of these disorders have additional localized signs and symptoms, whereas others are systemic. The economic and social costs of these diseases are staggering and will increase steadily as "baby boomers" continue to age. Patient care usually requires an interprofessional approach, including medicine, nursing, rehabilitation therapy, pharmacy, case management, and/or surgery.

Arthritis means inflammation of one or more joints. However, in clinical practice arthritis is categorized as either noninflammatory or inflammatory. The major exemplar for the concept of MOBILITY is osteoarthritis (OA), a noninflammatory, localized disorder. OA is not an autoimmune disease. The major exemplar for IMMUNITY is rheumatoid arthritis (RA), a systemic, inflammatory disorder. These priority concepts are reviewed briefly in Chapter 2.

❊ MOBILITY CONCEPT EXEMPLAR Osteoarthritis

❖ PATHOPHYSIOLOGY

Osteoarthritis is the most common arthritis and a major cause of impaired MOBILITY and disability among adults in the United States and the world. It is sometimes referred to as *osteoarthrosis* or *degenerative joint disease (DJD)*, although osteoarthritis is not always degenerative.

Osteoarthritis is the progressive deterioration and loss of cartilage and bone in one or more joints. Articular cartilage, also known as *hyaline cartilage,* contains water and a matrix of:
- Proteoglycans (glycoproteins containing chondroitin, keratin sulfate, and other substances)
- Collagen (elastic substance)
- Chondrocytes (cartilage-forming cells)

As people age or experience joint injury, proteoglycans and water decrease in the joint. The production of synovial fluid, which provides joint lubrication and nutrition, also declines because of the decreased synthesis of hyaluronic acid and less body fluid in the older adult (McCance et al., 2014).

In patients of any age with OA, enzymes such as stromelysin break down the articular matrix. In early disease the cartilage changes from its normal bluish white, translucent color to an opaque and yellowish brown appearance. As cartilage and the bone beneath the cartilage begin to erode, the joint space narrows, and osteophytes (bone spurs) form (Fig. 18-1). As the disease progresses, fissures, calcifications, and ulcerations develop; and the cartilage thins. Inflammatory cytokines (enzymes) such as interleukin-1 (IL-1) enhance this deterioration. The body's normal repair process cannot overcome the

rapid process of degeneration (McCance et al., 2014). Secondary joint inflammation can occur when joint involvement is severe.

Eventually the cartilage disintegrates, and pieces of bone and cartilage "float" in the diseased joint, causing crepitus, a grating sound caused by the loosened bone and cartilage. The resulting joint pain and stiffness can lead to decreased MOBILITY and muscle atrophy. Muscle tissue helps support joints, particularly those that bear weight (e.g., hips, knees).

Etiology and Genetic Risk

The cause of OA is a combination of many factors. For patients with *primary* OA, the disease is caused by aging and genetic factors. Weight-bearing joints (hips and knees), the shoulders, the vertebral column, and the hands are most commonly affected, probably because they are used most often or bear the mechanical stress of body weight and many years of use.

Secondary OA occurs less often than primary disease and results from joint injury and obesity. Injury to the joints from excessive use, trauma, or other joint disease (e.g., rheumatoid arthritis) predisposes a person to OA. Heavy manual occupations (e.g., carpet laying, construction, farming) cause high-intensity or repetitive stress to the joints. The risk for hip and knee OA is increased in professional and amateur athletes, especially football players, runners, and gymnasts. Fractures or other joint tissue injuries can lead to OA years after the trauma. Certain metabolic diseases (e.g., diabetes mellitus, Paget's disease of the bone) and blood disorders (e.g., hemophilia, sickle cell disease) can also cause joint degeneration.

Obesity is a common contributing factor to OA. Weight-bearing joints such as hips and knees are most often affected in obese people.

Incidence and Prevalence

The prevalence of OA varies among different populations but is a universal problem. Most people older than 60 years have joint changes that can be seen on x-ray examination, although not all of these adults actually develop the disease. According to the Arthritis Foundation (2016a) estimates, 27 million people in the United States have symptomatic OA.

▨ GENDER HEALTH CONSIDERATIONS
Patient-Centered Care QSEN

More men than women younger than 55 years have OA caused by athletic injuries. After age 55 women have the disease more often than men. Although the cause for this difference is not known, contributing factors may include increased obesity in women after having children and broader hips in women than men (Arthritis Foundation, 2016a).

Lesbian women have a high risk for OA because they are more likely to be overweight or obese when compared with other groups of women. Although the reason for this difference is not known, it is possible that lesbian women use food as a coping strategy because many have fears and concerns about "coming out" about their sexual orientation, especially to health care professionals and family members (Pettinato, 2012). Be sure to assess all patients in the hospital or community-based setting, particularly those who are older and obese, for signs and symptoms of OA.

Health Promotion and Maintenance

Based on the etiology of OA, teach patients to:
- Maintain proper nutrition to prevent obesity.
- Take care to avoid injuries, especially those that can occur from professional or amateur sports.

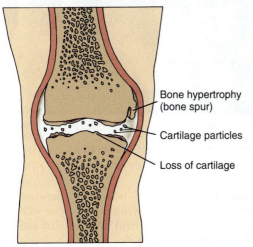

Bone hypertrophy (bone spur)

Cartilage particles

Loss of cartilage

FIG. 18-1 Joint changes in osteoarthritis.

- Take adequate work breaks to rest joints in jobs where repetitive motion is common.
- Stay active and maintain a healthy lifestyle.

❖ INTERPROFESSIONAL COLLABORATIVE CARE

◆ Assessment: Noticing

History. Patients with OA usually seek medical attention in ambulatory care settings for their joint pain. However, you will also care for those who have OA as a secondary diagnosis in acute and chronic care facilities. Ask the patient about the course of the disease. Collect information specifically related to OA such as the nature and location of joint pain and how much pain and suffering he or she is experiencing. *Remember that older patients may underreport pain, resulting in inadequate management.* Use a 0-to-10 scale or other assessment tool to assess pain intensity. Chapter 4 discusses pain assessment in detail.

Other questions to ask include:

- If joint stiffness has occurred, where and for how long?
- When and where has any joint swelling occurred?
- How much discomfort are you having?
- How much is your impaired COMFORT disrupting your daily life?
- What do you do to control the discomfort, pain, or stiffness?
- Do you have any loss of MOBILITY or difficulty in performing ADLs?

Because this disease occurs more often in older women, age and gender are important factors for the nursing history. Ask patients about their occupation, nature of work, history of injury (including falls), weight history, and current or previous involvement in sports. A history of obesity is significant, even for those currently within the ideal range for body weight. Document any family history of arthritis. Determine whether the patient has a current or previous medical condition that may cause joint symptoms.

Physical Assessment/Signs and Symptoms. In the early stage of the disease the signs and symptoms of OA may appear similar to those of rheumatoid arthritis (RA). The distinction between OA and RA becomes more evident as the disease progresses. Table 18-1 compares the major characteristics of both diseases and their common drug therapy.

The typical patient with OA is a middle-age or older woman who reports *chronic joint pain and stiffness.* Early in the course of the disease, the pain diminishes after rest and worsens after activity. Later, impaired COMFORT occurs with slight motion or even when at rest. Because cartilage has no nerve supply, the pain is caused by joint and soft-tissue involvement and spasms of the surrounding muscles. During the joint examination the patient may have tenderness on palpation or when putting the joint through range of motion. Crepitus may be felt or heard as the joint goes through range of motion. One or more joints may be affected. The patient may also report joint stiffness that usually lasts *less than* 30 minutes after a period of inactivity.

On inspection the joint is often enlarged because of bony hypertrophy. The joint feels hard on palpation. The presence of inflammation in patients with OA indicates a secondary synovitis. About half of patients with hand involvement have Heberden's nodes (bony nodules at the distal interphalangeal [DIP] joints) and Bouchard's nodes (bony nodules at the proximal interphalangeal [PIP] joints) (Fig. 18-2). Although OA is *not* typically a bilateral, symmetric disease, these large bony nodes appear on both hands, especially in women. The

TABLE 18-1   Differential Features of Rheumatoid Arthritis and Osteoarthritis

CHARACTERISTIC	RHEUMATOID ARTHRITIS	OSTEOARTHRITIS
Typical onset (age)	35-45 yr	Older than 60 yr
Gender affected	Female (3:1)	Female (2:1)
Risk factors or cause	Autoimmune (genetic basis) Emotional stress (triggers exacerbation) Environmental factors	Aging Genetic factor (possible) Obesity Trauma Occupation
Disease process	Inflammatory	Likely degenerative with secondary inflammation
Disease pattern	Bilateral, symmetric, multiple joints Usually affects upper extremities first Distal interphalangeal joints of hands spared Systemic	May be unilateral, single joint Affects weight-bearing joints and hands, spine Metacarpophalangeal joints spared Nonsystemic
Laboratory findings	Elevated rheumatoid factor, antinuclear antibody, and ESR	Normal or slightly elevated ESR
Common drug therapy	NSAIDs (short-term use) Methotrexate Leflunomide (Arava) Corticosteroids Biological response modifiers Other immunosuppressive agents	NSAIDs (short-term use) Acetaminophen Other analgesics

ESR, Erythrocyte sedimentation rate.

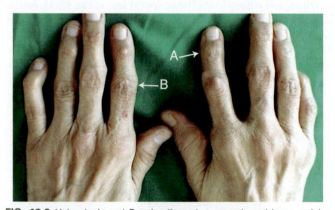

FIG. 18-2 Heberden's and Bouchard's nodes are enlarged bony nodules affecting the joints of the hand. (From Sainani, G. S. [2010]. *Manual of clinical and practical medicine.* New Delhi: Elsevier India.)

nodes may be painful and red. Some patients experience impaired COMFORT when developing nodes or when nodes are palpated. These deformities tend to be familial and are often a cosmetic concern to patients.

Joint effusions (excess joint fluid) are common when the knees are inflamed. Observe any *atrophy of skeletal muscle* from disuse. The vicious cycle of the disease discourages the movement of painful joints, which may result in contractures, muscle atrophy, and further pain. *Loss of function* or decreased MOBILITY may result, depending on which joints are involved. Hip or knee pain may cause the patient to limp and restrict walking distance.

OA can affect the spine, especially the lumbar region at the L3-4 level or the cervical region at C4-6 (neck). Compression of spinal nerve roots may occur as a result of vertebral facet bone spurs. The patient typically reports radiating pain, stiffness, and muscle spasms in one or both extremities.

Severe pain and deformity interfere with ambulation and self-care. In addition to performing a musculoskeletal assessment, collaborate with the physical and occupational therapists to conduct a functional assessment. Assess the patient's MOBILITY and ability to perform ADLs. Chapter 6 describes functional assessment.

Psychosocial Assessment. OA is a chronic condition that may cause permanent changes in lifestyle. An inability to care for oneself in advanced disease can result in role changes and other losses. Constant pain interferes with quality of life, including sexuality. Patients may not have the energy for sexual intercourse or may find positioning uncomfortable.

Patients with continuous pain from arthritis may develop depression or anxiety. The patient may also have a role change in the family, workplace, or both. To identify changes that have been or need to be made, ask about his or her roles before the disease developed. Identify coping strategies to help live with the disease. Ask the patient about his or her expectations regarding treatment for OA.

In addition to role changes, joint deformities and bony nodules often alter body image and self-esteem. Observe the patient's response to body changes. Does he or she ignore them or seem overly occupied with them? Ask patients directly how they perceive their body image. Document your assessment findings in the interprofessional health record per agency policy.

Laboratory Assessment. The primary health care provider uses the history and physical examination to make the diagnosis of OA. The results of routine laboratory tests are usually normal but can be helpful in screening for associated conditions. The erythrocyte sedimentation rate (ESR) and high-sensitivity C-reactive protein (hsCRP) may be slightly elevated when secondary synovitis occurs. The ESR also tends to rise with age, infection, and other inflammatory disorders.

Imaging Assessment. Routine x-rays are useful in determining structural joint changes. Specialized views are obtained when the disease cannot be visualized on standard x-ray film but is suspected. Magnetic resonance imaging (MRI) and computed tomography (CT) may be used to determine vertebral or knee involvement.

◆ *Analysis: Interpreting*

The priority collaborative problems for patients with osteoarthritis (OA) include:
1. Chronic pain due to joint swelling and deterioration
2. Potential for decreased MOBILITY due to joint pain and muscle atrophy

◆ *Planning and Implementation: Responding*

In 2010 the Osteoarthritis Research Society International (OARSI) committee updated its evidence-based expert consensus guidelines for patients with knee, hand, and hip OA (Zhang et al., 2010). These interprofessional best practice guidelines

remain the most current except for nonsurgical management for OA of the knee, which were updated in 2014 (McAlindon et al., 2014). The OARSI clinical guidelines have major implications for nursing care as described in the following section.

Managing Chronic Pain

Planning: Expected Outcomes. The patient with OA is expected to have a COMFORT level that is acceptable to the patient (e.g., at a 3 or less on a pain intensity scale of 0 to 10).

Interventions. No drug therapy can influence the course of OA. Optimal management of patients with OA requires a multimodal approach (combination of therapies) to manage pain. Perform a pain assessment before and after implementing interventions.

Nonsurgical Management. Management of chronic joint pain can be challenging for both the patient and the health care professional. Drug therapy and a variety of nonpharmacologic therapies are used to manage the patient with OA. Chapter 4 elaborates on interventions for chronic noncancer pain.

Drug Therapy. The purpose of drug therapy is to reduce pain and inflammation caused by cartilage destruction, muscle spasm, and/or synovitis. The American Pain Society, American Geriatrics Society, and OARSI committee recommend regular *acetaminophen* (Tylenol, Atasol) as the primary drug of choice because OA is not a primary anti-inflammatory disorder (Lilley et al., 2014).

! NURSING SAFETY PRIORITY QSEN

Drug Alert

The standard ceiling dose of acetaminophen is 4000 mg each day. However, patients may be at risk for liver damage if they take more than 3000 mg daily, have alcoholism, or have liver disease. *Older adults are particularly at risk because of normal changes of aging such as slowed excretion of drug metabolites.* Remind patients to read the labels of over-the-counter (OTC) or prescription drugs that could contain acetaminophen before taking them. Teach them that their liver enzyme levels may be monitored while taking this drug.

Topical drug applications may help with temporary relief of impaired COMFORT. Prescription lidocaine 5% patches (Lidoderm) have been approved by the Federal Drug Administration (FDA) for postherpetic neuralgia (nerve pain) but may also relieve joint pain (especially the knee) for some patients. Teach the patient to apply the patch on clean, intact skin for 12 hours each day. Up to three patches may be applied to painful joints at one time. Remind him or her that Lidoderm can cause skin irritation. Teach the patient that the lidocaine patch is contraindicated in patients taking class I antidysrhythmics. Topical salicylates such as OTC Aspercreme patch, gel, or cream, are useful for some patients as a temporary pain reliever, especially for knee pain. Buspirone HCl (Buspar) topical cream may also relieve local joint pain for some patients.

If acetaminophen or topical agents do not relieve discomfort, the analgesic drug class of choice is *NSAIDs* if the patient can tolerate them. These traditional drugs supported by OARSI guidelines include oral COX-2 nonselective and selective NSAIDs and topical NSAIDs.

Before beginning oral NSAID therapy, baseline laboratory information is obtained, including a complete blood count (CBC) and kidney and liver function tests. Celecoxib (Celebrex), a COX-2 inhibitor, is usually the first choice unless the patient has hypertension, kidney disease, or cardiovascular disease.

! **NURSING SAFETY PRIORITY** QSEN

Drug Alert

All of the COX-2 inhibiting drugs are thought to cause cardiovascular disease such as myocardial infarction and kidney problems. Older NSAIDs such as ibuprofen can cause severe GI side effects, bleeding, and acute kidney failure. Therefore they are prescribed at the lowest effective dose for a short period of time. Teach your patient about adverse effects from NSAIDs and the need to report them to his or her primary health care provider. Examples include having dark, tarry stools; shortness of breath; edema; frequent dyspepsia (indigestion); hematemesis (bloody vomitus); and changes in urinary output.

Topical NSAIDs are considered to be safe and effective non-systemic drugs for pain relief. For example, the diclofenac-epolamine patch and diclofenac solution are used for patients with signs and symptoms associated with knee OA.

When topical or systemic drugs are not effective and for temporary relief of pain in a single joint, the primary health care provider may inject an individual joint with *cortisone,* a commonly used steroid. Patients may have the same joint injected up to four times a year, or once every 3 months. Frequently injected joints include the knee, base of the thumb, shoulder, and trochanteric bursa, which people often call the *hip.*

Hyaluronic acid (HA) is an alternative injection for knee and hip pain associated with OA. This lubricating synthetic joint fluid replaces or supplements the body's natural hyaluronic acid, which is broken down by inflammation and aging. The effectiveness of these agents varies, depending on the patient. Current evidence supporting the use of HA is controversial but suggests that it is *least* likely to help patients who are obese, have severe OA, are over 65, and/or have had previous knee injections (Arthritis Foundation, 2016a).

Other oral drugs that can be given to patients with OA include muscle relaxants and weak opioids. Muscle relaxants such as cyclobenzaprine hydrochloride (Flexeril) are sometimes given for painful muscle spasms, especially those occurring in the back from OA of the vertebral column. *These drugs should be used with caution in older adults because they can cause acute confusion. Remind any patient not to drive or operate dangerous machinery when taking muscle relaxants.* Weak opioid drugs such as tramadol (Ultram or Ultram ER) may also be given for patients with OA. Chapter 4 discusses drug therapy for pain relief in more detail.

? **NCLEX EXAMINATION CHALLENGE 18-1**

Physiological Integrity

The primary health care provider prescribes acetaminophen for a client with osteoarthritis. Which health teaching will the nurse provide for the client regarding this drug? **Select all that apply.**
A. "Don't take more than 3000-4000 mg of this drug each day."
B. "Stop taking the drug if unusual bleeding occurs and call your primary health care provider."
C. "Tell your primary health care provider if you notice any yellowing of your skin or eyes."
D. "Expect fluid accumulation in your legs and feet that usually gets worse during the day."
E. "Check over-the-counter drugs to see if they contain acetaminophen."

Nonpharmacologic Interventions. In addition to analgesics, many nonpharmacologic measures can be used for patients with OA such as rest balanced with exercise, joint positioning, heat or cold applications, weight control, and a variety of complementary and integrative therapies. In addition, *stem cell therapy* is being used for knee OA to repair damaged cartilage.

Teach the patient to *position joints in their functional position.* For example, when in a supine position (recumbent), he or she should use a small pillow under the head or neck but avoid the use of other pillows. The use of large pillows under the knees or head may result in flexion contractures. Remind him or her to use proper posture when standing and sitting to reduce undue strain on the vertebral column. Teach the patient to wear supportive shoes; foot insoles may help relieve pressure on painful metatarsal joints. Collaborate with the physical therapist (PT) to plan a program for muscle-strengthening exercises to better support the joints.

Many patients apply *heat* or *cold* for temporary relief of pain. Heat may help decrease the muscle tension around the tender joint and thereby decrease pain and stiffness. Suggest hot showers and baths, hot packs or compresses, and moist heating pads. *Regardless of treatment, teach him or her to check that the heat source is not too heavy or so hot that it causes burns.* A temperature just above body temperature is adequate to promote COMFORT.

If needed, collaborate with the PT to provide special heat treatments such as paraffin dips, diathermy (using electrical current), and ultrasonography (using sound waves). A 15- to 20-minute application usually is sufficient to temporarily reduce pain, spasm, and stiffness. Cold packs or gels that feel hot and cold at the same time may also be used.

Cold therapy has limited use for most patients in promoting COMFORT. Cold works by numbing nerve endings and decreasing secondary joint inflammation, if present.

! **NURSING SAFETY PRIORITY** QSEN

Action Alert

Teach the patient to use ice packs that are not too heavy. Do not place them directly on skin; instead wrap them in a towel or soft cloth and apply for a maximum of 20 minutes at a time.

Gradual *weight loss* for obese patients may lessen the stress on weight-bearing joints, decrease pain, and perhaps slow joint degeneration. If needed, collaborate with the registered dietitian to provide more in-depth teaching and meal planning or make referrals to community resources.

Complementary and Integrative Health. Some patients with OA have reported that a variety of integrative therapies are useful. However, the evidence supporting their effectiveness is often inconsistent and inconclusive.

Topical *capsaicin* products are safe over-the-counter (OTC) drugs. They work by blocking or modifying substance P and other neurotransmitters for pain. Tell the patient using capsaicin to expect a burning sensation for a short time after applying it. Recommend the use of plastic gloves for application. To prevent burning of eyes or other body areas, wash hands immediately after applying the substance.

Dietary supplements may complement traditional drug therapies. Glucosamine and chondroitin are widely used and

---

CHART 18-1   Patient and Family Education: Preparing for Self-Management

Considerations for Taking Glucosamine Supplements

- Tell your primary health care provider if you decide to take glucosamine.
- Do not take glucosamine if you have hypertension.
- Do not take glucosamine if you are pregnant or breast-feeding.
- Monitor for bleeding if you take chondroitin with glucosamine or chondroitin alone if you are on anticoagulant therapy.
- If you have diabetes, monitor your blood glucose levels carefully because taking glucosamine for a prolonged time can increase them.
- Be aware that glucosamine can cause adverse effects such as a rash; GI disturbances, especially diarrhea; drowsiness; and headache.
- Be sure to take the recommended dosage based on your weight.
- Read drug labels to ensure that you do not take too much glucosamine for your weight; some drug names may not indicate they contain glucosamine (e.g., Bioflex, Arth-X Plus, Nutri-Joint).

---

are the most effective nonprescription supplements taken to decrease pain and improve functional ability. However, the evidence to support their use is inconsistent (Fouladbakhsh, 2012). These natural products are found in and around bone cartilage for repair and maintenance. Glucosamine may decrease inflammation, and chondroitin may play a role in strengthening cartilage. These supplements are used topically or taken in oral form. Chart 18-1 summarizes what you should teach your patients about glucosamine, with or without chondroitin.

Surgical Management. Surgery may be indicated when conservative measures and/or drug therapy no longer provide pain control, when MOBILITY becomes so restricted that the patient cannot participate in activities he or she enjoys, and when he or she cannot maintain the desired quality of life. The most common surgical procedure for OA is total joint arthroplasty (TJA) (surgical creation of a functional joint), also known as total joint replacement (TJR). Almost any synovial joint of the body can be replaced with a prosthetic system that consists of at least two parts—one for each joint surface. The hip and knee are most often replaced, but shoulder arthroplasty is becoming increasingly common as a result of advances in technology. TJAs are expected to increase as baby boomers age over the next 20 years.

TJA is a procedure used most often to manage the pain of OA and improve MOBILITY, although other conditions causing cartilage destruction may require the surgery. These disorders include rheumatoid arthritis (RA), congenital anomalies, trauma, and osteonecrosis. Osteonecrosis is bone death secondary to lack of or disruption in blood supply to the affected bone, usually from trauma or chronic steroid therapy. The affected bone site is most commonly the femoral or humeral head, distal femur, and proximal tibia.

The *contraindications* for TJA are active infection anywhere in the body, advanced osteoporosis, and rapidly progressive inflammation. An active infection elsewhere in the body or from the joint being replaced can result in an infected TJA and subsequent prosthetic failure. Advanced osteoporosis can cause bone fracture during insertion of the prosthetic device. Severe medical problems such as uncontrolled diabetes or hyperten-

sion put the patient at risk for major postoperative complications and possible death.

Total Hip Arthroplasty. The number of total hip arthroplasty (THA) procedures (also known as *total hip replacement [THR]*) has steadily increased over the past 35 years. If the patient has a joint replacement for the first time, it is referred to as primary arthroplasty. If the implant loosens or fails for any reason, revision arthroplasty may be performed. Availability of improved joint implant materials and better custom design features allow longer life of a replaced hip. Although patients of any age can undergo THA, the procedure is performed most often in those older than 60 years. *The special needs and normal physiologic changes of older adults often complicate the perioperative period and may result in additional postoperative complications.*

Preoperative Care. As with any surgery, preoperative care begins with assessing the patient's level of understanding about the surgery and his or her ability to participate in the postoperative plan of care. The surgeon explains the procedure and postoperative expectations (including possible complications) during the office visit, but this patient education may have occurred weeks or months before the scheduled surgery. Some patients may not know which questions to ask or may forget the important information that was taught. Information may be provided in a notebook or DVD format that the patient can take home to review and share with family. This is particularly useful to patients with poor reading skills or poor memory.

⊕ CULTURAL/SPIRITUAL CONSIDERATIONS

Patient-Centered Care

Written materials or other media provided in the language appropriate for the patient's educational level and culture are essential. If an interpreter is needed to be sure that the information is understood, one needs to be provided at each appointment, while in the hospital, and when discharged with home or inpatient rehabilitation services.

Additional preoperative education may be provided, depending on office, hospital, or Joint Replacement Center protocols. In some settings the physical therapist (PT) may teach the patient transfers, positioning, and ambulation and/or assist in building muscle strength before surgery. An occupational therapist (OT) may assess needs for assistive/adaptive equipment that will be needed after surgery. The cost of durable medical equipment (DME) is usually covered by most insurance companies, both Medicare and commercial. The items usually paid for following THA to prevent hip dislocation and promote recovery are a walker and a commode chair. Younger patients may be taught the use of crutches for gait assistance. Any additional equipment such as shower chairs and grab bars is usually not covered by third-party payers but can be privately purchased in medical supply stores or most pharmacies.

Patients need to have any necessary dental procedures done at least 2 weeks before surgery. Once the new joint has been inserted, the patient must take extreme care to avoid or receive immediate care for an infection that could migrate to the surgical area and cause prosthetic failure. *Remind the patient to tell any future health care provider that he or she has had any total joint arthroplasty.*

In addition to usual preoperative laboratory tests, the surgeon may ask the patient with RA to have a cervical spine x-ray if he or she is having general anesthesia. Those with RA often have cervical spine disease that can lead to subluxation during intubation. Hip x-rays, CT scan, and/or MRI may be done to assess the operative joint and surrounding soft tissues, especially if the patient is undergoing a robotic-assisted THA.

Because venous thromboembolism (VTE) is a serious post-operative complication, especially after hip surgery, assess the patient's risk factors for CLOTTING problems, including history of previous clotting, obesity, smoking, limited preoperative MOBILITY, and advanced age. *Teach patients that drugs that increase the risks for clotting and bleeding such as NSAIDs and vitamins C be discontinued 5 to 10 days before surgery, depending on surgeon instructions.* The concept of CLOTTING is reviewed in Chapter 2 of this text.

Current blood bank standards do not recommend either donor or autologous blood storage before surgery unless the patient's blood type or antibody profile is difficult to cross-match. Devices such as intraoperative cell savers and postoperative reinfusion blood collection systems can be used to assist in maintaining acceptable hemoglobin and hematocrit levels. A cell saver system allows for collection of the person's own red blood cells during surgery, which is then reinfused directly back to the patient via a closed system. A reinfusion system allows for collection of red blood cells from a joint drain over a specific time frame, which then can be reinfused directly back into the patient's systemic circulation.

For some patients who have a tendency for anemia or who have a low blood count before surgery, the surgeon may prescribe several weeks of epoetin alfa (Epogen, Procrit, Eprex) with or without iron to prevent anemia that can occur after hip or knee replacement. Epoetin alfa is recombinant human erythropoietin, a substance that is essential for developing red blood cells. This drug is particularly useful for older adults who frequently have mild anemia before surgery or for patients who for religious or personal reasons would not accept a blood transfusion.

Remind patients that they will likely be instructed to take a shower with special antiseptic soap 1 to 3 nights before and the morning of surgery, based on hospital or provider policy, to decrease bacteria that could cause infection. Teach them to wear clean nightwear after their shower and sleep on clean linen. Review which drugs are safe to take or necessary the morning of the operation such as antihypertensives and which ones should be avoided. Medication should be taken with a very small amount of water to prevent vomiting and aspiration during surgery. If an insulin pump is part of the drug therapy for the patient with diabetes, remind him or her to check with his or her primary health care provider about adjusting the insulin dosage on the morning of surgery. See Chapter 14 for additional preoperative care for any type of surgery.

Operative Procedures. Similar to other orthopedic surgeries, the patient receives an IV antibiotic, usually a cephalosporin such as cefazolin (Ancef), within an hour before the initial surgical incision per the Surgical Care Improvement Project (SCIP) Core Measures to help prevent infection. Chapter 14 discusses these measures in detail.

Several different types of anesthesia are used for THA surgeries and are administered by an anesthesiologist or nurse anesthetist. These options include general anesthesia, neuraxial (spinal) anesthesia, regional nerve blocks, or a combination of these agents. Patients receiving neuraxial or regional anesthetics may also be given IV moderate sedation to keep them unaware of their environment during the procedure. The benefit of a regional block is that the patient may receive extended pain relief, often up to 24 hours after surgery.

Some patients are candidates for *minimally invasive surgery* (MIS) using a smaller incision with special instruments to reduce muscle cutting and stretching. This newer technique cannot be used for patients who are obese or those with osteoporosis. It is done only for primary THAs, not for revision surgeries. Like those of any MIS, the benefits of minimally invasive THA are decreased soft tissue damage and postoperative pain. Patients often have a shorter hospital stay and quicker recovery. They are generally satisfied with the cosmetic appearance of the incision because there is less scarring. Postoperative complications are not as common in patients having minimally invasive ("mini") hip replacements when compared with those having the traditional technique.

Hip resurfacing is an alternative to total hip replacement surgery. This procedure is most often performed for younger patients or for those with early-stage cartilage loss of the weight-bearing surface of the femoral head. Instead of completely removing the femoral head and inserting the stem into the femoral canal, the surgeon removes the cartilage from the surface, and a metal cap is placed over the existing natural femoral head.

Two components are used in the THA—the acetabular component and the femoral component (Fig. 18-3). A noncemented prosthesis is most often used. Bone surfaces are smoothed as they are prepared to receive the artificial components. The noncemented components are press-fitted into the prepared bone. The acetabular cup may be placed using computer- or robotic-assisted guidance. If the prosthesis is cemented, polymethyl methacrylate (an acrylic fixating substance) is used. The hybrid technique usually involves a cemented femoral component and a noncemented acetabular component. A closed wound drainage system may be placed alongside the wound before the surgeon closes the incision.

Considerations of a noncemented prosthesis include protection of weight-bearing status to allow bone to grow into the

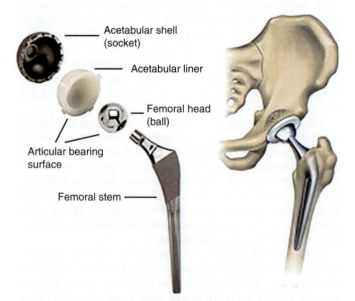

FIG. 18-3 Two major components of total hip arthroplasty. (From Zhang, Y., Zhu, J., Wang, Z., Zhou, Y., & Zhang, X. [2015]. Constructing a 3D-printable, bioceramic sheathed articular spacer assembly for infected hip arthroplasty. *Journal of Medical Hypotheses and Ideas, 9*[1], 13-19.)

TABLE 18-2 Nursing Interventions to Prevent Major Complications of Lower-Extremity Total Joint Arthroplasty

COMPLICATION	PREVENTION/INTERVENTION
Dislocation (hip)	Position correctly. Keep legs slightly abducted (for posterior surgical approach). Prevent hip flexion beyond 90 degrees (for posterior surgical approach). Prevent hip hyperextension (for anterior surgical approach). Assess for acute pain, rotation, and extremity shortening. Perform frequent neurovascular assessments, at least every 4 hours for the first 24 hours or per agency protocol. Report dislocation immediately to the surgeon.
Infection	Use aseptic technique for wound care and emptying of drains. Wash hands thoroughly when caring for patient. Culture drainage fluid, if change. Monitor temperature. Report excessive inflammation or drainage to surgeon.
Venous thromboembolism	Have patient wear elastic stockings and/or sequential compression device per agency policy. Teach leg exercises to patient. Encourage fluid intake. Observe for signs of deep vein thrombosis (redness, swelling, or pain). Observe patient for changes in mental status. Administer anticoagulant as prescribed. Do not massage legs. Do not flex knees for a prolonged period of time.
Hypotension, bleeding, or infection	Take vital signs at least every 4 hours for the first 24 hours or per agency protocol. Observe patient for bleeding. Report excessively low blood pressure or bleeding to physician.

CHART 18-2 Nursing Focus on the Older Adult

Postoperative Care of the Older Adult With a Total Hip Arthroplasty

- For patients who had a *posterior surgical approach*, use an abduction pillow or splint to prevent adduction after surgery if the patient is very restless or has an altered mental state. For patients with an *anterior surgical approach*, no abduction pillow is needed.
- Keep the patient's heels off the bed to prevent pressure injuries.
- Do not rely on fever as a sign of infection; older patients often have infection without fever. Be alert to decreasing mental status and/or elevated white blood cell count as indicators of infection.
- When assisting the patient out of bed, move him or her slowly to prevent orthostatic (postural) hypotension. Allow the patient to sit on the side of the bed for a brief period of time before standing; have him or her stand for a brief period before beginning ambulation.
- Encourage the patient to deep breathe and cough and to use the incentive spirometer every 2 hours to prevent atelectasis and pneumonia.
- As soon as permitted, get the patient out of bed to a recliner chair to prevent complications of immobility.
- Anticipate the patient's need for pain medication, especially if he or she cannot verbalize the need for pain control. For patients on a multimodal pain protocol, assess the need to medicate for break-through pain (see Chapter 4).
- Expect a temporary change in mental state immediately after surgery as a result of the anesthetic and unfamiliar sensory stimuli. Reorient the patient frequently.

! NURSING SAFETY PRIORITY (QSEN)

Action Alert

Teach patients to maintain correct positioning of the hip joint and leg at all times. When the patient returns from the postanesthesia care unit (PACU), place him or her in a supine position with the head slightly elevated. For the patient who had a *posterior surgical approach*, place a regular or abduction pillow between the legs to prevent adduction beyond the midline of the body according to agency policy or surgeon preference.

prosthesis and decreased problems with loosening of the prosthesis. With a cemented prosthesis, cement can fracture or deteriorate over time, leading to loosening of the prosthesis, which causes pain and can lead to the need for a revision arthroplasty. In revision arthroplasty the old prosthesis is removed, and new components are replaced. Bone graft may be placed if bone loss is significant. Outcomes from revision arthroplasty may not be as positive as with primary arthroplasty.

Postoperative Care. In addition to providing the routine postoperative care discussed in Chapter 16, assess for and help prevent possible postoperative complications. Table 18-2 summarizes these complications, including nursing measures for prevention, assessment, and intervention. Chart 18-2 highlights special concerns for the care of older adults in the postoperative period. Collaborate with your patient and his or her family to become safety partners to prevent "failure to rescue" events.

In some hospitals abduction devices with straps are placed on patients who are restless or cannot follow instructions, especially older adults with delirium or dementia. One or two regular bed pillows are used in most cases to remind patients to keep their legs abducted. For devices with straps, be sure to loosen the straps every 2 hours and check the patient's skin for irritation or breakdown. Patients having the *anterior surgical approach* do not require the use of the abduction pillow.

Place and support the affected leg in neutral rotation. *Keep the patient's heels, particularly those of older adults, off the bed to prevent skin breakdown.* The procedure for postoperative turning is not universal and is specified by agency policy or surgeon preference. Turning the patient to the operative side provides "splinting" of the operative hip but may be too painful for some patients. If the patient is turned to the nonoperative side, the operative leg needs to be fully supported with pillows to prevent slipping of the leg into a position that can lead to dislocation.

Teach the patient and family about other precautions to prevent dislocation as outlined in Chart 18-3. In addition to

CHART 18-3 Patient and Family Education: Preparing for Self-Management

Care of Patients With Total Hip Arthroplasty After Hospital Discharge

Hip Precautions
- Do not sit or stand for prolonged periods.
- Do not cross your legs beyond the midline of your body.
- For *posterior surgical approach* patients: Do not bend your hips more than 90 degrees.
- For *anterior surgical approach* patients: Do not hyperextend your operative leg behind you.
- Do not twist your body when standing.
- Use the prescribed ambulatory aid such as a walker when walking.
- Use assistive/adaptive devices as needed (e.g., sock aids, shoehorns, dressing sticks, reachers [also see Chapter 6]).
- Do not put more weight on your affected leg than allowed and intructed.
- Resume sexual intercourse as usual on the advice of your surgeon.

Pain Management
- Report increased hip or anterior thigh pain to the surgeon immediately.
- Take oral analgesics as prescribed and only as needed.
- Do not overexert yourself; take frequent rests.
- Use ice as needed to operative hip to decrease or prevent swelling and minimize pain.

Incisional Care
- Follow the instructions provided regarding dressing changes. Some surgeons use specialty dressings that do not need to be changed. No dressing may be needed if a skin sealant was used.
- Inspect your hip incision every day for redness, heat, or drainage; if any of these are present, call your surgeon immediately.
- Do not bathe the incision or apply anything directly to the incision unless instructed to do so. Shower according to the surgeon's instructions.

Other Care
- Continue walking and performing the leg exercises as you learned them in the hospital. Do not increase the amount of activity unless instructed to do so by the therapist or surgeon.
- Do not cross your legs to help prevent blood clots.
- Report pain, redness, or swelling in your legs to your surgeon immediately.
- Call 911 for acute chest pain or shortness of breath (could indicate pulmonary embolus).
- If you are taking an anticoagulant, follow the precautions learned in the hospital to prevent bleeding; avoid using a straight razor, avoid injuries, and report bleeding or excessive bruising to your surgeon immediately.
- Follow up with visits to the surgeon's office as instructed.

preventing adduction, remind them that the patient who had a *posterior approach* should avoid flexing the hips more than 90 degrees at all times. For patients having the *anterior approach*, teach them to avoid hyperextension of the operative hip and external rotation of the leg. Use diagrams or demonstrate correct positioning to help reinforce this information before the patient gets out of bed (Fig. 18-4).

If the hip is dislocated, the surgeon may be able to manipulate and relocate it after the patient receives moderate sedation. If the hip does not reduce into position, the patient may have surgical reduction in the operating room (OR). Following reduction, the hip is usually immobilized by an abduction splint or other device until healing occurs—usually in about 6 weeks.

As with other musculoskeletal surgery, *monitor neurovascular assessments* frequently for a possible compromise in circulation to the affected distal extremity.

! NURSING SAFETY PRIORITY QSEN
Action Alert

Check and document color, temperature, distal pulses, capillary refill, movement, and sensation.

The procedure for performing a thorough lower-extremity neurovascular assessment is described in detail in Chapter 51. Remember to compare the operative leg with the nonoperative leg. These assessments are performed at the same time the vital signs are checked. Report any changes in neurovascular assessment to the surgeon and carefully monitor for changes. Early detection of changes in neurovascular status can prevent permanent tissue damage.

The most potentially life-threatening complication after THA is venous thromboembolism (VTE), which includes deep venous thrombosis (DVT) and pulmonary embolism (PE). *Older patients are especially at increased risk for VTE because of age and decreased circulation before surgery. Obese patients and those with a history of VTE are also at high risk for thrombi.*

Preventive postoperative measures include applying bilateral sequential compression devices (SCDs) and/or antiembolism stockings and anticoagulant therapy. Anticoagulants such as warfarin (Coumadin, Warfilone ✦), subcutaneous low-molecular-weight heparin (LMWH), or factor Xa inhibitors are effective in preventing VTE to patients having a THA. Patients are usually on anticoagulants for 10 days to several weeks after surgery, depending on surgeon preference and the patient's response and risk factors. Patients on warfarin require frequent monitoring of prothrombin time (PT) and international normalized ratio (INR).

The use of subcutaneous LMWH has markedly increased for patients with total hip replacements. Examples include enoxaparin (Lovenox) and dalteparin (Fragmin). As an alternative to LMWH, subcutaneous fondaparinux (Arixtra), a factor Xa inhibiting agent, may be prescribed for some patients undergoing hip and knee arthroplasty. A newer Xa inhibitor, rivaroxaban (Xarelto), is given orally once a day. Recently oral apixaban (Eliquis) has received FDA approval for VTE prophylaxis in patients having a THA. You do not need to monitor the PT or INR for patients receiving these drugs because they do not affect coagulation values. However, for other anticoagulants, patients are at risk for bleeding due to impaired CLOTTING. A complete discussion of nursing care associated with patients taking anticoagulants and who have VTE is found in Chapter 36. The Joint Commission's *VTE Core Measures* are also discussed in that chapter.

Early ambulation and exercise help prevent VTE. Teach the patient about leg exercises, which should begin in the immediate postoperative period and continue through the rehabilitation period. These exercises include plantar flexion and dorsiflexion (heel pumping), circumduction (circles) of the feet, gluteal and quadriceps muscle setting, and straight-leg raises (SLRs). Teach the patient to perform gluteal exercises by pushing the heels into the bed and achieve quadriceps-setting exercises ("quad sets") by straightening the legs and pushing

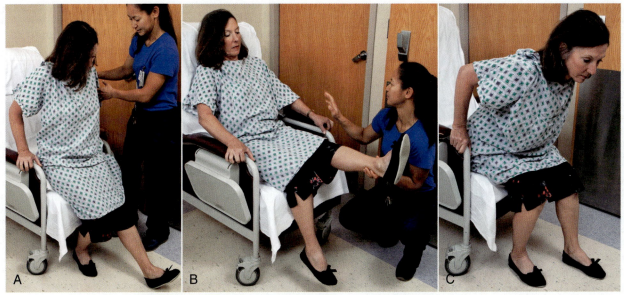

FIG. 18-4 Correct **(A, B)** and incorrect **(C)** hip flexion after a total hip replacement.

the back of the knees into the bed. In addition to preventing clots, these exercises improve muscle tone, which helps restore the function of the extremity.

Monitor the surgical incision and vital signs carefully—every 4 hours for the first 24 hours and every 8 to 12 hours thereafter, following facility and surgeon protocols. Observe for signs of infection such as an elevated temperature, increased redness around the incision, and excessive or foul-smelling drainage from the incision. *An older patient may not have a fever with infection but instead may experience an altered mental state.* If you suspect this problem, obtain a sample of any drainage for culture and sensitivity to determine the causative organisms and the antibiotics that may be needed for treatment.

Managing Postoperative Pain. Although hip arthroplasty is performed to relieve joint pain, patients experience varying levels of pain related to the surgical procedure. Many state that their pain is different and less severe than before surgery. Pain control protocols vary, depending on the region of the country, anesthesiologist/nurse anesthetist, and surgeon. Immediate pain control may be achieved by extended-release epidural morphine (EREM), regional blocks, patient-controlled analgesia (PCA), or IV push, typically with morphine or hydrocodone. Acetaminophen, ketorolac, and/or celecoxib are usually given as adjunct analgesics. For some patients, IV acetaminophen (Ofirmev) may be the *only* analgesic required to relieve mild-to-moderate pain, which avoids the risks of side effects from opioids and other NSAIDs. Chapter 4 contains information on the nursing care associated with these acute pain modalities.

Regardless of the pain management method used, most patients do not require parenteral analgesics after the first day. Oral opioids such as hydrocodone plus acetaminophen (Norco) and tramadol (Ultram) are then commonly prescribed until the pain can be controlled by NSAIDs such as celecoxib (Celebrex) or oral acetaminophen.

Nonpharmacologic methods for acute and chronic pain control can also be used to decrease the amount of drug therapy used (see Chapter 4).

Promoting Postoperative Mobility and Activity. Depending on the time of day that the surgery is performed, the patient with a

THA gets out of bed with assistance the night of surgery to prevent problems related to impaired MOBILITY (e.g., atelectasis, pneumonia), especially in older adults.

> ⚠ **NURSING SAFETY PRIORITY** QSEN
>
> ### Action Alert
>
> Be sure to assist the patient the first time he or she gets out of bed to prevent falls and observe for dizziness. When getting the patient out of bed, put a gait belt on him or her and then stand on the same side of the bed as the affected leg. After the patient sits on the side of the bed, remind him or her to stand on the unaffected leg and pivot to the chair with guidance. If the patient has been instructed by PT to use stretch bands, reinforce the correct use of this device to support and help in proper positioning of the operative leg. *To avoid injury, do not lift the patient!*

Remind the patient who had a *posterior approach for surgery* to avoid flexing the hips beyond 90 degrees as discussed earlier (see Fig. 18-4). Raised toilet seats and reclining chairs help prevent hyperflexion. Remind patients having the *anterior surgical approach* to avoid hyperextension of the operative hip. Be sure to teach all THA patients to also *avoid* twisting the body or crossing their legs to prevent hip dislocation.

The surgeon, type of prosthesis, and surgical procedure determine the amount of weight bearing that can be applied to the affected leg. A patient with a cemented implant is usually allowed immediate weight bearing as tolerated (WBAT). Typically only "toe-touch" or minimal weight bearing is permitted for patients with noncemented prostheses. When x-ray evidence of bony ingrowth can be seen, the patient can progress to partial weight bearing (PWB) and then to full weight bearing (FWB).

In collaboration with the physical therapist (PT), teach the patient how to follow weight-bearing restrictions. Most patients use a walker, but younger adults may use crutches. They are usually advanced to a single cane or crutch if they can walk without a severe limp 4 to 6 weeks after surgery. When the limp disappears, they no longer need an ambulatory/assistive device and may be permitted to sit in chairs of normal height, use regular toilets, and drive a car. Timing of driving may be slightly longer in a patient who has had surgery on the right hip because of patient safety concerns.

NCLEX EXAMINATION CHALLENGE 18-2
Physiological Integrity

A client had a left anterior total hip arthroplasty 2 days ago. Which precautions will the nurse teach the client to prevent surgical complications? **Select all that apply.**
A. "Avoid extending your left hip behind you when you sit."
B. "Do not flex your hips more than 90 degrees when toileting."
C. "You may cross your legs to be more comfortable in a chair."
D. "Avoid twisting your body when moving or performing ADLs."
E. "Stand on your right leg and pivot into the chair when getting out of bed."

Promoting Postoperative Self-Management. The hospital's occupational therapy department may supply assistive/adaptive devices to help with ADLs, especially for those having traditional surgery. Particularly important are devices designed for reaching to prevent patients from bending or stooping and flexing the hips more than 90 degrees. Extended handles on shoehorns and dressing sticks may be very useful to achieve ADL independence. Third-party payers may or may not pay for these devices, depending on the patient's status.

With the increase in Joint Replacement Center programs that emphasize a structured approach and recovery, the length of stay in the acute care hospital is typically 3 days or fewer if there are no postoperative complications. McCann-Spry et al. (2016) reported a quality improvement project in which the patient's length of stay was reduced to 2.5 days for a 2-night stay rather than the typical 3-night stay (see the Quality Improvement box). Patients experiencing postoperative complications often stay longer. Medicare patients need a 3-day qualifying hospital stay to receive rehabilitation in a skilled inpatient unit. Discharge from the acute care facility may be to the home, a rehabilitation unit, a transitional care unit, or a skilled unit or long-term care facility for continued rehabilitation before discharge to home. The interprofessional team provides written instructions for posthospital care and reviews them with patients and their family members (see Chart 18-3). Be sure to provide a copy of these instructions for the patient.

Acute rehabilitation usually takes several weeks, depending on the patient's age and progress and the type of prosthesis used. However, it often takes 6 weeks or longer for complete recovery. Some patients who are discharged to their home are able to attend physical therapy sessions in an office or ambulatory care setting. Others have no means or cannot use community resources and need physical therapy in the home, depending on their health insurance coverage. *Collaborate with the case manager to determine which option is best for your patient.*

Total Knee Arthroplasty. As the population ages, more adults are undergoing total knee arthroplasty (TKA, also known as *total knee replacement [TKR]*). Continued improvements in total knee implants have increased the expected life of a TKA to 20 years or more, depending on the age and activity level of the patient. Options for *total* knee replacements include medial compartment replacement and robotic-assisted partial knee replacement. Partial knee replacements are used most often in patients with minimal cartilage loss in specified areas of the

QUALITY IMPROVEMENT (QSEN)
Can Hospital Length of Stay Be Shortened for Patients Having Joint Replacements?

McCann-Spry, L., Pelton, J., Grandy, G., & Newell, D. (2016). An interdisciplinary approach to reducing length of stay in joint replacement patients. *Orthopaedic Nursing, 35*(5), 279–300.

Demand for total joint replacement surgeries is increasing as baby boomers become older adults. One large hospital in a northern U.S. state developed a process for decreasing postoperative hospital length of stay (LOS) using an interprofessional collaborative approach. Four interventions were implemented: (1) improve communication for primary health care providers (surgeons), including a letter explaining the goal of reducing LOS from 3 nights to 2 nights; (2) develop a script for staff conversations with the patient and family for each hospital day; (3) standardize the risk assessment and prediction for reducing LOS; and (4) initiate physical therapy the day of surgery. As a result of this quality improvement project, patient LOS was reduced an average of 0.5 days per patient for primary hip and knee replacement surgeries. This reduction was very cost-effective without negatively affecting patient and family satisfaction.

Commentary: Implications for Research and Practice
This QI project was very successful at improving financial outcomes and increasing collaboration and communication among interprofessional health care team members and improving staff-patient communication. Nurses play a major role in care coordination and discharge teaching for patients and their families. More QI projects and interventions are needed in additional joint replacement centers to achieve these positive outcomes.

involved knee and are typically done more often in younger patients. Minimally invasive surgery (MIS) is also an option for either partial or total knee replacements. Severe bone loss, obesity, and previous knee surgeries are contraindications for this type of surgery. Patients who have MIS procedures have less pain and blood loss and greater range of motion to promote a faster postoperative recovery.

Preoperative Care. TKA, like hip replacement, is performed when joint pain cannot be managed by conservative measures. When limited MOBILITY severely prevents patients from participating in work or activities they enjoy, this procedure can restore a high quality of life. The preoperative care and teaching for patients undergoing a TKA are similar to that for total hip replacement. However, precautions for positioning are not the same because joint dislocation is not a common complication. Differences in patient and family teaching depend on the procedure used by the orthopedic surgeon.

All patients are given verbal and either written or video preoperative instructions, which include the activity protocol to follow after surgery. The PT and OT provide information about transfers, ambulation, postoperative exercises, and ADL assistance. Patients may practice walking with walkers or crutches to prepare them for ambulation after TKA. Teach patients about the possible need for assistive/adaptive devices to assist with ADLs, including an elevated toilet seat, safety handrails, and dressing devices like a long-handled shoehorn. Some third-party payers cover these devices, depending on the patient's condition and age; however, other insurers may not pay for them. Teach the patient and family how and where this equipment can be obtained to have it available after surgery. Case managers or social workers may arrange for needed items to be delivered to the patient's room before discharge.

Routine diagnostic testing is requested and any additional tests such as cervical spine x-rays for patients with rheumatoid arthritis (RA) to determine if the patient can be intubated for anesthesia. Knee x-rays, CT scan, and/or MRI may be done to assess the joint and surrounding soft tissues.

Teach patients that they will need to shower with a special antiseptic soap 1 to 3 nights before surgery and the morning of surgery to decrease bacteria on the skin that could cause infection. Remind them to wear clean nightwear and sleep on clean linen. Ask them to check with their surgeon about which medications they can take the morning of surgery with a small amount of water, including antihypertensives, thyroid hormone supplements, and corticosteroids (taken by many patients with RA). Some medications such as NSAIDs are discontinued 5 to 10 days before surgery to prevent surgical bleeding. See Chapter 14 for additional preoperative care for any type of surgery.

Operative Procedures. As with the hip, the knee can be replaced with the patient under a variety of anesthetic agents, including general or neuraxial (epidural or spinal) anesthesia. One of the more recent advances in postoperative pain management for knee joint replacements is the use of peripheral nerve blocks (PNB), most commonly sciatic, femoral, or adductor canal blocks using a local anesthetic. An IV moderate sedation agent is used in addition to the neuraxial or PNB drug. PNB may be either a single injection or continuous infusion by a portable pump (e.g., **continuous femoral nerve blockade** or CFNB). In addition, other local medications may be injected into the knee or surrounding tissues to assist in the reduction of severe pain that usually occurs after knee surgery and to minimize perioperative bleeding.

An antibiotic, usually an IV cephalosporin or vancomycin, is given shortly before the surgical incision per the SCIP Core Measures to aid in the prevention of infection. In the *traditional surgery* the surgeon makes a central longitudinal incision about 6 to 8 inches (15 to 20 cm) long. Osteotomies of the femoral and tibial condyles and of the posterior patella are performed, and the surfaces are prepared for the prosthesis. The femoral component is often noncemented (using a press-fit) with the tibial component being cemented. The surgeon may insert a surgical drain, depending on the amount of expected postoperative bleeding. A compression (pressure) dressing is applied from the toes to the thigh to decrease edema and bleeding.

Minimally invasive TKA may be performed using a shorter incision and special instruments to spare muscle and other soft tissue. Computer-guided or robotic equipment may be used to ensure accurate positioning of the knee implants.

Postoperative Care. Provide the usual postoperative care needed for any patient who has surgery (see Chapter 16). Specific nursing care of the patient with a TKA is similar to that for the patient with a total hip arthroplasty as described in the previous section.

Since joint dislocation is rare after TKA, there are no special positioning precautions required to prevent adduction. Maintain the operative leg in a neutral position, avoiding both internal and external rotation. Do not place a pillow under the replaced knee or hyperextend the knee.

Although not as commonly used today, the surgeon may prescribe a continuous passive motion (CPM) machine, which can be applied in the postanesthesia care unit (PACU) or soon after the patient is admitted to the postoperative unit (Fig. 18-5). The CPM machine keeps the prosthetic knee in motion and may prevent the formation of scar tissue, which could

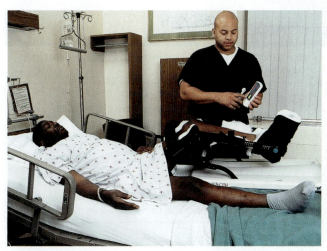

FIG. 18-5 A continuous passive motion (CPM) machine in use.

! NURSING SAFETY PRIORITY QSEN

Critical Rescue

If the patient has a continuous femoral nerve blockade (CFNB), perform and document neurovascular assessment every 2 to 4 hours, or according to hospital protocol. Be sure that patients can perform dorsiflexion and plantar flexion motions of the affected foot without pain in the lower leg. In addition, monitor these patients for signs and symptoms that indicate absorption of the local anesthetic into the patient's system, including:

- Metallic taste
- Tinnitus
- Nervousness
- Slurred speech
- Bradycardia
- Hypotension
- Decreased respirations
- Seizures

Document and report these new-onset signs and symptoms to the surgeon and anesthesiologist/nurse anesthetist immediately and carefully continue to monitor the patient for any changes.

---

decrease knee MOBILITY and increase postoperative pain. Observe and document the patient's response to the device and follow the surgeon's protocol for settings. Chart 18-4 outlines your responsibility when caring for a patient using the CPM machine. This device may also be used for other types of orthopedic surgery.

In the immediate postoperative period, the surgeon also typically prescribes some form of cryotherapy (cold application) to decrease swelling, hematoma formation, and pain at the surgical site. These problems are more common with this type of surgery than with hip surgery. Several types of cryotherapy are used, including ice/gel pack compression and circulating cold water cryotherapy devices. A recent study comparing these two cryotherapy methods for 100 randomized subjects found that the less expensive ice-gel packs were as effective as the circulating cold water devices in managing pain and swelling. Patient satisfaction was the same for both study groups (Schinsky, et al., 2016).

In general, pain control measures for patients with TKA are similar to those with total hip arthroplasty. Many patients report high ratings on the pain intensity scale and require

CHART 18-4 Best Practice for Patient Safety & Quality Care QSEN

The Patient Using a Continuous Passive Motion (CPM) Machine

- Ensure that the machine is well padded.
- Check the cycle and range-of-motion settings at least once every 8 hours.
- Ensure that the joint being moved is properly positioned on the machine.
- If the patient is confused, place the controls to the machine out of his or her reach.
- Assess the patient's response to the machine.
- Turn off the machine while the patient is having a meal in bed.
- When the machine is not in use, do not store it on the floor.

opioid medications longer than patients with THA, particularly if they have had bilateral surgery. However, for other patients, IV acetaminophen is very effective in managing TKA pain. *Be sure to manage your patient's pain to provide comfort, increase his or her participation in physical therapy, and improve joint mobility.*

Some complications that affect patients with THA may also affect those having TKA such as venous thromboembolism, infection, anemia, and neurovascular compromise. Assessments and interventions associated with these complications are described in the Postoperative Care section of the discussion of Total Hip Arthroplasty.

The desired outcome for discharge from the acute hospital unit is that the patient can walk with crutches or a walker and has adequate flexion in the operative knee for ambulation, including walking up and down stairs. Patients are able to bear weight as tolerated unless the prosthesis is not cemented. Patients may be discharged to their home or to an acute rehabilitation unit, transitional care unit, or skilled unit in a long-term care facility for therapy. For many patients home care services can provide physical therapy and nursing care for 1 to 2 weeks followed by outpatient therapy only if their insurance approves this plan and they have family support. *Collaborate with the case manager to determine which option is best for your patient.*

During the home rehabilitation phase, the use of a stationary bicycle or CPM machine may help gain flexion. These patients can return to work and other usual activities in 6 weeks, depending on their age, type of surgery, and other health status factors. Total recovery from a TKA surgery takes 6 weeks or longer, especially for those older than 75 years.

? NCLEX EXAMINATION CHALLENGE 18-3

Safe and Effective Care Environment

A nursing assistant (NA) is assigned to care for a client who had a cemented total knee arthroplasty. Which statement by the NA indicates a need for further teaching and supervision by the nurse?
A. "I'll keep an abduction pillow in place at all times."
B. "I'll tell the client not to place a pillow under the surgical knee."
C. "I'll apply ice packs to decrease swelling in the knee as ordered."
D. "I'll check to make sure the client's leg is not rotated."

Other Joint Arthroplasties. The shoulder and other upper-extremity joints do not bear weight and therefore tend to have

less degeneration and subsequent pain. Preoperative teaching for patients having any of these surgeries depends on the surgeon's technique and postoperative protocols.

Total shoulder arthroplasty (TSA) has gained popularity as newer prostheses and technology have been developed. This procedure usually decreases arthritic or traumatic pain and increases the patient's ability to perform ADLs. Because the shoulder joint is complex and has many **articulations** (joint surfaces), **subluxation** (partial dislocation) or complete dislocation is a major potential complication. Usually the glenohumeral joint, created by the glenoid cavity of the shoulder blade (scapula) and the head of the humerus, is replaced because it moves the most and is therefore most affected by arthritis. A cemented or noncemented **hemiarthroplasty** (replacement of part of the joint), typically the humeral component, may be performed as an alternative to TSA.

After surgery the patient is placed in an abduction immobilizer or pillow device to protect the joint from excessive motion until rehabilitation therapy begins. *Do not remove these devices unless instructed to do so by the surgeon.*

In addition to the potential for dislocation, postoperative complications are similar to those for other total joint replacements and include infection and neurovascular compromise. *As for any other total joint arthroplasty, perform frequent neurovascular assessments at least every 4 to 8 hours.* The procedure for performing a thorough upper-extremity neurovascular assessment is described in detail in Chapter 51. Document and report any significant changes to the surgeon immediately. The hospital stay for TSA is shorter than for a total hip or knee replacement. Rehabilitation with an OT generally takes several months.

Improving Mobility

Planning: Expected Outcomes. The patient with osteoarthritis (OA) is expected to maintain or improve a level of MOBILITY and activity that allows him or her to function independently with or without an assistive ambulatory device.

Interventions. Management of the patient with OA often requires an interprofessional health team effort. If needed, consult and collaborate with the physical therapist (PT) and occupational therapist (OT) to meet the outcome of independent function and MOBILITY. Major interventions include therapeutic exercise and the promotion of ADLs and ambulation by teaching about health and the use of assistive devices.

Certain recreational activities may also be therapeutic such as swimming to enhance chest and arm muscles. Aerobic exercises (e.g., walking, biking, swimming, aerobic dance) are also recommended. Exercises may be prescribed by rehabilitation therapists for the patient with OA, but you will need to reinforce their techniques and principles. The ideal time for exercise is immediately after the application of heat. To prevent further joint damage, teach patients to carefully follow the instructions for exercise outlined in Chart 18-5.

Collaborate with the PT to evaluate the patient's need for ambulatory aids such as canes, walkers, or platform crutches. Although some patients do not like to use these aids or may forget how to use them, they can help prevent further joint deterioration and pain. Collaborate with the OT, if needed, to provide suggestions and devices for assistance for ADLs. Chapter 6 discusses rehabilitation therapies in more detail.

Care Coordination and Transition Management

The patient with OA is not usually hospitalized for the disease itself but is admitted for surgical management. Expect that any

---

CHART 18-5 **Patient and Family Education: Preparing for Self-Management**

Exercises for Patients With Osteoarthritis or Rheumatoid Arthritis

- Follow the exercise instructions that have been prescribed specifically for you. There are no universal exercises; your exercises have been specifically tailored to your needs.
- Do your exercises on both "good" and "bad" days. Consistency is important.
- Respect pain. Reduce the number of repetitions when the inflammation is severe and you have more pain.
- Use active rather than active-assist or passive exercise whenever possible.
- Do not substitute your normal activities or household tasks for the prescribed exercises.
- Avoid resistive exercises when your joints are severely inflamed.

CHART 18-6 **Patient and Family Education: Preparing for Self-Management**

Evidence-Based Instructions for Joint Protection

- Use large joints instead of small ones; for example, place your purse strap over your shoulder instead of grasping the purse with your hand.
- Do not turn a doorknob clockwise. Turn it counterclockwise to avoid twisting your arm and promoting ulnar deviation.
- Use two hands instead of one to hold objects.
- Sit in a chair that has a high, straight back.
- When getting out of bed, do not push off with your fingers; use the entire palm of both hands.
- Do not bend at your waist; instead bend your knees while keeping your back straight.
- Use long-handled devices such as a hairbrush with an extended handle.
- Use assistive/adaptive devices such as Velcro closures and built-up utensil handles to protect your joints.
- Do not use pillows in bed except a small one under your head.
- Avoid twisting or wringing your hands.

---

patient older than 60 years will have some degree of arthritis and possibly chronic pain that need to be managed.

Home Care Management. If weight-bearing joints are severely involved, the patient may have difficulty going up or down stairs. Making arrangements to live on one floor with accessibility to all rooms is often the best solution. A home care nurse or case manager may collaborate with a rehabilitation therapist to assess the need for structural alterations to the home to accommodate ambulatory aids and enable the patient to perform ADLs. For example, a kitchen counter may need to be lowered, or a seat and handrails may need to be installed in the shower. If the patient has undergone a total hip replacement, an elevated toilet seat is necessary for several weeks after surgery to prevent excessive hip flexion. Patients who have TKAs may also find elevated toilet seats easier to use. Throw rugs and other environmental hazards should be removed to prevent tripping and falls.

Self-Management Education. Self-management education (SME) is an effective psychosocially focused nonpharmacologic intervention. Learning how to protect joints is the most important part of patient and family education. Preventing further damage to joints slows the progression of OA and minimizes pain. Explain the general principles of joint protection and give practical examples (Chart 18-6).

As with other diseases in which drugs and nutritional therapy are used, teach the patient and family the drug therapy protocol, desired effects and potential side effects, and toxic effects. Emphasize the importance of reducing weight and eating a well-balanced diet to promote tissue healing.

Many patients with arthritis look for a cure after becoming frustrated and desperate about the course of the disease and treatment. Better control of arthritis is possible, but cure is not yet available. Unfortunately tabloids, books, media, and the Internet often report "curative" remedies. People spend billions of dollars each year on quackery, including liniments, special diets, and copper bracelets. More hazardous substances such as snake venom and industrial cleaners are also advertised as remedies. Refer the patient to the Arthritis Foundation for up-to-date information about these "cures." The practice of wearing a copper bracelet will not cure arthritis, but it will not cause harm. However, if the patient is using a potentially harmful substance or method, reinforce the need to avoid the unproven

remedy and explain why it should not be used. Respect the patient's preferences, values, and beliefs for using benign remedies that do not cause harm.

With most types of arthritis and connective tissue disease (CTD), patients must live with a chronic, unpredictable, and painful disorder. Their roles, self-esteem, and body image may be affected by these diseases. Body image is often not as devastating in OA as in the inflammatory arthritic diseases such as RA. The psychosocial component associated with having arthritis is discussed in more detail later in this chapter in the Rheumatoid Arthritis section.

Health Care Resources. The patient who has undergone surgery may need help from community resources. After an arthroplasty, he or she may need assistance with MOBILITY. The patient may be discharged to home or an inpatient unit. Collaborate with the case manager and surgeon to determine the best placement. If the patient is discharged to home, home care nurses may be approved for third-party payment for several visits, depending on the presence of any existing systemic diseases. A home care aide may visit the home to help with hygiene-related needs, and a PT may work with ambulatory and MOBILITY skills. For older patients, a family member, significant other, or other caregiver should be in the home for at least the first few weeks when the patient needs the most assistance. Emphasize the need for patient safety, especially interventions to prevent falls as described in Chapter 3.

Provide written instructions about the required care, regardless of whether the patient goes home or to another inpatient facility. As required by The Joint Commission's National Patient Safety Goals (NPSGs) and other health care accrediting organizations, hand-off communication with the new care provider is essential for seamless continuity of care and care coordination.

The Arthritis Foundation (www.arthritis.org) is an important community resource for all patients with arthritis and other CTDs. This organization provides information to lay people and health care professionals and refers patients and their families to other resources as needed. Local support groups can help them cope with these diseases.

◆ *Evaluation: Reflecting*

Evaluate the care of the patient with OA on the basis of the identified priority problems. The expected outcomes are that he or she:

- Achieves pain control to a pain intensity level of 3 to 4 on a scale of 0 to 10 or at a level that is acceptable to the patient
- Moves and functions in his or her own environment independently with or without assistive devices

✳ IMMUNITY CONCEPT EXEMPLAR
Rheumatoid Arthritis

❖ PATHOPHYSIOLOGY

Rheumatoid arthritis (RA) is a chronic, progressive, systemic inflammatory autoimmune disease process that affects primarily the synovial joints. **Systemic** means this disease affects the body system, affecting many joints and other tissues.

In RA transformed autoantibodies (rheumatoid factors [RFs]) are formed that attack healthy tissue, especially synovium, causing inflammation. The disease then begins to involve the articular cartilage, joint capsule, and surrounding ligaments and tendons. IMMUNITY and inflammatory factors cause cartilage damage in patients with RA (Crawford & Harris, 2015; McCance et al., 2014):

- CD4 T–helper cells and other immune cells in synovial fluid promote cytokine release, especially interleukin-1 (IL-1) and tumor necrosis factor–alpha (TNFA), which attack cartilage.
- Neutrophils and other inflammatory cells in the joint are activated and break down the cartilage.
- Immune complexes deposit in synovium, and osteoclasts are activated.
- B- and T-lymphocytes of the immune system are stimulated and increase the inflammatory response. (Also see Chapter 17 for a complete discussion of the inflammatory response.)

The synovium then thickens and becomes hyperemic, fluid accumulates in the joint space, and a pannus forms. The pannus is vascular granulation tissue composed of inflammatory cells; it erodes articular cartilage and eventually destroys bone. As a result, in late disease fibrous adhesions, bony ankyloses (abnormal fusion of bones in the joint), and calcifications occur; bone loses density, and secondary osteoporosis occurs.

Permanent joint changes may be avoided if RA is diagnosed early. Early and aggressive treatment to suppress synovitis may lead to a remission. RA is a disease characterized by natural remissions and exacerbations. Interprofessional health care team management helps control the disease to decrease the intensity and number of exacerbations. Preventing flares helps prevent joint erosion and permanent joint damage.

Because RA is a systemic disease, areas of the body besides the synovial joints can be affected. Inflammatory responses similar to those occurring in synovial tissue may occur in any organ or body system in which connective tissue is prevalent. If blood vessel involvement (**vasculitis**) occurs, the organ supplied by that vessel can be affected, leading to eventual failure of the organ or system in late disease.

Etiology and Genetic Risk

The etiology of RA remains unclear, but research suggests a *combination of environmental and genetic factors*. Some researchers also suspect that female reproductive hormones influence the development of RA because it affects women more often than men—usually young to middle-age women. Others suspect that infectious organisms may play a role, particularly the Epstein-Barr virus (McCance et al., 2014). Physical and emotional stresses have been linked to exacerbations of the disorder and may be contributing factors or "triggers" to its development.

GENETIC/GENOMIC CONSIDERATIONS
Patient-Centered Care QSEN

Research has shown that there is a strong association between RA and several human leukocyte antigen (HLA)–*DR* alleles. The cause of this association is not clear, but most HLA diseases are autoimmune (McCance et al., 2014). *DR* alleles, especially *DR4* and *DRB1*, are the primary genetic factors contributing to the development of RA. *DR4* is associated with more severe forms of the disease. Other contributing factors are being researched.

Incidence and Prevalence

RA affects over 1.3 million people, and Euro-Americans have the disease more often than other groups (Arthritis Foundation, 2016b). The cause for this trend is not known.

❖ INTERPROFESSIONAL COLLABORATIVE CARE
◆ Assessment: Noticing

The onset of rheumatoid arthritis (RA) may be acute and severe or slow and progressive; patients may have vague symptoms that last for several months before diagnosis. The onset of the disease is more common in the winter months than in the warmer months. The manifestations of RA can be categorized as early or late disease and as articular (joint) or extra-articular (Chart 18-7).

Physical Assessment/Signs and Symptoms

Early Signs and Symptoms. In the early stage of RA the patient typically reports joint inflammation, generalized weakness, and fatigue. Anorexia, weight loss of about 2 to 3 lb (1 kg), and persistent low-grade fever are common. In patients with early disease, the upper-extremity joints are involved initially—often

---

>> **CHART 18-7**   **Key Features**

The Patient With Rheumatoid Arthritis

Early Signs and Symptoms	Late Signs and Symptoms
Joint	**Joint**
• Inflammation	• Deformities (e.g., swan neck or ulnar deviation)
	• Moderate-to-severe pain and morning stiffness
Systemic	
• Low-grade fever	
• Fatigue	**Systemic**
• Weakness	• Osteoporosis
• Anorexia	• Severe fatigue
• Paresthesias	• Anemia
	• Weight loss
	• Subcutaneous nodules
	• Peripheral neuropathy
	• Vasculitis
	• Pericarditis
	• Fibrotic lung disease
	• Sjögren's syndrome
	• Kidney disease
	• Felty's syndrome

the proximal interphalangeal (PIP) and metacarpophalangeal (MCP) joints of the hands. These joints may be slightly reddened, warm, stiff, swollen, and tender or painful, particularly on palpation (caused by synovitis). The typical pattern of joint involvement in RA is bilateral and symmetric (e.g., both wrists). The number of joints involved usually increases as the disease progresses. In early disease the patient may report migrating symptoms known as migratory arthritis.

The presence of only *one* hot, swollen, painful joint (out of proportion to the other joints) may mean that the joint is infected. *Refer the patient to the primary health care provider (generally the rheumatologist) immediately if this is the case.* Single hot, swollen joints are considered infected until proven otherwise and require immediate long-term antibiotic treatment.

Late Signs and Symptoms. As the disease worsens, the joints become progressively inflamed and very painful. The patient usually has frequent morning stiffness (also called the gel phenomenon), which can last for several hours after awakening. On palpation the joints feel soft and look puffy because of synovitis and effusions (joint swelling with fluid, especially the knees). The fingers often appear spindle-like. Note any muscle atrophy (which can result from disuse secondary to joint pain) and a decreased range of motion in the affected joints.

Most or all synovial joints are eventually affected. The temporomandibular joint (TMJ) may be involved in severe disease, but such involvement is uncommon. When the TMJ is affected, the patient may have pain when chewing or opening the mouth.

When the spinal column is involved, the cervical joints are most likely to be affected. During clinical examination gently palpate the posterior cervical spine and identify it as cervical pain, tenderness, or loss of motion.

> ### ! NURSING SAFETY PRIORITY QSEN
> #### Critical Rescue
>
> Cervical RA may result in subluxation (partial joint dislocation), especially of the first and second vertebrae. This complication may be life threatening because branches of the phrenic nerve that supply the diaphragm are restricted and respiratory function may be compromised. The patient is also in danger of becoming quadriparetic (weak in all extremities) or quadriplegic (paralyzed in all extremities). If cervical pain (may radiate down one arm) or loss of range of motion is present in the cervical spine, keep the neck straight in a neutral position to prevent permanent damage to the spinal cord or spinal nerves. *Notify the primary health care provider immediately about these neurologic changes!*

Joint deformity occurs as a late, articular manifestation, and secondary osteoporosis can cause bone fractures. Observe common deformities, especially in the hands and feet (Fig. 18-6). Extensive wrist involvement can result in carpal tunnel syndrome (see Chapter 51 for assessment and management of carpal tunnel syndrome).

Gently palpate the tissues around the joints to elicit pain or tenderness associated with other rheumatoid complications, unless the patient is having severe joint pain. For example, Baker's cysts (enlarged popliteal bursae behind the knee) may occur and cause tissue compression and pain. Tendon rupture is also possible, particularly rupture of the Achilles tendon.

Numerous extra-articular signs and symptoms are associated with advanced disease. Assess the patient to ascertain systemic involvement. In addition to increased joint swelling and tenderness, *moderate-to-severe weight loss, fever,* and *extreme fatigue* are common in late disease exacerbations, often called

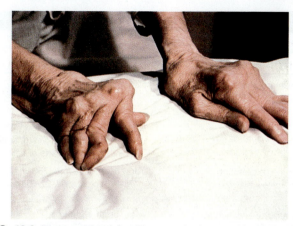

FIG. 18-6 Common joint deformities seen in rheumatoid arthritis. (From Damjanov I. [2006[. *Pathophysiology for the health professions* [3rd ed.]. Philadelphia: Saunders.)

flare-ups. Some patients have the characteristic round, movable, nontender subcutaneous nodules, which usually appear on the ulnar surface of the arm, on the fingers, or along the Achilles tendon. These nodules can disappear and reappear at any time and are associated with severe, destructive disease. Rheumatoid nodules usually are not a problem themselves; however, they occasionally open and become infected and may interfere with ADLs. Accidentally bumping the nodules may cause discomfort. Occasionally nodules occur in the lungs.

Inflammation of the blood vessels results in *vasculitis,* particularly of small to medium-size vessels. When arterial involvement occurs, major organs can become ischemic and malfunction. Assess for ischemic skin lesions that appear in groups as small, brownish spots, most commonly around the nail bed (periungual lesions). Monitor the number of lesions, note their location each day, and report vascular changes to the health care provider. Increased lesions indicate increased vasculitis, and a decreased number indicates decreased vasculitis. Also carefully assess any larger lesions that appear on the lower extremities. These lesions can lead to ulcerations, which heal slowly as a result of decreased circulation. Peripheral neuropathy associated with decreased circulation can cause footdrop and paresthesias (burning and tingling sensations), usually in older adults.

Respiratory complications may manifest as *pleurisy, pneumonitis, diffuse interstitial fibrosis,* and *pulmonary hypertension.* Cardiac complications include *pericarditis* and *myocarditis.* These health problems are discussed elsewhere in this text. Assess for eye involvement, which typically manifests as *iritis* and *scleritis.* If either of these complications is present, the sclera of one or both eyes is reddened, and the pupils have an irregular shape. Visual disturbances may occur.

Several syndromes are seen in patients with advanced RA. The most common is Sjögren's syndrome, which includes a triad of:

- Dry eyes (keratoconjunctivitis sicca [KCS], or the sicca syndrome)
- Dry mouth (xerostomia)
- Dry vagina (in some cases)

Note the patient's report of dry mouth or dry eyes. Some patients state that their eyes feel "gritty," as if sand is in their eyes. Inspect the mouth for dry, sticky membranes and the eyes for redness and lack of tearing.

Psychosocial Assessment. Rheumatoid arthritis (RA) and other inflammatory types of arthritis are chronic diseases that

CHART 18-8 Laboratory Profile

Connective Tissue Disease

TEST	NORMAL RANGE FOR ADULTS	SIGNIFICANCE OF ABNORMAL FINDINGS
Rheumatoid factor	Negative	Positive or increase indicative of possible RA or other CTD; may also be elevated in leukemia, liver disease, and kidney disease
ANA (total)	Negative (if positive, types of ANA identified [e.g., anti-ENA, anti-Smith, anti–SS-a (Ro)] to indicate what parts of cells are involved)	Elevations common in SLE, SSc, RA, and other inflammatory CTDs (5% of healthy adults have positive ANA results)
Serum complement	*Total:* 30-75 units/mL (75-160 kU/L) (*C3:* 75-175 mg/dL; *C4:* 22-45 mg/dL)	Decreased values indicative of active autoimmune disease such as SLE and other problems such as anemia, infection, and malnutrition
Erythrocyte sedimentation rate (ESR)	*Male:* up to 15 mm/hr *Female:* up to 20 mm/hr	Increased in inflammatory diseases such as RA, SLE, PMR, temporal arteritis; also elevated in patients with bacterial infections or severe anemias
SPEP	*Total:* 6.4-8.3 g/dL (64-83 g/L)	
Albumin	3.5-5.0 g/dL (35-50 g/L)	Decreased level occurs with chronic inflammation or infection; also decreased in malnutrition and advanced cirrhosis
Globulin	2.3-3.4 g/dL (23-34 g/L)	
Alpha₁ globulin	0.1-0.3 g/dL (1-3 g/L)	Increased level possible in RA
Alpha₂ globulin	0.6-1.0 g/dL (6-10 g/L)	
Beta globulin	0.7-1.1 g/dL (7-11 g/L)	
Gamma globulin	0.8-1.6 g/dL (8-16 g/L)	Increased levels indicative of CTD (inflammatory type)
HLA testing (*HLA-B27*)	None	Presence of *HLA-B27* indicative of Reiter's syndrome or ankylosing spondylitis

ANA, Antinuclear antibody; *CTD,* connective tissue disease; *ENA,* extractable nuclear antigens; *HLA,* human leukocyte antigen; *PMR,* polymyalgia rheumatica; *RA,* rheumatoid arthritis; *SLE,* systemic lupus erythematosus; *SPEP,* serum protein electrophoresis; *SSc,* systemic sclerosis.

can be disabling if not well controlled. Fear of becoming dependent, uncertainty about the disease process, altered body image, devaluation of self, frustration, and depression are common psychosocial problems. Physical limitations and chronic pain may limit MOBILITY. These limitations can result in role changes in the family and society. For example, the person may not be able to cook for the family or be an active sexual partner. In addition, extreme fatigue often causes patients to desire an early bedtime and may result in a reluctance to socialize.

Body changes caused by joint changes and drug therapy (if used) may also cause poor self-esteem and body image. Because many societies value people with physically fit, attractive bodies, the patient with RA may be embarrassed to be seen in public places. The patient may grieve or experience degrees of depression. He or she may have feelings of helplessness caused by a loss of control over a disease that can "consume" the body. Fortunately newer drugs have improved the treatment of RA and provide the patient with hope and better disease control. Only a small percentage of patients with RA become wheelchair dependent.

Living with a chronic disease and its associated impaired COMFORT is difficult for the patient and family. Chronic suffering and pain affect quality of life. Assess the patient's emotional and mental status in relation to the disease and its problems. Evaluate his or her support systems and resources. Patients who are knowledgeable about their disease and treatment options feel emotionally stronger to cope with their disease and better able to discuss treatment options with their primary health care provider.

Laboratory Assessment. Laboratory tests help support a diagnosis of RA, but no single test or group of tests can confirm

it. Chart 18-8 summarizes the most common laboratory tests that the primary health care provider may use for diagnosing connective tissue diseases.

The test for *rheumatoid factor (RF)* measures the presence of unusual antibodies of the immunoglobulins G (IgG) and M (IgM) types that develop in a number of connective tissue diseases. Many patients with RA have a positive titer (greater than 1:80), *especially in older adults* (Pagana et al., 2017). However, the presence of RF is not diagnostic for RA.

The newest laboratory test called the *anti-cyclic citrullinated peptide (anti-CCP)* is very specific and sensitive in detecting early RA. The presence of anti-CCP is also a marker for aggressive and erosive late-stage disease.

The *antinuclear antibody (ANA)* test measures the titer of a group of antibodies that destroy the nuclei of cells and cause tissue death in patients with autoimmune disease. The fluorescent method is sometimes referred to as *FANA.* If this test result is positive (a value higher than 1:40), various subtypes of this antibody are identified and measured.

When RA patients also have Sjögren's syndrome (SS) or if the syndrome occurs as a separate disease, several unusual anti–SS antibody types may be present. In particular, *anti–SS-a (Ro)* and *anti–SS-b (La)* antibodies are present in about 60% to 70% of those with Sjögren's syndrome or those with secondary Sjögren's and RA (Pagana et al., 2017).

An elevated *erythrocyte sedimentation rate (ESR),* or "sed rate," can confirm inflammation or infection anywhere in the body. An elevated ESR helps support a diagnosis of an unspecified inflammatory disease. The test is most useful to monitor the course of a disease, especially for inflammatory autoimmune diseases. In general the more severe the disease gets, the higher the ESR rises; as the disease improves or goes into remission, the ESR level decreases.

The *high-sensitivity C-reactive protein,* or *hsCRP,* is another useful test to measure inflammation and may be done with or instead of the ESR. As the name implies, it is more sensitive to inflammatory changes than the ESR. It is also very useful for detecting infection anywhere in the body.

The presence of most chronic diseases usually causes mild-to-moderate anemia, which contributes to the patient's fatigue. Therefore monitor the patient's complete blood count (CBC) for a low hemoglobin, hematocrit, and red blood cell (RBC) count. An increase in white blood cell (WBC) count is consistent with an inflammatory response. A decrease in the WBC count may indicate Felty's syndrome, a complication associated with late RA. Thrombocytosis (increased platelets) can also occur in patients with late RA. Additional laboratory tests may be performed, depending on the body systems and organs that may be affected by the disease. For example, if heart involvement is suspected, the primary health care provider may request cardiac enzymes.

Other Diagnostic Assessment. A standard x-ray is used to visualize the joint changes and deformities typical of RA. A CT scan may help determine the presence and degree of cervical spine involvement.

An *arthrocentesis* is an invasive procedure that may be used for patients with joint swelling caused by excess synovial fluid (effusion). It may be performed at the bedside or in a health care provider's office or clinic. After administering a local anesthetic, the provider inserts a large-gauge needle into the joint (usually the knee) to aspirate a sample of synovial fluid to relieve pressure. The fluid is analyzed for inflammatory cells and immune complexes, including RF. Fluid from patients with RA typically reveals increased WBCs, cloudiness, and volume.

Teach the patient to use ice and rest the affected joint for 24 hours after arthrocentesis. Often the primary health care provider will recommend acetaminophen as needed for discomfort. If increased pain or swelling occurs, teach the patient or family to notify the primary health care provider immediately.

> ### ! NURSING SAFETY PRIORITY QSEN
> **Action Alert**
>
> After an arthrocentesis, monitor the insertion site for bleeding or leakage of synovial fluid. Notify the health care provider if either of these problems occurs.
>
> A bone scan or joint scan can also assess the extent of joint involvement. MRI may be performed to assess spinal column disease or other joint involvement.
>
> Because RA can affect multiple body systems, tests to diagnose specific systemic manifestations are performed as necessary. For example, nerve conduction studies help confirm peripheral neuropathy. Pulmonary function tests help determine the presence of lung involvement.

◆ Analysis: Interpreting

The priority collaborative problems for patients with rheumatoid arthritis (RA) include:
1. Chronic inflammation and pain due to systemic autoimmune disease process
2. Potential for decreased mobility due to joint deformity, muscle atrophy, and fatigue

> ### ? NCLEX EXAMINATION CHALLENGE 18-4
> **Physiological Integrity**
>
> Which assessment findings will the nurse expect for the client with late-stage rheumatoid arthritis? **Select all that apply.**
> A. Bony nodes in finger joints
> B. Subcutaneous nodules
> C. Severe weight loss
> D. Joint deformity
> E. Thrombocytosis

3. Potential for decreased self-esteem image due to joint deformity

◆ Planning and Implementation: Responding

Patients who have RA are managed in the community under the supervision of a qualified health care provider. The goal of management is that the disease goes into remission and its progression slows to decrease pain, prevent joint destruction, and increase MOBILITY. When patients with RA are admitted to the inpatient acute care or long-term care facility, it is usually for health problems other than for complications of arthritis. Whether the patient is in a facility or community, be sure to plan interventions to manage his or her chronic pain and inflammation and the potential for decreased mobility and decreased self-esteem.

Managing Chronic Inflammation and Pain

Planning: Expected Outcomes. The patient with RA is expected to have a COMFORT level that is acceptable to the patient (e.g., at a 3 on a pain intensity scale of 0 to 10). A major focus of pain management is drug therapy to modify or prevent the progression of the disease, thereby decreasing joint and systemic inflammation.

Interventions. As in other types of arthritis, the interprofessional health care team manages pain by using a combination of pharmacologic and nonpharmacologic measures. A synovectomy to remove inflamed synovium may be needed for joints such as the knee or elbow. Total joint arthroplasty (TJA) may be indicated when other measures fail to relieve pain. TJA is discussed in the Osteoarthritis section of this chapter.

Drug Therapy. Some drugs prescribed for RA have anti-inflammatory and/or analgesic actions. For example, NSAIDs are sometimes used for RA to help promote COMFORT and decrease inflammation. The choice of which one to prescribe depends on the patient's needs and tolerance and the scientific evidence supporting the drug therapy. To decrease GI problems, the NSAID may be given with an H_2-blocking agent such as ranitidine (Zantac) or misoprostol (Cytotec). If there is no clinical change after 6 to 8 weeks, the health care provider may discontinue the current NSAID and try another one or change to a different drug class.

It was once thought that celecoxib (Celebrex), a COX-2 inhibiting NSAID, should be given rather than the older NSAIDs such as ibuprofen. However, all COX-2 inhibiting drugs have recently been associated with cardiovascular disease such as myocardial infarction, and some have been taken off the market. The risk for GI bleeding is also high in patients taking Celebrex, and the drug cannot be given to those who have had recent open-heart surgery.

Other drugs are immunosuppressive and disease modifying, which may cause remission of the illness and prevent erosive joint changes. Biological response modifiers make up the newest class of disease-modifying drugs that help reduce signals for the immune system to cause inflammation. Patients with inflammatory diseases other than RA are also using various biological response–modifying drugs successfully. Although RA is a chronic disease and no cure is yet available, drugs now used can better control the disease and prevent further deterioration. Adjustments in drug therapy are recommended every 3 to 6 months until the expected outcome or disease remission is met.

The primary health care provider, often a rheumatologist, makes decisions about appropriate drug therapy for patients with rheumatoid disease based on the severity of the disease. Initially most patients are managed with disease-modifying antirheumatic drugs (DMARDs). As the name implies, these drugs are given to slow the progression of the disease. For best results, they should be started early in the disease process.

First-Line Disease-Modifying Antirheumatic Drugs. Methotrexate (MTX) (Rheumatrex), an immunosuppressive medication, in a low, once-a-week dose (generally 25 mg or less per week orally) is the mainstay of therapy for RA because it is effective and relatively inexpensive. It is a slow-acting drug, taking 4 to 6 weeks to begin to control joint inflammation. Observe for desired therapeutic drug effects such as a decrease in joint discomfort and swelling.

Monitor patients for potential adverse effects such as decreasing WBCs and platelets (as a result of bone marrow suppression) or elevations in liver enzymes or serum creatinine.

> **⚠ NURSING SAFETY PRIORITY** QSEN
>
> **Drug Alert**
>
> Patients taking MTX are at risk for infection caused by impaired or decreased drug-induced IMMUNITY. Teach them to avoid crowds and people who are ill. Remind patients to avoid alcoholic beverages while taking MTX to prevent liver toxicity. Teach them to observe and report other side and toxic effects, which include mouth sores and acute dyspnea from pneumonitis. Although not commonly occurring, lymph node tumor (lymphoma) and pneumonitis (lung inflammation) have been associated in those who have RA and are taking MTX. Folic acid, one of the B vitamins, is often given to those who are taking MTX to help decrease some of the drug's side effects.

Pregnancy is not recommended while taking methotrexate because birth defects are possible. *Strict birth control is recommended for childbearing women who are in need of MTX to control their RA.* If pregnancy is ever desired, instruct the patient to consult the rheumatologist and an obstetric/gynecologic (OB/GYN) health care provider. Generally the health care provider will discontinue the drug at least 3 months before planned pregnancy. MTX may be restarted after birth if the patient does not breast-feed (Lilley et al., 2014).

Leflunomide (Arava) may be prescribed for some patients. It is a slow-acting immune-modulating medication that helps diminish inflammatory symptoms of joint swelling and stiffness and improves MOBILITY. The drug is generally prescribed as a loading dose of 100 mg orally daily for 3 days followed by 20 mg orally daily thereafter. Inform the patient that Arava takes 4 to 6 weeks and sometimes up to 3 months before maximum benefit is realized.

Arava is a potent medication that is generally tolerated; but side effects of hair loss, diarrhea, decreased WBCs and platelets, or increased liver enzymes have been reported. *Teach patients to report these changes and monitor laboratory results carefully.*

Remind them to avoid alcohol. Inform them that Arava can cause birth defects; therefore recommend strict birth control to women of childbearing age. Tell patients to contact their primary health care provider immediately if pregnancy occurs while taking the drug.

Another DMARD sometimes used for RA is hydroxychloroquine. This drug slows the progression of mild rheumatoid disease before it worsens. It is an antimalarial drug that helps decrease joint and muscle pain. Patients generally tolerate hydroxychloroquine quite well. In a few cases mild stomach discomfort, light-headedness, or headache has been reported.

> **⚠ NURSING SAFETY PRIORITY** QSEN
>
> **Drug Alert**
>
> The most serious adverse effect of hydroxychloroquine is retinal damage. Teach patients to report blurred vision or headache. Remind them to have an eye examination before taking the drug and every 6 months to detect changes in the cornea, lens, or retina. If this rare complication occurs, the primary health care provider discontinues the drug (Lilley et al., 2014).

Biological Response Modifiers. As a group, biological response modifiers (BRMs), sometimes called biologics, are one of the newest classes of DMARDs. Most BRMs neutralize the biologic activity of tumor necrosis factor–alpha (TNFA) by inhibiting its binding with TNF receptors. Any one of the BRMs may be tried. If one drug is not effective, the health care provider prescribes another drug in the same class. All these drugs are extremely expensive at this time, and insurance companies may not completely pay for their use. Some patients receive one of these drugs in addition to the drugs in this Drug Therapy section.

Teach patients receiving any one of the BRMs that they are at a high risk for developing impaired IMMUNITY and subsequent infection. Instruct them to stay away from people with infections and to avoid large crowds if possible. Remind patients with multiple sclerosis (MS), tuberculosis (TB), or a positive TB test that they should not receive TNF inhibitors because they make patients susceptible to flare-ups of these diseases. Determine whether the patient has had a recent negative purified protein derivative (PPD) test for TB. If not, a PPD skin test is typically administered, and the selected BRM is not started until a negative test result is confirmed. Collaborate with the health care provider to ensure that this process is complete. Chart 18-9 provides specific examples of BRMs and associated nursing implications. Most of these medications are given parenterally and require health teaching for self-administration.

Other Drugs. A few drugs may be given as adjuncts to or instead of the previously described drugs. It is not unusual for a patient to be taking several disease-modifying drugs such as methotrexate, a BRM, and an adjunct medication. Each drug works differently to relieve symptoms and slow the progression of the disease.

Glucocorticoids (steroids)—usually prednisone (Deltasone)—are given for their fast-acting anti-inflammatory and immunosuppressive effects. Prednisone may be given in high dose for short duration (pulse therapy) or as a low chronic dose. Moderate-dose short-term tapering bridge therapy may be used when inflammation is symptomatic and other RA medications are insufficient or have not yet had an effect.

Chronic steroid therapy can result in numerous complications such as:

CHART 18-9 Common Examples of Drug Therapy

Biological Response Modifiers Used for Rheumatoid Arthritis and Other Connective Tissue Diseases*

COMMON DRUGS	PURPOSE OF DRUG/DRUG CLASSIFICATION	NURSING IMPLICATIONS
For *all* biological response modifiers (BRMs) (also called *biologics*)	Neutralize biologic activity of tumor necrosis factor–alpha (TNFA), interleukins (IL), T-lymphocytes, or tyrosine kinase (TK) to decrease immune response and inflammation	Do not give BRMs if patient has a serious infection, TB, or MS *because they may exacerbate these health problems.* Teach patients taking BRMs *to avoid getting live vaccines.* Teach patient to avoid crowds and people with infections *because serious infections, especially respiratory infections, can lead to hospitalization or cause death.*
Etanercept (Enbrel)	TNFA inhibitor	Teach patient to report site reaction, *which may indicate a local allergic response and cause pain.* Teach patient how to self-administer drug.
Infliximab (Remicade)	TNFA inhibitor	Refrigerate all BRMs, except infliximab, *to prevent drug decomposition.* Teach patient to report chest pain or difficulty breathing during infusion, *which could indicate a severe allergic response;* monitor blood pressure and infusion site.
Adalimumab (Humira)	TNFA inhibitor	Teach patient to report site reaction, *which may indicate local allergic response.*
Anakinra (Kineret)	IL-1 receptor antagonist	Teach patient to monitor site for reaction (*occurs more commonly when compared with other BRMs*). Monitor WBC count *because the drug can cause a severe decrease in WBC count and make the patient very susceptible to infection.* Teach the patient to report respiratory symptoms such as cough and fever. Teach him or her that malignancies can result from taking this drug.
Abatacept (Orencia)	Selective T-lymphocyte co-stimulator modulator (T-cell inhibitor)	Report cough, dizziness, and sore throat; do not receive live vaccines while taking the drug. Monitor for dyspnea, wheezing, flushing, itching, *which may indicate a mild-to-moderate allergic reaction.*
Rituximab (Rituxan)	Monoclonal antibody	Observe for infusion reaction as for etanercept. *Drug has a* **black box warning** *about serious infections from opportunistic pathogens that can lead to hospitalizations or death.*
Golimumab (Simponi)	TNFA inhibitor	Teach patient to report signs and symptoms of infection, including fever and malaise; teach patient to avoid live vaccines while taking drug. Teach patient about adverse drug effects, including hypertension, GI distress, and infection from opportunistic pathogens; report signs and symptoms of these problems to the health care provider.
Tocilizumab (Actemra)	IL-6 inhibitor	Teach patient the importance of having frequent WBC, platelet, and liver enzyme testing. *This drug can cause decreased WBCs and platelets and liver dysfunction.*

MS, Multiple sclerosis; *TB,* tuberculosis; *TNF,* tumor necrosis factor; *WBC,* white blood cell.
*This is not a comprehensive list; this chart lists only the common biological response modifiers (BRMs) used for rheumatoid arthritis and other connective tissue diseases.

- Diabetes mellitus
- Impaired or decreased IMMUNITY
- Fluid and electrolyte imbalances
- Hypertension
- Osteoporosis
- Glaucoma

Some drug effects are dose related, whereas others are not. Observe the patient for complications associated with chronic steroid therapy and report them to the primary health care provider. For example, if blood pressure becomes elevated or significant laboratory values change, notify the primary health care provider.

Instruct patients taking chronic steroids to take calcium, 1200 to 1500 mg daily, plus vitamin D, 400 mg daily, to help prevent osteoporosis. Bisphosphonate drugs may also be prescribed. Bone-density measurements (DEXA [dual-energy x-ray absorptiometry] scans) are done every 2 to 3 years to monitor for bone loss.

Patients with RA may experience one or a few joints that have more pain and inflammation than the others. Cortisone injections in single joints may be used to relieve local pain and inflammation. Have the patient ice and rest the joint for 24

hours after the procedure. Oral analgesics also are sometimes needed during that time.

Nonpharmacologic Interventions. Adequate rest, proper positioning, and ice and heat applications are important in pain management. If acute inflammation is present, ice packs may be applied to "hot" joints for pain relief until the inflammation lessens. The ice pack should not be too heavy. At home the patient can use a small bag of frozen peas or corn as an ice pack.

Heated paraffin (wax) dips may help increase COMFORT of arthritic hands. Finger and hand exercises are often done more easily after paraffin treatment. To relieve morning stiffness or the pain of late-stage disease, recommend a hot shower rather than a sponge bath or a tub bath. It is often difficult for the patient with RA to get into and out of a bathtub, although special hydraulic lifts and tub chairs are available to allow him or her to bathe. Safety (grab) bars and nonskid tread in the tub or shower floor are important safety features to discuss with all patients. Some older adults prefer using shower chairs and a walk-in shower that does not have a ledge that could cause falls.

Hot packs applied directly to involved joints may be beneficial. Most physical therapy departments have machines that keep hot packs ready anytime they are needed. Teach patients to use the microwave or stovetop heating instructions to warm heat packs at home. Remind them to follow the instructions given with each heating device used.

Plasmapheresis (sometimes called *plasma exchange*) is an in-hospital procedure prescribed by a health care provider in which the patient's plasma is treated to remove the antibodies causing the disease. Although not commonly done, this procedure may be combined with steroid pulse therapy for patients with severe, life-threatening disease.

Complementary and Integrative Health. Some patients may have pain relief from hypnosis, acupuncture, imagery, music therapy, or other techniques. Stress management is also popular as a pain relief intervention. Chapter 4 discusses these therapies in more detail.

Adequate nutrition is an important part of the management of RA. Obesity should be avoided or treated if present. The inflammatory state may place a greater burden on the metabolism of some essential nutrients. This catabolic state may be related to increased cytokine production, specifically tumor necrosis factor.

According to the Arthritis Foundation (2016b), no one food causes or cures RA; however, healthy nutrition in general is important. Refer the patient to the Arthritis Foundation's pamphlet regarding diet and arthritis. Refer him or her to the dietitian for vitamin- and nutrition-specific questions or recommendations. Teach patients to take any herbal or nutrition supplement under the supervision of a qualified health care provider to prevent adverse events and drug-food or drug-drug interactions.

Other integrative therapies are safe and have been scientifically proven to be effective to help control RA pain for most people. Examples include mind-body therapies such as relaxation techniques, imagery, and spiritual practices. For information about these techniques, see Chapter 4.

Promoting Mobility

Planning: Expected Outcomes. Patients with RA often have decreased MOBILITY related to multiple joint deformities and muscle atrophy. Fatigue and generalized weakness also contribute to decreased mobility. The expected outcome is that the patient will be able to independently perform ADLs with or without ambulatory and assistive devices.

Interventions. Although the physical appearance of a patient with severe RA may create the image that ADL independence is not possible, a number of alternative and creative methods can be used to perform these activities. *Do not perform these activities for the patient unless asked. Those with RA do not want to be dependent.* For example, hand deformities often prevent a patient from opening packages of food such as a box of crackers; however, he or she may prefer to use the teeth to open the crackers rather than depend on someone else.

In the hospital or long-term care facility, a patient may not eat because of the barriers of heavy plate covers, milk cartons, small packages of condiments, and heavy containers. Styrofoam or paper cups may bend and collapse as he or she attempts to hold them. A china or heavy plastic cup with handles may be easier to manipulate. Collaborate with the dietitian to help with access to food and total independence in eating.

When fine-motor activities (e.g., squeezing a tube of toothpaste) become impossible, larger joints or body surfaces can substitute for smaller ones. For example, teach how to use the palm of the hand to press the paste onto the brush. Devices such as long-handled brushes can help patients brush their hair;

dressing sticks can assist with putting on pants. These examples illustrate the need to assess the problem area, suggest alternative methods, and refer the patient to an OT or PT for special assistive and adaptive devices if necessary.

Additional nursing interventions depend in part on identifying the factors contributing to fatigue. For example, decreased or impaired COMFORT, sleep disturbances, and weakness are associated with increased fatigue. Anemia may also be a contributing factor and may be treated with iron (if an iron deficiency anemia is present), folic acid, or vitamin supplements prescribed by the health care provider. Chronic normochromic or chronic hypochromic anemia often occurs in most chronic systemic diseases. Assess for drug-related blood loss such as that caused by NSAIDs by checking the stool for gross or occult blood. *Older white women are the most likely to experience GI bleeding as a result of taking these medications. The reason for this trend is not known.*

If fatigue and decreased MOBILITY result from muscle atrophy, the health care provider prescribes an aggressive physical therapy program to strengthen muscles and prevent further atrophy. Patients also experience increased fatigue when pain prevents them from getting adequate rest and sleep. Measures to facilitate sleep include promoting a quiet environment, giving warm beverages, and administering hypnotics or relaxants as prescribed if necessary.

In addition to identifying and managing specific reasons for fatigue, determine the patient's usual daily activities and teach principles of **energy conservation,** including:

- Pacing activities
- Allowing rest periods
- Setting priorities
- Obtaining assistance when needed

Chart 18-10 lists specific suggestions for conserving energy and thus increasing activity tolerance and mobility.

Enhancing Self Esteem

Planning: Expected Outcome. The patient with RA often has multiple joints that are inflamed or deformed, causing a potential for decreased self-esteem. Therefore the expected outcome is that the patient will verbalize a positive perception of self as a result of interprofessional interventions.

Interventions. Body image and self-esteem may be affected by both the disease process and drug therapy. Steroids can cause a moonfaced appearance, acne, striae, "buffalo humps," and weight gain. Determine the patient's perception of these changes and the impact of the reactions of family and significant others. The most important intervention is communicating acceptance of the patient. When a trusting relationship is established, encourage him or her to express personal feelings.

CHART 18-10 Patient and Family Education: Preparing for Self-Management

Energy Conservation for the Patient With Arthritis

- Balance activity with rest. Take one or two naps each day.
- Pace yourself; do not plan too much for one day.
- Set priorities. Determine which activities are most important and do them first.
- Delegate responsibilities and tasks to your family and friends.
- Plan ahead to prevent last-minute rushing and stress.
- Learn your own activity tolerance and do not exceed it.

As a reaction to body changes and joint deformity and the presence of a chronic, painful disease, some patients display behaviors indicative of loss. They may use coping strategies that range from denial or fear to anger or depression. In an attempt to regain control over the effects of the disease process, they may appear to be "manipulative and demanding" and sometimes may be referred to as having an "arthritis personality." *This personality, which represents a negative label, is a myth; avoid using these terms.* Patients are trying to cope with the effects of their illness and should be treated with patience and understanding. Continually assess and accept these behaviors but remain realistic in discussing goals to improve self-esteem and body image. Emphasize their strengths and help them identify previously successful coping strategies. If needed, consult with mental health professionals or religious/spiritual leaders to help patients cope with this potentially debilitating chronic disease.

Care Coordination and Transition Management

Patients with rheumatoid arthritis (RA) are usually managed at home but in a few cases may be institutionalized in a long-term care facility if they become restricted to bed or a wheelchair. Some patients may be transferred to a rehabilitation facility for several weeks to help develop strategies, techniques, and skills for independent living at home. Chapter 6 discusses the rehabilitation process in detail.

Home Care Management. The amount of home care preparation depends on the severity of the disease. Structural changes may be necessary if there are deficits in performing ADLs or MOBILITY. Doors must be wide enough to accommodate a wheelchair or walker if one is used. Ramps are needed to prevent the patient in a wheelchair from becoming homebound. If the person cannot use stairs, he or she must have access to facilities for all ADLs on one floor. Handrails should be available in the bathroom and halls.

To promote continued homemaking functions, countertops and appliances may require structural changes. The patient may also require handrails and elevated chairs and toilet seats, which facilitate transfers (Fig. 18-7). *These devices are especially important for older adults with arthritis.*

Self-Management Education. Self-management education (SME) is a vital role for nurses in collaborative management of arthritis. Many people have signs and symptoms of joint inflammation but do not seek medical attention. Teach them to

seek professional health care to reduce pain and prevent disability.

Teach patients to discuss any questions with their health care provider before trying any over-the-counter or home remedies. Some remedies may be harmful. Check with the Arthritis Foundation for the latest information on arthritis myths and quackery (www.arthritis.org).

Provide information to the patient and family about drug therapy, joint protection, energy conservation, rest, and exercise. This SME is summarized in Charts 18-5, 18-6, and 18-10.

Assess the patient's coping strategies. The patient with RA often reports being on an "emotional roller coaster" from coping with a chronic illness every day. Control over one's life is an important human need. The patient with an unpredictable chronic disease may lose this control, and this lowers self-esteem. Health care providers must allow the patient to make decisions about care. Families and significant others must also include him or her in decision making. Although the patient's behavior may be perceived as demanding or manipulative, his or her self-esteem cannot be improved without this important aspect of interpersonal relationships.

Increased dependency also affects a sense of control and self-esteem. Some people ignore their health needs and portray a tough image for others by insisting that they need no assistance. Emphasize to the patient and family that asking for help may be the best decision at times to prevent further joint damage and disease progression.

RA may also affect work and social roles. The patient may have physical difficulty doing tasks that require lifting, climbing, grasp, or gross- or fine-motor activities. The severity of RA disease may cause difficulty with total number of hours worked. Some people with RA can do their jobs well without problem; others may have varying degrees of difficulty. Those who can no longer do their job at work may need to discuss with their employer having a lighter workload, but some may need to file for disability with their company and Social Security office.

Health Care Resources. The need for health care resources for the patient with RA is similar to that for the patient with osteoarthritis. A home care nurse or aide, physical therapist, or occupational therapist may be needed during severe exacerbations or as the disease progresses. In collaboration with the case manager, identify these resources and make sure that they are available as needed. The Arthritis Foundation is an excellent source of information and support.

Arthritis support groups and self-help courses provide the education and support that patients, families, and friends need. Refer the patient to a psychological counselor or religious or spiritual leader for emotional support and guidance during times of crisis or as needed. Identify and recommend other support systems within the family and community when necessary.

◆ Evaluation: Reflecting

Evaluate the care of the patient with RA on the basis of the identified priority problems. The expected outcomes are that he or she:

- Achieves pain control to a pain intensity level of 3 to 4 or less on a scale of 0 to 10 or at a level that is acceptable to the patient
- Moves and functions in his or her own environment independently with or without assistive devices
- Verbalizes increased self-esteem and positive perception of self

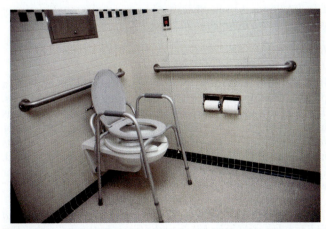

FIG. 18-7 Handrails and an elevated toilet seat make transfers easier for the patient.

CLINICAL JUDGMENT CHALLENGE 18-1
Teamwork and Collaboration; Safety QSEN

An 83-year-old woman with RA has been controlled with methotrexate (MTX) and prednisone for many years. Recently she was admitted to the acute care hospital for difficulty breathing and extreme weakness. She walked with a walker at home and rarely left her apartment. After a 9-day stay in the hospital for treatment of pneumonitis and congestive heart failure, she was transferred to a rehabilitation unit in a long-term care facility to regain her strength and ambulation ability. She was not ambulated during her entire hospital stay. Both medications being used to manage her long-term RA were discontinued.

1. What problems do you anticipate the patient will have and why?
2. Why do you think her medications were discontinued?
3. With which members of the health care team might you collaborate as part of her plan of care in rehabilitation and why?
4. Which home and community assessment might be needed to ensure her safety and provide continuity of care?
5. Which self-management education will she need before discharge from the rehabilitation setting? Will the patient be able to return to her apartment to live independently as she did before her hospital admission?

LUPUS ERYTHEMATOSUS

❖ PATHOPHYSIOLOGY

The two main classifications of lupus are discoid lupus erythematosus (DLE) and systemic lupus erythematosus (SLE). A small percentage of patients with lupus have the DLE type, which affects only the skin.

Unlike DLE, **systemic lupus erythematosus** is a chronic, progressive, inflammatory connective tissue disorder that can cause major body organs and systems to fail. Like RA, it is characterized by spontaneous remissions and **exacerbations** ("flare-ups"), and the onset may be acute or insidious (slow). The condition is potentially fatal, but most patients with SLE live many years after diagnosis and lead productive lives. Improvements in determining the cause, diagnosis, and treatment of lupus account for the prolonged survival.

Lupus is thought to be an autoimmune process. Antinuclear antibodies (ANAs) primarily affect the DNA, ribonucleic acid (RNA), and other components within the cell nuclei. As a result, immune complexes form in the serum and organ tissues, which cause inflammation, damage, and destruction (McCance et al., 2014). These complexes invade organs directly or cause **vasculitis** (vessel inflammation), which deprives the organs of arterial blood and oxygen.

Autoimmune complexes in SLE tend to be most attracted to the glomeruli of the kidneys. Therefore many of these patients have some degree of kidney involvement, called *lupus nephritis*—the leading cause of death from the disease. Other causes of death are cardiac and central nervous system involvement.

CULTURAL/SPIRITUAL CONSIDERATIONS
Patient-Centered Care QSEN

Lupus affects women 10 times more often than men; women of color are affected far more often than Euro-Americans. The reason for this difference is unknown (McCance et al., 2014). The disease also occurs among American Indians, Asian Americans, and Hispanics (Lupus Foundation of America, 2016).

CHART 18-11   Key Features
Systemic Lupus Erythematosus (SLE) and Systemic Sclerosis (SSc)

SYSTEMIC LUPUS ERYTHEMATOSUS	SYSTEMIC SCLEROSIS
Skin Manifestations	
Inflamed, red rash	Inflamed
Discoid lesions	Fibrotic
	Sclerotic
	Edematous
Renal Manifestations	
Nephritis	Kidney failure
Cardiovascular Manifestations	
Pericarditis	Myocardial fibrosis
Raynaud's phenomenon	Raynaud's phenomenon
	Deep vein thrombosis
Pulmonary Manifestations	
Pleural effusions	Interstitial fibrosis
Pneumonia	Pulmonary hypertension
Neurologic Manifestations	
CNS lupus	Not common
GI Manifestations	
Abdominal pain	Esophagitis
	Ulcers
	GERD
Musculoskeletal Manifestations	
Joint inflammation (polyarthritis)	Arthralgia
Myositis	Myositis
Other Manifestations	
Fever (indicates exacerbations)	Fever
Fatigue	Fatigue
Anorexia	Anorexia
Weight loss	Vasculitis
Generalized weakness	
Vasculitis	

CNS, Central nervous system; *GERD,* gastroesophageal reflux disease.

The onset of the disease occurs most often during the child-bearing years (ages 20 to 40 years), but it has been reported in young children and older adults. A genetic predisposition is based on the trend to develop the disease in some twins and the occurrence of autoimmune disease in some families of patients who have lupus. However, it is not the only basis of the disease. Like RA, lupus is probably caused by a complex *combination of genetic and environmental factors.*

❖ INTERPROFESSIONAL COLLABORATIVE CARE
◆ Assessment: Noticing

It is impossible to describe a typical textbook picture of a patient with lupus because of the extreme range of symptoms. There is no classic presentation of this disease. When lupus is in remission, the patient may appear healthy and have few or no activity limitations. When the disease flares, some patients may be so ill that admission to a critical care unit is needed. Chart 18-11 highlights the signs and symptoms that can occur with systemic lupus.

Physical Assessment/Signs and Symptoms

Skin Involvement. *The major skin manifestation of DLE and SLE is a dry, scaly, raised rash on the face* ("butterfly" rash) (Fig.

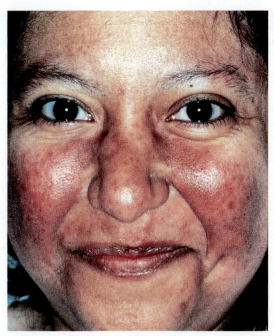

FIG. 18-8 The characteristic "butterfly" rash of systemic lupus erythematosus.

18-8). This rash may also appear on other sun-exposed areas. It is initially nonscarring and may increase in a lupus flare and disappear when the disease is in remission.

Individual round **discoid** (coinlike) **lesions** are the scarring lesions of discoid lupus. The lesions are especially evident when the patient is exposed to sunlight or ultraviolet light. Alopecia is also common in lupus. Observe and document all skin changes and monitor them daily while the patient is in an acute care setting or during an ambulatory care or home visit. Mouth ulcers are not uncommon.

Other Signs and Symptoms. In addition to skin changes, *polyarthritis* occurs in most patients with SLE. The early joint changes are similar to those seen in rheumatoid arthritis (RA), but severe deformities are not common even in late disease. Small joints and the knees are most commonly inflamed. **Osteonecrosis** (bone necrosis from lack of oxygen) is often seen in those who have been treated for at least 5 years with steroids like prednisone. Chronic steroid therapy may cause the constriction of small blood vessels supplying the joint, which causes the tissue to die. The hip is most commonly affected, and reports of pain and decreased MOBILITY result. As a result, a total hip arthroplasty may be done.

Because SLE is an inflammatory condition, *fever* and *fatigue* are common findings. *Fever is the classic sign of a flare, or exacerbation.* Various degrees of generalized weakness, fatigue, anorexia, and weight loss may occur. These signs may be the only evidence of disease, which makes diagnosis by the health care provider difficult. Therefore some patients have a diagnosis of "probable SLE." Additional signs and symptoms of SLE are listed in Chart 18-11.

Psychosocial Assessment. The psychosocial results of lupus can be devastating. With either DLE or SLE, the rash can be disfiguring and embarrassing. Young adult women who never had a blemish are confronted with a rash that cannot be completely covered with makeup. If chronic steroid therapy is used, side effects such as acne, striae, fat pads, and weight gain intensify the problem of an already altered body image.

Chronic fatigue and generalized weakness may prevent the patient from being as active as in the past. He or she may avoid social gatherings and may withdraw from family activities. The unpredictability and chronicity of SLE can cause fear and anxiety. Fear may increase if the patient knows another person with the disease, particularly if the other person has more advanced severe disease. Unfortunately the myth that lupus is fatal is still common. Inform the patient and family that control of lupus is generally possible with regular medical monitoring, medications, and healthy practices such as limiting sun exposure to prevent exacerbation of the disease.

Assess the patient's and family's feelings about the illness to identify areas requiring intervention. Determine their usual coping mechanisms and support systems before developing a plan of care. See the Psychosocial Assessment section of the Rheumatoid Arthritis section for additional information.

Laboratory Assessment. Because discoid lupus erythematosus (DLE) is not a systemic condition, the only significant test is a *skin biopsy.* The physician gently scrapes skin cells from the rash for microscopic evaluation. The characteristic lupus cell and a number of inflammatory cells confirm the diagnosis.

Some of the immunologic-based laboratory tests used to diagnose SLE are the same as those performed for rheumatoid arthritis (RA): rheumatoid factor, antinuclear antibody, erythrocyte sedimentation rate, serum protein electrophoresis, serum complement (especially C3 and C4), and immunoglobulins (see Chart 18-8). A false-positive Venereal Disease Research Laboratory (VDRL) syphilis test is common with lupus (Pagana et al., 2017).

More specific immunologic tests such as anti–SS-a (Ro), anti–SS-b (La), anti-Smith (anti-Sm), anti-DNA, and extractable nuclear antigens (ENAs) are also performed (Pagana et al., 2017). High titers of some of these antibodies are associated with lupus.

A complete blood count (CBC) commonly shows **pancytopenia** (a decrease of all cell types), probably caused by direct attack of the blood cells or bone marrow by immune complexes. Serum electrolyte levels, kidney function, cardiac and liver enzymes, and CLOTTING factors are also routinely assessed to determine other body system functioning.

◆ **Interventions: Responding**

The primary health care provider often prescribes potent drugs that are used topically and systemically. In addition, precautions are taken to prevent further skin impairment and exacerbations. Many of the skin lesions do not disappear, even with treatment, but they usually fade when the disease is in remission.

Managing Lupus With Drug Therapy. With DLE the patient's major concern is the rash or discoid lesions. Patients with SLE are also concerned about skin changes. Topical cortisone preparations help reduce inflammation and promote fading of the skin lesions. Acetaminophen (Tylenol) or NSAIDs may be used to treat joint and muscle pain and inflammation.

In addition, the health care provider may prescribe the anti-malarial agent *hydroxychloroquine* for some patients. Hydroxychloroquine decreases the absorption of ultraviolet light by the skin and therefore decreases the risk for skin lesions.

Teach patients to have frequent eye examinations (before starting the drug and every 6 months thereafter) if they are receiving hydroxychloroquine.

The primary health care provider often prescribes chronic steroid therapy to treat the systemic disease process. For renal or central nervous system lupus, he or she may also prescribe immunosuppressive agents such as methotrexate (Rheumatrex) or azathioprine (Imuran). Although signs and symptoms typically improve during remission, maintenance doses of these drugs are usually continued to prevent further exacerbations of the disease. These drugs make patients susceptible to decreased IMMUNITY.

! NURSING SAFETY PRIORITY (QSEN)

Drug Alert

When patients are taking steroids and/or immunosuppressants, stress the importance of avoiding large crowds and people who are ill. Teach patients to report any early sign of infection to their health care provider. Observe for side effects and toxic effects of these drugs and report their occurrence immediately. Remind patients to take their medication early in the morning before breakfast because that is the time when the body's natural corticosteroid level is the lowest.

For severe renal involvement, immunosuppressants may be given in combination with steroids. For patients who do not respond to this regimen, a high-dose IV bolus of glucocorticoids, cyclophosphamide, and plasmapheresis may be tried for 3 consecutive days. Kidney transplantation has been successful for some patients.

The first drug approved for SLE in 60 years is *belimumab (Benlysta)*. In SLE abnormal B-cells contribute to autoantibodies. Belimumab is an IV human monoclonal antibody (mAb) that prevents B-lymphocyte stimulator protein from binding to B-cell receptor sites, thus decreasing B-cell survival. It is given with other drugs to treat SLE. Like for other biologics, teach patients that the drug increases their risk for serious infections. Teach them not to receive live vaccines for 30 days before treatment.

Protecting the Skin. Teach patients to protect their skin to prevent an exacerbation of the disease.

! NURSING SAFETY PRIORITY (QSEN)

Action Alert

Instruct patients to avoid prolonged exposure to sunlight and other forms of ultraviolet lighting, including certain types of fluorescent light. Remind them to wear long sleeves and a large-brimmed hat when outdoors. Patients should use sun-blocking agents with a sun protection factor (SPF) of 30 or higher on exposed skin surfaces.

In addition, teach patients to clean the skin with mild soap (e.g., Ivory) and to avoid harsh, perfumed substances. The skin should be rinsed and dried well and lotion applied. Excess powder and other drying substances should be avoided. Cosmetics must be selected carefully and should include moisturizers and sun protectors. If desired, refer the patient to a medical cosmetologist who specializes in applying makeup for skin lesions of all types.

▣ CHART 18-12 Patient and Family Education: Preparing for Self-Management

Evidence-Based Practice for Skin Protection in Patients With Lupus Erythematosus

- Cleanse your skin with a mild soap such as Ivory.
- Dry your skin thoroughly by patting rather than rubbing.
- Apply lotion liberally to dry skin areas.
- Avoid powder and other drying agents such as rubbing alcohol.
- Use cosmetics that contain moisturizers.
- Avoid direct sunlight and any other type of ultraviolet lighting, including tanning beds.
- Wear a large-brimmed hat, long sleeves, and long pants when in the sun.
- Use a sun-blocking agent with a sun protection factor (SPF) of at least 30.
- Inspect your skin daily for open areas and rashes.

Patients' hair should receive special attention because alopecia (hair loss) is common. Recommend the use of mild protein shampoos and the avoidance of harsh treatments (e.g., permanents or highlights) until the hair regrows during remission.

Care Coordination and Transition Management

Community-based and continuing care for the patient with lupus is similar to that for RA. In general the patient is home but may need repeated hospitalizations during exacerbations of disease. He or she usually does not need rehabilitation unless having surgery, because severe joint deformity and prolonged immobility are not common in lupus.

Two major differences exist between SLE and RA in terms of education of the patient and family or significant others. First, instruct patients with SLE how to protect the skin (Chart 18-12). Second, teach them to monitor body temperature. Fever is the major sign of an exacerbation, during which they can become seriously ill. Teach the importance of reporting any other unusual or new signs and symptoms to the primary health care provider immediately.

Many patients become frustrated that family members, significant others, and lay people do not have a thorough understanding of lupus. When lupus is in complete remission, patients appear to be healthy; however, an exacerbation can lead to a critical care admission. This unpredictability disrupts the patient's life and can cause fear and anxiety. Help him or her identify coping strategies and support systems that can help with functioning in the community.

Teach the possible effects of the disease, including fatigue, on lifestyle. Women of childbearing age need to know that pregnancy can be a stressor and can cause an exacerbation of the disease, either during pregnancy or after delivery. The pregnant woman also has an increased risk for miscarriage, stillbirth, or premature birth. Pregnancy is not recommended for those with cardiac, renal, or central nervous system involvement.

The Arthritis Foundation is a general resource for all patients with connective tissue disease. The Lupus Foundation (www .lupus.org) is a resource specific for patients with lupus. It is a national organization and has chapters in every state to provide information and assistance for patients with lupus and their families. Local support groups and services are offered free of charge.

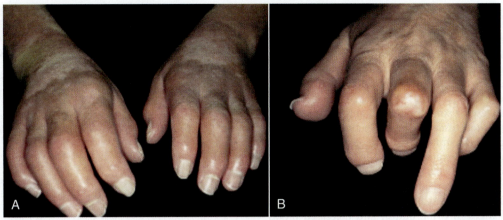

FIG. 18-9 Late-stage skin changes seen in patients with systemic sclerosis. (From Goldman, L., & Ausiello, D. [2007]. *Cecil medicine* [23rd ed.]. Philadelphia: Saunders.)

💡 NCLEX EXAMINATION CHALLENGE 18-5

Health Promotion and Maintenance

Which health teaching by the nurse is important for clients diagnosed with systemic lupus erythematosus? **Select all that apply.**
A. "Take frequent rest periods to prevent fatigue."
B. "Avoid green leafy vegetables to prevent bleeding."
C. "Avoid sun exposure to prevent disease flare-ups."
D. "Report fever to your health care provider immediately"
E. "Use a mild soap for bathing to prevent skin irritation."

SYSTEMIC SCLEROSIS

❖ PATHOPHYSIOLOGY

Systemic sclerosis (SSc), also called *scleroderma*, is another chronic, inflammatory, autoimmune connective tissue disease. Systemic sclerosis has been described in people of all races and in all geographic areas and affects over 300,000 people in the United States. Women are affected more often than men. The onset of the disease is usually between 25 and 55 years of age, with most women getting it in their 40s (Scleroderma Foundation, 2016).

Formerly called *progressive systemic disease,* or *PSS,* this illness is not always progressive. **Scleroderma** means hardening of the skin, which is only one sign of the problem. Some patients, often children, have only skin involvement, or localized scleroderma (also called *linear scleroderma*). However, adults usually have skin and other body system involvement. SSc is less common than systemic lupus erythematosus (SLE) but is associated with a higher mortality rate. See Chart 18-11 for a comparison of the key features of these two diseases. The signs and symptoms for both diseases vary widely from person to person.

Patients with the *limited* form of the disease often have the CREST syndrome:
- **C**alcinosis (calcium deposits)
- **R**aynaud's phenomenon (first symptom that occurs)
- **E**sophageal dysmotility
- **S**clerodactyly (scleroderma of the digits)
- **T**elangiectasia (spider-like hemangiomas)

Little is known about the cause of SSc, but autoimmunity is suspected. The occurrence of more than one case per family is uncommon, but other connective tissue diseases may be noted in the family history. At this time specific genetic causes have not been confirmed.

❖ INTERPROFESSIONAL COLLABORATIVE CARE

◆ Assessment: Noticing

Physical Assessment/Signs and Symptoms. **Arthralgia** (joint pain) and stiffness are common manifestations that you can assess during the musculoskeletal examination. The acute joint inflammation that occurs with rheumatoid arthritis (RA) is not common, and deformities are rare.

Findings on inspection of the skin depend on the stage of the scleroderma. Typically a painless, symmetric, pitting edema of the hands and fingers is present, especially in patients with the diffuse form of the disease. The edema may progress to include the entire upper and lower extremities and face. In this phase the fingers are described as *sausage-like*. The skin is taut, shiny, and free of wrinkles. If diffuse scleroderma occurs, swelling is replaced by tightening, hardening, and thickening of skin tissue; this phase is sometimes called the *indurative phase* (Fig. 18-9). The skin loses its elasticity, and range of motion is markedly decreased; ulcerations may occur. Joint contractures may develop, and the patient may be unable to perform ADLs independently.

Major organ damage is likely to develop with diffuse scleroderma, specifically affecting the renal and cardiopulmonary systems. The initial gastroesophageal reflux disease (GERD) symptoms progress into other problems, especially affecting the esophagus. The esophagus loses its motility, resulting in *dysphagia (difficulty swallowing). Assess for the ability of the patient to swallow before allowing him or her to drink or eat food!* Reflux of the gastric contents can cause esophagitis and subsequent ulceration, particularly in the lower two thirds of the esophagus. Intestinal changes are similar to those of the esophagus. Peristalsis is diminished, which causes signs and symptoms similar to a partial bowel obstruction. Malabsorption is a common complication, causing malodorous *diarrheal stools*.

In addition to assessing problems of the digestive tract, observe for *cardiovascular manifestations. Raynaud's phenomenon* occurs in various degrees in most patients with SSc. On exposure to cold or emotional stress, the small arterioles in the digits of both hands and feet rapidly constrict, which causes decreased blood flow. In severe cases the patient experiences digit necrosis, excruciating pain, and autoamputation of the distal digits (the tips of the digits fall off spontaneously). In many patients vasculitic lesions, often around the nail beds (periungual lesions), are evident. *Myocardial fibrosis,* another common problem, is evidenced by electrocardiographic (ECG) changes, cardiac dysrhythmias, and chest pain.

Lung involvement in the patient with SSc may go undetected until late in the disease or sometimes until autopsy. *Fibrosis of the alveoli and interstitial tissues* is present in almost all cases of the disease, but signs and symptoms may not be present. Patients with scleroderma and *pulmonary arterial hypertension* have a more serious prognosis. *Renal involvement* is an important aspect of the overall disease process and often causes malignant hypertension and death. Assess for signs of impending organ failure such as changes in urine output and increased blood pressure.

Laboratory Assessment. The laboratory findings for SSc are similar to those for SLE. Clinical findings and the patient's response to drug therapy help the health care provider differentiate between the two diseases. Additional tests depend on which organs seem to be affected. Upper and lower GI series are commonly performed because of the frequency of GI signs and symptoms.

◆ Interventions: Responding

The medical management of SSc aims to force the disease into remission and thus slow disease progression. The primary health care provider prescribes drug therapy primarily for this purpose, but it is often unsuccessful. Systemic steroids and immunosuppressants are used in large doses and often in combination. Another desired outcome of disease management is to identify early organ involvement and treat it before it becomes severe and irreversible. For example, a patient who has lung involvement receives aggressive respiratory therapy and other treatments as the condition requires.

Recently bosentan (Tracleer), the first of a new class of drugs called *endothelin receptor antagonists,* demonstrated improved walk tests for patients with class III or class IV pulmonary arterial hypertension. Various doses improved patients' breathing during exercise, but the potential for liver injury at the highest dose caused recommended doses to be lowered. Teach the patient the desired and potential adverse effects, including liver toxicity and birth defects. Remind him or her of the importance of follow-up testing for liver enzyme levels.

New oral tyrosine kinase inhibitors (TKIs), including nilotinib (Tasigna) and imatinib mesylate (Gleevec), are being tested in the United States for use for patients with systemic sclerosis, and the results are very promising. These drugs work to decrease inflammation and slow the progression of the disease. They are currently approved in the United States for use in certain types of cancer.

Local skin protective measures can help maintain skin integrity. Teach the patient to use mild soap and lotions and gentle cleaning techniques. Inspect the skin for further changes or open lesions. Skin ulcers are treated according to their type and location.

In addition to drug therapy to control the overall disease process, specific measures can provide COMFORT. The patient with SSc not only experiences chronic joint discomfort but also has severe, acute pain during episodes of Raynaud's phenomenon. Remind unlicensed nursing personnel to use a bed cradle and foot board to keep bed covers away from the skin in severe

---

⊚ CHART 18-13 Best Practice for Patient Safety & Quality QSEN

Care of the Patient With Systemic Sclerosis and Esophagitis

- Keep the patient's head elevated at least 60 degrees during meals and for at least 1 hour after each meal.
- Provide small, frequent meals rather than three large meals each day.
- Give the patient small amounts of food for each bite and explain the importance of chewing each bite carefully before swallowing.
- Provide semisoft foods such as mashed potatoes and pudding or custard; liquids are most likely to cause choking.
- Collaborate with the dietitian about the patient's diet.
- Teach the patient to avoid foods that increase gastric secretion such as caffeine, pepper, and other spices.
- Give antacids or histamine antagonists as needed.

---

cases. Adjust the room temperature to prevent chilling, which can precipitate digit vasospasm. The patient who can tolerate touching the affected areas can wear gloves and socks to increase warmth. Because cigarette smoking and extreme emotional stress can also cause symptoms to recur, teach the patient to avoid or minimize these factors as much as possible.

If the patient has esophageal involvement, collaborate with the speech and language pathologist to schedule a swallowing study. The patient may need small, frequent meals rather than the traditional three meals daily. He or she should minimize the intake of foods and liquids that stimulate gastric secretion (e.g., spicy foods, caffeine, alcohol). Teach the patient to keep his or her head elevated for 1 to 2 hours after meals. He or she may need to be in this position continuously. Histamine antagonists and antacids help reduce and neutralize gastric acid. To help prevent choking, collaborate with the dietitian for dietary changes (Chart 18-13).

Nursing care for the patient with joint pain and decreased MOBILITY is very similar to that for rheumatoid arthritis (see the Interventions section of the Rheumatoid Arthritis section).

Continuing and community-based care for the person with SSc is similar to that for lupus. The patient is treated at home but may need frequent hospitalizations if major organ involvement occurs during exacerbations. The Arthritis Foundation (www.arthritis.org) and Scleroderma Foundation (www.scleroderma.org) are excellent resources for more information about the disease and how to manage it.

GOUT

❖ PATHOPHYSIOLOGY

Gout, or gouty arthritis, is a systemic disease in which urate crystals deposit in the joints and other body tissues, causing inflammation. It is the most common acute inflammatory arthritis in older adults. The cause and treatment of gout have been firmly established. The classic case of well-advanced disease is seldom seen today unless the patient does not adhere to the therapeutic regimen. The two major types of gout are primary and secondary.

Primary gout is the most common type and results from one of several inborn errors of purine metabolism. An end product of purine metabolism is uric acid, which is usually excreted by the kidneys. In primary gout the production of uric acid exceeds the excretion capability of the kidneys. Sodium urate is deposited in synovium and other tissues, resulting in inflammation. For some patients primary gout is inherited as an X-linked trait; males are affected through female carriers. A number of patients have a family history of gout. Primary gout affects middle-age and older men and postmenopausal women. The peak time of onset in men is between 40 and 50 years of age (McCance et al., 2014).

Secondary gout involves hyperuricemia (excessive uric acid in the blood) caused by another disease or factor. Secondary gout affects people of all ages. Renal insufficiency, diuretic therapy, "crash" diets, and certain chemotherapeutic agents decrease the normal excretion of uric acid and other waste products. Disorders such as multiple myeloma and certain carcinomas result in increased production of uric acid because of a greater turnover of cellular nucleic acids. Treatment involves management of the underlying disorder.

Hyperuricemia and gout are often seen in older patients with cardiovascular health problems, obese people, and postmenopausal women. The incidence of gout is increasing as the baby boomer generation reaches 65 years of age.

The three clinical stages of the primary disease process are asymptomatic hyperuricemia, acute gouty arthritis, and chronic or tophaceous gout (McCance et al., 2014). The patient is usually unaware of the *asymptomatic hyperuricemic stage* unless he or she has had a serum uric acid level determination. The serum level is elevated, but no obvious signs of the disease are present. No treatment is needed in this stage.

The first "attack" of gouty arthritis begins the *acute stage*. The patient experiences excruciating pain and inflammation in one or more small joints, usually the metatarsophalangeal joint of the great toe, called podagra. The erythrocyte sedimentation rate (ESR) is usually increased as a result of the inflammatory process. Months or years may pass before additional attacks occur. The patient is asymptomatic, and no abnormalities are found during examination of the joints.

After repeated episodes of acute gout, deposits of urate crystals develop under the skin and within the major organs, particularly in the renal system. The patient is then classified as having *chronic tophaceous gout.* In chronic gout urate kidney stone formation is more common than renal insufficiency. Chronic gout can begin anywhere between 3 and 40 years after the initial gout symptoms occur (McCance et al., 2014).

❖ INTERPROFESSIONAL COLLABORATIVE CARE
◆ Assessment: Noticing

Note the patient's age, gender, and family history of gout. A complete history is needed to determine whether gout has been caused by another problem. Some women overuse diuretics, which can lead to secondary gout.

Overt manifestations are present in the acute and chronic phases of gout. You will likely encounter a patient with acute gout, but chronic gout is not as common in the United States today. *Joint inflammation is the most common finding of acute gout. The joint is usually so painful that the patient seeks medical care immediately.* Inspect the inflamed area; it is usually too painful and swollen to be touched or moved.

The primary health care provider requests a serum uric acid level to check for hyperuricemia. Because the level can be altered by food intake, several measurements may be obtained. A consistent level of more than 6.5 mg/dL is generally considered abnormal, depending on the laboratory test used. Urinary uric acid levels are also measured; an overproduction of uric acid is

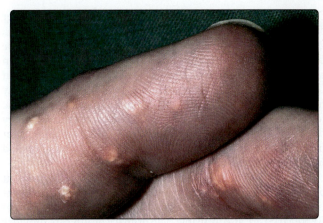

FIG. 18-10 Typical appearance of tophi, which may occur in chronic gout on an index finger. (From Currie, G., & Douglas, G. [2011]. *Flesh and bones of medicine*. Edinburgh: Mosby Ltd.)

confirmed by an excretion of more than 750 mg/24 hr (Pagana et al., 2017).

The primary health care provider may request kidney function tests such as blood urea nitrogen (BUN) and serum creatinine levels to monitor possible kidney involvement. A definitive diagnostic test for the disease is synovial fluid aspiration (arthrocentesis) to detect the needle-like crystals in the affected joint that are characteristic of the disorder.

With *chronic* gout inspect the skin for tophi, or deposits of sodium urate crystals (Fig. 18-10). Although tophi are rarely seen today, they may appear on the outer ear, arms, and fingers near the joints. The tophi are hard on palpation and irregular in shape. When the skin over the tophi is irritated, it may break open, and a yellow, gritty substance is discharged. Infection may result.

Other manifestations of chronic gout include signs of renal calculi (stones) or renal dysfunction such as severe pain or changes in urinary output. In some cases urate kidney stones occur before the arthritis is present.

◆ Interventions: Responding

Gout is one of the easiest diseases for the primary health care provider to diagnose and treat in its early phases. If the patient receives treatment and adheres to drug therapy, he or she should experience no further symptoms and no change in body image or lifestyle. The patient with gout is treated on an ambulatory basis, but hospitalized patients may have a secondary diagnosis of the disease.

Drug Therapy. Drug therapy is the key to managing patients with gout. In acute gouty "attacks," the inflammation subsides spontaneously within 3 to 5 days; however, most patients cannot tolerate the pain for that long. The drugs used for acute gout are different from those used for chronic gout. The health care provider typically prescribes a combination of colchicine (Colcrys) and an NSAID such as indomethacin (Indocin, Novomethacin ✚) or ibuprofen (Motrin, Amersol) for acute gout. IV colchicine works within 12 hours. The patient takes oral medications until the inflammation subsides, usually for 4 to 7 days.

For patients with repeated acute episodes or chronic gout, the health care provider prescribes drugs on a continuous, maintenance basis to promote uric acid excretion or reduce its production. Allopurinol (Zyloprim, Purinol) or febuxostat

(Uloric) is the drug of choice. Febuxostat may cause a greater risk to cardiovascular health than allopurinol (Lilley et al., 2014). As xanthine oxidase inhibitors, these drugs prevent the conversion of xanthine to uric acid. Teach patients to take them after meals and drink a glass of water with each dose to prevent GI distress. Drinking at least eight glasses of water each day helps prevent renal dysfunction. Remind patients that periodic follow-up laboratory tests, including liver enzymes, kidney function studies, and complete blood count, are important because xanthine oxidase inhibitors cause liver dysfunction and bone marrow suppression.

Probenecid can also be effective as a uricosuric drug in gout because it promotes the excretion of excess uric acid. Combination drugs that contain probenecid and colchicine (e.g., Col-BENEMID) are also available. The primary health care provider and nurse monitor serum uric acid levels to determine the effectiveness of these medications. Aspirin should be avoided because it inactivates the effects of the drug.

For patients with severe gout who do not respond to other drugs (refractory gout), pegloticase (Krystexxa) can be prescribed as an IV dose every 2 weeks. This drug is an enzyme that works directly on uric acid and converts it to allantoin, which can be excreted by the kidneys. Monitor patients carefully for allergic reactions, including anaphylaxis, during and immediately after drug administration because pegloticase is a protein that is foreign to the body.

Nutrition Therapy and Lifestyle Recommendations. The American College of Rheumatology best practice guidelines recommend a strict low-purine diet and suggest that patients avoid foods such as organ meats, shellfish, and oily fish with bones (e.g., sardines). Some primary health care providers and dietitians believe that limiting protein foods, especially red and organ meats, is sufficient. However, it is well known that excessive alcohol intake and fad "starvation" diets can cause a gouty attack. *Teach patients to determine which foods precipitate acute attacks and try to avoid them.*

In addition to food and beverage restrictions, patients with gout should avoid all forms of aspirin and diuretics because they may precipitate an attack. Likewise, excessive physical or emotional stress can exacerbate the disease. Surgery or acute illness such as a myocardial infarction can also trigger an attack. Stress-management techniques may be helpful for the patient with gout.

Teach the patient to drink plenty of fluids to prevent the formation of urinary stones. Increasing fluid intake helps dilute urine and prevents sediment formation.

> ### ? NCLEX EXAMINATION CHALLENGE 18-6
> #### Physiological Integrity
> The nurse is preparing to give medications to a group of clients. Which drug is not appropriate to treat the disease with which it is matched?
> A. Rheumatoid arthritis—leflunomide
> B. Osteoarthritis—acetaminophen
> C. Acute gout—allopurinol
> D. Systemic lupus erythematosus—prednisone

LYME DISEASE

Lyme disease is a reportable systemic infectious disease caused by the spirochete *Borrelia burgdorferi* and results from the bite of an infected deer tick, also known as the *black-legged tick.* It is the most common vector-borne disease in the United States and Europe. Most cases of the disease in the United States are seen in New England; the mid-Atlantic states, including Maryland and Virginia; the upper Midwest, including Wisconsin and Minnesota; and northern California, especially during the summer months.

In the early and *localized stage I,* the patient appears with *flu-like symptoms,* **erythema migrans** (round or oval, flat or slightly raised rash), and *pain and stiffness in the muscles and joints.* Most patients in the United States tend to have only one lesion, sometimes referred to as a *bull's-eye lesion.* Symptoms begin within 3 to 30 days of the tick bite, but most present in 7 to 14 days. Antibiotic therapy such as doxycycline or amoxicillin is prescribed during this uncomplicated stage for 14 to 21 days. Erythromycin can be used for patients who are allergic to penicillin. Without treatment these symptoms may disappear in about 4 to 5 weeks.

If not treated or if treatment is not successful, the patient may progress to the more serious complications of Lyme disease. *Stage II (early disseminated stage)* occurs 2 to 12 weeks after the tick bite. The patient may develop *carditis* with *dysrhythmias, dyspnea, dizziness, or palpitations* and central nervous system disorders such as *meningitis, facial paralysis* (often misdiagnosed as Bell's palsy), and *peripheral neuritis.* For severe disease, IV antibiotics (e.g., ceftriaxone or cefotaxime) are given for at least 30 days.

If Lyme disease is not diagnosed and treated in the earlier stages, later chronic complications (e.g., *arthritis, chronic fatigue, memory/thinking problems*) can result. This *late stage III (chronic persistent stage)* occurs months to years after the tick bite. *For some patients the first and only sign of Lyme disease is arthritis.* In some cases the disease may not respond to antibiotics in any stage, and the patient develops permanent damage to joints and the nervous system. *Prevention is the best strategy for Lyme disease.* Teach patients to follow the measures outlined in Chart 18-14 to prevent Lyme and other tick-borne diseases. Tell them about community resources such as the Lyme Disease Foundation (www.lyme.org) for more information.

DISEASE-ASSOCIATED ARTHRITIS

Arthritis can occur as a symptom of a number of diseases and other health disorders (see Tables 18-3 and 18-4). One of the most common disorders in which arthritis occurs is in patients who have psoriasis. **Psoriatic arthritis (PsA)** affects some people who have psoriasis—a skin condition characterized by a scaly, itchy rash, usually on the elbows, knees, and scalp. Fingernail and toenail lifting and pitting may also occur. The joint pain associated with psoriasis is often associated with stiffness, especially in the morning. Neck and back pain are particularly common, but various forms of the disease can cause small joint arthritis or involvement of the sacroiliac joints of the spine.

PsA occurs most often in people between 30 and 50 years of age in men and women of all races. Nail symptoms are common in patients who have the associated arthritis. Causes may include genetic and environmental factors, infectious agents, and immune system dysfunction.

Most patients do not experience destructive and deforming arthritis affecting more than three joints; but for those who do, the experience has a major impact on their quality of life.

CHART 18-14 Patient and Family Education: Preparing for Self-Management

Prevention and Early Detection of Lyme Disease

- Avoid heavily wooded areas or areas with thick underbrush, especially in the spring and summer months.
- Walk in the center of the trail.
- Avoid dark clothing. Lighter-colored clothing makes spotting ticks easier.
- Use an insect repellent (DEET) on your skin and clothes when in an area where ticks are likely to be found.
- Wear long-sleeved tops and long pants; tuck your shirt into your pants and your pants into your socks or boots.
- Wear closed shoes or boots and a hat or cap.
- Bathe immediately after being in an infested area and inspect your body for ticks (about the size of a pinhead); pay special attention to your arms, legs, and scalp.
- Check your pets for ticks.
- Gently remove with tweezers or fingers covered with tissue or gloves any tick that you find (do not squeeze). Dispose of the tick by flushing it down the toilet (burning a tick could spread infection).
- After removal, clean the tick area with an antiseptic such as rubbing alcohol.
- Wait 4 to 6 weeks after being bitten by a tick before being tested for Lyme disease (testing before this time is not reliable).
- Report symptoms such as a rash or influenza-like illness to your primary health care provider immediately.

TABLE 18-3 Common Health Disorders Associated With Arthritis

- Psoriasis
- Crohn's disease
- Ulcerative colitis
- Tuberculosis
- Hemophilia
- Whipple's disease
- Intestinal bypass surgery
- Hyperparathyroidism
- Hyperthyroidism
- Diabetes mellitus
- Sickle cell anemia crisis
- Infection

Treatment is focused on managing joint pain and inflammation, controlling skin lesions, and slowing the progression of the disease. Health teaching for skin care is similar to that for lupus. Management of joint inflammation is similar to that for rheumatoid arthritis as described earlier in this chapter. Methotrexate (Rheumatrex), sulfasalazine (Azulfidine), and biological response modifiers (also called *biologics*) such as etanercept (Enbrel), ustekinumab (Stelara), and golimumab (Simponi) are being used with success.

Teach the patient or family member how to self-administer Enbrel injections. Injection site reactions and infections (especially respiratory) are possible adverse effects. Ice and hydrocortisone 1% cream can be used if a red, itchy rash at the injection site develops.

Golimumab (Simponi) is the first biologic that is administered only once each month for psoriatic arthritis. Teach patients that this drug has a black box warning for serious infections that may lead to hospitalization or death from opportunistic pathogens (Lilley et al., 2014).

Several newer types of biologics have also been approved for psoriatic arthritis. Ustekinumab (Stelara) targets the cytokines *interleukin (IL)-12* and *IL-23* to decrease inflammation. Alefacept (Amevive) is an IV immunosuppressive drug (T-cell blocker) that is reserved for moderate-to-severe disease. Teach

patients taking these drugs about their risk for decreased IMMUNITY. Remind them to avoid crowds and anyone with an infection.

Acitretin (Soriatane) is an oral retinoid given for patients with severe disease. Teach patients to take the drug once a day with a meal and follow up with laboratory testing for liver enzymes.

The National Psoriasis Foundation (www.psoriasis.org) is an excellent community resource for patients and their families.

FIBROMYALGIA SYNDROME

Fibromyalgia syndrome (FMS), also referred to as simply *fibromyalgia*, is a chronic pain syndrome, not an inflammatory disease. However, arthritis and other comorbidities are commonly present in patients diagnosed with FMS. Pain, stiffness, and tenderness are located at specific sites in the back of the neck, upper chest, trunk, low back, and extremities. These tender points are also known as **trigger points** and can typically be palpated to elicit pain in a predictable, reproducible pattern. The pain is typically described as burning and gnawing. Increased muscle tenderness may be caused by the inability to tolerate pain, possibly related to dysfunction in the brain, especially the thalamus and hypothalamus (McCance et al., 2014).

The pain and tenderness tend to come and go but typically worsen in response to stress, increased activity, and weather conditions. The patient reports mild-to-severe fatigue, and sleep disturbances are common. Some people report numbness or tingling in their extremities; and others are sensitive to noxious odors, loud noises, and bright lights. Headaches and jaw pain are also common. Secondary FMS can accompany any connective tissue disease (CTD), particularly lupus and rheumatoid disease, and may not necessarily be related to sleep patterns.

Other symptoms include:
- GI, including abdominal pain, diarrhea and constipation, and heartburn
- Genitourinary, including dysuria, urinary frequency, urgency, and pelvic pain
- Cardiovascular, including dyspnea, chest pain, and dysrhythmias
- Visual, including blurred vision and dry eyes
- Neurologic, including forgetfulness and concentration problems

Many with these symptoms become frustrated because they are not properly diagnosed and are in constant pain and discomfort (Menzies, 2016).

Most patients are women between 30 and 50 years of age. It is unlikely that the disease is caused by one factor. Possible precipitating factors include CFS, Lyme disease, trauma, and flu-like illness (McCance et al., 2014). FMS may also be aggravated by deep-sleep deprivation. Teach patients to limit caffeine, alcohol, or other unnecessary substances that could interfere with deep sleep. Establish a regular sleep pattern.

Selected anticonvulsants such as gabapentin (Neurontin) and pregabalin (Lyrica) and selective norepinephrine reuptake inhibitors (SNRIs, a class of antidepressants) such as duloxetine HCl (Cymbalta) and milnacipran (Savella) may improve fibromyalgia nerve pain (Menzies, 2016). Teach the patient that these drugs can cause drowsiness and sleepiness and that alcohol should be avoided while taking them.

TABLE 18-4 **Other Less Common Connective Tissue Diseases That Affect Joints**

DISEASE	DESCRIPTION/ PATHOPHYSIOLOGY	ASSESSMENT/SIGNS AND SYMPTOMS	COLLABORATIVE INTERVENTIONS
Polymyositis/ dermatomyositis	Autoimmune, inflammatory disease that causes symmetric muscle atrophy; when skin rash is also present, disease is called *dermatomyositis (DM)*; women between 30 and 60 years affected most often	Severe muscle weakness Dysphagia (difficulty swallowing) Periorbital edema and lilac eyelid rash (DM) Malignant neoplasms in older patients	Comfort measures Swallowing precautions Nutritional support PT/OT support Immunosuppressant agents and/or chronic steroid therapy (Teach about risk for infection.) Health teaching about progression of disease, comfort measures, and dietary needs
Systemic necrotizing vasculitis	A group of autoimmune diseases that result in arteritis (inflammation of arterial walls) causing ischemia in the tissues or organs that are supplied by the arteries	Peripheral arterial disease causing severe pain and necrosis of toes or fingers Signs and symptoms of organ dysfunction or failure such as kidney or heart failure; also can cause strokelike symptoms	Chronic steroid therapy and other immunosuppressants Vasodilators, depending on type of vasculitis Management of organ dysfunction or failure
Polymyalgia rheumatica (PMR) and temporal arteritis (TA)	Autoimmune, genetic-based disease affecting middle-age and older women most often that causes proximal muscle weakness (shoulder and pelvic girdles) (PMR) (TA [also known as *giant cell arteritis*] may occur as a separate disease or with PMR.)	Shoulder, neck, pelvic, and hip weakness; stiffness; joint aches; low-grade fever; fatigue; and weight loss caused by inflammation (PMR) Headache and visual disturbances (TA)	Responds well to high-dose steroid therapy to cause remission of disease Symptom management Short-term PT/OT as needed Health teaching about medication and pain modalities such as heat application for joints
Ankylosing spondylitis	Autoimmune, inflammatory disease affecting the spine that is thought to be genetic (strongly associated with specific variations in the *HLA-27* allele on chromosome 6) Can occur in both men and women, but white men younger than 40 years most commonly affected	Chronic back pain Compromised respiratory function caused by rigid chest wall Visual disturbances caused by iritis (inflammation of the iris) Joint pain and aching Malaise Weight loss	Chronic pain management modalities NSAIDs DMARD such as methotrexate and biologic response modifiers Symptom management
Reiter's syndrome	Complex syndrome associated with the *HLA-27* allele causing a triad of arthritis, conjunctivitis, and urethritis (inflammation of the urethra) Triggered by exposure to infection, especially sexually transmitted disease or intestinal infection	Joint pain Eye infection causing redness, pain, and drainage Pain or burning on urination and changes in urinary pattern	Antibiotic therapy to manage infection Pain management NSAIDs Other symptom management
Marfan syndrome	Autosomal-dominant disorder resulting from mutations in the *fibrillin I* gene (FBNI) Fibrillin important in limiting the stretch of elastic connective tissues and allowing them to return to their original resting shape Shortens life expectancy, often with death in the 30s	Excessive height Elongated hands and feet Joint discomfort or pain Scoliosis Visual problems such as decreased visual acuity or glaucoma Cardiovascular problems such as mitral valve prolapse and aortic aneurysm, leading to heart failure or death	Symptom management Frequent echocardiography monitoring and physical examinations to detect heart problems Genetic counseling

DMARDs, Disease-modifying antirheumatic drugs; *OT,* occupational therapy; *PT,* physical therapy.

Tricyclic antidepressive agents such as amitriptyline (Elavil, Apo-Amitriptyline) or nortriptyline (Pamelor) may promote sleep and reduce pain or muscle spasm. These drugs should be used with caution in older adults because they can cause confusion and orthostatic hypotension. Trazodone (Desyrel) may be preferred for this population because of its minimal side effects. Tramadol (Ultram) is also effective for managing fibromyalgia. This drug has tricyclic effects and opioid properties to help relieve pain (see Chapter 4).

Physical therapy along with NSAIDs and possibly muscle relaxants may also be prescribed to help promote COMFORT.

Instruct the patient to exercise regularly. Home exercise should include stretching, strengthening, and low-impact aerobic exercise. Walking, swimming, rowing, biking, and water exercise are good examples of low-impact exercise. Integrative therapies such as tai chi, acupuncture, hypnosis, and stress management may help some patients with symptom relief. Refer patients to the land, water, and walking exercise pamphlets produced by the Arthritis Foundation (www.arthritis.org). Inform them about the National Fibromyalgia Association for additional information and patient and family support (www.fmaware.org).

GET READY FOR THE NCLEX® EXAMINATION!

KEY POINTS

Review these Key Points for each NCLEX Examination Client Needs Category.

Safe and Effective Care Environment

- Collaborate with the health care team to manage chronic pain and increase MOBILITY for patients with arthritis and other CTDs. **QSEN: Teamwork and Collaboration**
- Prioritize care for patients with systemic lupus erythematosus (SLE) and systemic sclerosis (SSc) by monitoring for life-threatening complications such as kidney failure.

Health Promotion and Maintenance

- Provide information about community resources for patients, especially professional organizations such as the Arthritis Foundation and Lupus Foundation.
- Teach patients to prevent joint trauma and reduce weight as needed to help prevent osteoarthritis. **QSEN: Evidence-Based Practice**
- Recall that a combination of environmental, genetic, and immune risk factors can cause arthritis and other connective tissue diseases.
- Reinforce the importance of good health practices such as adequate sleep, proper nutrition, regular exercise, and stress-management techniques for patients with arthritis and other CTDs.
- Teach patients with arthritis which exercises to do (Chart 18-5), joint protection techniques (Chart 18-6), and energy conservation guidelines (Chart 18-10). **QSEN: Evidence-Based Practice**
- Teach patients with SLE to avoid sunlight; exacerbations of the disease may be triggered.
- Remind patients with gout to avoid factors that trigger an attack such as aspirin, organ meats, and alcohol. **QSEN: Evidence-Based Practice**
- Teach people ways to prevent or detect early Lyme disease as listed in Chart 18-14.

Psychosocial Integrity

- Recognize that patients with rheumatoid arthritis (RA) may have body image disturbance as a result of potentially deforming joint involvement and nodules.
- Encourage patients with arthritis and connective tissue diseases to discuss their chronic illness and identify coping strategies that have previously been successful. **QSEN: Patient-Centered Care**
- Be aware that chronic, painful diseases affect the patient's quality of life and role performance.
- Recognize that patients with fibromyalgia syndrome (FMS) are often frustrated because they have not been diagnosed or have been misdiagnosed.

Physiological Integrity

- Be aware that most of the connective tissue diseases and arthritic disorders have a genetic basis as part of their etiology; most are also classified as autoimmune diseases and have remissions and exacerbations.

- Differentiate OA as primarily a joint problem that can affect one or more joints and RA as a systemic disease that presents as a bilateral symmetric joint inflammation.
- Realize that older patients have OA more than younger patients; younger patients have RA more than older adults. Other differences between the two diseases are summarized in Table 18-1.
- Teach patients who have osteoarthritis (OA) or are prone to the disease to lose weight (if obese), avoid trauma, and limit strenuous weight-bearing activities. **QSEN: Evidence-Based Practice**
- Instruct patients with arthritic pain to use multiple modalities for pain relief, including ice/heat, rest, positioning, integrative therapies, and drug therapy as prescribed.
- Teach patients to monitor and report side and adverse effects of drugs used to treat OA and other connective tissue diseases. **QSEN: Safety**
- Assess patients with rheumatoid arthritis for early or late signs and symptoms as listed in Chart 18-7.
- Teach patients who are taking hydroxychloroquine to have frequent (every 6 months) eye examinations to monitor for retinal changes. **QSEN: Safety**
- Remind patients to avoid crowds and other possible sources of infection when they are taking drugs that decrease IMMUNITY. **QSEN: Safety**
- Implement interventions for patients having total joint arthroplasty (TJA) to prevent venous thromboembolitic complications (e.g., anticoagulants, exercises, sequential compression devices); observe the patient for bleeding when he or she is taking anticoagulants. **Clinical Judgment**
- Be careful when positioning a patient after a total hip arthroplasty (THA) to prevent dislocation; do not hyperflex the hips or adduct the legs (see Chart 18-3). **QSEN: Safety**
- Be aware that disease-modifying antirheumatic drugs (DMARDs) and biological response modifiers (BRMs) slow the progression of connective tissue diseases, especially RA and SLE.
- Teach patients receiving BRMs and other disease-modifying agents to avoid crowds and people with infections; opportunistic pathogens may cause serious infections or death. Check the patient's PPD test or history of tuberculosis before starting any of these drugs (see Chart 18-9). **QSEN: Safety**
- Monitor and interpret laboratory test results for patients with autoimmune connective tissue diseases as highlighted in Chart 18-8.
- Differentiate signs and symptoms of patients with systemic lupus erythematosus (SLE) versus systemic sclerosis (SSc) as listed in Chart 18-11.
- Prioritize care by assessing for swallowing ability in patients who have SSc; collaborate with the dietitian for food modifications if needed. **QSEN: Teamwork and Collaboration**
- Monitor for acute joint pain and inflammation in patients with a history of gout; the great toe and other small joints are most typically affected.
- Be aware that arthritis often accompanies other diseases such as psoriasis and Crohn's disease.

SELECTED BIBLIOGRAPHY

Asterisk indicates a classic or definitive work on this subject.

Arthritis Foundation. (2016a). *Osteoarthritis.* www.arthritis.org/about-arthritis/types/osteoarthritis/what-is-osteoarthritis.php.

Arthritis Foundation. (2016b). *Rheumatoid arthritis.* www.arthritis.org/about-arthritis/types/rheumatoid-arthritis.php.

Catanzaro, J., & Dinkel, S. (2014). Sjögren's syndrome: The hidden disease. *Medsurg Nursing, 23*(4), 219–223.

Crawford, A., & Harris, H. (2015). Understanding the effects of rheumatoid arthritis. *Nursing, 45*(11), 32–38.

Firestein, G. S., Budd, R. C., Gabriel, S. E., McInnes, I. B., & O'Dell, J. R. (2013). *Kelley's textbook of rheumatology* (9th ed.). Philadelphia: Saunders.

*Fouladbakhsh, J. (2012). Complementary and alternative modalities to relieve osteoarthritis symptoms. *Orthopaedic Nursing, 31*(2), 115–121.

Harris, H., & Crawford, A. (2015). Recognizing and managing osteoarthritis. *Nursing, 45*(1), 36–43.

Jarvis, C. (2016). *Physical examination & health assessment* (7th ed.). St. Louis: Elsevier.

Lachner, K. D. (2016). Caring for the patient with limited systemic sclerosis. *Orthopaedic Nursing, 35*(1), 5–12.

Lilley, L. L., Collins, S. R., & Snyder, J. S. (2014). *Pharmacology and the nursing process* (7th ed.). St. Louis: Mosby.

Lupus Foundation of America. (2016). *What is lupus?* http://www.lupus.org/answers/entry/what-is-lupus.

Marchese, N. M., & Primer, S. R. (2013). Targeting Lyme disease. *Nursing, 43*(5), 28–33.

McAlindon, T. E., Bannuru, R. R., Sullivan, M. C., Arden, N. K., Berenbaum, F., Bierma-Zeinstra, S. M., et al. (2014). OARSI guidelines for the non-surgical management of knee osteoarthritis. *Osteoarthritis and Cartilage, 22*, 363–388.

McCance, K., Huether, S., Brashers, V., & Rote, N. (2014). *Pathophysiology: The biologic basis for disease in adults and children* (7th ed.). St. Louis: Mosby.

McCann-Spry, L., Pelton, J., Grandy, G., & Newell, D. (2016). An interdisciplinary approach to reducing length of stay in joint replacement patients. *Orthopaedic Nursing, 35*(5), 279–300.

McFadden, B. (2013). Is there a safe coital position after a total hip arthroplasty? *Orthopaedic Nursing, 32*(4), 223–228.

Menzies, V. (2016). Fibromyalgia syndrome: Current considerations in symptom management. *The American Journal of Nursing, 116*(1), 24–32.

Pagana, K. D., Pagana, T. J., & Pagana, T. N. (2017). *Mosby's diagnostic and laboratory test reference* (13th ed.). St. Louis: Mosby.

*Pettinato, M. (2012). Providing care for GLBTQ patients. *Nursing, 42*(12), 22–28.

Regan, E. R., Phillips, F., & Magri, T. (2013). Get a leg (or two) up on total knee arthroplasty. *Nursing, 43*(7), 32–37.

Schinsky, M. F., McCune, C., & Bonomi, J. (2016). Multifaceted comparison of two cryotherapy devices used after total knee arthroplasty: Cryotherapy device comparison. *Orthopaedic Nursing, 35*(5), 317–324.

Scleroderma Foundation. (2016). *What is scleroderma?* www.scleroderma.org/site/PageServer?pagename=patients_whatis#.Ur0aYbSJI5M.

*Zhang, W. W., Nuki, G., Moskowitz, R., Abramson, S., Altman, R. D., Arden, N. K., et al. (2010). OARSI recommendations for the management of hip and knee osteoarthritis, Part III: Changes in evidence following systematic cumulative update of research published through January 2009. *Osteoarthritis and Cartilage, 18*(4), 476–499.

CHAPTER 19

Care of Patients With Problems of HIV Disease

James G. Sampson and M. Linda Workman

ℯ http://evolve.elsevier.com/Iggy/

PRIORITY AND INTERRELATED CONCEPTS

The priority concept for this chapter is IMMUNITY.

✳ The IMMUNITY concept exemplar for this chapter is HIV Infection and AIDS, below.

The interrelated concepts for this chapter are:
- GAS EXCHANGE
- TISSUE INTEGRITY
- NUTRITION

LEARNING OUTCOMES

Safe and Effective Care Environment

1. Collaborate with the interprofessional team to coordinate high-quality care to patients with impaired IMMUNITY.
2. Prevent human immune deficiency virus (HIV) transmission to yourself and others.
3. Teach the patient and caregiver(s) how impaired IMMUNITY affects home safety.

Health Promotion and Maintenance

4. Identify community resources for patients with impaired IMMUNITY.
5. Assess all adults for high-risk behaviors related to HIV infection.

Psychosocial Integrity

6. Implement evidence-based nursing interventions to help the patient and family cope with the psychosocial impact caused by impaired IMMUNITY.

Physiological Integrity

7. Use signs, symptoms, and laboratory data to assess for impaired IMMUNITY and its complications.
8. Teach the patient and caregiver(s) about common drugs used for impaired IMMUNITY, HIV prevention, or HIV disease and its complications.

As described in Chapter 2 and explained in Chapter 17, IMMUNITY is protection from illness or disease that is maintained by the body's physiologic defense mechanisms. Provided by the cells, products, and actions of the immune system, immunity prevents the growth of infectious organisms and disease development, despite exposure to invading organisms. Immunity also detects body cells that undergo changes to become cancer cells. Impaired immunity can result in life-threatening infection and an increased risk for cancer development.

✳ IMMUNITY CONCEPT EXEMPLAR
HIV Infection and AIDS

❖ *PATHOPHYSIOLOGY*

Human immune deficiency virus (HIV) infection and disease can progress to acquired immune deficiency syndrome (AIDS). This common chronic disorder of impaired immunity is a serious worldwide epidemic (World Health Organization [WHO], 2015).

Etiology and Genetic Risk

The cause of HIV infection is a virus—the human immune deficiency virus. This virus, just like all other viruses, is an intracellular parasite because it must use the infected cell's resources to reproduce. The HIV can infect a cell and take over its functions to force the cell to make more copies of the virus (viral particles). These new viral particles are able to infect more cells, repeating the cycle as long as there are new host cells to infect.

The HIV Infectious Process. *Viral particle features* include an outer envelope with special "docking proteins," known as gp41 and gp120, which assist in finding a host (Fig. 19-1). Inside, the virus has genetic material along with the enzymes *reverse transcriptase (RT)* and *integrase*. To infect, HIV must first enter the

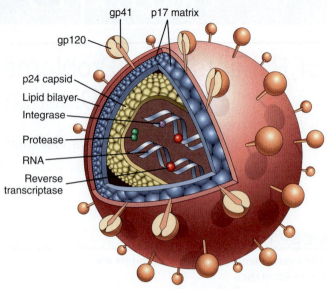

FIG. 19-1 The human immune deficiency virus (HIV). (From Kumar, V., Abbas, A., & Fausto, N. [2010]. *Robbins & Cotran pathologic basis of disease* (8th ed.). Philadelphia: Saunders.)

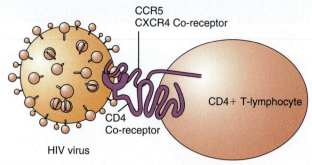

FIG. 19-2 The HIV "docking" proteins and the successful interaction of these proteins with the CD4+ T-lymphocyte receptors.

host's bloodstream and then "hijack" certain cells, especially the *CD4+ T-cell*, also known as the *CD4+ cell*, *helper/inducer T-cell*, or *T4-cell* (see Chapter 17). This cell directs IMMUNITY and regulates the activity of all immune system cells. When HIV enters a CD4+ T-cell, it can then create more virus particles (McCance et al., 2014).

Virus-host interactions are needed after infection for disease development. When an adult is infected with HIV, the virus randomly "bumps" into many cells. The docking proteins on the outside of the virus must find special receptors on a host cell to which the virus can bind and then enter the cell. The CD4+ T-cell has surface receptors known as *CD4, CCR5*, and *CXCR4* (Fig. 19-2). The gp120 and gp41 proteins on the HIV particle surface recognize these receptors on the CD4+ T-cell. For the virus to enter this cell, *both* the gp120 and the gp41 must bind to the receptors. The gp120 first binds to the primary CD4 receptor, which changes its shape and allows the gp120 to bind to either the CCR5 co-receptor or the CXCR4 co-receptor. Once co-receptor binding occurs, gp41 inserts a fusion peptide into the T-cell membrane, boring a hole to allow insertion of viral genetic material and enzymes into the host cell. This attachment allows the virus to then enter the CD4+ T-cell (McCance et al., 2014) (see Fig. 19-2). *Viral binding to the CD4 receptor and to either of the co-receptors is needed to enter the cell.* (The drug class known as *entry inhibitors* works here to prevent the interaction needed for entry of HIV into the CD4+ T-cell.)

After entering a host cell, HIV must insert its genetic material into the host cell's DNA. HIV is a **retrovirus**, which is able to insert its single-stranded ribonucleic acid (ss-RNA) genetic material into the host's DNA. The HIV enzyme *reverse transcriptase (RT)* converts HIV's RNA into DNA, which makes the viral genetic material the same as human DNA. (The drug classes known as *nucleoside reverse transcriptase inhibitors [NRTIs]* and *non-nucleoside reverse transcriptase inhibitors [NNRTIs]* work here to prevent viral replication [Fig. 19-3] by reducing how well reverse transcriptase can convert HIV genetic material into human genetic material.) HIV then uses its enzyme *integrase* to get its DNA into the nucleus of the host's

CD4+ T-cell and insert it into the host's DNA (McCance et al., 2014). This action completes the infection of the CD4+ T-cell. (The drug class known as *integrase inhibitors* works here to prevent viral DNA from integrating into the host's DNA.)

HIV particles are made within the infected CD4+ T-cell, using the metabolic machinery of the host cells. The new virus particle is made in the form of one long protein strand. The strand is clipped by the enzyme *HIV protease* into smaller functional pieces. These pieces are formed into a new finished viral particle. (The drug class known as *protease inhibitors* works here to inhibit HIV protease.) Once the new virus particle is finished, it fuses with the infected cell's membrane and then buds off in search of another CD4+ T-cell to infect (see Fig. 19-3).

> ### ❓ NCLEX EXAMINATION CHALLENGE 19-1
> #### *Physiological Integrity*
>
> Which part of the HIV infection process is disrupted by the antiretroviral drug class of entry inhibitors?
> A. Activating the viral enzyme "integrase" within the infected host's cells
> B. Binding the virus to the CD4+ receptor and either of the two co-receptors
> C. Clipping the newly generated viral proteins into smaller functional pieces
> D. Fusing the newly created viral particle with the infected cell's membrane

Effects of HIV infection are related to the new genetic instructions that now direct CD4+ T-cells to change their role in immune system defenses. The new role is to be an "HIV factory," making up to 10 billion new viral particles daily. The immune system is made weaker by removing some CD4+ T-cells from circulation. In early HIV infection before HIV disease is evident, the immune system can still attack and destroy most of the newly created virus particles. However, with time the number of HIV particles overwhelms the immune system. Gradually CD4+ T-cell counts fall, viral numbers *(viral load)* rise, and without treatment, the patient eventually dies of opportunistic infection or cancer (McCance et al., 2014).

Everyone who has AIDS has HIV infection; however, not everyone who has HIV infection has AIDS (Centers for Disease Control and Prevention [CDC], 2015b). The distinction is the number of CD4+ T-cells and whether any opportunistic infections have occurred. A healthy adult usually has at least 800 to 1000 CD4+ T-cells per cubic millimeter (mm^3) of blood. This number is reduced in HIV disease.

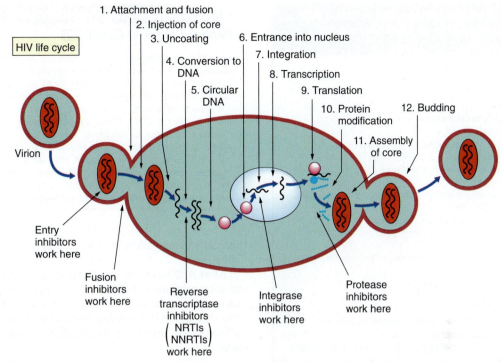

FIG. 19-3 The life cycle of the HIV and sites of action for anti-HIV therapy. (From McCance, K. L., & Huether, S.E. [2002]. *Pathophysiology: The biologic basis for disease in adults and children* [4th ed.]. St. Louis: Mosby.)

Some adults develop an acute infection within 4 weeks of first being infected. Symptoms of this acute HIV infection can be fever, night sweats, chills, headache, and muscle aches, which are similar to those of any viral infection—not just HIV. A sore throat and rash also may be present. With time these symptoms cease, and the patient feels well again, although a "war is going on" between HIV and the immune system. Even in this early phase of the disease, the viral numbers in the bloodstream and genital tract are high, and sexual transmission is possible (Grimes et al., 2016).

As time passes, more CD4+ T-cells are infected and taken out of immune system service. The count decreases, and those that remain function poorly. Poor CD4+ T-cell function leads to these IMMUNITY abnormalities:

- Lymphocytopenia (decreased numbers of lymphocytes)
- Increased production of incomplete and nonfunctional antibodies
- Abnormally functioning macrophages

As the CD4+ T-cell level drops, the patient is at risk for bacterial, fungal, and viral infections, as well as opportunistic cancers. Opportunistic infections are those caused by organisms that are present as part of the body's microbiome and usually are kept in check by normal IMMUNITY (see Chapter 5 for an explanation of the microbiome). The profound reduced immunity in the adult with AIDS allows these usually harmless organisms to overgrow and cause infection.

A diagnosis of AIDS requires that the adult be HIV positive and have either a CD4+ T-cell count of less than 200 cells/mm³ (0.2 × 10⁹/L) or less than 14% (even if the total CD4+ count is above 200 cells/mm³[0.2 × 10⁹/L]) or an opportunistic infection. Once AIDS is diagnosed, even if the patient's T-cell count goes higher than 200 cells/mm³ (0.2 × 10⁹/L), or if the percentage rises above 14%, or the infection is successfully treated, the AIDS diagnosis remains.

HIV Classification. The Centers for Disease Control and Prevention (CDC) defines five stages of HIV disease (CDC, 2015b). In this definition laboratory confirmation of HIV infection (by fourth-generation antigen/antibody testing or enzyme-linked immunosorbent assay [ELISA] and Western blot analysis) plus CD4+ T-lymphocyte count or percentage and the presence or absence of the 27 AIDS-defining conditions (Table 19-1) determine the classification (CDC, 2015b). *The adult with HIV infection can transmit the virus to others at all stages of disease, but the recently infected adult with a high viral load and those at end-stage without drug therapy can be particularly infectious.*

Stage 0 CDC Case Definition describes a patient who develops a first positive HIV test result within 6 months after a negative HIV test result. Changing the patient's status to stage 1, 2, or 3 does not occur until 6 months have elapsed since the stage 0 designation, even when CD4+ T-cell counts decrease or an AIDS-defining condition is present.

Stage 1 CDC Case Definition describes a patient with a CD4+ T-cell count of greater than 500 cells/mm³ (0.5 × 10⁹/L) or a percentage of 29% or greater. An adult at this stage has no AIDS-defining illnesses.

Stage 2 CDC Case Definition describes a patient with a CD4+ T-cell count between 200 and 499 cells/mm³ (0.2 to 0.449 × 10⁹/L) a percentage between 14% and 28%. An adult at this stage has no AIDS-defining illnesses.

Stage 3 CDC Case Definition describes any patient with a CD4+ T-cell count of less than 200 cells/mm³ (0.2 × 10⁹/L) or a percentage of less than 14%. An adult who has higher CD4+ T-cell counts or percentages but who also has an AIDS-defining illness meets the Stage 3 CDC Case Definition.

Stage Unknown CDC Case Definition is used to describe any patient with a confirmed HIV infection but no

TABLE 19-1 Centers for Disease Control and Prevention Classification of AIDS-Defining Conditions in Adults

- Bacterial infections, multiple or recurrent
- Candidiasis of bronchi, trachea, or lungs
- Candidiasis of esophagus
- Cervical cancer, invasive
- Coccidioidomycosis, disseminated or extrapulmonary
- Cryptococcosis, extrapulmonary
- Cryptosporidiosis, chronic intestinal (>1-month duration)
- Cytomegalovirus disease (other than liver, spleen, or nodes)
- Cytomegalovirus retinitis (with loss of vision)
- Encephalopathy, HIV-related
- Herpes simplex: chronic ulcers (>1-month duration) or bronchitis, pneumonitis, or esophagitis
- Histoplasmosis, disseminated or extrapulmonary
- Isosporiasis, chronic intestinal (>1-month duration)
- Kaposi's sarcoma
- Lymphoid interstitial pneumonia or pulmonary lymphoid hyperplasia complex
- Lymphoma, Burkitt's (or equivalent term)
- Lymphoma, immunoblastic (or equivalent term)
- Lymphoma, primary, of brain
- *Mycobacterium avium* complex or *Mycobacterium kansasii,* disseminated or extrapulmonary
- *Mycobacterium tuberculosis* of any site, pulmonary, disseminated, or extrapulmonary
- *Mycobacterium,* other species or unidentified species, disseminated or extrapulmonary
- *Pneumocystis jiroveci* pneumonia
- Pneumonia, recurrent (two instances within 12 months)
- Progressive multifocal leukoencephalopathy
- *Salmonella* septicemia, recurrent
- Toxoplasmosis of brain
- Wasting syndrome attributed to HIV

From Schneider, E., Whitmore, S., Glynn, K. M., Dominguez, K., Mitsch, A., McKenna, M.T.: Centers for Disease Control and Prevention. (2008). Revised surveillance case definitions for HIV infection among adults, adolescents, and children aged <18 months and for HIV infection and AIDS among children aged 18 months to <13 years—United States, 2008. *Morbidity and Mortality Weekly Report: Recommendations and Reports, 57*(RR-10), 9; www.cdc.gov/mmwr/preview/mmwrhtml/rr5710a2.htm.

information regarding CD4+ T-cell counts, CD4+ T-cell percentages, and AIDS-defining illnesses is available.

HIV Progression. The time from the beginning of HIV infection to development of AIDS ranges from months to years. The range depends on how HIV was acquired, which additional health problems the patient has, personal factors, and interventions. For example, for adults who have been transfused with HIV-contaminated blood, AIDS often develops quickly. For those who become HIV positive as a result of a single sexual encounter, progression to AIDS takes much longer. Other personal factors that influence progression to AIDS include frequency of re-exposure to HIV, presence of other sexually transmitted infections (STIs), NUTRITION status, and stress.

Incidence and Prevalence

Since the beginning of the epidemic in the United States, more than 658,507 people have died of AIDS. Currently about 50,000 people are diagnosed annually, and more than 1,200,000 people in the United States are living with HIV/AIDS (CDC, 2015a). Worldwide about 2 million people per year are newly infected with HIV, at least 34 million deaths from AIDS have occurred since the start of the epidemic, and 37 million people are

GENETIC/GENOMIC CONSIDERATIONS
Patient-Centered Care QSEN

About 1% of adults with HIV infection are *long-term nonprogressors (LTNPs)* who have been infected with HIV for at least 10 years and have remained asymptomatic, with CD4+ T-cell counts within the normal range and a viral load that is either undetectable or very low.

A genetic difference for this group is that their CCR5/CXCR4 co-receptors on the CD4+ T-cells are nonfunctional as a result of gene mutations for these co-receptors. The mutation creates defective co-receptors that do not bind to the HIV docking proteins, and these cells successfully resist the entrance of HIV. Adults who have only one mutated co-receptor gene allele have fewer normal co-receptors and can be infected with HIV, but progression is slow. Remind patients that even with low viral levels, they can still transmit the disease to others.

currently living with HIV (World Health Organization [WHO], 2015).

Most AIDS cases in North America occur among men who have sex with men (MSM) or adults of either gender who have used injection drugs (16%) (CDC, 2015a). *However, the perception that HIV/AIDS is only a problem for homosexual white men is false. The highest rates of new infections occur among adults of color.*

CULTURAL/SPIRITUAL CONSIDERATIONS
Patient-Centered Care QSEN

Most new HIV infections reported in the United States and Canada occur in racial and ethnic minorities, particularly among blacks/African Americans and Hispanics (CDC, 2015b). More culturally sensitive efforts targeted at these groups for prevention and treatment are needed.

GENDER HEALTH CONSIDERATIONS
Patient-Centered Care QSEN

About 25% of newly diagnosed cases are women. In less affluent countries 50% of cases occur in women (WHO, 2015). The largest risk factor is sexual exposure. Women with HIV disease have a poorer outcome, with shorter mean survival time than that of men. This outcome may be the result of late diagnosis and social or economic factors that reduce access to medical care. Encourage all women to monitor their HIV status.

Gynecologic problems, especially persistent or recurrent vaginal candidiasis, may be the first signs of HIV disease in women. Other problems include pelvic inflammatory disease, genital herpes, other sexually transmitted infections (STIs), and cervical dysplasia or cancer.

The effect of HIV on pregnancy outcomes includes higher incidence of premature delivery, low-birth-weight infants, and transmission of the disease to the infant. Appropriate antiretroviral drug therapy during pregnancy reduces the risk for transmitting the infection to the infant. (See the discussion in the Perinatal Transmission section.)

Health Promotion and Maintenance

AIDS has a high morbidity and mortality rate when untreated. Although there is no current cure for HIV/AIDS, the conscientious and continued use of antiretroviral therapy allows HIV patients to live long and healthy lives. The foci for health care

CONSIDERATIONS FOR OLDER ADULTS
Patient-Centered Care QSEN

> Infection with HIV can occur at any age. Assess the older patient for risk behaviors, including a sexual and drug use history. Age-related decline in IMMUNITY increases the likelihood that the older adult will develop the infection after an HIV exposure.

worldwide are prevention of HIV infection and antiretroviral treatment for all who are HIV positive (WHO, 2015).

HIV is in the blood, semen, vaginal secretions, breast milk, amniotic fluid, urine, feces, saliva, tears, cerebrospinal fluid, lymph nodes, cervical cells, corneal tissue, and brain tissue of infected patients. The fluids with the highest concentrations of HIV are semen, blood, breast milk, and vaginal secretions. Contact with tears, saliva, and sweat is considered low risk for transmission unless obvious blood is present. HIV is transmitted most often in these three ways:

- Sexual: genital, anal, or oral sexual contact with exposure of mucous membranes to infected semen or vaginal secretions
- Parenteral: sharing of needles or equipment contaminated with infected blood or receiving contaminated blood products
- Perinatal: from the placenta, from contact with maternal blood and body fluids during birth, or from breast milk from an infected mother to child

Teach all adults about the transmission routes and ways to reduce their exposure (discussed next). Also stress that HIV is not transmitted by casual contact in the home, school, or workplace. Sharing household utensils, towels and linens, and toilet facilities does not transmit HIV. HIV is not spread by mosquitos or other insects.

! NURSING SAFETY PRIORITY QSEN
Action Alert

> Teach all adults, regardless of age, gender, ethnicity, or sexual orientation, that they are susceptible to HIV infection.

HIV Status

About 1.2 million people are currently living with HIV infection in the United States, and about 75,000 are living with HIV infection in Canada (CDC, 2015a; Government of Canada, 2015). In both countries about 20% of those infected are unaware of their HIV infection. Many new transmission events come from those who are HIV positive and unaware of their diagnosis. Early identification and diagnosis allows for early treatment and preventive care. Once an adult is placed on combination antiretroviral therapy (cART), reducing the viral load to undetectable levels significantly reduces the risk that HIV will be transmitted, a concept known as *treatment as prevention (TAP)*.

The recommendations for HIV screening have been expanded to include a one-time screen for all adults between the ages of 15 and 65, an annual screening of those who are at heightened risk for HIV infection, routine prenatal screening, and frequent testing in adults with repeated high-risk exposures.

HIV testing requires interpretation, counseling, and confidentiality. Testing plays a role in prevention because tests are a

CHART 19-1 Patient and Family Education: Preparing for Self-Management

CDC Recommendations for Annual HIV Testing and One-Time Screening

You should be tested annually for HIV if you:
- Have a sexually transmitted infection
- Use injection drugs
- Consider yourself at risk
- Are a woman of childbearing age with identifiable risks, including:
  - Used injection drugs
  - Engaged in sex work
  - Had sexual partners who were infected or at risk
  - Had sexual contact with men from countries with high HIV prevalence
- Received a transfusion between 1978 and 1985
- Plan to get married
- Are undergoing medical evaluation or treatment for symptoms that may be HIV related
- Are in correctional institutions such as jails and prisons
- Are a sex worker or have had sex with a sex worker

In the absence of any of the above conditions, you should be tested (screened) once:
- If you are between the ages of 18 and 65 years
- As part of routine prenatal screening when you are pregnant

Modified from *CDC*, Centers for Disease Control and Prevention, 2015a.

♥ VETERANS' HEALTH CONSIDERATIONS
Patient-Centered Care QSEN

> The Veteran's Health Administration (VHA) is a major health care provider in the United States and has found that a significant number of veterans have undiagnosed HIV disease. As a result, in 2009 the VHA eliminated the need for written consent for including HIV screening as part of routine testing. Despite the directive, only about 9% of veterans treated annually at VHA facilities have ever been tested (Gant-Clark et al., 2015). When asked, most veterans believed that they were HIV negative because they thought the test had already been done as part of routine testing and that the VHA would have notified them of positive results. This false sense of security has major implications because of the high prevalence of risky behaviors such as substance abuse and unsafe sexual practices among the VHA patient population. When interacting with veterans and discussing the issue of being aware of their HIV status as part of disease prevention, be sure to inform them that HIV screening is available to them through the VHA.

way of diagnosing HIV infection before immune changes or disease symptoms develop. A major health care focus for testing is to teach those who test positive to modify their behaviors to prevent transmission to others. *Therefore all sexually active adults should know their HIV status.* Chart 19-1 lists conditions for which HIV testing is advised.

Pretest and post-test counseling must be performed by personnel trained in HIV issues. These counselors may be nurses, physicians, social workers, health educators, or lay educators who have specialized training. Counseling helps the patient make an informed decision about testing and provides an opportunity to teach risk-reduction behaviors. Post-test counseling is needed to interpret the results, discuss risk reduction, provide psychological support, and provide health promotion information for the patient with a positive test result. The newly diagnosed adult should be linked to care within an infectious disease practice or clinics. Adults who test positive should also be counseled on how to inform sexual partners and those with whom they have shared needles. Testing methods are listed in the Laboratory Assessment section.

Sexual Transmission

Safer sex methods of *A,* abstinence; *B,* be faithful (monogamous); and *C,* condom use can reduce HIV transmission. Abstinence and mutually monogamous sex with a noninfected partner are the *only* absolutely safe methods of preventing HIV infection from sexual contact. Many forms of sexual expression can spread HIV infection if one partner is infected. *The risk for becoming infected from a partner who is HIV positive is always present, although some sexual practices are more risky than others.* Because the virus concentrates in blood and seminal fluid and is also present in vaginal secretions, risk differs by gender, sexual act, and the viral load of the infected partner.

Gender affects HIV transmission, and the infection is more easily transmitted from infected male to uninfected female than vice versa. This is because HIV is most easily transmitted when infected body fluids come into contact with mucous membranes or nonintact skin. The vagina has more mucous membrane (surface area) than does the urethra of the penis. Teach women the importance of always either using a vaginal or dental dam or female condom or having their male partners use a condom.

Sexual acts or practices that permit infected seminal fluid to come into contact with mucous membranes or nonintact skin are the most risky for sexual transmission of HIV. The practice with the highest risk is anal intercourse with the penis and seminal fluid of an infected adult coming into contact with the mucous membranes of the uninfected partner's rectum. *Anal intercourse in which the semen depositor (inserting or active partner [top]) is infected is a very risky sexual practice, regardless of whether the semen receiver (receiving partner [bottom]) is male or female.* Anal intercourse allows seminal fluid to make contact with the rectal mucous membranes and also tears the mucous membranes, making infection more likely. Teach patients who engage in anal intercourse that the semen depositor needs to wear a condom during this act.

🌐 CULTURAL AND SPIRITUAL CONSIDERATIONS

Patient-Centered Care QSEN

In certain cultures anal receptive intercourse for male to female intercourse is a form of contraceptive practice. Because this act increases the risk for HIV transmission, instruct such couples to use condoms, regardless of whether intercourse is vaginal or anal.

Viral load, or the amount of virus present in blood and other body fluids, affects transmission. The higher the blood level of HIV (viremia), the greater the risk for sexual and perinatal transmission. Current combination antiretroviral therapy (cART) (formerly known as HAART-highly active antiretroviral therapy) has caused the viral load of some infected patients to drop below detectable levels. *Although there is less virus in seminal or vaginal fluids of patients receiving cART, the risk for transmission still exists.*

Safer sex practices are those that reduce the risk for nonintact skin or mucous membranes coming in contact with infected body fluids and blood. Teach all adults the importance of consistently using these safer sex practices:

- A latex or polyurethane condom for genital and anal intercourse
- An appropriate water-based lubricant with a latex condom
- A condom or latex barrier (dental dam) over the genitals or anus during oral-genital or oral-anal sexual contact
- Latex gloves for finger or hand contact with the vagina or rectum

Pre-Exposure Prophylaxis. Pre-exposure prophylaxis (PrEP) to HIV is the use of HIV-specific anti-retroviral drugs in an HIV-uninfected adult for the purpose of preventing HIV infection. The approved drug combination for PrEP is Truvada (tenofovir 300 mg/emtricitabine 300 mg), one oral tablet daily (Volk et al., 2015).

PrEP is for a select population that is at high risk for acquiring HIV infection. This includes men who have sex with men, heterosexually active men and women, injecting drug users, and those in serodiscordant relationships (one partner HIV positive, one partner HIV negative). Risk assessment is determined by asking focused questions about sexual and drug-injecting activities. After an adult has been identified as at risk (has screened positive for increased risk of acquiring HIV infection), specific blood and urine testing is done to make sure that it is safe to use PrEP. First ensure that the adult is HIV negative (often using a fourth-generation HIV antigen/antibody test and an HIV viral load test). Other necessary tests include renal function tests; estimated glomerular filtration rate (GFR); tests for other sexually transmitted infections such as syphilis, gonorrhea, and chlamydia; and hepatitis A, B, and C serologies. If the adult is found to have active hepatitis B, do not initiate PrEP but refer to an infectious disease specialist, because both tenofovir and emtricitabine have activity against hepatitis B and should be used appropriately.

After starting Truvada, ongoing testing of renal function and HIV infection is performed at specified intervals, usually every 3 months. The person using Truvada for PrEP is not protected until 4 days of consistent dosing leading to a steady-state blood drug level is achieved. Once the initial protection period is completed, one dose can be missed, and protection is still adequate; however, two consecutively missed doses significantly reduce protection. The patient needs to start over (before being exposed to HIV) with another 4 day-lead in period until a new steady state can be achieved. When Truvada is used consistently and correctly, it is very effective in HIV infection prevention (Mayer & Krakower, 2015). However, it has no effect in preventing the contraction of any other sexually transmitted infection (STI).

New studies are testing the efficacy of Truvada using various alternative dosing models; however, at present Truvada is the only drug approved for PrEP, and the once-daily dosing is the only approved dosing regimen. Two new injectable formulations of PrEP (rilpivirine and cabotegravir) administered once every 12 weeks are being explored for effectiveness as an alternative to daily Truvada.

Postexposure Prophylaxis. Using cART as postexposure prophylaxis (PEP) generally falls into one of three exposure categories for adults: those who have had an occupational exposure (such as a needlestick injury); those who have had a nonoccupational exposure (such as a consensual sexual exposure with an adult of unknown HIV status); and those who have suffered a sexual assault. In all cases, starting cART as soon as possible (preferably within the first 24 to 36 hours) is critical to preventing HIV infection. The current recommendations are

! NURSING SAFETY PRIORITY QSEN

Drug Alert

Pre-exposure prophylaxis does not replace the standard safer sex practices recommended to prevent HIV transmission. If this drug therapy is used in patients who become infected with HIV-1, the risk for developing drug resistance greatly increases. Therefore remind adults prescribed Truvada to use the safer sex practices described previously and to adhere to an every-3-month HIV testing schedule along with monitoring for side effects of this drug.

that significant exposures should be treated with the same three-drug regimen for 28 days or until the HIV status of the source has been determined to be negative (Fig. 19-4A).

Occupational exposure is defined as contact between blood, tissue, or selected body fluids (e.g., blood, cerebrospinal fluid [CSF], pleural fluid, synovial fluid, peritoneal fluid, pericardial fluid, breast milk, amniotic fluid, semen, and vaginal secretions) from a patient who is positive for HIV (*source patient*) and the blood, broken skin, or mucous membranes of a health care professional. Bodily substances not considered infectious for HIV unless obviously bloody (e.g., feces, nasal secretions, sputum, saliva, sweat, tears, urine, vomit) do not require prophylaxis.

In the case of an occupational exposure, a percutaneous needlestick with a hollow-bore or solid needle is the most common occurrence necessitating PEP. The other common exposure is fluid contact with mucous membranes (e.g., eyes, nose, mouth). For sharps injuries, initial steps include "bleeding" the wound, washing the wound carefully for at least 1 full minute, and immediately contacting employee health (or the emergency department during hours when employee health is not open) to begin the documentation, testing, and prophylaxis process.

Once the exposure has been discovered, three-drug cART within 2 hours of the exposure has the best possible outcome in preventing HIV infection. *The window of opportunity for best outcome closes when prophylaxis is started after 72 hours. Thus the exposed health care professional is started on cART before all test results are known.* The professional receiving prophylaxis must return for periodic HIV testing at 1, 3, and 6 months and electrolytes, creatinine, and complete blood counts 2 weeks after starting cART.

Nonoccupational exposure generally refers to consensual and nonconsensual sexual exposures, involving insertive and receptive types of sex with oral, vaginal, or anal contact. Other types of contact can include the sharing of needles and inadvertent percutaneous or mucosal contact in the home.

Exposure to HIV as a result of sexual assault also includes testing for gonorrhea, chlamydia, and syphilis. For women of childbearing age, emergency contraception is offered.

Parenteral Transmission

Preventive practices to reduce transmission among injection drug users (IDUs) include the use of proper cleaning of "works" (needles, syringes, other drug paraphernalia). Instruct IDUs to clean a used needle and syringe by first filling and flushing them with clear water. Next the syringe should be filled with ordinary household bleach. The bleach-filled syringe should be shaken for 30 to 60 seconds. Advise IDUs to carry a small container with this solution whenever sharing needles or to participate in community needle-exchange programs, if they are available.

The risk for HIV transmission through transfusion of banked blood and blood products is very low. All donated blood in North America is screened for the HIV antibody, and blood that is positive for HIV antibodies is not used for transfusion purposes. Because of the time lag in antibody production after exposure to HIV, infected blood can test negative for HIV antibodies. Inform patients that there is a small but real possibility of HIV transmission through blood and blood products.

Perinatal Transmission

HIV transmission can occur across the placenta during pregnancy, with infant exposure to blood and vaginal secretions during birth, or with exposure after birth through breast milk. Inform women of childbearing age with HIV infection about the risks for perinatal transmission. The risk for transmission to infants from pregnant women with HIV infection who are not using HIV drug therapy is about 25%. It is about 8% for women who are using HIV drug therapy. Encourage HIV-positive women who are pregnant to continue the therapy or, if they are not on antiviral therapy, to start the therapy as soon as possible.

Transmission and Health Care Workers

Needlestick or "sharps" injuries are the main means of occupation-related HIV infection for health care workers (Mitchell & Parker, 2015b). In addition, health care workers can be infected through exposure of nonintact skin and mucous membranes to blood and body fluids (Mitchell & Parker, 2015a). **The best prevention for health care professionals is the consistent use of Standard Precautions for all patients as recommended by the CDC and required by The Joint Commission's (TJC) National Patient Safety Goals (NPSG)** (see Chapter 23). Fig. 19-14B shows the recommended actions for prevention of HIV infection after a needlestick or other occupational exposure (postexposure prophylaxis [PEP]). When the source patient is known to be HIV negative, PEP is not recommended.

To prevent HIV transmission to patients, health care workers should wear gloves when in contact with patients' mucous membranes or nonintact skin. Infected workers with weeping dermatitis or open lesions must wear gloves or not perform direct patient care. The CDC guidelines for preventing HIV transmission by health care workers during exposure-prone invasive procedures are listed in Chart 19-2. These include any procedure in which there is a risk for broken skin injury to the health care worker and the worker's blood is likely to make contact with the patient's body cavity, subcutaneous tissues, or mucous membranes.

❓ NCLEX EXAMINATION CHALLENGE 19-2

Safe and Effective Care Environment

With which activities does the nurse teach unlicensed assistive personnel (UAP) and nursing students caring for a client who is HIV positive to wear gloves to prevent disease transmission? **Select all that apply.**
A. Applying lotion during a back rub
B. Brushing the client's teeth
C. Emptying a Foley catheter reservoir
D. Feeding the client
E. Filing the client's fingernails
F. Providing perineal care

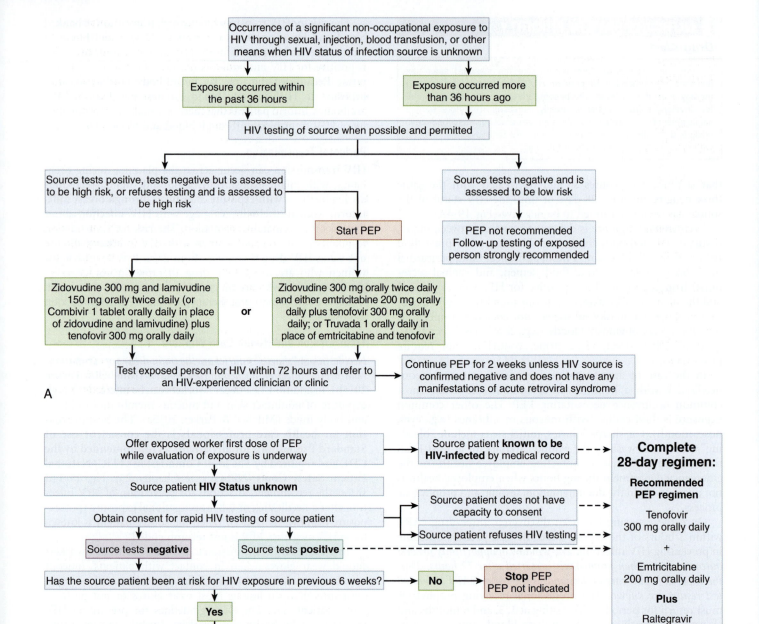

FIG. 19-4 New York State Health Department HIV guidelines. *PEP,* postexposure prophylaxis. **A,** Recommendations for nonoccupational postexposure prophylaxis for HIV infection. **B,** Recommendations for occupational postexposure prophylaxis for HIV infection. (**A** adapted from New York State Department of Health AIDS Institute. Clinical Guidelines Development Program. [2013]. *Recommendations for non-occupational postexposure prophylaxis for HIV infection.* New York: Author. www.hivguidelines.org. **B** adapted from New York State Department of Health AIDS Institute. Clinical Guidelines Development Program. [2012]. *Recommendations for occupational postexposure prophylaxis for HIV infection.* New York: Author. www.hivguidelines.org.)

❖ *INTERPROFESSIONAL COLLABORATIVE CARE*

With treatment HIV disease is chronic but manageable (Starr & Bradley-Springer, 2014). The usual disease course includes intermittent acute infections and periods of relative wellness. This period is often followed by chronic, progressive debilitation. Because of the cyclic nature of HIV disease and AIDS, the patient spends long periods at home between hospital admissions. During this time the patient must practice adequate self-care. New techniques and strategies to promote self-care, known as mHealth, include the use of mobile devices

CHART 19-2   Best Practice for Patient Safety & Quality Care QSEN

Recommendations for Preventing HIV Transmission by Health Care Workers

- Workers should adhere to Standard Precautions.
- Workers with exudative lesions or weeping dermatitis should not perform direct patient care or handle patient care equipment and devices used in invasive procedures.
- Workers must follow guidelines for disinfection and sterilization of reusable equipment used in invasive procedures.
- Workers infected with HIV are not restricted from practice of non–exposure-prone procedures, as long as they comply with Standard Precautions and sterilization and disinfection recommendations.
- Workers should identify exposure-prone procedures by institutions where they are performed.
- Workers who perform exposure-prone procedures should know their HIV antibody status.
- Workers who are infected with HIV should seek advice from an expert review panel before performing exposure-prone procedures to determine under which circumstances they may continue to practice these procedures. These circumstances would include notification of prospective patients of HIV positivity.

Adapted from Centers for Disease Control and Prevention. (1991). Recommendations for preventing transmission of human immunodeficiency virus and hepatitis B virus to patients during exposure-prone invasive procedures. *Morbidity and Mortality Weekly Report: Recommendations and Reports, 40*(RR-8), 1-9.

for reminders and information. This strategy appears to be helpful for some populations, but more information is needed to determine how to modify it for best use among minority populations (see the Evidence-Based Practice box).

In the acute care setting, the disease is best managed using an interprofessional team approach. Team members include physicians, nurses, registered dietitians, infectious disease specialists, social workers, mental health professionals, and wound care specialists among others.

◆ Assessment: Noticing

The adult who has HIV disease is monitored on a regular basis for changes in IMMUNITY or health status that indicate disease progression and the need for intervention. The frequency of monitoring varies from every 2 to 6 months based on disease progression and responses to treatment. Continuing assessment is crucial to ensure that the drugs continue to work optimally because the patient may have medication issues or problems related to disease in many organ systems. Assess for subtle changes so any problems can be found early and treated.

History. Ask about age, gender, occupation, and where the patient lives. Thoroughly assess the current illness, including when it started, the severity of symptoms, associated problems, and any interventions to date. Ask the patient about when the HIV infection was diagnosed and which symptoms led to

EVIDENCE-BASED PRACTICE QSEN

mHealth Technology as a Strategy for HIV Self-Management Among African-American Women

Adams-Tufts, K., Johnson, K., Shepherd, J., Lee, J., Bait-Ajzoon, M., Mahan, L., et al. (2015). Novel interventions for HIV self-management in African-American women: A systematic review of mHealth interventions. *Journal of the Association of Nurses in AIDS Care, 26*(2), 139-150.

HIV is now considered a chronic disease when antiretroviral drug therapy is used appropriately, which relies heavily on the very effective intervention of self-management. In addition to drug therapy, self-management includes adhering to scheduled medical visits, healthy diet, regular exercise, stress reduction, and self-monitoring of ongoing health status. However, even though about 45% of Americans newly diagnosed as HIV positive are African-American women, culturally appropriate strategies for promoting HIV self-management among this population are lacking. Without self-management skills, HIV-positive patients live shorter, less healthy lives and may contribute to greater HIV transmission.

mHealth, which is the use of mobile devices with software applications to provide access to health services, manage patient information, provide specific health knowledge, and assist skill development for health promotion and condition management, is now widely used to promote self-management of a variety of chronic conditions. The purpose of this study was to explore the use of mHealth technology for self-management of HIV disease and to determine the existence of culturally appropriate applications for HIV-positive African-American women.

This study was a systematic review of 411 completed analyses and 39 ongoing clinical trials reviewing the effectiveness of all types of mHealth and general self-management education programs for HIV. The majority of studies were conducted with men, and few used true mHealth technologies. Those that did include women who were focused more on HIV prevention rather than the skills needed to

successfully live with HIV. No completed studies were found that were specifically designed and culturally tailored for use among African-American women living with HIV/AIDS. The ongoing studies included several mHealth HIV intervention studies that were focused on women of all ethnicities but did not address the unique needs of African-American women.

Level of Evidence: 1

This study is an exhaustive meta-analysis of previous research studies on the use of electronic media, specifically mHealth, technologies to assist in self-management of HIV as a chronic disease. The methods used were appropriate for the purposes of the study, and the inclusion of results from ongoing randomized clinical trials added credible evidence to support study results.

Commentary: Implications for Practice and Research

mHealth provides a strategy that has been successfully used for self-management of many chronic diseases. The strategy is most successful when tailored to the specific needs of a population. Its use was previously limited to adults with the financial means to acquire and maintain mobile devices. This limitation has been ameliorated by specific programs providing cell phones and other mobile devices to adults with low incomes. Thus the remaining limitation is designing an mHealth application that addresses the specific needs (including cultural differences) related to African-American women living with HIV/AIDS. Although both qualitative and quantitative studies focused on this topic are needed, nurses caring for adults living with HIV/AIDS can make contributions by asking African-American women with HIV/AIDS specifically what could help them with medication management, keeping clinical appointments, and other aspects of living with this chronic disease.

that diagnosis. Ask him or her to give a chronologic history of infections and problems since the diagnosis. Assess the patient's health history, including whether he or she received a blood transfusion between 1978 and 1985 in the United States or Canada (before routine blood testing for HIV contamination). Ask the immigrant patient about his or her history of transfusion therapy before coming to North America.

Ask the patient about sex practices, sexually transmitted infections (STIs), and major infectious diseases, including tuberculosis and hepatitis. If the patient has hemophilia, ask about treatment with clotting factors. Determine whether the patient has engaged in past or present injection drug usage. Assess the patient's cognitive function and knowledge level of the diagnosis, symptom management, diagnostic tests, treatments, community resources, and modes of HIV transmission. Also assess his or her understanding and use of safer sex practices and provide the appropriate patient teaching.

Physical Assessment/Signs and Symptoms. HIV disease and AIDS progress on a continuum. The patient with HIV disease may either have few symptoms and problems or may have problems that are acute rather than chronic. However, as the disease progresses, more severe health problems occur. Assess for clusters of symptoms that may indicate disease progression (Chart 19-3).

 CHART 19-3 Key Features

AIDS

Immunologic Signs and Symptoms
- Low white blood cell counts:
  - CD4+/CD8+ ratio <2
  - CD4+ count <200/mm³ (0.2 × 10⁹/L)
- Hypergammaglobulinemia
- Opportunistic infections
- Lymphadenopathy
- Fatigue

Integumentary Signs and Symptoms
- Dry skin
- Poor wound healing
- Skin lesions
- Night sweats

Respiratory Signs and Symptoms
- Cough
- Shortness of breath

GI Signs and Symptoms
- Diarrhea
- Weight loss
- Nausea and vomiting

Central Nervous System Signs and Symptoms
- Confusion
- Dementia
- Headache
- Fever
- Visual changes
- Memory loss

- Personality changes
- Pain
- Seizures

Opportunistic Infections
- Protozoal infections:
  - Toxoplasmosis
  - Cryptosporidiosis
  - Isosporiasis
  - Microsporidiosis
  - Strongyloidiasis
  - Giardiasis
- Fungal infections:
  - Candidiasis
  - *Pneumocystis jiroveci* pneumonia
  - Cryptococcosis
  - Histoplasmosis
  - Coccidioidomycosis
- Bacterial infections:
  - *Mycobacterium avium* complex infection
  - Tuberculosis
  - Nocardiosis
- Viral infections:
  - Cytomegalovirus infection
  - Herpes simplex virus infection
  - Varicella-zoster virus infection

Malignancies
- Kaposi's sarcoma
- Non-Hodgkin's lymphoma
- Hodgkin's lymphoma
- Invasive cervical carcinoma

Opportunistic Infections. The patient with HIV/AIDS often develops pathogenic infections and opportunistic infections. *Pathogenic infections* are caused by virulent organisms and occur even among adults with normal IMMUNITY. *Opportunistic infections* are those caused by overgrowth of the patient's microbiome (normal flora). Only when IMMUNITY is depressed are such organisms capable of causing infection.

Opportunistic infections occur because of the profound reduced IMMUNITY of the adult with HIV disease. They may result from primary infection or reactivation of a latent infection. Opportunistic infections account for many of the signs and symptoms observed in HIV/AIDS and can be protozoan, fungal, bacterial, or viral. More than one infection may be present at the same time. The presence of opportunistic infections may represent disease progression or a temporary further reduction of immunity. *These infections can result in death if appropriate treatment is not started quickly.* Priority nursing actions when caring for a patient who is HIV positive are continually assessing for and documenting the presence of an opportunistic infection and monitoring the patient's response to therapy. Report to the primary health care provider any signs and symptoms that may indicate an infection.

Opportunistic infections do not pose a threat to the immunocompetent health care worker caring for a patient with HIV disease or AIDS. However, when the patient with HIV disease or AIDS has a pathogenic infection, health care personnel must use precautions appropriate to the specific disease to prevent disease spread. For example, when the adult with HIV/AIDS also has tuberculosis at a transmissible stage, Airborne Precautions are needed in addition to Standard Precautions. See Chapter 23 for a more complete discussion on Transmission-Based Precautions for specific infectious diseases.

Protozoal and fungal infections are common among patients with AIDS. *Pneumocystis jiroveci* pneumonia (PCP) is a common opportunistic infection in adults infected with HIV. This organism is now considered a soil fungus. Assess for dyspnea on exertion, tachypnea, a persistent dry cough, and a persistent low-grade fever. The patient may report fatigue and weight loss. Auscultate breath sounds for crackles.

Toxoplasmosis encephalitis, caused by *Toxoplasma gondii,* is acquired through contact with contaminated cat feces or by ingesting infected undercooked meat. Assess the patient for subtle changes in mental status, neurologic deficits, headaches, and fever. Additional changes may include difficulties with speech, gait, and vision; seizures; lethargy; and confusion. Perform a comprehensive mental status examination and monitor the patient to detect subtle changes.

Cryptosporidiosis is an intestinal infection caused by *Cryptosporidium* organisms. In AIDS this illness ranges from a mild diarrhea to a severe wasting with electrolyte imbalance. Diarrhea may result in fluid loss of up to 15 to 20 L/day. Ask the patient about the presence of diarrhea and whether he or she has had an unplanned weight loss of 5 lb or more.

Fungal infection usually occurs by overgrowth of normal body flora. *Candida albicans* is part of the intestinal tract's natural flora. In the adult with AIDS, candidiasis (overgrowth of the *Candida* fungus) occurs because the reduced IMMUNITY can no longer control fungal growth. *Candida* stomatitis or esophagitis occurs often in AIDS. Patients may report food tasting "funny," mouth pain, difficulty in swallowing, and pain behind the sternum. On examination of the mouth and throat, you may see cottage cheese–like, yellowish white plaques and inflammation (Fig. 19-5). Esophagitis is diagnosed by

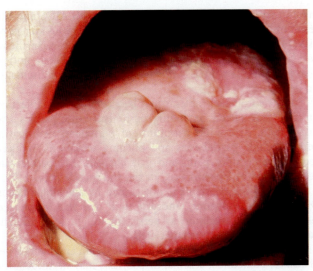

FIG. 19-5 Oral candidiasis (thrush). (From Marks, J., & Miller, J. [2006]. *Lookingbill & Marks' principles of dermatology* [4th ed.]. Philadelphia: Saunders.)

endoscopic examination with biopsy and culture. Women with HIV disease or AIDS may have persistent vaginal candidiasis with severe pruritus (itching), perineal irritation, and a thick, white vaginal discharge.

Cryptococcosis, caused by *Cryptococcus neoformans,* is a debilitating meningitis and can be a widely spread infection in AIDS. Ask about fever, headache, blurred vision, nausea and vomiting, neck stiffness, confusion, and other mental status changes. Patients may have seizures and other neurologic problems, or they may have mild malaise, fever, and headaches.

Histoplasmosis, caused by *Histoplasma capsulatum,* begins as a respiratory infection and progresses to widespread infection in the adult with AIDS. Assess for dyspnea, fever, cough, and weight loss. Check for enlargement of lymph nodes, the spleen, or the liver.

Bacterial infections are acquired from other people or sources and as overgrowth of skin flora. *Mycobacterium avium* complex (MAC) is a common bacterial infection with AIDS and is caused by *M. intracellulare* or *M. avium,* which infects the respiratory or GI tract of patients with AIDS. MAC is a systemic infection. Assess for fever, debility, weight loss, malaise, and sometimes swollen lymph glands or organ disease.

Tuberculosis (TB), caused by *Mycobacterium tuberculosis,* occurs in 2% to 10% of adults with AIDS (CDC, 2009). More than 50% of all patients with AIDS and TB have extrapulmonary disease sites. Ask about cough, dyspnea, chest pain, fever, chills, night sweats, weight loss, and anorexia. Symptoms of extrapulmonary infection vary with the site. *The adult with TB and a CD4+ T-cell count below 200/mm³ may not have a positive TB skin test (purified protein derivative [PPD]) because of an inability to mount an immune response to the antigen, a condition known as* anergy. Blood analysis by the fully automated nucleic acid amplification test (NAAT) for TB with results available in less than 2 hours is the most sensitive and rapid test for the presence of *M. tuberculosis*. It is very useful in the acute care setting to determine whether a symptomatic patient actually has TB. Other diagnostic tests include a chest x-ray, acid-fast sputum smear, and sputum culture.

TB is spread by airborne routes. When particles from the patient's respiratory tract are aerosolized, anyone near him or her is at risk for inhaling the particles and the bacillus. Therefore

! **NURSING SAFETY PRIORITY** QSEN
Action Alert

Maintain Airborne Precautions along with Standard Precautions for a patient with AIDS who also has TB symptoms until parameters other than a skin test come back negative for TB.

the interprofessional team member who gives cough-inducing aerosol treatments such as pentamidine isethionate to patients with AIDS should be screened every 6 months to determine whether he or she has been infected with TB.

Pneumonia from bacterial infection recurs often among patients with AIDS, and two or more episodes of any type of bacterial pneumonia in a 12-month period are an AIDS case definition. Assess for chest pain, productive cough, fever, and dyspnea.

Viral infection from a virus other than HIV is common among adults with HIV disease that has progressed to AIDS. Cytomegalovirus (CMV) can infect many sites in adults with AIDS, including the eye (CMV retinitis), respiratory and GI tracts, and the central nervous system. CMV infection causes many nonspecific problems such as fever, malaise, weight loss, fatigue, and swollen lymph nodes. CMV retinitis impairs vision, ranging from slight impairment to total blindness. CMV can also cause diarrhea, abdominal bloating and discomfort, and weight loss. Ask the patient whether he or she has any of these symptoms. CMV can cause encephalitis, pneumonitis, adrenalitis, hepatitis, and disseminated infection.

Herpes simplex virus (HSV) infections in adults with HIV disease or AIDS occur in the perirectal, oral, and genital areas. The symptoms are more widespread and of longer duration than among adults who have full IMMUNITY. Numbness or tingling at the site of infection occurs up to 24 hours before blisters form. Lesions are painful, with chronic open areas after blisters rupture. Assess for fever, pain, bleeding, and enlarged lymph nodes in the affected area. Also assess for headache, myalgia, and malaise.

Varicella-zoster virus (VZV) infection *(shingles)* is not a new infection for adults with AIDS. This virus causes chickenpox and then remains present in the nerve ganglia. When adults who have had chickenpox previously have reduced IMMUNITY, VZV leaves the nerve ganglia and enters other tissue areas, causing shingles. Ask whether the patient has pain and burning along sensory nerve tracts (see Chapter 41 for the dermatomes of sensory nerve locations), headache, and low-grade fever. Examine the skin for fluid-filled blisters with or without crusts.

Malignancies. Weakened IMMUNITY increases the risk for some cancers. These include Kaposi's sarcoma, lymphomas, invasive cervical cancer, lung cancer, GI cancer, and anal cancer.

Kaposi's sarcoma (KS) is the most common AIDS-related malignancy. The risk for KS is related to co-infection with human herpes virus-8.

KS develops as small, purplish brown, raised lesions on skin and mucous membranes that are usually not painful or itchy (Fig. 19-6). In some patients lesions develop in the lymph nodes, mouth and throat, intestinal tract, or lungs. KS is diagnosed by biopsy examination of the lesion. Assess KS lesions for number, size, location, and whether they are intact and monitor their progression.

Malignant lymphomas occurring with AIDS are Hodgkin's lymphoma, non-Hodgkin's B-cell lymphomas such as Burkitt's lymphoma, immunoblastic lymphoma, and primary brain

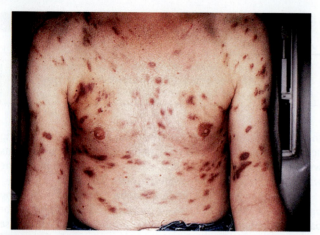

FIG. 19-6 Kaposi's sarcoma lesions. (From Leonard, P. C. [2012]. *Building a medical vocabulary* [8th ed.]. St. Louis: Saunders.)

lymphoma. Symptoms include swollen lymph nodes, weight loss, fever, and night sweats.

Human papilloma virus (HPV) infection results in multiple types of malignancies and symptoms, but the most common in HIV infection are cervical and anal cancers. Cervical Papanicolaou (Pap) testing every 6 months is the standard of care for HIV-positive patients. In patients having anal intercourse, an anal Pap test, using the same medium as for a cervical Pap test, is used for the early detection and treatment of anal cancers.

Endocrine Complications. Patients with HIV disease may have disease-related and treatment-related endocrine problems such as gonadal dysfunction, body shape changes, adrenal insufficiency, diabetes mellitus, and elevated triglycerides and cholesterol (which increase the risk for cardiovascular problems).

Many HIV-positive men have low testosterone levels, and HIV-positive women often have irregular menstrual cycles. With this gonadal dysfunction comes a decrease in body muscle mass for both genders, with a decrease in weight and a change in libido, accompanied by a decrease in energy and an increase in fatigue.

Body shape changes from fat redistribution or fat deposition (known as lipodystrophy) are common in patients receiving antiretroviral therapies, especially protease inhibitors and nucleoside reverse transcriptase inhibitors. Symptoms include "buffalo humps" or cervical (neck) fat development and large abdominal fat accumulations. Other body areas such as the face, arms, and legs have a wasted appearance and show prominent vein patterns or sunken facial cheeks from loss of subcutaneous fat, known as *lipoatrophy*.

Adrenal dysfunction can result from the glands being infected by opportunistic infections, resulting in adrenal insufficiency. This problem causes fatigue, weight loss, nausea, vomiting, low blood pressure, and electrolyte disturbances and can be life threatening.

Patients taking protease inhibitors have a higher-than-expected incidence of type 2 diabetes mellitus and hyperlipidemia. These problems are seen even among patients who have no other risks for these health problems.

Other Symptoms. All body systems are affected in AIDS. HIV-associated neurocognitive disorder (HAND) and *AIDS dementia complex (ADC)* (also called *HIV-associated dementia complex*) refer to symptoms of central nervous system involvement. ADC occurs in many adults with AIDS and is a result of infection of cells within the central nervous system by HIV. HAND and ADC cause cognitive and motor impairments and behavioral changes. Symptoms range from barely noticeable to severe dementia. (See Chapter 42 for more discussion on dementia.)

Some neurologic problems may be a result of HIV infection or drug side effects, including peripheral neuropathies and myopathies. Assess for symptoms of peripheral neuropathy, which include paresthesias and burning sensations, reduced sensory perception, pain, and gait changes. Myopathies are accompanied by leg weakness, ataxia, and muscle pain.

AIDS wasting syndrome is not caused by any single factor. Diarrhea, malabsorption, anorexia, and oral and esophageal lesions can all contribute to persistent weight loss; and the patient may appear quite emaciated.

Skin changes include dry, itchy, irritated skin and many types of rashes. Folliculitis, eczema, or psoriasis may occur. Ask the patient about skin sensation changes and examine any rash or irritation. When the platelet count is low, petechiae or bleeding gums may be present.

Kidney problems, including HIV-associated nephropathy (HIVAN) are common. These problems range from discrete glomerular injury to acute and chronic kidney diseases. Compared with the general population, patients with HIV have a far higher risk for requiring a renal replacement intervention.

Psychosocial Assessment. Psychosocial data collection for a patient with AIDS is very important. Ask about the patient's social support system, including family, significant others, and friends. To protect confidentiality, learn who in this support system is aware of the diagnosis so it is not mentioned inadvertently. Health care professionals must respect the patient's choices as much as possible without compromising care. Offer resources to help with disclosure to sexual partners or significant others.

The patient may be closest to a lover or a friend who is not legally recognized as next of kin. Obtain the name and telephone number of that person and determine whether a health care proxy or durable power-of-attorney document has been signed.

Ask about the patient's ADLs and any changes that may have occurred since the diagnosis. Assess his or her employment status and occupation, immigration status, social activities and hobbies, living arrangements, and financial resources, including health insurance. Ask whether he or she uses drugs, including tobacco, alcohol, supplements, opioids, benzodiazepines, cocaine, crystal methamphetamine, or injection drugs.

To plan care and monitor changes, assess the patient's feelings, thoughts, and behaviors, which include such areas as anxiety level, mood, cognitive ability, energy, and activity level. Ask about any experiences with discrimination and how they were handled. After assessing the patient's level of self-concept, work with him or her to identify strengths and coping strategies. Ask about any feelings of depression; suicidal ideation, intent, or plan, as well as other psychosocial concerns. Also ask about the use of support groups or other community resources.

The patient with HIV disease has less energy as the disease progresses. Pace interviews, assessments, and interventions to match his or her energy level. When the patient is greatly fatigued, postpone or eliminate nonurgent tests or care activities. Document psychosocial assessment and the patient's use of interventions using his or her own words. Communicate this information to all members of the interprofessional team.

Laboratory Assessment

Lymphocyte Counts. Lymphocyte counts are performed as part of a complete blood count (CBC) with differential (see Chapter 17). The normal white blood cell (WBC) count is between 5000 and 10,000 cells/mm³ (5 and 10×10^9/L), with a differential of about 30% to 40% lymphocytes (an absolute number of 1500 to 4500 [1.5 to 4.5 10×10^9/L]). Patients with AIDS are often leukopenic, with a WBC count of less than 3500 cells/mm³, and lymphopenic (<1500 lymphocytes/mm³ [<1.5 × 10^9/L]).

CD4+ T-cell and CD8+ T-cell counts and percentages are part of an IMMUNITY profile. Adults with HIV disease and AIDS usually have a lower-than-normal number of CD4+ T-cells, whereas the number of CD8+ T-cells remains normal. The normal ratio of CD4+ to CD8+ T-cells is 2:1. In HIV disease and AIDS, because of the low number of CD4+ T-cells, this ratio is low. Low CD4+ T-cell counts and a low ratio are associated with more disease symptoms.

Antibody-Antigen Tests. Antibody tests are used to measure the patient's response to the virus (the antigen) rather than parts of the virus. When the body is infected with HIV, it makes an antibody to the virus, usually within 3 weeks to 3 months after the infection first occurs. In some adults antibodies are not detectable until 36 months after initial infection. Measuring antibodies is an indirect test for HIV. *If an adult has a positive test result for HIV antibodies, it does not mean that he or she has HIV disease or AIDS—only that he or she has been infected with the virus.*

HIV antibodies can be measured by enzyme-linked immunosorbent assay (ELISA) and Western blot analysis, which is an older testing algorithm. This algorithm was the gold standard for many years and, while highly accurate, is more time consuming and expensive than fourth-generation testing. Using a third-generation test looks specifically for HIV IgG antibodies. When a positive test result is found, a confirmatory Western blot test is done, which is more sensitive and specific for HIV (co-infection with influenza A can cross-react with the third-generation test, leading to a false positive result). HIV antibodies are not detected for at least 21 days after exposure, and the confirmatory Western blot requires an additional 7 days before results can confirm infection. This time frame is known as the "window period" in which an adult is first infected with the virus and when viral replication is occurring but the immune system has not yet started making antibodies. Using this older algorithm, the period from the point of suspected infection to confirmation can take up to 28 days. *Therefore if the patient has unprotected sex with an HIV-positive adult one night and comes in for testing a week later, the ELISA will be negative, even though the patient may have active HIV. Thus testing during the window does not provide useful information* (Grimes et al., 2016; Taylor et al., 2015).

New technology allows for faster and more accurate initial diagnosis of HIV infection. The CDC now recommends the use of fourth-generation HIV assays that will detect HIV-IgM and IgG antibodies (positive in 21 days) and detect the presence of the p24 antigen (an HIV capsid protein) in serum (positive in 14 days). This type of testing reduces the window period in which false negatives are often reported. If the sample is negative, no further testing is required. If the sample is positive, step 2 in the new algorithm will be to differentiate between HIV-1 and HIV-2. If an indeterminate step 2 result is found, HIV-1 NAT (nucleic acid test) testing is done to detect HIV RNA, not only antibodies and antigens specific for HIV. If the sample is HIV-1 NAT+, it indicates acute HIV-1 infection. If HIV-1 NAT–, this sample is negative for HIV infection.

Viral Load Testing. *Viral load testing* directly measures the actual amount of HIV viral RNA particles present in 1 mL of blood. An uninfected adult has no viral load for HIV. A positive viral load test can measure as few as 40 particles/mL. High viral loads can be greater than 80,000 HIV particles/mL. The higher the viral load, the greater the risk for transmission. Current tests are not sensitive enough to measure viral loads less than 40/mL. An HIV-positive adult with an undetectable viral load can still transmit the virus, although this is less likely and transmission requires greater or multiple exposures. This test is the fastest way to determine HIV infectivity and therapy effectiveness.

In a newly infected adult a viral load is expressed about 10 days after infection (Taylor et al., 2015). HIV viral loads can be processed in as little as 24 hours. If positive, this is a clear diagnosis of HIV infection. One caution is that some immune systems can be strong enough to control the viral replication to report out an undetectable viral load. So in addition to running an HIV RNA, the fourth-generation testing should also be done, and the results reported out together. If the viral load is negative and the fourth-generation testing is negative, the specimen then is truly negative.

Some HIV testing uses techniques that are not blood based, and testing can be done anywhere, even at home. One test involves oral testing for HIV antibody. This test uses a device that is placed against the gum and cheek for 2 minutes. Fluid (called transmucosal exudate, not saliva) is drawn into an absorbable pad, which, in an HIV-positive adult, contains HIV-specific antibodies. The pad is placed in a solution; a positive result shows a change similar to a positive result in a urine pregnancy test. Total testing time is about 20 minutes. This test has the same accuracy as blood testing and can provide results quickly. If results are positive, a blood test is needed for confirmation.

Some home test kits require that a drop of blood be placed on a test card with a special code number. The card is mailed to a laboratory where the blood is tested for HIV antibodies. A special telephone number is called, and the code entered. Test results are then given. The OraQuick In-Home HIV Test uses oral transmucosal exudate, and results are ready at home in 20 to 40 minutes. The manufacturer recommends that the test be performed at least 3 months after a risk event has occurred. A positive result indicates the need for additional testing.

Other Laboratory Assessment. Other laboratory tests monitor the patient's overall health and detect or diagnose any infections or other problems related to HIV disease. These tests include blood chemistries; a CBC with differential and platelets; toxoplasmosis antibody titer; liver function tests; a serologic test for syphilis (STS); antigens and antibodies to hepatitis viruses A, B, and C; lipid profile; QuantiFERON TB testing or PPD; and cervical and anal Pap testing. Additional tests to evaluate the immune profile may include bone marrow aspiration with biopsy and cultures. Other tests may be performed to monitor toxicities from antiretroviral drugs.

Other Diagnostic Assessments. Other diagnostic tests are performed on the basis of the patient's symptoms. These may include testing stool for ova and parasites; biopsies of the skin, lymph nodes, lungs, liver, GI tract, or brain; a chest x-ray; gallium scans; bronchoscopy, endoscopy, or colonoscopy; liver and spleen scans; CT scans; pulmonary function tests; and arterial blood gas (ABG) analysis.

Patient-Centered Care QSEN

The HIV genotype test is used before starting antiretroviral drugs to determine whether any mutations causing drug resistance exist in the strain of HIV that has infected the patient. This test helps the clinician choose which antiretroviral drugs are most likely to be effective against viral replication. It is also useful in patients who demonstrate initial success in antiretroviral therapy and then have rapid disease progression. Ensure that newly diagnosed patients also have a genotype test performed.

The human leukocyte antigen (HLA) B5701 allele test is a genetic test to determine how an adult will respond to a drug. Patients with a variant of this gene allele have a hypersensitivity reaction to abacavir (Ziagen) that ranges from mild fever, rash, nausea, and vomiting to fatal anaphylaxis. Abacavir should not be used without first testing for B5701; if positive, abacavir is never used either as a single drug or in combination drug preparations.

The Trofile Test is a blood test to determine the degree of expression of the CCR5 receptor on CD4+ cells. This test is needed before starting drug therapy with maraviroc, which is a CCR5 antagonist drug in the entry inhibitor class. If no CCR5 receptors are present, the drug is ineffective.

🔍 **CLINICAL JUDGMENT CHALLENGE 19-1**

Patient-Centered Care, Evidence-Based Practice, Safety QSEN

A patient at an STI clinic is a worried-looking 28-year-old gay man who until a month ago was in a long-term mutually monogamous relationship. He became inebriated at a party last night and went home with a new acquaintance. Consensual unprotected sex occurred several times, and the patient was both a top and bottom partner. On awakening the partner was gone. This morning the patient is concerned about STI and HIV risks. His last HIV test, performed 2 weeks ago, was negative. He does not know how to contact the partner from last night, and he asks whether he should have another ELISA or that new "fast test" performed today.

1. Does the patient have cause for concern? Why or why not?
2. What will you tell him about testing today?
3. Is he a candidate for pre-exposure prophylaxis today? Why or why not?
4. Is he a candidate for postexposure prophylaxis today? Why or why not?
5. What other teaching or considerations are needed at this time?

◆ Analysis: Interpreting

The priority collaborative problems for patients with AIDS are:

1. Potential for infection due to reduced IMMUNITY
2. Inadequate GAS EXCHANGE due to anemia, respiratory infection (*P. jiroveci* pneumonia [PCP], cytomegalovirus [CMV] pneumonitis), pulmonary Kaposi's sarcoma (KS), or anemia
3. Pain due to neuropathy, myelopathy, cancer, or infection
4. Inadequate NUTRITION due to increased metabolic need, nausea, vomiting, diarrhea, difficulty chewing or swallowing, or anorexia
5. Diarrhea due to infection, food intolerance, or drugs
6. Potential for reduced TISSUE INTEGRITY due to KS, infection, reduced NUTRITION, incontinence, immobility, hyperthermia, or cancer

7. Cognitive decline due to AIDS dementia complex (ADC), central nervous system infection, or cancer
8. Potential for psychosocial distress due to living with a life-threatening chronic disease that affects all aspects of life

◆ Planning and Implementation: Responding

Preventing Infection. The patient with AIDS is susceptible to opportunistic infections because of reduced IMMUNITY. Initial management focuses on supporting the patient's immunity by controlling the HIV infection with antiretroviral therapy. When the patient's immunity declines, management includes both prophylaxis and treatment of opportunistic infections.

Planning: Expected Outcomes. The patient is expected to remain free of opportunistic *diseases* and other infection. Indicators include:

- Absence of chills, fever, or temperature instability
- Absence of purulent drainage or sputum
- Absence of diarrhea
- Absence of chest x-ray infiltration
- Maintenance of white blood cell (WBC) count within the patient's normal range

Interventions. The adult who has HIV infection with reduced IMMUNITY is at greater risk for any type of infection. Teach him or her to avoid exposure to infection (Chart 19-4). Chart 19-5 lists best practices for prevention of infection in a hospitalized patient with reduced immunity.

Drug Therapy. All currently licensed antiretroviral drugs have excellent activity against HIV; however, *it is important to remember that antiretroviral therapy only inhibits viral replication and does not kill the virus.* Treatment with only one antiretroviral agent *(monotherapy)* promotes drug resistance and does not improve life span. Instead multiple drugs from different classes are used in combinations. This approach, termed *combination antiretroviral therapy (cART),* has reduced viral load, improved CD4+ T-cell counts, and slowed disease progression (Starr & Bradley-Springer, 2014). Tell patients that they must take the drugs correctly 90% of the time, making sure that, out of 10 doses, 9 are taken on time and correctly.

An important issue with cART is the development of drug-resistant mutations in the HIV organism. When resistance develops, viral replication is no longer suppressed by the drugs. Testing is now possible to determine whether a strain of HIV has developed resistance to specific drugs (see the Genetic/Genomic Considerations box). Several factors contribute to the development of drug resistance to cART, with the most important being missed doses of drugs. When doses are missed, the blood drug concentrations become lower than those needed for inhibition of viral replication. The HIV then can replicate and produce new viral particles that are resistant to the drugs being used.

An important understanding about HIV resistance to one or more drugs is that, once a patient has HIV with resistant mutations, the resistant virus is stored in the body indefinitely, a process known as *archiving.* The drugs to which the virus is resistant are no longer used for that patient. Even years later, if the drug to which the HIV demonstrated resistance is tried again, the viruses with the resistant mutation come out of archival storage to defeat the drug.

The main actions of each drug category and representative drugs in each category are presented in Chart 19-6.

CHART 19-4 Patient and Family Education: Preparing for Self-Management

Prevention of Infection

During the times when your white blood cell counts are low:
- Avoid crowds and other large gatherings of people who might be ill.
- Do not share personal toilet articles such as toothbrushes, tooth-paste, washcloths, or deodorant sticks with others.
- If possible, bathe daily, using an antimicrobial soap. If total bathing is not possible, wash the armpits, groin, genitals, and anal area twice a day with an antimicrobial soap.
- Clean your toothbrush at least weekly by either running it through the dishwasher or rinsing it in liquid laundry bleach (and then rinsing out the bleach with hot running water).
- Wash your hands thoroughly with an antimicrobial soap before you eat or drink, after touching a pet, after shaking hands with anyone, as soon as you come home from any outing, and after using the toilet.
- Avoid eating salads; raw fruits and vegetables; undercooked meat, fish, and eggs; and pepper and paprika.
- Wash dishes between use with hot, sudsy water or use a dishwasher.
- Do not drink water, milk, juice, or other cold liquids that have been standing for longer than an hour.
- Do not reuse cups and glasses without washing.
- Do not change pet litter boxes. If unavoidable, use gloves and wash hands immediately.
- Avoid turtles and reptiles as pets.
- Do not feed pets raw or undercooked meat.
- Take your temperature at least once a day and whenever you do not feel well.
- Report any of these indications of infection to your primary health care provider immediately:
  - Temperature greater than 100°F (37.8°C)
  - Persistent cough (with or without sputum)
  - Pus or foul-smelling drainage from any open skin area or normal body opening
  - Presence of a boil or abscess
  - Urine that is cloudy or foul smelling or that causes burning on urination
- Take all prescribed drugs.
- Do not dig in the garden or work with houseplants.
- Wear a condom (if you are a man) when having sex. If you are a woman having sex with a male partner, ensure that he wears a condom or use a female vaginal polyurethane condom.
- Avoid travel to areas of the world with poor sanitation or less-than-adequate health care facilities.

CHART 19-5 Best Practice for Patient Safety & Quality Care QSEN

Care of the Hospitalized Patient With Reduced Immunity

- Place the patient in a private room whenever possible.
- Use good handwashing technique or alcohol-based hand rubs before touching the patient or any of his or her belongings.
- Ensure that the patient's room and bathroom are cleaned at least once each day.
- Do not use supplies from common areas for neutropenic patients. For example, keep a dedicated box of disposable gloves in his or her room and do not share this box with any other patient. Provide single-use food products, individually wrapped gauze, and other individually wrapped items.
- Limit the number of personnel entering the patient's room.
- Monitor vital signs, including temperature, every 4 hours.
- Inspect the patient's mouth at least every 8 hours.
- Inspect the patient's skin and mucous membranes (especially the anal area) for the presence of fissures and abscesses at least every 8 hours.
- Inspect open areas such as IV sites every 4 hours for signs of infection.
- Change gauze-containing wound dressings daily.
- Obtain specimens of all suspicious areas for culture (as specified by the agency) and promptly notify the primary health care provider.
- Help the patient perform coughing and deep-breathing exercises.
- Encourage activity at a level appropriate for the patient's current health status.
- Keep frequently used equipment in the room for use with this patient only (e.g., blood pressure cuff, stethoscope, thermometer).
- Limit visitors to healthy adults.
- Use strict aseptic technique for all invasive procedures.
- Avoid the use of indwelling urinary catheters.
- Keep fresh flowers and potted plants out of the patient's room.
- Teach the patient to eat a low-bacteria diet (e.g., avoiding raw fruits and vegetables; undercooked meat, eggs, and fish; pepper and paprika as seasonings sprinkled on food right before eating).

! NURSING SAFETY PRIORITY QSEN

Drug Alert

Ensure that cART drugs are not missed, delayed, or administered in lower-than-prescribed doses in the inpatient setting. Teach patients the importance of taking the cART drugs exactly as prescribed to maintain their effectiveness. Even a few missed doses per month can promote drug resistance (remember the 90% rule).

CHART 19-6 Common Examples of Drug Therapy

HIV Infection

DRUG CATEGORY	NURSING IMPLICATIONS
Nucleoside Reverse Transcriptase Inhibitors (NRTIs)—These drugs have a structure similar to the four nucleoside bases of DNA, making them "counterfeit" bases. They fool the HIV enzyme *reverse transcriptase* into using these counterfeit bases so viral DNA synthesis and replication are suppressed.	
Abacavir (Ziagen) Didanosine (Videx EC) Emtricitabine (Emtriva) Lamivudine (Epivir) Stavudine (Zerit) Tenofovir (Viread) Zidovudine (Retrovir)	Remind patients to avoid fatty and fried foods with these drugs *because they cause digestive upsets and may lead to pancreatitis when combined with NRTIs.* Teach patients to use precautions to prevent injury *because these drugs induce peripheral neuropathy.* Teach patients taking abacavir to report flu-like symptoms to the provider immediately *because these symptoms may indicate a hypersensitivity reaction that requires discontinuing the drug.* Instruct patients to avoid or severely limit alcoholic beverages *to reduce the risk for liver damage while on these drugs.* Do not give abacavir to a patient who tests positive for the HLA-B 5701 tissue type *because fatal allergic responses are likely.*

Continued

⬦ CHART 19-6   **Common Examples of Drug Therapy—cont'd**

HIV Infection

DRUG CATEGORY	NURSING IMPLICATIONS

Non-Nucleoside Reverse Transcriptase Inhibitors (NNRTIs)—These drugs work by binding directly to the HIV-1 enzyme *reverse transcriptase,* preventing viral cell DNA replication, RNA replication, and protein synthesis. This action suppresses viral replication of the HIV-1 virus but does not affect HIV-2 viral replication.

Delavirdine (Rescriptor) Efavirenz (Sustiva) Etravirine (Viramune) Rilpivirine (Edurant)	Check laboratory values for increases in liver enzymes and decreased red blood cells *because the most common side effects are anemia and liver toxicity.* Teach patients to take these drugs at least 1 hour before or 2 hours after taking an antacid *to avoid inhibiting GI absorption.* Instruct patients to notify the prescriber if a sore throat, fever, different types of rashes, blisters, or multiple bruises develop *because these are indications of a serious adverse drug effect.* Do not give delavirdine or efavirenz to pregnant women *because these two drugs have the potential to cause birth defects and developmental problems.*

Protease Inhibitors (PIs)—These drugs competitively block the HIV protease enzyme, preventing viral replication and release of viral particles. The HIV initially produces all of its proteins in one long strand, which must be broken down into separate smaller proteins by HIV protease to be active. Thus, when inhibited, viral proteins are not functional, and viral particles cannot leave the cell to infect other cells.

Atazanavir (Reyataz) Darunavir (Prezista) Fosamprenavir (Lexiva) Indinavir (Crixivan) Lopinavir/ritonavir (Kaletra) Nelfinavir (Viracept) Saquinavir (Invirase) Tipranavir (Aptivus)	Instruct patients to not chew or crush these drugs *because this action may cause the drug to be absorbed too rapidly and increase the risk for side effects.* Teach patients to report jaundice, nausea and vomiting, or severe abdominal pain *because these drugs can induce liver toxicity.* Instruct patients to keep all appointments for laboratory work *because these drugs increase blood lipid levels and increase the risk for atherosclerosis and pancreatitis.* Remind patients to avoid St. John's wort while taking these drugs *because the supplement reduces the effectiveness of all PIs.* Teach patients taking atazanavir and ritonavir to check their pulse daily and report low heart rate to the prescriber *because these two drugs can impair electrical conduction and lead to heart block.* Do not give darunavir or fosamprenavir to patients who have a known sulfa allergy *because these two drugs contain sulfa.*

Integrase Inhibitors—These drugs inhibit the HIV enzyme *integrase,* which the virus uses to insert the viral DNA into the host cell's human DNA. Without this action viral proteins are not made, and viral replication is inhibited.

Dolutegravir (TIVICAY) Elvitegravir (EVG) Raltegravir (Isentress)	Warn patients that diarrhea, nausea, rash, insomnia, and abdominal pain are common side effects of these drugs *because knowing the expected side effects decreases anxiety when they appear.* Suggest that patients take the drug with food *to reduce the GI side effects.* Instruct patients to not chew or crush these drugs *because this action may cause the drug to be absorbed too rapidly and increase the risk for side effects.* Instruct patients to report new-onset muscle pain or weakness *because these drugs can cause muscle breakdown (rhabdomyolysis), especially in adults taking a "statin" type of lipid-lowering drug.* Teach patients with diabetes to closely monitor blood glucose levels *because these drugs increase hyperglycemia.* Do not give raltegravir to pregnant women *because it is associated with an increased risk for birth defects.*

Fusion Inhibitors—These drugs block the fusion of HIV with a host cell by blocking the ability of *gp41* to fuse with the host cell's CD4 receptor. Without fusion, infection of new cells does not occur.

Enfuvirtide (Fuzeon)	Teach patients how to prepare and inject the drug subcutaneously *to ensure correct dosage and effectiveness.* Assess injection sites for warmth, swelling, redness, skin hardening, or bump formation *because these are indications of injection site reactions.* Instruct patients to report pain or numbness in the hands or feet *because this drug can induce peripheral neuropathy.* Teach patients to report jaundice, nausea and vomiting, or severe abdominal pain *because this drug can induce liver toxicity.* Teach patients to observe for and report cough, shortness of breath, fever, and purulent mucus *because this drug increases the risk for severe respiratory infections, including pneumonia.*

Entry Inhibitors/CCR5 Antagonists—These drugs prevent cellular infection with HIV by blocking the *CCR5* receptor on CD4+ T-cells. (The virus's *gp120* must bind to the CD4 receptor, and its *gp41* must bind to the *CCR5* receptor or to the *CXCR4* receptor for entry into host cells.

Maraviroc (Selzentry)	Instruct patients to not chew or crush this drug *because this action may cause the drug to be absorbed too rapidly and increase the risk for side effects.* Teach patients to change positions slowly *because hypotension is a common side effect, especially orthostatic hypotension.* Teach patients to report jaundice, nausea and vomiting, or severe abdominal pain *because these drugs can induce liver toxicity.* Instruct patients to report pain or numbness in the hands or feet *because this drug can induce peripheral neuropathy.*

Combination Products—Each ingredient has the same mechanism of action and nursing implications as the parent drug class.

Atripla (emtricitabine, tenofovir, & efavirenz)
Combivir (lamivudine & zidovudine)
Complera (emtricitabine, rilpivirine, & tenofovir)
Epzicom (lamivudine & abacavir)
Genvoya (elvitegravir, cobicistat*, emtricitabine, & tenofovir)
Stribild (elvitegravir, cobicistat*, emtricitabine, & tenofovir)
Truvada (emtricitabine & tenofovir)
Triumeq (dolutegravir, abacavir, & lamivudine)

*Cobicistat is a metabolizing enzyme inhibitor that allows other drugs in the combination to remain active longer, boosting their pharmacologic action. It is not a specific antiretroviral agent.

These categories are nucleoside reverse transcriptase inhibitors (NRTIs), nonnucleoside reverse transcriptase inhibitors (NNRTIs), protease inhibitors (PIs), integrase inhibitors, fusion inhibitors, and entry inhibitors. Drawbacks to cART include the expense of the drugs, food and timing requirements, and the number of daily drugs. Newer combination drug formulations have reduced the number of tablets and capsules that need to be taken daily. However, the daily regimen continues to be lifelong and burdensome.

Most antiretroviral drugs have significant side effects and many drug interactions. Be sure to consult a drug reference book for usual dosages, side effects, and nursing interventions.

An interesting complication of effective cART in some patients whose CD4+ T-cell counts rise and IMMUNITY returns to normal is the development of immune reconstitution inflammatory syndrome (IRIS). As the drugs begin to suppress HIV replication and the T4-cells slowly begin to rebound, the T4-cells "recognize" several opportunistic infections (e.g., tuberculosis, cryptococcosis, *Mycobacterium avium* complex, pneumocystis pneumonia, cytomegalovirus, hepatitis) that were present before but not recognized because of severe immunosuppression. With the T4-cells now in sufficient numbers and active, they begin to sound the alarm about the presence of these opportunistic infections. The T4-cells generate an inflammatory reaction with high fever, chills, and, depending on which infection the immune system is reacting against, worsening disease. For example, IRIS is common with those co-infected with HIV and TB. TB symptoms initially become much worse after starting cART. Because some symptoms are similar to those of drug therapy side effects and other problems, IRIS may go undiagnosed and untreated, increasing the risk for death. When IRIS is recognized, short-term therapy with corticosteroids can reduce the inflammatory responses.

Complementary and Integrative Health. Complementary therapies are often used by adults with HIV/AIDS, although the effectiveness of these therapies has not been established. Some products alter the effects of prescription drugs. Ask the patient which botanical or homeopathic agents he or she is using and check with the pharmacist to determine known drug interactions with cART therapy.

❓ NCLEX EXAMINATION CHALLENGE 19-3

Safe and Effective Care Environment

A client diagnosed with AIDS who is receiving combination antiretroviral therapy (cART) now has a CD4+ T-cell count of 525 cells/mm³. How will the nurse interpret this result?
A. The client can reduce the dosages of the prescribed drugs.
B. The virus is resistant to the current combination of drugs.
C. The client no longer has AIDS.
D. The drug therapy is effective.

Enhancing Gas Exchange
Planning: Expected Outcomes. The patient is expected to maintain adequate GAS EXCHANGE with oxygenation and perfusion and to have minimal dyspnea. Indicators include:
- Rate and depth of respiration within the normal range
- Pulse oximetry within the normal range
- Absence of cyanosis or pallor and abnormal breath sounds

Interventions. The nurse or respiratory therapist uses drug therapy, respiratory support and maintenance, comfort, and rest to enhance GAS EXCHANGE.

Drug therapy is a mainstay for GAS EXCHANGE problems resulting from infection. Drug therapy is started after an infectious cause for respiratory difficulty is identified. A common respiratory infection in adults with HIV disease is *P. jiroveci* pneumonia (PCP). The treatment of choice for PCP is trimethoprim with sulfamethoxazole (Apo-Sulfatrim ♣, Bactrim, Cotrim, Septra). Many patients have adverse reactions to this drug, including nausea, vomiting, hyponatremia, rashes, fever, leukopenia, thrombocytopenia, and hepatitis.

Pentamidine isethionate (Pentacarinat ♣, Pentam), usually given IV or IM, is also used to treat PCP. Aerosolized pentamidine isethionate is used as prophylaxis for patients with CD4+ T-cell counts below 200 (0.2×10^9/L) or 14% and for those who have already had PCP.

Other drug therapies include bronchodilators to improve airflow, as well as dapsone (Avlosulfon) and atovaquone (Mepron), which can be used as alternative therapies to trimethoprim-sulfamethoxazole for existing PCP or as prophylaxis. For moderate-to-severe PCP, steroids may be used to reduce the inflammation.

Respiratory support and maintenance help maintain GAS EXCHANGE and avoid complications. Assess the respiratory rate, rhythm, and depth, breath sounds, and vital signs and monitor for cyanosis at least every 8 hours. Apply oxygen and humidify the room as prescribed. Also monitor mechanical ventilation, perform suctioning and chest physical therapy as needed, and evaluate blood gas results.

Comfort can help improve GAS EXCHANGE. Assess the patient's comfort. The patient with difficulty breathing is often more comfortable with the head of the bed elevated. Pace activities to reduce shortness of breath and fatigue.

Rest and activity changes are needed when GAS EXCHANGE is impaired. Most patients with HIV/AIDS have fatigue, especially when respiratory problems also are present. Consult with the patient to pace activities to conserve energy. Schedule non–time-critical activities such as bathing so he or she is not fatigued at mealtime.

Managing Pain. The patient with severe HIV disease or AIDS often has pain from many causes. Pain can result from enlarged organs stretching the viscera or compressing nerves. Tumor invasion of bone and other tissues can cause pain, as can compression of nerves from swollen lymph nodes. Many patients with AIDS have peripheral neuropathy–induced pain from the disease or drug therapies (Anastasi et al., 2013). Many have generalized joint and muscle pain.

Planning: Expected Outcomes. The patient is expected to achieve an acceptable level of comfort and pain reduction. Indicators include:
- Reporting that pain is controlled to a level that is acceptable to him or her
- Absence of indicators of acute pain (increased heart rate and blood pressure)
- Absence of facial grimacing, teeth clenching
- Willingness to move and participate in self-care

Interventions. Drug therapy and other approaches are used together to manage pain in the patient with HIV/AIDS, depending on the cause of the pain.

Comfort measures include the use of pressure-relieving mattress pads, warm baths or other forms of hydrotherapy, massage, and applying heat or cold to painful areas to reduce pain levels, with or without drug therapy. Take care when moving or assisting the patient. Use lift sheets to avoid pulling or grasping the patient with joint pain. The patient may be thin and have poor circulation, contributing to pain and discomfort. Help him or her change positions often.

Drug therapy with different drug classes is used to manage different types of pain. For arthralgia and myalgia, NSAIDs may reduce inflammation and increase comfort. Pregabalin (Lyrica) may provide some relief from muscle and joint pain. Neuropathic pain may respond to tricyclic antidepressants such as amitriptyline (Elavil) or to anticonvulsant drugs such as gabapentin (Neurontin), phenytoin (Dilantin), or carbamazepine (Tegretol), although these drugs often interact with antiretroviral drugs. These drugs may take days to weeks before a full effect is seen. During this time opioids may be needed to control pain.

When opioids are used, assess the patient for pain intensity and quality. Mild-to-moderate pain is treated with weaker opioids such as hydrocodone or codeine. More intense pain is treated with stronger opioids such as oxycodone, morphine, hydromorphone (Dilaudid), or fentanyl transdermal (Duragesic). Combinations of weak and strong opioids along with nonopioid drugs may be used to provide the best sustained pain relief and allow the patient to participate in activities to the extent that he or she wishes.

Complementary and integrative therapies are used by many patients with pain from HIV/AIDS. These include acupuncture, massage, guided imagery, distraction, progressive relaxation, body-talk, and biofeedback. Integrative therapies can be used with traditional and pharmacologic measures to improve comfort.

Enhancing Nutrition. Many patients with AIDS have difficulty maintaining their weight and NUTRITION status, and a registered dietitian is part of the interprofessional health care team. This problem may be caused by fatigue, anorexia, nausea and vomiting, difficult or painful swallowing, diarrhea, intestinal malabsorption, or wasting syndrome.

Planning: Expected Outcomes. The patient is expected to maintain optimal weight through adequate NUTRITION and hydration. Indicators include:

- Selecting foods high in calories and protein
- Maintaining current weight or gaining weight
- Drinking at least 2 to 3 L of fluids per day
- Maintaining normal blood levels of ferritin, albumin, prealbumin, and hemoglobin

Interventions. Because there are many factors for poor NUTRITION in AIDS, diagnostic procedures are needed to determine the cause. Once the cause is determined, appropriate therapy is initiated. For example, in candidal esophagitis, nutrition is affected by swallowing difficulties.

Drug therapy can include ketoconazole (Nizoral) or fluconazole (Diflucan) orally, or IV amphotericin B (Fungizone). Administer the drug as prescribed and monitor for side effects such as nausea and vomiting, which also affect NUTRITION. Provide mouth care and ice chips and keep unpleasant odors out of the patient's environment. Antiemetics are used as needed.

Nutrition therapy includes monitoring weight, intake and output, and calorie count. Assess food preferences and dietary cultural or religious practices. Collaborate with the dietitian to teach the patient about the need for a high-calorie and high-protein diet. Encourage him or her to avoid dietary fat, because fat intolerance often occurs as a result of the disease and as a side effect of some antiretroviral drugs. Other strategies include providing small, frequent meals that are often better tolerated than large meals. Supplemental vitamins and fluids are indicated in some cases. For the patient who cannot achieve adequate NUTRITION through food, tube feedings or total parenteral nutrition may be needed.

Mouth care can improve appetite. When this nursing action is delegated to unlicensed assistive personnel (UAP), instruct them to offer the patient rinses of sodium bicarbonate with sterile water or normal saline several times a day. Explain to UAP the reason the patient needs to use a soft toothbrush and the need to drink plenty of fluids. For oral pain general analgesics or oral anesthetic gels and solutions may be needed. Avoid the use of alcohol-based mouthwashes.

Minimizing Diarrhea. Patients with AIDS often suffer from diarrhea. Sometimes an infectious cause (e.g., *Giardia, Cryptosporidium,* or amoeba) can be determined and treated; or the cause is determined, but no effective therapy is available. Many patients are lactose intolerant, and HIV disease worsens the condition. Diarrhea may occur as a side effect of drug therapy. In some cases no cause can be identified.

Planning: Expected Outcomes. The patient is expected to have decreased diarrhea; to maintain fluid, electrolyte, and NUTRITION status; and to reduce incontinence. Indicators include:

- Has a stool amount and character that are appropriate for the diet
- Recognizes urge to defecate
- Maintains control of stool passage

Interventions. For most patients with AIDS and diarrhea, symptom management is all that is available. Antidiarrheals such as diphenoxylate hydrochloride (Diarsed ✦, Lomotil) or loperamide (Imodium), given on a regular schedule, provide some relief. Consult with the dietitian and teach about appropriate foods. Recommended dietary changes include less roughage; less fatty, spicy, and sweet food; and no alcohol or caffeine. Some patients obtain relief when they eliminate dairy products or eat smaller amounts of food more often and drink plenty of fluids, especially between meals. If dehydration accompanies diarrhea, IV fluid infusions may be needed.

Assess the perineal skin every 8 to 12 hours for a change in skin TISSUE INTEGRITY. Provide a bedside commode or a bedpan if the patient cannot reach the bathroom in time. Teach UAP performing this care to provide the patient with privacy, support, and understanding. Explain the need to keep the patient's perineal area clean and dry and to wear gloves during this care. Instruct UAP to report any skin changes in the perineal area, including persistent redness, rashes, blisters, or open areas. Collaborate with a wound care specialist for more interventions to manage anal excoriation and discomfort.

Restoring Skin Integrity. Impaired TISSUE INTEGRITY in AIDS may be related to Kaposi's sarcoma (KS) of the skin, mucous membranes, and internal organs. Lesions may be localized or widespread. Large lesions can cause pain, restrict movement, and impede circulation, causing open, weeping, painful lesions. Another cause of impaired tissue integrity may be skin infection with herpes simplex virus (HSV) or varicella zoster virus (VZV) (shingles).

Planning: Expected Outcomes. The patient is expected to have healing of any existing lesions and avoid increased skin breakdown or secondary infection. Indicators include:

- Absence of new lesions or open skin areas
- Existing lesions become smaller in diameter
- Absence of pus, induration, or redness in, from, or around skin lesions

Interventions. Often KS responds well to effective antiretroviral drug therapy. With time and cART, many lesions disappear. For lesions that do not respond to cART, KS can be treated with local radiation, intralesional or systemic chemotherapy, systemic interferon, cryotherapy, or topical retinoids.

Treatment of painful KS lesions includes analgesics and comfort measures. Keep open, weeping KS lesions clean and dressed to prevent infection. Many patients with KS are concerned about their appearance and the risk for being identified as HIV positive. Makeup (if lesions are closed), long-sleeved shirts, and hats may help maintain a normal appearance.

For the patient with a herpes simplex virus (HSV) outbreak, provide good skin care directly or delegate this care to UAP. Stress the importance of keeping the area clean and dry. Teach UAP to clean abscesses at least once per shift with normal saline and allow them to air-dry. This infection is painful and requires analgesics, assistance with position, and other comfort measures. Modified Burow's solution (Domeboro) soaks promote healing for some patients. HSV infection is treated with acyclovir (Zovirax) or valacyclovir (Valtrex).

Enhancing Cognition. Neurologic changes and confusion are major areas of concern for patients with HIV disease or AIDS. These changes may be due to psychological stressors accompanying the disease or organic disorders caused by opportunistic infections, cancer, or HIV encephalitis.

Planning: Expected Outcomes. The patient is expected to show improved mental status. Indicators include that the patient demonstrates these behaviors:

- Identifies self and significant others
- Identifies correct month and year
- Recalls immediate, recent, and remote information accurately

Interventions. Patients with AIDS suffer from enormous loss and psychological stress, which complicates the assessment of changes in behavior or affect. Assess baseline neurologic and mental status by using neurologic assessment tools (see Chapter 41) to compare any changes. Evaluate the patient for subtle changes in memory, ability to concentrate, affect, and behavior. It is important to determine whether the cause of the neurologic changes is treatable.

Reorient the confused patient to person, time, and place as needed. Coordinate with all members of the interprofessional team to ensure that reorientation methods are performed by everyone who interacts with the patient. Remind the patient of your identity and explain what is to be done at any given time. Give simple directions; use short, uncomplicated sentences; explain activities in simple language; and involve him or her in daily planning. Ask significant others to bring in familiar items from home. When possible, arrange all items in the patient's environment in the same location as at home. Calendars, clocks, radios, and putting the bed close to a window may help keep the patient oriented.

Drug therapy is used for different conditions that can cause confusion in the adult with AIDS. Psychotropic drugs are used to manage ongoing behavioral problems or emotional disorders. Antidepressants and anxiolytics may be prescribed.

Safety measures are crucial to the well-being of the confused patient. He or she may not be aware of activities or surroundings and may need help with bathing, dressing, eating, ambulating, and other ADLs. Make the environment, whether a hospital room or long-term care facility, safe and comfortable.

Some patients with AIDS have seizures. Institute seizure precautions, including keeping side rails in the up position and having oxygen and suctioning equipment available. Anticonvulsants may be added to the drug therapy.

Assess the patient with neurologic symptoms for increased intracranial pressure (ICP). If not recognized and managed early, ICP can lead to permanent brain damage and death. Increased ICP in patients with HIV disease is most commonly managed with corticosteroids.

> **! NURSING SAFETY PRIORITY** QSEN
>
> *Critical Rescue*
>
> Assess the patient frequently to recognize any changes in level of consciousness (one of the earliest signs of increased ICP), vital signs, pupil size or reactivity, or limb strength. If any of these are present, respond by reporting them immediately to the primary health care provider for appropriate intervention.

Support the family and friends of the patient who has neurologic impairment. There is great trauma in seeing a loved one unable to care for himself or herself or showing childlike behavior. Teach UAP, the family, and significant others how to reorient the patient. Encourage them to continue to provide the patient with news of family happenings or current events. Coordinate with the social worker to identify community resources for the patient and family.

Addressing Psychosocial Distress. As discussed earlier, patients diagnosed with HIV disease have many issues that can lead to psychosocial distress in the forms of depression, anxiety, fear, isolation, and loss. The disease is chronic, debilitating, and fatal. Treatments are expensive, and both the disease and the associated drug therapy induce changes in function and appearance. The disease carries social stigma, regardless of how it was acquired.

The psychosocial issues of a patient with HIV/AIDS are usually ongoing and require many coping adaptations. The role of the medical-surgical nurse in addressing these issues is a more basic continuation of comprehensive therapy. Having a mental health professional as part of the interprofessional care team is essential. The role of this person is extensive and beyond the scope of this chapter.

Planning: Expected Outcomes. The patient is expected to express his or her personal strengths and self-worth.

Interventions. Being supportive, honest, caring, and open to the patient's thoughts and feelings form the basis of addressing psychosocial issues. Acceptance of the patient is key to respectful communication. Listen to what he or she has to say about his or her perspectives on the disease and on the reason for this hospitalization.

Be attuned to indications of depression and follow up by asking whether the patient is considering hurting himself or herself. If you believe the patient does have suicidal ideation, communicate this to the interprofessional team immediately. Ask whether he or she would like you to contact his or her usual mental health professional or any other person who usually provides emotional support.

Approach all interactions with the patient in a caring and professional manner. Whenever possible, without violating Standard Precautions, use bare-handed touch while providing care or any other interaction. Using touch during back rubs, hair care, administering medications, or even just shaking hands communicates acceptance. Ensure that unlicensed assistive personnel (UAP) are approaching the patient with the same attitude they approach all other patients. Reiterate with UAP which specific actions do not require wearing gloves.

Spending time with the patient also communicates acceptance. Even just a few minutes beyond what is needed to administer medications or perform an assessment demonstrates caring rather than fear. Allow for privacy, but do not isolate the patient. Encourage self-care, independence, control, and decision-making by helping him or her to set short-term, attainable goals and offering praise when goals are achieved.

At times drug therapy with antidepressants or anxiolytics may be needed long term or for situational issues. If the patient uses such drug therapies on a regular basis, be certain that they are prescribed during the hospitalization. If a new drug is started, record the patient's responses to the therapy.

Care Coordination and Transition Management

The management of HIV/AIDS as a chronic disease occurs in many settings, most often at home. Hospitalizations occur during periods of severe infection or other acute exacerbations of symptoms. As the illness becomes more severe, the patient may need referral to a long-term care facility, home care agency, or hospice. In collaboration with the social worker, dietitian, and others, work with patients to plan what will be needed and how they will manage at home with self-care and ADLs.

Home Care Management. Before the patient is discharged to home, assess his or her status, ability to perform self-care activities, and plans to maintain communication with primary health care providers. Home care can range from help with ADLs for those with weakness, debility, or limited function to around-the-clock nursing care, drugs, and NUTRITION support for severely ill patients. Assess available resources, including family members and significant others willing and able to be caregivers. Help the family make arrangements for outside caregivers or respite care, if needed. Patients may need referrals or help in planning housing, finances, insurance, legal services, and spiritual counseling. Coordinate with the case manager to ensure that these issues are addressed.

Usually a home care nurse makes an initial visit to the patient with AIDS for assessment purposes, and care is followed up by home care aides. Reassessment is needed if the patient becomes more debilitated. Chart 19-7 lists assessment areas for the patient with AIDS at home.

Self-Management Education. Teaching the patient, family, and friends is a high priority when preparing for discharge. Instruct about modes of transmission and preventive behaviors (e.g., guidelines for safer sex; not sharing toothbrushes, razors, and other potentially blood-contaminated articles). Caregivers also need instruction about best practices for Infection Control Precautions to prevent transmission while caring for the patient in the home (Chart 19-8), nursing techniques to use in the home, and coping or support strategies.

Teach the patient, family, and friends how to protect the patient from infection, how to identify the presence of

CHART 19-7 Focused Assessment

The Person With AIDS

Assess cardiovascular and respiratory status:
- Vital signs
- Presence of acute chest pain or dyspnea
- Presence of cough
- Presence of fever
- Activity tolerance

Assess nutrition status:
- Food intake
- Weight loss or gain
- General condition of skin
- Financial resources

Assess neurologic status:
- Cognitive changes
- Motor changes
- Sensory disturbances

Assess GI status:
- Mouth and oropharynx
- Presence of dysphagia
- Presence of abdominal pain
- Presence of nausea, vomiting, diarrhea, constipation

Assess psychological status:
- Feelings, thoughts, and behaviors
- Presence of anxiety, fear, or depression
- Suicide ideation, intent, or plan
- Support systems within the family and community

Assess activity and rest:
- ADLs
- Mobility and ambulation
- Fatigue
- Sleep pattern
- Presence of pain

Assess home environment:
- Safety hazards
- Structural barriers affecting functional ability

Assess patient's and caregiver's adherence and understanding of illness and treatment, including:
- Symptoms to report to nurse
- Medication schedule and side or toxic effects

Assess patient's and caregiver's coping skills.

infections, and what to do if these appear. Teach about the use of self-care strategies such as good hygiene, balanced rest and exercise, skin care, mouth care, and safe administration and potential side effects of all prescribed drugs. During diet teaching stress good NUTRITION; the need to avoid raw or rare fish, fowl, or meat; thorough washing of fruits and vegetables; and proper food refrigeration.

Teach the patient to avoid large crowds, especially in enclosed areas; not to travel to countries with poor sanitation; and to avoid cleaning pet litter boxes. Chart 19-4 lists more strategies to teach the patient and family how to avoid infection.

Psychosocial Preparation. Patients with AIDS often fear social stigma and rejection. Help patients identify strengths and coping strategies for difficult situations. Support family members and friends in efforts to help the patient and provide protection from discrimination.

Encourage patients to continue as many usual activities as possible. Except when too ill or too weak, they can continue to work and participate in most social activities. Support them in their selection of friends and relatives with whom to discuss the diagnosis. Stress that sexual partners and care providers should be informed; beyond that, it is up to the patient. Some patients

CHART 19-8 Best Practice for Patient Safety & Quality Care **QSEN**

Infection Control for Home Care of the Person With AIDS

Direct Care
- Follow Standard Precautions and good handwashing techniques.
- Do not share razors or toothbrushes.

Housekeeping
- Wipe up feces, vomit, sputum, urine, or blood or other body fluids and the area with soap and water. Dispose of solid wastes and solutions used for cleaning by flushing them down the toilet. Disinfect the area by wiping with a 1:10 solution of household bleach (1 part bleach to 10 parts water). Wear gloves during cleaning.
- Soak rags, mops, and sponges used for cleaning in a 1:10 bleach solution for 5 minutes to disinfect them.
- Wash dishes and eating utensils in hot water and dishwashing soap or detergent.
- Clean bathroom surfaces with regular household cleaners and then disinfect them with a 1:10 solution of household bleach.

Laundry
- Rinse clothes, towels, and bedclothes if they become soiled with feces, vomitus, sputum, urine, or blood. Dispose of the soiled water by flushing it down the toilet. Launder these clothes with hot water and detergent with 1 cup of bleach added per load of laundry.
- Keep soiled clothes in a plastic bag.

Waste Disposal
- Dispose of needles and other "sharps" in a labeled puncture-proof container such as a coffee can with a lid or empty liquid bleach bottle, using Standard Precautions, to avoid needlestick injuries. Decontaminate full containers by adding a 1:10 bleach solution. Then seal the container with tape and place it in a paper bag. Dispose of the container in the regular trash.
- Remove solid waste from contaminated trash (e.g., paper towels or tissues, dressings, disposable incontinence pads, disposable gloves); then flush the solid waste down the toilet. Place the contaminated trash items in tied plastic bags and dispose of them in the regular trash.

have depression or anxiety about the future. Almost all feel the burden of having a fatal disease widely considered unacceptable and feel compelled to maintain some secrecy about the illness. Referrals to community resources, mental health professionals, and support groups can help the patient verbalize fears and frustrations and cope with the illness.

Health Care Resources. In many cities community groups and volunteers assist adults with AIDS. The types and number of services vary by agency and city, but many include HIV testing and counseling, clinic services, buddy systems, support groups, respite care, education and outreach, referral services, and housing. Patients may need referrals to other local resources such as home care agencies, companies that provide home IV therapy, community mental health/behavioral health agencies, Meals on Wheels, transportation services, and others. In addition, educational materials and support groups are available through Internet access.

◆ Evaluation: Reflecting

The overall outcomes for care of patients with AIDS are to maintain the highest possible level of function for as long as possible, reduce infections, and maintain quality of life and dignity during the course of progressive illness. Evaluate the care of the patient with AIDS on the basis of the identified priority problems. Expected outcomes include that he or she will:

- Adhere to the prescribed drug therapy regimen at least 90% of the time
- Practice safer sex techniques all of the time
- Remain free from opportunistic infections
- Have adequate GAS EXCHANGE
- Achieve an acceptable level of physical comfort
- Attain adequate weight and NUTRITION and fluid status
- Maintain TISSUE INTEGRITY
- Remain oriented
- Identify personal strengths
- Use effective coping strategies
- Maintain a support system and involvement with others

? CLINICAL JUDGMENT CHALLENGE 19-2

Ethics; Patient-Centered Care; Teamwork and Collaboration **QSEN**

During morning rounds, one of the unlicensed assistive personnel (UAP) makes a comment to another UAP that she is glad not to be assigned to that "nasty" patient with AIDS today. The patient has also requested not to be assigned to this UAP because she wears gloves for all actions and tries to provide care without touching him.
1. How will you address this issue with the UAP?
2. Should you force this UAP to provide care to this patient? Why or why not?
3. What should you say to the patient?
4. Which, if any, ethical issues are in play here? (You may need to review the principles of ethics in Chapter 1).

GET READY FOR THE NCLEX® EXAMINATION!

KEY POINTS

Review these key points for each NCLEX Client Needs Category.

Safe and Effective Care Environment
- Use Standard Precautions for all patients, regardless of age, gender, race or ethnicity, sexual orientation, education level, and profession. **QSEN: Safety**

- Follow the best practices outlined in Chart 19-5 to protect the hospitalized immunosuppressed patient from infection. **QSEN: Safety**
- Use correct handwashing techniques before providing any care to a patient who has reduced IMMUNITY. **QSEN: Safety**
- Teach unlicensed assistive personnel (UAP) to use Standard Precautions. **QSEN: Teamwork and Collaboration**

- Collaborate with the primary health care provider, registered dietitian, respiratory therapist, pharmacist, social worker, and case manager to individualize patient care for the adult with HIV disease and AIDS in any care setting. **QSEN: Teamwork and Collaboration**
- Teach the patient and family to protect against infection transmission by following the recommendations in Chart 19-4. **QSEN: Safety**
- Teach the patient and family about the signs of infection and when to seek medical advice. **QSEN: Safety**

Health Promotion and Maintenance
- Urge all patients who are HIV positive to use condoms and other precautions during sexual intimacy even if the partner is also HIV positive. **QSEN: Evidence-Based Practice**
- Teach patients with protein-calorie malnutrition which foods to include in the diet to promote better NUTRITION. **QSEN: Patient-Centered Care**
- Urge patients to adhere to their antiviral drug regimen. **QSEN: Evidence-Based Practice**
- Refer patients newly diagnosed with HIV infection to local resources and support groups. **QSEN: Patient-Centered Care**

Psychosocial Integrity
- Urge all patients who are HIV positive to inform their sexual partners of their HIV status. **QSEN: Patient-Centered Care**
- Respect the patient's right to inform or not to inform family members about his or her HIV status. **Ethics**
- Ensure the confidentiality of the patient's HIV status. **Ethics**

- Use a nonjudgmental approach when discussing sexual practices, sexual behaviors, and recreational drug use. **QSEN: Patient-Centered Care**
- Encourage the patient to express his or her feelings about a change in health status or the diagnosis of an "incurable" disease. **QSEN: Patient-Centered Care**
- Allow patients who have a change in physical appearance to express feelings of loss and mourn this change. **QSEN: Patient-Centered Care**

Physiological Integrity
- Use prescribed oxygen therapy, drug therapy, and respiratory support to improve GAS EXCHANGE for the patient with respiratory problems related to reduced IMMUNITY. **QSEN: Evidence-Based Practice**
- Use pharmacologic and nonpharmacologic therapies to reduce pain for the patient with HIV disease and AIDS. **QSEN: Patient-Centered Care**
- Teach the patient and caregivers the schedule, side effects, and possible drug interactions of combination antiretroviral therapy (cART). **QSEN: Patient-Centered Care**
- Pace nonurgent health care activities to reduce the risk for fatigue for patients with AIDS. **QSEN: Patient-Centered Care**
- Assess the patient with impaired IMMUNITY every shift for signs of infection. Document the assessment findings and report any indication of infection immediately to the primary health care provider. **QSEN: Safety**
- Assess the TISSUE INTEGRITY of the perianal region of a patient with AIDS-related diarrhea after every bowel movement. **QSEN: Evidence-Based Practice**

SELECTED BIBLIOGRAPHY

Asterisk indicates a classic or definitive work on this subject.

Adams-Tufts, K., Johnson, K., Shepherd, J., Lee, J., Bait-Ajzoon, M., Mahan, L., et al. (2015). Novel interventions for HIV self-management in African-American women: A systematic review of mHealth interventions. *Journal of the Association of Nurses in AIDS Care, 26*(2), 139–150.

Anastasi, J., Capili, B., & Chang, M. (2013). HIV peripheral neuropathy and foot care management: A review of assessment and relevant guidelines. *The American Journal of Nursing, 113*(12), 34–40.

*Centers for Disease Control and Prevention (CDC). (1987). Public Health Service guidelines for counseling and antibody testing to prevent HIV infection and AIDS. *Morbidity and Mortality Weekly Report, 36*(31), 509–515.

*Centers for Disease Control and Prevention (CDC). (1991). Recommendations for preventing transmission of human immunodeficiency virus and hepatitis B virus to patients during exposure-prone invasive procedures. *Morbidity and Mortality Weekly Report, 40*(RR-8), 1–9.

*Centers for Disease Control and Prevention (CDC). (2005). Updated Public Health Service guidelines for the management of health-care worker exposure to HIV and recommendations for postexposure prophylaxis. *Morbidity and Mortality Weekly Report, 54*(RR-9), 1–22.

*Centers for Disease Control and Prevention (CDC). (2009). Guidelines for prevention and treatment of opportunistic infections in HIV-infected adults and adolescents. *Morbidity and Mortality Weekly Report, 58*(RR-4), 1–207.

Centers for Disease Control and Prevention (CDC). (2015a). *HIV in the United States: At a glance.* https://www.cdc.gov/hiv/pdf/statistics_basics_ataglance_factsheet.pdf.

Centers for Disease Control and Prevention (CDC). (2015b). *HIV surveillance report, 2014* (vol. 26). From: http://www.cdc.gov/hiv/pdf/library/reports/surveillance/cdc-hiv-surveillance-report-us.pdf.

Centers for Disease Control and Prevention (CDC). (2015c). *Preexposure prophylaxis (PrEP).* From: www.cdc.gov/hiv/risk/prep/index.html.

Costello, J., Carpentier, M., Slinely, A., MacLeod, C., Young, K., & Flanigan, T. (2016). Evaluation of a nurse-initiated routine HIV testing pilot on a medical-surgical unit. *Medsurg Nursing, 25*(1), 36–43.

Government of Canada (2015). *Summary: Estimates of HIV incidence, prevalence and proportion undiagnosed in Canada, 2014.* From: healthycanadians.gc.ca/publications/diseases-conditions-maladies-affections/hiv-aids-estimates-vih-sida-estimations/alt/hiv-aids-estimates-2014-vih-sida-estimations-eng-pdf.

Gant-Clark, V., Skipper, J., McCrackin, M., Gaillard, S., & Coxe, D. N. (2015). Veterans and HIV screening rates: What veterans are not getting tested, a veterans affairs nursing academic partnership (VANAP). *Journal of the Association of Nurses in AIDS Care, 26*(4), 485–491.

Grimes, R., Hardwicke, R., Grimes, D., & DeGarmo, S. (2016). When to consider acute HIV infection in the differential diagnosis. *The Nurse Practitioner, 41*(1), 1–5.

Keithley, J., & Swanson, B. (2013). HIV-associated wasting. *Journal of the Association of Nurses in AIDS Care, 24*(1S), S103–S111.

Kwong, J., & Gabler, S. (2015). Counseling, screening, and therapy for newly-diagnosed HIV patients. *The Nurse Practitioner, 40*(10), 34–43.

Lanier, Y., & Sutton, M. (2013). Reframing the context of preventive health care services and prevention of HIV and other sexually transmitted infections for young men: New opportunities to reduce racial/ethnic sexual health disparities. *American Journal of Public Health, 103*(2), 262–269.

Mayer, K., & Krakower, D. (2015). Scaling up antiretroviral preexposure prophylaxis: Moving from trials to implementation. *Clinical Infectious Diseases: An Official Publication of the Infectious Diseases Society of America, 61*(10), 1598–1600.

McCance, K., Huether, S., Brashers, V., & Rote, N. (2014). *Pathophysiology: The biologic basis for disease in adults and children* (7th ed.). St. Louis: Mosby.

Mitchell, A., & Parker, G. (2015a). Preventing blood and body fluid splashes and splatters. *American Nurse Today, 10*(11), 25–26.

Mitchell, A., & Parker, G. (2015b). Preventing needlestick and sharps injuries. *American Nurse Today, 10*(9), 29–30.

New York State Department of Health AIDS Institute. (2014). *Free compilation of current guidelines for clinical practice.* From: www.hivguidelines.org.

Pagana, K., Pagana, T. J., & Pagana, T. N. (2017). *Mosby's diagnostic and laboratory test reference* (13th ed.). St. Louis: Mosby.

Pagana, K., Pagana, T., & Pike-MacDonald, S. (2013). *Mosby's Canadian manual of diagnostic and laboratory tests.* St. Louis: Mosby.

Rhyne, D., Byrd, E., & Klibanov, O. (2014). Dolutegravir (Tivicay) for HIV infection. *The Nurse Practitioner Journal, 39*(6), 11–15.

Starr, M., & Bradley-Springer, L. (2014). Nursing in the fourth decade of the HIV epidemic. *The American Journal of Nursing, 114*(3), 38–47.

Taylor, D., Durigon, M., Davis, H., Archibald, C., Konrad, B., Coombs, D., et al. (2015). *International Journal of STD & AIDS, 26*(4), 215–224.

Volk, J., Marcus, J., Phengrasamy, T., Bleckinger, D., Nguyen, D., Follansbee, S., et al. (2015). No new HIV infections with increasing use of HIV preexposure prophylaxis in a clinical practice setting. *Clinical Infectious Diseases: An Official Publication of the Infectious Diseases Society of America, 61*(10), 1601–1603.

World Health Organization (WHO). (2015). *HIV/AIDS Fact Sheet.* From: http://www.who.int/mediacentre/factsheets/fs360/en/#.

Care of Patients With Hypersensitivity (Allergy) and Autoimmunity

M. Linda Workman

 http://evolve.elsevier.com/Iggy/

PRIORITY AND INTERRELATED CONCEPTS

The priority concept for this chapter is IMMUNITY.

✳ The IMMUNITY concept exemplar for this chapter is Angioedema, p. 361.

The interrelated concept for this chapter is GAS EXCHANGE.

LEARNING OUTCOMES

Safe and Effective Care Environment

1. Collaborate with the interprofessional team to coordinate high-quality care and protect the patient experiencing problems of overactive IMMUNITY, including allergic reactions and autoimmunity.
2. Teach the patient and caregiver(s) how overactive IMMUNITY affects home safety.

Health Promotion and Maintenance

3. Teach patients with allergies how to protect themselves against harm from a hypersensitivity reaction and from therapies used to treat overactive IMMUNITY.

Psychosocial Integrity

4. Implement nursing interventions to help the patient and family cope with the psychosocial impact caused by hypersensitivity or autoimmunity.

Physiological Integrity

5. Apply knowledge of anatomy and physiology to assess patients who have health problems related to overactive IMMUNITY.
6. Teach the patient and caregiver(s) about common drugs used for control of autoimmunity and other forms of overactive IMMUNITY.

Usually IMMUNITY with inflammation is a protective and helpful response. However, when the response is overactive (excessive) or when it is directed against normal body tissues, damage can result (Abbas et al., 2015; McCance et al., 2014).

HYPERSENSITIVITIES/ALLERGIES

Hypersensitivity or allergy is overactive IMMUNITY with inflammation occurring in response to the presence of an antigen (foreign protein or allergen) to which the patient usually has been previously exposed. It can cause problems that range from being uncomfortable (e.g., itchy, watery eyes, or sneezing) to life threatening (e.g., allergic asthma, angioedema, anaphylaxis, bronchoconstriction, or circulatory collapse). The terms *hypersensitivity* and *allergy* are used interchangeably. Hypersensitivity reactions are classified into four basic types, determined by differences in timing, pathophysiology, and symptoms (Table 20-1). Each type may occur alone or along with one or more of the other types (McCance et al., 2014).

TYPE I: RAPID HYPERSENSITIVITY REACTIONS

Type I, or rapid hypersensitivity, also called *atopic allergy,* is the most common type of hypersensitivity from overactive IMMUNITY. It results from the increased production of the immunoglobulin E (IgE) antibody class. Acute inflammation occurs when IgE responds to an antigen such as pollen and causes the release of histamine and other vasoactive amines from basophils, eosinophils, and mast cells. Examples of type I reactions include angioedema, anaphylaxis, and allergic asthma (discussed in Chapter 30); atopic allergies such as hay fever and allergic rhinosinusitis; and allergies to substances such as latex, bee venom, peanuts, iodine, shellfish, drugs, and many other allergens. Allergens can be contacted in these ways:
- Inhaled (plant pollens, fungal spores, animal dander, house dust, grass, ragweed)
- Ingested (foods, food additives, drugs)
- Injected (bee venom, drugs, biologic substances such as contrast dyes)

- Skin or mucous membrane contacted (latex, pollens, foods, environmental proteins)

Some reactions occur just in the areas exposed to the antigen such as the mucous membranes of the nose and eyes, causing symptoms of rhinorrhea, sneezing, and itchy, red, watery eyes. Other reactions may involve all blood vessels and bronchiolar smooth muscle, causing widespread blood vessel dilation, decreased cardiac output, and bronchoconstriction. This condition is known as anaphylaxis, which is a medical emergency and must be treated immediately (see the Anaphylaxis section).

The mechanism for type I reactions is the same, regardless of whether they are widespread and severe, or localized and annoying. On first exposure to an allergen, the patient initially responds by making antigen-specific IgE. This IgE binds to the surface of basophils and mast cells (Fig. 20-1). These cells have many granules containing vasoactive amines (including histamine) that are released when stimulated. Once the antigen-specific IgE is formed, the patient is sensitized to that allergen.

When the sensitized patient is re-exposed to the allergen, the resulting response has a primary phase and a secondary phase. In the primary phase, the allergen binds to two adjacent IgE molecules on the surface of a basophil or mast cell, which alters the cell membrane. The membrane opens and releases the vasoactive amines into tissue fluids (see Fig. 20-1).

The most common vasoactive amine is *histamine,* a short-acting biochemical. Histamine causes capillary leak, nasal and conjunctival mucus secretion, and pruritus (itching), often occurring with erythema (redness). These symptoms of inflammation last for about 10 minutes after histamine is first released. When the allergen is continuously present, mast cells continuously release histamine and other inflammatory proteins, prolonging the response.

The secondary phase results from the release of other cellular proteins. These other proteins draw more white blood cells to the area and stimulate a more general inflammatory reaction through actions of leukotriene and prostaglandins (other mediators of inflammation; see Chapter 17). This reaction occurs in addition to the allergic reaction stimulated in the primary phase. The resulting inflammation increases the symptoms and continues the response.

The production of high IgE levels in response to antigen exposure is genetically based on the inheritance of many genes. Although allergic tendencies are inherited, specific allergies are *not* inherited. For example, a woman who has an allergy to penicillin but not to peanuts may have a child with an allergy to peanuts but not to penicillin.

✳ IMMUNITY CONCEPT EXEMPLAR Angioedema

❖ *PATHOPHYSIOLOGY*

Angioedema is a severe type I hypersensitivity reaction that involves the blood vessels and all layers of the skin, mucous membranes, and subcutaneous tissues in the affected area (Abbas et al., 2015). Unlike the superficial responses of allergic rhinosinusitis, the angioedema response is a deep-tissue problem of IgE-mediated release of inflammatory proteins.

Although angioedema can occur in any part of the body, it is most often seen in the lips, face, tongue, larynx, and neck (Fig. 20-2). Intestinal angioedema can also occur, with problems of severe abdominal pain, cramping, nausea, and vomiting. It can be difficult to differentiate this problem from any other acute abdominal problem.

Exposure to any ingested drug or chemical can cause the problem. The most common drugs associated with angioedema are angiotensin-converting enzyme inhibitors (ACEIs) used for

---

TABLE 20-1	**Mechanisms and Examples of Types of Hypersensitivities**
MECHANISM	**CLINICAL EXAMPLES**
Type I: Rapid or Immediate	
Reaction of IgE antibody on mast cells with antigen, which results in release of mediators, especially histamine	Hay fever (rhinosinusitis) Allergic asthma Anaphylaxis Angioedema
Type II: Cytotoxic	
Reaction of IgG with host cell membrane or antigen adsorbed by host cell membrane	Autoimmune hemolytic anemia Goodpasture's syndrome Myasthenia gravis
Type III: Immune Complex–Mediated	
Formation of immune complex of antigen and antibody, which deposits in walls of blood vessels and results in complement release and inflammation	Serum sickness Vasculitis Systemic lupus erythematosus Rheumatoid arthritis
Type IV: Delayed	
Reaction of sensitized T-cells with antigen and release of lymphokines, which activates macrophages and induces inflammation	Poison ivy Graft rejection Positive TB skin tests Sarcoidosis

IgE, Immunoglobulin E; *IgG,* immunoglobulin G; *TB,* tuberculosis.

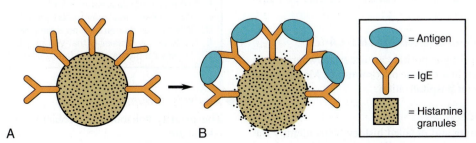

FIG. 20-1 Degranulation and histamine release. **A,** Mast cell with IgE. **B,** Mast cell degranulation and histamine release when allergen binds to IgE.

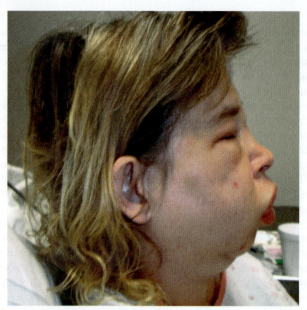

FIG. 20-2 Angioedema of the face, lips, and mouth. (From Auerbach, P. (2008). *Wilderness medicine* (5th ed.). Philadelphia: Mosby; courtesy Sheryl Olson.)

hypertension (United States Food and Drug Administration [FDA], 2014) and NSAIDs. Although only about 1 in 1000 adults taking these drugs develops angioedema, they are commonly prescribed, which accounts for the high incidence of the response among users of ACEIs and NSAIDs.

Although the greatest risk for angioedema from ACEIs is within the first 24 hours after taking the first dose, the reaction can occur after days, months, and even years of therapy (Chan & Soliman, 2015). This delay in onset of symptoms is confusing to patients who may not understand the association of the angioedema with the drug or drugs they have been taking.

⊕ CULTURAL/SPIRITUAL CONSIDERATIONS
Patient-Centered Care **QSEN**

Black adults, especially African Americans, have a higher incidence of angioedema and laryngeal edema from ACEIs (FDA, 2014). In a large study of ACEI-induced angioedema, 55% of fatalities occurred among blacks (Kim et al., 2014). Any ACEI should be used cautiously in black patients. Be sure to observe the patient carefully for any signs and symptoms of angioedema and laryngeal edema after the first dose. Teach black patients taking a drug from this category about the signs and symptoms of angioedema and the importance of going to an emergency department or calling 911 immediately if symptoms appear.

❖ INTERPROFESSIONAL COLLABORATIVE CARE

Angioedema from a drug exposure can occur anywhere but is more likely to happen in the home or community. Management requires at least a brief hospitalization.

◆ Assessment: Noticing

History. An accurate and detailed history helps identify the possible cause of angioedema. Ask the patient to list all drugs taken on a regular basis, especially drugs for blood pressure

control. Although more information can be helpful, intervention is critically important because laryngeal edema can cause the patient to lose his or her airway. Defer further history until interventions have been implemented.

Often a patient may have only lip swelling or a slight itching in the back of the throat from time to time before a fully developed case of angioedema occurs. Ask the patient specifically about whether he or she has had such a problem, when it occurred, how long it lasted, and whether any drugs were taken to reduce the symptoms. Also ask about any other allergies the patient may have. Not all patients with angioedema have a history of other allergic reactions. Because a tendency toward type I allergic responses can be inherited, ask about the presence of allergies among parents and siblings.

Physical Assessment/Signs and Symptoms. The patient with angioedema (with or without laryngeal edema) has deep, firm swelling of the face, lips, tongue, and neck. He or she may have difficulty speaking or drinking because the lips are so stiff from swelling. The face can be so distorted that friends and relatives may not recognize the patient. Often nasal swelling interferes with breathing through the nose. When swelling occurs around the eyes and eyelids, the patient may not be able to see. Some patients may have urticaria (hives), but many do not. Problems that indicate a need for immediate intervention are the inability to swallow, the feeling of a lump in the throat, or stridor.

Psychosocial Assessment. The patient with angioedema is often anxious and frightened. These feelings worsen if breathing is impaired. The rapid change in appearance is also disturbing to patients and families.

Diagnostic Assessment. Usually the patient is diagnosed based on the signs and symptoms. No specific test can diagnose angioedema, and valuable time should not be wasted in laboratory testing during an acute episode. For patients who have recurring angioedema not associated with a particular drug exposure, a blood test for C1-INH may be performed to determine whether a genetic deficiency of this substance may be the cause. This problem is known as *hereditary angioedema* and is rare. C1-INH is an enzyme that controls the C1 type of complement (see Chapter 17). When too little of this enzyme is present, complement proteins are easily activated and can cause inappropriate inflammatory reactions.

⍰ NCLEX EXAMINATION CHALLENGE 20-1
Safe and Effective Care Environment

Which questions are **most important** for the nurse to first ask a client who comes to the emergency department with signs of severe angioedema? **Select all that apply.**
A. "Are you able to swallow?"
B. "When did you last eat or drink?"
C. "Do you have an allergy to cortisone?"
D. "What drugs do you take on a daily basis?"
E. "Is there any possibility that you may be pregnant?"
F. "Do any members of your family also have allergies?"

◆ Analysis: Interpreting

The priority collaborative problems for patients with angioedema are:
1. Potential for airway obstruction due to mucosal swelling
2. Anxiety due to cerebral hypoxia and threat of death

◆ *Planning and Implementation: Responding*

Maintaining a Patent Airway. Interventions focus on stopping the reaction and ensuring an adequate airway.

Planning: Expected Outcomes. The patient with angioedema is expected to maintain a patent airway and adequate GAS EXCHANGE. Indicators include:

- End tidal carbon dioxide level within the normal range
- Rate and depth of respiration within the normal range
- Pulse oximetry within the normal range

Interventions. Prompt intervention can reverse angioedema before laryngeal edema forms and intubation is needed. Oxygen by nasal cannula is applied to help maintain GAS EXCHANGE. Because the reaction is mediated through antibodies and release of vasoactive amines (especially bradykinin), useful drugs include corticosteroids, diphendydramine, and epinephrine. Indications for intubation are the presence of stridor and the inability of the patient to swallow.

Drug therapy may need to continue for several hours after angioedema has initially resolved. Usually the agent that caused the angioedema has a longer half-life than the drugs used to treat it. This means that initial drug therapy can successfully shrink the facial, oral, and airway edema to the extent that symptoms are no longer felt or observed. However, if drug therapy is completely stopped at this point, the agent still circulating can cause angioedema to redevelop. Once drug therapy has stopped, the IV access remains, and the patient is closely monitored for 2 to 6 hours. If the angioedema does not recur, the patient is usually discharged to home.

If laryngeal edema forms and intubation is not possible, an emergency tracheostomy is needed. Location of the tracheotomy (incision into the trachea) must be below the level of the edema to ensure adequate airflow to the site of GAS EXCHANGE. Mechanical ventilation is usually not needed. The tracheostomy tube is discontinued when the patient can easily breathe around the tube. (See Chapter 28 for detailed information about tracheostomy.)

Minimizing Anxiety

Planning: Expected Outcomes. The patient with angioedema is expected to have decreased anxiety as the angioedema resolves. Indicators include that the patient:

- Verbalizes reduced anxiety
- Displays no distress or facial tension

Interventions. Anxiety is made worse by any breathing difficulty. Stay with the patient and assure him or her that proper treatment is occurring. Apply oxygen and monitor patient responses to drug and oxygen therapy. Continually assess pulse oximetry, respiratory status, and the patient's ability to swallow. Reassure the patient that, with drug therapy, the swelling will resolve and his or her appearance will return to normal within 6 to 12 hours.

Care Coordination and Transition Management

Severe angioedema is an acute emergency. With successful management the patient is discharged to resume his or her usual activities. The most important aspects of care coordination are to determine the cause of the angioedema, teach the patient to avoid the offending agent, and ensure that he or she knows to seek emergency care as soon as any signs or symptoms of the problem occur.

◆ *Evaluation: Reflecting*

Evaluate the care of the patient with angioedema based on the identified priority patient problems. The expected outcomes are that the patient:

- Maintains a patent airway
- Has anxiety reduced
- Knows what to do should angioedema recur

ANAPHYLAXIS

❖ *PATHOPHYSIOLOGY*

Anaphylaxis, the most life-threatening example of a type I hypersensitivity reaction, occurs rapidly and systemically. It affects many organs within seconds to minutes after allergen exposure. Anaphylaxis episodes can vary in severity and can be fatal. *The major factor in fatal outcomes for anaphylaxis is a delay in the administration of epinephrine* (Crawford & Harris, 2015a). Almost any substance can trigger anaphylaxis in a susceptible adult. Drugs and dyes are often causes of anaphylaxis in acute care settings; food and insect stings or bites are common causes in community settings.

Health Promotion and Maintenance

Anaphylaxis has a rapid onset and a potentially fatal outcome (even with appropriate intervention); thus prevention and early intervention are critical. *Teach the patient with a history of allergic reactions to avoid known allergens whenever possible, to wear a medical alert bracelet, and to alert health care personnel about specific allergies.* Some patients must carry an emergency anaphylaxis kit (e.g., a kit with injectable epinephrine, sometimes called a *bee sting kit*) or an epinephrine injector such as the AnaPen ♣, EpiPen, or Twinject automatic injector. The EpiPen is a spring-loaded injector that delivers 0.3 mg of epinephrine per 2-mL dose directly into the subcutaneous tissue (Fig. 20-3). Teach patients how to care for and use the device (Chart 20-1).

⚠ NURSING SAFETY PRIORITY QSEN

Action Alert

The medical records (paper or electronic) of patients with a history of anaphylaxis should prominently display the list of specific allergens. Ask the patient about drug allergies before giving any drug or agent. If he or she has a known allergy, be sure to document the allergen and the typical response produced and communicate the allergy and its response to other members of the interprofessional care team. Be aware of common cross-reacting agents. For example, a patient who is allergic to penicillin is also likely to react to cephalosporins because both have a similar chemical structure.

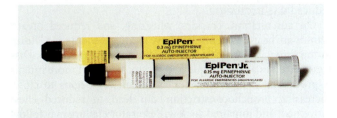

FIG. 20-3 EpiPen and EpiPen Jr. self-injectors for epinephrine. (Courtesy Dey, Napa, CA)

🏛️ **CHART 20-1** **Patient and Family Education: Preparing for Self-Management**

Care and Use of Automatic Epinephrine Injectors

- Practice assembly of injection device with a non–drug-containing training device provided through the injection device manufacturer.
- Keep the device with you at all times.
- When needed, inject the drug into the top of your thigh, slightly to the outside, holding the device so the needle enters straight down.
- You can inject the drug right through your pants; just avoid seams and pockets where the fabric is thicker.
- Use the device when *any* symptom of anaphylaxis is present and call 911. It is better to use the drug when it is not needed than to not use it when it is needed!!!
- Whenever you need to use the device, get to the nearest hospital for monitoring for at least the next 4 to 6 hours.
- Have at least two drug-filled devices on hand in case more than one dose is needed.
- Protect the device from light and avoid temperature extremes.
- Carry the device in the case provided by the manufacturer.
- Keep safety cap in place until you are ready to use the device.
- Check the device for:
  - Expiration date—If the date is close to expiring or has expired, obtain a replacement device.*
  - Drug clarity—If the drug is discolored, obtain a replacement device.
  - Security of cap—If the cap is loose or comes off accidently, obtain a replacement device.

*Some manufacturers have an automatic notification service to let you know your device is about to expire.

Take precautionary measures if a drug or agent must be used despite a history of allergic reactions. Start an IV and place intubation equipment and a tracheostomy set at the bedside. The patient is often premedicated with diphenhydramine (Benadryl, Allerdryl ♦) or a corticosteroid.

❖ INTERPROFESSIONAL COLLABORATIVE CARE

◆ Assessment: Noticing

A major problem with anaphylaxis management is that initial symptoms may be subtle, such as sudden severe abdominal cramping and diarrhea. A set of three criteria, listed in Chart 20-2, is used for diagnosis of anaphylaxis. A patient is considered to have anaphylaxis whenever any *one* of these three criteria is met, and interventions are started immediately.

Patients often have feelings of apprehension, weakness, and impending doom early in the reaction and are anxious and frightened. These feelings are followed quickly by generalized itching and urticaria (hives). Erythema and angioedema of the eyes, lips, or tongue may occur next. Intensely itchy hives may appear and may merge to form large, red blotches.

Histamine and other mediators cause inflammation, bronchoconstriction, mucosal edema, and excess mucus production. Respiratory symptoms include congestion, rhinorrhea, dyspnea, and increasing respiratory distress with audible wheezing with reduced GAS EXCHANGE.

On auscultation, crackles, wheezing, and reduced breath sounds are heard. Patients may have laryngeal edema as a "lump in the throat," hoarseness, and stridor (a crowing sound). Distress increases as the tongue and larynx swell and more mucus is produced. Stridor increases as the airway begins to close. Increasing bronchoconstriction can lead to reduced chest movement and impaired airflow. Respiratory failure may follow from laryngeal edema, suffocation, or lower airway constriction causing hypoxemia (poor blood oxygenation).

➤➤ **CHART 20-2** **Key Features**

Anaphylaxis

Clinical Criteria 1

Onset within minutes to hours of skin or mucous membrane problems involving swollen lips, tongue, soft palate, uvula; widespread hives; pruritus; or flushing along with any *one* of these new-onset symptoms:
- Respiratory distress or ineffectiveness:
  - Dyspnea
  - Bronchospasms
  - Wheezes
  - Stridor
  - Hypoxia
  - Cyanosis
  - Peak expiratory rate flow lower than the patient's usual rate
- Hypotension or any indication of reduced perfusion resulting in organ dysfunction:
  - Loss of consciousness
  - Incontinence
  - Hypotonia
  - Absent deep tendon reflexes

Clinical Criteria 2

Onset within minutes to hours of *two* or more of these symptoms after a patient has been exposed to a potential allergen:
- Skin or mucous membrane problems involving swollen lips, tongue, soft palate, uvula; widespread hives; pruritus; or flushing
- Respiratory distress or ineffectiveness as evidenced by any dyspnea, bronchospasms, wheezes, stridor, hypoxia, cyanosis, or peak expiratory rate flow lower than the patient's usual
- Hypotension or any indication of reduced perfusion resulting in organ dysfunction such as loss of consciousness, incontinence, hypotonia, or absent deep tendon reflexes
- Persistent GI problems such as nausea or vomiting, cramping, abdominal pain

Clinical Criteria 3

Onset within minutes to hours of hypotension with systolic blood pressure lower than 90 mm Hg or 30% lower than the patient's baseline systolic pressure.

Adapted from Simons, E., Ardusso, L., Bilo, M. B., El-Gamal, Y., Ledford, D., Ring, J., et al. (2011). World Allergy Organization guidelines for the assessment and management of anaphylaxis. *WAO Journal, 4*(2), 13-37.

The patient is hypotensive and has a rapid, weak, irregular pulse from extensive capillary leak and vasodilation. He or she is faint and diaphoretic with increasing anxiety and confusion.

❗ **NURSING SAFETY PRIORITY** **QSEN**

Critical Rescue

Closely monitor any patient receiving a drug that is associated with anaphylaxis to recognize symptoms early. If you suspect anaphylaxis, respond by immediately notifying the Rapid Response Team because most anaphylaxis deaths occur from dysrhythmias, shock, and cardiopulmonary arrest that are related to treatment delay.

◆ Interventions: Responding

Assess GAS EXCHANGE first. Emergency respiratory management is critical during an anaphylactic reaction because the severity of the reaction increases with time. The upper and lower airways become bronchoconstricted, which quickly impairs airflow and leads to arrest. Establish or stabilize the airway. If an IV drug is

CHART 20-3 Best Practice for Patient Safety & Quality Care QSEN

Emergency Care of the Patient With Anaphylaxis

- Immediately assess the respiratory status, airway, and oxygen saturation of patients who show any symptom of an allergic reaction.
- Call the Rapid Response Team.
- Ensure that intubation and tracheotomy equipment is ready.
- Apply oxygen using a high-flow, nonrebreather mask at 90% to 100%.
- Immediately discontinue the IV drug or infusing solution of a patient having an anaphylactic reaction to that drug or solution. **Do not** discontinue the IV, but change the IV tubing and hang normal saline.
- If the patient does not have an IV, start one immediately and run normal saline.
- Be prepared to administer epinephrine IV (preferred) or IM.
  - Epinephrine 1:1000 concentration, 0.3 to 0.5 mL IV push or IM
  - Repeat drug administration as needed every 5 to 15 minutes until the patient responds.
- Keep the head of the bed elevated about 10 degrees if hypotension is present; if blood pressure is normal, elevate the head of the bed to 45 degrees or higher to improve ventilation.
- Raise the feet and legs.
- Stay with the patient.
- Reassure the patient that the appropriate interventions are being instituted.

suspected to be causing the anaphylaxis, stop the drug immediately but do not remove the venous access because restarting an IV is difficult when the patient is severely hypotensive. Change the IV tubing and hang normal saline. Additional emergency interventions for patients with anaphylaxis are listed in Chart 20-3.

The patient with anaphylaxis is usually anxious or frightened and often expresses a sense of impending doom. Stay with the patient and reassure him or her that the appropriate interventions are being instituted.

Epinephrine (1:1000) 0.3 to 0.5 mL is the first-line drug for anaphylaxis. It is given IM or IV when symptoms appear (see Chart 20-3). This drug constricts blood vessels, improves cardiac contraction, and dilates the bronchioles. The same dose may be repeated every 5 to 15 minutes if needed (Vacca & McMahon-Bowen, 2013).

! NURSING SAFETY PRIORITY QSEN

Critical Rescue

Monitor susceptible patients for signs and symptoms of anaphylaxis. When you recognize anaphylaxis, respond by administering epinephrine as quickly as possible. Most deaths from anaphylaxis are related to delay in epinephrine administration.

Antihistamines such as diphenhydramine (Benadryl, Allerdryl ✦) 25 to 100 mg are second-line drugs and are given IV or IM for angioedema and urticaria. Other drugs used to support cardiovascular function during anaphylaxis are the same as those used in hypovolemic shock (see Chapter 37). If needed, an endotracheal tube may be inserted, or an emergency tracheostomy may be performed.

If the patient can breathe independently, give oxygen to reduce hypoxemia and promote GAS EXCHANGE. Start oxygen therapy via a high-flow nonrebreather facemask at 90% to

100% *before* arterial blood gas results are obtained. Monitor pulse oximetry to determine gas exchange adequacy. Arterial blood gases may be drawn to determine therapy effectiveness. Use suction to remove excess mucus and other secretions, if indicated. Continually assess the respiratory rate and depth, and assess breath sounds continually for bronchospasm, wheezing, crackles, and stridor. Elevate the bed to 45 degrees unless severe hypotension is present.

For bronchospasms the patient may be given an inhaled beta-adrenergic agonist such as metaproterenol (Alupent) or albuterol (Proventil) via high-flow nebulizer every 2 to 4 hours. Corticosteroids are added to emergency interventions, but they are not effective immediately. Oral steroids are continued (at lower doses) after the anaphylaxis is under control to prevent the late recurrence of symptoms.

Continually assess for changes in any system or for effects of drug therapy. For severe anaphylaxis the patient is admitted to an ICU for cardiac, pulmonary arterial, and capillary wedge pressure monitoring. Observe for fluid overload from the rapid drug and IV fluid infusions and report changes to the primary health care provider immediately. The patient is discharged from the hospital when respiratory and cardiovascular functions have returned to normal.

ALLERGIC RHINOSINUSITIS

❖ PATHOPHYSIOLOGY

Allergic rhinosinusitis, or *hay fever,* is triggered by IMMUNITY and inflammatory reactions to airborne allergens, especially plant pollens, molds, dust, animal dander, wool, food, and air pollutants. Some acute episodes are "seasonal," recurring at the same time each year and lasting only a few weeks. It can also occur continuously when an adult is exposed to certain allergens. Unlike angioedema, this form of type I reaction usually involves only superficial layers of the skin and mucous membranes and their associated blood vessels.

Symptoms of allergic rhinosinusitis are the same as those for rhinosinusitis caused by infection (see Chapter 31). These include pain over the cheek radiating to the teeth, tenderness to percussion over the sinuses, referred pain to the temple or back of the head, and general facial pain that is worse when bending forward.

❖ INTERPROFESSIONAL COLLABORATIVE CARE

Management first focuses on symptom relief and patient education. Teach the patient about correct use of the drug therapy prescribed. When the specific allergen is identified, such as animal dander, teach him or her to avoid coming into contact with the allergen. If symptoms do not respond to typical drug therapy or if they are severe and chronic, the patient may need immunotherapy for greater relief.

Drug therapy for symptom relief can be effective in reducing the allergic response and making the patient more comfortable. Drugs commonly include decongestants and intranasal steroid spray. *Antihistamines, leukotriene inhibitors,* and *mast cell stabilizers* block or reduce the amount of chemical mediators in nasal and sinus tissues and prevent local edema and itching. *Decongestants* constrict blood vessels and decrease edema. Analgesics may be given for pain.

Immunotherapy, also known as *desensitization therapy* or *allergy shots,* involves subcutaneous injections of very dilute solutions of the identified allergens. Thus allergy testing by skin testing or intradermal testing must be performed first to correctly identify the allergens. A 0.05-mL dose of this solution is injected subcutaneously. Usually an increasing dose is given weekly until the patient is receiving a 0.5-mL dose. The patient is then started on the lowest dose of the next higher concentration of allergen solution. The process is repeated with increasing concentrations of allergen solutions until the patient is receiving the maximum dose of the greatest concentration (usually 1:100), depending on his or her response. The recommended full course of treatment is about 5 years.

Immunotherapy appears to reduce allergic responses by competition. In theory, the very small amounts of allergen first injected are too low to bind to the IgE already present but are enough to induce immunoglobulin G (IgG) production against that allergen. IgG is not attached to either mast cells or basal cells, and allergens that bind to IgG do not trigger allergic responses. IgG then clears the allergen from the body. By gradually increasing the allergen injection, large amounts of IgG are produced against the allergen. When the patient is then exposed to the allergen in the environment, the IgG binds to it and clears it from the body before IgE can bind to it and trigger an allergic reaction. Because so much more IgG can be produced compared with IgE, IgG is successful in the competition to bind the allergen (Abbas et al., 2015).

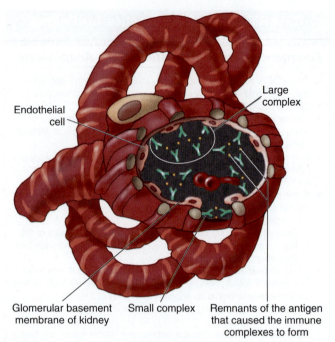

FIG. 20-4 An immune complex in a type III hypersensitivity reaction.

Labels: Endothelial cell — Large complex — Glomerular basement membrane of kidney — Small complex — Remnants of the antigen that caused the immune complexes to form

Complications such as hemolytic crisis and kidney failure can be life threatening.

TYPE III: IMMUNE COMPLEX REACTIONS

In a type III reaction excess antigens cause immune complexes to form in the blood (Fig. 20-4). These circulating complexes then lodge in small blood vessels of the kidneys, skin, and joints. The complexes trigger inflammation, and tissue or vessel damage results.

Many immune complex disorders (mostly autoimmune disorders) are caused by type III reactions. For example, the symptoms of rheumatoid arthritis are caused by immune complexes that lodge in joint spaces followed by tissue destruction, scarring, and fibrotic changes. Systemic lupus erythematosus (SLE) has immune complexes lodged in blood vessels (vasculitis), the glomeruli (glomerulonephritis), the joints (arthralgia, arthritis), and other organs and tissues.

Serum sickness is a group of symptoms that occurs after receiving serum or certain drugs. Immune complexes are deposited in blood vessel walls of the skin, joints, and kidneys and cause tissue damage. Common causes of serum sickness are penicillin, other antibiotics, and some animal serum-based drugs.

The patient with serum sickness has fever, arthralgia (achy joints), rash, malaise, lymphadenopathy (enlarged lymph nodes), and possibly polyarthritis and nephritis about 7 to 12 days after receiving the causative agent. Teach him or her about the possibility of serum sickness and what symptoms to look for whenever you give a foreign serum. Also keep emergency equipment and drugs close at hand in case he or she has an anaphylactic reaction.

Serum sickness is usually self-limiting, and symptoms subside after several days. Management is symptomatic; antihistamines are given for itching, and aspirin is given for arthralgias. Prednisone is given for severe symptoms.

? CLINICAL JUDGMENT CHALLENGE 20-1

Safety; Patient-Centered Care **QSEN**

Your 52-year-old next-door neighbor comes to your house and tells you that he woke up an hour ago with swollen lips and swelling of his lower face. He tells you that in the past hour his tongue also has become swollen, making it difficult for him to speak clearly. He is supposed to leave in 2 hours for the airport for a week-long business trip. When you ask him whether this has ever happened to him before, he says "No," and wonders if he is "coming down with something." When you ask him which medications he has taken today, he tells you that he took his usual 81 mg of aspirin and his usual lisinopril 10 mg on arising this morning. He asks whether he should just take diphenhydramine (Benadryl) and head for the airport.

1. What should your first assessment be? Provide a rationale for your answer.
2. Do you think he has angioedema or anaphylaxis? Explain your choice.
3. Are either of his usual medications associated with this type of response?
4. Should you advise him to take the diphenhydramine and go on his trip as planned? Why or why not?
5. What should your next action be?

TYPE II: CYTOTOXIC REACTIONS

In a type II (cytotoxic) reaction the body makes autoantibodies directed against self cells that have some form of foreign protein attached to them. The autoantibody binds to the self cell and forms an immune complex (see Fig. 17-10). The self cell is then destroyed along with the attached protein. Examples of type II reactions include immune hemolytic anemias, immune thrombocytopenic purpura, hemolytic transfusion reactions (when a patient receives the wrong blood type during a transfusion), and drug-induced hemolytic anemia.

Management of type II reactions begins with discontinuing the offending drug or blood product. *Plasmapheresis* (filtration of the plasma to remove specific substances) to remove autoantibodies may be beneficial. Otherwise treatment is symptomatic.

TYPE IV: DELAYED HYPERSENSITIVITY REACTIONS

In a type IV reaction the reactive cell is the T-lymphocyte (T-cell). Antibodies and complement are not involved (Abbas et al., 2015). Sensitized T-cells (from a previous exposure) respond to an antigen by releasing chemical mediators and triggering macrophages to destroy the antigen. A type IV response typically occurs hours to days after exposure. It consists of edema, induration, ischemia, and tissue damage at the site of the exposure.

An example of a small type IV reaction is a positive purified protein derivative (PPD) test for tuberculosis (TB). In a patient previously exposed to TB, an intradermal injection of this agent causes sensitized T-cells to clump at the injection site, release lymphokines, and activate macrophages. Induration and erythema at the injection site appear after about 24 to 72 hours.

Other examples of type IV reactions include contact dermatitis such as poison ivy skin rashes, local response to insect stings, tissue transplant rejections, and sarcoidosis.

The reaction is self-limiting in 5 to 7 days, and the patient is treated symptomatically. Monitor the reaction site and sites distal to the reaction for circulation adequacy. Histamine (H$_1$) antagonists such as diphenhydramine (Benadryl) are not useful for type IV reactions because histamine is not the main mediator. Because IgE does not cause this type of reaction, desensitization does not reduce the response. Corticosteroids can reduce the discomfort and help resolve the reaction more quickly.

AUTOIMMUNITY

❖ PATHOPHYSIOLOGY

Autoimmunity is a process whereby an inappropriate IMMUNITY develops to an adult's own tissues. In this response the body's antibodies or lymphocytes are directed against the body's own healthy normal cells and tissues, not just against invaders. The immune system essentially loses some ability to tolerate self cells and tissues. (Chapter 17 discusses the principles of immunity self-tolerance.) Examples of diseases that have an autoimmune cause are listed in Table 20-2. Some diseases such as type 1 diabetes mellitus may have multiple causes, one of which is autoimmune. Autoimmune diseases are

TABLE 20-2 Disorders With an Autoimmune Basis

- Ankylosing spondylitis (AS)
- Autoimmune hemolytic anemia
- Autoimmune thrombocytopenic purpura
- Celiac disease (CeD)
- Crohn's disease (CD)
- Diabetes (type 1)
- Dermatomyositis
- Erythema nodosum leprosum (ENL)
- Glomerulonephritis
- Goodpasture's syndrome
- Grave's disease
- Hashimoto's thyroiditis
- Idiopathic Addison's disease
- Irritable bowel disease (IBD)
- Multiple sclerosis (MS)
- Myasthenia gravis
- Pernicious anemia
- Psoriasis (PS)
- Psoriatic arthritis (PSA)
- Rheumatoid arthritis (RA)
- Reiter's syndrome
- Scleroderma
- Sjögren's syndrome (SS)
- Systemic lupus erythematosus (SLE)
- Ulcerative colitis (UC)
- Uveitis
- Vasculitis

common, chronic, progressive, and self-perpetuating (Abbas et al., 2015).

Development of autoimmune disease with failure of some immunity components to tolerate self is complex, involving genetic susceptibility or predisposition and environmental interactions. The incidence of autoimmunity within the general population is about 5% (Abbas et al., 2015; Jorde et al., 2016). However, the incidence is far higher in some families than in others.

GENDER HEALTH CONSIDERATIONS
Patient-Centered Care QSEN

Virtually all autoimmune disorders, especially rheumatic disorders, occur much more commonly among women than men (McCance et al., 2014). The risk for autoimmune disease among women compared with men ranges from 5:1 to 20:1 (Abbas et al., 2015).

GENETICS/GENOMICS CONSIDERATIONS
Patient-Centered Care QSEN

There is a strong genetic component to autoimmune disease development. Twin studies confirm the link between genetic inheritance and autoimmunity. For dizygotic twins (fraternal twins), when one twin is diagnosed with an autoimmune disease, the incidence of autoimmune disease development in the other twin is about 6%, nearly the same as the general population. For monozygotic twins (identical twins), when one twin is diagnosed with an autoimmune disease, the incidence of autoimmune disease development in the other twin is about 50% (Abbas et al., 2015; Jorde et al., 2016).

Specific tissue types (determined by genetic inheritance) are much more associated with autoimmunity. Susceptible tissue types, known as *human leukocyte antigens (HLAs),* include DR2, DR3, DRB, DQA, DQB, and Cw6. Ask any patient diagnosed with autoimmune disease whether other family members have an autoimmune disease.

As normal IMMUNITY develops, most immune system cells recognize the body's own cell surface antigens and learn to tolerate them without initiating any immunologic response. Those immune system cells that do not tolerate self cells and become self-reacting are either eliminated early from the immune system or are held in check by suppressive elements. A variety of immune system cells and cell products regulate these self-reactive IMMUNITY components to prevent attack and damage of normal, healthy self cells. Among these is a substance known as *cytotoxic T lymphocyte-associated protein 4 (CTLA4)*. CTLA4 binds to receptors on T-lymphocytes and helps prevent them from becoming self-reactive.

In some adults, for unknown reasons the immune system regulation of self-reacting cells fails to recognize certain tissues as self, and immune reactions are inappropriately triggered. As a result, both antibody- and cell-mediated responses and products are directed against normal body cells (McCance et al., 2014). (Antibodies directed against self tissues or cells are known as autoantibodies.) Immune system cells that cause inflammatory responses can be triggered to continue cell division and continue producing inflammatory mediators through the actions of intracellular enzymes known as *janus kinases (JAKs)*. These enzymes transmit signals from the cells' surfaces to the nucleus so that genes responsible for making inflammatory mediators are expressed and more mediators are produced.

Self-reactions can form against one type of cell and cause problems only for a specific tissue, organ, or system. A classic example of this type of selective autoimmune disease is myasthenia gravis in which the person makes antibodies against the acetylcholine receptor on muscle cells. As a result, transmission of nerve impulses to the skeletal muscles for contraction does not occur. Breathing and movement are impaired, and death can occur if the disease is not continually managed.

Self-reactions can also be directed against a specific tissue component or multiple components that are present in many organs or tissues, resulting in widespread problems or symptoms. An example of this type of autoimmunity is systemic lupus erythematosus (SLE) in which autoantibodies are produced against many cellular proteins and almost all organs are affected to some degree.

All autoimmune diseases have inflammation as part of the reaction that can damage tissues. Unregulated immune system cells and products stimulate the production of pro-inflammatory cytokines, especially interleukins 12, 17, and 23 (IL-12, IL-17, IL-23); gamma interferon; and tumor necrosis factor (TNF). These substances not only cause direct damage to tissues but also increase the cell growth rate for skin cells (inducing the scaling lesions of psoriasis) and inflammatory white blood cells (especially macrophages), which then continue the attack on self-tissues. TNF has several subtypes, and each subtype binds to its specific receptors to induce tissue-damaging actions. In addition to immune system cells producing TNF, some cells within joints such as synovial cells and epithelial cells also produce TNF (Crawford & Harris, 2015b).

❖ INTERPROFESSIONAL COLLABORATIVE CARE

There is no cure for autoimmune diseases. Management depends on the organ or organs affected. For example, in type 1 diabetes the patient uses insulin to manage the disease and its complications, not drugs that alter IMMUNITY. For other autoimmune diseases, such as rheumatoid arthritis or psoriasis in which controlling the immune response is the best way to manage the disorder, anti-inflammatory drugs and immunosuppressive drugs are commonly used along with symptomatic treatment to suppress the overactive immunity. Drug therapy often involves a combination of general immunosuppressant agents and selective immunosuppressive agents. Patient responses to therapy drive the types and combinations of drugs used. Regardless of the specific agents used, the desired outcomes of drug therapy for autoimmune disease are:

- Self-reacting, immune-mediated tissue-damaging actions slow or stop.
- Symptoms of autoimmune disease are reduced.
- The patient retains enough IMMUNITY to prevent serious infections.

General Immunosuppressive Therapy

The two drug categories of general immunosuppressive therapy for autoimmune diseases are corticosteroids and cytotoxic drugs. These two drug categories have many systemic harmful side effects and can lead to profound general immunosuppression. With the development of more specific immunosuppressant drugs, these less specific agents now have smaller roles in therapy for autoimmune diseases.

Corticosteroids. Corticosteroids are drugs similar to natural cortisol that suppress bone marrow production of all white blood cells (WBCs) and inhibit immune responses, as well as inflammation. Because the corticosteroids cause such a general immunosuppression and can greatly increase the patient's risk for infection, they now are used more sparingly than in years past. Chapter 62 discusses the side effects of corticosteroids and the associated nursing care and patient education.

Cytotoxic Drugs. *Cytotoxic drugs* are those with actions that purposely destroy cells. They are used most commonly as cancer chemotherapy with the intent of killing off cancer cells. Because any rapidly dividing cells are more sensitive to the killing effects of these drugs, WBCs are suppressed. For this action cytotoxic drugs such as methotrexate and cyclophosphamide have been used in lower dosages than required for cancer therapy to suppress cell division of WBCs, which then reduces the overactive IMMUNITY experienced by patients with various autoimmune diseases. For some patients these drugs are still used along with selective immunosuppressive therapy to control severe autoimmune diseases. Chapter 22 discusses the side effects of cytotoxic drugs and the associated nursing care and patient education.

Selective Immunosuppressive Therapy

Selective immunosuppressive therapy with single drugs may be used successfully to control autoimmune diseases for some patients. For others, drugs from more than one category of selective immunosuppressant agents are used along with more general immunosuppressant drugs. Patient responses guide therapy and often are highly individual. The classes for drugs used to manage autoimmune diseases are the antiproliferative agents, calcineurin inhibitors, and disease-modifying antirheumatic drugs (DMARDS).

> **! NURSING SAFETY PRIORITY** QSEN
> **Drug Alert**
>
> All selective immunosuppressants reduce protective IMMUNITY to some degree and increase the patient's risk for new infections and reactivation of dormant infections such as tuberculosis. These drugs are not to be started on any patient with a current infection. Tuberculosis testing is usually performed before starting any selective immunosuppressant. Teach patients taking these drugs to avoid crowds and people who are ill. Also teach them to contact their primary health care provider at the first sign of an infection.

Antiproliferative Drugs. *Antiproliferative drugs* slow the growth of immune system cells responsible for autoimmune diseases in several ways. Azathioprine, although somewhat less selective than other antiproliferatives, inhibits the metabolism of purines, which are important in DNA synthesis and cell division. It suppresses the actions of the lymphocytes that cause tissue damage in some autoimmune diseases.

Mycophenolate is more selective in suppressing lymphocyte activity than azathioprine. This drug reversibly inhibits an enzyme needed for lymphocyte reproduction. It also prevents T-lymphocytes already present from being active. Both actions selectively suppress the immune responses most associated with autoimmune tissue destruction.

Sirolimus selectively inhibits T-lymphocyte activation and reproduction by blocking the signal transduction pathways, especially mTOR, that promote movement of T-lymphocytes through the cell cycle for cell division. This drug also interferes with the ability of B-lymphocytes to mature into antibody-producing cells. The overall amount of antibodies produced, including autoantibodies, is significantly reduced.

Everolimus acts in a similar way to sirolimus. It also inhibits the mTOR pathway important to cell division and proliferation in lymphocytes. This drug greatly reduces protein synthesis and cell division in immune system cells that attack self cells.

⚠ NURSING SAFETY PRIORITY QSEN

Drug Alert

All antiproliferative drugs are associated with poor pregnancy outcomes, and pregnancy is an absolute contraindication for their use. Teach sexually active women in childbearing years to use two reliable methods of contraception during therapy with antiproliferatives and for 12 weeks after they are discontinued. Breast-feeding while taking these drugs is also contraindicated.

Calcineurin Inhibitors. *Calcineurin inhibitors* bind to proteins that normally promote T-lymphocyte activation and gene expression that causes increased production of pro-inflammatory cytokines (especially interleukins and tumor necrosis factor) and increased production of macrophages and other white blood cells. The calcineurin inhibitors form a complex with these proteins that suppresses T-lymphocyte activation, resulting in fewer pro-inflammatory cytokines and inflammatory white blood cells. These actions result in less damage to tissues and organs. The two drugs in this class are cyclosporine and tacrolimus. Although these drugs are used more in the prevention of transplant rejection (see Chapter 17), they are also used in the management of psoriasis and Sjögren syndrome.

Disease-Modifying Antirheumatic Drugs. *Disease-modifying antirheumatic drugs (DMARDs)* are drugs that reduce the progression and tissue destruction of the inflammatory disease process largely by inhibiting tumor necrosis factor (TNF) or its receptors. Some also have effects against other substances needed in the inflammatory tissue-destruction pathway(s). There are a variety of drugs in this category with different mechanisms of action. See Chart 20-4 for a listing of DMARDs and the associated nursing implications.

Biologic DMARDs. The biologic DMARDs are monoclonal antibodies directed against inflammatory cells or their receptors or products that attack and destroy healthy self cells. The monoclonal antibodies are administered intravenously or subcutaneously.

Some biologic DMARDs are directed against one or more subtypes of TNF, preventing it from binding to its receptors and stimulating tissue-destructive actions. These drugs include adalimumab (Humira), certolizumab (Cimzia), etanercept (Enbrel), golimumab (Simponi), and infliximab (Remicade). Although TNF is the primary target of these drugs, the resulting actions also decrease many other pro-inflammatory cytokines as a secondary response. Most DMARDs with this mechanism of action are approved for management of rheumatoid arthritis

(RA), psoriasis, ankylosing spondylitis, Crohn's disease, and ulcerative colitis.

Some DMARDs work by competing with interleukin-1 (IL-1), which is a pro-inflammatory cytokine. These drugs resemble parts of IL-1 and bind to the IL-1 receptor but do not activate it. The response is decrease inflammatory reactions. Drugs in this category include anakinra (Kineret) and canakinumab (Ilaris). Both drug are approved for management of RA.

Tocilizumab (Actemra) is a monoclonal antibody that binds to the interleukin-6 (IL-6) receptor, preventing the pro-inflammatory cytokine IL-6 from binding to it. The response is decreased inflammatory responses. It is approved to manage RA.

Ustekinumab (Stelara) is a monoclonal antibody to a protein (p40) found on the surface of many T-lymphocytes. When the drug binds to p40, the cell is unable to bind with interleukin-12 (IL-12) or interleukin-23 (IL-23). When these substances do not bind to lymphocytes, less TNF and gamma interferon are produced. As a result, inflammation and tissue damage are reduced. This drug is approved to manage psoriasis and psoriatic arthritis.

Secukinumab (Cosentyx) is an antibody that binds to the inflammatory cytokine interleukin-17 (IL-17) and prevents its interaction with receptors on lymphocytes. Lymphocytes are less active and then produce less TNF. This drug is approved to manage psoriasis, psoriatic arthritis, and ankylosing spondylitis.

Abatacept (Orencia) is a DMARD with a different mechanism of action. This drug is a fusion protein like an antibody that is very similar to CTLA4, which is an inhibitor of T-lymphocyte activation. When abatacept is administered, it acts like a synthetic CTLA4, reducing the number of activated T-lymphocytes, which results in less production of TNF, alpha interferon, autoantibodies, and pro-inflammatory interleukins. It is approved to manage RA.

Nonbiologic DMARDs. Nonbiologic DMARDs are those drugs that interfere with some critical pathway in inflammatory responses but are not monoclonal antibodies. The drugs in this class in current use include thalidomide, apremilast, and tofacitinb.

Thalidomide (Thalomid) is an oral DMARD that inhibits an enzyme important in the activation and expression of the TNF gene. Thus it reduces the amount of TNF produced. Currently its approved use is limited to the management of erythema nodosum leprosum (ENL). Thalidomide is in clinical trials for management of Crohn's disease.

Apremilast (Otezla) is an oral DMARD that reduces pro-inflammatory cytokines by inhibiting the enzyme phosphodiesterase 4 (PPD4). When this enzyme is inhibited, lymphocytes contain more of a substance (cAMP) that inhibits cytokine production. It is currently approved for management of psoriatic arthritis.

Tofacitinib (Xeljanz) is an oral DMARD that inhibits the janus kinase (JAK) enzymes. These enzymes are responsible for transmitting signals from immune system cell surfaces to the nucleus that activate the genes responsible for making some pro-inflammatory cytokines. By inhibiting the JAK enzymes, there is less inflammation and tissue damage. This drug is approved to manage RA.

CHART 20-4 **Common Examples of Drug Therapy**

Biologic Disease-Modifying Antirheumatic Drugs (DMARDs)

DRUG CATEGORY	NURSING IMPLICATIONS
Monoclonal antibodies to tumor necrosis factor (TNF) Common drug class examples: • Adalimumab (Humira) • Certolizumab (Cimzia) • Etanercept (Enbrel) • Golimumab (Simponi) • Infliximab (Remicade)	Ask the patient whether he or she has ever had tuberculosis (TB), hepatitis B (HVB), or cancer. *The immunosuppression caused by these drugs can reactivate TB and HVB and have been associated with cancer recurrence. These conditions are contraindications to the use of these drugs.* The first dose of any monoclonal antibody to TNF must be administered in a setting equipped to handle allergic reactions and anaphylaxis. *Although these reactions are rare, the antibodies are proteins that can trigger such reactions.* After administering the first dose, observe the patient for at least 2 hours to determine whether an adverse reaction, especially a severe allergic reaction, occurs. Indications of an adverse reaction include hypotension; rapid thread pulse, and decreased oxygen saturation. *Adverse reactions are most likely to occur within the first 60 to 90 minutes of receiving the drug.* Observe the patient for indications of heart failure *because these drugs are known to worsen existing heart failure and have caused new-onset heart failure.* Monitor subcutaneous injection sites for reactions (e.g., pain, redness, itching swelling), *which are common and may be painful but are not indications for stopping the drug because the reactions are localized and mild.* Document patient responses to the drug to use as a baseline for assessing future responses. Teach patients the proper technique for subcutaneous injection *because many patients will be able to self-inject the drug at home.* Ask women of child-bearing age whether they are pregnant. These drugs are not recommended during pregnancy *because they do cross the placenta and enter the fetus.* No controlled trials of the drugs have been conducted to ascertain the effect of these drugs on pregnancy outcomes. These drugs can be used during breast-feeding. *The drugs are large with high molecular weights and are unlikely to enter breast milk. In addition, they are poorly absorbed from the intestinal tract.*
Monoclonal antibodies to interleukin-1 (IL-1) Common drug class examples: • Anakinra (Kineret) • Canakinumab (Ilaris)	Ask whether the female patient is pregnant or breast-feeding before starting these drugs. *There are insufficient data to know how these drugs affect pregnancy and breast-feeding outcomes, and their use during pregnancy and breast-feeding is not recommended.* Ask the patient whether he or she has ever had TB, HVB, or cancer. *The immunosuppression caused by these drugs can reactivate TB and HVB and has been associated with cancer recurrence. These conditions are contraindications to the use of these drugs.* Just as for the monoclonal antibodies to TNF, monitor for hypersensitivity (anaphylaxis) and injection site reactions. These drugs are not to be administered by the intravenous route; *the formulation is for subcutaneous administration only.* Observe patients for a decreasing therapeutic effect over time *because many patients develop antibodies that neutralize the activity of these drugs.*
Monoclonal antibodies to interleukin-6 (IL-6) Common drug class examples: • Tocilizumab (Actemra)	Use during pregnancy and breast-feeding is the same as for monoclonal antibodies to IL-1. Infection and cancer precautions are the same as for monoclonal antibodies to TNF and IL-1. Precautions for hypersensitivity and injection site reactions are the same as for monoclonal antibodies to TNF and IL-1. Observe the patient for yellowing of the eyes and skin. Check results of liver function tests. *The drug is associated with hepatic toxicities.* May be injected intravenously or subcutaneously *because the formulation is approved for both types of administration.* Monitor blood pressure and lipid levels *because this drug is associated with development of hypertension and hyperlipidemia over time.*
Monoclonal antibodies to interleukin 17 (IL-17) Common drug class examples: • Secukinumab (Cosentyx)	Use during pregnancy and breast-feeding is the same as for monoclonal antibodies to IL-1. Infection and cancer precautions are the same as for monoclonal antibodies to TNF and IL-1. Precautions for hypersensitivity and injection site reactions are the same as for monoclonal antibodies to TNF and IL-1. Administer subcutaneously *because the formulation is not approved for the intravenous route.*
CTLA4 agonist Common drug class examples: • Abatacept (Orencia)	Use during pregnancy and breast-feeding is the same as for monoclonal antibodies to IL-1. Infection and cancer precautions are the same as for monoclonal antibodies to TNF and IL-1. Precautions for hypersensitivity and injection site reactions are the same as for monoclonal antibodies to TNF and IL-1. May be injected intravenously or subcutaneously *because the formulation is approved for both types of administration.*
Monoclonal antibodies to p40 Common drug class examples: • Ustekinumab (Stelara)	Use during pregnancy and breast-feeding is the same as for monoclonal antibodies to IL-1. Infection and cancer precautions are the same as for monoclonal antibodies to TNF and IL-1. Precautions for hypersensitivity and injection site reactions are the same as for monoclonal antibodies to TNF and IL-1. Administer subcutaneously *because the formulation is not approved for the intravenous route.*

GET READY FOR THE NCLEX® EXAMINATION!

KEY POINTS

Review these Key Points for each NCLEX Examination Client Needs Category.

Safe and Effective Care Environment

- Ensure that only latex-free products are used for a patient who has a known latex allergy. **QSEN: Safety**
- Verify that all allergies are documented in a prominent place in the patient's medical record or electronic health record. **QSEN: Safety**
- Keep emergency equipment and drugs (epinephrine, Benadryl, cortisol) in or near the room of a patient with known severe allergies or a history of anaphylaxis. **QSEN: Safety**
- Teach patients to remove common allergens from the home or avoid direct contact with them. **QSEN: Safety**

Health Promotion and Maintenance

- Urge all patients with severe allergies or those who have a history of anaphylaxis to wear a medical alert bracelet. **QSEN: Patient-Centered Care**
- Teach the patient and family about the symptoms of allergic reactions and when to seek medical help. **QSEN: Patient-Centered Care**
- Teach the patient who has a known drug allergy about which other drugs are likely to stimulate the same reactions. **QSEN: Patient-Centered Care**
- Teach the patient who carries an automatic epinephrine injector how to care for, assemble, and use the device. Obtain a return demonstration. **QSEN: Patient-Centered Care**

Psychosocial Integrity

- Explain all diagnostic procedures, restrictions, and follow-up care to the patient scheduled for tests related to hypersensitivities. **QSEN: Patient-Centered Care**
- Stay with the patient in anaphylaxis. **QSEN: Patient-Centered Care**
- Reassure patients who are in anaphylaxis that the appropriate interventions are being instituted. **QSEN: Patient-Centered Care**

Physiological Integrity

- Identify patients at risk for hypersensitivity reactions, especially anaphylaxis. **QSEN: Safety**
- Communicate a patient's allergies to all members of the interprofessional health care team. **QSEN: Safety**
- Immediately assess the respiratory status and airway of patients who show any symptoms of an allergic reaction. **QSEN: Evidence-Based Practice**
- Immediately discontinue the IV drug or solution of a patient having an anaphylactic reaction to that drug or solution. **Do not** discontinue the IV, but change the IV tubing and hang normal saline. **QSEN: Evidence-Based Practice**
- Hold the dose of any prescribed drug when a patient develops angioedema. **QSEN: Safety**
- Give oxygen to any patient in anaphylaxis. **QSEN: Evidence-Based Practice**

SELECTED BIBLIOGRAPHY

Abbas, A., Lichtman, A., & Pillai, S. (2015). *Cellular and molecular immunology* (8th ed.). Philadelphia: Saunders.

Burchum, J., & Rosenthal, L. (2016). *Lehne's pharmacology for nursing care* (9th ed.). St. Louis: Elsevier.

Caton, E., & Flynn, M. (2013). Management of anaphylaxis in the ED: A clinical audit. *International Emergency Nursing*, 21(1), 64–70.

Chan, N., & Soliman, A. (2015). Angiotensin converting enzyme inhibitor–related angioedema: Onset, presentation, and management. *Annals of Otology, Rhinology, & Laryngology*, 124(2), 89–96.

Crawford, A., & Harris, H. (2015a). Anaphylaxis: Rapid recognition and treatment. *Nursing Critical Care*, 10(4), 32–37.

Crawford, A., & Harris, H. (2015b). Understanding the effects of rheumatoid arthritis. *Nursing*, 45(11), 32–38.

Hohler, S. (2015). Latex allergies: Protecting patients and staff. *OR Nurse2015*, 9(1), 12–18.

Jorde, L., Carey, J., & Bamshad, M. (2016). *Medical genetics* (5th ed.). St. Louis: Elsevier.

Kim, S., Brooks, J., Sheikh, J., Kaplan, M., & Goldberg, B. (2014). Angioedema deaths in the United States: 1979-2010. *Annals of Allergy, Asthma, & Immunology*, 113(6), 630–634.

Krouse, H., & Krouse, J. (2014). Allergic rhinitis: Diagnosis through management. *The Nurse Practitioner*, 39(4), 20–29.

McCance, K., Huether, S., Brashers, V., & Rote, N. (2014). *Pathophysiology: The biologic basis for disease in adults and children* (7th ed.). St. Louis: Mosby.

Pagana, K., Pagana, T., & Pagana, T. (2017). *Mosby's diagnostic and laboratory test reference* (13th ed.). St. Louis: Mosby.

Pagana, K., Pagana, T., & Pike-MacDonald, S. (2013). *Mosby's Canadian manual of diagnostic and laboratory tests*. St. Louis: Mosby.

United States Food and Drug Administration (FDA). (2014). *Accupril*. Retrieved December 2015, from: http://www.accessdata.fda.gov/drugsatfda_docs/label/2014/019885s040lbl.pdf.

Vacca, V., & McMahon-Bowen, E. (2013). Anaphylaxis. *Nursing*, 43(11), 16–17.

Principles of Cancer Development

M. Linda Workman

http://evolve.elsevier.com/Iggy/

PRIORITY AND INTERRELATED CONCEPTS

The priority concept for this chapter is CELLULAR REGULATION.   *The interrelated concept for this chapter is* IMMUNITY.

LEARNING OUTCOMES

Health Promotion and Maintenance

1. Help adults identify behaviors that reduce the risk for cancer development.
2. Teach adults the recommended screening practices and schedules for specific cancer types.

Physiological Integrity

3. Apply knowledge of basic biology to understand the factors that allow or cause normal cells to lose CELLULAR REGULATION and become malignant, including the roles of oncogenes and suppressor genes.
4. Distinguish the features of normal cells from those of benign tumors and cancer cells.
5. Interpret cancer grading, ploidy, and staging reports.

Cancer is a common health problem in the United States and Canada. Over 1.8 million people are newly diagnosed with cancer each year (American Cancer Society [ACS], 2017; Canadian Cancer Society, 2016). Cancer is a life-threatening disease and without intervention leads to death. Every adult's risk for cancer differs. In addition, some types of cancer can be prevented; many have better cure rates if diagnosed early. As a nurse you can have a vital impact in educating the public about cancer prevention and early detection methods.

PATHOPHYSIOLOGY

During infancy and childhood orderly growth of cells and tissues must occur for body development and maturation. This growth and the continued cell growth needed to replace dead or damaged cells after maturation is complete are normal and controlled through CELLULAR REGULATION. As discussed in Chapter 2, cellular regulation is the process to control cellular growth, replication, and *differentiation* (maturation into a specific cell type) to maintain homeostasis. All steps in the process of cellular regulation are the result of gene interactions. Tissues that continue to grow by undergoing mitosis in adulthood include cells of the skin, hair, mucous membranes, bone marrow; and linings of organs such as the lungs, stomach, intestines, bladder, and uterus. These tissues are located in areas in which constant damage or wear is likely and continued cell growth is needed to replace dead tissues. In health this continued growth is controlled by cellular regulation to ensure that the right number of cells is always present in any tissue or organ.

For fully developed tissues and organs that stop growing by mitosis such as heart muscle, skeletal muscle, and neurons, damaged cells are replaced with scar tissue. Thus cardiac muscle cells in the heart do not undergo mitosis in adults, but fibroblastic scar tissue does.

Any new or continued cell growth not needed for normal development or replacement of dead and damaged tissues is called neoplasia. This cell growth is abnormal even if it causes no harm (is benign). Whether the new cells are benign or cancerous, neoplastic cells develop from normal cells (*parent cells*). Thus cancer cells were once normal cells but underwent genetic mutations to no longer look, grow, or function normally. The strict processes of CELLULAR REGULATION controlling normal growth and function have been lost (McCance et al., 2014). To understand how cancer cells grow, it is helpful to first understand the regulation and function of normal cells.

Biology of Normal Cells

Many different normal cells work together to make the whole body function at an optimal level. For optimal function, each cell must perform in a predictable manner. Normal cells have these characteristics:

- *Specific morphology* is the feature in which each normal cell type has a distinct and recognizable appearance, size, and shape, as shown in Fig. 21-1.

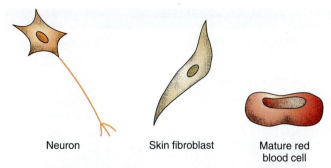

FIG. 21-1 Distinctive morphology of some normal cells.

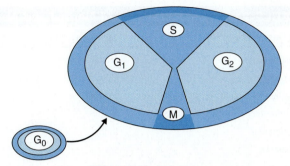

FIG. 21-2 The cell cycle.

- *A smaller nuclear-to-cytoplasmic ratio* means that the nucleus of a normal cell occupies a relatively small amount of space inside the cell. As shown in Fig. 21-1, the size of the normal cell nucleus is small compared with the size of the rest of the cell, including the cytoplasm.
- *Differentiated function* means that every normal cell has at least one function it performs to contribute to whole-body function. For example, skin cells make keratin, liver cells make bile, cardiac muscle cells contract, and red blood cells make hemoglobin.
- *Tight adherence* occurs because normal cells make proteins that protrude from the membranes, allowing cells to bind closely and tightly together. One such protein is fibronectin, which keeps most normal tissues bound tightly to each other. Exceptions are blood cells. Red blood cells and white blood cells produce no fibronectin and do not usually adhere together.
- *Nonmigratory* means that normal cells do not wander throughout the body (except for blood cells). This occurs in normal cells because they are tightly bound together, which prevents cells from wandering from one tissue into the next.
- *Orderly and well-regulated growth* or CELLULAR REGULATION is a very important feature of normal cells. They divide (undergo mitosis) for only two reasons: (1) to develop normal tissue or (2) to replace lost or damaged normal tissue. Even when they are capable of mitosis, normal cells divide only when body conditions are just right. Cell division (mitosis), occurring in a well-recognized pattern, is described by the cell cycle. Fig. 21-2 shows the phases of the cell cycle. Living cells not actively reproducing are in a reproductive resting state termed G_0. During the G_0 period, cells actively carry out their functions but do not divide. Normal cells spend most of their lives in the G_0 state rather than in a reproductive state.

    Mitosis makes one cell divide into two new cells that are identical to each other and to the cell that began mitosis. The steps of entering and completing the cell cycle are tightly controlled.

    Whether a cell enters and completes the cell cycle to form two new cells depends on the presence and absence of specific CELLULAR REGULATION proteins. Proteins that promote cells to enter and complete cell division are produced by oncogenes and are known as *cyclins*. When cyclins are activated by external or internal signaling, they allow a cell to leave G_0 and enter the cycle. These activated cyclins then drive the cell to progress through the different phases of the cell cycle and undergo cell division. Proteins produced by suppressor genes control the

amount of cyclins present and ensure that cell division occurs only when it is needed. *Thus cellular regulation of division is a balance between the oncogene protein products that promote cell division (cyclins) and the proteins that limit cell division (suppressor gene products).*
- *Contact inhibition* is CELLULAR REGULATION that stops further rounds of cell division when the dividing cell is completely surrounded and touched (contacted) by other cells. Of the normal cells that can divide, each cell divides only when some of its surface is not in direct contact with another cell. Once a normal cell is in direct contact on all surface areas with other cells, it no longer undergoes mitosis. Thus normal cell division is contact inhibited.
- *Apoptosis* is programmed cell death. Not only do normal cells have to divide only when needed and have to perform their specific differentiated functions, some cells also have to die at the appropriate time to ensure optimum body function. Thus normal cells have a finite life span. With each cell division the telomeric DNA at the ends of the cell's chromosomes shortens (see Chapter 5). When this DNA is gone, the cell responds to CELLULAR REGULATION signals for apoptosis. This ensures that each organ has an adequate number of cells at their functional peak.
- *Euploidy,* having a complete set of chromosomes, is a feature of most normal human cells. These cells have 23 pairs of chromosomes, the correct number for humans.

Biology of Abnormal Cells

Body cells are exposed to a variety of conditions that can alter how cells grow or function. When either cell growth or cell function is changed, the cells are considered abnormal. Table 21-1 compares features of normal, benign tumor, and cancer (malignant) cells.

Features of Benign Tumor Cells

Benign tumor cells are normal cells growing in the wrong place or at the wrong time as a result of a problem with CELLULAR REGULATION. Examples include moles, uterine fibroid tumors, skin tags, endometriosis, and nasal polyps. Benign tumor cells have these characteristics:
- *Specific morphology* occurs with benign tumors. They look like the tissues they come from, retaining the specific morphology of parent cells.
- *A smaller nuclear-to-cytoplasmic ratio* is a feature of benign tumors just like completely normal cells.
- *Specific differentiated functions* continue to be performed by benign tumors. For example, in endometriosis, a type of benign tumor, the normal lining of the uterus (endometrium) grows in an abnormal place (e.g., on

TABLE 21-1 Characteristics of Normal and Abnormal Cells

CHARACTERISTIC	NORMAL CELL	BENIGN TUMOR CELL	MALIGNANT CELL
Cell division	None or slow	Continuous or inappropriate	Rapid or continuous
Appearance	Specific morphologic features	Specific morphologic features	Anaplastic
Nuclear-to-cytoplasmic ratio	Smaller	Smaller	Larger
Differentiated functions	Many	Many	Some or none
Adherence	Tight	Tight	Loose
Migratory	No	No	Yes
Growth	Well regulated	Expansion	Invasion
Chromosomes	Diploid (euploid)	Diploid (euploid)	Aneuploid*
Mitotic index	Low	Low	High*

*Depends on the degree of malignant transformation.

an ovary or elsewhere in the abdominal or even the chest cavity). This displaced endometrium acts just like normal endometrium by changing each month under the influence of estrogen. When the hormone level drops and the normal endometrium sheds from the uterus, the displaced endometrium, wherever it is, also sheds.

- *Tight adherence* of benign tumor cells to each other occurs because they continue to make fibronectin.
- *No migration* or wandering of benign tissues occurs because they remain tightly bound and do not invade other body tissues.
- *Orderly growth* with normal growth patterns occurs in benign tumor cells even though their growth is not needed. The fact that growth continues beyond an appropriate time or occurs in the wrong place indicates some problem with CELLULAR REGULATION, but the rate of growth is normal. The benign tumor grows by expansion. *It does not invade.*
- *Euploidy* (normal chromosomes) are usually found in benign tumor cells, with a few exceptions. Most of these cells have 23 pairs of chromosomes, the correct number for humans.

Features of Cancer Cells

Cancer (**malignant**) cells are abnormal, serve no useful function, and are harmful to normal body tissues. Cancers commonly have these features:

- *Anaplasia* is the cancer cells' loss of the specific appearance of their parent cells. As a cancer cell becomes more malignant, it becomes smaller and rounded. Thus many different types of cancer cells look alike under the microscope.
- *A larger nuclear-cytoplasmic ratio* occurs because the cancer cell nucleus is larger than that of a normal cell and the cancer cell is smaller than a normal cell. The nucleus occupies much of the space within the cancer cell, especially during mitosis, creating a large nuclear-to-cytoplasmic ratio.
- *Specific functions are lost* partially or completely in cancer cells. *Cancer cells serve no useful purpose.*
- *Loose adherence* is typical for cancer cells because they do not make fibronectin. As a result, cancer cells easily break off from the main tumor.

- *Migration* occurs because cancer cells do not bind tightly together and have many enzymes on their cell surfaces. These features allow the cells to slip through blood vessel walls and between tissues, spreading from the main tumor site to many other body sites. The ability to spread (**metastasize**) is unique to cancer cells and is a major cause of death. Cancer cells invade other tissues, both close by and more remote from the original tumor. Invasion and persistent growth make untreated cancer deadly.
- *Contact inhibition does not occur* in cancer cells because of lost CELLULAR REGULATION, even when all sides of these cells are in continuous contact with the surfaces of other cells. This persistence of cell division makes the disease difficult to manage.
- *Rapid or continuous cell division* occurs in many types of cancer cells because they do not respond to check-point control of cell division because of gene changes that reduce the effectiveness of CELLULAR REGULATION and re-enter the cell cycle for mitosis almost continuously. In addition, these cells also do not respond to signals for apoptosis. Most cancer cells have a lot of the enzyme *telomerase,* which maintains telomeric DNA. As a result, cancer cells do not respond to apoptotic signals and have an unlimited life span (are "immortal").
- *Abnormal chromosomes* in which the chromosome number and/or structure is not normal (**aneuploidy**) are common in cancer cells as they become more malignant. Chromosomes are lost, gained, or broken; thus cancer cells can have more than 23 pairs or fewer than 23 pairs. Cancer cells also may have broken and rearranged chromosomes with mutated genes.

? NCLEX EXAMINATION CHALLENGE 21-1

Physiological Integrity

Which tumor features are **most** closely associated with malignant cells rather than benign cells? **Select all that apply.**
A. Aneuploidy
B. Growth by expansion
C. Highly differentiated
D. Large nuclear-to-cytoplasmic ratio
E. Migratory
F. Tight adhesion

CANCER DEVELOPMENT

Carcinogenesis/Oncogenesis

Carcinogenesis and oncogenesis are other names for cancer development. The process of changing a normal cell into a cancer cell is called malignant transformation, occurring through loss of CELLULAR REGULATION leading to the steps of initiation, promotion, progression, and metastasis (Jorde et al., 2016).

Initiation is the first step in carcinogenesis. Normal cells can become cancer cells if they lose CELLULAR REGULATION by having their genes promoting cell division (oncogenes) turn on excessively (are overexpressed) and produce more cyclins. Initiation is a change in gene expression caused by anything that can damage cellular DNA, leading to loss of cellular regulation. Such changes can activate oncogenes that should have only limited expression and can damage suppressor genes, which normally limit oncogene activity. Thus initiation leads to excessive cell division through DNA damage that results in loss of cellular regulation by either loss of suppressor gene function or enhancement of oncogene function. (Some researchers refer to genes promoting normal cell growth as *proto-oncogenes* and refer to oncogenes as mutated proto-oncogenes that are no longer well controlled. Others do not draw this distinction and refer to all genes promoting cell division as oncogenes.)

Initiation is an irreversible event that can lead to cancer development. After initiation a cell can become a cancer cell if the cellular regulation loss that occurred during initiation continues. *If growth conditions are right, widespread metastatic disease can develop from just one cancer cell.*

Substances that change the activity of a cell's genes so the cell becomes a cancer cell are carcinogens. Carcinogens may be chemicals, physical agents, or viruses. More than 56 agents, substances, mixtures, and exposures are known to cause cancer in humans; and about another 187 are suspected to be carcinogens (National Toxicology Program [NTP], 2016). The NTP's website (http://ntp.niehs.nih.gov/go/roc14/) lists these substances. Chapters presenting the care of patients with specific cancers discuss specific known carcinogens within the Etiology sections.

Promotion is the enhanced growth of an initiated cell by substances known as promoters. Once a normal cell has been initiated by a carcinogen and is a cancer cell, it can become a tumor if its growth is enhanced. Many normal hormones and body proteins, such as insulin and estrogen, can act as promoters and make cells divide more frequently. The time between a cell's initiation and the development of an overt tumor is called the latency period, which can range from months to years. Exposure to promoters can shorten the latency period.

Progression is the continued change of a cancer, making it more malignant over time. After cancer cells have grown to the point that a detectable tumor is formed (a 1-cm tumor has at least 1 billion cells in it), other events must occur for this tumor to become a health problem. First the tumor must develop its own blood supply. The tumor makes vascular endothelial growth factor (VEGF) that triggers nearby capillaries to grow new branches into the tumor, ensuring the tumor's continued nourishment and growth.

As tumor cells continue to divide, some of the new cells change features from the original, initiated cancer cell and form different groups. Some of the differences provide these cell groups with advantages (selection advantages) that allow them to live and divide no matter how the conditions around them change. These tumor changes may allow it to become more malignant. Over time the tumor cells have fewer and fewer normal cell features.

The original tumor is called the primary tumor. It is usually identified by the tissue from which it arose (parent tissue) such as in breast cancer or lung cancer. When primary tumors are located in vital organs such as the brain or lungs, they can grow and either lethally damage the vital organ or interfere with that organ's ability to perform its vital function. At other times the primary tumor is located in soft tissue that can expand without damage as the tumor grows. One such site is the breast. The breast is not a vital organ and, even with a large tumor, the primary tumor alone would not cause the patient's death. When the tumor spreads from the original site into vital areas, life functions can be disrupted, and death may follow.

Metastasis occurs when cancer cells move from the primary location by breaking off from the original group and establishing remote colonies. These additional tumors are called metastatic or secondary tumors. *Even though the tumor is now in another organ, it is still a cancer from the original altered tissue. For example, when breast cancer spreads to the lung and the bone, it is still breast cancer in the lung and bone—not lung cancer and not bone cancer.* Metastasis occurs through many steps, as shown in Fig. 21-3.

Tumors first extend into surrounding tissues by secreting enzymes that open up areas of surrounding tissue. Pressure, created as the tumor increases in size, forces tumor cells to invade new territory.

Spread to distant organs and tissues requires cancer cells to penetrate blood vessels. Bloodborne metastasis (tumor cell release into the blood) is the most common cause of cancer spread. Enzymes secreted by tumor cells also make large pores in the patient's blood vessels, allowing tumor cells to enter the blood and circulate. Because tumor cells are loosely held together, clumps of cells break off from the primary tumor into blood vessels for transport.

Tumor cells circulate through the blood and enter tissues at remote sites. Clumps of cancer cells can become trapped in capillaries. These clumps damage the capillary wall and allow cancer cells to leave the capillary and enter the surrounding tissue.

When conditions in the remote site can support tumor cell growth, the cells stop circulating (arrest) and invade the surrounding tissues, creating secondary tumors. Table 21-2 lists the common sites of metastasis for specific tumor types.

Another way cancers metastasize is by *lymphatic spread*. Lymphatic spread is related to the number, structure, and location of lymph nodes and vessels. Primary sites that are rich in lymphatics have earlier metastatic spread than areas with few lymphatics.

Cancer Classification

Cancers are classified by the type of tissue from which they arise (e.g., glandular, connective) (McCance et al., 2014), as described in Table 21-3. Other ways to classify cancer include biologic behavior, anatomic site, and degree of differentiation.

About 100 different types of cancer arise from various tissues or organs. Fig. 21-4 compares cancer distribution by site and gender. Cancers are either solid or hematologic. Solid tumors

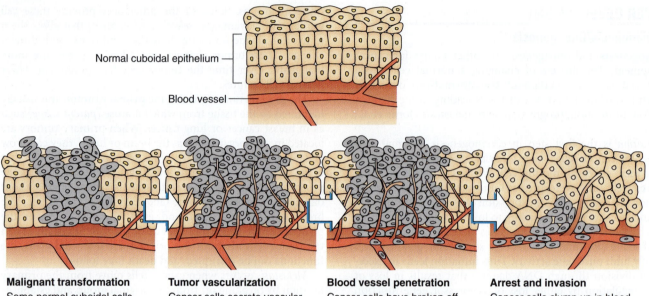

Malignant transformation
Some normal cuboidal cells have undergone malignant transformation and have divided enough times to form a tumorous area within the cuboidal epithelium.

Tumor vascularization
Cancer cells secrete vascular endothelial growth factor (VEGF), stimulating the blood vessels to bud and form new channels that grow into the tumor.

Blood vessel penetration
Cancer cells have broken off from the main tumor. Enzymes on the surface of the tumor cells make holes in the blood vessels, allowing cancer cells to enter blood vessels and travel around the body.

Arrest and invasion
Cancer cells clump up in blood vessel walls and invade new tissue areas. If the new tissue areas have the right conditions to support continued growth of cancer cells, new tumors (metastatic tumors) will form at this site.

FIG. 21-3 The steps of metastasis.

TABLE 21-2 Common Sites of Metastasis for Different Cancer Types

Breast Cancer
- Bone*
- Lung*
- Liver
- Brain

Lung Cancer
- Brain*
- Bone
- Liver
- Lymph nodes
- Pancreas

Colorectal Cancer
- Liver*
- Lymph nodes
- Adjacent structures

Prostate Cancer
- Bone (especially spine and legs)*
- Pelvic nodes

Melanoma
- GI tract
- Lymph nodes
- Lung
- Brain

Primary Brain Cancer
- Central nervous system

*Most common site of metastasis for the specific malignant neoplasm.

---

develop from specific tissues (e.g., breast cancer and lung cancer). Hematologic cancers arise from blood cell—forming tissues (e.g., leukemias and lymphomas).

Cancer Grading, Ploidy, and Staging

Systems of grading and staging have been developed to help standardize cancer diagnosis, prognosis, and treatment. Grading of a tumor classifies cellular aspects of the cancer. Ploidy classifies the number and structure of tumor chromosomes as normal or abnormal. Staging classifies clinical aspects of the cancer.

Grading is needed because some cancer cells are "more malignant" than others, varying in their aggressiveness and sensitivity to treatment. Some cancer cells barely resemble the mature tissue from which they arose (are "poorly differentiated"), are aggressive, and spread rapidly. These cells are a "high-grade" cancer. Less malignant cancer cells that are "well differentiated" and more closely resemble the mature tissue from which they arose are less aggressive. On the basis of cell appearance and activity, grading compares the cancer cell with the normal mature parent tissue from which it arose. It is a means of evaluating the patient with cancer for prognosis and appropriate therapy. Grading also allows health care professionals to evaluate the results of management.

Clinical groups have established specific grading systems for different types of cancer cells, but overall they resemble the standard system listed in Table 21-4. This system rates cancer cells with the lowest rating given to those cells that closely resemble normal cells and the highest rating given to cancer cells that barely resemble normal cells. Grading systems for different cancers are presented in the clinical chapters in which care is discussed.

Ploidy is the description of cancer cells by chromosome number and appearance. Normal human cells have 46 chromosomes (23 pairs), the normal diploid number (euploidy). When malignant transformation occurs, changes in the genes and chromosomes also occur. Some cancer cells gain or lose whole chromosomes and may have structural abnormalities of the remaining chromosomes, a condition called aneuploidy. The degree of aneuploidy increases with the degree of malignancy. Some chromosome changes are associated with specific cancers, and their presence is used for diagnosis and prognosis. One example is the "Philadelphia" chromosome abnormality often present in chronic myelogenous leukemia cells (see Chapter 40).

TABLE 21-3 Classification of Tumors by Tissue of Origin

PREFIX	TISSUE OF ORIGIN	BENIGN TUMOR	MALIGNANT TUMOR*
Adeno	Epithelial glands	Adenoma	Adenocarcinoma
Chondro	Cartilage	Chondroma	Chondrosarcoma
Fibro	Fibrous connective	Fibroma	Fibrosarcoma
Glio	Glial cells (brain)	Glioma	Glioblastoma
Hemangio	Blood vessel	Hemangioma	Hemangiosarcoma
Hepato	Liver	Hepatoma	Hepatocarcinoma
			Hepatoblastoma
Leiomyo	Smooth muscle	Leiomyoma	Leiomyosarcoma
Lipo	Fat/adipose	Lipoma	Liposarcoma
Lympho	Lymphoid tissues		Malignant lymphomas Hodgkin's lymphoma Non-Hodgkin's lymphoma Burkitt's lymphoma Cutaneous T-cell
Melano	Pigment-producing skin		Melanoma
Meningioma	Meninges	Meningioma	Malignant meningioma
			Meningioblastoma
Neuro	Nerve tissue	Neuroma Neurofibroma	Neurosarcoma Neuroblastoma
Osteo	Bone	Osteoma	Osteosarcoma
Renal	Kidney		Renal cell carcinoma
Rhabdo	Skeletal muscle	Rhabdomyoma	Rhabdomyosarcoma
Squamous	Epithelial layer of skin, mucous membranes, and organ linings	Papilloma	Squamous cell carcinoma of skin, bladder, lungs, cervix

*Carcinomas are tumors of glandular tissue; sarcomas are tumors of connective tissue; blastomas are tumors of less differentiated, embryonal tissues.

TABLE 21-4 Grading of Malignant Tumors

GRADE	CELLULAR CHARACTERISTICS
G_x	Grade cannot be determined.
G_1	Tumor cells are well differentiated and closely resemble the normal cells from which they arose. This grade is considered a low grade of malignant change. These tumors are malignant but are relatively slow growing.
G_2	Tumor cells are moderately differentiated; they still retain some of the characteristics of normal cells, but also have more malignant characteristics than do G_1 tumor cells.
G_3	Tumor cells are poorly differentiated, but the tissue of origin can usually be established. The cells have few normal cell characteristics.
G_4	Tumor cells are poorly differentiated and retain no normal cell characteristics. Determination of the tissue of origin is difficult and perhaps impossible.

Other gene changes in cancerous tumors alter the tumor's susceptibility to specific treatment. Some changes form the basis of "targeted therapy" for cancer (see Chapter 22).

Staging determines the exact location of the cancer and whether metastasis has occurred. Cancer stage influences selection of therapy. Staging is done by clinical staging, surgical staging, and pathologic staging. *Clinical staging* assesses the patient's symptoms and evaluates tumor size and possible spread. *Surgical staging* assesses the tumor size, number, sites, and spread by inspection at surgery. *Pathologic staging* is the most definitive type, determining the tumor size, number, sites, and spread by pathologic examination of tissues obtained at surgery.

The tumor, node, metastasis (TNM) system is used to describe the anatomic extent of cancers. The TNM staging systems have specific prognostic value for each solid tumor type. Table 21-5 shows a basic TNM staging system. TNM staging is not useful for leukemia or lymphomas (see Chapter 40). Additional specific staging systems include Dukes' staging of colon and rectal cancer and Clark's levels method of staging skin cancer.

Tumor growth is assessed in terms of doubling time (the amount of time it takes for a tumor to double in size) and mitotic index (the percentage of actively dividing cells within a tumor). The smallest detectable tumor is about 1 cm in diameter and contains 1 billion cells. A tumor with a mitotic index of less than 10% is a slower-growing tumor; a tumor with an index of 85% is faster growing. Different tumor types have a wide range of growth rates.

Cancer Etiology and Genetic Risk

Carcinogenesis usually takes years and depends on several tumor and patient factors (Boucher et al., 2014). Three interacting factors influence cancer development: exposure to carcinogens,

Leading Sites of New Cancer Cases and Deaths for the United States and Canada – 2014 Estimates*

Estimated New Cases*

Male

Prostate
182,960 (19%)

Lung and bronchus
131,390 (14%)

Colorectal
99,835 (11%)

Bladder
67,090 (7%)

Kidney and renal pelvis
44,710 (5%)

Leukemia
39,790 (4%)

Pancreas
30, 570 (3%)

Esophagus
15,160 (2%)

Other sites
327,495 (35%)

All sites
939,000 (100%)

Female

Breast
278,710 (29%)

Lung and bronchus
119,510 (13%)

Colorectal
89,800 (9%)

Uterine corpus and cervix
82,300 (9%)

Pancreas
28,300 (3%)

Leukemia
28,240 (3%)

Kidney and renal pelvis
25,680 (3%)

Ovary
25,240 (3%)

Bladder
20,640 (2%)

Esophagus
4,110 (<1%)

Other sites
249,600 (26%)

All sites
952,130 (100%)

Estimated Deaths

Male

Lung and bronchus
95,490 (27%)

Colorectal
36,370 (10%)

Prostate
30,780 (9%)

Pancreas
24,700 (7%)

Leukemia
15,950 (4%)

Esophagus
14,320 (4%)

Bladder
13,890 (4%)

Kidney and renal pelvis
10,670 (3%)

Other sites
117,960 (32%)

All sites
360,120 (100%)

Female

Lung and bronchus
81,080 (25%)

Breast
45,610 (14%)

Colorectal
32,540 (10%)

Pancreas
23,190 (7%)

Uterus corpus and cervix
16,630 (5%)

Ovary
15,830 (5%)

Leukemia
11,400 (4%)

Kidney and renal pelvis
5,590 (2%)

Bladder
5,300 (2%)

Esophagus
3,430 (1%)

Other sites
79,000 (25%)

All sites
319,600 (100%)

*Excludes basal and squamous cell skin cancers and in situ carcinoma except urinary bladder.
Note: Percentages may not total 100% due to rounding.

FIG. 21-4 Cancer incidence and death by site and sex. (Data from American Cancer Society, 2017, and Canadian Cancer Society, 2016.)

TABLE 21-5 Staging of Cancer—TNM Classification

Primary Tumor (T)

T_x	Primary tumor cannot be assessed
T_0	No evidence of primary tumor
T_{is}	Carcinoma in situ
T_1, T_2, T_3, T_4	Increasing size and/or local extent of the primary tumor

Regional Lymph Nodes (N)

N_x	Regional lymph nodes cannot be assessed
N_0	No regional lymph node metastasis
N_1, N_2, N_3	Increasing involvement of regional lymph nodes

Distant Metastasis (M)

M_x	Presence of distant metastasis cannot be assessed
M_0	No distant metastasis
M_1	Distant metastasis

genetic predisposition, and IMMUNITY. These factors account for variation in cancer development from one adult to another, even when each adult is exposed to the same hazards.

Oncogene activation is the main mechanism of carcinogenesis regardless of the specific cause. These oncogenes are turned on (expressed) under controlled conditions for CELLULAR REGULATION when cells divide for normal growth and replacement of dead or damaged tissues. At other times they are turned off, controlled, or suppressed by products of "suppressor genes."

When a normal cell is exposed to any carcinogen (initiator), the normal cell's DNA can be damaged and mutated. The mutations damage suppressor genes, preventing them from producing proteins that control CELLULAR REGULATION for the expression of oncogenes. As a result, the oncogenes are overexpressed and can cause the cells to change from normal cells to cancer cells. When oncogenes are overexpressed in a cell, excessive amounts of cyclins are produced and upset the balance between cell growth enhancement and cell growth limitation. The effect of the presence of these excessive cyclins is greater than the normal effect of the suppressor gene products, thus cell regulation is lost, allowing uncontrolled cell division.

Oncogenes are not abnormal genes but are part of every cell's normal makeup. Oncogenes become a problem only if they are overexpressed as a result of exposure to carcinogenic agents or events with loss of CELLULAR REGULATION. External and personal factors can activate oncogenes.

External Factors Causing Cancer

External factors, including environmental exposure, are responsible for about 80% of cancer in North America (ACS, 2017). Environmental carcinogens are chemical, physical, or viral agents that cause cancer (NTP, 2016).

Chemical carcinogenesis can occur from exposures to many known chemicals, drugs, and other products used in everyday life. Chemicals vary in how carcinogenic they are. For example, tobacco and alcohol appear to be only mildly carcinogenic. For these substances, chronic, long-term exposure to large amounts is required before CELLULAR REGULATION is lost and cancer develops. However, these two substances can act as *co-carcinogens,* meaning that when they are taken together, they enhance each other's carcinogenic activity.

Not all cells are susceptible to carcinogenesis to the same degree. Normal cells that have the ability to divide are at greater risk for cancer development than are normal cells that are not capable of cell division. For example, cancers commonly arise in bone marrow, skin, lining of the GI tract, ductal cells of the breast, and lining of the lungs. All of these cells normally undergo cell division. Cancers of nerve tissue, cardiac muscle, and skeletal muscle are rare. These cells do not normally undergo cell division.

About 30% of cancers diagnosed in North America are related to tobacco use (ACS, 2017; Canadian Cancer Society, 2016). Tobacco is the single most preventable source of carcinogenesis. It contains many carcinogens and co-carcinogens. The risk for cancer development from tobacco use depends on an adult's IMMUNITY, genetic susceptibility, and amount and types of tobacco exposure. Chapter 27 discusses the types of tobacco and tobacco smoke exposure.

Tissues at greatest risk for tobacco-induced cancer are those that have direct contact with tobacco or tobacco smoke such as the lungs and airways. Cigarette smoking and tobacco use also promote the development of pancreatic, oral and laryngeal, bladder, and cervical cancers.

> ### ♥ VETERANS' HEALTH CONSIDERATIONS
> #### Patient-Centered Care QSEN
>
> The incidence of tobacco-related cancers is high among military veterans. One reason is that at one time cigarette smoking was considered "manly" among military personnel. The cost of cigarettes was low in stores on military installations (no state taxes were applied). In addition, military field meals such as "C-rations" or "K-rations" included free cigarettes. Ask patients about their military service and whether cigarette smoking started, continued, or increased during that time.

Physical carcinogenesis from physical agents or events also causes cancer by DNA damage. Two physical agents that are known to cause cancer are radiation and chronic irritation.

Even small doses of radiation affect cells. Some effects are temporary and are self-repaired. Other effects cannot be repaired and may induce cancer in the damaged cells. Both ionizing and ultraviolet (UV) radiation can cause cancer. Some ionizing radiation is found naturally in radon, uranium, and radium found in rocks and soil. Other sources of ionizing radiation include x-rays for diagnosis and treatment of disease, as well as cosmic radiation. UV radiation is a type of solar radiation, coming from the sun. Other sources of UV radiation include tanning beds and germicidal lights. UV rays do not penetrate deeply, and the most common cancer type caused by UV exposure is skin cancer. Both ionizing and UV radiation exposure mutates genes.

Chronic irritation and tissue trauma are suspected to cause cancer. The incidence of skin cancer is higher in the scars of adults with burn scars or other types of severe skin injury. Chronically irritated tissues undergo frequent cell division and thus are at an increased risk for DNA mutation.

Viral carcinogenesis occurs when viruses infect body cells and break DNA strands. Viruses then insert their own genetic material into the human DNA. Breaking the DNA, along with viral gene insertion, mutates the cell's DNA and can either activate an oncogene or damage suppressor genes. Viruses that cause cancer are **oncoviruses**. Table 21-6 lists cancers of known viral origin.

Dietary factors related to cancer are poorly understood but are suspected to increase cancer risk. Suspected dietary factors include low fiber intake and a high intake of red meat or animal fat. Preservatives, preparation methods, and additives (dyes, flavorings, sweeteners) may have cancer-promoting effects. Chart 21-1 lists dietary habits that may help reduce cancer risk.

TABLE 21-6 Cancers Associated With a Known Viral Origin

VIRUS	MALIGNANCIES
Epstein-Barr virus	Burkitt's lymphoma, B-cell lymphoma, nasopharyngeal carcinoma
Hepatitis B virus	Primary liver carcinoma
Hepatitis C virus	Primary liver carcinoma, possibly B-cell lymphomas
Human papilloma virus	Cervical carcinoma, vulvar carcinoma, penile carcinoma, and other anogenital carcinomas
Human lymphotrophic virus type I	Adult T-cell leukemia
Human lymphotrophic virus type II	Hairy cell leukemia

Data from National Toxicology Program. (2016). *Report on carcinogens* (14th ed.). http://ntp.niehs.nih.gov/go.roc13.

> ### 🧍 CHART 21-1 Patient and Family Education: Preparing for Self-Management
> #### Dietary Habits to Reduce Cancer Risk
>
> - Avoid excessive intake of animal fat.
> - Avoid nitrites (prepared lunch meats, sausage, bacon).
> - Minimize your intake of red meat.
> - Keep your alcohol consumption to no more than one or two drinks per day.
> - Eat more bran.
> - Eat more cruciferous vegetables such as broccoli, cauliflower, Brussels sprouts, and cabbage.
> - Eat foods high in vitamin A (e.g., apricots, carrots, leafy green and yellow vegetables) and vitamin C (e.g., fresh fruits and vegetables, especially citrus fruits).

TABLE 21-7 The Seven Warning Signs of Cancer

C	**C**hanges in bowel or bladder habits
A	**A** sore that does not heal
U	**U**nusual bleeding or discharge
T	**T**hickening or lump in the breast or elsewhere
I	**I**ndigestion or difficulty swallowing
O	**O**bvious change in a wart or mole
N	**N**agging cough or hoarseness

Personal Factors and Cancer Development

Personal factors, including IMMUNITY, age, and genetic risk, also affect whether an adult is likely to develop cancer.

Immunity protects the body from foreign invaders and non-self cells (see Chapter 17). Non-self cells include cells that are not normal such as cancer cells. Cell-mediated immunity, especially natural killer (NK) cells and helper T-cells, provides immune surveillance (Abbas et al., 2015).

Cancer incidence increases among patients with reduced IMMUNITY. Adults older than 60 years have reduced immunity and a higher incidence of cancer compared with that of the general population. Organ transplant recipients taking immunosuppressive drugs to prevent organ rejection also have a higher incidence of cancer. In patients with acquired immune deficiency syndrome (AIDS), cancer incidence is very high (ACS, 2017).

Advancing age is the single most important risk factor for cancer (ACS, 2017). As an adult ages, immunity decreases and external exposures to carcinogens accumulate. Teach older adults to be aware of and report symptoms such as the seven warning signs of cancer (Table 21-7) to health care providers. Health care providers should investigate all symptoms suggestive of disease. Assessment considerations for the most common cancers that occur among older adult are listed in Chart 21-2.

🧬 GENETIC/GENOMIC CONSIDERATIONS

Patient-Centered Care 🆀🆂🅴🅽

A hereditary genetic risk for cancer occurs only in a small percent of the population; however, adults who have a genetic predisposition are at very high risk for cancer development (Jorde et al., 2016). Mutations in suppressor genes or oncogenes can be inherited when they occur in sperm and ova and are then passed on to one's children, in whom all body cells contain the inherited mutations. Thus for some adults tight CELLULAR REGULATION is lost as a result of a mutation in a suppressor gene, which reduces or halts its function and allows oncogene overexpression. In other adults the suppressor genes are normal, and the oncogene is mutated and does not respond to suppressor gene signals, thus reducing cellular regulation and increasing the risk for cancer development. Table 21-8 lists conditions associated with an increased genetic risk for cancer development. Be sure to include questions about these conditions when performing a family history and develop at least a three-generation pedigree.

Genetic testing for cancer predisposition is available to confirm or rule out an adult's genetic risk for some specific cancer types. (See Chapter 5 for explanation of genetic terminology.) These tests usually are performed on blood and are expensive. Genetic testing should not be performed unless a family history clearly

⬡ CHART 21-2 Nursing Focus on the Older Adult

Cancer Assessment

CANCER TYPE	ASSESSMENT CONSIDERATION
Colorectal cancer	Ask the patient whether bowel habits have changed over the past year (e.g., in consistency, frequency, color). Is there any obvious blood in the stool? Test at least one stool specimen for occult blood during the patient's hospitalization. Encourage the patient to have a baseline colonoscopy. Encourage the patient to reduce dietary intake of animal fats, red meat, and smoked meats. Encourage the patient to increase dietary intake of bran, vegetables, and fruit.
Bladder cancer	Ask the patient about the presence of: Pain on urination Blood in the urine Cloudy urine Increased frequency or urgency
Prostate cancer	Ask the patient about: Hesitancy Change in the size of the urine stream Pain in the back or legs History of urinary tract infections
Skin cancer	Examine skin areas for moles or warts. Ask the patient about changes in moles (e.g., color, edges, sensation).
Leukemia	Observe the skin for color, petechiae, or ecchymosis. Ask the patient about: Fatigue Bruising Bleeding tendency History of infections and illnesses Night sweats Unexplained fevers
Lung cancer	Observe the skin and mucous membranes for color. How many words can the patient say between breaths? Ask the patient about: Cough Hoarseness Smoking history Exposure to inhalation irritants Exposure to asbestos Shortness of breath Activity tolerance Frothy or bloody sputum Pain in the arms or chest Difficulty swallowing

indicates the possibility of increased genetic risk and the patient wants to have the test results. *These tests do not diagnose the presence of cancer; they only provide risk information.* Personal and family history facts that are considered "red flags" suggesting a genetic predisposition for cancer include:

- Cancer of any type appears in multiple members of every generation of a family, especially if an autosomal-dominant pattern of inheritance emerges
- Similar cancers appear in multiple first-degree relatives

TABLE 21-8 Conditions Associated With a Genetic Predisposition for Cancer

CONDITION	SPECIFIC CANCER TYPE
Inherited cancers*	Breast cancer
	Prostate cancer
	Ovarian cancer
Familial clustering	Breast cancer
	Melanoma
Bloom syndrome	Leukemia
Familial polyposis	Colorectal cancer
Chromosomal aberrations	
Down syndrome (47 chromosomes)	Leukemia
Klinefelter syndrome (47,XXY)	Breast cancer
Turner's syndrome (45,XO)	Leukemia
	Gonadal carcinoma
	Meningioma
	Colorectal cancer

*Not all breast, prostate, or ovarian cancers are inherited.

- Multiple instances of rare cancer types occur within a family
- Cancer occurs at ages several decades younger than the national average
- Cancer develops in both of paired organs (e.g., bilateral breast cancer)
- Breast cancer is present in a genetic male adult, regardless of gender identity

A variety of issues and potential problems exist with genetic testing for cancer risk. Correct interpretation of the results is critical. Ideally a genetic counselor is involved in giving the patient information *before* as well as after testing is performed. *When a patient tests positive for a known cancer-causing gene mutation, his or her risk for cancer development is greatly increased; however, the cancer still may never develop.* A negative result means that the particular gene mutation tested for is not present. In addition, testing might not find the particular mutation but may indicate a different mutation with an unknown significance. This result is particularly frustrating for patients and health care providers.

Other issues regarding genetic testing include who will have access to the information and whether to share the test results with family members. Genetic testing has implications for the entire family, not just the patient being tested. For more information on genetic testing, see Chapter 5.

🌐 CULTURAL/SPIRITUAL CONSIDERATIONS
Patient-Centered Care (QSEN)

The incidence of cancer varies among races. American Cancer Society (ACS) data (2015b, 2016) show that African Americans have a higher incidence of cancer than whites and the death rate is higher for African Americans. Since 1960 the overall incidence among African Americans has increased 27%, whereas for whites it has increased only 12%. Cancer sites and cancer-related mortality also vary by race. A possible reason for the difference is that more African Americans have less access to health care. They are more often diagnosed with later-stage cancer that is more difficult to cure or control. However, this disparity in access does not explain all differences.

When risks for cancer development are assessed, behavior and socioeconomic factors are assessed along with ethnicity and genetic predisposition. The American Cancer Society (2016) reports that cancer incidence and survival are often related to socioeconomic factors. These factors include the availability of health care services or the belief that seeking early health care has a positive effect on the outcome of cancer diagnosis.

❓ NCLEX EXAMINATION CHALLENGE 21-2
Health Promotion and Maintenance

Which statement by a client who has tested negative for a BRCA1 mutation (while her sister is positive) indicates to the nurse that the client has correct understanding of the results?
A. "I will continue to perform monthly breast self-examinations."
B. "It is a relief to know that I have no risk for breast cancer."
C. "After I have my next child, I will have my ovaries removed."
D. "I will wear softer bras to avoid putting pressure on or irritating my breasts."

CANCER PREVENTION

Cancer prevention activities focus on primary prevention and secondary prevention. **Primary prevention** is the use of strategies to prevent the actual occurrence of cancer. This type of cancer prevention is most effective when there is a known cause for a cancer type. **Secondary prevention** is the use of screening strategies to detect cancer early, at a time when cure or control is more likely.

Primary Prevention

Avoidance of known or potential carcinogens is an effective prevention strategy when a cause of cancer is known and avoidance is easily accomplished. For example, teach adults to use skin protection during sun exposure to avoid skin cancer. Most lung cancer can be avoided by not using tobacco and eliminating exposure to loose asbestos particles. Teach all adults about the dangers of cigarette smoking and other forms of tobacco use (see the Health Promotion and Maintenance feature in Chapter 27). Teach adults who are exposed to carcinogens in the workplace to use personal protective equipment that reduces direct contact with this substance. As more cancer causes are identified, avoidance may become even more effective.

Modifying associated factors appears to help reduce cancer risk. Absolute causes are not known for many cancers, but some conditions appear to increase risk. Examples are the increased incidence of cancer among adults who consume alcohol; the association of a diet high in fat and low in fiber with colon cancer, breast cancer, and ovarian cancer; and a greater incidence of cervical cancer among women who have multiple sexual partners (ACS, 2017). Modifying behavior to reduce the associated factor may decrease the risk for cancer development. Therefore teach all adults to limit their intake of alcohol to no more than one ounce per day and to include more fruits, vegetables, and whole grains in their diets. Instruct women about the importance of limiting the number of sexual partners and to use safer sex practices to avoid exposure to viruses that can increase the risk for cervical cancer (see Table 21-6 for a listing of cancer-causing viruses).

Removal of "at-risk" tissues reduces cancer risk for an adult who has a known high risk for developing a specific type of cancer. Examples include removing moles to prevent conversion to skin cancer, removing colon polyps to prevent colon cancer, and removing breasts to prevent breast cancer. Not all "at-risk" tissues can be removed (e.g., those that are part of essential organs).

Chemoprevention is a strategy that uses drugs, chemicals, natural nutrients, or other substances to disrupt one or more steps important to cancer development. These agents may be able to reverse existing gene damage or halt the progression of the transformation process. Only a few agents have been found effective for chemoprevention. These include the use of aspirin and celecoxib (Celebrex) to reduce the risk for colon cancer, the use of vitamin D and tamoxifen to reduce the risk for breast cancer, and the use of lycopene to reduce the risk for prostate cancer (ACS, 2017).

Vaccination is a newer method of primary cancer prevention. Currently the only vaccines approved for prevention of cancer are related to prevention of infection from several forms of the human papilloma virus (HPV). These vaccines are Gardasil and Cervarix. As more cancer-causing viruses are identified, it is hoped that vaccines will be developed to prevent those viral infections.

Secondary Prevention

Regular screening for cancer does not reduce cancer incidence but can greatly reduce some types of cancer deaths. Teach all adults the benefits of participating in specific routine screening techniques annually as part of health maintenance. General screening recommendations are listed in chapters discussing cancers by organ system. The age and type of participation in specific screening tests are different for adults who have an identified increased risk for a specific cancer type. In addition, there is some controversy about when the age and frequency for screening has the greatest benefit. Examples of recommended screenings include (ACS, 2017):

- The choice of annual mammography for women 40 to 44 years of age, annual mammography for women 45 to 54 years of age, and annual or biennial mammography for women over 55 years of age

- Annual clinical breast examination for women older than 40 years; every 3 years for women age 20 to 39 years.
- Colonoscopy at age 50 years and then every 10 years
- Annual fecal occult blood for adults of all ages
- Digital rectal examination (DRE) for men older than 50 years

Because cancer development clearly involves gene changes (either inherited gene mutations or acquired damage-induced gene mutations), adults can be screened for some gene mutations that increase the risk for cancer. A few examples of known gene mutations that increase cancer risk are found in the *BRCA1* gene, the *BRCA2* gene, and the *CHEK2* gene (which increase the risk for breast cancer) and mutations in the *APC*, *MLH1*, and *MSH2* genes (which increase the risk for colon cancer).

When a patient has a strong family history of either breast or colon cancer, create a three-generation pedigree to more fully explore the possibility of genetic risk. If a pattern of risk emerges, inform the person about the possible benefits of genetic screening and advise him or her to talk with an oncology health practitioner or genetics professional for more information. Genetic screening can help an adult at increased genetic risk for cancer to alter lifestyle factors, participate in early detection methods, initiate chemoprevention, or even have at-risk tissue removed. Genetic screening has some personal risks, as well as potential benefits (see Chapter 5).

❓ NCLEX EXAMINATION CHALLENGE 21-3

Health Promotion and Maintenance

Which actions does the nurse teach a client as **primary** cancer prevention strategies? **Select all that apply.**
A. Avoiding sun exposure
B. Having an annual digital rectal examination
C. Having genetic testing for specific colon cancer–causing genes
D. Performing monthly breast self-examinations
E. Quitting cigarette smoking
F. Having a mole surgically removed

GET READY FOR THE NCLEX® EXAMINATION

▌KEY POINTS

Review these Key Points for each NCLEX Examination Client Needs Category.

Health Promotion and Maintenance

- Teach adults to avoid tanning beds and to use sunscreen and wear protective clothing during sun exposure. **QSEN: Patient-Centered Care**
- Encourage patients to participate in the recommended cancer-screening activities for their age-group and cancer risk category. **QSEN: Patient-Centered Care**
- Assist adults interested in smoking cessation to find an appropriate smoking cessation program (see Chapter 27). **QSEN: Patient-Centered Care**
- Assess the patient's knowledge about causes of cancer and his or her screening/prevention practices. **QSEN: Patient-Centered Care**

- Ask all patients about their exposures to environmental agents that are known or suspected to impair CELLULAR REGULATION and increase the risk for cancer. **QSEN: Evidence-Based Practice**
- Obtain a detailed family history (at least three generations) and use this information to create a pedigree to assess the patient's risk for familial or inherited cancer. **QSEN: Patient-Centered Care**
- Teach anyone, especially older adults, the "seven warning signs of cancer" (see Table 21-7). **QSEN: Evidence-Based Practice**

Physiological Integrity

- Be aware of these facts regarding cancer risk and cancer development:
  - Cancer cells originate from normal body cells.

- Transformation of a normal cell into a cancer cell involves mutation of the genes (DNA) of the normal cell and results in the loss of CELLULAR REGULATION.
- Oncogenes that are overexpressed can cause a cell to develop into a tumor.
- Most tumors arise from cells that are capable of cell division.
- A key feature of cancer cells is the loss of CELLULAR REGULATION and apoptosis. These cells have an "infinite" life span.

- Tobacco use is a causative factor in 30% of all cancers.
- Adults with reduced IMMUNITY have a higher risk for cancer development.
- Tumors that metastasize from the primary site into another organ are still designated as tumors of the originating tissue.
- Cancer cells that are less differentiated and have a higher mitotic index are "more malignant" and harder to cure.

SELECTED BIBLIOGRAPHY

Abbas, A., Lichtman, A., & Pillai, S. (2015). Cellular and molecular immunology (8th ed.). Philadelphia: Saunders.

American Cancer Society (ACS). (2015a). *Cancer prevention and early detection: Facts & figures—2015-2016*. Report No. 8600.15. Atlanta: Author.

American Cancer Society (ACS). (2015b). *Cancer facts and figures for Hispanics/Latinos—2015-2017*. Report No. 862315. Atlanta: Author.

American Cancer Society (ACS). (2016). *Cancer facts and figures for African Americans—2016-2018*. Report No. 861416. Atlanta: Author.

American Cancer Society (ACS). (2017). *Cancer facts and figures—2017*. Report No. 00-300M–No. 500817. Atlanta: Author.

Boucher, J., Habin, K., & Underhill, M. (2014). *Cancer genetics and genomics: Essentials for oncology nurses. Clinical Journal of Oncology Nursing, 18*(3), 355–359.

Canadian Cancer Society, Statistics Canada. (2016). *Canadian Cancer Statistics, 2016*. Toronto, ON: Canadian Cancer Society. www.cancer.ca/~/media/cancer.ca/CW/cancer%20information/cancer%20101/Canadian%20cancer%20statistics/Canadian-Cancer-Statistics-2016-EN.pdf?la=en.

Jorde, L., Carey, J., & Bamshad, M. (2016). Medical genetics (5th ed.). Philadelphia: Elsevier.

Kannan, R., Madden, K., & Andrews, S. (2014). *Primer on immuno-oncology and immune response. Clinical Journal of Oncology Nursing, 18*(3), 311–317.

Mahon, S. (2014). *Breast cancer risk associated with CHEK2 mutations. Oncology Nursing Forum, 41*(6), 692–694.

McAllister, K., & Schmitt, M. (2015). *Impact of a nurse navigator on genomic testing and timely decision making in patients with breast cancer. Clinical Journal of Oncology Nursing, 19*(5), 510–512.

McCance, K., Huether, S., Brashers, V., & Rote, N. (2014). Pathophysiology: The biologic basis for disease in adults and children (7th ed.). St. Louis: Mosby.

National Toxicology Program (NTP). (2016). *Report on carcinogens* (14th ed.). Research Triangle Park, NC: US Department of Health and Human Services, Public Health Service. https://ntp.niehs.nih.gov/pubhealth/roc/index-1.html.

Care of Patients With Cancer

Constance G. Visovsky and Julie Ponto

http://evolve.elsevier.com/Iggy/

PRIORITY AND INTERRELATED CONCEPTS

The priority concept for this chapter is IMMUNITY.

The interrelated concepts for this chapter are:
- CELLULAR REGULATION
- CLOTTING
- GAS EXCHANGE
- SENSORY PERCEPTION

LEARNING OUTCOMES

Safe and Effective Care Environment

1. Collaborate with the interprofessional team to coordinate high-quality care to patients receiving cancer therapy.
2. Protect yourself and others from cytotoxic agents and radiation.
3. Teach the patient and caregiver(s) how impaired IMMUNITY, impaired CLOTTING, and other changes caused by cancer or cancer therapy affect home safety.

Health Promotion and Maintenance

4. Identify community resources for patients with cancer.

Psychosocial Integrity

5. Implement nursing interventions to help the patient and family cope with the psychosocial impact caused by cancer and cancer therapy.

Physiological Integrity

6. Apply knowledge of pathophysiology to assess patients with common problems and complications caused by cancer and cancer therapy, including oncologic emergencies.
7. Teach the patient and caregiver(s) about common drugs used for cancer therapy and its complications, including pain, impaired IMMUNITY, and impaired CLOTTING.
8. Prioritize interprofessional collaborative care for patients who experience an oncologic emergency.

With new treatment strategies resulting in more than 68% of people diagnosed with cancer being cured and thousands of others living 5 years or longer, cancer is considered a chronic illness (American Cancer Society [ACS], 2017; Canadian Cancer Society, 2016). Survivors may have exacerbations and remissions of the disease over their lifetimes. *Regardless of the treatment received, cancer has a negative impact on the adult's physical and psychological functioning and quality of life.*

Providing care to patients experiencing cancer and their families is complex, challenging, and best accomplished with an interprofessional team approach. This chapter describes the general interventions for cancer and the problems associated with cancer treatment. For treatments and patient problems that occur with specific cancer types, consult the chapters in which the cancer is described. Table 22-1 lists common cancer types and the specific locations within this text where the interventions are presented.

IMPACT OF CANCER ON PHYSICAL FUNCTION

Cancer can develop in any organ or tissue, reducing the function of that tissue or organ. Cancers that occur in nonvital tissues (such as the breast) can cause death by **metastasizing** (spreading) into vital organs (e.g., brain, liver, bone marrow) and disrupting critical physiologic processes (see Chapter 21). Advanced cancers often have an impact on:
- IMMUNITY and CLOTTING
- GI function
- Peripheral nerve SENSORY PERCEPTION
- Central motor and sensory function

TABLE 22-1 Text Location of Specific Cancer Content	
CANCER TYPE	CHAPTER
Bladder (urothelial)	66
Brain	45
Breast	70
Cervical	71
Colorectal	56
Esophageal	54
Head and Neck	29
Leukemia	40
Lung	30
Lymphoma	40
Ovarian	71
Prostate	72
Renal cell carcinoma	67
Skin	25
Stomach (gastric)	55

- Respiratory and cardiac function
- Comfort and quality of life

IMPAIRED IMMUNITY AND CLOTTING

Impaired IMMUNITY and blood-producing functions can occur when cancer starts in *or* invades the bone marrow, where blood cells are formed. Tumor cells enter the bone marrow and reduce the production and function of healthy white blood cells (WBCs) that are needed for normal immunity. Thus patients who have cancer, especially leukemia, are at an increased risk for infection (McCance et al., 2014). Some cancer treatments, especially chemotherapy, reduce neutrophil WBC numbers, making the patient more prone to infection.

Bone marrow invasion by cancer cells causes anemia by decreasing the number of red blood cells, and it causes thrombocytopenia (decreased number of platelets), resulting in impaired CLOTTING. These changes may be caused by the disease or by cancer treatment, especially chemotherapy. The patient with anemia usually has fatigue, shortness of breath, and tachycardia.

ALTERED GI FUNCTION

Tumors of the GI tract increase the metabolic rate and the need for nutrients; however, many patients suffer from disease-related and treatment-related appetite loss, and alterations in taste that have a negative impact on nutrition, leading to weight loss. Cachexia (extreme body wasting and malnutrition) develops from an imbalance between food intake and energy use (increased catabolism from cancer) and may occur despite adequate nutrition intake. Some patients experience early satiety or a sense of fullness even when only small volumes are ingested.

Nutrition support for the patient with cancer, especially one undergoing cancer therapy, is complex. There is no one recommended dietary approach to maintaining good nutrition during cancer treatment. Many approaches such as eating smaller, frequent meals, taking nutritional supplemental drinks between meals, and generally eating a healthy diet rich in complex carbohydrates (fiber) and protein are suggested. For patients who cannot take oral nutrition, enteral tube feeding or parenteral nutrition may be recommended. A registered dietitian is part of the interprofessional team and consulted for patients who have nutrition difficulties that accompany cancer and its treatment.

Abdominal tumors may obstruct or compress structures anywhere in the GI tract, reducing the ability to absorb nutrients and eliminate wastes. This problem needs to be addressed promptly to avoid complications such as a bowel obstruction.

Tumors that invade the liver have profound effects on this organ, which has many important metabolic functions. Liver damage has the potential to lead to malnutrition and death.

ALTERED PERIPHERAL NERVE FUNCTION

Although tumors in the spine can change peripheral nerve function, the more common cause is chemotherapy. Neurotoxic chemotherapy agents injure peripheral nerves, leading to peripheral neuropathy with reduced SENSORY PERCEPTION. Patients with chemotherapy-induced peripheral neuropathy (CIPN) report loss of sensation, especially in the lower extremities. Symptoms include numbness, tingling, neuropathic pain, and changes in gait and balance. Physical assessment of the degree of sensory perception loss can be performed using monofilaments as described in Chapter 64. Several instruments for self-report of CIPN and severity grading also are available (Curcio, 2016; Kaplow & Iyer, 2017).

For patients who already have peripheral neuropathy from problems such as diabetes or AIDS, chemotherapy increases its severity. CIPN is a dose-limiting toxicity of cancer chemotherapy treatment. This means that the development or increased severity of CIPN that has a negative impact on ADLs may result in a reduction of the optimum chemotherapy dose, potentially changing the outcome of cancer treatment.

MOTOR AND SENSORY DEFICITS

Motor and SENSORY PERCEPTION deficits occur when cancers invade bone or the brain or compress nerves. In patients with bone metastasis, the primary cancer started in another organ (e.g., lung, prostate, breast). Bones become thinner, with an increased risk for fractures that can occur with minimal trauma. Bone metastasis causes pain, fractures, spinal cord compression, and hypercalcemia, each of which reduces mobility. Spinal cord compression and hypercalcemia are *oncologic emergencies* and require immediate attention (see discussion of Oncologic Emergencies).

Patients have sensory perception changes if the spinal cord is damaged or if nerves are compressed. Sensory, motor, and cognitive functions are impaired when cancer spreads to the brain. Any tumor, malignant or benign, growing in the brain can destroy healthy brain tissue and lead to death.

CANCER PAIN

The patient with cancer may have pain, especially chronic pain. Pain does not always accompany cancer, but it can be a major problem. Cancer pain is best managed by an interprofessional team that includes an oncologist, advanced oncology nurse practitioner, certified oncology nurse, interventional radiologist, radiation oncologist, and pain management specialists. Patient education is needed to manage side effects of pain drugs, including constipation. Chapter 4 discusses the causes and management of pain.

ALTERED RESPIRATORY AND CARDIAC FUNCTION

Cancer can disrupt respiratory function, capacity, and GAS EXCHANGE and may result in death. Tumors that grow in the airways cause obstruction. If lung tissue is involved, lung capacity is decreased, leading to dyspnea and hypoxemia. Cancer cells thicken the alveolar membrane and damage lung blood vessels, both of which impair gas exchange. Patients are at risk for hypoxemia and hypoxia with either primary or metastatic lung tumors.

Tumors can also press on blood and lymph vessels in the chest, which results in airway compression and dyspnea. Superior vena cava syndrome is an oncologic emergency that results from compression of this vessel.

Both radiation therapy and certain chemotherapy agents can affect cardiac function. Following radiation to the chest, even with appropriate shielding, cardiac events may occur at a younger age in cancer patients compared with the general population. Cardiac conditions from radiation include pericarditis, coronary artery disease, myocardial dysfunction, and valvular heart disease. Higher risk for heart disease has been noted in patients with classic risk factors for cardiac problems such as hypertension, smoking, and hypercholesterolemia. Chemotherapy agents can also contribute to cardiac dysfunction through loss of myocardial muscle mass, leading to heart failure. These late effects of therapy are sometimes reversible but may be permanent.

CANCER MANAGEMENT

The purpose of cancer management is to cure or control the disease while minimizing the side effects of therapy. For certain cancer types such as leukemia, failure to treat the disease would result in death within weeks to months. Cancer therapy includes surgery, radiation, chemotherapy, immunotherapy (e.g., biological response modifiers, molecularly targeted therapy), photodynamic therapy, and hormonal therapy. These therapies may be used separately or in combination to kill cancer cells. The types of therapy used depend on the specific type of cancer, whether the cancer has spread, and the overall health and functional status of the patient. Treatment regimens (*protocols*) have been established for most types of cancer.

SURGERY

Overview

Surgery often plays a part in the diagnosis and/or management of cancer. Typically surgery is only one part of a comprehensive treatment approach for cancer therapy. It is used for prophylaxis, diagnosis, cure, control, palliation, assessment of therapy effectiveness, and tissue reconstruction.

Prophylactic surgery removes potentially cancerous tissue as a means of preventing cancer development. It is performed when a patient has either an existing premalignant condition or a strong predisposition for development of a specific cancer. For example, removing a benign polyp from the colon before it can develop into colon cancer is considered prophylactic surgery.

Diagnostic surgery (excisional biopsy) is the removal of all or part of a suspected lesion for examination and testing to confirm or rule out a cancer diagnosis. Exploratory surgery is a more extensive approach that may be performed if the suspicion of cancer cannot be confirmed by a less invasive means. Cancer treatment is not initiated without tissue confirmation of a cancer diagnosis.

Curative surgery removes all cancer tissue. Surgery alone can result in a cure when all visible and microscopic tumor is removed or destroyed. It is most effective for small localized tumors or noninvasive skin cancers such as basal cell lesions.

Cancer control or *cytoreductive surgery* removes part of the tumor when removal of the entire mass is not possible. It is also known as "debulking" surgery and decreases the size of the tumor and the number of cancer cells, which can alleviate symptoms and enhance the success of other types of cancer treatment, as well as increase survival time.

Palliative surgery focuses on providing symptom relief and improving the quality of life but is not curative. Examples include removal of tumor tissue that is causing pain, obstruction, or difficulty swallowing, and the treatment of neuropathic pain from bone metastasis (Roos, 2015).

Reconstructive or *rehabilitative surgery* increases function, enhances appearance, or both. Examples include breast reconstruction after mastectomy, reconstruction of the esophagus after surgical removal for esophageal cancer, bowel reconstruction, revision of scars, and cosmetic reconstruction in head and neck cancer.

Side Effects of Surgical Therapy

Cancer surgery often involves the loss of a body part or its function to ensure removal of all cancerous tissue. Sometimes whole organs are removed such as the kidney, lung, breast, testis, limb, or tongue. *Any organ loss reduces function.* Some cancer surgeries result in scarring or disfigurement. For example, the tongue and part of the mandible or larynx may be removed in patients with head and neck cancers (see Chapter 29). Often patients express the desire to have all cancerous tissue removed, which is not usually possible. Patients may not understand that cancer cells often escape from the original tumor, making cancer a systemic disease. Following some cancer surgeries, the removal of the affected area can cause profound changes in appearance or activity level and can lead to depression, grief, and decreased enjoyment of life.

❖ INTERPROFESSIONAL COLLABORATIVE CARE

The overall care needs following surgery for cancer are similar to the care required for patients who undergo surgery for other reasons (see Chapters 14, 15, and 16). For cancer surgery, additional priority care needs are psychosocial support and helping the patient achieve maximum functioning.

Often cancer surgery occurs shortly after the diagnosis, before the patient and family have time to adjust to a cancer diagnosis. The stress of the diagnosis can have a significant impact on the patient's and family's ability to understand any teaching provided at this time. Assess the patient's and family's ability to cope with the cancer diagnosis and its treatment and with the potential changes in body image and role. For example, surgery involving the genitals, urinary tract, colon, or rectum may permanently damage these organs, resulting in changes or losses that have an impact on sexual expression or control of elimination.

Coordinate with the interprofessional team to provide support and assistance to the patient and his or her family. Encourage the patient and family to ask questions and express their concerns. Help the patient accept changes in appearance or function by encouraging him or her to look at the surgical site, touch it, and participate in its care, including dressing changes. Provide information about support groups such as those sponsored by the ACS (www.cancer.org) and the Canadian Cancer Society (www.cancer.ca). Some organizations also have support groups for patients' spouses, caregivers, and children and may provide visits from cancer survivors who have coped with the same cancer or concerns. Such visits can help show the patient that many aspects of life can be the same after cancer treatment. For patients who have persistent anxiety or depression as a result of the cancer experience, initiation of drug therapy and/or inclusion of a mental health professional as part of the interprofessional team is indicated.

Physical rehabilitation to improve physical functioning may be indicated after cancer surgery. For example, a modified radical mastectomy for breast cancer can lead to shoulder muscle weakness and reduced arm function on the affected side. Performing specific exercises after surgery can reduce functional loss. Head and neck cancer surgery often requires therapy to improve swallowing and speech. Teaching patients about the importance of performing the exercises to regain as much function as possible and prevent complications is an important nursing function, even though therapy can be painful and challenging. The patient needs encouragement to perform the expected activities. The physical therapist and occupational therapist coordinate with other members of the interprofessional team to plan strategies individualized to each patient to regain or maintain optimal function.

The role of surgery in cancer care continues to change. Laparoscopic and other minimally invasive approaches with smaller incisions and robotic access to internal body cavities have reduced some risks (see Chapters 14 and 15). Regardless of the surgical approach, nurses have a critical role in the patient's recovery after surgery, such as reinforcing the importance of early mobility, pain management, and prevention of infection.

The use of surgery in combination with other therapies has increased and includes intraoperative radiation therapy, the placement of a radioactive source, or the administration of chemotherapy into a body cavity. Other uses include surgical placement of internal catheters into a specific vessel and placement of electronic pumps for chemotherapy or pain drugs.

RADIATION THERAPY

Overview

Radiation therapy (radiotherapy) uses high-energy radiation from gamma rays, radionuclides, or ionizing radiation beams to kill cancer cells, provide disease control, or relieve symptoms. The delivery of radiation should accomplish these actions with minimal damaging effects on the surrounding normal cells.

The effects of radiation are seen only in tissues within the radiation field or path; thus this type of therapy is a *local* treatment. For example, radiation to the chest for lung cancer causes skin changes and hair loss only on the chest area that is irradiated. There are no effects seen elsewhere on the body. When total body irradiation (TBI) is used, *all* body areas are affected. Other systemic radiation therapy uses a radioactive substance such as a radiolabeled monoclonal antibody that travels in the blood to tissues throughout the body to target cancerous cells. Radiation therapy has both short- and long-term effects, depending on the area(s) radiated. For example, a short-term effect is redness or desquamation of the skin, whereas a long-term effect can be pulmonary fibrosis from radiation of the chest.

When cancer cells are exposed to ionizing radiation, the cell's DNA is damaged directly, or DNA-damaging charged particles (free radicals) are formed, resulting in a change in CELLULAR REGULATION. These damaged cells usually can no longer reproduce or function, leading to cell death. However, normal cells in the field of radiation are also affected by radiation. Thus careful planning of the radiation field by a radiation physicist is necessary to minimize damage to normal tissues.

The energy produced by radioactive elements (gamma rays, alpha particles, beta particles) varies in its ability to penetrate tissues and damage cells (Fig. 22-1). *Gamma rays* are used most commonly for radiation therapy because of their ability to deeply penetrate tissues. *Beta particles* are weaker and must be placed within or very close to the cancer cells for cancer therapy (see discussion of brachytherapy in the Radiation Delivery Methods and Devices section).

The amount of radiation delivered to a tissue is the **exposure**; the amount of radiation absorbed by the tissue is the **radiation dose**. The dose is always less than the exposure because some energy is lost as it travels to the destination. The three factors determining the absorbed dose are the *intensity* of exposure, the *duration* of exposure, and the *closeness* (distance) of the radiation source to the cells. Absorbed radiation doses are described in units called **gray** (Gy). One Gy is equal to one joule of energy absorbed by 1 kg of a material. The total dose of radiation used depends on tumor size and location and on the radiation

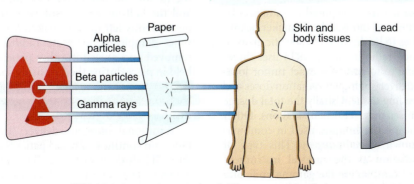

FIG. 22-1 Penetrating capacity of different types of radiation.

sensitivity of the tumor and nearby tissues. Some normal tissues are more sensitive than others to radiation. For example, breast tissue tolerates much higher doses of radiation than the liver does. A total dose of 50 to 60 Gy might be prescribed for a breast cancer. However, only 12 Gy might be prescribed for a liver tumor because a higher dose would destroy healthy liver cells as well as the tumor.

Radiation therapy usually is given as a series of divided doses (fractionation) because of the varying responses of all cancer cells within one tumor (Mitchell, 2013). Most often small doses of radiation are given on a daily basis for a set time period to allow greater destruction of cancer cells while reducing the damage to normal tissues.

The intensity of the radiation decreases with the distance from the radiation-emitting source. This factor is known as the *inverse square law*. For example, the radiation dose received at a distance of 2 meters from the radiation source is only one fourth of the dose received at a distance of 1 meter from the radiation source; the dose of radiation received at 3 meters is only one ninth of the dose received at 1 meter.

Cancer radiation therapy does not immediately kill all cells within a tumor because the cells absorb the radiation dose slightly differently and their overall response to the radiation is slightly different (Mitchell, 2013). A few tumor cells die immediately, and more die within the next few days. Some tumor cells are unable to divide as a result of a single treatment. Still other tumor cells repair the radiation-induced damage, recover, and continue to grow.

Radiation may be used as a stand-alone treatment or may be combined with other cancer therapies. Combining therapies requires careful planning of sequencing, timing, and dose of each therapy to maximize tumor kill and limit damage to normal cells. Often combining radiation with chemotherapy or immunotherapy involves first giving agents that radiosensitize to enhance the radiation damage and result in a greater cell kill than either therapy used alone.

Radiation Delivery Methods and Devices

Radiation cancer treatment can be delivered by external beam (teletherapy) or internal devices (brachytherapy). The type used depends on the patient's general health and on the shape, size, and location of the tumor. The ideal radiation dose is one that kills the cancer cells with an acceptable level of damage to normal tissues (damage to normal tissues cannot be avoided).

External beam or *teletherapy* is radiation delivered from a source outside of the patient. *Because the source is external, the patient is not radioactive, and there is no hazard to others.* The technique called *intensity-modulated radiation therapy* (IMRT) reduces the amount of normal tissue exposed to radiation by breaking up the single beam into thousands of smaller beams, allowing differing intensities to be delivered to specific areas of the tumor. Stereotactic body radiotherapy (SBRT) uses three-dimensional tumor imaging to identify the exact tumor location, which allows precise delivery of higher radiation doses and spares more of the surrounding tissue. Usually the total dosage is delivered in one to five separate treatment sessions. Other specialized radiation application techniques used in combination with surgery are known as *radiosurgery*. This type of surgery uses ionizing radiation as the surgical instrument instead of a cutting blade. Examples are the gamma knife and the CyberKnife that are used for the treatment of brain tumors

by carefully aiming the radiation target point within the brain, sparing normal brain tissue.

Regardless of the delivery method, the exact tumor location is first determined, and the area is fixated and/or the skin marked for therapy precision. The markings may be small, permanent "tattoos"; ink outlines on the skin; or a marked mask laid over the skin. Position-fixing devices include customized external body molds, foam-based body molds, and fiberglass splints. Once the pattern of radiation delivery is decided, the patient must always be in exactly the same position for all treatments. Radiation oncology nurses ensure the patient's ability to get into and maintain this position.

Brachytherapy, also known as internal radiotherapy, means "short" (close) therapy. The radiation source comes into direct, continuous contact with the tumor for a specific time period. This method provides a higher dose of radiation in the tumor over a specified time period, limiting the dose in surrounding normal tissues.

Brachytherapy uses radioactive isotopes either in solid form or within body fluids. Isotopes can be delivered to the tumor tissues in several ways. *With all types of brachytherapy, the radiation source is within the patient. Therefore the patient emits radiation for a period of time and is a potential hazard to others.* When the isotopes used are unsealed and suspended in a fluid, they are given by the oral or IV routes or instilled within body cavities. An example of brachytherapy with soluble isotopes is the ingestion or injection of the radionuclide iodine-131 (^{131}I) (an iodine base with a half-life of 8.05 days) to treat some thyroid cancers. The iodine concentrates in the thyroid gland and destroys the thyroid cancer cells.

> **⚠ NURSING SAFETY PRIORITY** QSEN
>
> ### Action Alert
>
> Unsealed isotopes enter body fluids and eventually are eliminated in waste products. These wastes are radioactive, and you must ensure that they are not directly touched by anyone. Handle the wastes according to guidelines established by the institution. During hospitalization for high-dose rate implant radiation, pregnant women and children are not allowed to visit the patient. After the isotope is completely eliminated from the body, neither the patient nor the body wastes are radioactive.

Solid or sealed radiation sources are implanted within or near the tumor. These sources can be temporary or permanent. Most implants emit continuous, low-energy radiation to tumors. Some devices (e.g., seeds or needles) can be placed into the tumor and stay in place by themselves. Seeds are so small and the half-life of the isotope is so short that this device is permanently left in place (often for prostate cancer) and, over time, completely loses its radioactivity. Other devices are removed and reused in other patients. Some sources must be held in place during therapy using special applicators. *While the solid implants are in place, the patient emits radiation but excreta are not radioactive. Thus at this time the patient poses a hazard to others, but the excreta do not.*

Traditional implants deliver "low-dose rates" (LDRs) of radiation continuously, and patients are hospitalized for several days. "High-dose rate" (HDR) implant radiation is another delivery type. The patient comes into the radiation therapy department several times a week, and a stronger radiation

CHART 22-1 Best Practice for Patient Safety & Quality Care QSEN

Care of the Patient With Sealed Implants of Radioactive Sources

- Assign the patient to a private room with a private bath.
- Place a "Caution: Radioactive Material" sign on the door of the patient's room.
- If portable lead shields are used, place them between the patient and the door.
- Keep the door to the patient's room closed as much as possible.
- Wear a dosimeter film badge at all times while caring for patients with radioactive implants. The badge offers no protection but measures a person's exposure to radiation. Each person caring for the patient should have a separate dosimeter to calculate his or her specific radiation exposure.
- Wear a lead apron while providing care. Always keep the front of the apron facing the source of radiation (do not turn your back toward the patient).
- If you are attempting to conceive, do not perform direct patient care, regardless of whether you are male or female.
- Pregnant nurses should not care for these patients; do not allow pregnant women or children younger than 16 years to visit.
- Limit each visitor to one-half hour per day. Be sure visitors stay at least 6 feet from the source.
- Never touch the radioactive source with bare hands. In the rare instance that it is dislodged, use a long-handled forceps to retrieve it. Deposit the radioactive source in the lead container kept in the patient's room.
- Save all dressings and bed linens in the patient's room until after the radioactive source is removed. After the source is removed, dispose of dressings and linens in the usual manner. Other equipment can be removed from the room at any time without special precautions and does not pose a hazard to other people.

TABLE 22-2 Acute and Late Site-Specific Effects of Radiation Therapy

ACUTE EFFECTS	LATE EFFECTS
Brain • Alopecia and radiodermatitis of the scalp • Ear and external auditory canal irritation • Cerebral edema • Nausea and vomiting • Somnolence syndrome	**Subcutaneous and Soft Tissue** • Radiation-induced fibrosis **Central Nervous System** • Brain necrosis • Leukoencephalopathy • Cognitive and emotional dysfunction • Pituitary and hypothalamic dysfunction • Spinal cord myelopathies
Head and Neck • Oral mucositis • Taste changes • Oral candidiasis • Oral herpes • Acute xerostomia • Dental caries • Esophagitis and pharyngitis	**Head and Neck** • Xerostomia and dental caries • Trismus • Osteoradionecrosis • Hypothyroidism
Breast and Chest Wall • Skin reactions • Esophagitis	**Lung** • Pulmonary fibrosis
Chest and Lung • Esophagitis and pharyngitis • Taste changes • Pneumonia	**Heart** • Pericarditis • Cardiomyopathy • Coronary artery disease
Abdomen and Pelvis • Anorexia • Nausea and vomiting • Diarrhea and proctitis • Cystitis • Vaginal dryness/vaginitis	**Breast/Chest Wall** • Atrophy, fibrosis of breast tissue • Lymphedema **Abdomen and Pelvis** • Small and large bowel injury
Eye • Conjunctival edema and tearing	

implant is placed for only an hour or so each time. The patient is radioactive only when the implant is in place. Chart 22-1 lists the best practices for the safety of the personnel providing care to the patient with a sealed radiation implant.

A recent study examined the effectiveness of a single treatment of CT-guided high-dose brachytherapy applied through a catheter to ablate liver metastases from 20 patients with pancreatic cancer. The rate of local tumor control was 91% for the patients in this study, showing this type of brachytherapy to be safe and effective for treating this type of liver metastases (Wieners et al., 2015).

Side Effects of Radiation Therapy

Radiation therapy can result in both acute and long-term side effects (Table 22-2). These side effects vary according to the radiation site and largely are limited to the areas exposed to radiation. Changes to the skin, known as *radiation dermatitis*, are the most common side effects of radiotherapy and can range from redness and rash to skin desquamation (Bauer, 2016). Multiple factors, including total radiation dose, duration of radiotherapy, and concurrent chemotherapy, can affect skin response to radiation. These changes may be permanent. Radiation to the head may result in permanent hair loss.

Some systemic side effects such as altered taste, fatigue, and bone marrow suppression may also occur. Taste changes are thought to be caused by metabolites released after cell death. Many patients develop an aversion to the taste of red meats. Fatigue may be related to the increased energy demands needed

to repair damaged cells. Regardless of the cause, radiation-induced fatigue can be debilitating and may last for months. Some degree of bone marrow suppression and reduced IMMUNITY occurs, regardless of the treatment site. The intensity of marrow suppression is related to the dose, site, and size of the area irradiated.

Radiation damage to normal tissues during therapy can start inflammatory responses that lead to tissue fibrosis and scarring. These effects may appear years after radiation treatment. For example, women who receive HDR therapy for uterine cancer may develop radiation-induced colon changes (which was in the radiation path) years later, resulting in constipation and obstruction. A recent study of 99 patients with gynecologic cancer who received pelvic radiation reported having the following acute GI side effects: diarrhea (64%), proctitis (55%), nausea (33.3%), and vomiting (16.2%) (Hafiz et al., 2015). Because radiation can damage and mutate normal cell DNA, which disrupts CELLULAR REGULATION, radiation therapy increases the risk for development of second malignancies.

Radiation therapy can contribute to the development of cardiovascular disease through effects on collateral blood flow and by increasing the risk for atherosclerosis over time. It is hypothesized that certain areas of the heart may be more susceptible to radiation. For example, women with left-sided breast tumors receiving radiation to the area have a fourfold to sevenfold higher incidence of left anterior descending artery stenosis compared with women who had right-sided tumors (Zagar et al., 2015).

Not all patients experience the same degree of side effects to normal tissues, even when receiving the same dose of radiation therapy. Genetic differences appear to influence how sensitive any person's normal tissues are to radiation damage (Proud, 2014).

❖ INTERPROFESSIONAL COLLABORATIVE CARE

Patients and family members are anxious about radiation and look to the nurse and radiation technician to explain the purpose and side effects of radiation therapy. Accurate information about radiation therapy helps patients cope with the treatment.

Skin in the radiation path becomes dry and may break down. Teaching patients about skin care needs during radiation therapy is a priority intervention. Instruct the patient to not remove temporary ink markings when cleaning the skin until radiation therapy is completed. There are no universal evidence-based interventions for skin care during radiation therapy. It is important to teach patients to avoid skin irritation from clothing.

Good skin hygiene involves washing the irradiated area with mild soap and water and avoiding skin scrubbing. The use of non–aluminum-containing deodorant is recommended. Limited evidence supports the use of any lotion or ointment to decrease radiation dermatitis (Bauer, 2016). Chart 22-2 is an example of an established skin-care protocol during external radiation therapy.

> **! NURSING SAFETY PRIORITY** **QSEN**
>
> **Action Alert**
>
> Skin in the radiation path becomes *photosensitive*, increasing the risk for sunburn and sun damage. Advise against direct skin exposure to the sun during treatment and for at least 1 year after completing radiation therapy.

The normal tissues most sensitive to external radiation are bone marrow cells, skin, mucous membranes, hair follicles, and germ cells (ova and sperm). When possible, these tissues are shielded from radiation during therapy. The long-term problems of radiotherapy vary with the location and dose received (see Table 22-2). For example, radiation to the throat and upper chest can cause difficulty in swallowing and can lead to reduced nutrition. A registered dietitian is part of the interprofessional oncology team. Head and neck radiation may damage the salivary glands and cause dry mouth (**xerostomia**), which has a negative impact on speaking, chewing, and swallowing, and increases the patient's lifelong risk for tooth decay. Interventions such as saliva-substitute sprays, lozenges, and mouth rinses may be helpful. Teach patients that regular dental visits are essential. Bone exposed to radiation therapy is less dense and breaks more easily (the cause of pathologic fractures). Fatigue remains a common and often persistent problem during and for some time after radiation therapy. Exercise and sleep interventions have shown some benefit in reducing fatigue. Teach about the symptoms that might be expected

---

> **[icon] CHART 22-2**   **Patient and Family Education: Preparing for Self-Management**
>
> **Skin Protection During Radiation Therapy**
>
> - Wash the irradiated area gently each day with either water or a mild soap and water as prescribed by your radiation therapy team.
> - Use your hand rather than a washcloth when cleansing the therapy site to be gentler.
> - Rinse soap thoroughly from your skin.
> - If ink or dye markings are present to identify exactly where the beam of radiation is to be focused, take care not to remove them.
> - Dry the irradiated area with patting rather than rubbing motions; use a clean, soft towel or cloth.
> - Use only powders, ointments, lotions, or creams that are prescribed by the radiation oncology department on your skin at the radiation site.
> - Wear soft clothing over the skin at the radiation site.
> - Avoid wearing belts, buckles, straps, or any type of clothing that binds or rubs the skin at the radiation site.
> - Avoid exposure of the irradiated area to the sun:
>   - Protect this area by wearing clothing over it.
>   - Try to go outdoors in the early morning or evening to avoid the more intense sun rays.
>   - When outdoors, stay under awnings, umbrellas, and other forms of shade during the times when the sun's rays are most intense (10 AM to 7 PM).
> - Avoid heat exposure.

---

from the specific location and dose of radiation (see Table 22-1 for the location of information within this text for different cancer types).

> **[icon] NCLEX EXAMINATION CHALLENGE 22-1**
>
> **Safe and Effective Care Environment**
>
> Which statements regarding care of the client receiving radiotherapy in the form of unsealed radioactive isotopes guides the nurse's care planning? **Select all that apply.**
> A. The client may have restrictions on who can visit and for how long.
> B. The client must be in total isolation while the isotopes are in place.
> C. When "seeds" are used for prostate cancer therapy, the client must have them removed before leaving the hospital.
> D. The client's urine and stool must be handled as radioactive material.
> E. The nurse must ensure that all personnel entering the client's room use appropriate precautions.
> F. Only female nurses who are past menopause can be assigned to care for this client.

CYTOTOXIC SYSTEMIC THERAPY

Cytotoxic systemic therapy refers to the use of antineoplastic (chemotherapy) drugs that are used to kill cancer cells and disrupt their CELLULAR REGULATION. Chemotherapy may be used as the only cancer treatment received, before or after other treatments, or in combination with other cancer treatments. Unlike surgery or radiation, cytotoxic chemotherapy kills cancer cells (and normal cells) throughout the body. Some areas of the body, such as the blood-brain barrier, are more difficult than others for chemotherapy agents to penetrate. In general chemotherapy agents can be used to shrink a tumor before surgery or radiation. This is called *neoadjuvant chemotherapy*. When chemotherapy is used to kill remaining cancer cells following surgery or radiation, it is known as *adjuvant chemotherapy*.

GENETIC/GENOMIC CONSIDERATIONS
Patient-Centered Care QSEN

It is now possible to check the patient's genetic profile to determine the likelihood of experiencing dangerous side effects from some cytotoxic agents. Genomic profiling, known as *pharmacogenomics*, allows a more individualized approach to chemotherapy selection and side effect management. In addition, checking the genetic profile of the tumor can determine its sensitivity to various chemotherapy and targeted therapy agents. This practice individualizes cancer therapy and improves therapy outcomes. Expected future outcomes include an economic advantage for cancer care because decisions for treatment can be based on likelihood of effectiveness for a given patient rather than on a tumor type or stage of disease. Remind patients that assessing genetic sensitivity can result in a selection of therapy that differs from that of other adults with the same cancer type.

Selection of specific agents to use as cytotoxic treatment of cancer is based on cellular kinetic concepts that include cell cycle, growth factors, and tumor burden. Most of the cytotoxic agents are not cancer-cell specific and thus potentially affect all cells in the body. This effect is especially seen on rapidly dividing cells such as those in the bone marrow. The time when bone marrow activity and white blood cell counts are at their lowest levels after cytotoxic therapy is the nadir. It occurs at different times for different drugs. To prevent greatly reduced IMMUNITY and immunosuppression, combination cytotoxic therapy avoids using drugs with nadirs that occur at or near the same time.

CHEMOTHERAPY
Overview

Chemotherapy, the treatment of cancer with chemical agents, is used to cure and to increase survival time. This killing effect on cancer cells is related to the ability of chemotherapy to damage DNA and interfere with cell division and CELLULAR REGULATION. Tumors with rapid growth are often more sensitive to chemotherapy.

As described in Chapter 21, cancer cells can separate from the original tumor, spread to new areas, and establish new cancers at distant sites (metastasize). Patients with metastatic cancer will die unless treatment eliminates the metastatic cancer cells along with the original cancer cells. Chemotherapy is useful in treating cancer because its effects are systemic, providing the opportunity to kill metastatic cancer cells that may have escaped local treatment. Drugs used for chemotherapy also exert their cell-damaging (cytotoxic) effects on healthy cells. The normal cells most affected by chemotherapy are those that divide rapidly, including skin, hair, intestinal tissues, spermatocytes, and blood-forming cells. These drugs are classified by the specific types of action they exert in the cancer cell (Table 22-3).

Chemotherapy Drug Categories

Alkylating agents cross-link DNA, making the DNA strands bind tightly together. This action prevents proper DNA and ribonucleic acid (RNA) synthesis, which inhibits cell division.

Antimetabolites are similar to normal metabolites needed for vital cell processes. Most cell reactions require metabolites to

TABLE 22-3 Categories of Chemotherapeutic Drugs

Antimetabolites	Alkylating Agents
Azacitidine (Vidaza)	Altretamine (Hexalen)
Capecitabine (Xeloda)	Bendamustine (Treanda)
Cladribine (Leustatin)	Busulfan (Busulfex)
Clofarabine (Clolar)	Carboplatin (Paraplatin)
Cytarabine (Cytosar, ara-C)	Carmustine (BiCNU, Gliadel)
Decitabine (Dacogen)	Chlorambucil (Leukeran)
Floxuridine (FUDR)	Cisplatin (Platinol)
5-Fluorouracil (Adrucil, Efudex, Fluoroplex)	Cyclophosphamide (Cytoxan, Procytox)
Fludarabine (Fludara, FLAMP)	Dacarbazine (DTIC)
Gemcitabine (Gemzar)	Estramustine (Emcyt, Estracyte)
6-Mercaptopurine (Purinethol)	Ifosfamide (Ifex)
Methotrexate (MTX, Mexate)	Lomustine (CCNU, CeeNU)
Nelarabine (Arranon)	Mechlorethamine (Mustargen)
Pemetrexed (Alimta)	Melphalan (Alkeran) (available in oral or IV form)
Pentostatin (Nipent)	Oxaliplatin (Eloxatin)
6-Thioguanine (Tabloid)	Streptozocin (Zanosar)
	Temozolomide (Temodar)
Antitumor Antibiotics	Thiotepa (Thioplex)
Bleomycin (Blenoxane)	
Dactinomycin (Cosmegen)	**Topoisomerase Inhibitors**
Daunorubicin (Cerubidine, Daunomycin)	Irinotecan (Camptosar)
Doxorubicin (Adriamycin, Rubex)	Topotecan (Hycamtin)
Doxorubicin liposomal (Doxil)	
Epirubicin (Ellence)	**Miscellaneous Agents**
Idarubicin (Idamycin)	Arsenic trioxide (Trisenox)
Mitomycin C (Mutamycin)	Asparaginase (Elspar)
Mitoxantrone (Novantrone)	Hydroxyurea (Droxia, Hydrea)
Valrubicin (Valstar)	Ixabepilone (Ixempra)
	Pegaspargase (Oncaspar)
Antimitotics/Mitosis Inhibitors	Procarbazine (Matulane, Natulan)
Cabazitaxel (Jevtana)	Vorinostat (Zolinza)
Docetaxel (Taxotere)	
Etoposide (VP-16, VePesid)	
Eribulin mesylate (Halaven)	
Paclitaxel (Taxol)	
Teniposide (Vumon)	
Vinblastine (Velban, Velbe, Velsar)	
Vincristine (Oncovin)	
Vinorelbine (Navelbine)	

Data from the US Food and Drug Administration website at www.fda.gov/cder/index.html; and MD Consult at www.mdconsult.com/php/82925233-2/homepage.

begin or continue the reaction. Antimetabolites closely resemble normal metabolites and act as "counterfeit" metabolites that fool cancer cells into using the antimetabolites in cellular reactions. Because antimetabolites cannot function as proper metabolites, their presence impairs CELLULAR REGULATION, especially cell division.

Antimitotic agents (also known as *mitosis inhibitors*) interfere with the formation and actions of microtubules so cells cannot complete mitosis during cell division. As a result the cancer cell either does not divide at all or divides only once.

Antitumor antibiotics are drugs that were originally developed as antibiotics that have effects on cancer cells. These drugs damage the cell's DNA and interrupt DNA or RNA synthesis. The exact mechanism of interruption varies with each agent.

Topoisomerase inhibitors disrupt an enzyme (topoisomerase) essential for DNA synthesis and cell division. When drugs disrupt the enzyme, proper DNA maintenance is prevented, resulting in increased DNA breakage and eventual cell death.

Miscellaneous chemotherapy drugs are those with mechanisms of action that are either unknown or do not fit those of other drug categories.

Combination Chemotherapy

Successful cancer chemotherapy often involves giving more than one type of anticancer drug in a timed manner (*combination chemotherapy*). Using more than one drug is more effective in killing cancer cells than using just one drug because of their different mechanisms of action. However, the side effects and damage caused to normal tissues also increase with combination chemotherapy.

Treatment Issues

Drugs selected for use with a given patient are based on the sensitivity of cancer cells to the drug and the stage or extent of disease. Selected treatment protocols have been developed for many cancers using well-established clinical guidelines for initial treatment and relapsed disease. Dosages for most chemotherapy drugs are calculated according to the patient's size, based on milligrams per square meter of body surface area (BSA), which considers the patient's height and weight at the time of chemotherapy administration.

Chemotherapy drugs are given on a regularly scheduled basis timed to maximize cancer cell kill and minimize damage to normal cells. Regimens vary for the number of days in a row for each round of drug delivery, the number of days or weeks between rounds of therapy, and the total number of rounds. The intent is to allow normal cells time to recover from any injury but prevent cancer cell recovery. **Dose-dense chemotherapy** protocols involve giving chemotherapy rounds closer together, supplemented with bone marrow growth factors to prevent neutropenia. Dose-dense therapy also results in more intense side effects. Maintaining the intended dosage and timing schedule to ensure that the patient receives the maximum recommended doses is a critical factor in the successful response to chemotherapy.

Patient and family education is critical in helping patients adhere to the prescribed schedule for best outcomes, reducing side effects, and preventing therapy complications. Side effects of chemotherapy are generally managed in the home. Therefore comprehensive and consistent patient education efforts by knowledgeable nurses are key to patient safety.

Many chemotherapy drugs are given IV, although other routes may be used. For specific cancer types, the chemotherapy may be infused or instilled into a body cavity. The *intrathecal* route delivers drugs into the spinal canal, and the *intraventricular* route delivers drugs directly into the ventricles of the brain. *Intraperitoneal* instillations place the drugs within the abdominal cavity, most often for ovarian cancer. Drugs for bladder cancer can be instilled directly into the bladder (*intravesicular* route). In some instances drugs may be applied as a *topical* preparation for skin lesions. *Intra-arterial* infusions may be used to deliver a higher dose locally. For example, with liver tumors an interventional radiologist places a catheter into the artery supplying the liver tumor. The concentrated chemotherapy drug, delivered in sponge-like beads, is infused, and the beads become trapped in the small arteries feeding the tumor. The techniques and care needs for different routes are described with the specific cancer type most commonly associated with the specific administration route. Regardless of the route, chemotherapy agents are designated

hazardous drugs (HDs) and must be handled as such (Callahan et al., 2016; Crickman & Finnell, 2017).

The IV route is the most common for traditional chemotherapy. The standard of care designated by the Oncology Nursing Society (ONS) and supported by the American Society of Clinical Oncology (ASCO) for safe administration of IV chemotherapy is that giving these drugs requires special education and handling (Callahan et al., 2016; Neuss et al., 2017). *Chemotherapy is to be given only by registered nurses who have completed an approved chemotherapy program and have demonstrated competence in administering these agents. However, responsibility for monitoring the patient during chemotherapy administration rests with all nurses providing patient care.*

Most chemotherapy drugs are absorbed through the skin and mucous membranes. As a result the interprofessional care workers who prepare or give these drugs (especially nurses and pharmacists) are at risk for absorbing them. Anyone preparing, giving, or disposing of chemotherapy drugs or handling excreta from patients within 48 hours of receiving IV chemotherapy must wear approved personal protective equipment (PPE) (Callahan et al., 2016; Neuss et al., 2017). Such equipment includes eye protection, masks, double gloves or "chemo" gloves, and gown. The Occupational Safety and Health Administration (OSHA) and the Oncology Nursing Society (ONS) have established practice guidelines and protective standards.

A serious complication of IV infusion is **extravasation**, which occurs when drug leaks into the surrounding tissues (also called *infiltration*). When the drugs given are **vesicants** (chemicals that damage tissue on direct contact), the results of extravasation can include pain, infection, and tissue loss (Fig. 22-2). Surgery is sometimes needed for severe tissue damage.

The most important nursing intervention for extravasation is prevention (Schulmeister, 2014). Small extravasations resolve

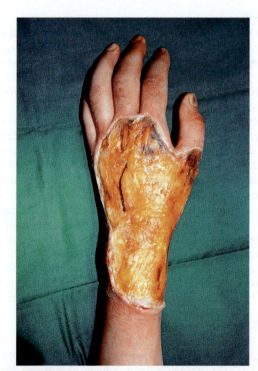

FIG. 22-2 Appearance of tissue damage and loss after chemotherapy extravasation. (From Weinzweig, J., & Weinzweig, N. [2005]. *The mutilated hand,* St. Louis: Mosby.)

without extensive treatment if less than 0.5 mL of the drug has leaked into the tissues. If a larger amount has leaked, extensive tissue damage occurs, and surgery may be needed. *Careful monitoring of blood return and the access site is critical during chemotherapy administration to prevent extravasation.* Institutions have established, evidence-based policies and procedures that are drug specific to guide extravasation management. With some drugs cold compresses to the area are prescribed; for other agents warm compresses are used. Antidotes may be injected into the site of extravasation. Coordinate with the oncologist and pharmacist to determine the specific antidote needed for the extravasated drug. When vesicants are part of therapy, the use of an implanted port or central line to decrease extravasation risk is recommended. Even with these devices, the nurse must observe closely for any indication of leakage and initiate management guidelines immediately.

Some anticancer drugs are available currently as oral agents (Table 22-4), and more are in development. Only a few oral agents are actually oral formulations of classic cytotoxic chemotherapy agents; more are classified as specific types of targeted therapy agents (discussed later). Oral drugs are more convenient for the patient and can be taken at home. However, there are many problems with oral anticancer drugs. One of the biggest problems is the misperception by patients and nononcology nurses that these drugs are less toxic than IV chemotherapy (Spoelstra & Rittenberg, 2015), which is **not** true. *Oral anticancer drugs are just as toxic to the patient taking the drug and to the person handling the drug as are standard chemotherapy drugs.*

TABLE 22-4 Current Oral Chemotherapeutic Drugs		
AGENT	**DRUG CATEGORY**	**CANCER TYPE**
Altretamine (Hexalen)	Alkylating agent	Ovarian cancer
Capecitabine (Xeloda)	Antimetabolite	Breast cancer Colorectal cancer
Chlorambucil (Leukeran)	Alkylating agent	Chronic lymphocytic leukemia; Hodgkin's lymphoma Non-Hodgkin's lymphoma
Dasatinib (Sprycel)	Tyrosine kinase inhibitor	Chronic myelogenous leukemia; acute myelogenous leukemia that is Philadelphia chromosome positive
Erlotinib (Tarceva)	Epidermal growth factor receptor inhibitor	Non–small-cell lung cancer Pancreatic cancer
Everolimus (Afinitor)	Angiogenesis inhibitor	Advanced renal cell carcinoma
Gefitinib (Iressa)	Epidermal growth factor receptor inhibitor	Non–small-cell lung cancer
Hydroxyurea (Droxia, Hydrea)	Miscellaneous agent	Chronic myelogenous leukemia Head and neck cancer Melanoma Ovarian cancer Sickle cell disease
Imatinib (Gleevec)	Tyrosine kinase inhibitor	Chronic myelogenous leukemia that is Philadelphia chromosome positive GI stromal tumors Myelodysplastic syndrome
Lapatinib (Tykerb)	Tyrosine kinase inhibitor	Breast cancer
Lenalidomide (Revlimid)	Angiogenesis inhibitor	Multiple myeloma; myelodysplastic syndrome
Lomustine (CCNU, CeeNU)	Alkylating agent	Hodgkin's lymphoma Malignant glioma
Melphalan (Alkeran)	Alkylating agent	Multiple myeloma Ovarian cancer
Mercaptopurine (Purinethol)	Antimetabolite	Acute lymphocytic leukemia
Nilotinib (Tasigna)	Tyrosine kinase inhibitor	Chronic myelogenous leukemia that is Philadelphia chromosome positive
Pazopanib (Votrient)	Multikinase inhibitor	Advanced renal cell carcinoma
Procarbazine (Matulane, Natulan)	Miscellaneous agent	Hodgkin's lymphoma
Sorafenib (Nexavar)	Multikinase inhibitor	Advanced renal cell carcinoma; hepatocellular carcinoma
Sunitinib (Sutent)	Multikinase inhibitor	Advanced renal cell carcinoma; gastrointestinal stromal tumor
Temozolomide (Temodar)	Alkylating agent	Brain tumors (primary)
Thioguanine (Tabloid)	Antimetabolite	Acute myelogenous leukemia
Topotecan (Hycamtin)	Topoisomerase inhibitor	Small cell lung cancer
Vorinostat (Zolinza)	Histone inhibitor	Cutaneous T-cell lymphoma

The responsibility for administering these drugs often shifts from the oncology clinic to the home or to nononcology acute care settings, and issues of protection, correct administration, adherence, and recognition and management of side effects are major concerns. There is a critical need for patient education and support to self-manage this therapy, including the accidental ingestion by another person. Not all patients are able to accept the responsibility of self-management, and this must be considered during patient selection for oral chemotherapy (Spoelstra & Sansoucie, 2015).

Because these oral agents can be absorbed through skin and mucous membranes and exert toxic effects, the person who handles and administers them needs to use PPE in the same way as during IV chemotherapy administration. This becomes a more critical issue when nononcology nurses are administering the drugs. The ONS practice guidelines stress nurse education for competence to administer these drugs. All nurses administering these drugs must know the indications for drug use, dosage ranges, side effects and adverse effects, schedules, and specific precautions (Thompson & Christian, 2016). *Oral agents must not be crushed, split, broken, or chewed.* These drugs are biohazardous and must be discarded in accordance with agency policy.

In the home environment it is important that the patient and family understand the importance of avoiding direct skin contact with oral chemotherapy agents and how to dispose of them properly. Teach patients or whoever prepares the dosages how to avoid touching the drugs. Tablets and capsules in blister packs are pressed into a small paper cup. Those in traditional medication bottles are "poured" first into the bottle cap and then into a paper cup. The patient then "drinks" the tablet/capsule from the cup into his or her mouth. These drugs are to be taken separately from all other drugs. Consult a drug handbook or a pharmacist for timing of the drug in relation to meals and what to do if a dose is missed. For many of these oral drugs, missed doses are **not** taken when remembered. The patient just takes the next scheduled drug dose.

Disposal of expired or discontinued oral chemotherapy agents can be problematic. Just like all other drugs, these agents are not to be flushed down the drain. Unlike many other drugs, disposal needs to consider that the drugs should not be directly touched. Taking them to a community drug disposal event or the police station can be hazardous to others. Instruct patients to (ideally) bring the expired or discontinued drugs back to the oncology clinic in the container in which they were dispensed. If this is not feasible, instruct patients to call the dispensing pharmacist about specific disposal methods.

Adherence to defined oral chemotherapy schedules and dosages is more of a problem than with IV administration (Spoelstra & Rittenberg, 2015). Even some highly motivated patients with cancer consider that skipping or reducing doses of oral drugs has only a minor impact. As with teaching other aspects of self-management, nurses have to be certain that patients and caregivers understand the implications of the decisions they make. Disrupting the schedule or reducing dosages has a negative impact on therapy outcomes and leads to drug resistance among cancer cells, disease progression, and reduced survival. Research on a variety of interventions to increase adherence is ongoing. The Quality Improvement box describes the effectiveness of an electronic intervention in promoting adherence (Spoelstra et al., 2015).

QUALITY IMPROVEMENT (QSEN)

Text Message Reminders Improve Adherence to Oral Anticancer Agents

Spoelstra, S., Given, C., Sikorskii, A., Coursaris, C., Majumder, A., DeKoekkoek, T., et al. (2015). Feasibility of a text-messaging intervention to promote self-management for patients prescribed oral anticancer agents. *Oncology Nursing Forum, 42*(6), 647–657.

Oral anticancer agents are becoming a common form of chemotherapy. They are convenient for the patient and are taken daily in the community environment. This change in delivery shifts responsibility for safe and consistent administration to the patient and family as part of self-management. A major issue with daily oral chemotherapy is consistent adherence to the prescribed schedule. Many patients have the false perception that an oral drug can't be very important to overall cancer therapy. The therapy schedule can be complex, with doses needed more than once daily and cycles changing over the course of a month. For patients who do not take other drugs on a daily or twice-daily basis, remembering to take the oral anticancer agent can be problematic. Whatever the cause, studies have shown that adherence to the prescribed schedule with an oral anticancer agent is less than 80%. Previous research has shown that a telephone reminder has helped some patients improve adherence. However, this intervention has limitations, especially when the telephone used is the patient's landline.

The current study sought to examine the utility of mHealth technology in improving self-management of patients taking oral anticancer agents, including schedule adherence and symptom management. mHealth, which is the use of mobile devices with software applications to provide access to health services, manage patient information, provide specific health knowledge, and assist skill development for health promotion and condition management, is now widely used to promote self-management of a variety of chronic conditions. The use of a text message (texting) has several advantages over a telephone reminder. Because a portable device is used, the patient can receive the message wherever he or she is. The message does not disturb others in the environment. Texting retains the ability of the patient to ask questions and receive responses in a timely manner.

The control group received and used a notebook-based toolkit for information, drug schedules, and symptom management techniques for 3 to 4 weeks. In addition to the toolkit, the intervention group received daily texts for adherence and weekly assessment of symptoms over the same time period.

The intervention group overall had a reduction in the number of symptoms and a higher adherence rate than did the control group. One patient in the intervention group reported that the texts were a burden.

Commentary: Implications for Research and Practice

The study design was a 10-week longitudinal, two-group, randomized control with a sample size of 80 adults newly prescribed oral anticancer agents. The methods were appropriate for the purpose of the study.

Future research is needed to determine how well the intervention performs and how acceptable it is over long-term therapy. In addition, texts were sent only once daily. More research is needed to determine the effectiveness on adherence when multiple texts per day are used. The increased use of mHealth techniques, even among older adults who may not be as comfortable with mobile devises as younger adults, necessitates ensuring that the techniques are personalized sufficiently and have an ease of use so users perceive them as helpful rather than a nuisance or burden.

Side Effects of Chemotherapy

Temporary and permanent damage can occur to normal tissues from chemotherapy because it is systemic and exerts its effects on all cells. Some problems include bladder toxicity (hemorrhagic cystitis), cardiac muscle damage, and loss of bone density. For some cancer drugs, agents that protect specific healthy cells (cytoprotectants or chemoprotectants) are given ahead of or with chemotherapy drugs to decrease the impact of these drugs on normal tissues. For example, amifostine (Ethyol) reduces DNA damage and is used to prevent kidney damage in patients receiving cisplatin; to reduce neutropenia; and to reduce radiation-induced xerostomia for patients receiving radiation therapy for head and neck cancer. Mesna (Mesnex) binds toxic metabolites to decrease bladder toxicity and prevent hemorrhagic cystitis from ifosfamide and high-dose cyclophosphamide use. Agents such as the anthracycline drug doxorubicin can result in cardiotoxicity, leading to heart failure. Loss of bone density is associated with the use of oral aromatase inhibitors for breast cancer treatment.

Serious short-term side effects occur with cytotoxic chemotherapy. The side effects on the hematopoietic (blood-producing) system can be life threatening and are the most common reason for changing the dosage or the treatment plan. The suppressive effects on the bone marrow blood-forming cells cause anemia (decreased numbers of red blood cells and hemoglobin); reduced IMMUNITY with neutropenia (decreased numbers of neutrophil white blood cells leading to immunosuppression); and thrombocytopenia (decreased numbers of platelets), which leads to impaired CLOTTING and bleeding. Common distressing side effects include nausea and vomiting, alopecia (hair loss), mucositis (open sores on mucous membranes), many skin changes, anxiety, sleep disturbance, altered bowel elimination, and changes in cognitive function. The impact of these side effects is referred to as *cancer therapy symptom distress*, which can vary from patient to patient. Cancer symptom distress is measured using the National Comprehensive Cancer Network® (NCCN®) Distress Thermometer (Fig. 22-3).

Drug therapy is used to reduce symptom distress from some of these side effects. For other problems such as alopecia, no evidence-based prevention strategies exist, but patients can use techniques to be more comfortable with its presence. Nonpharmacologic interventions for symptom distress include distraction, massage, guided imagery, and complementary therapies.

Psychosocial issues can occur during chemotherapy. For many chemotherapy regimens drugs are given over a period ranging from 30 minutes to 8 hours or longer. During this time the patient may be confined to a treatment area, which is a

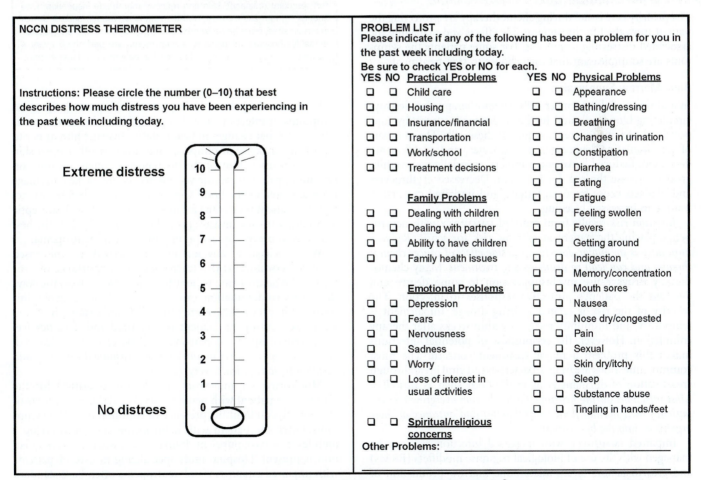

Version 2.2016. Reproduced with permission from the NCCN Clinical Practice Guidelines in Oncology (NCCN Guidelines®) for Distress Management V.2.2016. © 2016 National Comprehensive Cancer Network, Inc. All rights reserved. The NCCN Guidelines® and illustrations herein may not be reproduced in any form for any purpose without the express written permission of NCCN. To view the most recent and complete version of the NCCN Guidelines, go online to NCCN.org. The NCCN Guidelines are a work in progress that may be refined as often as new significant data becomes available. NCCN makes no warranties of any kind whatsoever regarding their content, use, or application and disclaims any responsibility for their application or use in any way.

FIG. 22-3 The NCCN Distress Thermometer for patients.

constant reminder of the disease and its treatment. Distraction methods such as virtual reality, guided imagery, reading, watching television, and talking with visitors may help reduce the sense of unpleasantness.

anti-infective drugs such as antibiotic, antifungal, and antiviral drugs. Just as for any other infection, anti-infective therapy is specific for the organism(s) causing the infection.

CLINICAL JUDGMENT CHALLENGE 22-1

Safety; Evidence-Based Practice; Patient-Centered Care QSEN

Mrs. G is a 67-year-old woman with colorectal cancer who has undergone a surgical resection of the tumor with anastomosis. She has returned for her follow-up visit to the oncologist, who has prescribed the oral chemotherapy agent capecitabine for her.

1. Which teaching concerning the handling of oral chemotherapy agents should be included in the care plan for Mrs. G?
2. Mrs. G calls the oncology clinic and tells you that she has accidentally skipped a dose. What would be your best response?
3. Mrs. G tells you that she dislikes taking pills and finds it easier to chew rather than swallow most medications. What would be your best response?

Mrs. G's oncologist has discontinued the capecitabine treatment because her disease has progressed.

4. What would be the best way to dispose of oral chemotherapy agents that are no longer needed?

❖ INTERPROFESSIONAL COLLABORATIVE CARE

The priority care issues during chemotherapy are protecting the patient from the life-threatening side effects and managing the associated distressing symptoms. For some patients the symptoms are so unpleasant that they choose to stop treatment.

Bone Marrow Suppression

In addition to killing cancer cells, chemotherapy also destroys circulating blood cells and further reduces IMMUNITY by suppressing bone marrow replacement of these cells. The numbers of all circulating leukocytes, erythrocytes, and platelets are decreased. Reduced leukocyte numbers, especially neutrophils, greatly increase the risk for infection. Decreased erythrocytes and platelets cause hypoxia, fatigue, and impaired CLOTTING, leading to increased bleeding.

Infection risk results from reduced IMMUNITY with neutropenia, placing the patient at extreme risk for sepsis. *Reduced immunity is the major dose-limiting side effect of cancer chemotherapy and can lead to death during treatment.* Many chemotherapy drugs cause myelosuppression to some degree and decrease the patient's protective responses to infection. The severity of the risk is related to drug dosage. Impairment is temporary, and immunity recovers within weeks after therapy completion. However, the seriousness of potential infections makes this problem a major treatment concern. The most common infections are fungal, bacterial, and viral breakthrough (reactivation of dormant virus in the body such as *varicella*). *Most infections during neutropenia result from overgrowth of the patient's own normal flora (microbiome) and entrance of these organisms into the bloodstream.*

Impaired IMMUNITY with increased infection risk can be managed with the use of biological response modifiers (BRMs) and growth factors to stimulate bone marrow production of immune system cells. Although not appropriate for all types of cancer, this supportive treatment can reduce the risk for infection during chemotherapy. This treatment is discussed in the Immunotherapy section. Actual infections are managed with

CONSIDERATIONS FOR OLDER ADULTS

Patient-Centered Care QSEN

Older adults are at even greater risk for chemotherapy-induced neutropenia because of age-related changes in bone marrow function (McCance et al., 2014). Using growth factors such as filgrastim (Neupogen) and pegfilgrastim (Neulasta) before neutropenia occurs rather than later can reduce the severity of neutropenia and the risk for infectious complications. Use frequent handwashing during times of immunosuppression. Be extra vigilant in assessing older adults for early indicators of infection.

NURSING SAFETY PRIORITY QSEN

Action Alert

The priority interventions for the patient with neutropenia are protecting him or her from infection within the health care system and teaching the patient and family how to reduce infection risk in the home. Total patient assessment, including a review of common symptoms associated with infection (e.g., fever, sore throat, urinary frequency or discomfort, purulent drainage), skin and mucous membrane inspection, lung sounds, mouth assessment, and inspection of venous access device insertion sites, must be performed on a scheduled basis by a registered nurse for hospitalized patients. Assessments are performed every 4 hours or as often as agency policy and the patient's condition warrant.

Explain to the patient the importance of reporting signs and symptoms of infection, any change in skin and mucous membranes, or other changes in health status. Instruct him or her to report the presence of pimples, sores, rash, or other open skin areas. Also teach him or her to report a cough, burning on urination, pain around the venous access site, or new drainage from any area of the body. Good handwashing before contact with the patient is essential for infection prevention. Use aseptic technique with any invasive procedure. Chart 22-3 lists the best practices to prevent infection in patients with neutropenia.

When delegating any nursing care activity to unlicensed assistive personnel (UAP), teach them the importance of protecting the neutropenic patient from infection. Stress the ways that cross-contamination can occur and how to avoid this source of infection. Also ensure that UAP understand that, even when the neutropenic patient is very tired and does not feel well, certain aspects of personal hygiene cannot be deferred. *Teach the importance of mouth care and washing the axillary and perianal regions at least every 12 hours.*

Monitoring for indicators of infection is critical for the hospitalized patient with neutropenia. The reduced numbers of neutrophils can limit the presence of common infection symptoms. Often the patient with neutropenia does not develop a high fever or have purulent drainage even when a severe infection is present. Hospital units specializing in care of patients with impaired IMMUNITY and neutropenia often have standard protocols that nurses initiate as soon as infection is suspected, *before* a primary health care provider examines the patient, because treatment delay can result in sepsis and death. These protocols specify which types of cultures to obtain (e.g., blood,

CHART 22-3 Best Practice for Patient Safety & Quality Care QSEN

Care of the Patient With Myelosuppression and Neutropenia

- Place the patient in a private room whenever possible.
- Use good handwashing technique or alcohol-based hand rubs before touching the patient or any of the patient's belongings.
- Ensure that the patient's room and bathroom are cleaned at least once each day.
- Do not use supplies from common areas for patients with myelosuppression and neutropenia. For example, keep a dedicated box of disposable gloves in his or her room and do not share this box with any other patient. Provide single-use food products, individually wrapped gauze, and other individually wrapped items.
- Limit the number of health care personnel entering the patient's room.
- Monitor vital signs every 4 hours, including temperature.
- Inspect the patient's mouth at least every 8 hours.
- Inspect the patient's skin and mucous membranes (especially the mouth and anal area) for the presence of fissures and abscesses at least every 8 hours.
- Inspect open areas such as IV sites every 4 hours for indications of infection.
- Change wound dressings daily.
- Obtain specimens of all suspicious areas for culture (as specified by the agency) and promptly notify the primary health care provider.
- Assist the patient in coughing and deep-breathing exercises.
- Encourage activity at a level appropriate for the patient's current health status.
- Change IV tubing daily or according to unit protocol.
- Keep frequently used equipment in the room for use with this patient only (e.g., blood pressure cuff, stethoscope, thermometer).
- Limit visitors to healthy adults.
- Use strict aseptic technique for all invasive procedures.
- Monitor the white blood cell count daily.
- Avoid the use of indwelling urinary catheters.
- Follow agency policy for restriction of fresh flowers and potted plants in the patient's room.

CHART 22-4 Patient and Family Education: Preparing for Self-Management

Prevention of Infection

During the times your white blood cell counts are low:
- Avoid crowds and other large gatherings of people who might be ill.
- Do not share personal toiletries such as toothbrushes, toothpaste, washcloths, or deodorant sticks with others.
- If possible, bathe daily with an antimicrobial soap. If total bathing is not possible, wash the armpits, groin, genitals, and anal area twice a day with an antimicrobial soap.
- Keep your toothbrush dry.
- Wash your hands thoroughly with an antimicrobial soap before you eat and drink, after touching a pet, after shaking hands with anyone, as soon as you come home from any outing, and after using the toilet.
- Follow the cancer center's instructions for eating fresh salads; raw fruits and vegetables; meat, fish and eggs; and pepper and paprika.
- Wash dishes between use with hot, sudsy water or use a dishwasher.
- Do not drink water, milk, juice, or other cold liquids that have been standing at room temperature for longer than an hour.
- Do not reuse cups and glasses without washing.
- Do not change pet litter boxes.
- Take your temperature at least once a day and whenever you do not feel well.
- Report any of these indications of infection to your oncologist immediately:
  - Temperature greater than 100° F (37.8° C)
  - Persistent cough (with or without sputum)
  - Pus or foul-smelling drainage from any open skin area or normal body opening
  - Presence of a boil or abscess
  - Urine that is cloudy or foul smelling or that causes burning on urination
- Take all prescribed drugs.
- Wear clean disposable gloves underneath gardening gloves when working in the garden or with houseplants.
- Wear a condom when having sex. If you are a woman having sex with a male partner, ensure that he wears a condom.

urine, sputum, central line, wound), which diagnostic tests to obtain (e.g., chest x-ray), and which antibiotics to start immediately.

NURSING SAFETY PRIORITY QSEN

Critical Rescue

Monitor patients with reduced IMMUNITY to recognize signs of infection. When any temperature elevation (>100° F or 37.8° C) is present, respond by reporting this to the health care provider immediately and implement standard infection protocols. When IV anti-infective drugs are started, the neutropenic patient is admitted to the hospital. The patient with neutropenia but no other symptoms of communicable disease is NOT an infection hazard to other people; however, other people can be an infection hazard to the patient.

Many patients remain at home during periods of neutropenia and are at continuing risk for infection. The focus remains on keeping the patient's own normal flora under control and preventing transmission of organisms from others. Teach patients and families self-care actions to reduce the risk for infection (Chart 22-4), especially handwashing.

Anemia and *thrombocytopenia* also result from the bone marrow suppression caused by some chemotherapy drugs.

Anemia causes patients to feel fatigued from a lack of adequate red blood cells to transport oxygen, and some tissues are hypoxic. Thrombocytopenia increases the risk for excessive bleeding from impaired CLOTTING. When the platelet count is less than $50,000/mm^3$ ($50 \times 10^9/L$), small trauma can lead to prolonged bleeding. With a count lower than $20,000/mm^3$ ($20 \times 10^9/L$), spontaneous and uncontrollable bleeding may occur. Both anemia and thrombocytopenia may require transfusion therapy.

The use of growth factors to stimulate production of red blood cells and platelets to improve CLOTTING is common. Erythropoiesis-stimulating agents (ESAs) such as darbepoetin alfa (Aranesp) and epoetin alfa (Epogen and Procrit) can prevent or improve anemia associated with chemotherapy and reduce the need for transfusions. These drugs increase the production of many blood cell types, not just erythrocytes, increasing the patient's risk for hypertension, blood clots, strokes, and heart attacks, especially among older adults. In addition, certain types of cancer cells, such as head and neck cancer cells, leukemias, and some lymphomas, grow faster in the presence of these ESAs; and their use may be restricted. Dosing is based on each patient's hemoglobin levels to ensure that enough red blood cells are produced to avoid the need for transfusion but not necessarily to bring hemoglobin or hematocrit levels up to normal.

CHART 22-5   Best Practice for Patient Safety & Quality Care QSEN

Prevention of Injury for the Patient With Thrombocytopenia

- Handle the patient gently.
- Use and teach unlicensed assistive personnel (UAP) to use a lift sheet when moving and positioning the patient in bed.
- Avoid IM injections and venipunctures.
- When injections or venipunctures are necessary, use the smallest-gauge needle for the task.
- Apply firm pressure to the needlestick site for 10 minutes or until the site no longer oozes blood.
- Apply ice to areas of trauma.
- Test all urine and stool for the presence of occult blood.
- Observe IV sites every 4 hours for bleeding.
- Instruct patients to notify nursing personnel immediately if any trauma occurs and if bleeding or bruising is noticed.
- Avoid trauma to rectal tissues:
  - Do not administer enemas.
  - If suppositories are prescribed, lubricate liberally and administer with caution.
- Instruct the patient and UAP that the patient should use an electric shaver rather than a razor.
- When providing mouth care or supervising others in providing mouth care:
  - Use a soft-bristled toothbrush or tooth sponges.
  - Do not use water-pressure gum cleaners.
  - Make certain that dentures and other dental devices fit and do not irritate the gums.
- Instruct the patient not to blow the nose or insert objects into the nose.
- Instruct UAP and the patient that the patient should wear shoes with firm soles whenever ambulating.
- Practice fall prevention strategies according to the agency's policies.
- Keep pathways and walkways clear and uncluttered.

CHART 22-6   Patient and Family Education: Preparing for Self-Management

Preventing Injury or Bleeding

During the time your platelet count is low:
- Use an electric shaver.
- Use a soft-bristled toothbrush.
- Do not have dental work performed without consulting your cancer health care provider.
- Do not take aspirin or any aspirin-containing products. Read the label to be sure that the product does not contain aspirin or salicylates.
- Do not participate in contact sports or any activity likely to result in your being bumped, scratched, or scraped.
- If you are bumped, apply ice to the site for at least 1 hour.
- Avoid hard foods that would scrape the inside of your mouth.
- Eat only warm, cool, or cold foods to avoid burning your mouth. Be especially cautious with cheese topping on pizza.
- Check your skin and mouth daily for bruises; swelling; or areas with small, reddish-purple marks that may indicate bleeding.
- Notify your cancer health care provider if you:
  - Are injured and persistent bleeding results
  - Have menstrual bleeding that is excessive for you
  - See blood in your vomit, urine, or bowel movement
- Avoid trauma with intercourse.
- Avoid anal intercourse.
- Take a stool softener to prevent straining during a bowel movement.
- Do not use enemas or rectal suppositories.
- Avoid bending over at the waist, which increases pressure in the brain.
- Do not wear clothing or shoes that are tight or that rub.
- Avoid blowing your nose or placing objects in your nose. If you must blow your nose, do so gently without blocking either nasal passage.
- Avoid playing musical instruments that raise the pressure inside your head such as brass wind instruments and woodwinds or reed instruments.

NCLEX EXAMINATION CHALLENGE 22-2

Health Promotion and Maintenance

The client who received combination chemotherapy 7 days ago for breast cancer calls the oncology clinic to report a temperature of 100.5° F (38.6° C) and has no other symptoms of infection. What is the nurse's **best** response?
A. "This is a normal immune-related response to the chemotherapy."
B. "Please go to the nearest emergency room for a full workup for infection."
C. "You are most likely dehydrated. Come to the clinic now for IV fluids."
D. "There is no concern at this time but call if your temperature reaches 101.5° F (38.6° C)."

An example of growth factor therapy for thrombocytopenia and reduced CLOTTING is the use of oprelvekin (Neumega). This drug increases the production of platelets. The drug may cause fluid retention and increase the risk for heart failure and pulmonary edema. Other side effects include conjunctival bleeding, hypotension, and tachycardia. Teach patients to weigh themselves daily and keep a record. Remind them to immediately report sudden weight gain or dyspnea to the health care provider.

The priority for nursing care for the patient with thrombocytopenia is to provide a safe environment. Chart 22-5 lists the best practices for Bleeding Precautions for impaired CLOTTING. Teach UAP the importance of using Bleeding Precautions and the need to report any evidence of bleeding immediately. Caregivers at home also need to know these practices.

Teach patients with thrombocytopenia and their families to avoid injury and excessive bleeding when discharge occurs before the platelet count has returned to normal. Chart 22-6 reviews precautions to teach patients to prevent bleeding and what to do if bleeding occurs.

Chemotherapy-Induced Nausea and Vomiting

Chemotherapy-induced nausea and vomiting (CINV) arises from a variety of GI and neural mechanisms. It may manifest as *anticipatory* (before receiving the chemotherapy, often triggered by thoughts, sights, and sounds related to the anticipated chemotherapy), *acute* (within the first 24 hours after chemotherapy), *delayed* (occurring after the first 24 hours), *breakthrough* (occurring intermittently during therapy for CINV), or a combination. Many cancer drugs are **emetogenic** (vomiting inducing), with some agents causing more nausea and vomiting than others. Although there are advances in prevention and control of CINV, it remains a common and distressing issue. Nausea often persists, even when vomiting is controlled. Current studies examining genetic factors in the metabolism of chemotherapy agents and antiemetics are ongoing to help identify adults at higher risk for CINV and to allow more precise therapies to manage it (Kiernan, 2016).

Acute CINV is the most common type. It may persist for 1 to 2 days after chemotherapy is given. A few drugs, such as dacarbazine (DTIC), may trigger CINV almost as soon as the drug is started. Other drugs, such as cisplatin (Platinol), induce delayed nausea and vomiting that can continue as long as 5 to 7 days after receiving it. Patients who have CINV during the first round of chemotherapy may begin to experience the same symptoms before the next dose as a result of sheer anticipation. Once considered the single most distressing side effect of chemotherapy, CINV often can be well controlled with appropriate evidence-based antiemetic therapy, especially with serotonin (5-HT3) antagonist drugs and the use of standardized protocols for its prevention and management.

Drug Therapy. Many antiemetics are available to relieve nausea and vomiting. These drugs vary in the side effects they produce and how well they control CINV. One or more antiemetics are usually given before, during, and after chemotherapy. Drugs commonly used short term to control CINV are listed in Chart 22-7. A new drug, Akynzeo, combines the 5-HT3 antagonist palonosetron with the drug netupitant to provide greater control of CINV (Aschenbrenner, 2015). Netupitant belongs to a new drug class, P/neurokinin-1 receptor antagonists. *Patient response to antiemetic therapy is variable, and the drug combinations are individualized for best effect (Barak et al., 2013).*

NURSING SAFETY PRIORITY QSEN
Drug Alert

Do not confuse the antiemetic drug Anzemet (dolasetron) with the diabetes drug Avandamet (a combination of metformin and rosiglitazone). The drugs have similar sounding names but totally different actions.

Regardless of which drugs are being used to prevent or reduce CINV, they are most effective when used in an evidence-based approach on a scheduled basis for prevention and management. Drug therapy for CINV works best when given *before* the nausea and vomiting begin. *The nursing priority is to coordinate with the patient and cancer health care provider to ensure adequate control of CINV. Ensure that antiemetics are given before chemotherapy and are repeated based on the response and duration of CINV.* When patients are receiving dose-dense chemotherapy, the intensity of CINV also increases, and more aggressive antiemetic therapy is needed. Teach patients to continue the therapy, even when CINV appears controlled. *When the patient stops taking the drug(s), teach him or her to start retaking the drug at the first sign of nausea to prevent it from becoming uncontrollable.*

CONSIDERATIONS FOR OLDER ADULTS
Patient-Centered Care QSEN

The older adult can become dehydrated more quickly than a younger adult if CINV is not controlled. Teach older adults to be proactive with taking their prescribed antiemetics and to contact their health care provider if the CINV either does not resolve within 12 hours or becomes worse.

Mucositis

Mucositis (sores in mucous membranes) is a dose-limiting side effect of cancer therapy and a common reason for stopping or delaying treatment. It often develops in the entire GI tract, especially in the mouth (stomatitis is a reaction that involves other tissues and structures in the oral cavity). Mucositis is a complex, multiphase process at the cellular level started

CHART 22-7 Common Examples of Drug Therapy
Chemotherapy-Induced Nausea and Vomiting

DRUG CATEGORIES	NURSING IMPLICATIONS
Serotonin Antagonists—Prevent CINV by blocking the 5-HT3 receptors of the chemotrigger zones in the brain and intestines. This action prevents serotonin from binding to the receptors and activating the nausea and vomiting centers.	
Ondansetron (Zofran) *Oral or IV* Granisetron (Kytril) *IV* Granisetron transdermal (Sancuso) *patch* Dolasetron (Anzemet) *Oral or IV* Palonosetron (Aloxi) *IV*	Teach patient to change positions slowly to avoid falls *because these drugs may induce bradycardia, hypotension, and vertigo.* Assess the patient for headache, which is *a common side effect of drugs from this class.*
Neurokinin Receptor Antagonists—Reduce CINV by blocking the substance P neurokinin receptor. When used together with a serotonin antagonist and a corticosteroid, both acute and delayed nausea and vomiting are controlled.	
Aprepitant (Emend) *Oral or IV*	Teach patients who are also taking warfarin (Coumadin) to have their INR checked before and after the 3 days of this therapy *because this drug interferes with warfarin effectiveness.* Teach women who are using oral contraceptives to use an additional form of birth control while on this drug *because it reduces the effectiveness of oral contraceptives, increasing the risk for an unplanned pregnancy.*
Corticosteroids—Reduce CINV by decreasing swelling in the brain's chemotrigger zone.	
Dexamethasone (Decadron) *Oral or IV*	Teach patients to reduce salt intake to about 4 g daily *because these drugs cause fluid retention and hypertension.*
Prokinetic Agents—Reduce CINV by blocking dopamine receptors in the brain's chemotrigger zone.	
Metoclopramide (Reglan) *IM or IV*	Teach the patient to avoid driving or operating heavy machinery *because these drugs induce drowsiness.*
Benzodiazepines—Reduce CINV by enhancing cholinergic effects and decreasing the patient's awareness.	
Lorazepam (Ativan) *Oral or IV*	Teach the patient and family that the patient should avoid driving, operating heavy machinery, making legal decisions, and going up and down staircases unassisted *because drugs from this class induce amnesia and profound drowsiness.*

CINV, Chemotherapy-induced nausea and vomiting; *INR,* international normalized ratio.

CHART 22-8 Patient and Family Education: Preparing for Self-Management

Mouth Care for Patients With Mucositis

- Examine your mouth (including the roof, under the tongue, and between the teeth and cheek) every 4 hours for fissures, blisters, sores, or drainage.
- If sores or drainage is present, contact your cancer health care provider to determine whether these areas need to be cultured.
- Brush the teeth and tongue with a soft-bristled brush or sponges every 8 hours and after meals.
- Avoid the use of mouthwashes that contain alcohol or glycerin.
- "Swish and spit" room-temperature tap water, normal saline, or salt and soda water on a regular basis (at least 4 times a day) and as needed according to changes in the oral cavity.
- Drink 2 or more liters of water per day if another health problem does not require limiting fluid intake.
- Take all drugs, including antibiotics and drugs for nausea and vomiting, as prescribed.
- Use topical analgesic drugs as prescribed.
- Take pain medications on schedule as needed.
- Apply a water-based moisturizer to your lips after each episode of mouth care and as needed.
- Use prescribed "artificial saliva" or mouth moisturizers as needed.
- Avoid using tobacco or drinking alcoholic beverages.
- Avoid spicy, salty, acidic, dry, rough, or hard food.
- Cool liquids to prevent burns or irritation.
- If you wear dentures, use them only during meals. When not in place, soak them in an antimicrobial solution. Rinse thoroughly before placing them in your mouth.

in response to cytotoxic chemotherapy. Mouth sores cause pain and interfere with eating, nutrition, and quality of life. Chart 22-8 lists patient education for self-management of mucositis.

Oral cryotherapy using ice water or ice chips can be used for the prevention of mucositis. Instruct patients to suck on ice chips or to hold ice-cold water in their mouths before, during, and after rapid infusions of specific mucositis-causing agents. It is believed that vasoconstriction caused by the cold temperature decreases exposure of the oral mucous membranes to the mucositis-causing agents. Other recommended treatments include low-level laser therapy, sodium bicarbonate rinses, and IV injections of palifermin (Kepivance), which stimulate the growth of mucous membrane cells in the mouth. For multiple mouth lesions, most patients require systemic pain medications.

Frequent mouth assessment and oral hygiene are key in managing mucositis. Stress the importance of good and frequent oral hygiene, including teeth cleaning and mouth rinsing. Because most patients with mucositis also have bone marrow suppression and are at risk for impaired CLOTTING with bleeding, they must take care to avoid traumatizing the oral mucosa. Instruct them to use a soft-bristled toothbrush or disposable mouth sponges. Recommendations include *gentle* flossing once daily. Encourage them to rinse the mouth with plain water or saline at frequent intervals during the day and night when awake. Frequency is guided by the intensity of the mucositis. Initially the rinses start after meals and at bedtime, then every 2 hours, and then progressing to hourly if needed for comfort. Teach patients to avoid mouthwashes that contain alcohol or other drying agents that may further irritate the mucosa.

Oral hygiene equipment must be kept clean. Remind patients not to share toothbrushes. Toothbrushes can be cleaned weekly by using a home dishwasher or by rinsing them with a solution of liquid bleach or hydrogen peroxide and then rinsing with hot water.

Alopecia

Alopecia, hair loss, may occur as whole-body hair loss or may be as mild as only a thinning of the scalp hair. When body hair loss includes pubic hair, patients may struggle with their body image and sexuality. Reassure patients that hair loss is temporary. Regrowth usually begins about 1 month after completion of chemotherapy; however, the new hair may differ from the original hair in color, texture, and thickness. No known evidence-based treatment safely prevents alopecia. The use of cold caps and cyclosporine for the prevention and treatment of chemotherapy-induced alopecia has recently been explored with some promising results; however, further research is needed to fully evaluate these therapies and the incidence of metastasis that may occur as a result of their use. *The priority nursing actions are to teach patients how to avoid scalp injury and to help them cope with this body image change.*

The hairless scalp is at risk for injury. Teach the patient to avoid direct sunlight on the scalp by wearing a hat or other head covering. Sunscreen use is essential to prevent sunburn because many drugs increase sun sensitivity, regardless of skin darkness. This skin can be damaged by helmets, headphones, headsets, wigs, and other items that rub the head. Teach the patient to wear a head covering underneath these items. Head coverings also are needed during cold weather and in cool environments to reduce body heat loss and prevent hypothermia.

Help patients select a type of head covering that suits their income and lifestyle. One recommendation is to coordinate wig purchases with the patient's hairdresser or barber. Having very short hair or a shaved head now is common and socially acceptable for men, and many men choose not to wear a wig during chemotherapy. Cutting the hair very short before chemotherapy begins will allow a better wig fit.

Suggest that patients obtain a wig before therapy begins and have their hairdresser shape it to mimic their usual hairstyle to reduce appearance changes. High-quality wigs are expensive but can look very much like the patient's own hair. Many local units of the ACS offers wigs at no cost that former patients have donated. Patients also can disguise hair loss with caps, scarves, and turbans. The ACS also provides instruction (Look Good–Feel Better) regarding makeup and the use of scarves, for example, to improve appearance and how patients feel about themselves.

Changes in Cognitive Function

Some patients receiving chemotherapy report changes in cognitive function, most commonly reduced ability to concentrate, memory loss, and difficulty learning new information during treatment and for months to years after treatment. This problem, termed *chemo brain,* is often reported in women undergoing chemotherapy for breast cancer, although it is not limited either to women or to breast cancer treatment. Cognitive impairment has been reported in up to 75% of patients with breast cancer and in patients with brain tumors and those treated with bone marrow transplantation after high-dose chemotherapy (Armstrong, 2016; Von Ah, 2015). Although most types of chemotherapy drugs do not cross the blood-brain barrier, they can induce inflammation and general biochemical changes that could reduce cognitive function, at least temporarily.

Comparisons of brain structure and cognitive function before, during, and after high-dose chemotherapy show some anatomic changes in brain white matter and gray matter. Most changes are not present at 3 years after completion of therapy. It is not known why all patients receiving high-dose chemotherapy do not develop the problem; however, genetic differences may be partly responsible. Not only is the exact cause of this side effect unclear, so are the personal risk factors. Cognitive training strategies may be effective in improving, maintaining, or restoring mental function through the repeated practicing of tasks that challenge thinking and problem solving (Bail & Meneses, 2016).

The priorities for nursing care are supporting the patient who reports this side effect and providing resources for cognitive training. Listen to the patient's concerns and tell him or her that other patients have also reported such problems. Warn patients against participating in other behaviors that could alter cognitive functioning, such as excessive alcohol intake, recreational drug use, and activities that increase the risk for head injury.

Chemotherapy-Induced Peripheral Neuropathy

Chemotherapy-induced peripheral neuropathy (CIPN) is the loss of SENSORY PERCEPTION or motor function of peripheral nerves associated with exposure to certain anticancer drugs (Smith et al., 2014). Some patients undergoing chemotherapy with nerve-damaging drugs (e.g., antimitotics and platinum-based drugs) have rapid onset of severe CIPN. The degree of CIPN is related to the dosage of the nerve-damaging drugs; higher doses lead to greater neuropathy. The results of CIPN on function are widespread, with the most common problems including loss of sensation in the hands and feet, impaired gait and balance, orthostatic hypotension, erectile dysfunction, neuropathic pain, loss of taste discrimination, and severe constipation. CIPN is a long-term consequence and may be permanent in some adults. No known evidence-based interventions are available to prevent CIPN; however, some patients have reduced pain and improved function and quality of life when taking duloxetine.

The priority for nursing care of patients experiencing CIPN is teaching them to prevent injury. Loss of SENSORY PERCEPTION increases the patient's risk for injury because he or she may not be aware of excessive heat, cold, or pressure. The risk for injury to the feet is very high. Falls are more likely because of changes in gait and balance, decreased sensation in the feet, and orthostatic hypotension. Chart 22-9 lists teaching priorities for the patient with CIPN.

Poor gait may be helped with devices such as orthotics and calf braces. Erectile dysfunction may be helped with drug therapy (see Chapter 72 for options for erectile dysfunction). Other issues are not correctable and affect quality of life. The loss of hand sensation may make some activities that require very fine motor skills (i.e., writing, buttoning clothing, playing a musical instrument) difficult or impossible. Assess the patient's ability to cope with these changes. Coordinate with an occupational therapist to help the patient adjust for SENSORY PERCEPTION deficits in performing activities.

IMMUNOTHERAPY: BIOLOGICAL RESPONSE MODIFIERS AND TARGETED THERAPIES

Biological response modifiers (BRMs) enhance or alter the patient's biologic responses to cancer cells. BRMs have a variety

---

CHART 22-9 Patient and Family Education: Preparing for Self-Management

Chemotherapy-Induced Peripheral Neuropathy

- Protect feet and other body areas where sensation is reduced (e.g., do not walk around in bare feet or stocking feet; always wear shoes with a protective sole).
- Be sure that shoes are long enough and wide enough to prevent creating sores or blisters.
- Buy shoes in the afternoon or evening to accommodate any size change needed for foot swelling.
- Provide a long break-in period for new shoes; do not wear new shoes for longer than 2 hours at a time.
- Avoid pointed-toe shoes and shoes with heels higher than 2 inches.
- Inspect your feet daily (with a mirror) for open areas or redness.
- Avoid extremes of temperature; wear warm clothing in the winter, especially over hands, feet, and ears.
- Test water temperature with a thermometer when washing dishes or bathing. Use warm water rather than hot water (less than 105°F or 40.6°C).
- Use potholders when cooking.
- Use gloves when washing dishes or gardening.
- Do not eat foods that are "steaming hot"; allow them to cool before placing them in your mouth.
- Eat foods that are high in fiber (e.g., fruit, whole grain cereals, vegetables).
- Drink 2 to 3 liters of fluid (nonalcoholic) daily unless your health care provider has told you to restrict fluid intake.
- Use the actions for "Falls Prevention" supplied by the cancer center during all activities.
- Get up slowly from a lying or sitting position. If you feel dizzy, sit back down until the dizziness fades before standing; then stand in place for a few seconds before walking or using the stairs.
- To prevent tripping or falling, look at your feet and the floor or ground where you are walking to assess how the ground, floor, or step changes.
- Avoid using area rugs, especially those that slide easily.
- Keep floors free of clutter that could lead to a fall.
- Use handrails when going up or down steps.

---

of effects. Some have direct antitumor activity (i.e., helping the body recognize cancer cells as foreign so the immune system destroys them). BRMs also can improve IMMUNITY and enhance the repair or replacement of cells damaged by cancer treatment. Targeted therapies used in cancer treatment are drugs that act on specific components needed for cellular function and reproduction. These therapies include monoclonal antibodies and small molecule drugs.

BRMs as Cancer Therapy

As discussed in Chapter 17, cytokines released from immune system cells are not usually cytotoxic alone but influence how immune system cells function. The cytokines include the interferons, interleukins, tumor necrosis factors, and colony-stimulating factors. Some cytokines enhance IMMUNITY, which plays a role in cancer prevention (see Chapters 17 and 21). Cytokines and other BRMs are used as cancer treatment because they stimulate the patient's immune system to recognize cancer cells and take actions to eliminate or destroy them. Some BRMs are used as supportive therapy during chemotherapy by enhancing recovery of bone marrow function after treatment-induced myelosuppression.

Two common types of BRMs for cancer therapy are interleukins and interferons. Some agents can stimulate specific immune system components to attack and destroy cancer cells; other agents block cancer cell access to an essential function or nutrient needed for cell survival.

Interleukins (ILs) are substances the body makes to help regulate inflammation and IMMUNITY. Some ILs are synthesized as anticancer drugs. In particular, ILs have been effective in treating renal cell carcinoma and melanoma. They help different immune cells recognize and destroy abnormal body cells. In particular, IL-1, IL-2, and IL-6 appear to boost IMMUNITY and enhance attacks on cancer cells by macrophages, natural killer (NK) cells.

Interferons (IFNs) are cell-produced proteins that have some effect in the treatment of melanoma, hairy cell leukemia, renal cell carcinoma, AIDS-related Kaposi's sarcoma, and lymphoma. IFNs can assist in cancer therapy by:

- Slowing tumor cell division
- Stimulating the growth and activation of NK cells
- Inducing cancer cells to resume a more normal appearance and function
- Inhibiting the expression of oncogenes

BRMs as Supportive Therapy

BRMs used for supportive therapy during cancer treatment are the colony-stimulating factors or "growth factors" (Table 22-5). These factors affect CELLULAR REGULATION and induce more rapid recovery of bone marrow cells after suppression by chemotherapy. This effect has two benefits. First, when impaired IMMUNITY and CLOTTING are shortened or less severe, patients are less at risk for life-threatening infections and bleeding. Second, because the growth factors allow more rapid bone marrow recovery, patients can receive their chemotherapy regimen as scheduled and may even be able to tolerate higher doses, potentially increasing the likelihood of a remission or cure.

TABLE 22-5 Common Biological Response Modifiers Used as Supportive Cancer Therapy

AGENT	CELL TYPE AFFECTED	INDICATIONS
Sargramostim (Leukine, Prokine)	All granulocytes Neutrophils Eosinophils Monocytes Macrophages	Chemotherapy-induced leukopenia
Filgrastim (Neupogen) Pegfilgrastim (Neulasta) Tbo-filgrastim (Granix)	Neutrophils	Chemotherapy-induced neutropenia
Epoetin alfa (Epogen, Procrit) Darbepoetin (Aranesp)	Erythrocytes	Chemotherapy-induced anemia Chemotherapy-induced fatigue Anemia induced by renal failure
Oprelvekin (Neumega)	Platelets	Chemotherapy-induced thrombocytopenia
Sipuleucel-T (Provenge) (product is a vaccine)	T-cells; antigen-processing cells (macrophages)	Hormone-refractory prostate cancer

Side Effects of Biological Response Modifier Therapy

Patients receiving interleukins have generalized and often severe inflammatory reactions. Fluid shifting from the intracellular space and capillary leak syndrome cause widespread edema formation. Tissue swelling affects the function of all organs and can be life threatening. Pulmonary, cardiovascular, and GI reactions can occur. Patients receiving high-dose BRM therapy may need to be in an ICU or on a monitored unit. These inflammatory effects occur during the days of active drug infusion and resolve after therapy completion.

Many BRMs and growth factors induce symptoms of inflammation during and just after receiving the drug, including fever, chills, rigors, and flu-like symptoms (general malaise). Problems are worse when higher doses are given, but they seem to become less severe over time. The nursing priorities for patients receiving BRMs include assessing for complications of systemic inflammation and making patients as comfortable as possible. Fever is treated with acetaminophen. Patients with severe rigors are managed with meperidine (Demerol). Patients may also experience nausea, vomiting, diarrhea, and anorexia. Antiemetics are helpful in the management of nausea and vomiting.

Neurologic symptoms associated with BRM use can be significant. These include confusion, fatigue, somnolence, irritation or agitation, hallucinations, vivid dreams, anxiety, and sleep disturbances. Some patients have psychosocial reactions of fear, tearfulness, depression, and mood swings. Early identification of these symptoms is an important nursing care activity.

Interferon therapy causes peripheral neuropathy. (See the Chemotherapy-Induced Peripheral Neuropathy section.)

Skin dryness, itching, and peeling occur with many types of BRM therapy. The skin problems are more severe with higher doses and when more than one type of BRM is used at the same time. Reactions are temporary but cause much discomfort and distress. Advise patients to apply moisturizers (unscented) to the skin and to use mild soap to clean the skin. Involved areas should be protected from the sun with clothing or the use of sunscreen agents. Teach patients to avoid swimming and to not use topical steroid creams on affected areas.

Monoclonal Antibodies

Monoclonal antibody therapy combines actions from immunotherapy and targeted therapy to help treat specific cancers. The body normally responds to foreign substances by producing antibodies. These proteins are then able to target the antigen when present in the body, attacking and destroying the foreign antigen (non–self cells). In cancer therapy human and/or mouse proteins are used to form antibodies against given targets known to be present in or on certain types of cancer cells.

Monoclonal antibodies bind to their target antigens, which are often specific cell surface membrane proteins. Binding prevents the protein from performing its functions. Some cancer cells express cell membrane surface proteins that are unique to cancer cells and have a role in cancer cell division. So by binding these proteins, monoclonal antibodies change CELLULAR REGULATION and prevent cancer cell division. Some monoclonal antibodies make tumor cells more sensitive to therapy and increase the effectiveness of immune system attacks on the cancer cells. A commonly used monoclonal antibody for targeted therapy is rituximab (Rituxan). It binds to the protein CD20, which is often overexpressed on the surface of non-Hodgkin's lymphoma cell membranes. This protein activates an early step of the cell cycle division process. Binding CD20 with rituximab prevents it from stimulating cell division in the non-Hodgkin's lymphoma cells.

Allergic reactions may occur in patients receiving monoclonal antibodies because of the incorporation of some nonhuman proteins. Most of these antibodies initially were developed in mice and express some mouse proteins. Now many of these antibodies have been "humanized," reducing the risk for allergic reactions. Nursing assessment is key for early recognition of a potentially life-threatening allergic reaction.

The monoclonal antibodies to the epidermal growth factor receptor (EGFR) bind to those specific receptors on normal and cancerous cells. Thus side effects also occur in the skin, mucous membranes, and lining of the GI tract.

SMALL MOLECULE INHIBITOR TARGETED THERAPY

Molecularly targeted therapies are technically biologic agents. However, their unique actions and roles in cancer therapy warrant separate discussion. These agents use the molecular features present in some cancer cells as specific targets, and by acting more specifically they have less of an impact on normal cells. In general, molecularly targeted therapies block the growth and spread of cancer by interfering with the specific cellular growth pathways or molecules involved in the CELLULAR REGULATION of growth and progression of cancer cells. These agents reflect the increased understanding of the biology of cancer cells and are becoming an effective treatment option that provides patients with a new sense of hope against a challenging disease.

As discussed in Chapter 21, normal cells have tightly controlled regulation over when and to what extent a cell divides; cancer cells have altered features that evade this normal control.

External events can indicate to a cell that cell division is needed (i.e., tissue loss, injury). However, these external events must be communicated to the cell's nucleus to activate the genes that promote cell division (oncogenes) and turn off the genes that normally suppress cell division (suppressor genes). The key to communicating the need for cell division is the presence and activation of signal transduction pathways. Fig. 22-4 shows a segment of a cell with one signal transduction pathway. When this pathway is activated at the cell surface by binding growth factors to their receptors, having certain drugs interact with the cell's plasma membrane, or by the binding of certain adhesion factors, the first result is an increase in the cell's production of a family of enzymes known as *tyrosine kinases (TKs)*. With increased TKs present, the pro–cell division signal activates transcription factors within the pathway. When the pro–cell division transcription factors reach the cell's nucleus, oncogenes are activated, suppressor genes are inactivated, and a variety of proteins are produced to make cell division occur.

When cell division is not needed, external signals such as growth factor inhibitors and the direct contact of a cell's plasma membrane with other cells send signals that inhibit activation of TKs and the signal transduction pathway. As a result, fewer transcription factors are produced, suppressor genes are expressed, and oncogenes are suppressed. The proteins needed for cell division are not produced, and cell division does not occur.

Overall cancer cells have more active signal transduction pathways and transcription factors that ultimately lead to excessive division of the cancer cells. Often the signaling pathways and receptors are overexpressed in cancer cells. Targeted therapies take advantage of differences in CELLULAR REGULATION for one or more parts of the signal transduction pathway to block it. Targeted therapies can disrupt the pathway and slow or stop cell division. They may work by blocking a growth factor receptor, by preventing the activation of tyrosine kinases, by limiting

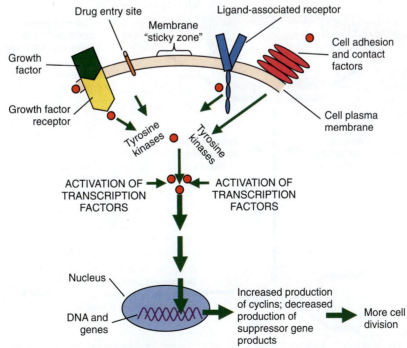

FIG. 22-4 Pro–cell division signal transduction pathway. (From Workman, M. L., & LaCharity, L. [2011]. *Understanding pharmacology: Essentials for medication safety.* St. Louis: Saunders.)

the production of transcription factors, and by other mechanisms that are not yet fully understood. Regardless of how a targeted therapy works, it will work only with cancer cells that have the actual target. The result is that the signal for turning on cell division genes (oncogenes) does not get through to the cell's nucleus (Fig. 22-5) (Santos et al., 2013).

Drugs for targeted therapy of some cancers are classified based on the mechanism of action, and some have more than one action (Table 22-6). *It is important to remember that these drugs will not work unless the cancer cell overexpresses the actual target substance. Thus not all patients with the same cancer type would benefit from the use of targeted therapy.* Each patient's cancer cells are evaluated to determine whether the cells have enough of a target to be affected by targeted therapy. Because of the varying mechanisms of action, a priority nursing action is careful assessment for adverse reactions to therapy.

! NURSING SAFETY PRIORITY (QSEN)

Drug Alert

Many targeted therapies, the small molecule therapies in particular, are administered as oral agents. Some patients minimize the potential effects of the drug because it is "just a pill." Emphasize with patients and their family members and caregivers the importance of taking the drugs as prescribed and using safe handling techniques. Teach them that only the patient should handle the oral chemotherapy and that, if the patient is unable, the family member or caregiver needs to wear gloves when handling the chemotherapy drug.

TABLE 22-6 Common Targeted Therapy Agents

CLASSIFICATION	AGENT
Tyrosine kinase inhibitors	Dasatinib (Sprycel)
	Erlotinib (Tarceva)
	Imatinib mesylate (Gleevec)
	Lapatinib (Tykerb)
	Nilotinib (Tasigna)
Epidermal growth factor/ receptor inhibitors (EGFRIs)	Cetuximab (Erbitux)
	Gefitinib (Iressa)
	Panitumumab (Vectibix)
	Trastuzumab (Herceptin)
Vascular endothelial growth factor/receptor inhibitors (VEGFRIs)	Bevacizumab (Avastin)
	Axitinib (Inlyta)
Multikinase inhibitors	Sorafenib (Nexavar)
	Sunitinib (Sutent)
	Pazopanib (Votrient)
	Crizotinib (Xalkori)
Proteasome inhibitors	Bortezomib (Velcade)
Angiogenesis/mTOR kinase inhibitors	Everolimus (Afinitor)
	Lenalidomide (Revlimid)
	Polamlidomide (Pomlyst)
	Temsirolimus (Torisel)
Monoclonal antibodies	Alemtuzumab (Campath)
	Ibritumomab (Zevalin)
	Rituximab (Rituxan)
	^{131}I tositumomab (Bexxar)

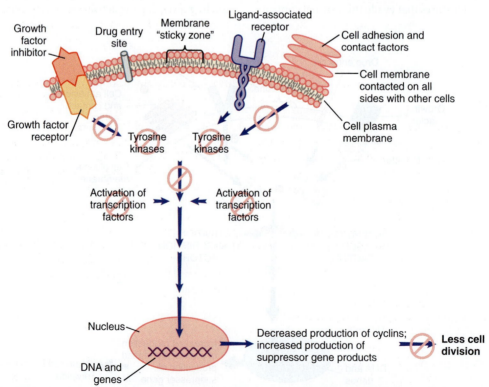

FIG. 22-5 Sites of action for targeted therapies that inhibit a signal transduction pathway and greatly reduce cell division. (From McCuistion, L., Kee, J., Hayes, E. [2015]. *Pharmacology: A nursing process approach* [8th ed.]. St. Louis: Saunders.)

Targeted therapy agents are classified based on their action. The first application of these agents was against estrogen in breast cancer (discussed in the Hormonal Manipulation section). Selective estrogen receptor modulators (SERMs) and aromatase inhibitors (AIs) have been developed to interfere with estrogen's ability to promote the growth of estrogen receptor–positive breast cancers. Discussion in this section focuses on the tyrosine kinase inhibitors (TKIs), epidermal growth factor/receptor inhibitors (EGFRIs), vascular endothelial growth factor/receptor inhibitors (VEGFRIs), multikinase inhibitors (MKIs), proteasome inhibitors, and angiogenesis inhibitors.

Tyrosine Kinase Inhibitors

Drugs with the main action of inhibiting activation of tyrosine kinases (TKs) are tyrosine kinase inhibitors (TKIs). There are many different TKs. Some are unique to the cell type; others may be present only in cancer cells that express a specific gene mutation. As a result, the different TKI drugs are effective in disrupting the CELLULAR REGULATION and growth of some cancer cell types and not others. An example of a TKI is imatinib mesylate (Gleevec, TEVA-Imatinib ✦). This drug binds to the energy site of the enzyme TK and prevents its activation. The drug is useful in cancers that overexpress the *ABL1* oncogene such as most types of chronic myeloid leukemia (CML) and metastatic GI stromal tumors (GISTs).

Side effects common to most TKIs include nausea, vomiting, fluid retention, electrolyte imbalances, and bone marrow suppression that reduces IMMUNITY with neutropenia, anemia, and thrombocytopenia. The problems associated with bone marrow suppression are further increased when the patient also receives traditional chemotherapy with drugs that suppress bone marrow.

Epidermal Growth Factor/Receptor Inhibitors

The epidermal growth factor/receptor inhibitors (EGFRIs) block epidermal growth factor from binding to its cell surface receptor. As shown in Fig. 22-5, when this receptor is blocked, it cannot activate tyrosine kinase. As a result, the signal transduction pathway for promotion of cell division is inhibited.

An example of an EGFRI drug is trastuzumab (Herceptin), which binds the excessive amounts of a certain type of EGFR produced by some breast and colon cancers in response to the activation of the *HER2/neu* gene. Binding this receptor prevents cancer cell division and increases the sensitivity to chemotherapy and immune system actions.

The most common side effects of EGFRIs include hypersensitivity reactions and a variety of skin reactions because skin cells also have EGFRs. These side effects may be as mild as a rash or result in excessive skin peeling and fissures (Wallner et al., 2016). Trastuzumab has been found to have adverse effects on the heart.

Vascular Endothelial Growth Factor/Receptor Inhibitors

An example of a vascular endothelial growth factor/receptor inhibitor drug is bevacizumab (Avastin). It binds to vascular endothelial growth factor (VEGF) and prevents the binding of VEGF with its receptors on the surfaces of endothelial cells present in blood vessels. This inhibits formation of new blood vessels within a tumor. As a result, tumor cells are poorly nourished and growth is inhibited. This drug is used with standard chemotherapy for many cancers that overexpress the receptor, such as colon, rectal, lung, and renal cell cancers.

The most common side effects are hypertension and impaired wound healing. Bone marrow suppression with reduced IMMUNITY and neutropenia and thrombocytopenia also occur, especially when the drug is used in combination with chemotherapy drugs that cause bone marrow suppression.

Multikinase Inhibitors

The multikinase inhibitors (MKIs) inhibit the activity of specific kinases in cancer cells and tumor blood vessels. An example of an MKI is sunitinib (Sutent). These drugs are most effective in preventing the activation of tyrosine kinases that have a specific gene mutation found most often in some renal cell carcinomas, GI stromal tumors, and pancreatic cancers.

A common side effect of this class of drugs is hypertension. Other side effects include nausea and vomiting, diarrhea, constipation, mucositis, erythematous rash on the hands and feet (palmar-plantar erythrodysesthesia), and mild neutropenia and thrombocytopenia.

Proteasome Inhibitors

Proteasome inhibitors prevent the formation of a large complex of proteins (a proteasome) in cells. The proteasome helps regulate the genes that promote cell division and prevent cell death. Proteasome inhibitors limit the amount of proteasome present, impairing the tumor's CELLULAR REGULATION and making its cells less likely to divide and more likely to respond to signals for cell death. The proteasome inhibitor bortezomib (Velcade) is used in the treatment of multiple myeloma. Proteasomes are present in normal and cancer cells, but cancer cells are much more sensitive to the effects of proteasome inhibition than are normal cells.

The most common side effects of bortezomib are nausea, vomiting, anorexia, abdominal pain, bowel changes, decreased taste sensation, and peripheral neuropathy. Other side effects include headache, rash, pruritus, back and bone pain, muscle aches, and tumor lysis syndrome.

Angiogenesis Inhibitors

Angiogenesis inhibitors target a specific protein kinase known as the *mammalian target of rapamycin (mTOR)*. An example of an angiogenesis inhibitor is temsirolimus (Torisel) used for renal cell cancer. When the drug binds to an intracellular protein, a protein-drug complex forms that inhibits the activity of mTOR. When mTOR is inhibited, the concentrations of vascular endothelial growth factor (VEGF) are greatly reduced, and many pro–cell division signal transduction pathways are disrupted.

Hyperglycemia and hypersensitivity reactions to these drugs are common. Bone marrow suppression is moderate to severe with anemia, neutropenia, and thrombocytopenia. Other general side effects include headache, nausea and vomiting, back pain, muscle and joint pain, mucositis, diarrhea, and skin problems.

PHOTODYNAMIC THERAPY

Overview

Photodynamic therapy (PDT) is the selective destruction of cancer cells through a chemical reaction triggered by high energy laser light. It can be used to destroy some cancers, reduce the size of tumors to allow subsequent complete surgical removal, and shrink tumors in airways or the esophagus to

CLINICAL JUDGMENT CHALLENGE 22-2

Safety; Evidence-Based Practice QSEN

A 70-year-old was diagnosed with colon cancer 3 years ago. At that time he underwent IV combination chemotherapy. He responded to the chemotherapy regimen until about 6 months ago when his colon cancer returned. His oncologist has now prescribed an oral chemotherapy, which has been effective for some colon cancers. When you talk with the patient, his comment to you is that "this new drug will be a breeze. I'll just take it like my other pills. My wife puts those out for me to take."

1. What concerns do you have about this man's response to his oral chemotherapy and why?
2. How will you respond to the man's comments about his oral chemotherapy drug?

TABLE 22-7 **Common Agents Used for Hormonal Manipulation of Cancer**

TYPE OF AGENT	EXAMPLE
Hormone Agonists	
Androgen	Fluoxymesterone (Halotestin)
	Testolactone (Teslac)
Estrogen	Chlorotrianisene (Tace)
	Conjugated equine estrogen (Premarin)
	Diethylstilbestrol (DES, Stilphostrol)
	Ethinyl estradiol (Estinyl)
Progestin	Medroxyprogesterone (Amen, Provera)
	Megestrol (Megace)
Luteinizing hormone–releasing hormone (LHRH)	Leuprolide (Eligard, Lupron, Viadur)
	Goserelin (Zoladex)
Hormone Antagonists	
Antiandrogens	Bicalutamide (Casodex)
	Flutamide (Eulexin)
Antiestrogens	Fulvestrant (Faslodex)
	Raloxifene (Evista)
	Tamoxifen (Nolvadex)
	Toremifene (Fareston)
Hormone Inhibitors	
	Aminoglutethimide (Cytadren, Elipten)
	Anastrozole (Arimidex)
	Exemestane (Aromasin)
	Letrozole (Femara)

relieve obstruction. PDT is used most often for nonmelanoma skin cancers, ocular tumors, GI tumors, and cancers located in the upper airways. PDT use in patients with noninvasive bladder cancer is being explored.

An agent that sensitizes cells to light is injected IV along with a dye to achieve cell death with exposure to specific wavelengths of laser light administered later. These agents enter all cells but leave normal cells more rapidly than cancer cells. Usually within 48 to 72 hours, most of the drug has collected in high concentrations in cancer cells. At this time a laser light is focused on the tumor. The light activates a chemical reaction, inducing irreversible cell damage in the cells retaining the sensitizing drug. Some cells die and slough immediately; others continue to slough for several days. Some lesions require only one exposure to the laser, and others must be re-exposed several days after the first treatment.

❖ INTERPROFESSIONAL COLLABORATIVE CARE

PDT is typically performed in the outpatient setting, but at times the patient may require short-term ICU monitoring for airway management when the upper airways are treated. The photosensitizer dose, laser light exposure, and depth of tissue penetration by the light are items to be considered depending on the tumor type. Laser light exposure following photosensitizer administration leads to multiple chemical reactions that result in death of malignant tumor cells and the ultimate destruction of the vascular bed that fed the tumor. The application of PDT is contraindicated in patients with known tumor involvement of a major blood vessel because of the triggering of a severe or fatal episode of bleeding.

The risks associated with PDT are increased in patients who have had prior radiation or a history of coagulation disorders. The patient may be instructed to avoid sunlight exposure for 24 to 48 hours or longer, depending on the type and dose of photosensitizing agent. Patient and family teaching regarding sun and other types of light exposure are important for safety.

HORMONAL MANIPULATION

Hormonal manipulation involves changing the body's usual hormone responses. Hormones are chemicals secreted by endocrine glands and taken up by capillaries where they then circulate to all areas of the body. Hormones exert their effects only on their specific target tissues. Some hormones cause hormone-sensitive tumors to grow more rapidly, thus decreasing the amount of these hormones that reach hormone-sensitive tumors can slow cancer growth.

Hormonal manipulation may include the use of steroids, steroid analogues, and enzyme inhibitors (aromatase inhibitors, gonadotropin-releasing hormone analogues, anti-androgens, and antiestrogens). Many of these agents are used to block receptors and thus affect CELLULAR REGULATION by preventing the cancer cells from receiving normal hormonal growth stimulation. Hormonal manipulation can help control or slow the growth of some cancers for years but does not cure the disease. If a tumor depends on hormone A for growth and a large quantity of hormone B (similar to A) is given to the patient, hormone B will interfere with the tumor's uptake of hormone A or will limit the amount produced. As a result, tumor growth is slowed, and survival time increases. Table 22-7 lists drugs used in hormonal manipulation for cancer therapy.

Some drugs are *hormone antagonists* that compete with natural hormones at the receptors. When hormone antagonists are given, they bind to the specific hormone receptors on or in the tumor cell and prevent the needed hormone from binding to its receptors. If a tumor needs a certain hormone to grow and the hormone can enter or activate the cell only through receptors, hormone antagonists can alter CELLULAR REGULATION and slow tumor growth.

The hormone inhibitors also are used for hormonal therapy. These drugs inhibit the normal organ production of some specific hormones. For example, the aromatase inhibitor anastrozole (Arimidex) prevents the production of estrogen in the adrenal gland and reduces the blood level of estrogen, which results in slower growth of some breast cancers.

Side effects of hormonal manipulation are different from those of other types of chemotherapy. Androgens and the antiestrogen receptor drugs cause masculinizing effects in women. Chest and facial hair may develop, menstrual periods stop, and breast tissue shrinks. Patients may have some fluid retention. For men and women receiving androgens, acne and hypercalcemia are common, and liver dysfunction may occur with prolonged therapy. Women receiving estrogens or progestins may have irregular menses, fluid retention, and breast tenderness. All patients who take estrogen or progestins are at increased risk for venous thromboembolism (VTE).

Feminine manifestations appear in men who take estrogens, progestins, or antiandrogen receptor drugs. Facial hair thins, facial skin is smoother, body fat is redistributed, and breast development (gynecomastia) can occur. Bone loss is common, which increases the risk for osteoporosis and pathologic bone fractures (Limburg et al., 2014). Testicular and penile atrophy also occur to some degree. Teach patients and families about expected side effects. Encourage them to express their feelings about body changes. Refer them for counseling if needed.

ONCOLOGIC EMERGENCIES

With improvements in cancer treatments, many cancers have become a chronic disease. However, acute complications from the cancer or its treatment can occur at any time. This chapter presents select acute complications of cancer or cancer therapy, including sepsis and disseminated intravascular coagulation, syndrome of inappropriate antidiuretic hormone, spinal cord compression, hypercalcemia, superior vena cava syndrome, and tumor lysis syndrome as emergencies. Early diagnosis and immediate intervention of these emergency conditions are essential to avoid life-threatening situations. The role of the nurse is to implement interventions to prevent and detect these complications early for immediate treatment.

SEPSIS AND DISSEMINATED INTRAVASCULAR COAGULATION

Sepsis, or *septicemia,* is a condition in which organisms enter the bloodstream (bloodstream infection [BSI]) and can result in septic shock, a life-threatening condition. Adults with cancer who have low white blood cell counts (WBCs) (neutropenia) and impaired IMMUNITY from cancer therapy are at risk for infection and sepsis. Chapter 37 describes the pathophysiology of sepsis and septic shock. Adults with neutropenia do not have enough WBCs to always produce the typical signs and symptoms of infection (i.e., erythema, swelling, warmth, high fever). Often a low-grade fever (100.4°F or 38°C) is the only sign of infection. Infection and sepsis have a high mortality rate in adults with neutropenia (Shelton et al., 2016).

Disseminated intravascular coagulation (DIC) is a problem with the blood-CLOTTING process. DIC is triggered by many severe illnesses, including cancer. In patients with cancer DIC often is caused by gram-negative sepsis, although viral and other bacterial infections can trigger it. A patient's normal bacterial flora enter the bloodstream through any site of skin breakdown and cause a severe infection, especially when neutropenia is present. Other causes of sepsis include liver disease, intravascular hemolysis, prosthetic devices, or metabolic acidosis.

Extensive, abnormal CLOTTING occurs throughout the small blood vessels of patients with DIC. This widespread clotting depletes circulating clotting factors and platelets. As this happens, extensive bleeding occurs. Bleeding from many sites is the most common problem and ranges from oozing to fatal hemorrhage. Clots block blood vessels and decrease blood flow to major body organs and result in pain, ischemia, strokelike symptoms, dyspnea, tachycardia, reduced kidney function, and bowel necrosis.

! NURSING SAFETY ALERT QSEN
Critical Rescue

DIC is a life-threatening problem with a high mortality rate, even when proper therapies are instituted. *Thus the best management of sepsis and DIC is prevention. Identify patients at greatest risk for sepsis and DIC. Practice strict adherence to aseptic technique during invasive procedures and during contact with nonintact skin and mucous membranes. Teach patients and families the early indicators of infection and to seek prompt assistance.*

When sepsis is present and DIC is likely, management focuses on reducing the infection and halting the DIC process. IV antibiotic therapy is initiated. During the early phase of DIC, anticoagulants (especially heparin) are given to limit CLOTTING and prevent the rapid consumption of circulating clotting factors. When DIC has progressed and hemorrhage is the primary problem, clotting factors are given. See Chapter 37 for a detailed discussion of DIC.

? NCLEX EXAMINATION CHALLENGE 22-3
Safe and Effective Care Environment

Which assessment findings in a client who has neutropenia from cancer chemotherapy indicate to the nurse that severe disseminated intravascular coagulation (DIC) is present? **Select all that apply.**
A. The client is bleeding from the nose, IV sites, and rectum.
B. The client's temperature is 99°F (37.2°C).
C. The client's pulse rate is 130 beats per minute.
D. The client's respiratory rate is 24 breaths per minute.
E. The client's white blood cell count is 3200/mm3 (3.2 × 109/L)
F. The client's hourly urine output is 100 mL.

SYNDROME OF INAPPROPRIATE ANTIDIURETIC HORMONE

In healthy adults antidiuretic hormone (ADH) is secreted by the posterior pituitary gland only when more fluid (water) is needed in the body, such as when plasma volume is decreased. Certain conditions induce ADH secretion when not needed by the body, which leads to syndrome of inappropriate antidiuretic hormone (SIADH).

Cancer is a common cause of SIADH, especially small cell lung cancer. SIADH also may occur with other cancers, including head and neck, melanoma, GI, prostate, and hematologic malignancies, especially when metastatic tumors are present in the brain. Some cancers make and secrete ADH, whereas others stimulate the posterior pituitary to secrete ADH. Drugs used for cancer therapy or supportive therapy also can cause SIADH (e.g., cyclophosphamide, morphine sulfate).

In SIADH water is reabsorbed in excess by the kidneys and put into systemic circulation. The retained water dilutes blood sodium levels, causing hyponatremia. Mild symptoms include weakness, muscle cramps, loss of appetite, and fatigue. Serum sodium levels range from 115 to 120 mEq/L (mmol/L) or lower (normal range is 135 to 145 mEq/L [mmol/L]). With greater fluid retention, weight gain, nervous system changes, personality changes, confusion, and extreme muscle weakness occur. As the sodium level drops toward 110 mEq/L (mmol/L), seizures, coma, and death may follow depending on how rapidly hyponatremia occurs.

SIADH is managed by treating the condition and the cause. Nursing priorities focus on patient safety, restoring normal fluid balance, and providing supportive care. Management includes fluid restriction, increased sodium intake, and drug therapy. Immediate cancer therapy with radiation or chemotherapy may cause enough tumor regression that ADH production returns to normal. Effective treatment of the cancer triggering the syndrome is the only cure for SIADH. See Chapter 62 for a detailed discussion of SIADH management.

> **⚠ NURSING SAFETY PRIORITY** **QSEN**
>
> *Critical Rescue*
>
> Monitor patients at least every 2 hours to recognize signs and symptoms of increasing fluid overload (bounding pulse, increasing neck vein distention (jugular venous distention [JVD]), presence of crackles in lungs, increasing peripheral edema, reduced urine output) because pulmonary edema can occur very quickly and lead to death. When symptoms indicate that the fluid overload from SIADH either is not responding to therapy or is becoming worse, respond by notifying the health care provider immediately.

SPINAL CORD COMPRESSION

Spinal cord compression (SCC) is an oncologic emergency that requires immediate intervention to relieve pain and prevent neurologic damage. Damage from SCC occurs either when a tumor directly enters the spinal cord or spinal column or when the vertebrae collapse from tumor degradation of the bone. Tumors metastasizing from the lung, prostate, breast, and colon account for most SCC. Primary tumors of the spinal cord causing compression are less common. The most frequent area for SCC is the thoracic spine.

The symptoms of SCC can vary depending on the severity and location of the compression. Back pain is a common first symptom and occurs before other problems or nerve deficits. Other symptoms include weakness, loss of sensation, urinary retention, and constipation. Loss of or reduced deep tendon reflexes along with reduced pinprick and vibratory sensations are other findings that may be present on physical assessment. Neurologic problems are specific to the level of spinal compression and can lead to paralysis, which is usually permanent if the compression is not alleviated promptly.

Early recognition and treatment of spinal cord compression are key to a positive outcome. Assess for back pain that worsens over time; neurologic changes; muscle weakness or a sensation of heaviness in the arms or legs; numbness or tingling in the hands or feet; inability to distinguish pinprick, touch, or hot and cold sensation; and an unsteady gait. Depending on how low the compression occurs, constipation, incontinence, and difficulty starting or stopping urination also may be present. Teach patients and families to recognize and report the symptoms of early SCC, and instruct them to seek help immediately.

An MRI is used to confirm a diagnosis of SCC; however, if SCC is suspected by clinical symptoms, treatment should begin immediately to preserve function. Treatment is often palliative, with high-dose corticosteroids given first as an IV bolus to reduce swelling around the spinal cord and relieve symptoms, followed by a tapered dose over time. High-dose radiation may be used to reduce the size of the tumor in the area and relieve compression. Surgery may be performed to remove the tumor and trim the bony tissue so less pressure is placed on the spinal cord or to repair the spine if the spinal column is unstable. External back or neck braces may be used to reduce the weight borne by the spinal column and to reduce pressure on the spinal cord or spinal nerves.

HYPERCALCEMIA

Hypercalcemia (increased serum calcium level) occurs in up to a third of patients with cancer. It is a metabolic emergency and can lead to death. Breast, lung, and renal cell carcinomas; multiple myeloma; and adult T-cell leukemia and lymphoma are the most common causes among cancer patients. These cancers can secrete parathyroid hormone, causing bone to release calcium. Bone metastasis can stimulate bone breakdown (osteoclast activity) and bone resorption, which releases more calcium from bone and leads to hypercalcemia. In addition, systemic secretion of vitamin D analogues by the tumor can also cause elevated calcium levels in the bloodstream. Dehydration worsens hypercalcemia.

Early symptoms of hypercalcemia are nonspecific. Common symptoms include skeletal pain, kidney stones, abdominal discomfort, and altered cognition that can range from lethargy to coma. Additional symptoms include fatigue, loss of appetite, nausea, vomiting, constipation, and increased urine output. More serious problems include severe muscle weakness, loss of deep tendon reflexes, paralytic ileus, dehydration, and electrocardiographic (ECG) changes. Symptom severity depends on how high the calcium level is and how quickly it rose (see Chapter 11).

Cancer-induced hypercalcemia often develops slowly for many patients, which allows the body time to adapt to this electrolyte change. As a result, symptoms of hypercalcemia may not be evident until the serum calcium level is greatly elevated.

For patients who have elevated serum calcium levels and symptoms of hypercalcemia, vigorous IV hydration with normal saline at an infusion rate for 500 mL/hour (if cardiovascular function is normal) is used. Correcting the dehydration that often accompanies hypercalcemia restores urine output. Loop diuretics can promote calcium loss in urine. Thiazide diuretics are avoided because they can increase calcium reabsorption from urine. Many drugs such as bisphosphonates (which block bone resorption of calcium), calcitonin, and oral glucocorticoids can temporarily lower serum calcium levels. Treatment of the cancer is needed for long-term calcium control. When cancer-induced hypercalcemia is life threatening or occurs with kidney disease, dialysis can temporarily reduce serum calcium levels.

SUPERIOR VENA CAVA SYNDROME

The superior vena cava (SVC), which returns all blood from the head, neck, and upper extremities to the heart, has thin walls, and compression or obstruction by tumor growth or by clots in the vessel leads to congestion of the blood (Fig. 22-6). This is known as *superior vena cava syndrome (SVCS)* and can occur quickly or develop gradually over time. With gradual development physiologic adaptation occurs that allows the development of collateral circulation to handle the blood flow. SVCS occurs most often in patients with lymphomas (especially with tumors in the mediastinum), thymoma, right-sided lung cancer, and breast cancer.

Compression of the SVC is painful and can be life threatening. Symptoms result from the blockage of venous return from the head, neck, and upper trunk. Early signs and symptoms include edema of the face, especially around the eyes (periorbital edema) on arising in the morning, and tightness of the collar. As the compression worsens, the patient develops engorged blood vessels and erythema of the upper body (Fig. 22-7), edema in the arms and hands, and dyspnea. The development of stridor (a high-pitched crowing sound) indicates narrowing of the pharynx or larynx and is an alarming sign of rapid SVCS progression. Symptoms are more apparent when the patient is in the supine position. Late symptoms include hemorrhage, cyanosis, mental status changes, decreased cardiac

output, and hypotension. Imaging with CT or MRI is essential for diagnosis and treatment planning. Death results if compression is not relieved.

SVC syndrome is often associated with late-stage disease when the tumor is widespread. Occasionally SVCS occurs with obstruction in an indwelling vascular device by a blood clot. This type of obstruction can be treated successfully with fibrinolytic drugs. High-dose radiation therapy to the upper chest area may be used to provide temporary relief of airway obstruction. Chemotherapy may be the only option for long-term control of the cancer causing the compression. Surgery is rarely performed for this condition. A metal stent can be placed in the vena cava in an interventional radiology department to relieve swelling. Follow-up angioplasty can keep this stent open for a longer period.

> **? NCLEX EXAMINATION CHALLENGE 22-4**
>
> ### *Safe and Effective Care Environment*
>
> Which client report indicates to the nurse that spinal cord compression may be present?
> A. The client reports having a headache for the past 7 hours.
> B. The client has reduced breath sounds in the left lung.
> C. The client has worsening mid-thoracic back pain.
> D. Pedal edema is now present bilaterally.

TUMOR LYSIS SYNDROME

In tumor lysis syndrome (TLS) large numbers of tumor cells are destroyed rapidly. The intracellular contents of damaged cancer cells, including potassium and purines (DNA components), are released into the bloodstream faster than the body can eliminate them (Fig. 22-8). Unlike other oncologic emergencies, TLS is a positive sign that cancer treatment is effective in destroying cancer cells.

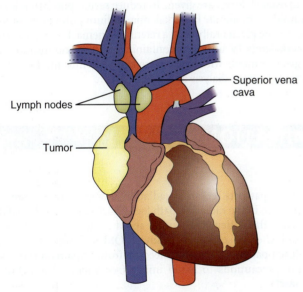

FIG. 22-6 Compression of the superior vena cava by lymph nodes and tumors in superior vena cava syndrome.

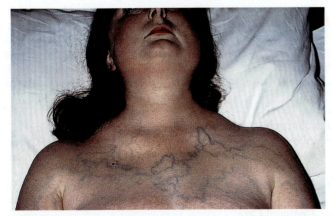

FIG. 22-7 Appearance of the face, neck, upper arms, and chest in a patient with superior vena cava syndrome. (From Forbes, C. D., & Jackson, W. F. [2003[. *Colour atlas and text of clinical medicine* [3rd ed.]. London: Mosby.)

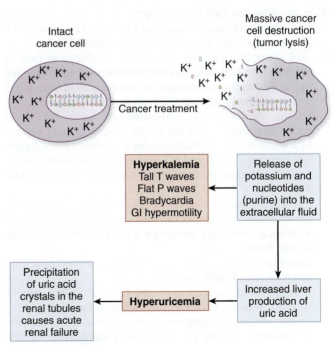

FIG. 22-8 Pathway of tumor lysis syndrome.

Severe or untreated TLS can cause tissue damage, acute kidney injury (AKI), and death (Wang et al., 2015). Serum potassium levels can increase to the point of hyperkalemia, causing cardiac dysfunction (see Chapter 11). The large amounts of purines form uric acid, causing hyperuricemia. These uric acid crystals precipitate in the kidney, blocking kidney tubules and leading to AKI. Sudden development of hyperkalemia, hyperuricemia, and hyperphosphatemia has life-threatening effects on the heart muscle, kidneys, and central nervous system.

TLS is usually seen in patients with high-grade cancers that are growing quickly and in extensive cancers that are very responsive to treatment (Kaplow & Iyere, 2016). Adults receiving radiation or chemotherapy for cancers that are very sensitive to these therapies are at risk for TLS. Common cancers likely to cause TLS include acute leukemia, high-grade lymphomas, small cell lung cancer, germ cell tumors, inflammatory breast cancer, melanoma, and multiple myeloma. Chemotherapy drugs most likely to cause TLS include paclitaxel, fludarabine, etoposide, thalidomide, bortezomib, zoledronic acid, and hydroxyurea. In addition, TLS is more likely to occur in older adults undergoing cancer treatment (Sleutel et al., 2016). Early symptoms of TLS include lethargy, nausea, vomiting, anorexia, flank pain, muscle weakness, cramps, seizures, edema, and altered mental status.

Hydration prevents and manages TLS by diluting the serum potassium level and increasing the kidney flow rates. These actions prevent the precipitation of uric acid crystals, increase the excretion of potassium, and flush any kidney precipitates.

With tumors known to be very sensitive to cancer therapy, instruct patients to drink at least 3000 mL (5000 mL is more desirable) of fluid the day before, the day of, and for 3 days after treatment. Some fluids should be alkaline (e.g., sodium bicarbonate) to help prevent uric acid precipitation. Stress the importance of keeping fluid intake consistent throughout the 24-hour day, and help patients draw up a schedule of fluid intake.

Because some patients have nausea and vomiting after cancer therapy and may not feel like drinking fluids, stress the importance of following the antiemetic regimen. Instruct patients to contact the oncologist immediately if nausea prevents adequate fluid intake so parenteral fluids can be started.

Prophylaxis is essential for high-risk patients receiving cancer therapy that is expected to reduce tumor burden quickly. Monitor daily weights and serum electrolyte values. Management becomes more aggressive for patients who become hyperkalemic or hyperuricemic. In addition to fluids, diuretics (especially osmotic types) are given to increase urine flow through the kidney. These agents are used cautiously to avoid dehydration. Drugs that promote purine excretion, such as allopurinol (Aloprim, Zyloprim), rasburicase (Elitek), or febuxostat (Uloric) are given. To reduce serum potassium levels for mild-to-moderate hyperkalemia, sodium polystyrene sulfonate can be given orally or as a retention enema. For more severe hyperkalemia IV infusions containing glucose and insulin may be given. Patients who have severe hyperkalemia and hyperuricemia may need dialysis and intensive care.

GET READY FOR THE NCLEX® EXAMINATION!

▌ KEY POINTS

Review these Key Points for each NCLEX Examination Client Needs Category.

Safe and Effective Care Environment

- Use aseptic technique during care for open skin areas or any invasive procedure to prevent infection. **QSEN: Safety**
- Perform good handwashing before providing any care to patients with neutropenia. **QSEN: Evidence-Based Practice**
- Assess the venous access device at least every 30 to 60 minutes during chemotherapy administration. **QSEN: Safety**
- During chemotherapy administration, verify the blood return after every 2 to 5 mL for IV push drugs and every 5 to 10 minutes for short continuous infusions. **QSEN: Safety**
- Use Bleeding Precautions for any patient with thrombocytopenia and impaired CLOTTING (see Chart 22-5). **QSEN: Safety**
- Use appropriate personal protection equipment (gowns, gloves, masks, eye protection) when handling the excreta of a patient receiving chemotherapy and for 48 hours afterward. **QSEN: Safety**
- Inspect the oral mucosa of patients with neutropenia at least every 8 hours. **QSEN: Safety**
- Report any temperature over 100°F (37.8°C) in a patient with neutropenia. **QSEN: Evidence-Based Practice**
- Ensure proper shielding and waste disposal when patients in inpatient settings are receiving brachytherapy. **QSEN: Safety**

- Teach patients receiving radiation therapy how to care for the skin in the radiation path (see Chart 22-2). **QSEN: Safety**
- Teach the patient and family about symptoms of infection and when to seek medical advice. **QSEN: Safety**
- Teach patients at risk for bleeding from impaired CLOTTING the precautions to avoid injury (see Chart 22-6). **QSEN: Safety**
- Instruct patients to contact the oncologic pharmacist or oncology clinic to determine the proper disposal of expired or discontinued oral chemotherapy agents. **QSEN: Safety**

Health Promotion and Maintenance

- Assist patients and families experiencing cancer to find appropriate community resources such as the American Cancer Society and the Canadian Cancer Society for support, supplies, care, and other assistance. **QSEN: Patient-Centered Care**

Psychosocial Integrity

- Allow the patient and family the opportunity to express concerns regarding the diagnosis of cancer or the treatment regimen. **QSEN: Patient-Centered Care**
- Encourage the patient to verbalize feelings about changes in appearance resulting from cancer therapy. **QSEN: Patient-Centered Care**
- Encourage patients to use strategies to improve their appearance when alopecia occurs. **QSEN: Patient-Centered Care**

Physiological Integrity

- Perform a total assessment each time the patient with cancer is seen to determine the level of cancer treatment side effects and whether an oncologic emergency exists. **QSEN: Patient-Centered Care**
- Assess the patient's pain level on a regular basis. **QSEN: Patient-Centered Care**
- Use pharmacologic and nonpharmacologic therapies to reduce pain for the patient with cancer. **QSEN: Patient-Centered Care**
- Explain all procedures, restrictions, drugs, and follow-up care to the patient and family. **QSEN: Patient-Centered Care**
- Instruct patients to use prescribed antiemetic drugs on a schedule for maximum relief of nausea and vomiting. **QSEN: Evidence-Based Practice**
- Work with other members of the interprofessional oncology care team to ensure the implementation of a personalized pain management and symptom control regimen. **QSEN: Teamwork and Collaboration**

- Assess the patient receiving chemotherapy for infection at least every 8 hours. **QSEN: Patient-Centered Care**
- Assess the patient with thrombocytopenia and impaired CLOTTING for bleeding. **QSEN: Patient-Centered Care**
- Assess the patient receiving hormonal therapy for evidence of inappropriate CLOTTING and blood clot formation. **QSEN: Patient-Centered Care**
- Closely monitor patients receiving any type of targeted therapy for severe side effects or adverse drug reactions. **QSEN: Patient-Centered Care**
- Stress the importance of adhering to the prescribed schedule for oral chemotherapy agents. **QSEN: Evidence-Based Practice**
- Demonstrate to the patient and whomever prepares oral chemotherapy agents at home how to do so without touching the tablets or capsules. **QSEN: Patient-Centered Care**
- Teach patients and families the symptoms of oncologic emergencies and when to notify the health care provider. **QSEN: Patient-Centered Care**

SELECTED BIBLIOGRAPHY

American Cancer Society. (2017). *Cancer facts and figures—2017.* Report No. 00-300M–No. 500817. Atlanta: Author.

Armstrong, K. (2016). Chemobrain: Physiological predisposing factors. *Medsurg Nursing, 25*(4), 215–218.

Aschenbrenner, D. (2015). New antiemetic for chemotherapy-induced nausea. *American Journal of Nursing, 115*(2), 20.

Bail, J., & Meneses, R. (2016). Computer-based cognitive training for chemotherapy-related cognitive impairment in breast cancer survivors. *Clinical Journal of Oncology Nursing, 20*(5), 504–509.

Barak, F., Amoyal, M., & Kalichman, L. (2013). Using a simple diary for management of nausea and vomiting during chemotherapy. *Clinical Journal of Oncology Nursing, 17*(5), 479–481.

Bauer, C. (2016). Understanding radiation dermatitis. *American Nurse Today, 11*(1), 13–15.

Bauer, C., Laszewski, P., & Magnan, M. (2015). Promoting adherence to skin care practices among patients receiving radiation therapy. *Clinical Journal of Oncology Nursing, 19*(2), 196–203.

Beck, M. (2015). Radiation safety in the management of patients undergoing radioactive iodine ablation therapy. *Clinical Journal of Oncology Nursing, 19*(1), 44–46.

Boucher, J., Habin, K., & Underhill, M. (2014). Cancer genetics and genomics: Essentials for oncology nurses. *Clinical Journal of Oncology Nursing, 18*(3), 355–359.

Burhenn, P., & Smudde, J. (2015). Using tools and technology to promote education and adherence to oral agents for cancer. *Clinical Journal of Oncology Nursing, 19*(3Suppl), 53–59.

Callahan, A., Ames, N., Manning, M., Touchton-Leonard, K., Yang, L., & Wallen, G. (2016). Factors influencing nurses' use of hazardous drug safe-handling precautions. *Oncology Nursing Forum, 43*(3), 342–349.

Canadian Cancer Society, Statistics Canada. (2016). *Canadian cancer statistics, 2016.* Toronto, ON: Canadian Cancer Society. www.cancer.ca/~/media/cancer.ca/CW/cancer%20information/cancer%20101/Canadian%20cancer%20statistics/Canadian-Cancer-Statistics-2016-EN.pdf?la=en.

Crickman, R., & Finnell, D. (2017). Chemotherapy safe handling. *Clinical Journal of Oncology Nursing, 21*(1), 73–78.

Curcio, K. (2016). Instruments for assessing chemotherapy-induced peripheral neuropathy: A review of the literature. *Clinical Journal of Oncology Nursing, 20*(2), 144–151.

Fenton-Kerimian, M., Cartwright, F., Peat, E., Florentino, R., Maisonet, O., Budin, W., et al. (2015). Optimal topical agent for radiation dermatitis during breast radiotherapy: A pilot study. *Clinical Journal of Oncology Nursing, 19*(4), 451–455.

Foster, M. (2014). Reevaluating the neutropenic diet: Time to change. *Clinical Journal of Oncology Nursing, 18*(2), 239–241.

Hafiz, A., Abbasi, A. N., Ali, N., Kahn, K. A., & Qureshi, B. M. (2015). Frequency & severity of acute toxicity of pelvic radiotherapy for gynecological cancer. *Journal of the College of Physicians and Surgeons–Pakistan, 25*(11), 802–806.

Irwin, M., & Johnson, L. (2015). Factors influencing oral adherence: Qualitative metasummary and triangulation with quantitative evidence. *Clinical Journal of Oncology Nursing, 19*(3Suppl), 6–30.

Kaplow, R., & Iyere, K. (2016). Recognizing and preventing tumor lysis syndrome. *Nursing, 46*(11), 26–32.

Kaplow, R., & Iyere, K. (2017). Grading chemotherapy-induced peripheral neuropathy in adults. *Nursing, 17*(2), 67–68.

Kiernan, J. (2016). Genetic influence on chemotherapy-induced nausea and vomiting. *Oncology Nursing Forum, 43*(3), 389–393.

Limburg, C., Maxwell, C., & Mautner, B. (2014). Prevention and treatment of bone loss in patients with nonmetastatic breast or prostate cancer who receive hormone ablation therapy. *Clinical Journal of Oncology Nursing, 18*(2), 223–230.

McCance, K., Huether, S., Brashers, V., & Rote, N. (2014). *Pathophysiology: The biologic basis for disease in adults and children* (7th ed.). St. Louis: Mosby.

Mitchell, G. (2013). The rationale for fractionation in radiotherapy. *Clinical Journal of Oncology Nursing, 17*(4), 412–417.

National Cancer Institute. (2015). *Photodynamic therapy for cancer.* www.cancer.gov/cancertopics/factsheet/Therapy/photodynamic.

Neuss, M., Gilmore, T., Belderson, K., Billett, A., Conti-Kalchik, T., Harvey, B., et al. (2017). 2016 updated American Society of Clinical Oncology/Oncology Nursing Society chemotherapy administration safety standards, including standards for pediatric oncology. *Oncology Nursing Forum, 44*(1), 31–43.

Polovich, M., Olsen, M., & LeFebvre, K. B. (2014). *Chemotherapy and biotherapy guidelines and recommendations for practice* (4th ed.). Pittsburgh, PA: Oncology Nursing Society.

Proud, C. (2014). Radiogenomics: The promise of personalized treatment in radiation oncology? *Clinical Journal of Oncology Nursing, 18*(2), 185–189.

Roos, D. (2015). Radiotherapy for neuropathic pain due to bone metastases. *Annals of Palliative Medicine, 4*(4), 220–224.

Santos, E. M. M., Edwards, Q. T., Floria-Santos, M., Rogatto, S. R., Achatz, M. I. W., & MacDonald, D. J. (2013). Integration of genomics in cancer care. *Journal of Nursing Scholarship, 45*(1), 43–51.

Schulmeister, L. (2014). Safe management of chemotherapy: Infusion-related complications. *Clinical Journal of Oncology Nursing, 18*(3), 283–287.

Shelton, B., Stanik-Hutt, J., Kane, J., & Jones, R. (2016). Implementing the surviving sepsis campaign in an ambulatory clinic for patients with hematologic malignancies. *Clinical Journal of Oncology Nursing, 20*(3), 281–288.

Sleutel, M., Brown, W., & Wells, J. (2016). Preventing tumor lysis syndrome: Two case studies of unexpected outcomes. *Clinical Journal of Oncology Nursing, 20*(2), 195–200.

Smith, E. M., Campbell, G., Tofthagen, C., Kottschade, L., Collins, M., Warton, C., et al. (2014). Nursing knowledge, practice patterns, and learning preferences regarding chemotherapy-induced peripheral neuropathy. *Oncology Nursing Forum, 41*(6), 669–679.

Spoelstra, S., Given, C., Sikorskii, A., Coursaris, C., Majumder, A., DeKoekkoek, T., et al. (2015). Feasibility of a text-messaging intervention to promote self-management for patients prescribed oral anticancer agents. *Oncology Nursing Forum, 42*(6), 647–657.

Spoelstra, S., & Rittenberg, C. (2015). Assessment and measurement of medication adherence: Oral agents for cancer. *Clinical Journal of Oncology Nursing, 19*(3Suppl), 47–52.

Spoelstra, S., & Sansoucie, H. (2015). Putting evidence into practice: Evidence-based interventions for oral agents for cancer. *Clinical Journal of Oncology Nursing, 19*(3Suppl), 60–72.

Thompson, N., & Christian, A. (2016). Oral chemotherapy: Not just an ordinary pill. *American Nurse Today, 11*(9), 16–20.

Von Ah, D. (2015). Cognitive changes associated with cancer and cancer treatment: State of the science. *Clinical Journal of Oncology Nursing, 19*(1), 47–56.

Von Ah, D., Jansen, C., & Allen, D. (2014). Evidence-based interventions for cancer- and treatment-related cognitive impairment. *Clinical Journal of Oncology Nursing, 18*(6), 17–25.

Wallner, M., Kock-Hodi, S., Booze, S., White, K., & Mayer, H. (2016). Nursing management of cutaneous toxicities from epidermal growth factor receptor inhibitors. *Clinical Journal of Oncology Nursing, 20*(5), 529–536.

Wang, L., Jian, Y., Yang, G., Gao, W., Wu, Y., & Zuo, L. (2015). Management of tumor lysis syndrome in patients with multiple myeloma during bortezomib treatment. *Clinical Journal of Oncology Nursing, 19*(1), E4–E7.

Wieners, G., Schippers, A. C., Collettini, F., Schnapauff, D., Hamm, B., Wust, P., et al. (2015). CT-guided high-dose brachytherapy in the interdisciplinary treatment of patients with liver metastases of pancreatic cancer. *Hepatobiliary Pancreatic Disease International, 14*(5), 530–538.

Williams, A., Mowlazadeh, B., Sisler, L., & Williams, P. (2015). Self-reported assessment of symptoms and self-care within a cohort of U.S. veterans during outpatient care for cancer. *Clinical Journal of Oncology Nursing, 19*(5), 595–602.

Yeboa, D. N., & Evans, S. B. (2016). Contemporary breast radiotherapy and cardiac toxicity. *Seminars in Radiation Oncology, 26*(1), 71–78.

Yu, H., Friedlander, D. R., Patel, S., & Hu, J. C. (2013). The current status of robotic oncologic surgery. *CA: A Cancer Journal for Clinicians, 63*(1), 45–56.

Zagar, T. M., Cardinale, D. M., & Marks, L. B. (2015). Breast cancer therapy–associated cardiovascular disease. *Nature Reviews. Clinical Oncology*, doi:10.1038/nrclinonc.2015.171. [Epub ahead of print].

CHAPTER 23

Care of Patients With Infection

Donna D. Ignatavicius

 http://evolve.elsevier.com/Iggy/

PRIORITY AND INTERRELATED CONCEPTS

The priority concept for this chapter is IMMUNITY.

✳ The IMMUNITY concept exemplar for this chapter is Infection, below.

The interrelated concept for this chapter is TISSUE INTEGRITY.

LEARNING OUTCOMES

Safe and Effective Care Environment

1. Use clinical judgment to determine infection control measures, such as hand hygiene and Transmission-Based Precautions.
2. Apply current principles of infection prevention and control to ensure safe, patient-centered care.

Health Promotion and Maintenance

3. Outline health teaching for patients, families, and staff about infection control measures.

Psychosocial Integrity

4. Explain the importance of assessing the patient's emotional response to having an infection.

Physiological Integrity

5. Determine patients most at risk for infection, including older adults and others with impaired IMMUNITY.

6. Teach the patient and family about drug therapy for infections, including the need for adherence.
7. Describe common causes of infection, including impaired TISSUE INTEGRITY.
8. Identify common signs and symptoms of infection.
9. Interpret laboratory test findings related to infections.
10. Evaluate evidence-based interprofessional collaborative interventions for management of the patient with an infection.
11. Explain why multidrug-resistant organisms are increasing and how genetic/genomic research is helping to fight them.
12. Identify examples of common emerging diseases and bioterrorism agents.
13. Discuss nursing implications for the patient having a fecal microbiota transplantation (FMT) for recurrent *C. difficile* infections.

The human body has many systems that promote homeostasis. Physiologic mechanisms are the structural and functional defenses that maintain IMMUNITY and protect people from stressors such as infection. When these mechanisms fail to work properly or are overcome with microbes, infection can result.

Infections and infectious diseases have been the major cause of millions of deaths worldwide for centuries. Threats of bioterrorism have been added to the concerns about multidrug-resistant and emerging infections. Global travel and migration have increased exposure to a wider variety of infectious agents than in the past.

Advancing technology and invasive procedures also introduce microorganisms into the body, often resulting in infection. In other environments these microorganisms are harmless. This chapter provides an overview of infection and general principles

for prevention and management. Specific infections and their management are described elsewhere in this text.

✳ IMMUNITY EXEMPLAR Infection

A **pathogen** is any microorganism (also called an *agent*) capable of producing disease. Infections can be **communicable** (transmitted from person to person [e.g., influenza]) or not communicable (e.g., peritonitis). Microorganisms with differing levels of **pathogenicity** (ability to cause disease) surround everyone. **Virulence** is a term for pathogenicity. However, virulence is related more to the frequency with which a pathogen causes disease (degree of communicability) and its ability to invade and damage a host. It can also indicate the severity of the disease.

GENETIC/GENOMIC CONSIDERATIONS
Patient-Centered Care **QSEN**

A current related issue in IMMUNITY and genomics is the microbiome. As described in Chapter 5, the **microbiome** for an adult is genomes of all the microorganisms that coexist in and on him or her. Many microorganisms live in or on the human host without causing disease and may be beneficial. These include the organisms that live in the mouth, the rest of the GI tract, the nose and sinuses, the vagina, and on the skin. Most of these organisms are part of our normal flora, which differ somewhat from person to person. **Normal flora** are mostly nonpathogenic (non–disease causing) when they remain confined to the expected area. However, when they manage to escape their normal human habitat and move elsewhere, they may be pathogenic in the new environment. For example, when GI organisms get into the urinary tract or the blood, serious infections can result. In some instances microorganisms that are often pathogenic may be present in the tissues of the host and yet not cause symptomatic disease because of normal flora; this process is called **colonization**.

TABLE 23-1 Host Factors That Influence the Development of Infection

HOST FACTOR	INCREASED RISK FOR INFECTION
Natural immunity	Congenital or acquired immune deficiencies
Normal flora	Alteration of normal flora by antibiotic therapy
Age	Infants and older adults
Hormonal factors	Diabetes mellitus, corticosteroid therapy, and adrenal insufficiency
Phagocytosis	Defective phagocytic function, circulatory disturbances, and neutropenia
Skin/mucous membranes/ normal excretory secretions	Break in skin or mucous membrane integrity; interference with flow of urine, tears, or saliva; interference with cough reflex or ciliary action; changes in gastric secretions
Nutrition	Malnutrition or dehydration
Environmental factors	Tobacco and alcohol consumption and inhalation of toxic chemicals
Medical interventions	Invasive therapy such as endoscopy, urinary catheters, IVs; chemotherapy, radiation therapy, and steroid therapy (suppress immune system); surgery

In the United States, the Centers for Disease Control and Prevention (CDC) collects information about the occurrence and nature of infections and infectious diseases. It then recommends guidelines to health care agencies for infection control and prevention. Certain diseases such as tuberculosis must be reported to health departments and the CDC. In Canada the Public Health Agency of Canada also provides guidelines for infection control and for prevention of common infections. The infection control practitioner (ICP) for each health care organization is responsible for tracking infections (**surveillance**) and ensuring compliance with federal, provincial, and local requirements and accreditation standards.

Transmission of Infectious Agents

Transmission of infection requires three factors:
- Reservoir (or source) of infectious agents
- Susceptible host with a portal of entry
- Mode of transmission

Reservoirs (sources of infectious agents) are numerous. Animate reservoirs include people, animals, and insects. Inanimate reservoirs include soil, water, handheld mobile devices (especially cell phones), and medical equipment (e.g., IV solutions, urine collection devices). Stethoscopes used for auscultation by many health care professionals carry *Staphylococcus aureus* from the skin of one patient to another. These devices should be cleaned with an antibacterial solution between patients (Alspach, 2014). The host's body can be a reservoir; pathogens colonize skin and body substances (e.g., feces, sputum, saliva, wound drainage). A person with an active infection or an asymptomatic **carrier** (one who harbors an infectious agent without active disease) is a reservoir. Examples of *community* reservoirs include sewage, stagnant or contaminated water, and improperly handled foods.

Bacteria such as *Neisseria meningitidis* can exist in the respiratory tract while causing no illness. If the bacteria invade the bloodstream or cerebrospinal fluid, they become extremely pathogenic. Another example is *Enterococcus,* which lives as normal flora in the GI system, where it is nonpathogenic and assists in the digestive process. If it enters the bloodstream, *Enterococcus* can cause disease.

Continued multiplication of a pathogen is sometimes accompanied by toxin production. **Toxins** are protein molecules released by bacteria to affect host cells at a distant site. *Exotoxins* are produced and released by certain bacteria into the surrounding environment. Botulism, tetanus, diphtheria, and *Escherichia coli* 0157:H7–related systemic diseases are attributed to exotoxins. *Endotoxins* are produced in the cell walls of certain bacteria and released only with cell lysis. For example, typhoid and meningococcal diseases are caused by endotoxins.

Host factors influence the development of infection (Table 23-1). Host defenses provide the body with an efficient system for IMMUNITY against pathogens. Breakdown of these defense mechanisms may increase the **susceptibility** (risk) of the host for infection.

The patient's *immune status* plays a large role in determining risk for infection. Congenital abnormalities and acquired health problems (e.g., renal failure, steroid dependence, cancer, acquired immune deficiency syndrome [AIDS]) can result in numerous immunologic deficiencies. Depression of IMMUNITY may make the host more susceptible to infection or impair the ability to combat organisms that have gained entry.

Immunity is resistance to infection; it is usually associated with the presence of antibodies or cells that act on specific microorganisms. **Passive immunity** is of short duration (days or months) and either natural by transplacental transfer from the mother or artificial by injection of antibodies (e.g., immunoglobulin). **Active immunity** lasts for years and is natural by infection or artificial by stimulation of the body's immune defenses (e.g., vaccination). Chapter 17 discusses the immune system and IMMUNITY in detail.

Environmental factors can also influence patients' immune status and thus their susceptibility to or ability to fight infection. Examples include alcohol consumption, nicotine use, inhalation of bone marrow–suppressing toxic chemicals, and certain vitamin deficiencies. Malnutrition, especially protein-calorie

CHART 23-1 Nursing Focus on the Older-Adult

Factors That May Increase Risk for Infection in the Older Patient

FACTOR	AGING-ASSOCIATED CHANGES OR CONDITIONS
Immune system	Decreased antibody production, lymphocytes, and fever response
Integumentary system	Thinning skin, decreased subcutaneous tissue, decreased vascularity, slower wound healing
Respiratory system	Decreased cough and gag reflexes
GI system	Decreased gastric acid and intestinal motility
Chronic illness	Diabetes mellitus, chronic obstructive pulmonary disease, neurologic impairments
Functional/cognitive impairments	Immobility, incontinence, dementia
Invasive devices	Urinary catheters, feeding tubes, IV devices, tracheostomy tubes
Institutionalization	Increased person-to-person contact and transmission

QUALITY IMPROVEMENT QSEN

Reducing Catheter-Associated Urinary Tract Infections

Mori, C. (2014). A-voiding catastrophe: Implementing a nurse-driven protocol. *Medsurg Nursing, 23*(1), 15–21, 28.

In spite of the move to decrease the use of indwelling urinary catheters (e.g., Foley catheters), catheter-associated urinary tract infections (CAUTIs) remain a major cause of sepsis and increased hospital costs. The Centers for Medicare and Medicaid Services (CMS) recently began to link health care reimbursement to quality improvement efforts to prevent CAUTIs.

An interdisciplinary team led by a clinical nurse specialist in a Midwestern community hospital implemented a protocol that decreased the use of urinary catheters and ensured best practices for patients for whom the catheters were indicated. Using a screening checklist, each patient was assessed to determine the need for a Foley catheter. If certain criteria were not met, the catheter was removed by a nurse using a specific protocol during and after removal. For patients who had to have a Foley catheter, the nurse provided care to minimize the chance for urinary infection, including checking that the:

- Catheter was secure
- Tamper-evident seal was intact
- Catheter tubing was not twisted or had a dependent loop
- Catheter bag was positioned lower than the bladder level
- Drainage bag did not touch the floor or was not overfilled

Commentary: Implications for Practice and Research

Research demonstrates that decreasing the use of indwelling urinary catheters is the most important intervention to prevent hospital-acquired CAUTIs. This project used this research and showed how an interdisciplinary team led by a Clinical Nurse Specialist (CNS) in a community hospital could improve the quality of care by decreasing urinary tract infections. In addition, nurses provided evidence-based care for patients who needed urinary catheters to ensure adequate urinary flow.

A limitation of the project was that incremental changes or strategies to maintain the positive changes were not discussed. More quality improvement activities at a unit or health care agency are needed to use current research, sustain a change in nursing practice, and achieve positive patient outcomes.

---

malnutrition and obesity, places patients at increased risk for infection. Diseases such as diabetes mellitus also predispose a patient to infection. Older adults have decreased IMMUNITY and other physiologic changes that make them very susceptible to infection (Chart 23-1).

Medical and surgical interventions may impair normal immune response. Steroid therapy, chemotherapy, and anti-rejection drugs increase the risk for infection. Medical devices (e.g., intravascular or urinary catheters, endotracheal tubes, synthetic implants) may also interfere with normal host defense mechanisms. Surgery, trauma, radiation therapy, and burns result in impaired TISSUE INTEGRITY. *The body's skin is one of the best barriers or defenses against infection.* When this barrier is broken, infection often results. Microorganisms may enter the body in a variety of ways, including the respiratory tract, GI tract, genitourinary tract, skin and mucous membranes, and bloodstream.

Routes of Transmission

Pathogens may enter the body through the *respiratory tract*. Microbes in droplets are sprayed into the air when people with infected oral or nasal tissues talk, cough, or sneeze. A susceptible host then inhales droplets, and pathogens localize in the lungs or are distributed via the lymphatic system or bloodstream to other areas of the body. Microorganisms that enter the body by the respiratory tract and produce distant infection include influenza virus, *Mycobacterium tuberculosis*, and *Streptococcus pneumoniae*.

Other pathogens enter the body through the *GI tract*. Some stay there and produce disease (e.g., *Shigella* causing self-limited disease). Others invade the GI tract to produce local and distant infection (e.g., *Salmonella enteritidis*). Some produce limited GI symptoms, causing systemic infection (e.g., *Salmonella typhi*) or profound involvement of other organs (e.g., hepatitis A

virus). Millions of foodborne illness cases occur each year in the United States. This type of illness results in many hospitalizations and deaths.

Microorganisms also enter through the *genitourinary tract*. *Urinary tract infection (UTI) is one of the most common health care–associated infections (HAIs).* Indwelling urinary catheters are a primary cause of *catheter-associated urinary tract infections (CAUTIs),* especially in older adults. CAUTIs can increase hospital costs by prolonging the patient's length of stay and complicating his or her recovery. In many settings nurse-driven protocols have helped decrease the use of urinary catheters and associated infections (see the Quality Improvement box).

Although intact skin is the best barrier to prevent most infections, some pathogens such as *Treponema pallidum* can enter the body through intact *skin* or *mucous membranes.* However, most pathogens enter through breaks in these normally effective surface barriers. Sometimes a medical procedure causes impaired TISSUE INTEGRITY or a break in mucous membranes, as in catheter-acquired **bacteremia** (bacteria in the bloodstream) and surgical-site infections (SSIs). *Fragile skin of older patients and of those receiving prolonged steroid therapy increases infection risk.*

Microorganisms can gain direct access to the *bloodstream,* especially when invasive devices or tubes are used. The incidence of bloodstream infections (BSIs) continues to increase in hospitals throughout the United States. Central venous catheters (CVCs) are a primary cause of these infections (see Chapter 13 for more discussion of CVC-related BSIs). In the community setting biting insects can inject organisms into the bloodstream, causing infection (e.g., Lyme disease, West Nile viral encephalitis).

Methods of Transmission

For infection to be transmitted from an infected source to a susceptible host, a transport mechanism is required. Microorganisms are transmitted by several routes:

- Contact transmission (indirect and direct)
- Droplet transmission
- Airborne transmission

Contact transmission is the usual mode of transmission of most infections. Many infections are spread by direct or indirect contact. With *direct contact* the source and host have physical contact. Microorganisms are transferred directly from skin to skin or from mucous membrane to mucous membrane. Often called *person-to-person transmission,* direct contact is best illustrated by the spread of the "common cold."

Indirect contact transmission involves the transfer of microorganisms from a source to a host by passive transfer from a contaminated object. Contaminated articles or hands may be sources of infection. For example, patient-care devices such as glucometers and electronic thermometers may transmit pathogens if they are contaminated with blood or body fluids. Uniforms, laboratory coats, and isolation gowns used as part of personal protective equipment (PPE) may be contaminated as well.

Indirect transmission may involve contact with infected secretions or *droplets.* Droplets are produced when a person talks or sneezes; the droplets travel short distances. Susceptible hosts may acquire infection by contact with droplets deposited on the nasal, oral, or conjunctival membranes. Therefore the CDC recommends that staff stay at least 3 feet (1 m) away from a patient with droplet infection. An example of droplet-spread infection is influenza.

Airborne transmission occurs when small airborne particles containing pathogens leave the infected source and enter a susceptible host. These pathogens can be suspended in the air for a prolonged time. The particles carrying pathogens are usually contained in droplet nuclei or dust; they are usually propelled from the respiratory tract by coughing or sneezing. A susceptible person then inhales the particles directly into the respiratory tract. For example, tuberculosis is spread via airborne transmission.

Preventing the spread of microbes that are transmitted by the airborne route requires the use of special air handling and ventilation systems in an airborne infection isolation room (AIIR). *M. tuberculosis* and the varicella-zoster virus (chickenpox) are examples of airborne agents that require one of these systems. In addition to the AIIR, respiratory protection using a certified **powered air-purifying respirator (PAPR)** is recommended for health care personnel entering the patient's room. This device has a high-efficiency particulate air (HEPA) filter and battery to promote positive-pressure airflow and is more effective than N95 respirators.

Other sources of infectious agents include the environment such as contaminated food, water, or vectors. *Vectors* are insects that carry pathogens between two or more hosts such as the deer tick that causes Lyme disease and, a more current concern, the mosquito that carries the Zika virus.

The **Zika virus** has affected people in over a dozen countries, including the United States, and can cause microcephaly (abnormally small heads) in newborns and Guillain-Barré syndrome and other neurologic diseases in adults (Simon & Carpenetti, 2016). In addition to vector transmission, the virus can be transmitted via sexual transmission, blood transmission, and prenatal transmission from mother to fetus. Teach patients to apply liberal amounts of insect repellent to prevent getting bitten by insects. One in five people with the virus have mild, self-limiting flu-like symptoms such as muscle and joint pain, fever, headaches, and fatigue. Treatment is supportive with rest, hydration, and acetaminophen (Simon & Carpenetti, 2016).

The *portal of exit* completes the chain of infection. Exit of the microbe from the host often occurs through the portal of entry. An organism such as *M. tuberculosis* enters the respiratory tract and then exits the same tract as the infected host coughs. Some organisms can exit from the infected host by several routes. For example, varicella-zoster virus can spread through direct contact with infective fluid in vesicles and by airborne transmission.

Physiologic Defenses for Infection

Strong and intact host defenses can prevent microbes from entering the body or destroy a pathogen that has entered. Impaired host defenses may be unable to defend against microbial invasion, allowing entry of organisms that can destroy cells and cause infection. Common defense mechanisms include:

- Body tissues
- Phagocytosis
- Inflammation
- Immune systems

Intact skin forms the first and most important physical barrier to the entry of microorganisms. In addition to providing a mechanical barrier, the skin's slightly acidic pH (resulting from breakdown of lipids into fatty acids), together with normal skin flora, creates an unfriendly environment for many bacteria.

Mucous membranes' mucociliary action provides some mechanical protection against pathogenic invasion. More important, however, mucous membranes are bathed in secretions that inactivate many microorganisms. Lysozymes, which dissolve the cell walls of some bacteria, are present in large quantities in many body secretions, particularly in tears and nasal mucus.

Other body systems provide natural barriers to infection. For instance, the healthy respiratory tract clears most of all inhaled material by upper airway filtration, humidification, mucociliary transport, and coughing. Peristaltic action mechanically empties the GI tract of pathogenic organisms. Stomach acid, intestinal secretions, pancreatic enzymes, and bile, together with the competition from normal bowel flora, provide an environment that protects the GI tract from invasion by harmful organisms. In the genitourinary tract, the flushing action of urine eliminates pathogenic organisms. The low pH of urine also maintains a sterile environment, although some microorganisms, such as *E. coli,* can thrive in an acid medium.

Phagocytosis occurs when a foreign substance evades the first-line mechanical barriers and enters the body. Various leukocyte types function differently in the immune reaction, but neutrophils bear primary responsibility for phagocytosis. This process of engulfing, ingesting, killing, and disposing of an invading organism is an essential mechanism in host defense. Phagocytic dysfunction dramatically increases a patient's risk for infection.

Inflammation is another important nonspecific defense mechanism for preventing the spread of infection. It occurs when tissue becomes damaged or impaired. Damaged cells release enzymes, and polymorphonuclear (PMN) leukocytes (neutrophils) are attracted to the infected site from the bloodstream. One important substance, histamine, increases the permeability of the capillaries in inflamed tissues, thus allowing fluid, proteins, and white blood cells to enter an inflamed area. Other enzymes activate fibrinogen, which causes leaked fluid to clot and prevents its flow away from the damaged site into unaffected tissue, essentially "walling off" the inflamed tissue. The process of phagocytosis disposes of the invading microorganism and often dead tissue. If inflammation is caused by infection, the end products of inflammation form pus, which is then absorbed or exits the body through a break in the skin. Chapter 17 discusses the process of inflammation in more detail.

Specific defense responses to specific microorganisms are provided by antibody- and cell-mediated IMMUNITY. The antibody-mediated immune system produces antibodies directed against certain pathogens. These antibodies inactivate or destroy invading microorganisms and protect against future infection from that microorganism. Resistance to other microorganisms is mediated by the action of specifically sensitized T-lymphocytes and is called cell-mediated immunity. The components of the immune system work both independently and together to protect against infection. Chapter 17 describes the function of the immune system in detail.

Health Promotion and Maintenance

Infections occur most often in high-risk patients such as older adults and those who have inadequate or impaired IMMUNITY (immunocompromised). Implement interventions to prevent infection and detect signs and symptoms as early as possible. Chart 23-2 summarizes nursing interventions for infection prevention and control.

◎ **CHART 23-2   Best Practice for Patient Safety & Quality Care** QSEN

Nursing Interventions for the Patient at Risk for Infection

- Assess patients for risk for infections.
- Monitor for signs and symptoms of infection.
- Monitor laboratory tests results such as cultures and white blood cell (WBC) count and differential.
- Screen all visitors for infections or infectious disease.
- Inspect skin and mucous membranes for redness, heat, pain, swelling, and drainage.
- Promote sufficient nutritional intake, especially protein for healing.
- Encourage fluid intake to treat fever.
- Teach the patient and family the signs and symptoms of infections and when to report them to the primary health care provider.
- Teach the patient and family how to avoid infections in health care agencies and the community.

Infection Control in Health Care Settings

Infection acquired in the inpatient health care setting (not present or incubating at admission) is termed a health care–associated infection (HAI). When occurring in a hospital setting, it is sometimes referred to as a *hospital-acquired infection,* but the former term is more accurate. HAIs can be *endogenous* (from a patient's flora) or *exogenous* (from outside the patient, often from the hands of health care workers, tubes, or implants). HAIs, including surgical site infections (SSIs), cause increased health care costs and many deaths (see discussion in Chapter 16). These infections tend to occur most often because health care workers do not follow basic infection control principles.

Infection control within a health care facility is designed to reduce the risk for HAIs and thus reduce morbidity and mortality, as recommended in The Joint Commission's National Patient Safety Goals (NPSGs). This expected outcome is consistent with the desire for health care facilities to create a *culture of safety* within their environments (see Chapter 1). Infection control and prevention are interprofessional efforts and include:

- Health organization–specific and department-specific infection control policies and procedures
- Surveillance and analysis
- Patient and staff education
- Community and interprofessional collaboration
- Product evaluation with an emphasis on quality and cost savings
- Bioengineering for designing health care facilities that help control the spread of infections

The infection control program of a hospital is coordinated and implemented by a health care professional certified in infection control (CIC) who has clinical and administrative experience. The Centers for Disease Control and Prevention (CDC) recommends one person with CIC credentials for every 100 occupied acute care beds. Long-term care facilities may not have a practitioner who specializes in infection control. However, every facility must designate a health care professional to be responsible for coordinating and implementing an infection prevention and control program.

Long-term care facilities are unique in that they have a large group of older adults who are together in one setting for weeks to years. Nursing homes in particular are required to provide a homelike environment in which residents can move and interact freely. Therefore infection control in these settings can be challenging. As a result, many infectious outbreaks may occur such as pneumonia, *Clostridium difficile,* and multidrug-resistant organisms (discussed in the Multidrug-Resistant Organism Infections and Colonizations section).

Ambulatory and home health care are the fastest-growing segments of the health care system. Infection remains a common cause of death for dialysis patients. Little information is available about acquired infections in home health settings because data are not systematically collected, surveillance programs are not established, and best practices for infection prevention and control do not yet exist.

Methods of Infection Control and Prevention

All health care workers who come in contact with patients or care areas are involved in some aspect of the infection control

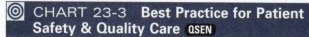

CHART 23-3 Best Practice for Patient Safety & Quality Care QSEN

Hand Hygiene

- When hands are visibly soiled or contaminated with proteinaceous material or visibly soiled with blood or other body fluids, wash hands with soap and water.
- If hands are not visibly soiled, use an alcohol-based hand rub (ABHR) for decontaminating hands or wash hands with soap and water.
- Use either ABHR or wash with soap and water (decontaminate hands) before having direct contact with patients.
- Decontaminate hands before donning sterile gloves to perform a procedure such as inserting an invasive device (e.g., indwelling urinary catheter).
- Decontaminate hands after contact with a patient's intact skin (e.g., taking a pulse) or with body fluids or excretions/secretions.
- Decontaminate hands after removing gloves.
- Decontaminate hands after contact with inanimate objects (including medical equipment) in the immediate vicinity of the patient.

program of the agency. According to the CDC, infections can be prevented or controlled in several ways:

- Hand hygiene
- Disinfection/sterilization
- Standard Precautions
- Transmission-Based Precautions
- Staff and patient placement and cohorting

Hand Hygiene

Health care workers' hands are the primary way in which infection is transmitted from patient to patient or staff to patient. Hand hygiene refers to both handwashing and alcohol-based hand rubs (ABHRs) ("hand sanitizers").

In 2002 the U.S. CDC released the classic document entitled "CDC Hand Hygiene Recommendations." These recommendations are summarized in Chart 23-3. *Handwashing is still an important part of hand hygiene, but it is recognized that in some health care settings, sinks may not be readily available.* Despite years of education, health care workers do not wash their hands or perform hand hygiene on a consistent basis.

Effective handwashing includes wetting, soaping, lathering, applying friction under running water for at least 15 seconds, rinsing, and adequate drying. Friction is essential to remove skin oils and disperse transient bacteria and soil from hand surfaces. Performing adequate handwashing takes time that health care workers (HCWs) may not think they have. Handwashing can also cause dry skin; therefore hand moisturizers are essential to maintain good hand health and hygiene.

Alcohol-based hand rubs (ABHRs) allow care providers to spend less time seeking sinks and more time delivering care. However, these hand rubs have their limitations.

The classic CDC guidelines (CDC, 2002) also address the issue of artificial fingernails, which have been linked to a number of outbreaks because of poor fingernail health and hygiene. The guidelines recommend that artificial fingernails and extenders not be worn while caring for patients at high risk for infections, such as those in ICUs or operating suites. Most health care agencies have banned artificial nails for all health care workers providing direct patient care and require that natural nails be short. Some agencies also ban the use of nail polish or gel.

NURSING SAFETY PRIORITY QSEN
Action Alert

If your hands are visibly dirty or soiled or feel sticky or if you have just toileted, *wash your hands instead of using ABHRs.* Keep in mind that ABHRs are also ineffective against spore-forming organisms such as *Clostridium difficile,* a common cause of health care–associated diarrhea, especially in older adults. Do not use an ABHR before inserting eyedrops, ointments, or contact lenses because alcohol can irritate the patient's eyes, causing burning and redness. The Joint Commission's National Patient Safety Goals require that health care agencies monitor handwashing practices and the use of ABHRs to make sure that HCWs are performing hand hygiene on a regular basis.

The CDC recommends using antiseptic solutions such as chlorhexidine for handwashing in caring for patients who are at high risk for infection (e.g., those with impaired IMMUNITY).

Sterilization and Disinfection

Sterilization and disinfection have helped invasive procedures become much more common and safe. Sterilization means destroying all living organisms and bacterial spores. Many invasive procedures, such as inserting vascular access devices (VADs) and urinary catheters, require sterile technique. Sterile technique in the operating suite is discussed in detail in Chapter 15.

All items that invade human tissue where bacteria are not commonly found should be sterilized. Disinfection does not kill spores and only ensures a reduction in the level of disease-causing organisms. High-level disinfection is adequate when an item is going inside the body where the patient has resident bacteria or normal flora (e.g., GI and respiratory tracts). As with sterilization, no high-level disinfection can occur without first cleaning the item. This can be especially difficult with items that have narrow lumens in which organic debris can become trapped and is not easily visible. For example, endoscopes have been especially challenging to clean and have been linked to a number of infectious outbreaks.

Standard Precautions

The classic 2007 guidelines from the CDC focus on transmission mechanisms and the precautions needed to prevent the spread of infection. Included in these guidelines are Standard Precautions and Transmission-Based Precautions, including Airborne, Droplet, and Contact Precautions (Tables 23-2 and 23-3).

Standard Precautions are based on the belief that all body excretions, secretions, and moist membranes and tissues, excluding perspiration, are potentially infectious. As barriers to potential or actual infections, personal protective equipment (PPE) is used. PPE refers to gloves, isolation gowns, face protection (masks, goggles, face shields), and powered air-purifying respirators (PAPRs) or N95 respirators (Fig. 23-1).

NURSING SAFETY PRIORITY QSEN
Action Alert

Remember that gloves are an essential part of infection control and should always be worn as part of Standard Precautions. Either handwashing or use of alcohol-based hand rubs should be done before donning and after removing gloves. The combination of hand hygiene and wearing gloves is the most effective strategy for preventing infection transmission!

TABLE 23-2 Recommendations for Application of Standard Precautions for the Care of All Patients in All Health Care Settings

COMPONENT	RECOMMENDATIONS
Hand hygiene	Perform hand hygiene after touching blood, body fluids, secretions, excretions, contaminated items; immediately after removing gloves; between patient contacts
Personal protective equipment (PPE)	Use appropriate PPE, including:
• Gloves	• For touching blood, body fluids, secretions, excretions, contaminated items; for touching mucous membranes and nonintact skin
• Gown	• During procedures and patient-care activities when contact of clothing/exposed skin with blood/body fluids, secretions, and excretions is anticipated
• Mask, eye protection (goggles), face shield*	• During procedures and patient-care activities likely to generate splashes or sprays of blood, body fluids, secretions, especially suctioning, endotracheal intubation
Soiled patient-care equipment	Handle in a manner that prevents transfer of microorganisms to others and to the environment; wear gloves if visibly contaminated; perform hand hygiene
Environmental control	Develop procedures for routine care, cleaning, and disinfection of environmental surfaces, especially frequently touched surfaces in patient-care areas
Textiles and laundry	Handle in a manner that prevents transfer of microorganisms to others and to the environment
Needles and other sharps	Do not recap, bend, break, or hand manipulate used needles; use safety features such as needleless systems when available; place used sharps in puncture-resistant container
Patient resuscitation	Use mouthpiece, resuscitation bag, other ventilation devices to prevent contact with mouth and oral secretions
Patient placement	Prioritize for single-patient room if patient is at increased risk for transmission, is likely to contaminate the environment, does not maintain appropriate hygiene, or is at increased risk for acquiring infection or developing adverse outcome following infection
Respiratory hygiene/cough etiquette (source containment of infectious respiratory secretions in symptomatic patients, beginning at initial point of encounter [e.g., triage and reception areas in emergency departments and physician offices])	Instruct symptomatic people to cover mouth/nose when sneezing/coughing; use tissues and dispose in no-touch receptacle; observe hand hygiene after soiling of hands with respiratory secretions; wear surgical mask if tolerated or maintain spatial separation, >3 feet if possible

*During aerosol-generating procedures on patients with suspected or proven infections transmitted by respiratory aerosols, wear a powered air-purifying respirator (PAPR) (most effective) or N95 mask in addition to gloves, gown, and face/eye protection.

Health care settings in the United States and Canada have switched from latex to nonlatex gloves. The U.S. National Institute for Occupational Safety and Health (NIOSH) issued a public warning about potential allergic reactions to those exposed to latex in gloves and other medical products. Reactions include rashes, nasal or eye symptoms, asthma, and (rarely) shock. People with latex allergy usually have an allergy to foods such as bananas, kiwis, and avocados. Health care workers (HCWs) have not been as strict with wearing gloves as they should because of poor fit or skin dryness, irritation, and dermatitis. One possible solution to dry skin is the use of aloe vera–coated gloves or moisturizers such as Eucerin or AmLactin products.

The respiratory hygiene/cough etiquette (RH/CE) requirement is directed at patients and visitors with signs of respiratory illness such as sinus or chest congestion, cough, or rhinorrhea ("runny nose"). The elements for RH/CE include:

- Patient, staff, and visitor education
- Posted signs
- Hand hygiene
- Covering the nose and mouth with a tissue and prompt tissue disposal or using surgical masks (or sneezing/coughing into a shirt sleeve rather than the hand)
- Separation from the person with respiratory infection by more than 3 feet (1 m)

Transmission-Based Precautions

Transmission-Based Precautions may also be referred to as *Isolation Precautions.* But the word *isolation* implies that the

patient is physically separated from everyone, which is not always the case.

Airborne Precautions are used for patients known or suspected to have INFECTIONS transmitted by the airborne transmission route. These infections are caused by organisms that can be suspended in air for prolonged periods. Negative-airflow rooms are required to prevent airborne spread of microbes. Enclosed booths with high-efficiency particulate air (HEPA) filtration or ultraviolet light may be used for sputum induction procedures. Tuberculosis, measles (rubeola), and chickenpox (varicella) are examples of airborne diseases.

Droplet Precautions are used for patients known or suspected to have INFECTIONS transmitted by the droplet transmission route. Such infections are caused by organisms in droplets that may travel 3 feet but are not suspended for long periods. Examples of infectious conditions requiring Droplet Precautions include influenza, mumps, pertussis, and meningitis caused by either *Neisseria meningitidis* or *Haemophilus influenzae* type B.

Contact Precautions are used for patients known or suspected to have INFECTIONS transmitted by direct contact or contact with items in the environment. Patients with significant multidrug-resistant organism (MDRO) infection or colonization, such as methicillin-resistant *Staphylococcus aureus* (MRSA) or vancomycin-resistant *Enterococcus* (VRE), are placed on Contact Precautions. Other infections requiring Contact Precautions include pediculosis (lice), scabies, respiratory syncytial virus (RSV), and *C. difficile.*

TABLE 23-3 Transmission-Based Infection Control Precautions

PRECAUTIONS (IN ADDITION TO STANDARD PRECAUTIONS)	EXAMPLES OF DISEASES IN CATEGORY

Airborne Precautions
1. Private room required with monitored negative airflow (with appropriate number of air exchanges and air discharge to outside or through HEPA filter); keep door(s) closed
2. Special respiratory protection:
  • Wear PAPR for known or suspected TB
  • Susceptible people not to enter room of patient with known or suspected measles or varicella unless immune caregivers are not available
  • Susceptible people who must enter room must wear PAPR or N95 HEPA filter*
3. Transport: patient to leave room only for essential clinical reasons, wearing surgical mask
	Diseases that are known or suspected to be transmitted by air:
	• Measles (rubeola)
	• *Mycobacterium tuberculosis,* including multidrug-resistant TB (MDRTB)
	• Varicella (chickenpox)†; disseminated zoster (shingles)†

Droplet Precautions 1. Private room preferred: if not available, may cohort with patient with same active infection with same microorganisms if no other infection present; maintain distance of at least 3 feet from other patients if private room not available 2. Mask: required when working within 3 feet of patient 3. Transport: as for Airborne Precautions	Diseases that are known or suspected to be transmitted by droplets: • Diphtheria (pharyngeal) • Streptococcal pharyngitis • Pneumonia • Influenza • Rubella • Invasive disease (meningitis, pneumonia, sepsis) caused by *Haemophilus influenzae* type B or *Neisseria meningitidis* • Mumps • Pertussis
Contact Precautions 1. Private room preferred: if not available, may cohort with patient with same active infection with same microorganisms if no other infection present 2. Wear gloves when entering room 3. Wash hands with antimicrobial soap before leaving patient's room 4. Wear gown to prevent contact with patient or contaminated items or if patient has uncontrolled body fluids; remove gown before leaving room 5. Transport: patient to leave room only for essential clinical reasons; during transport, use needed precautions to prevent disease transmission 6. Dedicated equipment for this patient only (or disinfect after use before taking from room)	Diseases that are known or suspected to be transmitted by direct contact: • *Clostridium difficile* • Colonization or infection caused by multidrug-resistant organisms (e.g., MRSA, VRE) • Pediculosis • Respiratory syncytial virus • Scabies

HEPA, High-efficiency particulate air; *MRSA,* methicillin-resistant *Staphylococcus aureus; PAPR,* powered air-purifying respirator; *TB,* tuberculosis; *VRE,* vancomycin-resistant *Enterococcus.*
*Before use: training and fit testing required for personnel.
†Add Contact Precautions for draining lesions.

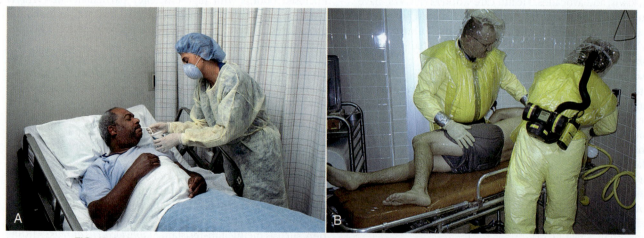

FIG. 23-1 A, Nurse in personal protective equipment (PPE) caring for a patient in a private room. **B,** Powered air-purifying respirator (PAPR). (**A** From deWit, S. C. [2014]. *Fundamental concepts and skills for nursing* [4th ed.]. Philadelphia: Saunders; **B** from Currance, P. [2006]. *Medical response to weapons of mass destruction.* Philadelphia: Mosby/JEMS.)

Staff and Patient Placement and Cohorting

Adequate staffing of nurses is an essential method for preventing infection. In addition to a ratio of one infection control practitioner to 100 occupied acute care beds, nurse staffing is critical. When possible, bedside nurse staffing should consist of full-time nurses assigned regularly to the unit to ensure consistent practices.

Patient placement has been used as a way to reduce the spread of infection. The CDC does not mandate that all patients with infections have a private room. It does recommend that private rooms always be used for patients on Airborne Precautions and those in a protective environment (PE). A PE is architecturally designed and structured to prevent infection from occurring in patients who are at extremely high risk, such as those having stem cell therapy. The CDC also prefers private rooms for patients who are on Contact and Droplet Precautions. If private rooms are not available, keep these patients at least 3 feet apart. Many hospitals are becoming totally private-room facilities. Large health care systems have biomedical engineers to assist in designing the best environment to reduce the spread of infection, including ventilation systems and physical layout.

Cohorting is another method of patient placement. Cohorting is the practice of grouping patients who are colonized or infected with the same pathogen. This method has been used the most with patients who have an outbreak of a multidrug-resistant organism such as methicillin-resistant *Staphylococcus aureus* (MRSA). It is particularly effective in long-term care settings.

Infection control principles for *patient transport* include limiting movement to other areas of the facility, using appropriate barriers such as covering infected wounds, and notifying other departments or agencies who are receiving the patient about the necessary precautions. **Accurate hand-off communication between agencies is also very important to prevent the spread of infection, according to The Joint Commission's National Patient Safety Goals.**

Protection of Visitors of Patients on Transmission-Based Precautions

Many agencies have policies regarding visitors of patients who are on Transmission-Based Precautions. However, visitors are seldom monitored to ensure that they are following these policies. Munoz-Price et al. (2015) made the following recent recommendations for visitors:

- Use proper hand hygiene before and after the patient visit. (Health care organizations should provide conveniently located alcohol-based rub stations.)
- Wear gowns and gloves (Contact Precautions) to prevent the spread of enteric pathogens or drug-resistant organisms.
- Wear a surgical mask if visiting a patient on Droplet or Airborne Precautions.
- Do not visit patients if you have an active cough or fever.

MULTIDRUG-RESISTANT ORGANISM INFECTIONS AND COLONIZATIONS

Antibiotics have been available for many years. Unfortunately these drugs were commonly prescribed for conditions that did not need them or were given at higher doses and for longer periods of time than were necessary. As a result, a number of microorganisms have become resistant to certain

---

❓ NCLEX EXAMINATION CHALLENGE 23-1

Safe and Effective Care Environment

Which statements by a nursing student indicate a need for further teaching by the nurse regarding infection control measures needed to care for a client who has possible tuberculosis? **Select all that apply.**
A. "I'll wear an isolation gown when providing direct care."
B. "I'll wear gloves when emptying the bed pan."
C. "I'll wear a mask each time I enter the client's room."
D. "I'll use a hand sanitizer when I can't wash my hands."
E. "I'll wear goggles to protect my eyes."

antibiotics; that is, drugs that were once useful no longer control these infectious agents (multidrug-resistant organisms [MDROs]). New antibiotics are not keeping up with preventing antimicrobial-resistant infection (ARI); therefore patients are at risk for increased morbidity and mortality because of health care–associated infections (HCAIs) (Plavskin, 2016). For this reason, a culture of safety related to infection control has been mandated by the CDC, the Institute for Healthcare Improvement (IHI), and The Joint Commission. Standard Precautions must be strictly followed today in all health care settings to prevent more of these difficult and deadly infections.

One of the newest discoveries to explain the increase in HCAIs, especially the rise in drug-resistant infections, is the formation of biofilms. A biofilm, also called *glycocalyx*, is a complex group of microorganisms that functions within a "slimy" gel coating on medical devices such as urinary catheters, orthopedic implants, and enteral feeding tubes; on parts of the body such as the teeth (plaque) and tonsils; and in chronic wounds. These reservoirs become sources of infection for which antibiotics and disinfection are not effective. Antibiotic therapy may increase the growth of microbes within biofilms.

Biofilms are extremely difficult to treat, and mechanical disruption strategies are the mainstay of management and research. Studies on biofilms that cause the most common HCAIs, such as catheter-associated urinary tract infections (CAUTIs) and wound infections, continue to be conducted. Many specific biofilms have been identified, and methods to remove or disrupt them are being researched.

🧬 GENETIC/GENOMIC CONSIDERATIONS

Evidence-Based Practice **QSEN**

A new area of research is the study of genetics and genomics of pathogens to help fight drug-resistant organisms and reduce ARIs. For example, genomic bacterial analysis can provide information about sources of infection and how they can be controlled. Population genetic studies can track pathogen transmission and identify infection prevalence and incidence. Transmission mapping can help identify the characteristics of infectious agents, how they are spread, and where carriers of infections are likely to occur within an institution. Research in the genetics and genomics of pathogens is ongoing and can help the interprofessional team promote patient safety by preventing and treating ARIs (Plavskin, 2016).

The most common MDROs are methicillin-resistant *Staphylococcus aureus,* vancomycin-resistant *Enterococcus,* and carbapenem-resistant *Enterococcus.* Other infections such as vancomycin-intermediate *S. aureus* (VISA) and vancomycin-resistant *S. aureus* (VRSA) may also occur, which may be effectively treated with antibiotics such as linezolid (Zyvox) and quinupristin-dalfopristin (Synercid). In 2014 the *Shigella sonnei* bacterium showed signs of becoming more resistant to ciprofloxacin (Cipro) and other antibiotics. As a result, shigellosis has become another public health concern in the United States.

Methicillin-Resistant *Staphylococcus aureus* (MRSA)

Staphylococcus aureus (S. aureus) is a common bacterium found *on* the skin and perineum and in the nose of many people. It is usually not infectious when in these areas because the number of bacteria is controlled by good hygiene measures. However, when skin or mucous membranes are not intact, localized infection such as boils or conjunctivitis may occur. If the organism enters into deep wounds, surgical incisions, the lungs, or bloodstream, more serious or systemic infections occur that require strong antibiotics such as methicillin.

Within the past 40 years, more and more *S. aureus* infections have not responded to methicillin or other penicillin-based drugs. Known as *MRSA,* these infections are one of the fastest growing and most common in health care today. This type of infection is called *health care–associated MRSA,* or *HA-MRSA.* Patients who have HA-MRSA have increased hospital stays at a very high cost. To add to this problem, some patients may be colonized with the organism. Health care staff members may also colonize. Patients who develop HA-MRSA pneumonia, abscesses, or bacteremia (bloodstream infection [BSI]) can quickly progress to sepsis and death.

MRSA is spread by direct contact and invades hospitalized patients through indwelling urinary catheters, vascular access devices, open wounds, and endotracheal tubes. It is susceptible to only a few antibiotics, such as IV vancomycin (Lyphocin, Vancocin) and oral linezolid (Zyvox). A newer IV antibiotic, ceftaroline fosamil (Teflaro), is the first cephalosporin approved to treat MRSA.

Studies show that bathing hospitalized patients with premoistened cloths or warm water containing chlorhexidine gluconate (CHG) solution can significantly reduce MRSA infection by 23% to 32% (Kassakian et al., 2011; Powers et al., 2012). In 2013 the American Association of Critical Care published a recommendation that nurses use CHG to bathe patients in critical care settings as a way to reduce MRSA and other multidrug-resistant organisms.

! NURSING SAFETY PRIORITY QSEN

Action Alert

Patients most at risk for HA-MRSA are older adults and those who have suppressed IMMUNITY, have a long history of antibiotic therapy, or have invasive tubes or lines. ICU patients are especially at risk. Check with your agency policy regarding specific MRSA preventive measures. Examples include bathing patients with chlorhexidine wipes and administering nasal mupirocin ointment.

Although controversial, some health care facilities have a MRSA-surveillance program in which each patient's nose is swabbed and cultured for MRSA. Staff may also be cultured. All patients with HA-MRSA infection or colonization should be placed on Contact Precautions.

Community-associated MRSA, or *CA-MRSA,* causes infections in healthy, nonhospitalized people, especially those living in college housing and prisons. It is easily transmitted among family members and can cause serious skin and soft-tissue infections, including abscesses, boils, and blisters. The best way to decrease the incidence of this growing problem is health teaching, including:

- Performing frequent hand hygiene, including using hand sanitizers
- Avoiding close contact with people who have infectious wounds
- Avoiding large crowds
- Avoiding contaminated surfaces
- Using good overall hygiene

Minocycline (Minocin, Apo-Minocycline) and doxycycline (Doryx, Apo-Doxy) are usually effective in treating CA-MRSA.

? NCLEX EXAMINATION CHALLENGE 23-2

Safe and Effective Care Environment

A client is diagnosed with a foot ulcer infected with methicillin-resistant *Staphylococcus aureus* (MRSA) infection. Which personal protective equipment is appropriate when providing **direct** client care? **Select all that apply.**

A. Mask
B. Gloves
C. Shoe covers
D. Goggles
E. Gown

Vancomycin-Resistant *Enterococcus* (VRE)

Enterococci are bacteria that live in the intestinal tract and are important for digestion. When they move to another area of the body, such as during surgery, they can cause an infection, which is usually treatable with vancomycin. However, in recent years many of these infections have become resistant to the drug, and VRE results. Risk factors for this infection include prolonged hospital stays, severe illness, abdominal surgery, enteral nutrition, and immunosuppression. Place patients with VRE infections on Contact Precautions to prevent contamination from body fluids.

Unfortunately VRE can live on almost any surface for days or weeks and still be able to cause an infection. Contamination of toilet seats, door handles, and other objects is very likely for a lengthy period.

Carbapenem-Resistant *Enterobacteriaceae* (CRE)

Carbapenem antibiotics, most often given for abdominal infections such as peritonitis, have been used extensively for the past 15 years. Examples of this class of antibiotics include imipenem (Cilastin) and meropenem (Merrem IV).

Klebsiella and *Escherichia coli* (*E. coli*) are types of *Enterobacteriaceae* that are located within the intestinal tract. Carbapenem-resistant *Enterobacteriaceae* (CRE) is a family of pathogens that are difficult to treat because they have a high level of resistance to carbapenems caused by enzymes that break down the antibiotics. *Klebsiella pneumoniae* (KPC) and New Delhi metallo-beta-lactamase are examples of these enzymes. Patients who are high risk for CRE include those in ICUs or nursing homes and patients who are immunosuppressed, including older adults.

To prevent the transmission of this infection, place patients who are high risk on Contact Precautions. The CDC (2013) also recommends chlorhexidine (2% dilution) bathing to prevent

CRE or decrease colonization and other types of infections from MDROs.

OCCUPATIONAL AND ENVIRONMENTAL EXPOSURE TO SOURCES OF INFECTION

The U.S. Occupational Safety and Health Administration (OSHA) is a federal agency that protects workers from injury or illness at their place of employment. Unlike the voluntary guidelines developed by the CDC, OSHA regulations are law. Employers can be fined or disciplined for noncompliance with OSHA regulations. The regulation for prevention of exposure to bloodborne pathogens, such as hepatitis B and hepatitis C or the human immune deficiency virus (HIV), is one example of an OSHA regulation.

Reduction of skin and soft-tissue injuries (e.g., needlesticks) is essential to reduce bloodborne pathogen transmission to health care personnel. *OSHA mandates that sharp objects ("sharps") and needles be handled with care.* Many contaminated sharp-object exposures involve nurses. Needleless devices have helped decrease these exposures, especially when caring for patients receiving infusion therapy (see Chapter 13).

Other infection control concerns that nurses and other HCWs have are the possibilities of pandemic influenza or biologic agent exposure. A large outbreak of one of the MDROs is also worrisome, especially if no drug is sensitive enough for successful management. Nurses may fear that they will accidentally bring the infectious agent to their homes and families.

> ### ❗ NURSING SAFETY PRIORITY QSEN
> #### *Action Alert*
>
> To help prevent the transmission of an MDRO, wear scrubs and change clothes before leaving work. Keep work clothes separate from personal clothes. Take a shower when you get home, if possible, to rid your body of any unwanted pathogens. Be careful not to contaminate equipment that is commonly used such as your stethoscope.

Another environmental source for infection is animals or insects. For example, *hantaviruses* are caused by exposure to rodent-infected areas such as old sheds or cabins. Lyme disease can be caused by deer ticks (see Chapter 18).

Saliva and excrement from mice and rats living in the southwestern part of the United States are the primary sources of hantaviruses. While not a common infection, patients can die from complications such as *hantavirus pulmonary syndrome,* a severe and potentially lethal respiratory disease. Teach patients to avoid exposure to potential hantaviruses by avoiding rodent-infested areas. If infested areas need to be cleaned, teach patients to wear rubber or nonlatex gloves and either a tight-seal negative-pressure respirator or a positive-pressure powered air-purifying respirator equipped with N100 or P100 filters (Ly, 2013).

PROBLEMS RESULTING FROM INADEQUATE ANTIMICROBIAL THERAPY

Inadequate antimicrobial therapy may range from an incorrect choice of drug to inadequate drug dosing. Drug regimen noncompliance (deliberate failure to take the drug) or nonadherence (accidental failure to take the drug) also contributes to resistant-organism development.

Some diseases such as tuberculosis (TB) have legal sanctions that require that a patient complete treatment. Patients who are at risk for noncompliance or nonadherence with an anti-TB drug regimen may be placed on *directly observed therapy (DOT).* This means that a health care worker must observe and validate patient compliance with the drug regimen. DOT has been very effective at reducing the spread of multidrug-resistant TB.

Serious complications of infection may also result from incomplete or inadequate antibiotic therapy. Local infections that could be cured without complications such as cellulitis and pneumonia may progress to abscess formation or systemic infection if appropriate drug therapy is not continued. Although drug therapy does not always prevent abscess, early therapy may prevent or limit the size of an abscess.

In addition to abscess formation, inadequate therapy or a missed diagnosis may lead to systemic spread, or sepsis. *Sepsis is the number one cause of hospitalized patient deaths (Lopez-Bushnell et al., 2014; Plavskin, 2016).* If the infection is not resolved or if it is treated with drugs that are ineffective for the offending microorganism, the pathogen may enter the bloodstream (referred to as septicemia or bloodstream infection [BSI]). Inadequately treated local infections may also lead to widespread sepsis with leukocytosis (increased white blood cell count) and inflammation (systemic inflammatory response syndrome [SIRS]). In severe or advanced cases, leukopenia (decreased white blood cell count) and life-threatening disseminated intravascular coagulation (DIC) may occur. After pathogens invade the bloodstream, no site is protected from invasion.

BSI may progress to septic shock, more accurately called *sepsis-induced distributive shock.* In septic shock, insufficient cardiac output is compounded by hypovolemia. Inadequate blood supply to vital organs leads to hypoxia (lack of oxygen) and multiple organ failure. Chapter 37 describes sepsis, septic shock, and management in detail.

❖ INTERPROFESSIONAL COLLABORATIVE CARE

◆ Assessment: Noticing

History. The patient's age, history of tobacco or alcohol use, current illness or disease (e.g., diabetes), past and current drug use (e.g., steroids), and poor nutritional status may place him or her at increased risk for infection. Patients with impaired IMMUNITY as a result of disease or therapies such as chemotherapy and radiation are also at a high risk for infection. Ask the patient about previous vaccinations or immunizations, including the dates of administration.

Ask the patient if he or she has recently been in a hospital or nursing home as a patient or visitor. Inquire about any invasive testing, such as a colonoscopy, or recent surgery. Ask if the patient had an indwelling urinary catheter or IV line. These invasive treatments often are the source of infections.

Determine whether the patient has been exposed to infectious agents. A history of recent exposure to someone with similar clinical symptoms or to contaminated food or water, as well as the time of exposure, helps to identify a possible source of infection. This information helps determine the incubation period for the disease and thus provides a clue to its cause.

Contact with animals, including pets, may increase exposure to infection. Question the patient about recent animal contact at home or work or in leisure activities (e.g., hiking). Insect bites should be documented.

Obtain a travel history. Travel to areas both within and outside the patient's home country may expose a susceptible person to infectious organisms not encountered in the local community.

A thorough sexual history may reveal behavior associated with an increased risk for sexually transmitted diseases. Obtain a history of IV drug use and a transfusion history to assess the patient's risk for hepatitis B, hepatitis C, and HIV infections.

Identifying the type and location of symptoms may point to affected organ systems. The onset order of symptoms gives clues to the specific problem. Gathering a history of past infection or colonization with multidrug-resistant organisms will help determine which type of Transmission-Based Precautions is needed.

Physical Assessment/Signs and Symptoms. Disorders caused by pathogens vary depending on the infection cause and site. Common signs and symptoms are associated with specific sites of infection. Carefully inspect the skin for symptoms of *local* infection at any site *(pain, swelling, heat, redness, pus).* Wounds can easily become infected when TISSUE INTEGRITY is impaired (also see Chapter 2).

CONSIDERATIONS FOR OLDER ADULTS
Patient-Centered Care QSEN

Fever (generally a temperature above 101°F [38.3°C]), chills, and malaise are primary indicators of a systemic infection. Fever may accompany other noninfectious disorders; and infection can be present without fever, especially in patients who have impaired IMMUNITY. The older adult, whose normal temperature may be 1° to 2° lower than the normal temperature in younger adults, may have a fever at 99°F (37.2°C). In most patients with an infection, fever (hyperthermia) is a normal immune response that can help destroy the pathogen. Assess the patient for these signs and symptoms and carefully ask about their history and pattern.

Lymphadenopathy (enlarged lymph nodes), pharyngitis, and GI disturbance (usually diarrhea or vomiting) are often associated with infection. To detect enlargement, palpate the cervical, axillary, and other lymph nodes; examine the throat for redness. Ask about changes in stool and if the patient has had any nausea or vomiting.

Psychosocial Assessment. The patient with an infectious disease often has psychosocial concerns. Delay in diagnosis because of the need to await clinical test results produces anxiety. Assess the patient's and family's level of understanding about various diagnostic procedures and the time required to obtain test results. Plan education on infection risk reduction at a time when they are ready to learn.

Feelings of malaise and fatigue often accompany infection. Assess the patient's current level of activity and the impact of these symptoms on family, occupational, and recreational activities.

The potential spread of infection to others is an additional stress associated with the diagnosis. The patient may curtail family and social interactions for fear of spreading the illness. Determine the patient's and family's understanding of the infection, the mode of transmission, and mechanisms that may limit or prevent transmission. Special precautions,

although sometimes necessary for preventing transmission of the organism, can be emotionally difficult for the patient and family.

A number of transmissible infectious diseases, especially those identified with social stigmas (e.g., IV drug abuse), are associated with labeling. The patient may feel socially isolated or have guilt related to behavior that increased the risk for infection. Observe carefully for the patient's reaction to labels and how these feelings further affect socialization.

Laboratory Assessment. The definitive diagnosis of an infectious disease requires identification of a microorganism in the tissues of an infected patient. Direct examination of blood, body fluids (such as urine), and tissues under a microscope may not yield a definitive identification. However, laboratory assessment usually provides helpful information about organisms, such as amount, shape, motility, and reaction to staining agents. Even when direct microscopy does not provide a conclusive specific diagnosis, often enough information is obtained for starting appropriate antimicrobial therapy.

The best procedure for identifying a microorganism is culture, or isolation of the pathogen by cultivation in tissue cultures or artificial media. Specimens for culture can be obtained from almost any body fluid or tissue. The health care provider usually decides when and where the specimen for culture is taken.

Proper collection and handling of specimens for culture, using Standard Precautions, are essential for obtaining accurate results. Specimens collected must be appropriate for the suspected infection. Be sure that the specimen is of adequate quantity and is freshly obtained and placed in a sterile container to preserve the specimen and microorganism. Label the specimen properly, including the date and time it was collected. Follow your health care organization's policy if you have any questions about how to perform a culture.

After isolation of a microorganism in culture, antimicrobial sensitivity testing is performed to determine the effects of various drugs on that particular microorganism. For example, an agent that is killed by acceptable levels of an antibiotic is considered sensitive to that drug. An organism that is not killed by tolerable levels of an antibiotic is considered resistant to that drug. Preliminary results are usually available in 24 to 48 hours, but the final results generally take 72 hours. *Antimicrobial therapy should not begin until after the culture specimen is obtained.*

Rapid cultures or assays are used in ambulatory care settings to provide quicker assessments of infections. The most popular is the rapid antigen detection test for group A streptococci to rule out "strep throat" in patients who present with pharyngitis (sore, inflamed throat). Other examples of rapid testing are those for tuberculosis (TB) and influenza ("flu"), discussed in Chapter 31.

A *white blood cell (WBC) count with differential* is often done for the patient with a suspected infection. Five types of leukocytes (WBCs) are measured as part of the results:

- Neutrophils
- Lymphocytes
- Monocytes
- Eosinophils
- Basophils

In most active infections, especially those caused by bacteria, the total leukocyte count is elevated. Various infections are characterized by changes in the percentages of the different types of leukocytes. The differential count usually shows an increased number of immature neutrophils, or a **shift to the left** ("left shift"). However, a few infectious diseases such as malaria and infectious mononucleosis are associated with neutropenia (decreased neutrophils). See Chapter 17 for further discussion.

The *erythrocyte sedimentation rate (ESR)* measures the rate at which red blood cells fall through plasma. This rate is most significantly affected by an increased number of acute-phase reactants, which occurs with inflammation. Thus an elevated ESR (>20 mm/hr) indicates inflammation or infection somewhere in the body. Chronic infection, especially osteomyelitis and chronic abscesses, is commonly associated with an elevated ESR. The ESR is chronically elevated with inflammatory arthritis and other connective tissue diseases as well (see Chapter 18). The effectiveness of therapy is often determined by a decrease in this value.

Serologic testing is performed to identify pathogens by detecting antibodies to the organism. The antibody titer tends to *increase* during the acute phase of infectious diseases such as hepatitis B. The titer *decreases* as the patient improves. Other examples of testing for viruses include the enzyme-linked immunosorbent assay (ELISA) and the reverse transcriptase-polymerase chain reaction (RT-PCR).

Imaging Assessment. X-ray films may be obtained to determine activity or destruction by an infectious microorganism. Radiologic studies (e.g., chest films, sinus films, joint films, GI studies) are available for diagnosis of infection in a specific body site.

More sophisticated techniques for infection diagnosis include computed tomography (CT) scans and magnetic resonance imaging (MRI). CT and ultrasonography are helpful in assessing for abscesses. CT scans help identify suspected osteomyelitis and fluid collections that point to possible infection. MRI scans provide a cross-sectional assessment for infection.

Another diagnostic tool for the evaluation of a patient with an infectious disease is ultrasonography. This noninvasive procedure is particularly helpful in detecting infection involving the heart valves.

Scanning techniques using radioactive substances such as gallium can determine the presence of inflammation caused by infection. Inflammatory tissue is identified by its increased uptake of the injected radioactive material.

◆ **Analysis: Interpreting**

The priority collaborative problem for patients with an infection is *fever due to the immune response triggered by the pathogen*. In addition, the patient has a potential for developing severe sepsis, systemic inflammatory response syndrome (SIRS), and septic shock, which are discussed in detail in Chapter 37.

◆ **Planning and Implementation: Responding**

Managing Fever

Planning: Expected Outcomes. Patients with an infection are expected to have a body temperature within normal limits as a result of effective interprofessional collaborative care.

Interventions. The primary concern is to provide measures to eliminate the underlying cause of fever (also known as *hyperthermia*) and to destroy the causative microorganism. In collaboration with the interprofessional health care team, nurses use a variety of methods to manage fever.

Drug therapy plays a major role in interprofessional collaborative care of patients with infection. *Antimicrobials*, also called *anti-infective agents*, are the cornerstone of drug therapy. Antipyretics are used to decrease patient discomfort and reduce fever.

Antibiotics, antiviral agents, and antifungals are common types of antimicrobial drugs that are given for infection, depending on its type. Effective antibiotics are available to treat nearly all bacterial infections, but misuse of antibiotics has contributed to the development of multidrug-resistant organisms (MDROs) discussed earlier in this chapter. A few effective antifungal agents have been developed, but these drugs generally cause more toxicity than antibacterial agents.

Effective antimicrobial therapy requires delivery of an appropriate drug, sufficient dosage, proper administration route, and sufficient therapy duration. These four requirements ensure delivery of a concentration of drug sufficient to inhibit or kill infecting microorganisms. To ensure effectiveness of antibiotic therapy such as vancomycin, health care providers may require serum trough and peak levels to be drawn. A specimen for a *trough level* (lowest serum drug concentration) is drawn about 30 minutes before the next scheduled vancomycin dose. A specimen for a *peak level* (highest serum drug concentration) is drawn 30 to 60 minutes after medication administration (Rosini & Srivastava, 2013).

Primary health care providers collaborate on selecting drugs and dosing. Antimicrobials act on susceptible pathogens by:

- Inhibiting cell wall synthesis (e.g., penicillins and cephalosporins)
- Injuring the cytoplasmic membrane (e.g., antifungal agents)
- Inhibiting biosynthesis, or reproduction (e.g., erythromycin and gentamicin)
- Inhibiting nucleic acid synthesis (e.g., actinomycin)

> **! NURSING SAFETY PRIORITY** (QSEN)
>
> **Drug Alert**
>
> Before administering an antimicrobial drug, check to see that the patient is not allergic to it. Be sure to take an accurate allergy history before drug therapy begins to prevent possible life-threatening reactions, such as anaphylaxis!

Teach the drug's actions, side effects, and toxic effects to patients and their families. Observe and report side effects and adverse events. These reactions vary according to the specific classification of the drug. Most antibiotics can cause nausea, vomiting, diarrhea, and rashes. Stress the importance of completing the entire course of drug therapy, even if symptoms have improved or disappeared.

> **CONSIDERATIONS FOR OLDER ADULTS**
>
> **Patient-Centered Care** (QSEN)
>
> For older adults, be sure to teach the need to drink additional fluids if diarrhea occurs as result of antibiotic therapy. Observe older adults in inpatient facilities carefully for signs and symptoms of dehydration as described in Chapter 11. Acute confusion, hypotension, and tachycardia are common indicators of dehydration and require interventions such as IV fluids. Serum electrolyte levels may increase, causing additional risks to the older adult.

Antipyretic drugs such as acetaminophen (Tylenol, Ace-Tabs) are often given to reduce fever. Because these drugs mask fever, monitoring the course of the disease may be difficult. Therefore, unless the patient is very uncomfortable or if fever presents a significant risk (e.g., in the patient with heart failure, febrile seizures, or head injury), antipyretics are not always prescribed.

Teach patients that they may have waves of sweating after each dose. Sweating may be accompanied by a fall in blood pressure followed by return of fever. These unpleasant side effects of antipyretic therapy can often be alleviated by increasing fluid intake and regular scheduling of drug administration.

Other interventions to reduce fever may include external cooling and fluid administration. Perform a thorough assessment before and after interventions are implemented.

External cooling by hypothermia blankets or ice bags or packs can be effective mechanisms for reducing a high fever. Alternative cooling methods may be used. Sponging the patient's body with tepid water or applying cool compresses to the skin and pulse points to reduce body temperature is sometimes helpful. Ice packs and cooling blankets may be used for patients with extremely high temperatures. *Teach unlicensed assistive personnel (UAP) to observe for and report shivering during any form of external cooling. Shivering may indicate that the patient is being cooled too quickly.*

The use of fans is discouraged because they can disperse airborne- or droplet-transmitted pathogens. Fans can also disturb air balance in negative-pressure rooms, making them positive-pressure rooms and allowing possible transmission of the agent to those outside the room.

In patients with fever, fluid volume loss is increased from rapid evaporation of body fluids and increased perspiration. As body temperature increases, fluid volume loss increases.

Care Coordination and Transition Management

Patients with infections may be cared for in the home (group or individual), hospital, nursing home, or ambulatory care setting, depending on the type and severity of the infection. Infections among older adults in nursing homes and assisted-living facilities are common. Residents often have meals together in a communal dining room and participate in group activities. Confused residents may not wash their hands or may enter other resident rooms. Immunizing them against respiratory infections is highly recommended because these illnesses can cause severe complications or death in older adults.

Home Care Management. The patient with an infectious disease such as osteomyelitis may require continued, long-term antibiotic therapy at home or in a long-term care facility. Emphasize the importance of a clean home environment, especially for the patient who continues to have compromised IMMUNITY or who is uniquely susceptible to superinfection (i.e., reinfection or a second infection of the same kind) to reduce the chance of infection. Drugs often need to be refrigerated. Ensure that the patient has access to proper storage facilities, and teach him or her to check for signs of improper storage, such as discoloration of the drug.

Ask about the availability of handwashing facilities in the home and check that supplies and instructions are provided as needed. Most people do not know how to wash hands correctly. Demonstrate the procedure with the patient and family and request a repeat demonstration.

Self-Management Education. Explaining the disease and making certain that the patient understands what is causing the illness are the primary purposes of health teaching. Discuss whether the pathogen causing the infection can be spread to others and the modes of transmission.

If the patient has an infection that is potentially transmissible, teach the patient, family, and other home caregivers about precautions. Explain whether any special household cleaning is necessary and, if so, what those special steps include. If syringes with needles are used to administer drug therapy, explain how to dispose safely and legally of needles in the community. Clothing soiled with blood or other body fluids can be washed with bleach or disinfectant (e.g., Lysol). Recommended cleaning measures should be based on actual available equipment and facilities.

For the patient who is discharged to the home setting to complete a course of antimicrobial therapy, the importance of adherence to the planned drug regimen needs to be stressed. Explain the importance of both the timing of doses and the completion of the planned number of days of therapy. Teach the patient (and family as appropriate) how the agents need to be taken (e.g., before meals, with meals, without other agents) and the possible side effects. Side effects include those that are expected (e.g., gastric distress) and adverse reactions that are more severe (e.g., rash, fever, other systemic signs and symptoms). Teach the patient about allergic manifestations and the need to notify a primary health care provider if an adverse reaction occurs. Also discuss what to do if a drug dose is missed (e.g., doubling the dosage, waiting until the next dose time).

Many patients are discharged with an infusion device to continue drug therapy at home or in other inpatient facilities. The patient, family member, or home care nurse administers the drugs. Home care services are often used to teach appropriate administration of drug therapy in the patient's home. Health teaching and wound care may also be needed. These services have proven to be efficient, effective, psychologically supportive, and less expensive than hospitalization or skilled nursing facilities (SNFs).

The patient is often anxious and fearful that the infection will be transmitted to family members or friends. Teaching the patient and the family ways of preventing the spread of disease allays these fears. Pay careful attention to the patient's and family's concerns. Making concrete suggestions (e.g., "Your partner can wear gloves when changing your dressing") to address specific concerns may reduce these fears.

The patient with an infection associated with lifestyle behaviors such as sexual activity or IV drug abuse may have guilt related to the disease. Encourage discussion of feelings associated with the illness, and assist in locating support systems that may help alleviate these feelings, such as clergy or other spiritual or cultural leaders.

Health Care Resources. At times a patient who has been hospitalized for an infection may not be able to return to the home setting because of lack of caregiver support. In such cases temporary placement in an SNF may be needed. Document care requirements, patient history of infection or colonization with multidrug-resistant organisms, medication schedules, and personal needs and preferences on transfer forms. **Hand-off communication such as the SBAR between the two facilities is required to facilitate a smooth transition from the hospital to the intermediate care setting, according to The Joint Commission's National Patient Safety Goals.**

◆ *Evaluation: Reflecting*

Evaluating the care of the patient with an infection on the basis of the identified priority problems is important. The expected outcomes include that the patient:

- Has body temperature and other vital signs within baseline
- Adheres to drug therapy regimen

CRITICAL ISSUES: EMERGING INFECTIONS AND GLOBAL BIOTERRORISM

Additional current concerns related to infection and infection control are the risk for emerging infectious diseases and global bioterrorism. As for any pathogen, strict infection control measures can prevent transmission of these microbes to you and your patients. Some of the most serious infections are briefly described here.

The 2014 Ebola epidemic was labeled as the largest in history, with many West African countries affected (CDC, 2016). An epidemic occurs when new cases of a certain disease substantially exceed expectation during a given period. The ongoing struggle with the Ebola virus outbreak in West Africa became a concern within the United States when an individual who flew back from Liberia was diagnosed, although after initial discharge, at a Dallas hospital. That individual later died. Symptoms of Ebola, which can present from 2 to 21 days after exposure (with an average of 8 to 10 days), include fever greater than 101.5°F (38.6°C), severe headache, muscle pain, weakness, diarrhea, vomiting, abdominal pain, and unexplained hemorrhage (bleeding or bruising) (CDC, 2016). The virus is most commonly spread through exposure to bodily fluids of the infected individual and through needlesticks in which the needle has been contaminated with the virus. Recovery from this virus is contingent on appropriate clinical care and the immune response of the patient. Patients who recover from Ebola infection develop antibodies that can last for 10 years (CDC, 2016) (Table 23-4).

With the Dallas Ebola incident, there was reported to be a communication concern within the electronic medical record (EMR) in which the physician was unable to view the nurse's notes and see that the nurse had recorded the patient's recent return from West Africa. It is of vital importance that the nurse and primary health care provider be sure to communicate pertinent historical information both verbally and in the EMR so appropriate interventions for both the individual and the general public can be undertaken immediately.

Pandemic infections such as influenza are another threat to the population. As recently as the early 1900s, the "Spanish flu" killed millions of people throughout the world. Health care workers are encouraged to have annual influenza vaccines to prevent infection with common strains of the virus. The federal government and health care agencies around the United States include the risk for pandemic disease in their disaster planning (see Chapter 10).

Contaminated food is another source of infection. The incidence of foodborne infections has risen in the United States as contaminated fresh spinach, ground beef, and other foods were

---

TABLE 23-4 Care for Patients With Ebola Virus Disease

TRANSMISSION OF DISEASE	PREVENTION OF DISEASE	ASSESSMENT	PATIENT-CENTERED COLLABORATIVE CARE
The primary source of the Ebola virus is most likely contaminated bats or primates (apes and monkeys) in West Africa. Information that is known about transmission includes: • The Ebola virus cannot be transmitted unless a person is sick and has signs and symptoms of the disease. • The Ebola virus is not spread via air, water, or food. • Nurses can help identify people at high risk for having or transmitting the disease by taking a complete history, including asking about travel to West Africa or exposure to family and friends who have Ebola. • The disease can be transmitted by unprotected contact with people infected with the Ebola virus or with people who have died from Ebola. • Teach patients who recover from Ebola and their partners that the virus is present in semen for up to 3 months. Using a condom may prevent transmission.	Take special training *before* caring for patients with the Ebola virus. Use these precautions: • Avoid direct contact with body fluids (blood, feces, saliva, urine, vomit, and semen). • Use Standard, Contact, and Droplet Precautions, including appropriate PPE. • Isolate patient with Ebola in a single room. • Use dedicated or disposable medical equipment and supplies. • Practice proper sterilization measures.	Signs and symptoms occur 2-21 days after exposure to the Ebola virus. Assess for: • Fever • Severe headache • Muscle pain • Weakness • Fatigue • Diarrhea • Vomiting • Abdominal pain • Unexplained hemorrhage (bleeding and bruising)	No drug therapy or vaccine is yet FDA approved for Ebola. Remember that the virus can enter the body through broken skin or unprotected mucous membranes such as the eyes, nose, and mouth. Supportive care includes: • IV fluid and electrolyte replacement • Oxygen and ventilation support • Blood pressure support • Treatment of other infections • Care and comfort measures • Symptomatic care • Emotional support • Possible end-of-life care

Data from Centers for Disease Control and Prevention. (2014). *Ebola (Ebola virus disease).* www.cdc.gov/vhf/ebola/index/html.
FDA, Food and Drug Administration; *PPE*, personal protective equipment.

found to contain *E. coli* 0157:H7 and other pathogens. Major restaurant chains such as Chipotle have been the source of GI infections for many of their customers. Multiple illnesses and deaths in the United States have been caused by these infections. Safer food preparation practices and increased monitoring by federal agencies have resulted from demand for public safety, but more oversight is needed to prevent large outbreaks.

Another pathogen, *Clostridium difficile,* is associated with antibiotic therapy use, especially in older adults. Associated problems have led to the development of the diagnosis of *C. difficile–associated disease (CDAD)*. A new, more virulent strain of this pathogen has developed in the past decade as a result of the use of fluoroquinolone antibiotics such as cipro-floxacin (Cipro).

C. difficile is spread by indirect contact with inanimate objects such as medical equipment and commodes, and its toxins cause colon dysfunction and cell death from sepsis. CDAD is confirmed by stool culture. Patients who have three or more liquid stools per day for two or more days are suspected of having the infection. Fever and abdominal pain and cramping commonly occur with diarrheal stools. Oral metronidazole (Flagyl) and vancomycin have been the drugs of choice to treat CDAD. However, some patients experience recurrence of infection after treatment with these drugs. A new oral antibacterial drug available for specifically managing *C. difficile* is fidaxomicin (Dificid).

A recently approved treatment for CDAD is **fecal microbiota transplantation (FMT)** to place healthy normal flora into the lower GI system of the infected patient who does not respond to antibiotic therapy or has recurrent disease. Potential donors of fecal material should not have impaired IMMUNITY, history of drug abuse, chronic GI disorders, or recent exposure to potential pathogens such as those that could be present from tattooing or travel to endemic areas. Before the FMT, the donor is screened using a variety of blood and stool tests to rule out active or chronic infections such as hepatitis A, B, or C.

Fecal transplantation is most commonly performed by colonoscopy. Therefore the pre-procedure and follow-up care are the same as for any patient having a colonoscopy (see Chapter 52). FMT has been very successful for many patients with *C. difficile*. It is being investigated for use in patients who have other lower GI diseases such as inflammatory bowel disease and irritable bowel syndrome (Kelly et al., 2015).

In addition to concerns about emerging infections, preparation for and education about *bioterrorism* have been major focuses of the U.S. government since September 11, 2001 (Table 23-5). In some cases vaccines are no longer given for biologic agents such as smallpox. Many people in the United States have never been vaccinated, and those who had vaccinations many years ago are not guaranteed to have lifelong immunity. Anthrax, usually seen in animals, may be spread to the skin or inhaled. These infections have a high fatality rate in humans. Plague, once seen centuries ago, is one of the biggest threats because the survival rate is low. Vaccines are being researched and stockpiled by the U.S. government for some of the common biologic agents.

GET READY FOR THE NCLEX® EXAMINATION!

KEY POINTS

Review these Key Points for each NCLEX Examination Client Needs Category.

Safe and Effective Care Environment

- Handwashing and alcohol-based hand rubs are two methods of hand hygiene to prevent infection (see Chart 23-3). **QSEN: Safety; Quality Improvement**
- The Centers for Disease Control and Prevention (CDC) recommends a ban on artificial fingernails for health care professionals when they are caring for patients at high risk for infection. **QSEN: Evidence-Based Practice**
- Use clinical judgment to prevent or control infection through hand hygiene, disinfection/sterilization, personal protective equipment (PPE), patient placement, and adequate staffing. Proper hand hygiene and gloves are the most important interventions because health care workers' hands are the primary way in which disease is transmitted from patient to patient. **Clinical Judgment; QSEN: Evidence-Based Practice**
- Standard Precautions are used with all patients in health care settings, assuming that all body excretions and secretions are potentially infectious (see Table 23-2). **QSEN: Safety**
- Airborne Precautions are used for patients who have infections transmitted through the air such as tuberculosis.
- Droplet Precautions are used for patients who have infections transmitted by droplets such as influenza and certain types of meningitis.
- Contact Precautions are used for patients who have infections transmitted by direct contact or contact with items in the patient's environment.

Health Promotion and Maintenance

- Health teaching about signs and symptoms of infection and drug therapy is important for the patient with an infection being managed at home; some patients may need health care nursing services for IV antimicrobial therapy.
- Teach patients about antimicrobial therapy and protective measures to prevent infection transmission. **QSEN: Safety**
- Teach patients how to avoid community-acquired MRSA by performing frequent hand hygiene and by avoiding crowds and direct contact with others who have infections. **QSEN: Safety**
- Teach patients about how to prevent vector transmission of infection (e.g., using insect repellent to prevent tick and mosquito bites).

Psychosocial Integrity

- Help patients cope with feelings about having an infection through verbalization and collaboration with the health care team. **QSEN: Teamwork and Collaboration**

Physiological Integrity

- Patients at the highest risk for infection include older adults, health care professionals at risk for needlesticks, and patients who have chronic disease (e.g., diabetes) or impaired IMMUNITY. Patients who take long-term steroid therapy or have had invasive procedures or impaired TISSUE INTEGRITY are also at a high risk for infection.
- Multidrug-resistant organisms (MDROs) are the result of the overuse of antibiotic therapy and include methicillin-resistant

TABLE 23-5 Centers for Disease Control and Prevention* Examples of Bioterrorism Agents and General Clinical Management

PATHOGEN OR AGENT AND DISEASE INFORMATION	CLINICAL MANAGEMENT
Anthrax (Bacillus anthracis) **Cutaneous:** 1-7 days after contact; exposed skin itching, progressing to papular and vesicular lesions, eschar, edema, ulceration, and sloughing. If untreated, may spread to lymph nodes and bloodstream. Fatality 5%-20%. **Inhalation:** 48 hr after organism or spore inhalation; flu-like illness with possible brief improvement. 2-4 days from initial symptoms, abrupt onset of severe cardiopulmonary illness (dyspnea, tachycardia, fever, diaphoresis, thoracic edema, shock, and respiratory failure). If antibiotics delayed until onset of cardiopulmonary symptoms, mortality high. May be confused with common upper respiratory infection (URI). **Other forms:** GI, meningeal, and sepsis.	For cutaneous and inhaled anthrax: No person-to-person spread. Contact Precautions not needed unless patient presents directly from exposure. Standard Precautions for: • Prescribed wound cleansing and management of lesions • Ventilator support for respiratory failure • Postmortem care
Botulism (Clostridium botulinum and Neurotoxin) Toxin ingestion results in dysphasia, dry mouth, drooping eyelids, and blurred or double vision. Vomiting and constipation or diarrhea may be present initially, extending to symmetric flaccid paralysis in an alert person. Acute bilateral cranial nerve impairment and descending weakness or paralysis follow. Neurologic symptoms after 12-36 hr for foodborne botulism and 24-72 hr after aerosol exposure. Case fatality up to 10%. Recovery may take months.	Standard Precautions: decontamination of patient is not required. No person-to-person spread. Consider outbreak with suspicion of a single case. Consult with CDC and health departments. Advise careful cleanup and disposal of suspected contaminated food source *after* consultation with health department about any needed laboratory sampling. Interdisciplinary planning for nutrition and rehabilitation support during lengthy neuromuscular and respiratory recovery.
Plague (Yersinia pestis) **Lymphatic infection:** 2-8 days after bites from fleas of an infected rodent (rarely after infected tissue or body fluid contact), onset of fever and chills, painful lymphadenopathy (or bubo—usually inguinal, axillary, or cervical lymph nodes), headache, GI symptoms, and rapidly progressive weakness. 50%-60% fatality if untreated. **Pneumonic:** 1-3 days after aerosolized organism inhalation, fever and chills, productive cough, hemoptysis, rapidly progressive weakness, GI symptoms, and bronchopneumonia. Survival unlikely if not treated within 18 hr of symptom onset. **Other forms:** Sepsis with coagulopathy, rarely meningitis.	Droplet Precautions: required for pneumonic plague (until 72 hr of antibiotic therapy). Contact Precautions until decontamination is complete: • For any suspected gross contamination. See documentation information listed under Anthrax. • For prescribed management of bubo(s) if incised to drain. Community and other environmental modifications: • Apply insecticide to infested environment and pets (to kill fleas). • Reduce food and water supply for rodents. • Avoid sick or dead animals.
Smallpox (Variola Virus) (Variola Major and Minor) 10-17 days after droplet or airborne virus inhalation or contact with bleeding lesions, onset of severe myalgias, headache, and high fever. 2-3 days later, a papular rash appears on face and spreads to extremities (and palms and soles). The rash quickly (simultaneously) becomes vesicular and then painful and pustular (contrasted to varicella rash that crops and concentrates more on trunk with various stages of macules to vesicles seen at one time). Patients are infectious at onset of rash until scabs separate (3 weeks). Historically variola major kills 20%. May be confused with varicella.	Standard, Contact, and Airborne Precautions for patients with vesicular rash pending diagnosis. Same for varicella and variola. Also avoid contact with organism while handling contaminated clothes and bedding. Wear protective attire (gloves, gown, and N95 respirator). One case is a public health emergency—highly communicable. Consult CDC and health departments at earliest suspicion. Vaccine does not give reliable lifelong immunity. Previously vaccinated people are considered susceptible. *Following exposure:* Initiate Airborne Precautions and observe for unprotected contacts (from days 10-17). Vaccinate within 2-3 days of exposure.

Other Key Points

Assessment: Include account of symptoms, patient's incident (what, where, when, how, others exposed or ill, and officials aware).

Treatment: Antibiotic-resistance possible. Vaccine and postexposure prophylaxis are subject to change. If any of the above diseases are suspected, consult infection control practitioner for coordination with community health officials and CDC about current recommendations and specimen collection. *If bioterrorism suspected,* Federal Bureau of Investigation (FBI) will coordinate evidence collection and delivery.

Multiple exposures planning: Emergency and critical care managers must address availability and acquisition of stocks of medications, vaccines, equipment (e.g., ventilators), and communications with officials, as well as public information needs.

CDC, Centers for Disease Control and Prevention.
*Data from the CDC.

Staphylococcus aureus (MRSA), vancomycin-resistant *Enterococcus* (VRE), and carbapenem-resistant *Enterobacteriaceae* (CRE).

- A biofilm, also called *glycocalyx,* is a complex group of microorganisms that function within a "slimy" gel coating on medical devices such as urinary catheters, orthopedic implants, and enteral feeding tubes; on parts of the body such as the teeth (plaque) and tonsils; and in chronic wounds.
- Common signs and symptoms of infection include fever and lymphadenopathy. If infections are not treated or are inadequately treated by the interprofessional health care team, systemic sepsis (septicemia), septic shock, and disseminated intravascular coagulation (DIC) may result.
- A culture is the most definitive way to confirm and identify microorganisms; sensitivity testing determines which antibiotics will destroy the identified microbes. **QSEN: Evidence-Based Practice**
- The white blood cell differential count usually shows a shift to the left (increased number of immature neutrophils) during active infections.

- Antimicrobials and antipyretics are the most common types of drugs used when infection is accompanied by fever.
- Antipyretics are used only when the fever presents a significant risk or the patient is very uncomfortable because antipyretics may mask the disease. **QSEN: Evidence-Based Practice**
- Critical issues for the next decade include bioterrorism, emerging infectious diseases (such as Ebola), and multidrug-resistant organisms (MDROs).
- Foodborne infections are becoming increasingly common as a result of contaminated food consumed by restaurant customers.
- Fecal microbiota transplantation (FMT) is a recent therapy for managing chronic *Clostridium difficile*–associated disease (CDAD). Fecal transplantation restores normal flora to the infected patient. **QSEN: Evidence-Based Practice**

SELECTED BIBLIOGRAPHY

Asterisk indicates a classic or definitive work on this subject.

Alspach, J. G. (2014). About that health care icon dangling around your neck: Do we have some cleaning up to do? *Critical Care Nurse, 34*(4), 11–14.

Anderson, N., Johnson, D., & Wendt, L. (2015). Use of a novel teaching method to increase knowledge and adherence to isolation procedures. *Medsurg Nursing, 24*(3), 159–164.

Casey, D. (2015). A nurse's obligations to patients with Ebola. *Nursing, 45*(11), 47–49.

*Centers for Disease Control and Prevention (CDC). (2002). Guideline for hand hygiene in health-care settings: Recommendations of the Healthcare Infection Control Practices Advisory Committee and the HICPAC/SHEA/APIC/IDSA Hand Hygiene Task Force. *MMWR. Morbidity and Mortality Weekly Report, 51*(RR–16), 1–44.

Centers for Disease Control and Prevention (CDC). (2013). *2012 CRE toolkit: Guidance for control of carbapenem-resistant Enterobacteriaceae, Part 1: Facility-level CRE prevention.* www.cdc.gov/hai/organisms/cre/cre-toolkit/f-level-prevention-supmeasures.html.

Centers for Disease Control and Prevention (CDC). (2016). *Ebola (Ebola virus disease).* www.cdc.gov/vhf/ebola.

*Grossman, S., & Mager, D. (2010). *Clostridium difficile:* Implications for nursing. *Medsurg Nursing, 19*(3), 155–158.

*Kassakian, S. Z., Mermel, L. A., Jefferson, J. A., Parenteau, S. L., & Machan, J. T. (2011). Impact of chlorhexidine bathing on hospital-acquired infections among general medical patients. *Infection Control and Hospital Epidemiology, 32*(3), 238–243.

Kelly, C. R., Kahn, S., Kashyap, P., Laine, L., Rubin, D., Atreja, A., et al. (2015). Update on fecal microbiota transplantation 2015: Indications, methodologies, mechanisms, and outlook. *Gastroenterology, 149*(1), 223–237.

Lopez-Bushnell, K., Demaroy, W. S., & Jaco, C. (2014). Reducing sepsis mortality. *Medsurg Nursing, 23*(1), 9–14.

Ly, E. (2013). A closer look at hantavirus. *Nursing, 43*(9), 65–66.

Mori, C. (2014). A-voiding catastrophe: Implementing a nurse-driven protocol. *Medsurg Nursing, 23*(1), 15–21, 28.

Munoz-Price, L. S., Banach, D. B., Bearman, G., Gould, J. M., Leekha, S., Morgan, D. J., et al. (2015). Isolation Precautions for Visitors. *Infection Control and Hospital Epidemiology,* Available on CJO 2015 doi:10.1017/ice.2015.67.

Plavskin, A. (2016). Genetics and genomics of pathogens: Fighting infections with genome-sequencing technology. *Medsurg Nursing, 25*(2), 91–96.

*Powers, J., Peed, J., Burns, L., & Ziemba-Davis, M. (2012). Chlorhexidine bathing and microbial contamination in patients' bath basins. *American Journal of Critical Care, 21*(5), 338–342.

Powers, J., & Fortney, S. (2014). Bed baths: Much more than a basic nursing task. *Nursing, 44*(10), 67–68.

Rosini, J. M., & Srivastava, N. (2013). Understanding vancomycin levels. *Nursing, 43*(11), 66–67.

Shaffer, C., & Aymong, L. (2014). Administering vaccines. *Nursing, 44*(10), 46–50.

Simon, R. B., & Carpenetti, T. L. (2016). Zika virus: Facing a new threat. *Nursing, 46*(8), 24–33.

*Siegel, J. D., Rhinehart, E., Jackson, M., Chiarello, L., & Healthcare Infection Control Practices Advisory Committee. (2007). *Guidelines for isolation precautions: Preventing transmission of infectious agents in healthcare settings 2007.* Atlanta: CDC.

*Upshaw-Owens, M., & Bailey, C. A. (2012). Preventing hospital-associated infection: MRSA. *Medsurg Nursing, 21*(2), 77–80.

CHAPTER 24

Assessment of the Skin, Hair, and Nails

Janice Cuzzell

 http://evolve.elsevier.com/Iggy/

PRIORITY AND INTERRELATED CONCEPTS

The priority concept for this chapter is TISSUE INTEGRITY.

LEARNING OUTCOMES

Safe and Effective Care Environment
1. Protect patients from skin injury and loss of TISSUE INTEGRITY.

Health Promotion and Maintenance
2. Teach adults how to protect the skin from damage and cancer development.

Psychosocial Integrity
3. Implement nursing interventions to minimize stressors for the patient undergoing assessment and testing of the integumentary system.

Physiological Integrity
4. Apply knowledge of anatomy and physiology, genetic risk, and principles of aging to perform a focused assessment of the skin, hair, and nails.

The integumentary system is made of the skin, hair, and nails. Intact skin, the largest organ of the body, has barrier, alarm, and combat functions. Skin TISSUE INTEGRITY plays a major role in protection by protecting the body against invasion of pathogenic organisms by providing first, second, and third lines of defense. The normal flora on the surfaces of skin and mucous membranes repels some of the more harmful microorganisms. Specialized cells in the skin engulf foreign substances (antigens) that invade the body when TISSUE INTEGRITY is lost and then alert the immune system to the presence of the invader. Localized tissue inflammation and swelling work to contain the invading pathogen until white blood cells can respond and remove this threat.

Intact skin helps regulate body temperature and maintains fluid and electrolyte balance. Emotional stress, systemic disease, some drugs, and skin injury or disease can alter skin function, appearance, and texture. The skin's sensory function allows the use of touch as an intervention to provide comfort, relieve pain, and communicate caring.

ANATOMY AND PHYSIOLOGY REVIEW

Structure of the Skin

There are three skin layers: subcutaneous tissue (fat), dermis, and epidermis (Fig. 24-1). Each layer has unique properties that help the skin maintain its complex functions.

Subcutaneous fat (adipose tissue [fat]) is the innermost layer of the skin, lying over muscle and bone. Fat distribution varies with body area, age, and gender. Fat cells insulate the body and absorb shock, padding internal structures. Blood vessels go through the fatty layer and extend into the dermis, forming capillary networks that supply nutrients and remove wastes.

The dermis (corium) is the layer above the fat layer and contains no skin cells but does contain some protective mast cells and macrophages (see Chapter 17). The dermis is composed of interwoven collagen and elastic fibers that give the skin flexibility and strength.

Collagen, the main component of dermal tissue, is a protein produced by fibroblast cells. Its production increases in areas of

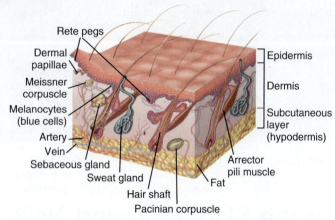

FIG. 24-1 Anatomy of the skin. (From Kumar., V et al: *Robbins & Cotran pathologic basis of disease* [8th ed.], St. Louis, 2009, Saunders.)

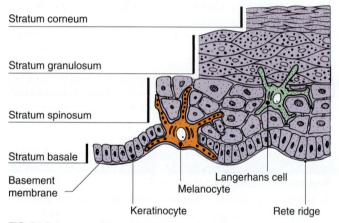

FIG. 24-2 Anatomy of the epidermis. (From Gawkrodger D., & Ardern-Jones, MR [2012]: *Dermatology*. (5th ed.). Philadelphia: Churchill Livingstone.)

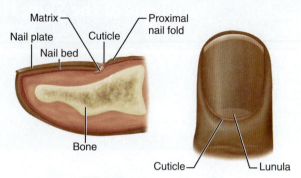

FIG. 24-3 Anatomy of the nail.

the outermost horny skin layer (**stratum corneum**). When these cells reach the stratum corneum (in 28 to 45 days), they are no longer living cells and are shed from the skin surface. **Keratin**, a protein produced by keratinocytes, makes the horny layer waterproof.

On the palms of the hands and soles of the feet an additional thick, clear layer of epidermis forms, known as the *stratum lucidum.* This layer of nonliving cells pads and protects the underlying dermal and epidermal structures in these vulnerable areas.

Vitamin D is activated in the epidermis by ultraviolet (UV) light, such as sunlight. Once activated, it is distributed by the blood to the GI tract to promote uptake of dietary calcium.

Melanocytes are pigment-producing cells found at the basement membrane. These cells give color to the skin and account for the ethnic differences in skin tone. Darker skin tones are not caused by increased numbers of melanocytes; rather, the size of the pigment granules *(melanin)* contained in each cell determines the color. Melanin protects the skin from damage by UV light, which stimulates melanin production. For this reason, people with dark skin (and thus more melanin) are less likely to develop sunburn than lighter-skinned people. Freckles, birthmarks, and age spots are lesions caused by patches of increased melanin production. Melanin production also increases in areas that have endocrine changes or inflammation.

Structure of the Skin Appendages

Hair differs in type and function in various body areas. Hair growth varies with race, gender, age, and genetic predisposition. Individual hairs can differ in both structure and rate of growth, depending on body location.

Hair follicles are located in the dermal layer of the skin but are actually extensions of the epidermal layer (see Fig. 24-1). Within each hair follicle, a round column of keratin forms the hair shaft. Hair color is genetically determined by an individual's rate of melanin production.

Hair growth occurs in cycles of a growth phase followed by a resting phase. Growth is dependent on a good blood supply and adequate nutrition. Stressors can alter the growth cycle and result in temporary hair loss. Permanent baldness, such as male pattern baldness, is inherited.

Nails protect and enhance sensation of the fingertips and toe tips, have cosmetic value, and are useful for grasping and scraping. Like hair follicles, the nails are extensions of the keratin-producing epidermal layers of the skin.

The white, crescent-shaped part of the nail at the lower end of the nail plate is the **lunula** and is where nail keratin is formed and nail growth begins (Fig. 24-3). Nail growth is a continuous

tissue injury and helps form scar tissue. Fibroblasts also produce **ground substance**, a gel-like substance the fills the spaces between cells and contributes to skin suppleness and turgor. Skin elasticity depends on the amount and quality of the dermal elastic fibers, which are primarily composed of elastin.

The dermis has capillaries and lymph vessels for the exchange of oxygen and heat. It is rich in sensory nerves that transmit the sensations of touch, pressure, temperature, pain, and itch.

The epidermis is the outermost skin layer. It is anchored to the dermis by fingerlike projections (**rete pegs**) that interlock with dermal structures called **dermal papillae**. Less than 1 mm thick, the epidermal layer is the first line of defense between the body and the environment.

The epidermis (Fig. 24-2) does not have its own blood supply. Instead it receives nutrients by diffusion from the blood vessels in the dermal layer. Attached to the basement membrane of the epidermis are the basal **keratinocytes**—skin cells that undergo cell division and differentiation to continuously renew skin TISSUE INTEGRITY and maintain optimal barrier function. As basal cells divide, keratinocytes are pushed upward and form the *spinous layer (stratum spinosum).* Together the basal layer and the spinous layer are referred to as the *germinative layer (stratum germinativum)* because these layers are responsible for new skin growth (McCance et al., 2014). The keratinocytes continue to enlarge and flatten as they move upward to form but slow process. Fingernail replacement requires 3 to 4 months. Toenail replacement may take up to 12 months.

The cuticle attaches the nail plate to the soft tissue of the nail fold. The nail body is translucent, and the pinkish hue reflects a rich blood supply beneath the nail surface. Nail growth and appearance are often altered during systemic disease or serious illness.

Sebaceous glands are distributed over the entire skin surface except for the palms of the hands and soles of the feet. Most of these glands are connected directly to the hair follicles (see Fig. 24-1).

Sebaceous glands produce sebum, a mildly bacteriostatic, fat-containing substance. Sebum lubricates the skin and reduces water loss from the skin surface.

Sweat glands of the skin are of two types: eccrine and apocrine. Eccrine sweat glands arise from the epithelial cells. They are found over the entire skin surface and are not associated with the hair follicle. The odorless, colorless secretions of these glands are important in body temperature regulation. This sweat and the resultant water evaporation can cause the body to lose up to 10 to 12 L of fluid in a single day.

Apocrine sweat glands are in direct contact with the hair follicle and are found mostly in the axillae, nipple, umbilical, and perineal body areas. The interaction of skin bacteria with the secretions of these glands causes body odor.

Functions of the Skin

The skin is a complex organ responsible for the regulation of many body functions throughout the life span (Table 24-1) (McCance et al., 2014). In addition to the skin's protective and regulatory functions, its location on the outside of the body makes it an important way to communicate a patient's state of health and body image.

Skin Changes Associated With Aging

The process of aging begins at birth. As changes in physiology progress with aging, the skin also undergoes age-related changes in structure and function (Chart 24-1). Figures 24-4 through 24-7 show age-related skin changes.

Individual differences exist in how quickly and to what degree the skin ages (Touhy & Jett, 2015). Although genetic factors, hormonal changes, and disease may change skin appearance over time, chronic sun exposure is the single most important factor leading to degeneration of the skin components.

ASSESSMENT: NOTICING AND INTERPRETING

Patient History

Take an accurate history from the patient so skin problems can be readily identified. Chart 24-2 highlights specific questions to ask during a skin assessment.

Demographic data include age, race, occupation, and hobbies or recreational activities. This information can help identify causative or aggravating factors for skin problems. Age is important because many changes in the skin, hair, and nails are normal for the aging process.

Ethnicity can also be important. Some variations in skin appearance are normal for patients of some ethnicities but are abnormal for those of other races or ethnicities.

Information about occupation and hobbies can provide clues to chronic skin exposure to chemicals, irritants, and other substances that can contribute to skin problems.

TABLE 24-1　Functions of the Skin

EPIDERMIS	DERMIS	SUBCUTANEOUS TISSUE
Protection		
Keratin provides protection from injury by corrosive materials	Provides cells for wound healing	Mechanical shock absorber
Inhibits proliferation of microorganisms because of dry external surface	Provides mechanical strength:	Energy reserve
Mechanical strength through intercellular bonds	Collagen fibers	Insulation
	Elastic fibers	
	Ground substance	
	Sensory nerve receptors signal skin injury and inflammation	
Homeostasis (Water Balance)		
Low permeability to water and electrolytes prevents systemic dehydration and electrolyte loss	Lymphatic and vascular tissues respond to inflammation, injury, and infection	No real function in water balance
Temperature Regulation		
Eccrine sweat glands allow dissipation of heat through evaporation of sweat secreted onto the skin surface	Cutaneous vasculature promotes or inhibits heat loss from the skin surface	Fat cells insulate and assist in retention of body heat
Sensory Organ		
Transmits a variety of sensations through the neuroreceptor system	Has many nerve receptors for relaying sensations to the brain	Contains large pressure receptors
Vitamin Synthesis		
Allows photo conversion of 7-dehydrocholesterol to active vitamin D	No function	No function
Psychosocial		
Body image alterations occur with many epidermal diseases	Body image alterations occur with many dermal diseases	Body image alterations may result from changes in body fat stores

CHART 24-1   Nursing Focus on the Older Adult

Changes in the Integumentary System Related to Aging

PHYSICAL CHANGES	CLINICAL FINDINGS	NURSING ACTIONS
Epidermis		
Decreased epidermal thickness	Skin transparency and fragility	Handle patients carefully to reduce skin friction and shear. Assess for excessive dryness or moisture. Avoid taping the skin.
Decreased cell division	Delayed wound healing	Avoid skin trauma and protect open areas.
Decreased epidermal mitotic homeostasis	Skin hyperplasia and skin cancers (especially in sun-exposed areas)	Assess non–sun-exposed areas for baseline skin features. Assess exposed skin areas for sun-induced changes.
Increased epidermal permeability	Increased risk for irritation	Teach patients how to avoid exposure to skin irritants.
Decreased immune system cells	Decreased skin inflammatory response	Do not rely on degree of redness and swelling to correlate with the severity of skin injury or localized infection.
Decreased melanocyte activity	Increased risk for sunburn	Teach patients to wear hats, sunscreen, and protective clothing. Teach patients to avoid sun exposure from 10 AM to 4 PM.
Hyperplasia of melanocyte activity (especially in sun-exposed areas)	Changes in pigmentation (e.g., liver spots, age spots)	Teach patients to keep track of pigmented lesions. Teach them which changes should be evaluated for malignancy.
Decreased vitamin D production	Increased risk for osteomalacia	Urge patients to take a multiple vitamin or a calcium supplement with vitamin D.
Flattening of the dermal-epidermal junction	Increased risk for shearing forces, resulting in blisters, purpura, skin tears, and pressure-related problems	Avoid pulling or dragging patients. Help patients confined to bed or chairs change positions at least every 2 hours. Avoid or use care when removing adhesive wound dressings.
Dermis		
Decreased dermal blood flow	Increased susceptibility to dry skin	Teach patients to apply moisturizers when the skin is still moist and to avoid agents that promote skin dryness.
Decreased vasomotor responsiveness	Increased risk for heat stroke and hypothermia	Teach patients to dress for the environmental temperatures.
Decreased dermal thickness	Paper-thin, transparent skin with an increased susceptibility to trauma	Handle patients gently and avoid the use of tape or tight dressings. Use lift sheets when positioning patients.
Degeneration of elastic fibers	Decreased tone and elasticity	Check skin turgor on the forehead or chest.
Benign proliferation of capillaries	Cherry hemangiomas	Teach patients that these are benign.
Reduced number and function of nerve endings	Reduced sensory perception	Tell patients to use bath thermometer and lower the water heater temperature to prevent scalds.
Subcutaneous Layer		
Thinning subcutaneous layer	Increased risk for hypothermia	Teach patients to dress warmly in cold weather.
	Increased risk for pressure injury	Help patients confined to bed or chairs change positions at least every 2 hours.
Hair		
Decreased number of hair follicles and rate of growth	Increased hair thinning	Suggest wearing hats to prevent heat loss in cold weather and to prevent sunburn.
Decreased number of active melanocytes in follicle	Gradual loss of hair color (graying)	Inform patients that hair color loss can occur at any age.
Nails		
Decreased rate of growth	Increased risk for fungal infections	Inspect the nails of all older adults. Teach patients to keep feet clean and dry.
Decreased nail bed blood flow	Longitudinal nail ridges	Use the oral mucosa to assess for cyanosis.
Thickening of the nail	Toenails thicken and may overhang the toes	Use fingernails to assess capillary refill. Cut toenails straight across. Do not use nail appearance alone to assess for a fungal infection. Assess skin next to the nail to determine whether the thick nail is irritating it.
Glands		
Decreased sebum production	Increased size of nasal pores; large comedones	Teach patients not to squeeze the pores or comedones to prevent skin trauma.
Decreased eccrine and apocrine gland activity	Increased susceptibility to dry skin	Urge patients to use soaps with a high fat content. Teach patients to avoid frequent bathing with hot water. Teach patients to apply moisturizers after bathing while skin is moist.
	Decreased perspiration with decreased cooling effect	Do not use sweat production as an indicator of hyperthermia.

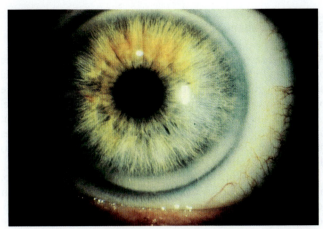

FIG. 24-4 Arcus senilis of the iris.

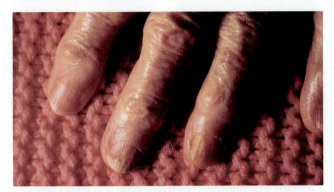

FIG. 24-5 Nail changes, longitudinal ridges and thickening.

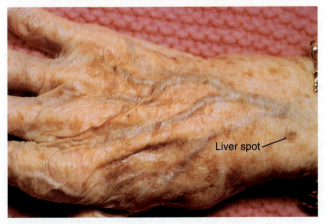

Liver spot

FIG. 24-6 Paper thin, transparent skin with actinic lentigo (liver spots).

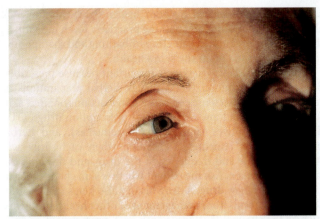

FIG. 24-7 Eyelid eversion, deepening of the eye orbit, and "bags" under the eye.

◎ **CHART 24-2 Best Practice for Patient Safety & Quality Care** QSEN

Questions to Obtain an Accurate Nursing History of the Patient With a Skin Problem

Medical-Surgical History
- Do you have any current or previous medical problems?
- Have you undergone any recent or previous surgical procedures?

Family History
- Is there any family tendency toward chronic skin problems?
- Do any members of your immediate family have skin problems?

Medication History
- Are you allergic to any drugs? If so, describe the reaction.
- What prescription drugs have you taken recently? When was the drug started? What is the dose or frequency of administration? When was the last dose taken?
- What over-the-counter drugs have you taken recently? When was the drug started? What is the dose or frequency of administration? When was the last dose taken?

Social History
- What is your occupation?
- What recreational activities do you enjoy?
- Have you traveled recently? If so, where?
- What is your nutrition status?
- Do you use tobacco or recreational drugs or drink alcohol?

Current Health Problem
- When did you first notice the skin problem?
- Where on the body did the problem begin?
- Has the problem gotten better or worse?
- Has a similar skin condition ever occurred before? If so, what was the course, and how was it treated?
- Is the problem associated with any itching, burning, stinging, numbness, pain, fever, nausea and vomiting, diarrhea, sore throat, cold, stiff neck, new foods, new soaps or cosmetics, new clothing or bed linens, or stressful situations?
- What seems to make the problem worse?
- What seems to make the problem better?

Socioeconomic status data can help identify environmental factors that might contribute to skin disease. Unhealthy or crowded living conditions promote the spread of contagious skin pathogens. Recent or frequent travel to tropical climates may be a source of unusual skin infections or infestations.

Regardless of skin color or ethnicity, always ask patients about the amount of time spent in the sun and tanning booths and identify skin problems caused by sun overexposure. Use this time to teach the patient about the harmful aspects of sun exposure and how to reduce risk by avoiding time in the sun and wearing sunscreen. Because one in five Americans is expected to develop skin cancer in their lifetime, simple actions such as these can make an impact in preventing this diagnosis (Roebuck et al., 2015). Also determine whether he or she regularly assesses the skin for lesion development or changes.

Skin problems caused by poor hygiene are common. Ask about living conditions and bathing practices. Teach individuals that keeping the skin and hair clean by bathing and shampooing regularly helps maintain the skin's health.

Information about drug use is important because prescribed drugs, over-the-counter (OTC) drugs, herbal preparations or remedies, and tobacco use can cause skin reactions or affect skin function. Ask about any recent use of prescription drugs, OTC drugs (e.g., laxatives, antacids, cold remedies), and herbal preparations or remedies. Determine when each drug was started, the dose and frequency of the drug, and the time the last dose was taken. Ask the patient whether skin changes began after starting a new drug. A drug history also helps identify skin changes that result from management of other health problems, such as the changes that occur with long-term steroid or anticoagulant therapy.

Allergies to environmental substances, whether a new onset or history thereof, often have skin implications. Ask about the use of any new personal care product (e.g., shaving products, perfumes, soap, shampoo, lotion, makeup, hair gel), laundry detergents and softeners, and home cleaning products. Ask whether the patient wears gloves to avoid direct contact with cleaning solutions. New clothing may contain chemicals that irritate the skin. Noting the body location(s) of the skin problem can help determine its cause.

Nutrition Status

Document the patient's weight, height, body build and fat distribution, and food preferences. Protein deficiencies, vitamin deficiencies, and obesity can increase the risk for skin lesions and delay wound healing. Fat-free diets and chronic alcoholism can lead to vitamin deficiencies and related skin changes. Skin problems such as chronic urticaria and acne may be worsened by certain foods or food additives.

Hydration influences overall skin health, and the skin reflects hydration status. Reduced fluid intake can lead to dry skin. Symptoms of severe fluid losses are seen as loose skin that tents when pinched together. Fluid overload with edema can stretch the skin, masking wrinkles and allowing the formation of skin "pits" (i.e., pitting edema) when pressure is applied to it.

Family History and Genetic Risk

Many skin problems (e.g., psoriasis, keloid formation, eczema) have a familial predisposition. Explore any family tendency of chronic skin problems. Ask about immediate family members' current health to identify a transmittable disorder (e.g., ringworm, scabies).

Current Health Problems

Begin by gathering information about skin changes and skin care practices (see Chart 24-2).

If a skin problem is identified, obtain more information about the specific problem, such as when the patient first noticed the rash or skin change, where the rash began, and whether the problem has improved or become worse.

If the problem has occurred before, ask the patient to describe the course of the skin lesion and how it was treated. Try to link the problem with symptoms, such as itching, burning, numbness, pain, fever, sore throat, stiff neck, or nausea and vomiting. Ask the patient to identify anything that seems to make the problem better or worse.

Skin Assessment

Inspection

A thorough assessment of the skin is best performed with the patient undressed. (Always provide privacy to maintain the patient's dignity.) Incorporate skin examination as a routine part of daily care during the bath or when assisting with hygiene.

Inspect the patient's skin surfaces in a well-lighted room; natural or bright fluorescent lighting makes subtle skin changes more visible. Use a penlight to closely inspect lesions and to illuminate the mouth.

Assess each skin surface systematically, including the scalp, hair, nails, and mucous membranes. Give particular attention to the skinfold areas. The moist, warm environment of skinfolds can harbor organisms such as yeast or bacteria. Observe and document obvious changes in color and vascularity, moisture presence or absence, edema, skin lesions, and skin integrity. Check the cleanliness of the various body areas to determine whether the patient's self-care activities need to be evaluated.

Skin color is affected by blood flow, gas exchange, body temperature, and pigmentation. The wide variation in skin tones requires different techniques for patients who have darker skin. (See the Cultural/Spiritual Considerations box for tips for assessing patients with darker skin.)

Describe and document changes in skin color by their appearance (Table 24-2). Include in your description whether the changes are general or confined to one body region. Color changes are more visible in the areas of least pigmentation, such as the oral mucosa, sclera, nail beds, and palms and soles. Inspect these areas to help confirm more subtle color changes of general body areas.

Lesions in skin disease are clinically described in terms of primary and secondary lesions (Fig. 24-8). **Primary lesions** develop as a direct result of a disease process. **Secondary lesions** evolve from primary lesions or develop as a consequence of the patient's activities. These changes occur with progression of an underlying disease or in response to a topical or systemic therapeutic intervention. For example, acute dermatitis often occurs as primary vesicles with associated **pruritus** (itching). Secondary lesions in the form of crusts occur as the patient scratches, the vesicles are opened, and the exudate dries. With chronic dermatitis, the skin often becomes **lichenified** (thickened) because of the patient's continual rubbing of the area to relieve itching.

Describe lesions by color, size, location, and shape. Note whether they are isolated or are grouped and form a distinct pattern. Table 24-3 defines terms used to describe lesions. Research continues on tools such as the WoundVision Scout, an imaging device designed to photograph and measure area of a wound (Langemo et al., 2015), and on other methods of digitized tracing and digital wound photography (Gabison et al., 2015). Methods such as these may increase accuracy of measurement as a wound is assessed over time.

Assess each lesion for these ABCDE features that are associated with skin cancer (The Skin Cancer Foundation, 2016):
- **A**symmetry of shape
- **B**order irregularity
- **C**olor variation within one lesion
- **D**iameter greater than 6 mm
- **E**volving or changing in any feature (shape, size, color, elevation, itching, bleeding, or crusting)

TABLE 24-2 Common Alterations in Skin Color

ALTERATION	UNDERLYING CAUSE	LOCATION	SIGNIFICANCE
White (pallor)	Decreased hemoglobin level	Conjunctivae	Anemia
	Decreased blood flow to the skin (vasoconstriction)	Mucous membranes Nail beds Palms and soles Lips	Shock or blood loss Chronic vascular compromise Sudden emotional upset Edema
	Genetically determined defect of the melanocyte (decreased pigmentation)	Generalized	Albinism
	Acquired patchy loss of pigmentation	Localized	Vitiligo, tinea versicolor
Yellow-orange	Increased total serum bilirubin level (jaundice)	Generalized Mucous membranes Sclera	Hemolysis of red blood cells Liver disorders
	Increased serum carotene level (carotenemia)	Perioral Palms and soles Ears and nose Absent in sclera and mucous membranes	Increased ingestion of carotene-containing foods (carrots) Pregnancy Thyroid deficiency Diabetes
	Increased urochrome level	Generalized Absent in sclera and mucous membranes	Chronic kidney disease (uremia)
Red (erythema)	Increased blood flow to the skin (vasodilation)	Generalized	Generalized inflammation (e.g., erythroderma)
		Localized (to area of involvement)	Localized inflammation (e.g., sunburn, cellulitis, trauma, rashes)
		Face, cheeks, nose, upper chest Area of exposure	Fever, increased alcohol intake Exposure to cold
Blue	Increase in deoxygenated blood (cyanosis)	Nail beds Mucous membranes Generalized	Cardiopulmonary disease Methemoglobinemia
	Bleeding from vessels into tissue:		
	Petechiae (1-3 mm)	Localized	Thrombocytopenia
	Ecchymosis (>3 mm)	Localized	Increased blood vessel fragility
Reddish blue	Increased overall amount of hemoglobin	Generalized	Polycythemia vera
	Decreased peripheral circulation	Distal extremities, nose	Inadequate tissue perfusion
Brown	Increased melanin production	Localized (to area of involvement) Pressure points, areolae, palmar creases, and genitalia	Chronic inflammation Exposure to sunlight Addison's disease
		Face, areolae, vulva, linea nigra	Pregnancy; oral contraceptives (melasma)
	Café au lait spots (tan-brown patches):		
	<6 spots	Localized	Nonpathogenic
	>6 spots	Generalized	Possible neurofibromatosis
	Melanin and hemosiderin deposits (bronze or grayish tan color)	Distal lower extremities	Chronic venous stasis
		Exposed areas or generalized	Hemochromatosis

Because of the continued rise of incidence of melanoma (Masterson, 2015), routinely teach patients signs of skin cancer and encourage them to perform skin self-examination on a monthly basis (American Cancer Society, 2015). High-risk patients may benefit from taking The Brief Skin Cancer Assessment Tool (BRAT) to self-assess their relative risk for developing melanoma (Gordon, 2014). *A patient who has a lesion with one or more of the ABCDE features should be evaluated by a dermatologist or surgeon.*

In describing location, determine whether lesions are generalized or localized. If the lesions are localized, identify the specific body areas involved. This information is important because some diseases have a specific pattern of skin lesions. For example, involvement of only the sun-exposed areas of the body is important when considering possible causes. Rashes limited to the skinfold areas (e.g., on the axillae, beneath the breasts, in the groin) may reflect problems related to friction, heat, and excessive moisture.

Edema causes the skin to appear shiny, taut (tightly stretched), and paler than uninvolved surrounding skin. During skin inspection, document the location, distribution, and color of areas of edema.

Primary lesions

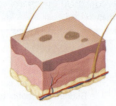

Macules
(such as *freckles, flat moles* or *rubella*) are flat lesions of less than 1 cm in diameter. Their color is different from that of the surrounding skin—most often white, red or brown.

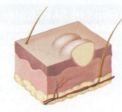

Nodules
(such as *lipomas*) are elevated marble-like lesions more than 1 cm wide and deep.

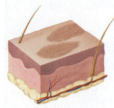

Patches
(such as *vitiligo* or *café au lait spots*) are macules that are larger than 1 cm in diameter. They may or may not have some surface changes—either slight scale or fine wrinkles.

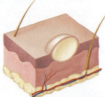

Cysts
(such as *sebaceous cysts*) are nodules filled with either liquid or semisolid material that can be expressed.

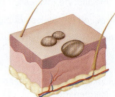

Papules
(such as *warts* or *elevated moles*) are small, firm, elevated lesions less than 1 cm in diameter.

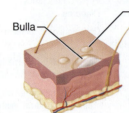

Bulla — Vesicle

Vesicles
(such as in *acute dermatitis*) and **Bullae** (such as *second-degree burns*) are blisters filled with clear fluid. Vesicles are less than 1 cm in diameter, and bullae are more than 1 cm in diameter.

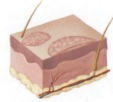

Plaques
(such as in *psoriasis* or *seborrheic keratosis*) are elevated, plateau-like patches more than 1 cm in diameter that do not extend into the lower skin layers.

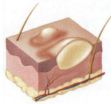

Pustules
(such as in *acne* and *acute impetigo*) are vesicles filled with cloudy or purulent fluid.

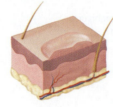

Wheals
(such as *urticaria* and *insect bites*) are elevated, irregularly shaped, transient areas of dermal edema.

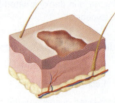

Erosions
(such as in *varicella*) are wider than fissures but involve only the epidermis. They are often associated with vesicles, bullae, or pustules.

Secondary lesions

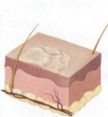

Scales
(such as in *exfoliative dermatitis* and *psoriasis*) are visibly thickened stratum corneum. They appear dry and are usually whitish. They are seen most often with papules and plaques.

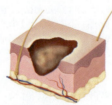

Ulcers
(such as *stage 3 pressure sores*) are deep erosions that extend beneath the epidermis and involve the dermis and sometimes the subcutaneous fat.

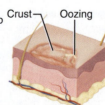

Crust — Oozing

Crusts and oozing
(such as in *eczema* and *late-stage impetigo*) are composed of dried serum or pus on the surface of the skin, beneath which liquid debris may accumulate. Crusts frequently result from broken vesicles, bullae, or pustules.

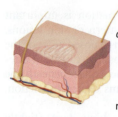

Lichenifications
(such as in *chronic dermatitis*) are palpably thickened areas of epidermis with accentuated skin markings. They are caused by chronic rubbing and scratching.

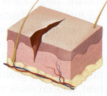

Fissures
(such as in *athlete's foot*) are linear cracks in the epidermis that often extend into the dermis.

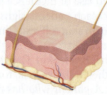

Atrophy
(such as *striae* [stretch marks] and *aged skin*) is characterized by thinning of the skin surface with loss of skin markings. The skin is translucent and paper-like. Atrophy involving the dermal layer results in skin depression.

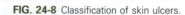

FIG. 24-8 Classification of skin ulcers.

TABLE 24-3 Terms Commonly Used to Describe Skin Lesion Configurations

annular Ringlike with raised borders around flat, clear centers of normal skin
circinate Circular
circumscribed Well-defined with sharp borders
clustered Several lesions grouped together
coalesced Lesions that merge with one another and appear confluent
diffuse Widespread, involving most of the body with intervening areas of normal skin; generalized
linear Occurring in a straight line
serpiginous With wavy borders, resembling a snake
universal All areas of the body involved, with no areas of normal-appearing skin

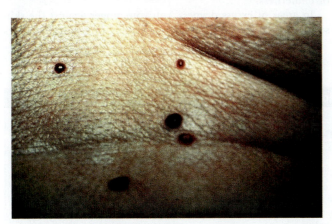

FIG. 24-9 Senile (cherry) angiomas.

Skin elasticity is affected by edema. Using moderate pressure, place the tip of a finger against edematous tissue to determine the degree of indentation, or pitting (see Chapter 11).

Moisture content is assessed by noting the thickness and consistency of secretions. Normally increased moisture in the form of sweat occurs with increased activity or elevated environmental temperatures. Dampness of skinfold areas occurs with reduced air circulation where the skin surfaces touch. Excess moisture can cause impaired TISSUE INTEGRITY with skin breakdown in bedridden and debilitated patients.

Overly dry skin is caused by a dry environment, poor skin lubrication, inadequate fluid intake, and the normal aging process. Dry skin usually has scaling and flaking and may be especially marked in areas of limited circulation such as the feet and lower legs. It is a common problem during the winter months when the air contains less moisture, for those living in geographic areas with little humidity, and in the hospital environment where humidity is often low.

Vascular changes or markings may be normal or abnormal, depending on the cause. Normal vascular markings include birthmarks, cherry angiomas (Fig. 24-9), spider angiomas, and venous stars. Bleeding into the skin is abnormal and results in purpura (bleeding under the skin that may progress from red to purple to brownish-yellow), petechiae, and ecchymosis.

Petechiae are small, reddish-purple lesions (<0.5 mm in diameter) that do not fade or blanch when pressure is applied (Fig. 24-10). They often indicate increased capillary fragility. Petechiae of the lower extremities often occur with stasis dermatitis, a condition usually seen with chronic venous insufficiency. Petechiae found below the nipple line may be indicative of a serious underlying medication problem such as disseminated intravascular coagulation (DIC).

Ecchymoses (bruises) are larger areas of hemorrhage. In older adults, bruising is common after minor trauma to the skin. Certain drugs (e.g., aspirin, warfarin, corticosteroids) and low platelet counts lead to easy or excessive bruising. Anticoagulants and decreased numbers of platelets disrupt clotting action, resulting in ecchymosis.

Skin TISSUE INTEGRITY is assessed by first examining areas with actual breaks or open areas. For example, skin tears are a common finding in older adults as a result of aging. The thin, fragile skin is easily damaged by friction or shearing forces, especially if bruising is already present. Look for skin tears where clothing rubs against the skin, on upper extremities where skin is grasped to assist in ambulation, and where adhesive tapes or dressings have been applied and removed. Check for the presence of multiple abrasions or early pressure-related skin changes. These changes may indicate unrecognized problems in mobility or sensory perception.

Document breaks in skin TISSUE INTEGRITY by describing their location, size, color, and distribution and by the presence and characteristics of drainage or infection. The evaluation of partial- and full-thickness wounds, including objective criteria that describe progress toward healing, is discussed in Chapter 25. A model such as the Skin Safety Model (SSM) or the Pathway to Assessment/Treatment of Skin Tears can help you thoroughly evaluate potential for skin injury and associated outcomes, especially for older adults (Campbell et al., 2016; LeBlanc et al., 2014).

Cleanliness of the skin is evaluated to learn about self-care needs. Inspect the hair, nails, and skin closely for excessive soiling and offensive odor. Depending on a patient's degree of self-care deficit, hard-to-reach areas (e.g., perirectal and inguinal skinfolds, axillae, feet) may be less clean than other skin surface areas.

Patients who have cognitive problems may not observe hygiene measures. Assess the cognition of any patient whose hygiene of the skin, hair, or nails appears inadequate.

Tattoos and piercings can cause or mask skin problems and must be examined carefully. Bruises and rashes may be difficult to see in tattooed areas. Examine newly pierced areas for inflammation or infection. Scars may be present in old tattoos or pierced areas and should be documented. Closely examine any areas where tattoos have been removed. Skin cancer is more likely to occur in these areas.

❓ NCLEX EXAMINATION CHALLENGE 24-1
Physiological Integrity

While performing skin assessment on an elderly client, the nurse observes an isolated brownish-purple lesion with irregular borders on the anterior chest wall. The lesion feels slightly raised on palpation, and crusted blood is visible at the lower edge. Which is the appropriate nursing intervention?

A. Wash the lesion gently with warm water to remove the crusts and teach not to pick it.
B. Document lesion's location, size, and characteristics and request a dermatology consult.
C. Reassure that the lesion is a common occurrence with aging, especially in sun-exposed areas.
D. Ask the patient about exposure to new lotions or perfumes that could cause an allergic reaction.

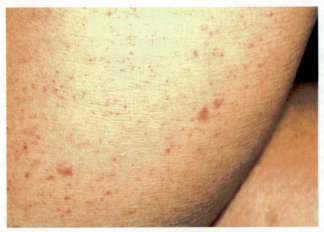

FIG. 24-10 Petechiae. (Modified from Marks, J., & Miller, J. [2013]. *Lookingbill and Marks' Principles of dermatology* (5th ed.). Philadelphia: Saunders.)

Palpation

Skin inspection can be misleading in areas of color changes, tattoos, and piercings. Use palpation to gather additional information about skin lesions, moisture, temperature, texture, and turgor (Table 24-4). Wash hands thoroughly before and after palpating a patient's skin. Use gloves to examine nonintact skin, and use Standard Precautions when skin areas are draining.

Palpation confirms lesion size and whether the lesions are flat or slightly raised. Consistency of larger lesions can vary from soft and pliable to firm and solid. Subtle changes, such as the difference between a fine macular (flat) rash and a papular (raised) rash, are best determined by palpating with your eyes closed. Ask the patient if skin palpation causes pain or tenderness.

In areas of excess dryness, rub your finger against the skin surface to determine the degree of flaking or scaling. Changes

TABLE 24-4 Common Clinical Findings in Skin Palpation

CLINICAL FINDINGS	CAUSE	LOCATION	EXAMPLES OF PREDISPOSING CONDITIONS
Edema			
Localized	Inflammatory response	Area of involvement	Trauma
Dependent or pitting	Fluid and electrolyte imbalance	Ambulatory: dorsum of foot and medial ankle	Congestive heart failure Kidney disease
	Venous and cardiac insufficiency	Bedridden: buttocks, sacrum, and lower back	Liver cirrhosis Venous thrombosis or stasis
Nonpitting	Endocrine imbalance	Generalized, but more easily seen over the tibia	Hypothyroidism (myxedema)
Moisture			
Increased	Autonomic nervous system stimulation	Face, axillae, skinfolds, palms, and soles	Fever, anxiety, activity Hyperthyroidism
Decreased	Dehydration Endocrine imbalance	Buccal mucous membranes with progressive involvement of other skin surfaces	Fluid loss Postmenopausal status Hypothyroidism Normal aging
Temperature			
Increased	Increased blood flow to the skin	Generalized	Fever, hypermetabolic states Neurotrauma
		Localized	Inflammation
Decreased	Decreased blood flow to the skin	Generalized	Impending shock, sepsis, anxiety Hypothyroidism
		Localized	Interference with vascular flow
Turgor			
Decreased	Decreased elasticity of the dermis (tenting when pinched)	Abdomen, forehead, or radial aspect of the wrist	Severe dehydration Sudden, severe weight loss Normal aging
Texture			
Roughness or thickness	Irritation, friction	Pressure points (e.g., soles, palms, elbows)	Calluses Chronic eczema
		Localized areas of pruritus	Atopic skin diseases
	Sun damage	Areas of sun exposure	Normal aging
	Excessive collagen production	Localized or generalized	Scleroderma Scars and keloids
Softness or smoothness	Endocrine disturbances	Generalized	Hyperthyroidism

in skin temperature are detected by placing the back of your hand on the skin surface. First, make certain to have warm hands. Cold hands interfere with accurate assessment and are uncomfortable for the patient.

Palpate skin surfaces to assess texture, which differs according to body area and exposure to irritants. For example, areas of long-term sun exposure have a rougher texture than protected skin surfaces. The patient who has repeated exposure to harsh soaps or chemicals may show skin changes related to this exposure. Increased skin thickness from scarring, lichenification, or edema usually decreases elasticity.

Turgor indicates the amount of skin elasticity. Skin turgor can be altered by water content and aging. Gently pinch the patient's skin between your thumb and forefinger and then release. If skin turgor is normal, the skin immediately returns to its original state when released. Poor skin turgor is seen as "tenting" of the skin, with a gradual return to the original state (see Chapter 11). Loss of elasticity with aging makes the assessment of skin turgor difficult in an older-adult patient. Although usually checked on the back of the hand, you may also check for turgor on the abdomen, forehead, or radial aspect of the wrist.

> ### ! NURSING SAFETY PRIORITY QSEN
> **Action Alert**
>
> To avoid mistaking dehydration for dry skin in an older adult, always assess skin turgor on the forehead or chest.

Hair Assessment

During the skin assessment, inspect and palpate the hair for general appearance, cleanliness, distribution, quantity, and quality. Hair is normally found in an even distribution over most of the body surfaces. The hair on the scalp, in the pubic region, and in the axillary folds is thicker and coarser than hair on the trunk, arms, and legs. Although color and growth patterns vary, sudden changes in hair characteristics may reflect an underlying disease. Check any abnormal findings by obtaining a detailed history of the change.

How well the hair is groomed, including the cleanliness of areas of thicker hair growth, can provide information about a patient's health care needs. If the patient has intense itching or scratches continually, examine the scalp and pubis for lice and **nits** (lice eggs). Inspect the scalp for scaling, redness, open areas, crusting, and tenderness.

Dandruff, a collection of patchy or diffuse white or gray scales on the surface of the scalp, is common. The flaking that occurs with dandruff causes many adults to mistakenly think the scalp is too dry; however, it is a problem of excessive oil production. Dandruff is a cosmetic problem, but a very oily scalp can induce inflammatory changes with redness and itching. Severe inflammatory dandruff can extend to the eyebrows and the skin of the face and neck. *If severe dandruff is not treated, alopecia (hair loss) can occur.* Teach the patient that dandruff is not caused by dryness and should be treated to prevent hair loss.

Although gradual hair loss occurs with aging, sudden asymmetric or patchy hair loss at any age is of concern. Assess the scalp for hair distribution and thickness, and document variations. Body hair loss, especially on the feet or lower legs, may occur with decreased blood flow to the area and also is a part of aging.

Hirsutism is excessive growth of body hair or hair growth in abnormal body areas. Increased hair growth across the face and chest in women is a sign of hirsutism. It may occur on the face of a woman as part of aging, is one sign of hormonal imbalance, and can also occur as a side effect of drug therapy. If hirsutism is present, look for changes in fat distribution and capillary fragility, which can occur in Cushing's disease, and for clitoral enlargement and deepening of the voice, which may indicate ovarian dysfunction.

Nail Assessment

Dystrophic (abnormal-appearing) nails may occur with a serious systemic illness or local skin disease involving the epidermal keratinocytes. Assess the fingernails and toenails for color, shape, thickness, texture, and the presence of lesions.

Many variations in color, texture, and grooming of the nails are influenced by factors unrelated to disease, such as occupation. When assessing the older adult, observe for minor variations associated with the aging process, such as a gradual thickening of the nail plate, the presence of longitudinal ridges, or a yellowish-gray discoloration.

Color of the nail plate depends on nail thickness and transparency, amount of red blood cells, arterial blood flow, and pigment deposits (Table 24-5). Fig. 24-11 shows normal variations in nail pigmentation. Changes in color can be caused by chemical damage that occurs with some occupations and with the long-term use of nail polish. Regardless of skin color, the healthy nail blanches (lightens) with pressure.

During examination, the patient's fingers and toes should be free of any surface pressure that interferes with local blood flow or alters the appearance of the digits. To differentiate between color changes from the underlying blood supply and those from pigment deposits, blanch the nail bed to see whether the color changes with pressure. Gently squeeze the end of the finger or toe, exerting downward pressure on the nail bed, and then release the pressure. Color caused by blood flow changes as pressure is applied and returns to the original state when pressure is released. Color caused by pigment deposits remains unchanged.

Nail shape changes may be related to systemic disease. For example, fingernail clubbing occurs with impaired gas exchange (see Fig. 30-10).

Assess nail shape by examining the curve of the nail plate and surrounding tissue from all angles. Palpate the fingertips to assess for sponginess, tenderness, or edema. Table 24-6 describes common variations in nail shape.

Thickness of the nail plate varies with age, trauma, dermatologic disease, or decreased arterial blood flow. In older patients, look for a "heaped-up" appearance of the toenails, which occurs with fungal infection (*onychomycosis*).

Consistency of the nail is described as hard, soft, or brittle. Nail plates become hard, with thickening. A warm-water soak is required to soften the nail plates before they can be trimmed. Soft nail plates, which are thin and bend easily with pressure, are associated with malnutrition, chronic arthritis, myxedema, and peripheral neuritis.

Brittle nails can split, as with onychomycosis or advanced psoriasis involving the fingers or toes. Splitting of the nail plate is caused by repeated exposure to water and detergents, which damage the plate over time.

Lesions can occur around, on, within, or under the nail. Separation of the nail plate from the nail bed (*onycholysis*)

TABLE 24-5   **Common Alterations in Nail Color**

ALTERATION	CLINICAL FINDINGS	SIGNIFICANCE
White	Horizontal white banding or areas of opacity	Chronic liver or kidney disease (hypoalbuminemia)
	Generalized pallor of nail beds	Shock Anemia Early arteriosclerotic changes (toenails) Myocardial infarction
Yellow-brown	Diffuse yellow-to-brown discoloration	Jaundice Peripheral lymphedema Bacterial or fungal infections of the nail Psoriasis Diabetes Cardiac failure Staining from tobacco, nail polish, or dyes Long-term tetracycline therapy Normal aging (yellow-gray color)
	Vertical brown banding extending from the proximal nail fold distally	Normal finding in dark-skinned patients Nevus or melanoma of nail matrix in light-skinned patients
Red	Thin, dark red vertical lines 1-3 mm long (splinter hemorrhages)	Bacterial endocarditis Trichinosis Trauma to the nail bed Normal finding in some patients
	Red discoloration of the lunula	Cardiac insufficiency
	Dark red nail beds	Polycythemia vera
Blue	Diffuse blue discoloration that blanches with pressure	Respiratory failure Methemoglobinuria Venous stasis disease (toenails)

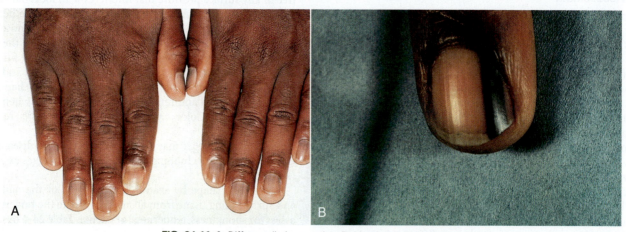

FIG. 24-11 A, Diffuse nail pigmentation. **B,** Linear nail pigmentation.

creates an air pocket beneath the plate. The pocket first appears as a grayish-white opacity. The color changes as dirt and keratin collect in the pocket, and the area begins to have a bad odor. This problem occurs with fungal infections and after trauma. Separation of the nail plate may also occur with psoriasis or with prolonged chemical contact.

Inspect the tissue folds around the nail plate for redness, heat, swelling, and tenderness. Acute paronychia (inflammation of the skin around the nail) often occurs with a torn cuticle or an ingrown toenail.

Chronic paronychia is common and is an inflammation that persists for months. Adults at risk for chronic paronychia are those with frequent exposure to water, such as homemakers, bartenders, laundry workers, and nurses.

🌐 **CULTURAL/SPIRITUAL CONSIDERATIONS**

Patient-Centered Care (QSEN)

Pallor, erythema, cyanosis, and other skin color changes are less visible in patients with naturally dark skin tones. Although physiologic processes are the same for both light-skinned and dark-skinned patients, the amount of skin pigmentation alters how the skin appears in response to physiologic alterations. Different assessment skills are needed to detect the more subtle color changes. Become familiar with the normal appearance of a dark-skinned patient's mucous membranes, nail beds, and skin tone so variations from baseline can be identified. Chart 24-3 lists assessment techniques to assess skin changes in people with dark skin.

TABLE 24-6 Common Variations in Nail Shape

NAIL SHAPE	CLINICAL FINDINGS		SIGNIFICANCE
Normal	Angle of 160 degrees between the nail plate and the proximal nail fold Nail surface slightly convex Nail base firm when palpated		Normal finding
Clubbing			
Early clubbing	Straightening of angle between the nail plate and the proximal nail fold to 180 degrees Nail base spongy when palpated		Hypoxia Lung cancer
Late clubbing	Angle between the nail plate and the proximal nail fold exceeds 180 degrees Nail base visibly edematous and spongy when palpated Enlargement of the soft tissue of the fingertips gives a "drumstick" appearance when viewed from above		Prolonged hypoxia Emphysema Chronic obstructive pulmonary disease Advanced lung cancer Cystic fibrosis Chronic heart disease
Spoon nails (koilonychia)			
Early koilonychias	Flattening of the nail plate with an increased smoothness of the nail surface		Iron deficiency (with or without anemia) Poorly controlled diabetes >15 yr in duration Local injury
Late koilonychias	Concave curvature of the nail plate		Psoriasis Chemical irritants Developmental abnormality
Beau's grooves	1-mm–wide horizontal depressions in the nail plates caused by growth arrest (involves all nails)		Acute, severe illness Prolonged febrile state Isolated periods of severe malnutrition
Pitting	Small, multiple pits in the nail plate May be associated with plate thickening and onycholysis Most often involves the fingernails (several or all)		Psoriasis Alopecia areata

Skin Assessment Techniques for Patients With Darker Skin

Pallor can be detected in people with dark skin by first inspecting the mucous membranes for an ash-gray color (Jarvis, 2016). If the lips and the nail beds are not heavily pigmented, they appear paler than normal for that patient. Use good lighting to assess for the absence of the underlying red tones that normally give heavily pigmented skin a healthy glow. With decreased blood flow to the skin, brown skin appears yellow-brown, and very dark brown skin is ash gray.

Cyanosis can be present when gas exchange is impaired. Examine the lips, tongue, nail beds, conjunctivae, and palms and soles for subtle color changes (Jarvis, 2016). In a patient with cyanosis, the lips and tongue are gray; and the palms, soles, conjunctivae, and nail beds have a bluish tinge. To support these findings, assess for other indicators of hypoxia, including tachycardia, hypotension, changes in respiratory rate, decreased breath sounds, and changes in cognition.

Inflammation in dark-skinned patients appears as excessive warmth and changes in skin consistency or texture (Jarvis, 2016). Use the back of your hand to palpate areas of suspected inflammation for increased warmth. With the fingertips, palpate for hardened areas deep in the tissue, which may give the skin a "woody" feeling. Inflamed skin is tender and edematous. If edema is extensive, the skin is taut and shiny.

Skin areas where inflammation has recently resolved appear *darker* than the patient's normal skin tone. This change is caused by stimulation of the melanocytes during the inflammatory process and the increased pigment production that continues after inflammation subsides. Deep skin injury with destruction of melanocytes (e.g., deep ulcer, full-thickness burn) may heal with color changes that are *lighter* than the normal skin tone. Chronic inflammatory changes are not tender. Scarred skin feels less supple, especially over the joints. If chronic inflammatory changes are suspected, ask the patient about a history of skin problems in that area.

CHART 24-3   Best Practice for Patient Safety & Quality Care QSEN

Assessing Changes in Dark Skin

Cyanosis
- Examine lips and tongue for gray color.
- Examine nail beds, palms, and soles for blue tinge.
- Examine conjunctiva for pallor.

Inflammation
- Compare affected area with nonaffected area for increased warmth.
- Examine the skin of the affected area to determine whether it is shiny or taut or pits with pressure.
- Compare the skin color of affected area with the same area on the opposite side of the body.
- Palpate the affected area and compare it with unaffected area to determine whether texture is different (affected area may feel hard or "woody").

Jaundice
- Check for yellow tinge to oral mucous membranes, especially the hard palate.
- Examine the sclera nearest to the iris rather than the corners of the eye.

Bleeding
- Compare the affected area with the same area on the unaffected body side for swelling or skin darkening.
- If the patient has thrombocytopenia, petechiae may be present on the oral mucosa or conjunctiva.

Jaundice in a patient with dark skin is best assessed by inspecting the oral mucosa, especially the hard palate, for yellow discoloration. Yellowness of the conjunctivae and adjacent sclera may be misleading because normal deposits of fat produce a yellowish hue that is visible in contrast to the dark skin around the eyes (Jarvis, 2016). Examine the sclera closest to the cornea for a more accurate determination of jaundice. The palms and soles of dark-skinned patients may appear yellow if they are calloused, even when jaundice is not present.

Skin bleeding with purpuric lesions may not be visible with deep pigmentation. Areas of ecchymoses appear darker than normal skin; they may be tender and easily palpable, depending on whether hematoma is present. Often the patient relates a history of trauma to the area that confirms the assessment. Petechiae are rarely visible in dark skin and may be seen only in the oral mucosa and conjunctiva.

Psychosocial Assessment

Skin changes, especially of the face, hair, and hands, often affect body image. Encourage the patient to express feelings about a change in appearance. Assess body language for clues indicating a disturbance in self-concept. The avoidance of eye contact or the use of clothing to cover the affected areas may suggest concern about appearance. Patients with chronic skin diseases often become socially isolated related to a fear of rejection by others or a belief that the skin problem is contagious.

Skin changes linked to poor hygiene are common among homeless individuals and those who have reduced cognitive functioning. Assess the patient's overall appearance for excessive soiling, matted hair, body odor, or other self-care deficits. Confirm unsanitary living conditions by obtaining a social

history. Patients may relate similar skin problems among family members, friends, and sexual contacts.

If skin problems related to poor hygiene are identified in older patients, also evaluate any physical limitations that might interfere with grooming. For example, visual or mobility problems can make it difficult for them to see or reach skin surfaces to clean them.

CLINICAL JUDGMENT CHALLENGE 24-1

Patient-Centered Care QSEN

You are a home health care nurse caring for an African-American patient following hospital discharge for an acute exacerbation of congestive heart failure. During your initial assessment, you observe that the patient's pulse is slightly elevated and mild dyspnea on exertion is noted. Both lower extremities are edematous and cool to the touch.
1. What skin changes suggest that the patient is hypoxic?
2. What other assessment findings may you notice that could indicate hypoxia?
3. How do you differentiate between tissue edema caused by altered cardiac perfusion and deep tissue inflammation?
4. What action(s) should you take at this time?

Diagnostic Assessment

Laboratory Tests

When a fungal, bacterial, or viral infection of the skin is suspected, confirmation by microscopic examination is necessary. *Always wear gloves (use Standard Precautions) when examining skin that is not intact.*

Cultures for fungal infection are obtained by using a tongue blade and gently scraping scales from skin lesions into a clean container. Collect fingernail clippings and hair in a similar manner. Waiting for culture results can delay treatment of a superficial fungal infection. For this reason, the specimen is also treated with a potassium hydroxide (KOH) solution and examined microscopically. A positive fungal infection shows branched hyphae when viewed under a microscope after treatment with KOH and may eliminate the need for a culture.

For deeper fungal infections, a piece of tissue is obtained for culture. The health care provider obtains the specimen by punch biopsy (see Skin Biopsy section). Check with the laboratory for any specific instructions related to specimen handling.

Cultures for bacterial infection are obtained from intact primary lesions (abscess, bullae, vesicles, or pustules), if possible. Express material from the lesion, collect it with a cotton-tipped applicator, and place it in a bacterial culture medium specified by the laboratory. For intact lesions, *unroofing* (lifting or puncturing of the outer surface) may be needed using a sterile small-gauge needle before the material can be easily expressed. If crusts are present, the nurse or other health care professional removes them with normal saline and swabs the underlying exudate to obtain a specimen for culture (Cross, 2014).

A biopsy of deep bacterial infections may be needed to obtain a specimen for culture. If bacterial cellulitis is suspected, the health care provider can inject nonbacteriostatic saline deep into the tissue and then aspirate it back; the aspirant is sent for culture.

Cultures for viral infection are indicated if a herpes virus infection is suspected. A cotton-tipped applicator is used to obtain vesicle fluid from intact lesions. Viral culture specimen tubes must be placed on ice immediately after specimens are obtained and are transported to the laboratory as soon as possible.

The presence of a viral infection can be confirmed by *Tzanck smear*, although the exact virus is not identified. A smear is obtained from the base of the lesion and examined under a microscope. The presence of multinucleated giant cells confirms a viral infection.

Other Diagnostic Tests

Other tests for diagnosis of skin problems include biopsy, special noninvasive examination techniques, and skin testing for allergy (discussed in Chapter 20).

Skin Biopsy. A small piece of skin tissue may be obtained for diagnosis or to assess the effectiveness of an intervention. Check with the health care provider to determine the number, location, and type of skin biopsies to be performed. Depending on the size, depth, and location of the skin changes, the health care provider may perform a punch biopsy, shave biopsy, or scalpel excision (excisional biopsy).

Punch biopsy is the most common technique. A small circular cutting instrument, or "punch," ranging in diameter from 2 to 6 mm, is used. After the site is injected with a local anesthetic, a small plug of tissue is cut and removed. The site may be closed with sutures or may be allowed to heal without suturing.

Shave biopsies remove only the part of the skin that rises above the surrounding tissue when injected with a local anesthetic. A scalpel or razor blade is moved parallel to the skin surface to remove the tissue specimen. Shave biopsies are usually indicated for superficial or raised lesions. Suturing is not needed.

Excisional biopsy is rarely used for skin problems. When needed, larger or deeper specimens are obtained by deep excision with a scalpel followed by closure with sutures. Excisional biopsies are more uncomfortable than punch or shave biopsies while healing.

⁇ NCLEX EXAMINATION CHALLENGE 24-2

Safe and Effective Care Environment

What is the appropriate nursing response when a client asks, "What is a punch biopsy?"
A. "The health care provider will use a scalpel to remove a portion of the skin."
B. "A circular cutting instrument will be used to remove a small plug of tissue."
C. "A deep specimen of skin will be taken, and then the health care provider will suture this area closed."
D. "A local anesthetic will be injected before a razor blade is moved parallel to the skin's surface to obtain a sample."

Patient Preparation. Explain to the patient what to expect and that a biopsy is a minor procedure with few anticipated complications. Obtain informed consent. If a punch or shave biopsy is planned, reassure the patient that only a small amount of skin is removed and scarring is minimal. For an excisional biopsy, teach that a scar similar to that of a healed surgical incision will result.

Procedure. Establish a sterile field and assemble all needed supplies and instruments. Local anesthesia is provided by local infiltration using a small-gauge (25-gauge) needle to reduce discomfort during injection. Preparation of the biopsy site differs by health care provider preference, but usually the skin is simply wiped with alcohol.

The injection of a local anesthetic agent, which produces a burning or stinging sensation, may be uncomfortable. Reassure the patient that the discomfort will subside as the anesthetic takes effect. Talking the patient through the procedure with a quiet voice along with a gentle touch may have a calming effect.

After removal, tissue specimens for pathologic study are placed in 10% formalin for fixation. Specimens for culture are placed in sterile saline solution. Bleeding of the site may be controlled by applying localized pressure, applying a topical hemostatic agent, or suturing.

Follow-up Care. After bleeding is controlled and any sutures are placed, the site is covered with an adhesive bandage or a dry gauze dressing. Instruct the patient to keep the dressing dry and in place for at least 8 hours. Teach him or her to clean the site daily after the dressing is removed. Tap water or saline is used to remove any dried blood or crusts. An antibiotic ointment may be prescribed to reduce the risk for infection. The site may be left open or covered for cosmetic reasons or because the site is an area often soiled. Instruct the patient to report any redness or excessive drainage. Sutures are usually removed 7 to 10 days after biopsy.

Wood's Light Examination. A handheld, long-wavelength ultraviolet (black) light or Wood's light may be used during physical examination. Exposure of some skin infections with this light produces a specific color, such as blue-green or red, that can be used to identify the infection. Hypopigmented skin is more prominent when it is viewed under black light, making evaluation of pigment changes in lighter skin easier. This examination is carried out in a darkened room and does not cause discomfort.

Diascopy. Diascopy is a painless technique to eliminate erythema caused by increased blood flow to the skin, thereby easing the inspection of skin lesions. A glass slide or lens is pressed down over the area to be examined, blanching the skin and revealing the shape of the lesions.

⁇ NCLEX EXAMINATION CHALLENGE 24-3

Safe and Effective Care Environment

Which are appropriate nursing interventions for a client who has poor personal hygiene? **Select all that apply.**
A. Obtain a social history.
B. Assist the client with bathing.
C. Tell the client that he or she smells bad.
D. Consult social services to assess the client's living conditions.
E. Teach client and family members how to help with personal hygiene.
F. Notify the health care provider of any suspected drug or alcohol addiction.
G. Assess for poor cognitive function or physical limitations that might interfere with grooming.
H. Instruct the client and family to use rubbing alcohol to cleanse skin areas with most visible amount of dirt.

GET READY FOR THE NCLEX® EXAMINATION!

KEY POINTS

Review these Key Points for each NCLEX Examination Client Needs Category.

Safe and Effective Care Environment

- Assist patients with limited mobility to change positions at least every 2 hours, noting any areas of compromised TISSUE INTEGRITY. **QSEN: Safety**
- Wash your hands before and after touching any areas of impaired skin TISSUE INTEGRITY. **QSEN: Safety**
- Use Standard Precautions when providing care to a patient who has areas of impaired skin TISSUE INTEGRITY or skin with an abnormal appearance. **QSEN: Safety**
- Use lift sheets when moving patients with fragile skin to avoid shearing. **QSEN: Safety**
- Position patients who are confined to bed to promote air circulation to skinfold areas and minimize pressure over bony prominences. **QSEN: Safety**

Health Promotion and Maintenance

- Teach adults to reduce sun exposure and exposure to ultraviolet (UV) light and to regularly use sunscreen. **QSEN: Safety**
- Teach adults to examine all skin areas on a monthly basis for new lesions and changes to existing lesions using the ABCDE method of checking lesions for signs of melanoma. **QSEN: Evidence-Based Practice**

- Teach and encourage patients to bathe, shampoo the hair, and keep fingernails clean and trimmed. **QSEN: Patient-Centered Care**

Psychosocial Integrity

- Use effective communication when teaching patients and family members about what to expect during tests and procedures associated with skin assessment. **QSEN: Patient-Centered Care**
- Reassure patients who have skin changes that are variations of normal. **QSEN: Patient-Centered Care**

Physiological Integrity

- Assess the cognitive function of any patient whose hygiene of the skin, hair, and nail hygiene appears inadequate.
- Modify techniques to assess skin changes in patients with dark skin. **QSEN: Evidence-Based Practice**
- Be aware of specific allergies that have skin indications. **QSEN: Patient-Centered Care**
- Ask any patient who has started taking a newly prescribed or over-the-counter drug whether skin changes have occurred since starting the drug. **QSEN: Patient-Centered Care**
- Distinguish between normal variations and abnormal skin signs and symptoms regarding skin color, texture, warmth, elastic turgor, and moisture. **Clinical Judgment**
- Use the ABCDE method of assessing skin lesions for cancer. **QSEN: Evidence-Based Practice**

SELECTED BIBLIOGRAPHY

American Cancer Society (2015). *Cancer facts and figures:2015*. Atlanta: Author.

Campbell, J., Coyer, F., & Osborne, S. (2016). The skin safety model: Reconceptualizing skin vulnerability in older patients. *Journal of Nursing Scholarship*, 48(1), 14–22.

Cross, H. H. (2014). Obtaining a wound swab culture specimen. *Nursing 2015*, 44(7), 68–69.

Gabison, S., McGillivray, C., Hitzig, S., & Nussbaum, E. (2015). A study of the utility and equivalency of 2 methods of wound measurement: Digitized tracing versus digital photography. *Advanced in Skin and Wound Care*, 28(6), 252–258.

Gordon, R. (2014). Skin cancer: Increasing awareness and screening in primary care. *The Nurse Practitioner*, 39(5), 49–54.

Jarvis, C. (2016). *Physical examination & health assessment* (7th ed.). St. Louis: Saunders.

Langemo, D., Spahn, J., & Snodgrass, L. (2015). Accuracy and reproducibility of the wound shape measuring and monitoring system. *Advances in Skin and Wound Care*, 28(7), 317–323.

LeBlanc, K., Baranoski, S., & the International Skin Tear Advisory Panel. (2014). Skin tears: Best practices for care and prevention. *Nursing 2014*, 44(5), 36–48.

Masterson, K. (2015). Skin cancer prevention. *Journal of the Dermatology Nurses' Association*, 7(2), 73–75.

McCance, K., Huether, S., Brashers, V., & Rote, N. (2014). *Pathophysiology: The biologic basis for disease in adults and children* (7th ed.). St. Louis: Mosby.

Roebuck, H., Moran, K., MacDonald, D., Shumer, S., & McCune, R. (2015). Assessing skin cancer prevention and detection educational needs: An andragogical approach. *The Journal for Nurse Practitioners*, 11(4), 409–416.

The Skin Cancer Foundation. (2016). *Understanding melanoma—Warning signs: The ABCDEs of melanoma*. www.skincancer.org/skin-cancer-information/melanoma.

Touhy, T., & Jett, K. (2015). *Ebersole & Hess' toward healthy aging* (9th ed.). St. Louis: Elsevier.

CHAPTER 25

Care of Patients With Skin Problems

Janice Cuzzell

 http://evolve.elsevier.com/Iggy/

PRIORITY AND INTERRELATED CONCEPTS

The priority concept for this chapter is TISSUE INTEGRITY.

✳ The TISSUE INTEGRITY concept exemplar for this chapter is Pressure Injuries, below.

The interrelated concept for this chapter is CELLULAR REGULATION.

LEARNING OUTCOMES

Safe and Effective Care Environment

1. Collaborate with the interprofessional team to coordinate high-quality care for patients with skin problems.
2. Protect patients from skin injury, loss of TISSUE INTEGRITY, and infection.

Health Promotion and Maintenance

3. Teach adults how to protect the skin from damage and cancer development.

Psychosocial Integrity

4. Implement nursing interventions to minimize stressors for the patient with changes in appearance or function of the integumentary system.

Physiological Integrity

5. Apply knowledge of anatomy and physiology to assess skin changes, lesions, and open wounds.
6. Prioritize nursing care for the patient with skin problems.

Skin TISSUE INTEGRITY helps to protect the entire body by providing a strong barrier, especially to invasion by harmful microorganisms and other foreign proteins (antigens). Problems associated with the skin are common, especially in older adults. Skin TISSUE INTEGRITY changes reduce protective function, and the cause of the change is often difficult to determine. The skin also reflects underlying medical conditions, so skin symptoms may indicate injury or underlying systemic disease.

Interventions and medications for any health problem can trigger a skin response. Skin problems can interfere with the management of other conditions. Age-related changes and problems caused by immobility, chronic disease, debility, and reduced immune function increase the older patient's risk for skin damage and loss of tissue integrity. Pressure injuries reflect one of the most concerning skin conditions with tissue integrity loss for which nurses provide care. Nurses coordinate the activities of an interprofessional team comprised of health care providers, wound care nurses, registered dietitians, and therapists to provide high-quality care for patients with skin concerns.

✳ TISSUE INTEGRITY CONCEPT EXEMPLAR
Pressure Injuries

❖ PATHOPHYSIOLOGY

A **pressure injury** (PrI) is a loss of TISSUE INTEGRITY caused when the skin and underlying soft tissue are compressed between a bony prominence and an external surface for an extended period. Although they commonly occur over the sacrum, hips, and ankles, *pressure injuries can occur on any body surface.* For example, nasal cannula tubing that is too tight can cause pressure injuries behind the ears or in the nares (Ambutas et al., 2014).

Tissue compression from pressure restricts blood flow to the skin, resulting in reduced tissue perfusion and gas exchange, which eventually leads to cell death. Ulcers occur most often in adults with limited mobility because they cannot change their position to relieve pressure. Patients who cannot feel or communicate the pain that occurs with unrelieved pressure are more likely to develop pressure injuries. Once formed, these chronic wounds are slow to heal, resulting in increased morbidity and health care costs. Complications include sepsis, kidney failure, infectious arthritis, and osteomyelitis.

Friction and shear are mechanical forces that impair skin TISSUE INTEGRITY and cause skin tears, which set the stage for skin breakdown (LeBlanc & Baranoski, 2014). Excessive skin moisture, such as urinary or fecal incontinence, also increases the risk for skin damage. Nutrition status is an important concern. Protein malnutrition makes normal tissue more prone to breakdown and also delays healing (Posthauer et al., 2015).

Mechanical Forces

Pressure occurs as a result of gravity. Dependent tissues in contact with a fixed surface experience varying degrees of pressure. Pressure is determined by the amount and distribution of weight exerted at the point of contact and the density of the contacting surface. Excessive or prolonged pressure compresses blood vessels at the point of contact, such as over bony prominences. Pressure occurs when the patient is positioned on a hard surface that does not redistribute the weight, such as when lying on a hard floor for hours after a fall or when remaining in the same position too long. Unrelieved pressure leads to ischemia, inflammation, and tissue necrosis.

Friction occurs when surfaces rub the skin and irritate or tear fragile epithelial tissue. Such forces are generated when the patient is dragged or pulled across bed linen.

Shearing forces are generated when the skin itself is stationary and the tissues below the skin (e.g., fat, muscle) shift or move (Fig. 25-1). The movement of the deeper tissue layers reduces the blood supply to the skin, leading to skin hypoxia, anoxia, ischemia, inflammation, and necrosis.

A shear ulcer usually occurs when a patient is in a wheelchair or in bed in a semi-sitting position and gradually slides downward. The skin over the sacrum may not slide down at the same pace as the deeper tissues, mechanically "shearing" the skin, causing blood vessels to stretch and break. Shearing leads to soft-tissue ischemia and deep-tissue ulcer, even though no external break in skin integrity is observed.

Incidence/Prevalence

Pressure injury development is a problem found among patients in any care setting, including the home. Although new products

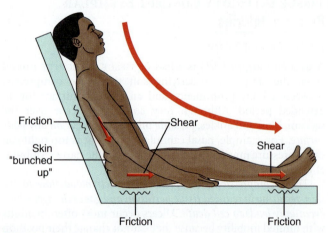

FIG. 25-1 Shearing forces pulling skin layers away from deeper tissue. The skin is "bunched up" against the back of the mattress while the rest of the bone and muscle in the area presses downward on the lower part of the mattress. Blood vessels become kinked, obstructing circulation and leading to tissue death.

CONSIDERATIONS FOR OLDER ADULTS
Patient-Centered Care QSEN

Older adults are at higher risk for skin tears and pressure injuries because of age-related skin changes. Flattening of cells at the dermal-epidermal junction predisposes older adults to skin tears from mechanical shearing forces such as tape removal and minor trauma. Skin moisture and irritation combined with friction over bony prominences can lead to skin destruction with loss of TISSUE INTEGRITY and pressure injury formation. Patients with cognitive impairments may not readily report discomfort from inadequate pressure relief. **If pressure is unrelieved, tissue destruction progresses to full-thickness ulcer.** Assess patients with cognitive impairments more frequently for loss of skin tissue integrity.

are available for prevention and treatment, many hospitalized patients still experience pressure injury formation, which contributes significantly to morbidity and mortality in this patient population (Paul et al., 2014; Roe & Williams, 2014).

Health Promotion and Maintenance

Pressure injuries can be prevented if the risk is recognized and intervention begins early (Chart 25-1) (National Pressure Ulcer Advisory Panel, 2016). Pressure injury prevention does not just happen, even with conscientious nursing care. Deliberate and consistent interventions, as described in the Evidence-Based Practice box, are needed to prevent pressure injuries across the health care continuum, particularly for critically ill patients. Key health care team members for pressure injury prevention and management are the certified wound care specialist and the dietitian. Involving unlicensed assistive personnel (UAP) in pressure injury prevention also enhances prevention program effectiveness.

A pressure injury prevention program consists of two steps: (1) early identification of high-risk patients, and (2) implementation of aggressive intervention for prevention with the use of pressure-relief or pressure-reduction devices. Pressure mapping with a computerized tool that measures pressure distribution during sitting or lying can identify specific body areas at risk for breakdown and can help plan interventions for patients who are bedridden or wheelchair bound. The map is displayed in colors on the computer screen based on temperature differences. Red indicates areas of greater heat production and increased pressure loads. Blue indicates cooler areas under lower pressure. When used in combination with risk assessment tools, pressure mapping helps identify problem areas before skin changes can be seen and allows for more targeted prevention strategies.

Effective risk identification and prevention measures include patient and caregiver education. Documentation of risk assessment, implementation of prevention measures, and education of all adults involved in the care of the patient at risk for pressure injury formation are key to the plan's success. Continuing evaluation and risk assessment are critical, especially when the patient's condition changes.

Identification of High-Risk Patients

As suggested by The Joint Commission's National Patient Safety Goals (NPSGs), all patients admitted to a health care facility or home care agency are to be assessed for pressure injury risk. The use of a risk assessment tool increases the chances of identifying patients at greater risk for skin

CHART 25-1   Best Practice for Patient Safety & Quality Care QSEN

Preventing Pressure Injuries

Positioning
- Pad contact surfaces with foam, silicone gel, air pads, or other materials with pressure-redistribution properties.
- Do not keep the head of the bed elevated above 30 degrees to prevent shearing.
- Use a lift sheet to move a patient in the bed. Avoid dragging or sliding him or her.
- When positioning a patient on his or her side, position at a 30-degree tilt.
- Re-position an immobile patient at a frequency consistent with assessed needs.
- Do not place a rubber ring or donut under the patient's sacral area.
- When moving an immobile patient from a bed to another surface, use a designated slide board well lubricated with talc or use a mechanical lift.
- Place pillows or foam wedges between two bony surfaces.
- Keep the patient's skin directly off plastic surfaces.
- Keep the patient's heels off the bed surface using bed pillow under ankles or a heel-suspension device.

Nutrition
- Ensure a fluid intake between 2000 and 3000 mL/day.
- Help the patient maintain an adequate intake of protein and calories.

Skin Care
- Perform a daily inspection of the patient's entire skin.
- Document and report any manifestations of skin infection.

- Use moisturizers daily on dry skin and apply when skin is damp.
- Keep moisture from prolonged contact with skin:
  - Dry areas where two skin surfaces touch, such as the axillae and under the breasts.
  - Place absorbent pads under areas where perspiration collects.
  - Use moisture barriers on skin areas where wound drainage or incontinence occurs.
- **Do not massage bony prominences.**
- Humidify the room.

Skin Cleaning
- Clean the skin as soon as possible after soiling occurs and at routine intervals.
- Use a mild, heavily fatted soap or gentle commercial cleanser for incontinence.
- Use tepid rather than hot water.
- In the perineal area, use a disposable cleaning cloth that contains a skin-barrier agent.
- While cleaning, use the minimum scrubbing force necessary to remove soil.
- Gently pat rather than rub the skin dry.
- Do not use powders or talc directly on the perineum.
- After cleaning, apply a commercial skin barrier to areas in frequent contact with urine or feces.

EVIDENCE-BASED PRACTICE QSEN

Using a Skin Integrity Care Bundle to Reduce Pressure Injuries

Coyer, F., et al. (2015). Reducing pressure injuries in critically ill patients by using a patient skin integrity care bundle (InSPiRE). *American Journal of Critical Care, 24*(3), 199-210.

This study sought to determine whether using a skin integrity bundle, the InSPiRE protocol, would reduce the incidence of pressure injuries in critically ill patients.

The sample included 207 patients in an Australian intensive care unit. Of the 207, 105 were part of the intervention group, and 102 were in the control group. Both groups had an average age of 55, a comparable average length of stay in intensive care, and similar Sequential Organ Failure Assessment (SOFA) scores. The InSPiRE protocol, used with the intervention group, included a bundle of processes, including ongoing skin assessment; intervention attention to hygiene, repositioning, and use of devices intended to lower pressure and friction; and focus on nutrition, mobility, and documentation. Within the intervention group, cumulative incidence of pressure injuries (skin and mucous) was significantly lower than that of the control group. Patients in the intervention group also developed significantly fewer pressure injuries over time than those in the control group.

Level of Evidence: 2
This research was designed as a prospective comparative study.

Commentary: Implications for Practice and Research
A significant reduction in the incidence of pressure injuries between the groups, from 30% in the control group to 18% in the intervention group, was noted. Use of protocols such as InSPiRE draws attention to the importance of diligence in ongoing interventions to prevent development of pressure injuries throughout the length of the patient's stay. As noted by the authors, nurses and all members of the interdisciplinary team benefit the patient by continually being aware of, and implementing, evidence-based strategies on a continual basis.

breakdown. The Braden scale (Fig. 25-2) is a commonly used valid skin risk assessment tool. Using it helps the nurse assess and document risk categories for pressure injury formation (e.g., mental status, activity and mobility, nutritional status, incontinence).

Mental status changes and decreased sensation determine whether the patient is a partner in pressure injury prevention. When the patient understands that turning and shifting of weight prevent tissue damage, the risk for pressure injuries decreases. Stroke, head injury, organic brain disease, Alzheimer's disease, sedation, or other cognitive problems increase the risk for pressure injuries.

Impaired mobility is a factor in the risk for pressure injury formation. Patients who have unimpaired mobility and can respond to pain are at lower risk for pressure injuries. *Regardless of age, any patient who requires assistance with turning and positioning or who is unable to verbalize discomfort is at higher risk for pressure injuries.* Those confined to bed or a chair also are at higher risk than a patient who requires assistance only with ambulation.

Nutrition status is a critical risk factor for pressure injury development and for successful healing (Posthauer et al., 2015). TISSUE INTEGRITY and wound healing depend on a positive nitrogen balance and adequate serum protein levels. The patient

Patient's name _____ Evaluator's name _____ Date of assessment

Category	1	2	3	4	Date of assessment
Sensory perception Ability to respond meaningfully to pressure-related discomfort	**1. Completely limited** Unresponsive to painful stimuli (does not moan, flinch, or grasp) because of diminished level of consciousness or sedation OR limited ability to feel pain over most of body surface	**2. Very limited** Responds only to painful stimuli; cannot communicate discomfort except by moaning or restlessness OR has a sensory impairment that limits the ability to feel pain or discomfort over half of the body	**3. Slightly limited** Responds to verbal commands but cannot always communicate discomfort or need to be turned OR has some sensory impairment that limits ability to feel pain or discomfort in one or two extremities	**4. No impairment** Responds to verbal commands; has no sensory deficit that would limit ability to feel or voice pain or discomfort	
Moisture Degree to which skin is exposed to moisture	**1. Constantly moist** Skin is kept moist almost constantly by perspiration, urine; dampness is detected every time the client is moved or turned	**2. Very Moist** Skin is often but not always moist; linen must be changed at least once a shift	**3. Occasionally moist** Skin is occasionally moist, requiring an extra linen change approximately once a day	**4. Rarely moist** Skin is usually dry; linen requires changing only at routine intervals	
Activity Degree of physical activity	**1. Bedfast** Confined to bed	**2. Chairfast** Ability to walk severely limited or nonexistent; cannot bear own weight and must be assisted into chair or wheelchair	**3. Walks occasionally** Walks occasionally during the day but for very short distances, with or without assistance; spends the majority of each shift in bed or chair	**4. Walks frequently** Walks outside the room at least twice a day and inside the room at least once every 2 hours during waking hours	
Mobility Ability to change or control body position	**1. Completely immobile** Does not make even slight changes in body or extremity position without assistance	**2. Very limited** Makes occasional slight changes in body or extremity position but unable to make frequent or significant changes independently	**3. Slightly limited** Makes frequent though slight changes in body or extremity position independently	**4. No limitations** Makes major and frequent changes in position without assistance	
Nutrition Usual food intake pattern	**1. Very poor** Never eats a complete meal; rarely eats more than a third of any food offered; eats two servings or less of protein (meat or dairy products) per day; takes fluids poorly; does not take a liquid dietary supplement OR is NPO or maintained on clear liquids or IV for more than 5 days	**2. Probably inadequate** Rarely eats a complete meal and generally eats only about half of any food offered; protein intake includes only three servings of meat or dairy products per day; occasionally will take a dietary supplement OR receives less than optimal amount of liquid diet or tube feeding	**3. Adequate** Eats over half of most meals; eats a total of four servings of protein (meat, dairy products) each day; occasionally will refuse a meal, but will usually take a supplement if offered OR is receiving tube feeding or total parenteral nutrition, which probably meets most nutritional needs	**4. Excellent** Eats most of every meal; never refuses a meal; usually eats a total of four or more servings of meat and dairy products; occasionally eats between meals; does not require supplementation	
Friction and shear	**1. Problem** Requires moderate to maximum assistance in moving; complete lifting without sliding against sheets is impossible; frequently slides down in bed or chair, requiring frequent repositioning with maximum assistance; spasticity, contractures, or agitation leads to almost constant friction	**2. Potential problem** Moves feebly or requires minimum assistance during a move; skin probably slides to some extent against sheets, chair, restraints, or other devices; maintains relatively good position in chair or bed most of the time but occasionally slides down	**3. No apparent problem** Moves in bed and in chair independently and has sufficient muscle strength to lift up completely during move; maintains good position in bed or chair at all times		Total score

Scoring system: 15-16 = mild risk, 12-14 = moderate risk, <11 = severe risk

FIG. 25-2 The Braden scale for predicting pressure ulcer risk. *IV*, Intravenous; *NPO*, nothing by mouth. (From Barbara Braden & Nancy Bergstrom. ©1988. Reprinted with permission.)

in negative nitrogen balance not only heals more slowly but also is at risk for accelerated tissue destruction. Draining wounds contribute to protein loss and require aggressive intervention.

Nutrition assessment includes laboratory studies; evaluation of weight and weight change; ability of the patient to consume an adequate diet; and the need for vitamin, mineral, or protein supplementation. Serum prealbumin levels are often used to monitor nutrition status. *Nutrition is considered inadequate when the serum prealbumin level is less than 19.5 g/dL, albumin level is less than 3.5 g/dL, or the lymphocyte count is less than 1800/mm³.* Because serum protein levels are affected by a number of other factors, laboratory values are useful only when supported by additional assessment information. Other indicators of inadequate nutrition include poor daily intake of food and fluids with a weight loss greater than 5% change in 30 days or greater than 10% change in 180 days (Posthauer et al., 2015).

A positive nitrogen balance requires an intake of 30 to 35 calories per kilogram of body weight daily with a protein intake of 1.25 to 1.5 g/kg/day. Up to 2 g/kg/day of protein may be needed when nutritional deficits are severe or protein loss is ongoing. Vitamin and mineral supplementations are based on the patient's nutrition status. Collaborate with a dietitian for all patients at risk for a pressure injury to perform a thorough nutrition assessment and plan interventions for nutrition deficits (National Pressure Ulcer Advisory Panel, European Pressure Ulcer Advisory Panel, & Pan Pacific Pressure Injury Alliance, 2014).

Incontinence results in prolonged contact of the skin with substances that irritate the skin, destroy TISSUE INTEGRITY, and predispose to skin breakdown (e.g., urea, bacteria, yeast, and enzymes in urine and feces). Excessive moisture macerates skin, further increasing the risk for breakdown. Daily inspection of the skin for any areas of redness, maceration, or loss of skin TISSUE INTEGRITY is a major part of pressure injury prevention. Maintenance of clean, dry, intact skin also assists in ulcer prevention. Wash the skin with a pH-balanced soap to maintain the normal acid level. Use creams or lotions to lubricate and moisturize the skin. Barrier ointments and zinc oxide–based creams help protect intact skin from urine and feces when incontinence is present. Change absorbent pads or garments immediately after each incontinence episode and avoid using adult briefs when patients are unable to communicate their needs to avoid prolonged skin contact with urine or feces.

> ### ! NURSING SAFETY PRIORITY QSEN
> #### *Action Alert*
>
> Teach all nursing care personnel and family members not to massage reddened skin areas directly or use donut-shaped pillows for pressure relief. These actions can damage capillary beds and increase tissue necrosis.

Pressure-Redistribution Techniques

Support Surfaces and Devices. The cornerstone in the prevention and management of pressure injuries is maintaining adequate pressure redistribution so pressure over bony prominences remains below the capillary closing pressure. Capillary closing pressure is the pressure needed to occlude skin capillary blood flow and normally ranges from 12 to 32 mm Hg. An effective pressure-redistribution surface or device keeps tissue interface pressure *below* the capillary closing pressure, thus promoting adequate tissue perfusion and gas exchange. *Most support surfaces and devices have a standardized guaranteed pressure-redistribution reading; however, these readings do not ensure that capillary blood flow for any given patient is adequate. Observe skin color, capillary refill, tissue integrity, and temperature directly to determine capillary flow adequacy.*

Products that redistribute tissue load are available in several forms: specialty bed replacements, mattress replacements, mattress overlays, seat cushion replacements, seat cushion overlays, and heel-suspension devices (McInnes et al., 2015). Choosing the correct product is important to the success of any prevention or treatment plan. Factors to consider when selecting a product include:

- Number and severity of existing pressure injuries
- Risk for developing new pressure injuries
- Patient's ability to reposition self to relieve pressure-related discomfort
- Need for microclimate control to help manage skin temperature and moisture
- Need to reduce shearing forces
- Compatibility of product with care setting

Support surfaces are classified as either nonpowered (*static*) or powered (*dynamic*). Static devices use gel, water, foam, or air to increase the body surface area that comes in contact with the surface and reduce interface pressure. A static high-specification reactive foam mattress with frequent repositioning is recommended for patients at high risk for pressure injury development and for management of those with existing Stage 1 or Stage 2 pressure injuries.

Dynamic systems are comprised of cells that inflate and deflate to continuously alter the area of the body that is bearing the load. Alternating pressure surfaces with small air cells are considered to be less effective than those with air compartments >10 cm. Consider the use of a dynamic support surface for immobile patients when manual repositioning is medically contraindicated; when the number and severity of existing pressure injuries limit turning options; for management of Stage 3, Stage 4, and unstageable pressure injuries (as in Chart 25-2); and for suspected deep-tissue injury when repositioning is ineffective.

Evaluate the surface daily for effectiveness in redistributing pressure, reducing discomfort, managing the microclimate and shear, and eliminating "bottoming out." Bottoming out occurs when the product is not providing adequate pressure redistribution for the patient's size and weight and the patient's bony prominences sink into the mattress or cushion. If the patient has a pressure injury involving the heel, use a heel-suspension device to elevate the heel and offload pressure completely without placing pressure on the Achilles tendon. Check heel-suspension devices periodically to assess skin integrity (National Pressure Ulcer Advisory Panel, European Pressure Ulcer Advisory Panel, & Pan Pacific Pressure Injury Alliance, 2014).

Pressure-redistribution devices lower pressure below that of a standard hospital mattress or chair surface but do not reduce pressure consistently below the capillary closing pressure. These devices are effective for preventing pressure injuries only when used together with a turning schedule and other preventive skin-care measures.

Positioning. *Frequent repositioning* of bedbound patients, as described in Chart 25-1, is critical in reducing pressure over bony prominences. A good plan for positioning is the 30-degree rule. This plan ensures that the patient is positioned

CHART 25-2   Key Features

Pressure Injuries

Suspected Deep-Tissue Injury
- The intact skin area appears purple or maroon.
- Blood-filled blisters may be present.
- Before the previously listed changes appeared, the tissue in this area may first have been painful.
- Other changes that may have preceded the discoloration include that the area may have felt more firm, boggy, mushy, warmer, or cooler than the surrounding tissue.

Stage 1
- Skin is intact.
- Area, usually over a bony prominence, is red and does not blanch with external pressure.
- For patients with darker skin that does not blanch, observe pressure-related alteration of intact skin; changes are compared with an adjacent or opposite area and include one or more of these:
  - Skin color (darker or lighted than the comparison area)
  - Skin temperature (warmth or coolness)
  - Tissue consistency (firm or boggy)
  - Sensation (pain, itching)
  - The ulcer appears as a defined area of persistent redness in lightly pigmented skin, whereas in darker skin tones, the ulcer may appear with persistent red, blue, or purple hues.

Stage 2
- Skin is not intact.
- There is partial-thickness skin loss of the epidermis or dermis.

- Ulcer is superficial and may be characterized as an abrasion, a blister (open or fluid-filled), or a shallow crater.
- Bruising is *not* present.

Stage 3
- Skin loss is full thickness.
- Subcutaneous tissues may be damaged or necrotic.
- Damage extends down to but not through the underlying fascia; bone, tendon, and muscle are *not* exposed.
- The depth can vary with anatomic location; areas of thin skin (e.g., the bridge of the nose) may show only a shallow crater, whereas thicker tissue areas with larger amounts of subcutaneous fat may show a deep, crater-like appearance.
- Undermining and tunneling may or may not be present.

Stage 4
- Skin loss is full thickness with exposed or palpable muscle, tendon, or bone.
- Often includes undermining and tunneling.
- Sinus tracts may develop.
- Slough and eschar are often present on at least part of the wound.

Unstageable
Skin loss is full thickness; and the base is completely covered with slough or eschar, obscuring the true depth of the wound.

Data from National Pressure Ulcer Advisory Panel. (2016). *NPUAP pressure injury stages.* Retrieved from http://www.npuap.org/resources/educational-and-clinical-resources/npuap-pressure-injury-stages/.

and propped so whatever part of the body is elevated is tilted back to no more than a 30-degree angle to the mattress rather than resting directly on a dependent bony prominence. This rule applies to side-lying and head-of-bed elevation positions. The patient who requires greater head elevation because of respiratory difficulties should be tilted up above 30 degrees with pillows behind the back to keep pressure off of the sacral/coccyx area. Often positioning is delegated to UAP. Teach UAP the importance of proper positioning, demonstrate how to perform it, and provide appropriate supervision. Also teach family members to use these techniques in the home.

The patient at risk for pressure injuries in bed is also at risk while sitting. Assess for proper chair cushioning. Collaborate with physical therapists and rehabilitation specialists for selection of these products. Periodically assist high-risk patients who are chair bound to a standing position to promote perfusion and prevent breakdown over the sacral area.

Even with an appropriate mattress or cushion, the patient needs to change or be helped to change positions periodically to prevent loss of skin TISSUE INTEGRITY. Many facilities require turning and positioning every 2 hours. *However, pressure can occur in less time, and the actual turning or repositioning schedule for each patient must be individualized.* When this action is delegated to UAP, teach them the importance of maintaining a repositioning schedule and supervise appropriately.

Use pillows and other positioning or heel-suspension devices to keep heels pressure free at all times for high-risk patients. Assess heel positioning every 4 hours to ensure that pressure is not redistributed to other high-risk areas, such as the ankles or side of the feet. Check heels even more often when devices that hide the feet (e.g., boots, heel protectors) are used, especially if the patient has a vascular problem. Also check knees and elbows regularly, especially when the patient is in a side-lying position.

❖ INTERPROFESSIONAL COLLABORATIVE CARE

Care of the patient with a pressure injury, depending on stage and associated health issues, can take place in a variety of settings: the hospital, long-term care center, or home. Members of the interprofessional team who collaborate most closely to care for the patient with pressure injury include the primary health care provider, who continually assesses the wound condition and prescribes treatment; the nurse; and the dietitian, who assesses nutrition status and recommends dietary modification to speed wound healing.

◆ Assessment: Noticing

History. When a patient already has a pressure injury, identify the cause of skin TISSUE INTEGRITY loss and factors that may impair healing. Ask about the circumstances of the skin loss. Patients with chronic pressure injuries may have a history of delayed healing or recurrence of the ulcer after healing has occurred. Assess for any of these contributing factors:
- Prolonged bedrest
- Immobility
- Incontinence
- Diabetes mellitus

- Inadequate nutrition or hydration
- Decreased sensory perception or cognitive problems
- Peripheral vascular disease

Physical Assessment/Signs and Symptoms. Inspect the entire body, including the back of the head, for areas of skin TISSUE INTEGRITY loss or pressure. Give special attention to bony prominences (e.g., the heels, sacrum, elbows, knees, trochanters, and posterior and anterior iliac spines) and areas with excessive moisture. Make sure that tubing and other medical devices are not under the patient, producing a pressure point. Assess the patient's general appearance for issues related to skin health, such as the proportion of weight to height. Obese and thin patients are at increased risk for malnutrition and pressure injuries. Check overall cleanliness of the skin, hair, and nails. Determine whether any loss of mobility or range of joint motion has occurred. *Do not delegate this assessment to UAP because it is beyond their scope of practice.*

Wound Assessment. The appearance of pressure injuries changes with the depth of the ulcer. Chart 25-2 lists the features of the six categories or stages of pressure ulceration, and Fig. 25-3 shows examples.

Assess wounds for location, size, color, extent of tissue involvement, cell types in the wound base and margins, exudate, condition of surrounding tissue, and presence of foreign bodies. Document this initial assessment to serve as a starting point for determining the intervention plan and its effectiveness. How often a wound is assessed is determined by the policies and procedures at the facility or agency. Weekly documented assessment is standard in many long-term care facilities. Daily assessment is needed when the patient is in an acute care setting. *Also assess the wound at each dressing change, comparing the existing wound features with those documented previously to determine the current state of healing or deterioration.*

Blanchable erythema of intact skin over a bony prominence is an early sign of pressure-related complications. In light-skinned patients, assess whether blanching is present by pressing the reddened area firmly with a gloved finger and releasing the pressure. An area that blanches (lightens) when pressure is briefly applied and reddens again when pressure is released suggests adequate capillary blood flow to the tissue. A reddened area that does not blanch indicates absence of capillary blood flow and early tissue damage (Stage 1 pressure injury). Redness and blanching may be difficult to detect in darker-skinned patients. Look for more subtle differences in the skin color and texture over the pressure point compared with the surrounding area. In addition to being painful, the skin may feel firmer, softer, warmer, or cooler than adjacent areas (Steven et al., 2015).

First record the location and size of the wound. Wounds are sized by length, width, and depth using millimeters or centimeters. For standardization in documentation, assess the wound as a clock face with the 12 o'clock position in the direction of the patient's head and the 6 o'clock position in the direction of the patient's feet (van Rijswijk, 2013). Using a disposable measuring device, always measure the length from the 12 o'clock position to the 6 o'clock position and the width between the 9 o'clock position and the 3 o'clock position. Measure depth as the distance from the deepest portion of the wound base to the skin level. Touch the bottom of the wound with a cotton-tipped applicator or swab and mark the place on the swab that is level with the skin surface to obtain wound depth. Then measure the area of the swab between the tip and the mark. When everyone uses this format, measurement is accurate, and progress can be determined.

Inspect the wound margins for *cellulitis* (inflammation of the skin and subcutaneous tissue) extending beyond the area of injury. Progressive tissue destruction, seen as an increase in the size or depth of the ulcer and increased wound drainage, may indicate an increased risk for infection if proper measures have not been taken to relieve pressure.

Inspect the wound for the presence or absence of necrotic tissue. Because of the depth of tissue destruction, a full-thickness pressure injury is often covered by a layer of black, gray, or brown collagen called wound **eschar**.

In the early stages of wound healing, the eschar is dry, leathery, and firmly attached to the wound. As the inflammatory phase of wound healing begins and removal of wound debris progresses, the eschar starts to lift and separate from the tissue beneath. This nonliving eschar is a good breeding ground for any bacteria on the skin surface. As bacteria increase, they release enzymes that cause the eschar to soften and become more yellow or tan in appearance. With bacterial colonization, wound exudate increases substantially; the color and odor of wound exudate indicate the major organism present. The features of wound exudate are listed in Table 25-1.

Beneath the dead tissue, granulation tissue appears. Early granulation is pale pink, progressing to a beefy red color as it grows and fills the wound. Palpate the wound to determine the granulation texture. Healthy granulation tissue is moist and has a slightly spongy texture. Wounds with a poor arterial blood supply or that have stopped healing appear dry with hard (fibrotic) granulation tissue on palpation. Venous obstruction causes a very moist ulcer surface with a deep reddish-purple color from the deoxygenated blood beneath the surface.

Pressure injuries may have more tissue destruction than is first seen on inspection. Deep, extensive tissue damage may be present under normal-appearing skin surrounding the wound, with separation of the skin layers from the underlying granulation tissue. This problem is known as **undermining**. Inspect undermined areas for gradual filling with healthy granulations and for wound-healing progress. Palpate the bony prominences for deep hardening of the surrounding soft tissue, which often occurs with deep-tissue ischemia.

TABLE 25-1	Types of Wound Exudate
CHARACTERISTICS	**SIGNIFICANCE**
Serosanguineous Exudate	
Blood-tinged amber fluid consisting of serum and red blood cells	Normal for first 48 hr after injury Sudden increase in amount precedes wound dehiscence in wounds closed by first intention
Purulent Exudate	
Creamy yellow pus	Colonization with *Staphylococcus*
Greenish-blue pus causing staining of dressings and accompanied by a "fruity" odor	Colonization with *Pseudomonas*
Beige pus with a "fishy" odor	Colonization with *Proteus*
Brownish pus with a "fecal" odor	Colonization with aerobic coliform and *Bacteroides* (usually occurs after intestinal surgery)

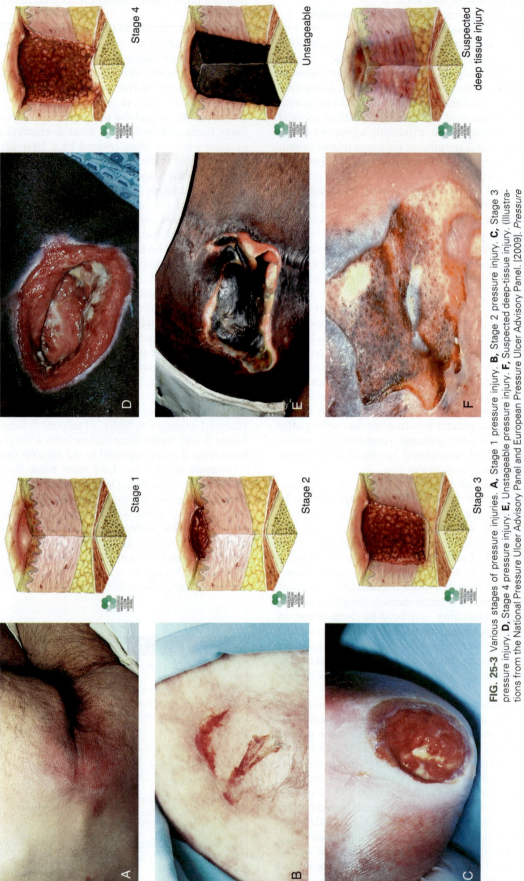

FIG. 25-3 Various stages of pressure injuries. **A,** Stage 1 pressure injury. **B,** Stage 2 pressure injury. **C,** Stage 3 pressure injury. **D,** Stage 4 pressure injury. **E,** Unstageable pressure injury. **F,** Suspected deep-tissue injury. (Illustrations from the National Pressure Ulcer Advisory Panel and European Pressure Ulcer Advisory Panel. [2009]. *Pressure ulcer prevention and treatment: Clinical practice guideline.* Washington, DC: NPUAP. Used with permission.)

After ischemia has occurred, continued pressure over the area increases tissue destruction from the deep-tissue layers toward the surface, resulting in the formation of tunnels. This "hidden" wound may have a small opening in the skin with purulent drainage. If such an opening is observed, use a cotton-tipped applicator to probe gently for a much larger tunnel or pocket of necrotic tissue beneath the opening. Additional tunnels may occur along the main wound. Check all wounds for tunneling and, if present, document the location and length of each tunnel.

In addition to recording regular wound assessments, serial photographs of the wound help document changes in wound appearance and progress toward healing. Policies on photographic documentation vary from facility to facility and require informed consent from the patient or responsible family member. New ways of assessing and managing wounds are emerging with advancing technology. For example, in rural or long-term care settings, facilities can use bidirectional video to consult with a wound specialist at the bedside and get recommendations on how to better manage nonhealing wounds (Chanussot-Deprez & Contreras-Ruiz, 2013).

Psychosocial Assessment. The patient with pressure injuries may have an altered body image. Many changes in lifestyle are needed for healing. Chronic injuries are often painful and costly to treat.

Assess the patient's and family's knowledge of the desired treatment outcomes during the healing process and adherence to the prescribed treatment regimen. Also assess the patient's skills in cleaning and dressing the wound. Poor adherence to pressure injury care procedures may reflect an inability to cope with the pain, cost, or potential scarring associated with prolonged healing. Depending on the patient's activity level and the ulcer location, family assistance or a home care nurse may be needed to provide pressure injury care at home.

Teach the patient and family specific changes in ADLs to relieve pressure and promote healing. Encourage increased activity whenever possible to enhance circulation to the affected tissue. Leg position changes may be needed for chronic leg ulcers, depending on whether vascular problems are present. For patients who have arterial insufficiency, keeping the legs and feet in a dependent position helps ensure adequate blood flow to the lower legs. When arterial blood flow is adequate but venous return is impaired, elevation of the legs may be needed for healing. When the patient is bedridden, frequent repositioning to relieve pressure can be labor intensive. In the home, repositioning, incontinence management, and dressing changes are often needed around the clock, not only increasing patient discomfort but also disrupting family routines and causing added stress.

Laboratory Assessment. An exposed chronic wound is always *colonized with microorganisms* but is not always *infected.* *Colonization* is the presence of one or more communities of organisms that attach to the wound surface in the form of a wound biofilm. Polymicrobial biofilms are composed of non-pathogenic, microbiome organisms that impede normal wound healing by producing a state of chronic inflammation without clinical infection (Cowan et al., 2014). Pathogenic organisms form biofilms that lead to wound infection. *Wound infection* is a state of critical colonization with pathogenic organisms to the degree that organism growth and spread cannot be controlled by the body's immune defenses. Wounds that are red and indurated with moderate-to-heavy exudate and an odor should be cultured to identify the organism and determine antibiotic sensitivity. *The presence of purulent exudate alone does not indicate an infection because pus forms whenever necrotic tissue liquefies and separates.*

If wounds are extensive, if the patient is severely immuno-compromised, or if local blood supply to the wound is impaired, bacterial growth exceeds the body's defenses against invasion into deeper tissues. The result is deep wound infection and eventually bacteremia and sepsis.

Swab cultures are helpful only in identifying the types of bacteria present on the ulcer surface and may not identify bacteria encapsulated within a mature biofilm or invading deeper tissues (Cross, 2014). Wound biopsies allow the numbers of bacteria to be analyzed, but these tests are time consuming, costly, and not always available. Clinical indicators of infection (cellulitis, progressive increase in ulcer size or depth, changes in the quantity and quality of exudate) and systemic signs of bacteremia (e.g., fever, elevated white blood cell [WBC] count) are used to diagnose an infection.

Other Diagnostic Assessments. Additional laboratory studies are performed based on the suspected cause of the wound. For example, noninvasive and invasive arterial blood flow studies are indicated if arterial occlusion is suspected in delayed healing of a pressure injury on the heel or ankle. Blood tests to determine nutritional deficiencies (e.g., prealbumin, albumin, total protein) are helpful in managing the debilitated, malnourished patient with a pressure injury.

? CLINICAL JUDGMENT CHALLENGE 25-1

Evidence-Based Practice QSEN

A 78-year-old man with hypertension, hyperlipidemia, osteoporosis, and urge incontinence is admitted to a long-term care facility after having an ischemic stroke. His wife tells you that, over the past 6 months, the patient has become progressively dependent on her to assist with ADLs. You observe the patient to be a slender, frail elderly male who appears alert and cooperative. He has significant left-sided weakness and requires assistance to transfer from the wheelchair to the bed. While helping him change clothes, you notice a large reddened area on his left hip that doesn't change color when you press it with your index finger.

1. What is the most probable cause of his reddened hip?
2. How would you stage this skin change?
3. Which risk factors does this patient have for pressure injury formation?
4. What other body areas do you need to inspect for skin breakdown?
5. Which support surface would be appropriate for this patient?

◆ *Analysis: Interpreting*

The priority collaborative problems for patients with pressure injuries include:

1. Compromised TISSUE INTEGRITY due to vascular insufficiency and trauma
2. Potential for wound deterioration due to insufficient wound management

◆ *Planning and Implementation: Responding*

The Concept Map addresses care issues related to patients who have or are at risk for pressure injuries.

Managing Wounds

Planning: Expected Outcomes. The patient with a pressure injury is expected to progress to complete wound healing and not develop new pressure injuries. Indicators include:

CONCEPT MAP

PRESSURE INJURY

TISSUE INTEGRITY

CELLULAR REGULATION

INTERVENTIONS—RESPONDING

1. Physical Assessment—Noticing Signs and Symptoms

- Identify cause of existing PIs and factors that impair healing: prolonged bedrest, immobility, incontinence, diabetes mellitus, inadequate nutrition or hydration, decreased sensory perception, and peripheral vascular disease. *Identifies risk factors to address for minimizing or eliminating risk of developing compromised TISSUE INTEGRITY.*
- Use an evidence-based risk assessment tool (e.g., Braden) to monitor for risk of skin breakdown. Ensure tubing and other medical devices are not placed underneath the patient to produce a pressure point. *Identifies early risks to develop PI and prevents and maintains TISSUE INTEGRITY.*
- Monitor mental status and vital signs. *Assesses overall condition—confusion can be caused from infection, dehydration, and fluid & electrolyte imbalance.*
- Determine loss of mobility or a decreased range of motion (ROM). *Provides clues about mobility as a risk factor for PIs.*
- Assess wounds at each dressing change; document initial assessment as a starting point for determining the intervention plan and its effectiveness. *Indicates current state of healing or deterioration.*

2. Wound Care Assessment

- Record the location and size of wounds measuring the length, width, and depth. *Accurately measures wounds for evidence of healing and effectiveness of treatment.*
- Elevate the heels off of support surfaces. *Stops the compression of blood vessels that result in ischemia, inflammation, and tissue necrosis.*
- Inspect wounds for necrotic tissue. *Assesses the need for débridement. Dead tissue supports bacterial growth, obstructs collagen deposition, and wound contraction.*
- Coordinate with a WOCN to select the best dressing that promotes an optimal environment for healing. *Promotes high quality care to protect new tissue and allow for wound healing.*
- Cleanse the sacral pressure injury with normal saline; remove existing dressing and allow for wound healing. *Decreases the risk of infection and promotes an environment of moist wound healing.*

3. Nursing Safety Priority: Action Alert!

- Change synthetic dressings when exudate causes the adhesive seal to break and leakage to occur. *Prevents skin maceration around the wound.*

4. Assessing for Infection and Inflammation

- Monitor for signs of infection (cellulitis, progressive increase in ulcer size or depth, changes in quantity and quality of exudate) and systemic signs of bacteremia (fever, elevated WBC count). *Helps prevent the slowing or stopping of wound healing.*
- Inspect wound margins for cellulitis. *Identifies signs of inflammation extending beyond area of injury which can indicate infection.*
- Use Standard Precautions to care for wounds and dispose of soiled dressings and linens. *Maintains a safe environment to help prevent wound infection and transmission to others.*

5. Reducing Mechanical Forces

- Obtain pressure reduction devices. *Protects against the mechanical forces of pressure, shear, friction, and moisture.*
- Perform daily inspection of the skin, especially bony prominences, skin folds, and perineal area for redness, maceration, or skin breakdown. *Prevents or minimizes mechanical forces that impair TISSUE INTEGRITY.*
- Keep skin clean and dry. *Excessive skin moisture, or urinary or fecal incontinence increases the risk for skin damage and macerates skin.*
- Wash skin with pH-balanced soap, use alcohol-free creams or lotions to lubricate skin, use barrier ointments with incontinence, and change absorbent pads or garments immediately. *Incontinence results in prolonged contact of the skin with irritating substances, destroys TISSUE INTEGRITY, and predisposes to skin breakdown.*

6. Nursing Safety Priority: Action Alert!

- Teach all interprofessional personnel and family members not to massage reddened skin areas directly. Use donut-shaped pillows for pressure relief. *Prevents damage to capillary beds and decreases risk of tissue necrosis.*

7. Interpreting Lab Values

- Evaluate WBCs, prealbumin, albumin, and total protein levels. *Indicates signs of infection and protein malnutrition which makes tissue prone to breakdown and delays healing.*

EXPECTED OUTCOMES

Restoration of TISSUE INTEGRITY - demonstrate progress to complete wound healing and no new development of pressure injuries (evidence of granulation tissue, decreased wound size, absence of new pressure injuries).

Prevent infection, inflammation and wound deterioration - remain free of wound infection or systemic sepsis (indicators: WBC within normal range, negative blood cultures, no purulent drainage, decrease in wound size or depth, and absence of fever).

Planning

PATIENT PROBLEMS

Compromised TISSUE INTEGRITY related to vascular insufficiency and deep tissue trauma.
Potential for wound deterioration related to insufficient wound management

Interpretation of Data

- Prolonged bedrest
- Immobility
- Incontinence
- Inadequate nutrition and dehydration
- Altered mental status (decreased sensory perception, cognitive problems)
- Diabetes mellitus
- Peripheral vascular disease

Risk Factors

Data Analysis Interpretation

NOTICE IN THE HISTORY

Older adult Tom McKnight has had a loss of tissue integrity and has developed a stage 3 sacral pressure injury (PI) and bilateral stage 1 heel pressure injuries. These pressure injuries are due to significant postoperative perfusion issues from cardiac surgery and resulting immobility.

NOTICING—Physical Assessment

- T 100° F; P 92; R 20; BP 130/80
- Stage 3 sacral PI (moderate drainage, no necrotic tissue, red base)
- Stage 1 bilateral heels
- Midsternal chest incision–wound edges approximated, slight redness, tender to touch, no drainage
- Labs - WBC 12,000; albumin 3.0; prealbumin 12 mg/dL

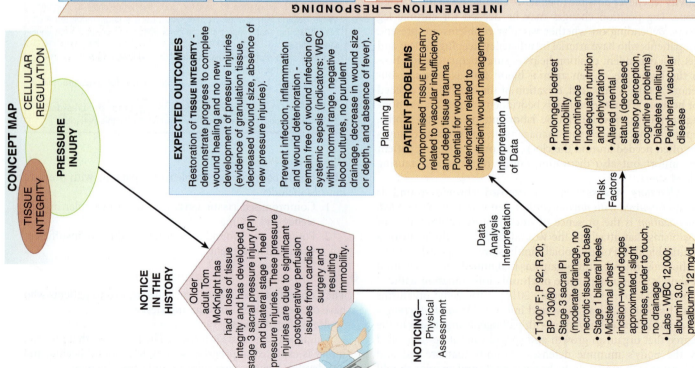

Concept Map by Deanne A. Blach, MSN, RN

- Presence of granulation, re-epithelialization, and scar tissue formation
- Decreased wound size
- Absence of new pressure injuries

Interventions. Wound care for pressure injuries varies according to each patient's needs and the health care provider's preferences. Surgery may be indicated for some patients, whereas a nonsurgical approach to ulcer débridement is preferred for a patient who has adequate defenses but is too ill or debilitated for surgery.

Nonsurgical Management. General interventions for wound management of pressure injuries are listed in Chart 25-3. Nonsurgical intervention of pressure injuries is often left to the discretion of the nurse, who coordinates with the primary health care provider and certified wound care specialist (if available) to select an appropriate method of wound dressing and management. Many agencies have guidelines for wound dressings based on wound size and depth and presence of drainage.

Dressings. A well-designed dressing helps healing by removing surface debris, protecting exposed healthy tissues, and creating a barrier until the ulcer is closed. *For a draining, necrotic ulcer, the dressing must also remove excessive exudate and loose debris without damaging healthy epithelial cells or new granulation tissue. Extensive necrosis and thick eschar require sharp surgical or chemical removal before débridement with dressings can be effective.* Different dressing materials help remove debris by mechanical débridement (mechanical entrapment and detachment of dead tissue), topical chemical débridement (topical enzyme preparations to loosen necrotic tissue), or natural chemical débridement (promoting self-digestion of dead tissues by naturally occurring bacterial enzymes [autolysis]) (Table 25-2).

After all the dead tissue has been removed, protection of exposed healthy tissues is critical to pressure injury care. The ideal healing environment is a clean, *slightly* moist ulcer surface with minimal bacterial colonization as evidenced by the absence of a wound biofilm, a shiny gel-like film on the surface of the wound. Heavy moisture from an excessively draining ulcer or a dressing that is too wet promotes the growth of organisms and causes maceration (mushiness) of healthy tissue. Likewise, if a clean ulcer surface is exposed to air or if highly absorbent dressing materials are used for prolonged periods, overdrying can dehydrate surface cells, form scabs, and convert the wound to a deeper injury. The right balance of moisture is the key to maintaining a healing environment. The type of dressing should change as wound features change with healing (Ayello & Baranoski, 2014; Krasner et al., 2014).

Assess the ulcer for necrotic tissue and amount of exudate. Coordinate with a wound care specialist to select a dressing material that promotes an optimal environment for healing. For example, a material that does not stick to the wound surface and does not remove new epithelial cells when it is changed is used for protecting new tissue. Depending on the amount of drainage, select either a hydrophobic or a hydrophilic material:

- A hydrophobic (nonabsorbent, waterproof) material is useful when the wound has little drainage and needs to be protected from external contamination.
- A hydrophilic (absorbent) material draws excessive drainage away from the injury surface, preventing maceration.

A variety of synthetic materials with different absorbent and antimicrobial properties are available. Unlike cotton gauze dressings, these may be left intact for extended periods. Biologic and synthetic skin substitutes are the newest materials being researched. Although useful, these "smart" dressings may be cost prohibitive for many patients.

The frequency of dressing changes depends on the amount of necrotic material or exudate. Dry gauze dressings are changed when "strike through" occurs (i.e., when the outer layer of the dressing first becomes saturated with exudate). Gauze dressings

---

⊚ **CHART 25-3** **Best Practice for Patient Safety & Quality Care** QSEN

Wound Management of Pressure Injuries

- If injury is covered, change dressing according to manufacturer's instructions, when dressing seal is compromised, when drainage is visible on the outer layer (gauze), or when the dressing becomes contaminated with body fluids.
- Measure wound size at greatest length and width using a disposable paper tape measure or, for asymmetric injuries, by tracing the wound onto a piece of plastic film or sheeting (plastic template) at least weekly or more often if the wound shows signs of deterioration.
- Compare all subsequent measurements against the initial measurement.
- Assess the injury for presence of necrotic tissue and amount of exudate.
- Assess and document the condition of the skin surrounding the pressure injury in terms of color, temperature, texture, moisture, and appearance.
- Remove or trim loose bits of tissue (may be done by a certified wound care specialist, physical therapist, advanced practice nurse, or other as specified by the agency and the state nurse practice act).
- Cleanse the injury with saline, nontoxic wound cleanser or a prescribed solution (after diluting it per manufacturer's directions or prescriber's instructions).
- Rinse and dry the injury surface.
- In collaboration with the certified wound care specialist, select and apply the dressing materials most appropriate for the volume of wound drainage.
- If possible, avoid positioning the patient on the pressure injury.
- Re-position frequently to prevent injury extension or generation of additional pressure injuries.
- Use prescribed pressure redistribution devices and techniques as described in Chart 27-2.

TABLE 25-2 **Common Dressing Techniques for Wound Débridement**

TECHNIQUE	MECHANISM OF ACTION
Wet-to-damp saline-moistened gauze	As with the wet-to-dry technique, necrotic debris is mechanically removed but with less trauma to healing tissue.
Continuous wet gauze	The wound surface is continually bathed with a wetting agent of choice, promoting dilution of viscous exudate and softening of dry eschar.
Topical enzyme preparations	Proteolytic action on thick, adherent eschar causes breakdown of denatured protein and more rapid separation of necrotic tissue.
Moisture-retentive dressing	Spontaneous separation of necrotic tissue is promoted by autolysis.

used for débridement of a wet wound (allowed to become damp and then removed) are changed often enough to take off any loose debris or exudate, usually every 4 to 6 hours.

> ### ⚠ NURSING SAFETY PRIORITY QSEN
> #### Action Alert
>
> Change synthetic dressings when exudate causes the adhesive seal to break and leakage to occur.

Before reapplying any dressing, gently clean the ulcer surface with saline or another wound cleanser as prescribed. If an antibacterial cleanser is prescribed, dilute the agent to reduce tissue toxicity and then rinse with tap water and dry the surface before applying the dressing.

Physical Therapy. Physical therapists are a valuable resource on the wound care team. Consult them to help plan and implement therapeutic strategies to redistribute and off-load pressure, maximize overall function, and improve quality of life for patients with chronic wounds. In addition to recommending assistive devices and facilitating ADLs, physical therapists typically administer modalities to promote healing, such as electrical stimulation and ultrasound (Aviles, 2014).

Drug Therapy. Clean, healthy granulation tissue has a blood supply and is capable of providing white blood cells and antibodies to the ulcer to combat infection. If extensive necrosis is present or if local tissue defenses are impaired, topical antibacterial agents or dressing materials are often needed to control bacterial growth (see Chart 26-5 for a list of topical antibacterial agents). Antibiotic use is avoided in the absence of infection to reduce the development of resistant bacterial strains.

Nutrition Therapy. Successful healing of pressure injuries depends on adequate intake of calories, protein, vitamins, minerals, and water. Nutrition deficiencies are common among chronically ill patients and increase the risk for skin breakdown and delayed wound healing. Severe protein deficiency inhibits healing and impairs host infection defenses.

Coordinate with the dietitian to help the patient eat a well-balanced diet, emphasizing protein, vegetables, fruits, whole grains, and vitamins. Fats also are needed to ensure formation of cell membranes. (See Chapter 60 for interventions to ensure adequate nutrition.) If the patient cannot eat sufficient amounts of food, other types of feedings may be needed to increase protein and caloric intake (see Chapter 60). Vitamin and mineral supplements are also indicated.

Technology-Based Therapies. For chronic injuries that remain open for months, new technologies have had some success. These include electrical stimulation, negative-pressure wound therapy, hyperbaric oxygen therapy, low-frequency ultrasound, topical growth factors, and skin substitutes.

Electrical stimulation is the application of a low-voltage current to a wound area to increase blood vessel growth and promote granulation. This treatment is usually performed by a physical therapist or certified wound care specialist. The voltage is delivered in "pulses" that may cause a "tingling" sensation. Usually this technique is performed for 1 hour a day, 5 to 7 days a week. It is not used with patients who have a pacemaker, a wound over the heart, or a skin cancer involving the wound or periwound skin.

Negative-pressure wound therapy (NPWT) can reduce or even close chronic injuries by removing fluids or infectious materials from the wound and enhancing granulation. This technique requires that a suction tube be covered by a special sponge and sealed in place. Per manufacturer's instructions, the foam dressing is changed every 48 to 72 hours (or at least three times weekly). Continuous low-level negative pressure is applied through the suction tube. Duration of the treatment is determined by the wound's response. It should not be used in areas of skin cancer. Failure of NPWT is often caused by the inability to maintain an adequate dressing seal (Rock, 2014).

Current evidence does not support greater effectiveness of NPWT in closing chronic wounds than more traditional methods. Serious bleeding and even deaths have occurred with NPWT, and these devices have received a warning from the Food and Drug Administration (FDA) to exclude high-risk patients from its use. Any patient who is receiving this therapy must be monitored at least every 2 hours for bleeding at or near the wound site.

> ### ⚠ NURSING SAFETY PRIORITY QSEN
> #### Critical Rescue
>
> Recognize that you do not use a continuous negative-pressure wound therapy device with any patient who is on anticoagulant therapy; has reduced tissue health near the wound (e.g., with radiation therapy or poor nutrition); or has any exposed blood vessels, nerves, or organs in the wound area. Respond by consulting with members of the interprofessional team, such as the primary health care provider and wound nurse, for appropriate methods of treatment.

Hyperbaric oxygen therapy (HBOT) is the administration of oxygen under high pressure, raising the tissue oxygen concentration. This type of therapy is usually reserved for life- or limb-threatening wounds such as burns, necrotizing infections, brown recluse spider bites, osteomyelitis, and diabetic ulcers. The patient is enclosed in a large chamber and exposed to 100% oxygen at pressures greater than normal atmospheric pressure. Systemic oxygen enhances the ability of white blood cells to kill bacteria and reduce swelling. Treatment usually lasts from 60 to 90 minutes. Smaller topical oxygen-delivery devices are also available. These devices are applied directly over an open wound to promote local tissue gas exchange; however, their effectiveness in promoting wound healing requires further study.

Topical growth factors are normal body substances that stimulate cell movement and growth. These factors are deficient in chronic wounds, and topical application is used to stimulate wound healing. For example, platelet-derived growth factor (PDGF) stimulates the movement of fibroblasts into the wound space. Use of this and other growth factors has been effective for healing of some clean granulating chronic wounds, but further study is needed (Cowan et al., 2014).

Skin substitutes are engineered products that aid in the closure of different types of wounds. These products vary widely in design and application and are used mainly for surgically débrided wounds before reconstruction with grafts or muscle flaps (Daugherty & Spear, 2015).

Ultrasound-assisted wound therapy (USWT) uses energy produced by low frequency (40 kHz) sound waves to cleanse and débride necrotic tissue over time, thus reducing microbial bioburden. USWT is administered with a disposable applicator, which is moved over the wound without coming in direct contact with tissue. Atomized saline mist serves as a conduit for delivery of the ultrasound energy. Additional benefits of non-contact low-frequency ultrasound therapy may include pain reduction, stimulation of granulation, and reduced rates of infection (Hakim & Heitzman, 2013).

The use of exogenous *electrical stimulation* (ES) has been shown to promote healing of chronic wounds that are stalled in the healing process. ES works by restoring the natural electric impulses found in healthy tissue and promoting more normal cellular function. Potential benefits include increased fibroblast activity to stimulate granulation, increased epithelial cell migration, enhanced macrophage activity, and reduced pain. Since electrical stimulation can also increase the activity of cancer cells, contraindications for use include basal or squamous cell carcinoma in the wound or periwound tissues or melanoma.

Surgical Management. Surgical management of a pressure injury includes removal of necrotic tissue and skin grafting or use of muscle flaps to close wounds that do not heal by re-epithelialization and contraction. Not all wounds are candidates for grafting. Those with poor blood flow are unlikely to have successful graft take and heal. The procedures are very similar to the surgical management of burn wounds. See the Surgical Interventions section of Managing Wound Care in Chapter 26.

Preventing Infection and Wound Deterioration

Planning: Expected Outcomes. The patient with a pressure injury is expected to remain free of wound infection or sepsis. Indicators include that the patient will have mild or no:

- White blood cell (WBC) elevation
- Positive blood culture
- Purulent or malodorous drainage
- Increase in wound size or depth
- Fever

Interventions. Priority nursing interventions focus on preventing wound infection and identifying it early to prevent complications.

Monitoring the ulcer's appearance using objective criteria allows evaluation of the response to treatment and early recognition of infection. If an ulcer shows no progress toward healing within 7 to 10 days or worsens, the treatment plan is re-evaluated. Chart 25-4 outlines objectives of monitoring wounds with and without tissue loss. Patients who are at highest risk for infection are those who are older, have diabetes, have WBC disorders, are receiving steroid therapy, or have wounds with a compromised blood supply.

Preventing infection and its complications starts with monitoring the ulcer's progress. Routinely check for signs and symptoms of wound infection: increased pain, tenderness, and redness at the wound margins, edema, and purulent and malodorous drainage. Report these changes to the primary health care provider:

- Sudden deterioration of the ulcer, with an increase in the size or depth of the lesion
- Changes in the color or texture of the granulation tissue
- Changes in the quantity, color, or odor of exudate

These changes may occur with or without signs and symptoms of bacteremia, such as fever, an elevated WBC count, and positive blood cultures. Use the previously described interventions to prevent the formation of new pressure injuries and to prevent early-stage injuries from progressing to deeper wounds (see Chart 25-1).

Maintaining a safe environment can help prevent wound infection. Because of the variety of organisms in the hospital environment, keeping an ulcer totally free of bacteria is impossible. Optimal ulcer management is based on maintaining acceptably low levels of organisms through meticulous wound care and reducing contamination with pathogenic organisms that could lead to sepsis and death. *Teach all personnel to use Standard Precautions and to properly dispose of soiled dressings and linens.*

❓ CLINICAL JUDGMENT CHALLENGE 25-2

Patient-Centered Care; Teamwork and Collaboration QSEN

An unlicensed assistive personnel (UAP) reports to you that an 86-year-old resident of the nursing home has what appears to be a large early-stage pressure injury over her "bum." Skin changes are evident on the buttocks, inner upper thighs, and labia. The patient has hemiparesis and urinary incontinence from a series of strokes and wears adult diapers for continence care. When you assess the client, you find the whole area to be bright red with a few small blisters on the very edges and an area on her upper, outer thigh to be brown and peeling. The reddened area appears slightly edematous and blanches when you touch it, and the client tells you that her "bum hurts and burns." The UAP asks whether the physical therapist should be called to obtain an air cushion to prevent the pressure injury from getting worse.

1. What is the most likely cause of the patient's skin problems?
2. Does this skin problem meet the criteria of any stage of pressure injury? Explain your rationale.
3. Should the physical therapist be asked to order a pressure-relieving device for the patient's wheelchair? Provide a rationale for your answer.
4. Which interventions are most likely to address this patient's skin problems?
5. Which other interprofessional team members would be helpful for this situation?

Care Coordination and Transition Management

Patients with pressure injuries may be in acute care, subacute care, long-term care, or home care settings. If pressure injury therapy requires hospitalization, most patients are discharged before complete wound closure is achieved. Discharge may be to the home setting or to a long-term care facility, depending on the degree of debilitation and other patient factors.

Home Care Management. Ulcer care in the patient's home is similar to care in the hospital. Most dressing supplies and pressure-relief devices can be obtained at a pharmacy or medical supply store. If ulcer débridement is needed, a handheld shower device or forceful irrigation of the wound with a 35-mL syringe and 19-gauge angiocatheter can be substituted for whirlpool therapy.

Many patients cannot change their own dressings because of wound location, distress over an altered body image, or the pain of dressing removal. Others depend on family members or support personnel because of limited physical mobility.

For some patients, drastic changes in daily activities are needed to promote healing. Patients with leg ulcers may need frequent rest periods with leg elevation to avoid or reduce edema. Immobile patients with pressure injuries require around-the-clock repositioning to prevent further breakdown, which takes its toll on caregivers. Explain the rationale for activity changes to the patient and family and explore ways of coping with these changes.

Some patients may need to continue the use of special beds or mattress overlays at home. Although these items can be expensive, home use can keep the patient out of more costly

⊚ CHART 25-4 Best Practice for Patient Safety & Quality Care QSEN

Monitoring the Wound

VARIABLE	FREQUENCY OF ASSESSMENT	RATIONALE
Wounds Without Tissue Loss		
Examples		
Surgical incisions and clean lacerations closed primarily by sutures or staples		
Observations (Using First Postoperative Dressing Change as Baseline)		
Check for the presence or absence of increased: • Localized tenderness • Swelling of the incision line • Erythema of the incision line >1 cm on each side of wound • Localized heat	At least every 24 hr until sutures or staples are removed	To detect cellulitis (bacterial infections)*
Check for the presence or absence of: • Purulent drainage from any portion of the incision site • Localized fluctuance (from fluid accumulation) and tenderness beneath a *portion* of the wound when palpated	At least every 24 hr until sutures or staples are removed	To detect abscess formation related to presence of foreign body (suture material) or deeper wound infection*
Check for the presence or absence of: • Approximation (sealing) of wound edges with or without serosanguineous drainage • Necrosis of skin edges	At least every 24 hr until sutures or staples are removed	To detect potential for wound dehiscence
Wounds With Tissue Loss		
Examples		
Partial- or full-thickness skin loss caused by pressure necrosis, vascular disease, trauma, etc., and allowed to heal by secondary intention		
Observations		
Wound Size		
Measure wound size at greatest length and width using a disposable paper tape measure or, for asymmetric ulcers, by tracing the wound onto a piece of plastic film or sheeting (plastic template) Measure depth of full-thickness wounds using cotton-tipped applicator Compare all subsequent measurements against the initial measurement	Once per week	To detect increase in wound size and depth secondary to infectious process (Expect an increase in wound size after débridement of necrotic tissue in deep wounds.)
Ulcer Base		
Check for the presence or absence of: • Necrotic tissue (loose or adherent) • Foul odor from wound when dressing is changed Note the frequency of dressing changes or dressing reinforcements owing to drainage	At least every 24 hr	To detect the need for débridement or the response to treatment (necrotic tissue) and to detect local wound infection (frequent dressing changes and foul odor)
Wound Margins		
Check for the presence or absence of: • Erythema and swelling extending outward >1 cm from wound margins • Increased tenderness at wound margins	At least every 24 hr or at each dressing change	To detect wound infection*
Systemic Response		
Check for the presence or absence of elevated body temperature or WBCs or positive blood culture	Check temperature daily; if elevated, check WBCs and blood culture	To detect bacteremia

WBCs, White blood cells.

*The wounds of patients who are severely immunosuppressed or wounds with compromised blood supply may not exhibit a typical inflammatory response to local wound infection.

health care settings. Consider both the space and power supply when choosing a pressure-relief device for home use. Coordinate with the case manager to work with the insurance company in providing these important aids for quality patient care.

Self-Management Education. Before the patient is discharged, have the patient or caregiver demonstrate competence in removing the dressing, cleaning the wound, and applying the dressing. When choosing a dressing to be used at home, consider the patient's or caregiver's ability to apply the dressing properly. If the patient's finances are limited, address the cost of the dressing material. At times, the more expensive dressing

materials that require less frequent changing may be preferred. Explain the signs and symptoms of wound infection and remind the patient and family to report their presence to the primary health care provider or wound care clinic.

Encourage the patient to eat a balanced diet, including high-protein snacks. Discuss diet preferences with the patient and consult a dietitian as needed to design a food plan to promote wound healing. Vitamin and mineral supplements may be needed to prevent or treat deficiencies.

If the patient is incontinent, emphasize the need to keep the skin clean and dry. If bowel and bladder training are not possible, discuss the use of absorbent underpads, briefs, and topical moisture barrier creams and ointments as methods to reduce skin exposure to urine and feces.

Health Care Resources. A home health nurse may be needed to follow wound progress after discharge. As indicated by The Joint Commission's NPSGs, the hospital nurse provides details of ulcer size and appearance and any special wound care needs in a hand-off report to the home care nurse, who can then accurately judge changes in ulcer appearance. Chart 25-5 is a guideline for a focused assessment of the patient with risk for pressure injuries.

To help decrease the cost of treatment, emphasize proper use of dressing materials. Clean tap water and nonsterile supplies are used for home management of chronic wounds and are less costly than sterile products. Stress the importance of properly cleaning reused items and of handwashing before touching any supplies.

CHART 25-5 Focused Assessment

The Patient at Risk for Pressure Injuries

Assess cardiovascular status:
- Presence or absence of peripheral edema
- Hand-vein filling in the dependent position
- Neck-vein filling in the recumbent and sitting positions
- Weight gain or loss

Assess cognition and mental status:
- Level of consciousness
- Orientation to time, place, and person
- Can the patient accurately read a seven-word sentence containing words of three syllables or fewer?

Assess condition of skin:
- Assess general skin cleanliness
- Observe all skin areas, paying particular attention to bony prominences and areas in greatest contact with the bed and other firm surfaces
- Measure and record any areas of redness or loss of integrity
- If possible, photograph areas of concern
- Note the presence or absence of skin tenting over the sternum or the forehead
- Note the moistness of skin and mucous membranes
- If wounds are present, remove dressings (noting condition of dressings), cleanse the wound, and compare with previous notations of wound condition:
  - Presence, amount, and nature of exudate
  - Use a disposable paper tape measure to measure wound diameter and depth
  - Amount (%) and type of necrotic tissue
  - Presence of granulation/epithelium
  - Presence or absence of cellulitis
  - Presence or absence of odor
  - Take patient's temperature to assess for fever

Assess the patient's understanding of illness and compliance with treatment:
- Signs and symptoms to report to primary health care provider
- Drug therapy plan (correct timing and dose)
- Ambulation or positioning schedule
- Dressing changes/skin care
- Nutrition modifications (24-hr diet recall)

Assess the patient's nutritional status:
- Change in muscle mass
- Lackluster nails, sparse hair
- Recent weight loss of more than 5% of usual weight
- Impaired oral intake
- Difficulty swallowing
- Generalized edema

The patient with activity restrictions may need daily assistance from a home health aide. Collaborate with a physical therapist or occupational therapist to help the patient and family continue rehabilitation efforts in the home.

◆ Evaluation: Reflecting

Evaluate the care of the patient with a pressure injury on the basis of the identified priority patient problems. The expected outcomes include that the patient will:
- Experience progress toward wound healing by second intention as evidenced by granulation, epithelialization, contraction, and reduction or resolution of wound size
- Re-establish skin TISSUE INTEGRITY and restore skin barrier function
- Remain infection free

MINOR SKIN IRRITATIONS

PRURITUS

❖ PATHOPHYSIOLOGY

Irritation of the skin is often associated with **pruritus** (itching), a distressing and often debilitating condition caused by stimulation of itch-specific nerve fibers. Physical or chemical agents either activate nerve fibers directly or stimulate the release of chemical mediators (i.e., histamine), which then act on itch receptors.

Itching can be localized or generalized and occur with or without a skin rash. It is estimated that over 50% of elderly patients have **xerosis** (dry skin), a condition often described generalized discomfort in the absence of skin lesions. Comorbid medical conditions such as diabetes can also lead to generalized pruritus. Certain localized pruritic skin diseases are more common among the older population, including scabies and bullous pemphigoid.

Itching is a subjective condition similar to pain, and severity of the sensation varies among patients. Regardless of the cause, patients often report that itching is worse at night when there are fewer distractions. Other conditions that make itching worse include skin dryness, increased temperature, perspiration, and emotional stress.

❖ INTERPROFESSIONAL COLLABORATIVE CARE

Care of the patient with minor skin irritations usually takes place in the outpatient setting. Members of the interprofessional team who collaborate most closely to care for this patient include the primary health care provider, who continually assesses the skin condition and prescribes treatment, and the nurse.

The priority nursing interventions focus on increasing patient comfort and preventing skin injury with loss of TISSUE INTEGRITY. Patients usually try to relieve itching by scratching or rubbing the skin, a response that further stimulates the itch receptors and causes the *"itch-scratch-itch" cycle* (McCance et al., 2014). Itching with skin lesions can often be relieved by treating the underlying skin disorder with topical or systemic drugs. Systemic diseases, such as liver and venous disorders, can also cause itching without skin lesions. Liver disease often increases the buildup of bilirubin in the skin, which stimulates itch receptors. Pruritus can also be caused by too little or too much blood flow to an area (especially the feet and legs).

CHART 25-6   Patient and Family Education: Preparing for Self-Management

Prevention of Dry Skin

- Use a room humidifier during the winter months or whenever the furnace is in use.
- Take a complete bath or shower only every other day (wash face, axillae, perineum, and any soiled areas with soap daily).
- Use tepid water.
- Use a superfatted, nonalkaline soap instead of deodorant soap.
- Rinse the soap thoroughly from your skin.
- If you like bath oil, add the oil to the water at the end of the bath.
- Take care to avoid falls; oil makes the tub slippery.
- Pat rather than rub skin surfaces dry.
- Avoid clothing that continuously rubs the skin, such as tight belts, nylon stockings, or pantyhose.
- Maintain a daily fluid intake of 3000 mL unless contraindicated for another medical condition.
- Do not apply rubbing alcohol, astringents, or other drying agents to the skin.
- Avoid caffeine and alcohol ingestion.

Plan care to promote comfort and prevent disruption of skin tissue integrity from vigorous scratching. Because dry skin worsens itching, emphasize interventions to prevent it (Chart 25-6). Encourage patients to keep the fingernails trimmed short, with rough edges filed to reduce damage from scratching and secondary infection. Wearing mittens or splints at night can help prevent scratching during sleep. If the patient cannot perform self-care, teach the family (for home care) and unlicensed assistive personnel (UAP) to trim the patient's fingernails and apply mittens or gloves. Stress the importance of not breaking the skin or digging into nail corners when trimming the nails of patients with diabetes.

A cool sleeping environment and comfort measures (e.g., cool shower, moisturizers) may help promote sleep. Using sleep-promoting herbal teas or sedating antihistamines at bedtime (when the side effect of drowsiness is welcome) may provide an uninterrupted night's sleep for some patients. Colloidal oatmeal or tar extract baths provide temporary relief.

If antihistamines are prescribed, monitor the patient's response so the dosage can be adjusted as needed. The effectiveness of topical steroid preparations and other topical agents is improved if the drug is applied to slightly damp skin. Using topical drugs under an occlusive dressing increases the dose being delivered. Avoid occluding treated areas unless specifically prescribed by the primary health care provider.

URTICARIA

Urticaria (hives) is a rash of white or red edematous papules or plaques of various sizes. This problem is usually caused by exposure to allergens, which releases histamine into the skin. Blood vessel dilation and plasma protein leakage lead to formation of lesions or wheals. Some common causes of urticaria include drugs, temperature extremes, foods, infection, diseases, cancer, and insect bites.

Management focuses on removal of the triggering substance and relief of symptoms. Because the skin reaction is caused by histamine release, antihistamines such as diphenhydramine (Benadryl) are helpful. Teach the patient to avoid overexertion, alcohol consumption, and warm environments, which further dilate blood vessels and make urticaria worse. Alcohol increases sedating effect of antihistamines, increasing the risk for falls.

COMMON INFLAMMATIONS

❖ PATHOPHYSIOLOGY

Skin inflammation can have many nonspecific signs and symptoms, including severe itching, lesions with indistinct borders, and different distribution patterns. The cause may not be identified. Rashes from inflammation can evolve from acute to chronic conditions.

Most skin inflammations are related to allergic immune responses. The responses may be triggered by external skin exposure to allergens or internal exposure to allergens and irritants. The result is tissue destruction or skin changes induced by the immune system. (A more detailed description of these immune mechanisms is presented in Chapter 17.)

The specific cause of skin inflammation is not always known. When this is the case, the catch-all diagnosis of *nonspecific eczematous dermatitis,* or *eczema,* is often used.

Contact dermatitis is an acute or chronic rash caused by direct contact with either an irritant or an allergen. Irritants cause a toxic injury to the skin. Allergens result in a cell-mediated immune reaction in the skin.

Atopic dermatitis is a chronic rash that occurs with allergies and atopic skin disease. It is made worse by dry or irritated skin, food allergies, chemicals, or stress. (Atopic reactions are described in Chapter 20.)

❖ INTERPROFESSIONAL COLLABORATIVE CARE

Because all skin eruptions from inflammation appear similar, personal data are needed to identify the cause. Inflammatory skin problems differ from eczematous dermatitis in chronicity, lesion distribution, and associated signs and symptoms. Chart 25-7 lists the symptoms of many types of inflammatory skin conditions.

If the cause of the rash is identified, avoidance therapy is used to reverse the reaction and clear the rash. For example, if a new soap for handwashing causes contact dermatitis of the hands, teach the patient to avoid that substance. Even when the cause is unclear, certain irritants may worsen the rash and increase discomfort. Additional interventions promote comfort through suppression of inflammation.

Steroid therapy with topical, intralesional, or systemic steroids is prescribed to suppress inflammation. Because a side effect of oral corticosteroids (e.g., prednisone) is adrenal suppression, patients receiving long-term systemic therapy must taper their drug dosages rather than stop them abruptly.

Remember that corticosteroids never cure the inflammation. During active disease, these drugs reduce symptoms and relieve discomfort. Moisten dressings with warm tap water and place them over topical steroids for short periods to increase absorption. Avoid applying topical steroids under occlusive dressings unless prescribed by the primary health care provider.

Avoid applying oil-based ointments and pastes to the sweaty skinfold areas to prevent blocking of pores and folliculitis. Water-soluble creams are better for these areas. Lotions and gels prevent matting of the hair and are more appropriate for the scalp and other hairy areas. Thick, stiff ointments or pastes (e.g., zinc oxide pastes) are applied to localized areas because they

CHART 25-7 Key Features
Common Inflammatory Skin Conditions

SIGNS AND SYMPTOMS	DISTRIBUTION
Nonspecific Eczematous Dermatitis	
Evolution of lesions from vesicles to weeping papules and plaques. Lichenification occurs in chronic disease.	Anywhere on the body; localized eczema commonly involves the hands or feet
Oozing, crusting, fissuring, excoriation, or scaling may be present.	
Itching is common.	
Contact Dermatitis	
Localized eczematous eruption with well-defined, geometric margins that are consistent with contact by an irritant or allergen.	Cosmetic/perfume allergy: head and neck
Usually seen in the acute form but may become chronic if exposure is repeated.	Hair product allergy: scalp Shoe/rubber allergy: dorsum of feet
Allergy to plants (e.g., poison ivy or oak) classically occurs as linear streaks of vesicles or papules.	Nickel allergy: earlobes Mouthwash/toothpaste allergy: perioral region Airborne contact allergy (e.g., paint, ragweed): generalized
Atopic Dermatitis	
Hallmark in adults is lichenification with scaling and excoriation.	Face, neck, upper chest, and antecubital and popliteal fossae
Extremely itchy.	
Face involvement is seen as dry skin with mild-to-moderate erythema, perioral pallor, and skinfolds beneath the eyes (Dennie-Morgan lines).	
Associated with linear markings on the palms.	
Drug Eruption	
Bright red erythematous macules and papules are found. Skin blisters in extreme cases.	Generalized Involvement begins on trunk, proceeds distally (legs are the last to be involved)
Lesions tend to be confluent in large areas.	
Moderately itchy.	
Fever is rare.	
Dehydration and hypothermia can occur with extensive involvement.	
Condition clears only after offending drug has been discontinued.	

cling to the skin where applied and resist spreading to uninvolved skin.

Antihistamines provide some relief of itching but may not keep the patient totally comfortable. The sedative effects of these drugs may be better tolerated if most of the daily dose is taken near bedtime. Teach patients to avoid driving or operating heavy machinery if these drugs are taken during the day.

> ## ! NURSING SAFETY PRIORITY QSEN
> ### Drug Alert
>
> Polypharmacy combined with the sedating effects of H₁-antihistamines [diphenhydramine (Benadryl), carbinoxamine (Clistin), clemastine (Tavist), chlorpheniramine (Chlor-Trimeton), and brompheniramine (Dimetane)] place older adults at increased risk for falls.

Comfort measures such as cool, moist compresses and lukewarm baths with bath additives have a soothing effect, decrease inflammation, and help débride crusts and scales. Colloidal oatmeal, tar extracts, cornstarch, or oils added to baths may relieve itching.

PSORIASIS

❖ PATHOPHYSIOLOGY

Psoriasis is a chronic autoimmune disorder affecting the skin with exacerbations and remissions. It results from overstimulation of the immune system (Langerhans' cells) in the skin that activates T-lymphocytes. These cells then target the keratinocytes, causing increased cell division (because some degree of CELLULAR REGULATION is lost) and plaque formation. Even though psoriasis cannot be cured, patients can often achieve control of symptoms with proper management.

Psoriasis lesions are scaled with underlying dermal inflammation from an abnormality in the growth of epidermal cells. Normally basal cells take about 28 days to reach the outermost layer where they are shed. In a person with psoriasis, the rate of cell division is speeded up so cells are shed every 4 to 5 days.

> ## 🧬 GENETIC/GENOMIC CONSIDERATIONS
> ### Patient-Centered Care QSEN
>
> A genetic predisposition is associated with psoriasis as indicated by the fact that, when one identical (monozygotic) twin develops the disease, the second twin also develops it about 70% of the time. Variation in many gene sequences, labeled PSORS1 through PSORS13, influences the development of this autoimmune disorder. It is likely that different variations of these gene loci also influence individual patient responses to therapy. Always ask about a family history of the disorder when assessing the patient with psoriasis (OMIM, 2017).

Many environmental factors lead to outbreaks and influence the severity of symptoms, but these vary from person to person. Triggering factors may be local or systemic. A psoriatic lesion may appear after skin trauma (i.e., Koebner's phenomenon, in which a previously injured area is more susceptible to development of cancer or chronic skin problems) such as surgery, sunburn, or excoriation.

Patients with psoriasis often improve with more exposure to sunlight. Systemic factors that can aggravate the disease include infection (severe streptococcal throat infection, *Candida* infection, upper respiratory infections), hormonal changes (e.g., puberty, menopause), stress, drugs (lithium, beta-blocking agents, indomethacin), obesity, and the presence of other diseases.

Some patients with psoriasis also develop debilitating *psoriatic arthritis*. This arthritis may lead to severe joint changes similar to those seen in rheumatoid arthritis and indicates that psoriasis is a systemic disorder (McCance et al., 2014). See Chapter 18 for more discussion of arthritis.

❖ INTERPROFESSIONAL COLLABORATIVE CARE

Care of the patient with psoriasis most often takes place in an outpatient setting. When a patient with psoriasis is hospitalized for another health problem, psoriasis therapy may continue in this setting. Members of the interprofessional team who collaborate most closely to care for the patient with psoriasis include the primary health care provider, who continually assesses the patient's condition and prescribes treatment, and the nurse.

◆ Assessment: Noticing

History. Ask the patient about any family history of psoriasis, including the age at onset, a description of the disease progression, and the pattern of recurrences. Have the patient describe the current flare-up of psoriasis, including whether the onset was gradual or sudden, where the lesions first appeared, whether there have been any changes in severity over time, and whether fever and itching are present. Explore possible precipitating factors and ask about the effectiveness of any previous interventions.

Physical Assessment/Signs and Symptoms. The appearance of psoriasis and its course vary among patients. Typically during flare-ups of the disease, lesions thicken and extend into new body areas. As psoriasis responds to treatment, lesions become thinner with less scaling.

Psoriasis vulgaris is the most common type of psoriasis, with thick, reddened papules or plaques covered by silvery white scales (Fig. 25-4). Borders between the lesions and normal skin are sharply defined. Patches are less red and moister in skinfold areas. Lesions are usually present in the same areas on both sides of the body (bilateral distribution). Common sites include the scalp, elbows, trunk, knees, sacrum, and outside surfaces of the limbs. Facial skin is rarely affected. The patient may have only a few lesions, or the entire skin surface may be affected.

Exfoliative psoriasis (erythrodermic psoriasis) is an explosively eruptive and inflammatory form with generalized erythema and scaling but no obvious lesions. Fluid loss with this severe inflammatory reaction can lead to dehydration and hypothermia or hyperthermia.

Palmoplantar pustulosis (PPP) is a type of psoriasis that forms pustules on the palms of the hands and soles of the feet along with reddened hyperkeratotic plaques. The course of the disease is cyclic, with new outbreaks of pustules occurring after older lesions have resolved. PPP is difficult to treat, and patients often have social and physical problems.

◆ Planning and Implementation: Responding

The three different approaches to therapy are based on the extent of disease, the patient's distress, and the response of the

psoriasis to treatment. Patients must understand that no cure for psoriasis exists yet. Therapy is aimed at reducing cell proliferation and inflammation. *Priority nursing strategies include teaching the patient about the disease and its treatment and providing emotional support for the changes in body image often experienced with psoriasis.*

Topical Therapy. The topical agents used to treat moderate-to-severe psoriasis are topical steroids, topical tar and anthralin preparations, and ultraviolet (UV) light.

Corticosteroids have anti-inflammatory actions. When applied to psoriatic lesions, they suppress cell division. The effectiveness of a topical steroid depends on its potency and ability to be absorbed into the skin. The more potent agents are used as therapy for patients with psoriasis. Examples of commonly prescribed topical corticosteroids include clobetasol (Temovate, Dermovate ❖), triamcinolone (Aristocort, Triaderm ❖), fluocinolone (Synalar, Fluoderm ❖), and betamethasone (Diprolene).

Teach patients to enhance the skin penetration of these drugs by applying the steroid directly to the skin. When prescribed, using warm, moist dressings and an occlusive outer wrap of plastic (film, gloves, booties, or similar garments) may enhance absorption. Avoid using high potency steroids on the face, scalp, or skinfold areas because of the potential for increased absorption and side effects.

Tar preparations applied to the skin suppress cell division from impaired CELLULAR REGULATION and reduce inflammation. These drugs are available as solutions, ointments, lotions, gels, and shampoos. The ointments are messy, cause staining, and have an unpleasant odor.

Topical therapy with anthralin (Zithranol, Anthraforte ❖, Drithocreme, Psoriatec), a hydrocarbon similar in action to tar, also relieves chronic psoriasis. These drugs can be used alone or in combination with coal tar baths and ultraviolet (UV) light.

Teach the patient to apply the high-potency anthralin, suspended in a stiff paste, to each lesion for short periods of time as directed by the physician. The drug is a strong irritant and can cause chemical burns if left on lesions too long or not washed off completely after each treatment. Remind the patient to check for local tissue reaction and to take care to prevent this drug from coming into contact with uninvolved skin.

Other topical therapies can be effective for many patients with mild-to-moderate psoriasis. These drugs include calcipotriene

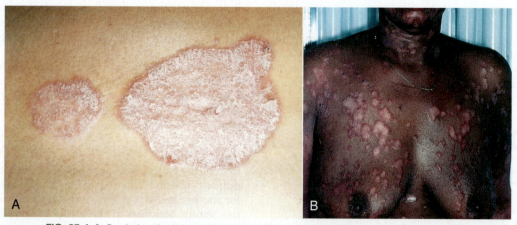

FIG. 25-4 A, Psoriasis vulgaris in a white patient. **B,** Psoriasis vulgaris in a patient with dark skin.

(Dovonex), a synthetic form of vitamin D that regulates skin cell division, and tazarotene (Avage, Tazorac), a derivative of vitamin A that slows cell division and reduces inflammatory responses. In some cases calcitriol (Vectical ointment) has been helpful but is very expensive.

! NURSING SAFETY PRIORITY QSEN
Drug Alert

Tazorac is **teratogenic** (can cause birth defects) even when used topically. Teach sexually active women of childbearing age using this drug to adhere to strict contraceptive measures.

Light Therapy. UV radiation is a physical agent commonly used as a topical therapy in many skin conditions, including psoriasis. Ultraviolet B (UVB) light, which produces more energy, is responsible for the obvious biologic effects of the sun such as burning. Although the sun is an inexpensive source of UV radiation, better availability and intensity control occur with the use of artificial light sources. These sources include lamps or cabinets containing UV tubes. *The use of commercial tanning beds is not recommended for the patient with psoriasis.*

UV therapy is limited by exposure time and effects on the surrounding normal skin. The time of exposure is gradually increased to achieve a mild suntan effect without burning or tenderness. The patient's skin pigmentation determines the exposure times. Because of the extremely high intensity of most artificial UVB light sources, therapy is measured in seconds of exposure, and patients must wear eye protection during treatment. Narrow-band UVB light therapy, although intense, can shorten the time to effectiveness and reduce the number of exposures needed to maintain the response.

Light therapy with lasers can be effective in controlling mild-to-moderate psoriasis. Laser sources, whether administered in a continuous or pulsed exposure, allow for better focus on the lesions and reduce exposure to the surrounding normal skin.

Teach patients to inspect the skin carefully each day for signs of overexposure. If tenderness on palpation occurs and severe erythema or blister formation develops, notify the primary health care provider before therapy is resumed.

Psoralen and ultraviolet A (UVA) (PUVA) therapy involves the ingestion of a photosensitizing agent (psoralen) 45 to 60 minutes before exposure to UVA light. Therapy sessions are limited to two or three times a week and are not given on consecutive days. Exposure is gradually increased until tanning occurs. Dosages are adjusted according to the erythema reaction of normal skin and the response of psoriatic lesions.

Teach the patient to check for redness with edema and tenderness. If these are present, treatment must be interrupted until they subside. Because psoralen is a strong photosensitizer, patients must wear dark glasses during treatment and for the rest of the day.

Systemic Therapy. Oral systemic agents are often prescribed when psoriasis fails to respond to topical treatment. Agents commonly used include acitretin (Soriatane), a vitamin A derivative, and apremilast (Otezla), a small molecule inhibitor that inhibits the spontaneous production of tumor necrosis factor alpha (TNF-α).

! NURSING SAFETY PRIORITY QSEN
Drug Alert

Both acitretin and bexarotene are teratogenic. Teach sexually active women of childbearing age using this drug to adhere to strict contraceptive measures.

A variety of biologic (immunomodulating) agents that alter the immune response and prevent overstimulation of keratinocytes from impaired CELLULAR REGULATION are now being used to manage moderate-to-severe plaque psoriasis. These agents may be prescribed when other drugs are not effective and when psoriatic arthritis is also present. Most of these drugs are given by IV infusion, IM injection, or subcutaneous injection. All of these agents induce some degree of immunosuppression, and patients are at an increased risk for serious infection.

! NURSING SAFETY PRIORITY QSEN
Drug Alert

Instruct patients to discontinue the biologic agent and notify the primary health care provider immediately if signs and symptoms of an active infection occur.

Biologics currently approved for the treatment of psoriasis are listed in Chart 25-8. These drugs should NOT be used by patients who are pregnant or breast-feeding.

Other less commonly used systemic drugs for the patient whose disease is resistant to topical therapy include methotrexate (Folex, Mexate), cyclosporine (Sandimmune), and azathioprine (Imuran). The many health risks associated with these therapies must be considered along with the potential benefits, especially in older adults.

Emotional Support. Often patients' self-esteem suffers because of the presence of skin lesions. Encourage the patient and family members to express their feelings about having an incurable skin problem that can alter appearance. Support groups for individuals with psoriasis are available in many communities. Urge patients and families to consider participating in these groups.

The use of touch takes on an added significance for patients with psoriasis. For example, shake the patient's hand during an introduction or place a hand on the patient's shoulder when explaining a procedure. *Do not wear gloves during these social interactions. Touch, more than any other gesture, communicates acceptance of the person and the skin problem.*

? NCLEX EXAMINATION CHALLENGE 25-1
Health Promotion and Maintenance

A 45-year-old client is receiving subcutaneous injections of a biologic therapy for plaque psoriasis. Which condition will the nurse **immediately** report to the health care provider?
A. Missed injection
B. Increased pruritus
C. Cough with fever
D. New plaques on leg

Chart 25-8   Common Examples of Drug Therapy

Plaque Psoriasis

DRUG	NURSING IMPLICATIONS
Adalimumab (Humira)	Given subcutaneously After loading dose given as two injections, maintenance dose given every other week starting week 1 after the loading dose for 16 weeks Black Box warning: active infections, risk of lymphomas/leukemias, tuberculosis
Etanercept (Enbrel)	Given subcutaneously Given twice weekly for 3 months Black Box warning: Should not be given to patients with hypersensitivity to product, latex needle cap, benzyl alcohol; can cause infection, lymphoma, neoplastic disease; patients on immunosuppressive therapy, corticosteroids, and/or methotrexate at greater risk
Infliximab (Remicade, Inflectra ✦)	Given IV Given at 0, 2, and 6 weeks; then every 8 weeks Black Box warning: infection, neoplastic disease, tuberculosis
Secukinumab (Cosentyx)	Given subcutaneously Given at weeks 0, 1, 2, 3, and 4, followed by maintenance dose every 4 weeks Although no Black Box warning, the nurse should monitor for signs of infection
Ustekinumab (Stelara)	Given subcutaneously Initial dose given, followed by a dose 4 weeks later and then every 12 weeks Although no Black Box warning, the nurse should monitor for signs of infection

SKIN INFECTIONS

❖ PATHOPHYSIOLOGY

Skin infection can be bacterial, viral, or fungal. Chart 25-9 lists key features and common locations of each type.

Bacterial Infections

Bacterial skin lesions usually start at the hair follicle, where bacteria easily collect and grow in the warm, moist environment. **Folliculitis** is a superficial infection involving only the upper part of the follicle and is often caused by *Staphylococcus*. The rash is raised and red and usually shows small pustules. **Furuncles** (boils) are also caused by *Staphylococcus*, but the infection is much deeper in the follicle (Fig. 25-5). This larger, inflamed, raised bump may or may not have a pustular "head" at its point. Cellulitis often occurs as a generalized infection with either *Staphylococcus* or *Streptococcus* and involves the deeper connective tissue.

Minor skin trauma usually occurs before the appearance of folliculitis and furuncles and may contribute to the development of cellulitis. Patients may spread the infection to other parts of their bodies by scratching or rubbing the skin. Furuncles most often occur in areas of heat and moisture, such as in the hair-bearing skinfold areas. Cellulitis can occur as a result of secondary bacterial infection of an open wound, or it may be unrelated to skin trauma.

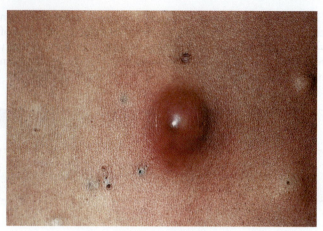

FIG. 25-5 A furuncle.

A common skin problem is infection with methicillin-resistance *Staphylococcus aureus* (MRSA). This infection can range from mild folliculitis to extensive furuncles. It is easily spread to other body areas and to other people by direct contact with infected skin and by contact with clothing, linens, athletic equipment, and other objects used by a person with MRSA. The infection does not respond to cleansing with antibacterial soaps or most types of topical and many oral antibiotic therapies. If MRSA infects a wound or enters the bloodstream, deep wound infection, sepsis, organ damage, and death can occur. The incidence is highest among adults living in communal environments, such as dormitories or prisons, and among patients in hospitals or other health care settings. (See Chapter 23 for a more detailed MRSA discussion.)

Cutaneous anthrax is an infection caused by the spores of the bacterium *Bacillus anthracis*. In the United States the most common risk factor is contact with an infected animal. Those most at risk for cutaneous anthrax include farm workers, veterinarians, and tannery and wool workers. This organism has now become a tool for terrorism.

! NURSING SAFETY PRIORITY QSEN
Action Alert

Consider the possibility of bioterrorism whenever lesions consistent with cutaneous anthrax appear in patients who do not have a history of exposure to infected animals.

The infection can be confined to the skin, or it may be systemic. At first a raised vesicle appears on an exposed body area such as the head or arms (Fig. 25-6). The lesion may itch and often resembles an insect bite. Within a few days, the center of the vesicle becomes hemorrhagic and sinks inward, starting an area of necrosis and ulceration. The tissue around the wound swells and can become very edematous. With necrosis, an eschar forms (see Fig. 25-6). The two features that distinguish anthrax lesions from insect bites or other skin lesions are that it is painless and that eschar forms, regardless of treatment. Patients may have only one lesion, or there may be multiple lesions, usually in the same body area.

Some patients develop systemic symptoms with cutaneous anthrax. The area becomes edematous and tender. Fever, chills,

CHART 25-9 Key Features

Common Skin Infections

SIGNS AND SYMPTOMS	DISTRIBUTION
Bacterial Infections	
Folliculitis	
Isolated erythematous pustules occur singly or in groups; hairs grow from centers of many of the lesions. Occasional papules are present. There is little or no associated discomfort. There is no residual scarring.	Areas of hair-bearing skin, especially buttocks, thighs, beard area, and scalp
Furuncle	
Small, tender, erythematous nodules become pus filled and more tender over time. Lesions may be single or multiple and also recurrent. Regional lymphadenopathy is sometimes present; fever is rare. Occasional scarring results.	Areas of hair-bearing skin, especially buttocks, thighs, abdomen, posterior neck regions, and axillae
Cellulitis	
Localized area of inflammation may enlarge rapidly if not treated. Redness, warmth, edema, tenderness, and pain are present. On rare occasions, blisters are present. Cellulitis is often accompanied by lymphadenopathy and fever.	Lower legs, areas of persistent lymphedema, and areas of skin trauma (e.g., leg ulcer, puncture wound)
Viral Infections	
Herpes Simplex	
Grouped vesicles are present on an erythematous base. Vesicles evolve to pustules, which rupture, weep, and crust. Older lesions may appear as punched-out, shallow erosions with well-defined borders. Lesions are associated with itching, stinging, or pain. Secondary bacterial infection with necrosis is possible in immunocompromised patients.	Type 1 classically on the face and type 2 on the genitalia, but either may develop in any area where inoculation has occurred; recurrent infections occur repeatedly in the same skin area
Herpes Zoster (Varicella Zoster)	
Lesions are similar in appearance to herpes simplex and also progress with weeping and crusting. Grouped lesions present unilaterally along a segment of skin following the pathway of a spinal or cranial nerve (dermatomal distribution). Eruption is preceded by deep pain and itching. Postherpetic neuralgia is common in older adults. Secondary infection with necrosis is possible in immunocompromised patients.	Anterior or posterior trunk following involved dermatome; face, sometimes involving trigeminal nerve and eye
Fungal Infections	
Dermatophytosis	
Annular or serpiginous patches are present with elevated borders, scaling, and central clearing. Itching is common. Lesions may be single or multiple.	Anywhere on the body
Candidiasis	
Erythematous macular eruption occurs with isolated pustules or papules at the border (satellite lesions). Candidiasis is associated with burning and itching. Oral lesions (thrush) appear as creamy white plaques on an inflamed mucous membrane. Cracks or fissures at the corners of the mouth may be present.	Skinfold areas: perineal and perianal region, axillae, beneath breasts, and between the fingers; under wet or occlusive dressings. Lesions possibly present on the oral or vaginal mucous membranes

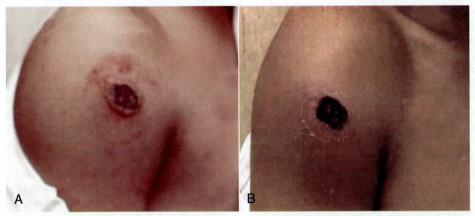

FIG. 25-6 Cutaneous anthrax. Note ulcer with vesicular ring, induration, and erythema **(A)**. As eschar forms, induration lessens, surrounding desquamation occurs, but erythema persists **(B)**. (From The Centers for Disease Control and Prevention, Atlanta, GA [https://www.cdc.gov/anthrax].)

and enlarged lymph nodes may be present. Diagnosis is made based on lesion features, a positive culture, or the presence of anthrax antibodies in the patient's blood. Cultures are obtained from patients who have a fever.

Oral antibiotics for 60 days are indicated for patients who have no edema or systemic symptoms and whose lesions are not located on the head or neck. The antibiotics of choice are ciprofloxacin (Cipro) or doxycycline (Doryx, Vibramycin). For patients who have a fever, have lesions on the head or neck, are pregnant, or have extensive edema, antibiotics are given IV and then followed by an oral course of 60 days (Weant et al., 2014).

Viral Infections

Herpes simplex virus (HSV) infection is the most common viral infection of adult skin and has two types. Type 1 (HSV-1) infections cause the classic recurring cold sore. The severity of the disease increases with age and is worse when the patient is immunosuppressed. Genital herpes, caused by type 2 infection (HSV-2), is also recurrent (see Chapter 74).

After the first infection the virus remains in a dormant state in the nerve ganglia, and the patient has no symptoms. Reactivation stimulates the virus to travel down sensory nerves to the skin, where lesions reappear. Recurrence of HSV infection in healthy people is triggered by stressors, such as dry lips, sunburn, trauma, fever, menses, and fatigue. The virus can also be spread by contact between an actively infected person and a susceptible host. *Autoinoculation,* or transfer of either viral type from one part of the body to another, is also possible.

The time span between episodes and the severity of each attack vary. Outbreaks of oral herpes simplex usually last 3 to 10 days. The patient may have tingling or burning of the lip before any lesion is evident. The patient sheds virus and is contagious for the first 3 to 5 days.

The clinical picture of HSV-1 infection is isolated or grouped painful vesicles on a red base. The infection can occur anywhere on the skin and may be spread by respiratory droplets or direct contact with an active lesion or virus-containing fluid (e.g., saliva).

Herpetic whitlow is a form of herpes simplex that occurs on the fingertips of health care personnel who come into contact with viral secretions. It can be spread easily to patients and can become severe in immunosuppressed patients.

Herpes zoster (shingles) is infection caused by reactivation of the varicella-zoster virus (VZV) in patients who have previously had chickenpox. The dormant virus resides in the dorsal root ganglia of sensory nerves. Multiple lesions occur in a segmental distribution on the skin area innervated by the infected nerve (Fig. 25-7). Herpes zoster eruptions usually occur after several days of discomfort, which may vary from minor irritation and itching to severe, deep pain. The eruption usually lasts several weeks. Postherpetic neuralgia (severe pain persisting after the lesions have resolved) is common in older patients. Early diagnosis of shingles and prompt treatment with antiviral drugs help decrease the duration and severity of postherpetic neuralgia.

Herpes zoster occurs most often in older adults or in anyone who is immunosuppressed. The disorder can be accompanied by fever and malaise. *It is contagious to people who have not previously had chickenpox and have not been vaccinated against the disease.* Reduce the risk of viral transmission by isolating patients with fluid-filled blisters and vesicles until the lesions have crusted over and are dry. Complications include

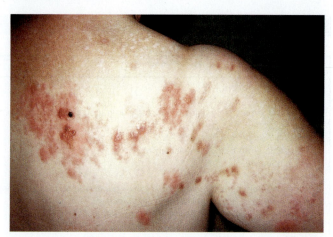

FIG. 25-7 Herpes zoster (shingles).

full-thickness skin necrosis, Bell's palsy, or eye infection, and scarring if the virus is introduced into the eye.

Fungal Infections

Dermatophyte infections, especially superficial infections, differ in lesion appearance, body location, and species of the organism. The term *tinea* is used to describe dermatophytoses; this term is then followed by the location description. For example, *tinea pedis* involves the foot (athlete's foot), *tinea manus* involves the hands, *tinea cruris* involves the groin (jock itch), *tinea capitis* involves the head, and *tinea corporis* involves the rest of the body (ringworm).

Depending on the species, dermatophytes live mainly in the soil, on animals, and on humans. Superficial infection can start only when the infecting organism comes in contact with impaired skin in a susceptible host. Infections are spread by direct contact with infected humans or animals. Some infections, such as tinea capitis and tinea corporis, can be transmitted by inanimate objects. For example, tinea capitis can be spread by sharing contaminated combs, hats, pillowcases, and other objects with individuals with poor personal hygiene.

Candida albicans, also known as *yeast infection,* is a common fungal infection of skin and mucous membranes. The organism is present almost everywhere and easily grows in a warm, moist environment. Risk factors for this infection include immunosuppression, long-term antibiotic therapy, diabetes mellitus, and obesity.

Infected skin has a moist, red, irritated appearance with itching and burning. Common areas for infection are the perineum, vagina, axillae, under the breasts, and in the mouth (where it is known as *thrush* or *oral candidiasis*).

Prevention is aimed at keeping skinfold areas clean and dry. Turning patients and positioning to enhance airflow also aid in prevention. When the infection is present, meticulous cleanliness and the use of topical antifungal agents are needed.

Health Promotion and Maintenance

Preventing skin infection, especially bacterial and fungal infections, involves avoiding the offending organism and practicing good hygiene to remove the organism before infection can occur. *Handwashing and not sharing personal items with others are the best ways to avoid contact with these organisms, including MRSA.* Chart 25-10 lists strategies to teach patients and family

CHART 25-10 Patient and Family Education: Preparing for Self-Management

Preventing the Spread of MRSA

- Avoid close contact with others, including participation in contact sports, until the infection has cleared.
- Take all prescribed antibiotics exactly as prescribed for the entire time prescribed.
- Keep the infected skin area covered with clean, dry bandages.
- Change the bandage whenever drainage seeps through it.
- Place soiled bandages in a plastic bag and seal it closed before placing it in the regular trash.
- Wash your hands with soap and warm water before and after touching the infected area or handling the bandages.
- Shower (rather than bathe) daily, using an antibacterial soap.
- Wash all uninfected skin areas before washing the infected area or use a fresh washcloth to wash the uninfected areas.
- Use each washcloth only once before laundering and avoid using bath sponges or puffs.
- Sleep in a separate bed from others until the infection is cleared.
- Avoid sitting on or using upholstered furniture.
- Do not share clothing, washcloths, towels, athletic equipment, shavers or razors, or any other personal items.
- Clean surfaces that may have come into contact with your infected skin, drainage, or used bandages (e.g., bathroom counters, shower/bath stalls, toilet seats) with household disinfectant or bleach water mixed daily (1 tablespoon of liquid bleach to 1 quart of water).
- Wash all soiled clothing and linens with hot water and laundry detergent. Dry clothing either in a hot dryer or outside on a clothesline in the sun.
- Urge family members and close friends to shower daily with an antibacterial soap.
- If another person helps you change the bandages, make certain that he or she uses disposable gloves, pulls them off inside out when finished, places them with the soiled bandages in a sealed bag, and washes his or her hands thoroughly.

MRSA, Methicillin-resistant *Staphylococcus aureus*.

members to prevent infection spread to other body areas and to others.

For older adults who have had chickenpox and therefore are at risk for shingles (herpes zoster), the vaccine Zostavax is available to prevent VZV reactivation and shingles. The Centers for Disease Control and Prevention (CDC) recommends the vaccine for anyone older than 50 years who has a healthy immune system. This one-time subcutaneous injection significantly reduces the incidence of shingles. Cost remains a factor in vaccination, and few insurance carriers currently include this coverage.

! NURSING SAFETY PRIORITY QSEN

Drug Alert

Zostavax is a live viral vaccine and should not be used in patients with severe immunosuppression because of the risk for viral dissemination. Always check with the prescriber before giving any live vaccines to severely immune compromised patients or those receiving biologic agents for autoimmune disease.

❖ INTERPROFESSIONAL COLLABORATIVE CARE

Depending on the type of infection and associated health issues, patients with skin infections may be treated in a hospital setting, long-term care facility, or home environment. Members of the interprofessional team who collaborate most closely to care for

this patient include the primary health care provider, who will assess the infection and prescribe treatment, and the nurse.

◆ Assessment: Noticing

History. Concentrate on risk factors for each type of infection. If the location and appearance of lesions suggest a bacterial infection, ask about a recent history of skin trauma or recent staphylococcal or streptococcal infections. Assess living conditions, home sanitation, personal hygiene habits, and leisure or sport activities. Ask whether fever and malaise are also present.

Lesions appearing on the lips, in the mouth, or in the genital region are more likely to be a possible viral infection. Ask about:
- A history of similar lesions in the same location
- Presence of burning, tingling, or pain
- Recent stress factors that preceded the outbreak
- Recent contact with an infected person

Information that the same type of lesions has occurred before is important in helping differentiate viral from bacterial lesions. Ask whether the patient has had chickenpox in the past and about a history of shingles. Also ask whether he or she has received the shingles vaccination Zostavax.

Obtain information about a probable dermatophyte infection based on lesion location. If tinea corporis or tinea capitis is present, assess the social and home factors that may contribute to infection, such as direct contact with an infected person, poor personal hygiene, or frequent contact with animals. If tinea cruris and tinea pedis are suspected, ask about the type and frequency of athletic activities.

Physical Assessment/Signs and Symptoms. *Because most skin infections are contagious, take precautions to prevent the spread of infection when performing a physical assessment.* Chart 25-9 lists the signs and symptoms of common skin infections.

Laboratory Assessment. When pustules are present in bacterial infections, the infecting organism is confirmed by swab culture of the purulent material (Cross, 2014). Blood cultures may be helpful if fever and malaise are present. Various cultures and other techniques are used to identify viral and fungal infections (see Chapter 24).

◆ Planning and Implementation: Responding

Most skin infections heal well with nonsurgical management. Surgery may be required when an infectious agent is present in deep-tissue layers. *Priority nursing interventions focus on patient and family education to prevent infection spread to other body areas or to other people* (see Chart 25-10). Meticulous skin care is needed for prevention of infection spread. In some instances drug therapy is needed.

Skin care with proper cleansing is the most effective intervention to prevent infection spread. Teach patients with bacterial infections to bathe daily with an antibacterial soap and to not squeeze any pustules or crusts. Teach patients to gently remove crusts before applying topical drugs so the drugs can be more easily absorbed. Teach the patient to apply warm compresses to furuncles or areas of cellulitis to increase comfort. Most superficial skin infections resolve more quickly if the involved skin dries between treatments. Excessive moisture, especially if occluded by dressings, clothing, or bedding, promotes organism growth. Position bedridden patients for optimal air circulation to the area and avoid occlusive dressings or garments.

Transmission-Based Precautions may be needed to reduce the infection spread to other people. For most superficial bacterial infections, proper handwashing prevents cross-contamination.

However, when hospitalized patients are colonized with antibiotic-resistant *Staphylococcus*, strict adherence to isolation procedures is necessary.

Of the dermatophyte infections, tinea capitis, tinea corporis, and tinea pedis are most easily transmitted to others. Teach patients to avoid sharing personal items, such as hairbrushes, articles of clothing, or footwear. Repeated infections transmitted by dogs or cats indicate that the pet also needs to be treated.

Drug therapy for superficial infection involves topical agents. Mild bacterial infections of the skin usually resolve with topical antibacterial treatment. Patients with extensive infections, especially if fever or lymphadenopathy is present, require systemic antibiotic therapy. The most common systemic drugs used for bacterial skin infections are the penicillins and cephalosporins. For those who are allergic to drugs from these classes, tetracyclines, macrolides, or aminoglycoside antibiotics may be used. For patients infected with MRSA or other drug-resistant organisms, drug therapy may involve IV vancomycin or oral linezolid or clindamycin.

Acyclovir (Zovirax, Xerese ✦), valacyclovir (Valtrex), or famciclovir (Famvir) is used for the treatment of viral infections. Topical treatment decreases the numbers of active viruses on the skin surface and reduces pain in herpetic infections and localized lesions in immunocompromised patients during an initial outbreak. Topical treatment is of little benefit in recurrent infection. IV administration is limited to severe primary infections, immunosuppressed patients with symptoms of systemic infection, and recurrent outbreaks.

Topical antifungal agents are used for patients with dermatophyte or yeast infections at least twice a day until the lesions have cleared. To prevent recurrence, therapy is usually continued for 1 to 2 weeks after clearing. In some instances antifungal powders may also help suppress fungal growth. For widespread or resistant fungal infections, systemic antifungal agents, such as ketoconazole (Nizoral), are given.

⚲ NCLEX EXAMINATION CHALLENGE 25-2

Health Promotion and Maintenance

Which statement, made by the student nurse, requires further teaching by the nurse preceptor?
A. "I will always remove crusts from bacterial lesions before applying topical antimicrobials."
B. "I will avoid using adult briefs for my bedridden incontinent client who has a perineal yeast infection."
C. "If signs and symptoms of a systemic infection are present, I will contact the health care provider to discuss ordering blood cultures."
D. "I will tell my client that transmission-based precautions are not necessary after the first dose of oral antiviral therapy for herpes zoster is taken."

PARASITIC DISORDERS

Parasitic skin disorders occur most often in patients with poor hygiene and in those who are homeless. Examine any patient who shows obvious signs of a self-care deficit for contagious parasitic infections.

Pediculosis

Pediculosis is a lice infestation: *pediculosis capitis* (head lice), *pediculosis corporis* (body lice), and *pediculosis pubis* (pubic, or crab, lice). Human lice are oval and 2 to 4 mm long. The female louse lays many eggs (*nits*) at the hair shaft base in hair-bearing areas.

The most common manifestation of pediculosis is itching (pruritus). Excoriation from scratching also may be present. Some parasites may carry disease (e.g., typhus).

Pediculosis capitis occurs more often in people with longer hair. Scalp itching from parasite bites is intense. A secondary infection may also be present from scratching (Simmons, 2015).

Because the louse is difficult to see, examine the scalp for visible white flecks of the nits attached to the hair shaft near the scalp. Matting and crusting of the scalp and a foul odor indicate a probable secondary infection.

Pediculosis corporis is caused by lice that live and lay eggs in the seams of clothing. The parasites also cause itching. The only visible sign of infestation may be excoriations on the trunk, abdomen, or extremities.

Pediculosis pubis causes intense itching of the vulvar or perirectal region. Pubic lice are more compact and crablike in appearance than body lice and can be contracted from infested bed linens or during sexual intercourse with an infected individual. Although these lice are usually found in the genital region, they can also infest the axillae, the eyelashes, and the chest.

The treatment of pediculosis is chemical killing of the parasites with topical sprays, creams, and shampoos. Agents used include permethrin (Elimite), lindane (Bio-Well, Kwell, Kwellada), or topical malathion (Ovide, Prioderm). Oral agents such as ivermectin (Stromectol) may also be used. In the case of pediculosis capitis, spinosad (Natroba, ParaPro) is a topical agent used as part of an overall lice-management program. Areas where the patient's head has rested (e.g., on pillows of chair backs) will also need to be treated. Clothing and bed linens should be washed in hot water with detergent or dry cleaned. The use of a fine-tooth comb helps remove nits but does not cure the infection. For any louse infestation, social contacts are treated when possible.

⚲ NCLEX EXAMINATION CHALLENGE 25-3

Physiological Integrity

The nurse is teaching a client how to treat pediculosis (lice). Which teaching will the nurse include? **Select all that apply.**
A. Use a fine-tooth comb to remove nits.
B. Chemical killing of these parasites is required.
C. Wash bed linens in cold water to remove lice and eggs.
D. Lice do not affect clothing items because they jump off of fabric.
E. Eggs of lice must be killed to reduce the risk for development of skin cancer.
F. Lice can infest hair on the head, in the genital region, in the axillae, on eyelashes, and on other body hair (e.g., arms, chest, legs).

Scabies

Scabies is a contagious skin infection caused by mite infestations. It is transmitted by close contact with an infested person or infested bedding. Infestation is common among patients with poor hygiene or crowded living conditions. The scabies mite is carried by pets and is found among homeless individuals and institutionalized older patients. Health care personnel are at risk for contracting scabies from contact with an infected patient or his or her bed linen (McGoldrick, 2015).

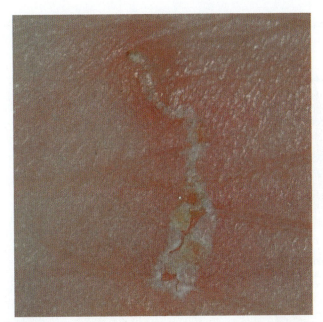

FIG. 25-8 Scabies. Note the lines indicating burrowing of the organism under the skin.

Curved or linear ridges in the skin are a feature of scabies (Fig. 25-8). The itching is very intense, and patients often report that it becomes unbearable at night.

The visible, horizontal white skin ridges are formed by burrowing of the mite into the outer skin layers. Examine the skin between the fingers and on the palms and inner aspects of the wrists, where these ridges are most common. A hypersensitivity reaction to the mite results in excoriated erythematous papules; pustules; and crusted lesions on the elbows, nipples, lower abdomen, buttocks, and thighs and in the axillary folds. Males can have lesions on the penis.

Infestation is confirmed by taking a scraping of a lesion and examining it under the microscope for mites and eggs. Close contacts also should be examined for possible infestation.

Treatment involves the use of scabicides, such as permethrin (Acticin), lindane (Kwell, Kildane, Scabene, Thionex), crotamiton (Eurax) or benzyl benzoate (Ascabiol). Laundering clothes and personal items with hot water and detergent is sufficient to eliminate the mites.

Bedbugs

A common parasite is the bedbug, *Cimex lectularius*. Infestations are increasingly common as a result of travel and resistance to pesticides. This pest does not live on humans; however, it feeds on human blood. The bite causes an itchy discomfort. The most common mode of infestation is carrying the "hitchhiking" bug home from an infested environment such as a hotel room. This problem is not related to socioeconomic level or to a lack of cleanliness.

The adult bedbug is about the size, shape, and color of an apple seed. After feeding, it may double in size and have a red or black color. The insect bites a human host at night and sucks blood for 3 to 10 minutes. The bite area resembles a mosquito or flea bite with a raised bite mark surrounded by a wheal. The degree of itching and redness is related to how allergic the individual is to the insect's saliva. All body areas are susceptible; and one insect can bite multiple times, resulting in clusters of bite marks (Barnes & Murray, 2013).

TABLE 25-3 Normal Wound Healing

Inflammatory Phase
- Begins at the time of injury or cell death and lasts 3 to 5 days.
- Immediate responses are vasoconstriction and clot formation.
- After 10 minutes, vasodilation occurs with increased capillary permeability and leakage of plasma (and plasma proteins) into the surrounding tissue.
- White blood cells (especially macrophages) migrate into the wound.
- Signs and symptoms of local edema, pain, erythema, and warmth are present.

Proliferative Phase
- Begins about the fourth day after injury and lasts 2 to 4 weeks.
- Fibrin strands form a scaffold or framework.
- Mitotic fibroblast cells migrate into the wound, attach to the framework, divide, and stimulate the secretion of collagen.
- Collagen, together with ground substance, builds tough and inflexible scar tissue.
- Capillaries in areas surrounding the wound form "buds" that grow into new blood vessels.
- Capillary buds and collagen deposits form the "granulation" tissue in the wound, and the wound contracts.
- Epithelial cells grow over the granulation tissue bed.

Maturation Phase
- Begins as early as 3 weeks after injury and may continue for a year or longer.
- Collagen is reorganized to provide greater tensile strength.
- Scar tissue gradually becomes thinner and paler in color.
- The mature scar is firm and inelastic when palpated.

Management of the patient with bedbug bites is symptomatic for discomfort from itching, usually with topical antihistamines. When the discomfort is more widespread or the allergic reaction is severe, systemic antihistamines or corticosteroids may be used. Because humans do not harbor the insect, the usual topical insecticides are not needed.

Bedbugs can live anywhere, hiding in cracks and crevices. They can live and lay their eggs in soft upholstery or in wooden crevices. Eradicating the infestation and preventing re-infestations require considerable effort and can be frustrating. Often the home environment needs the extensive eradication efforts of a licensed professional pest-control company with experience in the management of bedbugs (Barnes & Murray, 2013; Fulton, 2015).

TRAUMA

❖ PATHOPHYSIOLOGY

Skin trauma can vary from an aseptic surgical incision to a grossly infected, draining pressure injury with deep-tissue destruction. Injury to the skin starts a series of actions to repair the skin and restore TISSUE INTEGRITY to a protective barrier.

Phases of Wound Healing

Wound healing occurs in three phases: inflammatory phase, proliferative phase, and maturation phase. Table 25-3 lists the key events for each stage of normal wound healing. The length of each phase depends on the type of injury and degree of loss of TISSUE INTEGRITY, the patient's overall health, and whether the wound is healing by first, second, or third intention (Fig. 25-9).

The process of wound healing

▶ Healing by first intention

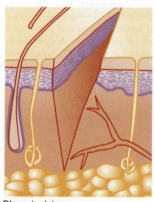
Clean incision

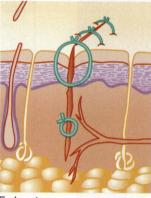
Early suture

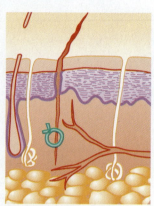
"Hairline" scar

An aseptically made wound with minimal tissue destruction and minimal tissue reaction begins to heal as the edges are approximated by close sutures or staples. No open areas or dead spaces are left to serve as potential sites of infection.

▶ Healing by second intention (granulation) and contraction

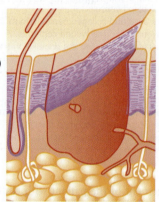
Gaping, irregular wound

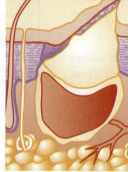
Granulation and contraction

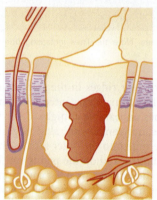
Growth of epithelium over scar

An infected or chronic wound or one with tissue damage so extensive that the edges cannot be smoothly approximated is usually left open and allowed to heal from the inside out. The nurse periodically cleans and assesses the wound for healthy tissue production. Scar tissue is extensive, and healing is prolonged.

▶ Healing by third intention (delayed closure)

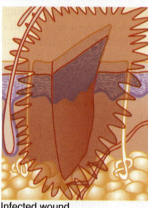
Infected wound

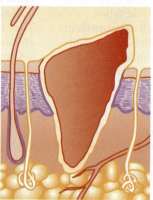
Granulation

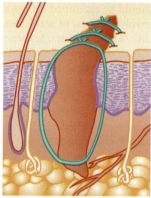
Closure with wide scar

A potentially infected surgical wound may be left open for several days. If no clinical signs of infection occur, the wound is then closed surgically.

FIG. 25-9 The process of wound healing.

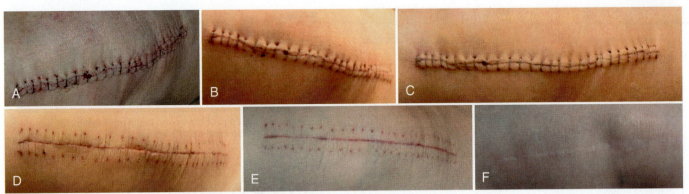

FIG. 25-10 Appearance of a normally healing surgical wound over time.

A wound without tissue loss, such as a clean laceration or a surgical incision, can be closed with sutures, staples, or adhesives. The wound edges are brought together with the skin layers lined up in correct anatomic position (approximated) and held in place until healing is complete. This type of wound represents healing by first intention, in which the closed wound eliminates dead space and shortens the phases of tissue repair. Inflammation resolves quickly, and connective tissue repair is minimal, resulting in less remodeling and a thin scar. Fig. 25-10 shows the appearance of a normally healing surgical wound over time.

Deeper-tissue injuries with greater loss of TISSUE INTEGRITY, such as a chronic pressure injury or venous stasis ulcer, result in a cavity that requires gradual filling in of the dead space with connective tissue. This represents healing by second intention and prolongs the repair process.

Wounds at high risk for infection, such as surgical incisions into a nonsterile body cavity or contaminated traumatic wounds, may be intentionally left open for several days. After debris (dead tissues) and exudate have been removed (débrided) and inflammation has subsided, the wound is closed by first intention. This type of healing represents delayed primary closure (third intention) and results in a scar similar to that found in wounds that heal by first intention. Healing can be impaired by many factors (Table 25-4).

Mechanisms of Wound Healing

When skin injury occurs, the body restores TISSUE INTEGRITY through three processes: re-epithelialization, granulation, and wound contraction. The depth of injury and extent of tissue integrity loss determine to what degree each process contributes to wound healing.

Partial-Thickness Wounds. Partial-thickness wounds are superficial with minimal loss of TISSUE INTEGRITY from damage to the epidermis and upper dermal layers. These wounds heal by re-epithelialization, the production of new skin cells by undamaged epidermal cells in the basal layer of the dermis, which also lines the hair follicles and sweat glands (Fig. 25-11). Injury is followed immediately by local inflammation that causes the formation of a fibrin clot and releases growth factors that stimulate epidermal cell division (mitosis). New skin cells move into open spaces on the wound surface where the fibrin clot acts as a frame to guide cell movement. Regrowth across the open area (resurfacing) is only one cell layer thick at first. As healing continues, the cell layer thickens, stratifies (forms layers), and produces keratin to resemble normal skin.

In a healthy adult, healing of a partial-thickness wound takes about 5 to 7 days. This process is more rapid in skin that is hydrated, well oxygenated, and has few microorganisms.

Full-Thickness Wounds. In deep partial-thickness wounds and full-thickness wounds, loss of tissue integrity and damage extend into the lower layers of the dermis and subcutaneous tissue. As a result, most of the epithelial cells at the base of the wound are destroyed, and the wound cannot heal by re-epithelialization alone. Removal of the damaged tissue results in a defect that must be filled with scar tissue (granulation) for healing to occur. During the second phase of healing, new blood vessels form at the base of the wound, and fibroblast cells begin moving into the wound space. These cells deposit new collagen to replace the lost tissue.

Fibroblasts also begin to pull the wound edges inward along the path of least resistance (contraction) (see Fig. 25-11). This causes the wound to decrease in size at a uniform rate. Complete wound closure by contraction depends on the mobility of the surrounding skin as tension is applied to it. If tension in the surrounding skin exceeds the force of wound contraction, healing will be delayed until undamaged epidermal cells at the wound edges can bridge the defect. The bridging of epithelial cells across a large area of granulation tissue results in an unstable barrier rather than near-normal skin. A venous leg ulcer is one example of a skin defect that heals poorly by contraction. Re-epithelialization of these chronic wounds often results in a thin epidermal barrier that is easily re-injured.

The natural healing processes of re-epithelialization, granulation, and contraction can slow and even stop in the presence of chronic infection, unrelieved pressure, or mechanical obstacles. For example, dead tissue not only supports bacterial growth but also obstructs collagen deposition and wound contraction. Once dead tissue is removed, 60% of chronic wounds remained colonized with communities of bacteria that grow together in an extracellular matrix on the wound surface in the form of a biofilm. Stress-response mediators and other factors alter the cutaneous microbiome, leading to chronic inflammation and allowing biofilm bacteria to become more virulent and resistant to antimicrobials (Holmes et al., 2015). Thus thorough wound cleansing and débridement are essential for healing. In the case of chronic wounds, healing may stop spontaneously without an obvious cause. In addition, infection in chronic wounds may not show the expected signs or symptoms. Often the only manifestation is an increase in wound size or failure of the wound to decrease in size. Nonhealing chronic wounds that remain open for extended periods are of particular

TABLE 25-4   Causes of Impaired Wound Healing

CAUSE	MECHANISM
Altered Inflammatory Response	
Local	
Arteriosclerosis	Reduced local tissue circulation, resulting in ischemia, impaired leukocytic response to wounding, and increased probability of wound infection
Diabetes	
Vasculitis	
Thrombosis	
Venous insufficiency	
Lymphedema	
Pharmacologic vasoconstriction	
Irradiated tissue	
Crush injuries	
Primary closure under tension	
Systemic	
Leukemia	Systemic inhibition of leukocytic response, resulting in impaired host resistance to infection
Prolonged administration of high-dose anti-inflammatory drugs:	
• Corticosteroids	
• Aspirin	
Impaired Cellular Proliferation	
Local	
Biofilm formation	Prolonged inflammatory response, which can result in low tissue oxygen tension and further tissue destruction
Wound infection	
Foreign body	
Necrotic tissue	
Repeated injury or irritation	
Movement of wound (e.g., across a joint)	
Wound desiccation or maceration	
Systemic	
Aging	Impaired cellular proliferation and collagen synthesis
Chronic stress	Decreased wound contraction
Nutritional deficiencies:	
• Calories	
• Protein	
• Vitamins	
• Minerals	
• Water	
Impaired oxygenation:	
• Pulmonary insufficiency	
• Heart failure	
• Hypovolemia	
Cirrhosis	
Uremia	
Prolonged hypothermia	
Coagulation disorders	
Cytotoxic drugs	

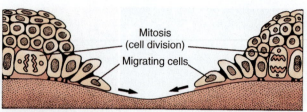

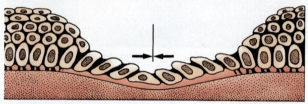

Skin cells at the edge of the wound begin multiplying and migrate toward the center of the wound.

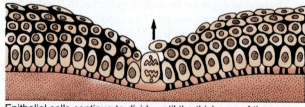

Once advancing epidermal cells from the opposite sides of the wound meet, migration halts.

Epithelial cells continue to divide until the thickness of the new skin layer approaches normal.

FIG. 25-11 Re-epithelialization and wound contraction. (Modified from Swaim, S. F. [1980]. *Surgery of traumatized skin.* Philadelphia: Saunders.)

⬤ CONSIDERATIONS FOR OLDER ADULTS
Patient-Centered Care QSEN

As skin ages, the process of wound healing is less efficient. Re-epithelialization and wound contraction slow, and replacement of connective tissue is reduced. Thus the strength of a healed wound in an older adult is reduced with poor TISSUE INTEGRITY, and the area is at greater risk for re-injury. When inadequate nutrition, incontinence, or immobility is present, any wound in an older adult has a high risk for becoming a chronic wound. Although prevention strategies provide the best outcome, aggressive treatment of any degree of loss of skin tissue integrity, no matter how small, should be started as soon as it is discovered in an older adult (Touhy & Jett, 2015).

surgical repair of an affected area; the primary health care provider, who assesses healing and prescribes treatment; and the nurse.

SKIN CANCER

❖ *PATHOPHYSIOLOGY*

Any skin cancer occurs as a result of failure of CELLULAR REGULATION over cell division. (See Chapter 21 for a discussion of the general mechanisms leading to changes in CELLULAR REGULATION and cancer development.) *Overexposure to sunlight is the major cause of skin cancer, although other factors also are associated.* Because sun damage is an age-related skin finding, screening for suspicious lesions is an important part of physical assessment of the older adult. The most common precancerous lesions are actinic (solar) keratosis, and the most common skin cancers are squamous cell carcinoma, basal cell carcinoma, and melanoma, as described in Table 25-5. A biopsy

concern. Although rare, these wounds are at higher risk for evolving into an aggressive malignancy (Marjolin ulcer) (Tobin & Sanger, 2014; Yu et al., 2013).

❖ INTERPROFESSIONAL COLLABORATIVE CARE

Collaborative management of skin trauma and the setting for care vary with the depth and type of injury. Interventions always focus on supporting a healing environment, enhancing wound healing, preventing infection, and restoring function to the area. Members of the interprofessional team who collaborate most closely to care for the patient with skin trauma include the surgeon (if indicated), who performs any necessary

TABLE 25-5   Common Premalignant Lesions and Skin Cancers

SIGNS AND SYMPTOMS	DISTRIBUTION	COURSE
Actinic (Solar) Keratosis (Premalignant) Small (1-10 mm) macule or papule with dry, rough, adherent yellow or brown scale Base may be erythematous Associated with yellow, wrinkled, weather-beaten skin Thick, indurated keratoses more likely to be malignant	Cheeks, temples, forehead, ears, neck, backs of hands, and forearms	May disappear spontaneously or reappear after treatment Slow progression to squamous cell carcinoma possible
Squamous Cell Carcinoma Firm, nodular lesion topped with a crust or a central area of ulceration Indurated margins Fixation to underlying tissue with deep invasion	Sun-exposed areas, especially head, neck, and lower lip Sites of chronic irritation or injury (e.g., scars, irradiated skin, burns, leg ulcers)	Rapid invasion with metastasis via the lymphatics in 10% of cases Larger tumors more prone to metastasis
Basal Cell Carcinoma Pearly papule with a central crater and rolled, waxy borders Telangiectasias and pigment flecks visible on close inspection	Sun-exposed areas, especially head, neck, and central portion of face	Metastasis rare May cause local tissue destruction; 50% recurrence rate related to inadequate treatment
Melanoma Irregularly shaped, pigmented papule or plaque Variegated colors, with red, white, and blue tones	Can occur anywhere on the body, especially where nevi (moles) or birthmarks are evident Commonly found on upper back and lower legs Soles of feet and palms in dark-skinned people	Horizontal growth phase followed by vertical growth phase Rapid invasion and metastasis with high morbidity and mortality

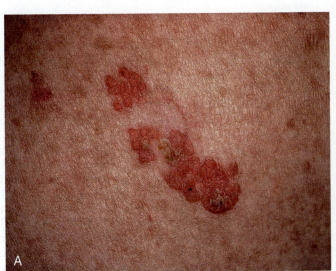

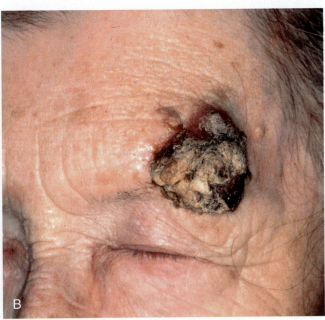

FIG. 25-12 A and **B,** Varying presentations of squamous cell carcinoma. (**A** and **B** from Bolognia, J. L., Jorizzo, J. L., & Schaffer, J. V. [2012]. *Dermatology* (3rd ed.). St. Louis: Saunders.)

of suspicious lesions is necessary to determine whether a skin lesion is malignant.

Etiology and Genetic Risk

Actinic (solar) keratoses are premalignant lesions of the cells of the epidermis. These lesions are common in adults with chronically sun-damaged skin. Progression to squamous cell carcinoma may occur if lesions are untreated.

Squamous cell carcinomas are cancers of the epidermis. They can invade locally and are potentially metastatic (Fig. 25-12). Chronic skin damage from repeated injury or irritation also predisposes to this malignancy. Chronic wounds that remain

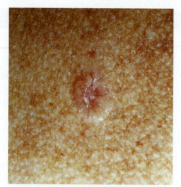

FIG. 25-13 Basal cell carcinoma.

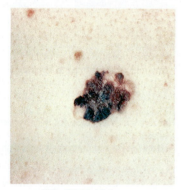

FIG. 25-14 Melanoma.

open for long periods are also at increased risk for malignant transformation to cancer.

Basal cell carcinomas arise from the basal cell layer of the epidermis (Fig. 25-13). Early lesions often go unnoticed; and, although metastasis is rare, underlying tissue destruction can occur. Genetic predisposition and chronic irritation are risk factors; however, UV exposure is the most common cause.

Melanomas are pigmented cancers arising in the melanin-producing epidermal cells (Fig. 25-14). Most often they start as the benign growth of a nevus (mole) (Skin Cancer Foundation, 2016). Normal nevi have regular, well-defined borders and are uniform in color, ranging from light colors to dark brown. The lesion's surface may be rough or smooth. Nevi with irregular or spreading borders and those with multiple colors are abnormal. Other suspicious features include sudden changes in lesion size and reports of itching or bleeding.

Risk factors include genetic predisposition, excessive exposure to UV light, and the presence of one or more precursor lesions that resemble unusual moles. *This skin cancer is highly metastatic, and a person's survival depends on early diagnosis and treatment.*

Incidence/Prevalence

The incidence of skin cancer is highest among light-skinned races and adults older than 55 years (ACS, 2015). Skin cancer occurs more often among those who work outdoors, live at higher altitudes or lower latitudes, or spend much time sunbathing. Occupational exposure to arsenic or other chemical carcinogens also increases risk. Melanoma reflects only 1% of total skin care cases but has one of the highest associated mortality rates (ACS, 2017).

CHART 25-11   Patient and Family Education: Preparing for Self-Management

Prevention of Skin Cancer

- Avoid sun exposure between 11 AM and 3 PM.
- Use sunscreens with the appropriate skin protection factor for your skin type.
- Wear a hat, opaque clothing, and sunglasses when you are in the sun.
- Keep a "body map" of your skin spots, scars, and lesions to detect when changes have occurred.
- Examine your body monthly for possibly cancerous or precancerous lesions.
- Seek medical advice if you note any of these:
  - A change in the color of a lesion, especially if it darkens or shows evidence of spreading
  - A change in the size of a lesion, especially rapid growth
  - A change in the shape of a lesion, such as a sharp border becoming irregular or a flat lesion becoming raised
  - Redness or swelling of the skin around a lesion
  - A change in sensation, especially itching or increased tenderness of a lesion
  - A change in the character of a lesion, such as oozing, crusting, bleeding, or scaling

GENETIC/GENOMIC CONSIDERATIONS

Patient-Centered Care QSEN

Genetic mutations in the CDKN2A and CDK4 have been identified for some cases of familial melanoma. These mutations in a suppressor gene result in loss of CELLULAR REGULATION for cell growth. Other genetic considerations for melanoma are that some specific mutations in the genes of the actual tumor cells increase the response of these cells to targeted therapy. All melanomas should be tested for mutations of the BRAF and KIT genes (OMIM, 2016). Always ask patients who have a diagnosed melanoma whether any other family members have ever had this disease.

Health Promotion and Maintenance

The most effective prevention strategy for skin cancer is avoiding or reducing skin exposure to sunlight. However, even when adults understand the cause of skin cancer and the seriousness of the disease, preventive behaviors are not always practiced. Common prevention practices are listed in Chart 25-11. *Teach all individuals to avoid tanning beds and salons.*

Secondary prevention (early detection) is critical to survival with melanoma. Teach adults to be aware of their skin markings. Keeping a total body spot and lesion map can provide baseline information about suspicious new lesions and help identify changes in existing lesions. Once a map is made, the person should systematically inspect his or her body monthly for new lesions and for changes in any existing lesions by performing thorough *skin self-examination (SSE)*. Some people find taking pictures of their skin on a regular basis makes identifying changes easier. Teach everyone to evaluate all skin lesions using the ABCDE guide for melanoma (see Chapter 24) and to consult his or her health care provider to examine any lesion having unusual features. When lesions such as moles are present, they should be monitored annually by a dermatologist or other health care professional.

❖ INTERPROFESSIONAL COLLABORATIVE CARE

Care of the patient with skin cancer, depending on the degree of cancer and associated health concerns, may be treated in the hospital, ambulatory surgical, or outpatient setting. Members of the interprofessional team who most often care for patients with skin cancer include the surgeon to remove cancerous lesions, the oncologist to manage radiation and/or chemotherapy, the pharmacist to dispense medication, the social worker to assist with care coordination and payer sources, the spiritual leader of the patient's choice to provide comfort, and the nurse.

◆ Assessment: Noticing

In addition to age and race, ask the patient about any family history of skin cancer and any past surgery for removal of skin growths. Recent changes in the size, color, or sensation of any mole, birthmark, wart, or scar are also significant. Ask in which geographic regions the patient has lived and where he or she currently resides. Obtain information about occupational and recreational activities in relation to sun exposure and any occupational history of exposure to chemical carcinogens (e.g., arsenic, coal tar, pitch, radioactive waste, radium). Ask whether any skin lesions are repeatedly irritated by the rubbing of clothing.

Skin that has been injured previously is at greater risk for cancer development, an effect known as *Koebner's phenomenon.* Ask the patient if he or she has ever experienced a severe skin injury that resulted in a scar. Examine all scarred skin areas for the presence of potentially cancerous lesions. A biopsy may be required to rule out cancer in a chronic open wound that fails to close with proper treatment.

Skin cancers vary in their appearance and distribution. Although most skin cancers appear in sun-exposed areas of the body, inspect the entire skin surface and any unusual lesions, particularly moles, warts, birthmarks, and scars. Also examine hair-bearing areas of the body, such as the scalp and genitalia. Palpate lesions to determine surface texture. Document the location, size, color, and features of all lesions and any reports of tenderness or itching. Use the ABCDE method of evaluating all lesions for possible melanoma (see Chapter 24).

◆ Planning and Implementation: Responding

Surgical and nonsurgical interventions are combined for the effective management of skin cancer. Treatment is determined by the size and severity of the malignancy, the location of the lesion, and the age and general health of the patient.

Surgical Management. Surgical intervention is needed to manage any type of skin cancer. It can range from local removal of small lesions to massive excision of large areas of the skin and underlying tissue for treatment of melanoma. Surgical types for skin cancer include:

- Cryosurgery—Cell destruction by the local application of liquid nitrogen (−200° C) to isolated lesions, causing cell death and tissue destruction.
- Curettage and electrodesiccation—Removal of cancerous cells with the use of a dermal curette to scrape away cancerous tissue, followed by the application of an electric probe to destroy remaining tumor tissue.
- Excisional biopsy—Total surgical removal of small lesions for pathologic examination.
- Mohs' surgery—A specialized form of excision usually for basal and squamous cell carcinomas. Tissue is sectioned horizontally in layers, and each layer is examined histologically to determine the presence of residual tumor cells.
- Wide excision—Deep skin resection often involving removal of full-thickness skin in the area of the lesion.

Depending on tumor depth, subcutaneous tissues and lymph nodes may also be removed.

Nonsurgical Management. Drug therapy may involve topical or systemic chemotherapy, biotherapy, or targeted therapy. Topical chemotherapy with 5-fluorouracil cream is used for treatment of multiple actinic keratoses or for widespread superficial basal cell carcinoma that would require several surgical procedures to eradicate. Therapy is continued for several weeks; and the treated areas become increasingly tender and inflamed as the lesions crust, ooze, and erode. Prepare the patient for an unsightly appearance during therapy and reassure him or her that the cosmetic result will be positive. Imiquimod (Aldara) is a newer topical treatment option for superficial basal cell carcinoma. This type of therapy stimulates the immune system to produce interferon, a chemical that attacks cancer cells.

Several systemic agents are indicated for treatment of locally advanced or metastatic squamous cell skin cancer. These include a platinum based-agent (Cisplatin or Carboplatin), 5-fluorouracil, and cetuximab (Erbitux) for advanced squamous cell carcinoma. Oral drugs approved for advanced basal cell carcinoma include vismodegib (Erivedge) and sonidigib (Odomzo).

Biotherapy with interferon, monoclonal antibodies, and targeted therapy are now accepted treatment for melanoma after surgical removal. Interferon is used for melanomas that are at stage 3 or higher. The patient is first started on high-dose IV interferon infusions daily for 5 days per week for 4 weeks. Maintenance doses, given subcutaneously, are then continued three times per week for 1 year. The patient must learn to self-inject the drug.

Monoclonal antibody therapy with ipilimumab (Yervoy), a drug that targets the CTLA4 (cytotoxic T-lymphocyte associated antigen 4) receptor and blocks it, leads to greater T-cell lymphocyte activity. (T-cells are a type of lymphocyte that can stimulate antitumor immune responses.) The side effects of this drug include significant inflammation in many tissues, including the pituitary gland, liver, skin, GI tract, and nervous system. Some of the side effects can be life threatening (Bryce & Passoni, 2013).

Targeted therapy is available for melanomas with specific mutations in the *BRAF* gene. Normally the *BRAF* gene is involved in CELLULAR REGULATION of growth. Mutations in this gene allow melanoma to grow and metastasize. When melanoma cells are positive for a specific *BRAF* mutation (V600E), the cells respond to the drug vemurafenib (Zelboraf). The drug inhibits an enzyme important in signaling cell division and prevents melanoma cell division. This oral drug interacts with a variety of other drugs, and allergic reactions are common.

Radiation therapy for skin cancer is limited to older patients with large, deeply invasive basal cell tumors and to those who are poor risks for surgery. Melanoma is relatively resistant to radiation therapy. Immune check inhibitors stimulate the immune system to recognize and destroy cancer cells more effectively. Pembrolizumab (Keytruda) and nivolumab (Opdivo) target a protein on the surface of T-cells (PD-1). Blocking PD-1 increases T-cell activation, which helps the body attack melanoma cells but can also stimulate the immune system to attack noncancerous tissue. To avoid serious side effects, teach patients to report any new symptoms to the health care team immediately (ACS, 2015).

NCLEX EXAMINATION CHALLENGE 25-4

Physiological Integrity

The nurse is performing an assessment on a female client and notices a large, irregularly shaped mole on her upper back. The client expresses concern about the cosmetic appearance of the lesion. What is the **priority** nursing intervention?
A. Refer to a dermatological health care provider.
B. Ask if there are any other lesions that bother her.
C. Perform a head-to-toe skin assessment and document the findings.
D. Teach about the importance of avoiding excessive sun exposure and tanning beds.

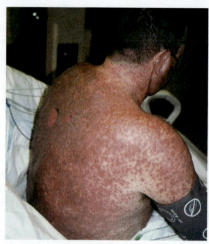

FIG. 25-15 Stevens-Johnson syndrome. (Courtesy Stevens Johnson Syndrome Foundation, Littleton, CO.)

OTHER SKIN DISORDERS

Toxic Epidermal Necrolysis and Stevens-Johnson Syndrome

Toxic epidermal necrolysis (TEN) and Stevens-Johnson Syndrome (SJS) (Fig. 25-15) are life-threatening cutaneous reactions to medications. Thought to be variations in severity of the same immune process, TEN/SJN is characterized by diffuse erythema and blister formation, often involving the mucous membranes. The most common causative drugs are allopurinol, antiepileptics, NSAIDs, chemotherapy agents, sulfonamides, pyrazolones, barbiturates, and antibiotics. Discontinuation of the drug is usually followed by gradual healing in 2 to 3 weeks, with widespread peeling of the epidermis (Dodiuk-Gad et al., 2015).

This problem can occur at any age and as a result of almost any drug therapy. However, older patients with cancer who are receiving chemotherapy, some targeted therapies, and immunotherapy are at greatest risk. Other precipitating factors include stem cell transplantation and neutropenia-induced infections.

The drug thought to be causing a toxic reaction is discontinued, and management focuses on systemic support and prevention of secondary infection. Patients are often admitted to burn units, where fluid and electrolyte balance, caloric intake, and hypothermia can be closely monitored. Topical antibacterial drugs are used to suppress bacterial growth until healing occurs.

GET READY FOR THE NCLEX® EXAMINATION!

KEY POINTS

Review these Key Points for each NCLEX Examination Client Needs Category.

Safe and Effective Care Environment
- Wash your hands before and after touching any skin lesions. **QSEN: Safety**
- Use Standard Precautions when providing care to a patient who has any areas of nonintact skin. **QSEN: Safety**
- Ensure that the skin of incontinent patients is kept clean and dry. **QSEN: Evidence-Based Practice**
- Assist patients with limited mobility to change positions while awake. Base frequency of repositioning on individual patient assessment criteria. **QSEN: Evidence-Based Practice**
- Use a structured approach (e.g., Braden scale or other validated tool) to evaluate the pressure injury risk for all patients on admission and regularly thereafter. **QSEN: Evidence-Based Practice**
- Use pressure-distribution devices for any patient who is identified to be at risk for pressure injury formation (i.e., requires prolonged bedrest, is an older adult, has some degree of immobility, is incontinent, has some degree of malnutrition, is dehydrated, has decreased sensory perception, or has an altered mental state). **QSEN: Safety**
- Use a lift sheet or mechanical lift to move immobilized older patients rather than pulling or dragging them across bed linens. **QSEN: Safety**

Health Promotion and Maintenance
- Teach the patient with mobility problems and caregivers how to redistribute skin pressure in the home environment. **QSEN: Patient-Centered Care**
- Encourage adults to reduce sun exposure and exposure to ultraviolet (UV) light. **QSEN: Patient-Centered Care**
- Teach adults how to examine all skin areas on a monthly basis for new lesions and changes to existing lesions and to keep a record or "body map" of skin lesions. **QSEN: Patient-Centered Care**
- Teach patients with skin scarring from a previous skin injury to examine this area at least monthly for changes. **QSEN: Patient-Centered Care**
- Urge patients to regularly bathe, shampoo the hair, and keep fingernails clean. **QSEN: Patient-Centered Care**
- Teach patients with infected skin lesions or infestations how to limit transmission. **QSEN: Safety**
- Teach patients the ABCDE method of evaluating a lesion for melanoma. **QSEN: Patient-Centered Care**

- Assess the patient's ability to see and reach the affected skin area and care for the problem. **QSEN: Patient-Centered Care**

Psychosocial Integrity

- Assess the patient's and family's feelings about how a skin, hair, or nails condition has affected body image. **QSEN: Patient-Centered Care**
- Support the patient and family in coping with changes in skin integrity and body image. **QSEN: Patient-Centered Care**
- Encourage the patient with a visible wound or other skin problem to participate in the care of the wound. **QSEN: Patient-Centered Care**
- Professionally demonstrate acceptance of the patient with skin changes. **Ethics**
- Encourage patients with chronic skin problems, especially those that alter appearance, to become involved in a community support group. **QSEN: Patient-Centered Care**

Physiological Integrity

- Keep skin well hydrated to promote TISSUE INTEGRITY. **QSEN: Evidence-Based Practice**
- Use appropriate risk assessment tools to perform a focused skin assessment and re-assessment to determine risk for pressure injury development and adequacy of the skin's protective functions. **Clinical Judgment**
- Keep skinfold areas clean and dry. **QSEN: Evidence-Based Practice**
- Ask the patient who has started taking a newly prescribed drug if skin changes have occurred since starting the drug. **QSEN: Patient-Centered Care**
- Evaluate any open skin area on a patient daily for size, depth, exudate, presence of infection, and indicators of healing. **Clinical Judgment**
- Differentiate the signs and symptoms for all pressure injury categories. **Clinical Judgment**
- Evaluate wounds for size, depth, presence of infection, and indications of healing. **Clinical Judgment**

SELECTED BIBLIOGRAPHY

Ambutas, S., Staffileno, B., & Fogg, L. (2014). Reducing nasal pressure ulcers with an alternative taping device. *MEDSURG Nursing, 23*(2), 96–100.

American Cancer Society (ACS). (2015). *Cancer facts and figures 2015.* http://www.cancer.org/acs/groups/content/@editorial/documents/document/acspc-044552.pdf.

American Cancer Society (ACS). (2017). *Melanoma skin cancer.* http://www.cancer.org/cancer/skincancer-melanoma/detailedguide/melanoma-skin-cancer-treating-immunotherapy.

Aviles, F. (2014). Determining the increased role of the physical therapist within the wound care industry. *Today's Wound Clinic, 8*(4).

Ayello, E., & Baranoski, S. (2014). Wound care and prevention. *Nursing 2014, 44*(4), 32–40.

Barnes, E., & Murray, B. (2013). Bedbugs: What nurses need to know. *AJN, 113*(10), 58–62.

Bryce, J., & Passoni, C. (2013). Nursing management of patients with metastatic melanoma receiving ipilimumab. *Oncology Nursing Forum, 40*(3), 215–218.

Chanussot-Deprez, C., & Contreras-Ruiz, J. (2013). Telemedicine in wound care: A review. *Advances in Skin & Wound Care, 26*(2), 78–82.

Cowan, L., Stechmiller, J., Phillips, P., & Schultz, G. (2014). Science of wound healing: Translation of bench science into advances for chronic wound care. In *Chronic Wound Care: The Essentials* (p. 25). Malvern, PA: HMP Communications, LLC.

Cross, H. H. (2014). Obtaining a wound swab culture specimen. *Nursing 2014, 44*(7), 68–69.

Daugherty, S., & Spear, M. (2015). Skin & skin substitutes—An overview. *Plastic Surgery Nursing, 35*(2), 92–97.

Dodiuk-Gad, R., Chung, W. H., Valeyrie-Allanore, L., & Shear, N. (2015). Stevens–Johnson syndrome and toxic epidermal necrolysis: An update. *American Journal of Clinical Dermatology, 16*(6), 475–493.

Fulton, M. J. (2015). Don't let the bedbugs bite. *Nursing 2016, 45*(7), 46–47.

Gould, L., Abadir, P., Brem, H., Carter, M., Conner Kerr, T., Davidson, J., et al. (2015). Chronic wound repair and healing in older adults: Current status and future research. *Wound Repair and Regeneration, 23*(1), 1–13.

Hakim, E., & Heitzman, J. (2013). Wound management in the presence of peripheral arterial disease. *Topics in Geriatric Rehabilitation, 29*(3), 187–194.

Holmes, C. J., Plichta, J. K., Gamelli, R. L., & Radek, K. A. (2015). Dynamic role of host stress responses in modulating the cutaneous microbiome: Implications for wound healing and infection. *Advances in Wound Care, 4*(1), 24–37.

Krasner, D., Sibbald, G., & Woo, K. (2014). Wound dressing product selection: A holistic, interprofessional, patient-centered approach. In *Chronic wound care: The essentials* (pp. 165–172). Malvern, PA: HMP Communications, LLC.

LeBlanc, K., & Baranoski, S. (2014). Skin tears: Best practices for care and prevention. *Nursing 2014, 44*(5), 36–46.

McCance, K., Huether, S., Brashers, V., & Rote, N. (2014). *Pathophysiology: The biologic basis for disease in adults and children* (7th ed.). St. Louis: Mosby.

McGoldrick, M. (2015). Scabies infestation. *Home healthcare now, 33*(9), 503–504.

McInnes, E., Jammali-Blasi, A., Bell-Syer, S., Dumville, J., Middleton, V., & Cullum, N. (2015). Support surfaces for pressure ulcer prevention. *The Cochrane Database of Systematic Reviews,* (9), Art. No.: CD001735, doi:10.1002/14651858.CD001735.pub5.

National Pressure Ulcer Advisory Panel, European Pressure Ulcer Advisory Panel, & Pan Pacific Pressure Injury Alliance (2014). *Prevention and treatment of pressure ulcers: Quick reference guide.* Perth, Australia: Cambridge Media. www.npuap.org/wp-content/uploads/2014/08/Quick-Reference-Guide-DIGITAL-NPUAP-EPUAP-PPPIA.pdf.

National Pressure Ulcer Advisory Panel. (2016). *NPUAP pressure injury stages.* http://www.npuap.org/resources/educational-and-clinical-resources/npuap-pressure-injury-stages/.

Online Mendelian Inheritance in Man (OMIM). (2016). *Susceptibility to cutaneous malignant melanoma.* www.omim.org/entry/155600.

Online Mendelian Inheritance in Man (OMIM). (2017). *Susceptibility to psoriasis.* www.omim.org/entry/177900.

Paul, R., McCutcheon, S., Tregarthen, J., Denend, L., & Zenios, S. (2014). Sustaining pressure ulcer best practices in a high-volume cardiac care environment. *American Journal of Nursing, 114*(8), 34–44.

Posthauer, M. E., Banks, M., Dorner, B., & Schols, J. M. (2015). The role of nutrition for pressure ulcer management: National Pressure Ulcer Advisory Panel, European Pressure Ulcer Advisory Panel, and Pan Pacific Pressure Injury Alliance White Paper. *Advances in Skin & Wound Care, 28*(4), 175–188.

Rock, R. (2014). Guidelines for safe negative-pressure wound therapy. *Wound Care Advisor, 3*(2), 29–33.

Roe, E., & Williams, D. (2014). Using evidence-based practice to prevent hospital-acquired pressure ulcers and promote healing. *American Journal of Nursing, 114*(8), 61–65.

Simmons, S. (2015). Taking a closer look at pediculosis capitis. *Nursing 2016, 45*(6), 57–58.

Skin Cancer Foundation. (2016). *Understanding melanoma—Warning signs: The ABCDEs of melanoma.* www.skincancer.org/skin-cancer-information/melanoma.

Steven, M., Struble, L., & Larson, J. (2015). Recognizing pressure injury in the darkly pigmented skin type. *Medsurg Nursing, 24*(4), 237–242, 267.

Tobin, C., & Sanger, J. R. (2014). Marjolin's ulcers: A case series and literature review. *Wounds: A Compendium of Clinical Research and Practice, 26*(8), 248–254.

Touhy, T., & Jett, K. (2015). *Ebersole and Hess' gerontological nursing healthy aging* (9th ed.). St. Louis: Mosby.

van Rijswijk, L. (2013). Measuring wounds to improve outcomes. *AJN, 113*(8), 60–61.

Ventura, M., Cassano, N., Romita, P., Vestita, M., Foti, C., & Vina, G. A. (2015). Management of chronic spontaneous urticaria in the elderly. *Drugs and Aging, 32*(4), 271–282.

Weant, K., Bailey, A., Fleishaker, E., & Justice, S. (2014). Being prepared: Bioterrorism and mass prophylaxis: Part I. *Advanced Emergency Nursing Journal, 36*(3), 226–238.

Yu, N., Long, X., Lujan-Hernandez, J., Hassan, K., Bai, M., Wang, Y., et al. (2013). Marjolin's ulcer: A preventable malignancy arising from scars. *World Journal of Surgical Oncology*, doi:10.1186/1477-7819-11-313. http://www.wjso.com/content/11/1/313.

CHAPTER 26

Care of Patients With Burns

Tammy Coffee

e http://evolve.elsevier.com/Iggy/

PRIORITY AND INTERRELATED CONCEPTS

The priority concepts for this chapter are:
- Tissue Integrity
- Fluid and Electrolyte Balance
- Perfusion
- Gas Exchange

The interrelated concepts for this chapter are:
- Nutrition
- Comfort
- Mobility

LEARNING OUTCOMES

Safe and Effective Care Environment
1. Collaborate with the interprofessional team to coordinate high-quality care for patients with burn injury.
2. Protect patients with burns from infection.

Health Promotion and Maintenance
3. Teach adults fire- and burn-prevention strategies.

Psychosocial Integrity
4. Implement nursing interventions to help patients and families cope with the psychosocial impact of burn injury.

Physiological Integrity
5. Ensure optimal pain control and increase COMFORT for the patient with a burn injury.
6. Prioritize nursing care for the patient with burns during the resuscitation, acute, and rehabilitation phases of burn injury to preserve TISSUE INTEGRITY, FLUID AND ELECTROLYTE BALANCE, and GAS EXCHANGE.

Physiologic, metabolic, and psychological changes take place with loss of TISSUE INTEGRITY associated with burns. These complex injuries can range from "sunburn" to major injuries involving all layers of the skin. The function of many body systems is changed when the skin is injured. The patient with burns needs comprehensive care for weeks to months to survive the injury, reduce complications, and return to the best functional status. Nurses coordinate the activities of an interprofessional team comprised of health care providers, nurses with burn specialty, registered dietitians, therapists, and religious and spiritual leaders (as requested by the patient) to provide the best care and patient outcomes.

INTRODUCTION TO BURN INJURY

❖ PATHOPHYSIOLOGY

Tissue destruction caused by a burn injury leads to local and systemic problems that affect FLUID AND ELECTROLYTE BALANCE and lead to protein losses; sepsis; and changes in metabolic, endocrine, respiratory, cardiac, hematologic, and immune functioning. The extent of problems is related to age, general health, extent of injury, depth of injury, and the specific body area injured. Even after healing, the burn injury may cause late complications such as contracture formation and scarring. Priorities of care are the prevention of infection and closure of the burn wound. A lack of or delay in wound healing is a key factor for all systemic problems and a major cause of disability and death among patients who are burned.

Skin Changes

Anatomic Changes. The skin is the largest organ of the body (see Chapter 24). Each of its two major layers, the epidermis and the dermis, has several sublayers. The epidermis is the outer layer of skin. It can grow back after a burn injury because the epidermal cells surrounding sweat and oil glands and hair follicles extend into dermal tissue and regrow to heal partial-thickness wounds. Together the sweat and oil glands and the hair follicles are the *dermal appendages,* which vary in depth in different body areas. For example, the sweat and oil glands in the palm of the hand and the sole of the foot extend deep into the dermis. This allows for healing of deep burns in these areas. The epidermis has no blood vessels, and nutrients must diffuse from the second layer of skin, the dermis.

The dermis is thicker than the epidermis and is made up of collagen, fibrous connective tissue, and elastic fibers. Within the dermis are the blood vessels, sensory nerves, hair follicles, lymph vessels, sebaceous glands, and sweat glands.

When burn injury occurs, skin can regrow as long as parts of the dermis are present. When the entire dermal layer is burned, all cells and dermal appendages are destroyed, and the skin can no longer restore itself. The subcutaneous tissue lies below the dermis and is separated from the dermis by the basement membrane, a thin, noncellular protein surface. With deep burns, the subcutaneous tissues may be damaged, leaving bones, tendons, and muscles exposed.

Functional Changes. The skin has many functions when TISSUE INTEGRITY is intact (see Table 24-1). It is a protective barrier against injury and microbial invasion. Burns break this barrier, greatly increasing the risk for infection.

The skin helps maintain the delicate FLUID AND ELECTROLYTE BALANCE essential for life. After a burn injury, massive fluid loss occurs through excessive evaporation. The rate of evaporation is in proportion to the total body surface area (TBSA) burned and the depth of injury.

The skin is an excretory organ through sweating. Full-thickness burns destroy the sweat glands, reducing excretory ability.

The sensations of pain, pressure, temperature, and touch are triggered on the skin in normal daily activities, which allows a person to react to changes in the environment. *All burn injuries are painful.* With partial-thickness burns, nerve endings are exposed, increasing sensitivity and pain. With full-thickness burns, nerve endings are completely destroyed. At first these wounds may not transmit sensation except at wound edges. Despite this destruction, patients often have dull or pressure-type pain in these areas.

Skin exposed to sunlight activates vitamin D. Partial-thickness burns reduce the activation of vitamin D, and this function is lost completely in areas of full-thickness burns.

The internal body temperature remains within a narrow range (about 84.2° to 109.4° F [29° to 43° C]) compared with the temperatures of the external environment. Skin TISSUE INTEGRITY is important in maintaining normal body temperature. Circulating blood in the skin both provides and dissipates heat efficiently. When heat is applied to the skin, the temperature under the dermis rises rapidly. As soon as the heat source is removed, compensatory processes quickly return the area to a normal temperature. If the heat source is not removed or if it is applied at a rate that exceeds the skin's capacity to dissipate it, cells are destroyed.

Physical identity is partly determined by the skin's cosmetic quality, which contributes to each individual's unique appearance. A patient who sustains a major burn often develops reduced self-image and other psychosocial problems as a result of appearance changes.

Depth of Burn Injury. The severity of a burn is determined by how much of the body surface area is involved and the depth of the burn. The degree of TISSUE INTEGRITY loss is related to the agent causing the burn, the temperature of the heat source, and how long the skin is exposed to it.

Differences in skin thickness in various parts of the body also affect burn depth. In areas where the skin is thin (e.g., eyelids, ears, nose, genitalia, tops of the hands and feet, fingers, and toes), a short exposure to high temperatures causes a deep burn injury. The skin is thinner in older adults (Touhy & Jett, 2015), which increases their risk for greater burn severity, even at lower temperatures of shorter duration.

Burn wounds are classified as superficial-thickness wounds, partial-thickness wounds, full-thickness wounds, and deep full-thickness wounds. The partial-thickness wounds are further divided into superficial and deep subgroups. Table 26-1 lists the differences of these burns.

Burns are classified as minor, moderate, or major, depending on the depth, extent, and location of injury (Table 26-2). Fig. 26-1 shows the tissue layers involved with different depths of injury.

Superficial-Thickness Wounds. Superficial-thickness wounds have the least damage because the epidermis is the only part of the skin that is injured. The epithelial cells and basement membrane, needed for total regrowth, remain present.

These wounds are caused by prolonged exposure to low-intensity heat (e.g., sunburn) or short (flash) exposure to

TABLE 26-1	Classification of Burn Depth				
CHARACTERISTIC	**SUPERFICIAL**	**SUPERFICIAL PARTIAL-THICKNESS**	**DEEP PARTIAL-THICKNESS**	**FULL-THICKNESS**	**DEEP FULL-THICKNESS**
Color	Pink to red	Pink to red	Red to white	Black, brown, yellow, white, red	Black
Edema	Mild	Mild to moderate	Moderate	Severe	Absent
Pain	Yes	Yes	Yes	Yes and no	Absent
Blisters	No	Yes	Rare	No	No
Eschar	No	No	Yes, soft and dry	Yes, hard and inelastic	Yes, hard and inelastic
Healing time	3-6 days	About 2 wk	2-6 wk	Weeks to months	Weeks to months
Grafts required	No	No	Can be used if healing is prolonged	Yes	Yes
Example	Sunburn, flash burns	Scalds, flames, brief contact with hot objects	Scalds; flames; prolonged contact with hot objects, tar, grease, chemicals	Scalds; flames; prolonged contact with hot objects, tar, grease, chemicals, electricity	Flames; electricity, grease, tar, chemicals

TABLE 26-2 Classification of Burn Injury and Burn Center Referral Criteria

CHARACTERISTICS	COMMENTS
Minor Burns Partial-thickness burns less than 10% TBSA Full-thickness burns less than 2% TBSA No burns of eyes, ears, face, hands, feet, or perineum No electrical burns No inhalation injury No complicated additional injury Patient is younger than 60 years and has no chronic cardiac, pulmonary, or endocrine disorder	Patients in this category should receive emergency care at the scene and be taken to a hospital emergency department. A special expertise hospital or designated burn center is usually not necessary.
Moderate Burns Partial-thickness burns 15%-25% TBSA Full-thickness burns 2%-10% TBSA No burns of eyes, ears, face, hands, feet, or perineum No electrical burns No inhalation injury No complicated additional injury Patient is younger than 60 years and has no chronic cardiac, pulmonary, or endocrine disorder	Patients in this category should receive emergency care at the scene and be transferred to either a special-expertise hospital or a designated burn center.
Major Burns Partial-thickness burns greater than 25% TBSA Full-thickness burns greater than 10% TBSA Any burn involving the eyes, ears, face, hands, feet, perineum Electrical injury Inhalation injury Patient is older than 60 years Burn complicated with other injuries (e.g., fractures) Patient has cardiac, pulmonary, or other chronic metabolic disorders	Patients who meet *any one* of the criteria for a major burn should receive emergency care at the nearest emergency department and then be transferred to a designated burn center as soon as possible.

TBSA, Total body surface area.

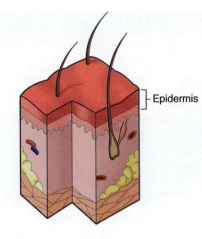

Superficial burns damage only the top layer of the skin—the epidermis. Healing occurs in 3-6 days.

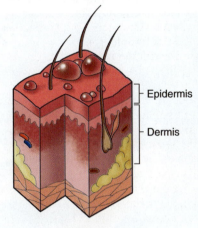

Superficial partial-thickness burns are those in which the entire epidermis and variable portions of the dermis layer of skin are destroyed. Uncomplicated healing occurs in 10-21 days.

Deep partial-thickness burns extend into the deeper layers of the dermis. Healing occurs in 2-6 weeks.

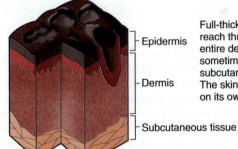

Full-thickness burns reach through the entire dermis and sometimes into the subcutaneous fat. The skin cannot heal on its own.

FIG. 26-1 Tissues involved in burns of various depths.

high-intensity heat. Redness with mild edema, alterations in COMFORT, and increased sensitivity to heat occurs as a result. Desquamation (peeling of dead skin) occurs 2 to 3 days after the burn. The area heals rapidly in 3 to 6 days without a scar or other complication.

Partial-Thickness Wounds. A partial-thickness wound involves TISSUE INTEGRITY loss of the entire epidermis and varying depths of the dermis. Depending on the amount of dermal tissue damaged, partial-thickness wounds are further subdivided into superficial partial-thickness and deep partial-thickness injuries.

Superficial partial-thickness wounds are caused by injury to the upper third of the dermis, leaving a good blood supply. These wounds are pink and moist and blanch (lighten) when pressure is applied (Fig. 26-2). The small vessels bringing blood to this area are injured, resulting in the leakage of large amounts of plasma, which in turn lifts the heat-destroyed epidermis, causing blister formation. The blisters continue to increase in size after the burn as cell and protein breakdown occur. Small blisters are often left

intact if they are not located over a joint. Large blisters usually are opened and débrided to promote healing.

Superficial partial-thickness wounds increase pain sensation. Nerve endings are exposed, and any stimulation (touch or temperature change) causes intense pain. With standard care, these burns heal in 10 to 21 days with no scar; but some minor pigment changes may occur.

Deep partial-thickness wounds extend deeper into the skin dermis, and fewer healthy cells remain. Blisters usually do not form because the dead tissue layer is thick, sticks to the underlying dermis, and does not readily lift off the surface. The wound surface is red and dry with white areas in deeper parts (dry because fewer blood vessels are patent). When pressure is applied to the burn, it blanches slowly or not at all (Fig. 26-3).

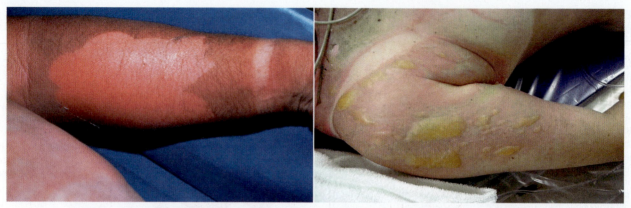

FIG. 26-2 Typical appearance of a superficial partial-thickness burn injury.

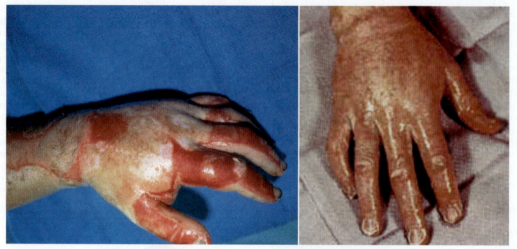

FIG. 26-3 Typical appearance of a deep partial-thickness burn injury.

Edema is moderate, and pain is less than with superficial burns because more of the nerve endings have been destroyed.

Blood flow to these areas is reduced, and progression to deeper injury can occur from hypoxia and ischemia. Adequate hydration, nutrients, and oxygen are needed for regrowth of skin cells and prevention of conversion to deeper burns. These wounds can convert to full-thickness wounds when tissue damage increases with infection, hypoxia, or ischemia. Deep partial-thickness wounds generally heal in 2 to 6 weeks, but scar formation results. Surgical intervention with skin grafting can reduce healing time.

Full-Thickness Wounds. A full-thickness wound occurs with destruction of the entire epidermis and dermis, leaving no skin cells to repopulate (Fig. 26-4). This wound does not regrow, and areas not closed by wound contraction (see Chapter 25) require grafting.

The full-thickness burn has a hard, dry, leathery *eschar* that forms from coagulated particles of destroyed skin. *The eschar is dead tissue; it must slough off or be removed from the wound before healing can occur.* These thick particles often stick to the lower tissue layers, making eschar removal difficult. Edema is severe under the eschar in a full-thickness wound. When the injury is **circumferential** (completely surrounds an extremity or the chest), blood flow and chest movement for breathing may be reduced by tight eschar. **Escharotomies** (incisions through the eschar) or **fasciotomies** (incisions through eschar and fascia)

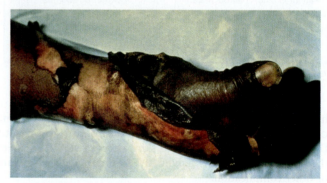

FIG. 26-4 Typical appearance of a full-thickness burn injury.

may be needed to relieve pressure and allow normal blood flow and breathing. (See the Surgical Management discussion in the Preventing Hypovolemic Shock and Inadequate Gas Exchange section.)

A full-thickness burn may be waxy white, deep red, yellow, brown, or black. Thrombosed and heat-coagulated blood vessels may be seen beneath the surface of the burn and leave the burned tissue without a blood supply. Sensation is reduced or absent because of nerve-ending destruction. Healing time depends on establishing a good blood supply in the injured areas. This process can range from weeks to months.

Deep Full-Thickness Wounds. Deep full-thickness wounds extend beyond the skin and damage muscle, bone, and tendons. These burns occur with flame, electrical, or chemical injuries. The wound is blackened and depressed, and sensation is completely absent (Fig. 26-5). All full-thickness burns need early excision and grafting. Grafting decreases pain and length of stay and hastens recovery. Amputation may be needed when an extremity is involved.

Vascular Changes

Circulation to the burned skin is disrupted immediately after injury by blood vessel occlusion. Macrophages in damaged tissues release chemicals that at first cause blood vessel constriction. Blood vessel thrombosis may occur, causing necrosis, which can lead to deeper injuries in these areas.

Fluid shift occurs after initial vasoconstriction as a result of blood vessels near the burn dilating and leaking fluids into the interstitial space (Fig. 26-6). This fluid shift, also known as *third spacing* or *capillary leak syndrome,* is a continuous leak of plasma from the vascular space into the interstitial space. The impaired FLUID AND ELECTROLYTE BALANCE leads to loss of plasma fluids and proteins, which decreases blood volume and blood pressure (McCance et al., 2014). Leakage of fluid and electrolytes from the vascular space continues, causing extensive edema, even in areas that were not burned. Fluid shift, with excessive weight gain, occurs in the first 12 hours after the burn and can continue for 24 to 36 hours.

The amount of fluid shifted depends on the extent and severity of injury. Capillary leak occurs in both burned and unburned areas when tissue damage is extensive (i.e., more than 25% total body surface area [TBSA]). Edema develops as plasma and electrolytes escape into the interstitial space. The proteins now in the interstitial space increase the movement of fluids out from the vascular space.

Profound disruptions of FLUID AND ELECTROLYTE BALANCE and acid-base balance occur as a result of the fluid shift and cell damage. These imbalances often include hypovolemia, metabolic acidosis, hyperkalemia (high blood potassium level), and hyponatremia (low blood sodium level). Hyperkalemia occurs as a result of direct cell injury that releases large amounts of cellular potassium. Sodium is retained by the body as a result of the endocrine response to stress. Aldosterone secretion increases, leading to increased sodium reabsorption by the kidney. However, this sodium quickly passes into the interstitial spaces of the burned area with the fluid shift. Thus, despite the increased amount of sodium in the body, most of the sodium is trapped in the interstitial space, and a sodium deficit occurs in the blood. Hemoconcentration (elevated blood osmolarity, hematocrit, and hemoglobin) develops from vascular dehydration. This problem increases blood viscosity, reducing blood flow and increasing tissue hypoxia.

Fluid remobilization starts at about 24 hours after injury, when the capillary leak stops. The diuretic stage begins at about 48 to 72 hours after the burn injury as capillary membrane integrity returns and edema fluid shifts from the interstitial spaces into the intravascular space. Blood volume increases, leading to increased kidney blood flow and diuresis unless kidney damage has occurred. Body weight returns to normal over the next few days as edema subsides.

During this phase, hyponatremia develops because of increased kidney sodium excretion and the loss of sodium from wounds. Hypokalemia (low blood potassium level) results from potassium moving back into the cells and also being excreted in urine. Anemia often develops as a result of hemodilution, but it is generally not severe enough to require blood transfusions. Transfusions are needed only if the patient's hematocrit is less than 20% to 25% and the patient has signs and symptoms of hypoxia. Protein continues to be lost from the wounds. Metabolic acidosis is possible because of the loss of bicarbonate in the urine and the increased rate of metabolism.

Cardiac Changes

Heart rate increases, and cardiac output decreases because of the initial fluid shifts and hypovolemia that occur after a burn injury. Cardiac output may remain low until 18 to 36 hours after the burn injury. It improves with fluid resuscitation and reaches normal levels before plasma volume is restored completely.

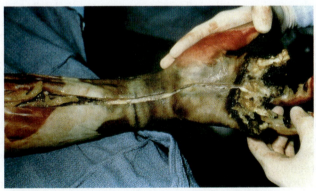

FIG. 26-5 Typical appearance of a deep full-thickness burn injury.

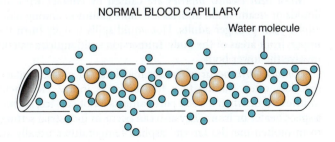

NORMAL BLOOD CAPILLARY

Water molecule

Water is the smallest molecule that can pass through the capillary pores.

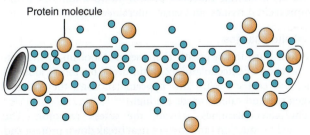

POSTBURN BLOOD CAPILLARY

Protein molecule

Permeability is drastically increased, which allows large molecules such as proteins to pass through the capillary pores easily.

FIG. 26-6 Capillary response to burn injury (early phase). This response is also known as "capillary leak syndrome."

Proper fluid resuscitation and support with oxygen prevent further complications.

Pulmonary Changes

Direct injury to the lungs from contact with flames rarely occurs. Rather, respiratory problems are caused by superheated air, steam, toxic fumes, or smoke. *Such problems are a major cause of death in patients with burns and are most likely to occur when the burn takes place indoors.* Respiratory failure with burn injuries can result from airway edema during fluid resuscitation, pulmonary capillary leak, chest burns that restrict chest movement, and carbon monoxide poisoning.

Respiratory damage from an inhalation injury can occur in the upper and major airways and the lung tissue. The upper airway is affected when inhaled smoke or irritants cause edema and obstruct the trachea. Heat can reach the upper airway, causing an inflammatory response that leads to edema of the mouth and throat with the potential of airway obstruction.

Chemicals and toxic gases produced during combustion can cause airway injury. The ciliated membranes lining the trachea normally trap foreign materials. Smoke and gases slow this activity, allowing particles to enter the bronchi. The lining of the trachea and bronchi may slough 48 to 72 hours after injury and obstruct the lower airways.

Lung tissue injuries result from toxic irritant damage to the alveoli and capillaries. Leaking capillaries cause alveolar edema, which can occur immediately or up to a week after the injury. The fluid that diffuses into the lung tissue spaces contains proteins that form fibrinous membranes and lead to respiratory distress. Progressive pulmonary failure develops, leading to acute pulmonary insufficiency and infection.

Gastrointestinal Changes

The fluid shifts and decreased cardiac output that occur after injury decrease blood flow to the GI tract. Gastric mucosal TISSUE INTEGRITY and motility are impaired. The sympathetic nervous system stress response increases secretion of epinephrine and norepinephrine, which inhibit GI motility and further reduce blood flow to the area. Peristalsis decreases, and a paralytic ileus may develop. Secretions and gases collect in the GI tract, causing abdominal distention.

Curling's ulcer (acute gastroduodenal ulcer that occurs with the stress of severe injury) may develop within 24 hours after a severe burn injury because of reduced GI blood flow and mucosal damage (McCance et al., 2014). The mucus lining the stomach normally protects the tissue from the hydrogen ions secreted into the stomach. With decreased gastric mucus production and increased hydrogen ion production, ulcers may develop. This complication is now less common because of the use of H_2 histamine blockers, proton pump inhibitors, drugs that protect GI tissues, and early enteral feeding.

Metabolic Changes

A serious burn injury greatly increases metabolism by increasing secretion of catecholamines, antidiuretic hormone, aldosterone, and cortisol. With this hypermetabolism, the patient's oxygen use and calorie needs are high.

The catecholamines activate the stress response. The increased production (and loss) of heat break down protein and fat *(catabolism)*, rapidly use glucose and calories, and increase urine nitrogen loss. The heat and water lost from the burn also increase metabolic rate and calorie needs. Depending on the extent of injury, the patient's calorie needs double or triple normal energy needs. These increased rates peak 4 to 12 days after the burn and can remain elevated for months until all wounds are closed.

The hypermetabolic condition also increases core body temperature. The patient loses heat through the burned areas. Core body temperature increases as a response to the adjustment in temperature regulation by the hypothalamus, resulting in a low-grade fever.

Immunologic Changes

Burn injury disrupts or destroys the protective skin tissue integrity, increasing the risk for infection. The injury activates the inflammatory response and often suppresses all types of immune functions. Antibiotic therapy and other interventions for burns further reduce immune function.

Compensatory Responses

Any injury is a stressor and can disrupt homeostasis. Two compensatory (adaptive) responses have immediate benefit: the inflammatory response and the sympathetic nervous system stress response. Together these responses cause changes that result in many of the signs and symptoms seen in the first 2 to 3 days after a burn injury.

Inflammatory compensation is helpful by triggering healing in the injured tissues and also is responsible for the serious problems that occur with the fluid shift. This compensation causes blood vessels to leak fluid into the interstitial space and white blood cells to release chemicals that trigger local tissue reactions. These responses cause the massive fluid shift, edema, and hypovolemia that are seen in the resuscitation phase (first 24 to 48 hours) after a burn injury. The extent of the inflammatory response depends on the burn severity. Chapter 17 explains inflammation and the inflammatory responses in detail.

Sympathetic nervous system compensation is the stress response that occurs when any physical stressors are present. Changes caused by sympathetic compensation are most evident in the cardiovascular, respiratory, and GI systems. Fig. 26-7 shows the results of sympathetic nervous system stimulation.

Etiology

Burn injuries are caused by dry heat (flame), moist heat (scald), contact with hot or rough surfaces, chemicals, electricity, and ionizing radiation. The cause of the injury affects both the prognosis and the treatment.

Dry heat injuries are caused by open flame in house fires and explosions. Explosions usually result in flash burns because they produce a brief exposure to very high temperatures.

Moist heat (scald) injuries are caused by contact with hot liquids or steam. Scald injuries are more common among older adults than younger adults. Hot liquid spills usually burn the upper, front areas of the body. Immersion scald injuries usually involve the lower body.

Contact burns occur when hot metal, tar, or grease contacts the skin, often leading to a full-thickness injury. Hot metal injuries occur when a body part contacts a hot surface, such as a space heater or iron. They also can occur in industrial settings from molten metals. Tar and asphalt temperatures usually are greater than 400° F (204.4° C), and deep injuries occur within seconds when the skin is immersed in or splashed with them. Hot grease injuries from cooking are usually deep because of the high temperature of the grease.

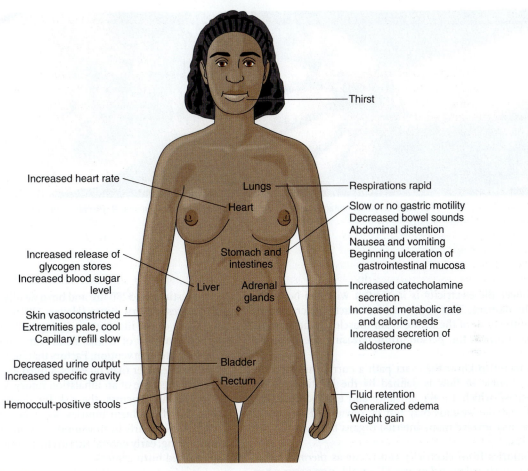

FIG. 26-7 Physiologic actions of the sympathetic nervous system compensatory responses to burn injury (early phase).

Chemical burns occur in home or industrial accidents or as the result of assault. Injury occurs when chemicals directly contact the skin and epithelial tissues or are ingested. The severity of the injury depends on the duration of contact, the concentration of the chemical, the amount of tissue exposed, and the action of the chemical.

Alkalis found in oven cleaners, fertilizers, drain cleaners, and heavy industrial cleaners damage the tissues by causing the skin and its proteins to liquefy. This allows for deeper spread of the chemical and more severe burns. Acids found in bathroom cleaners, rust removers, pool chemicals, and industrial drain cleaners damage TISSUE INTEGRITY by coagulating cells and skin proteins, which can limit the depth of tissue damage. Chemical disinfectants and gasoline are easily absorbed through the skin and have toxic effects on the kidneys and liver.

Electrical injuries are burns occurring when an electrical current enters the body (Fig. 26-8). These injuries have been called the "grand masquerader" of burns because the surface injuries may look small but the associated internal injuries can be huge. Tissue injury from electrical trauma results from electrical energy being converted to heat energy. The extent of injury depends on the type of current, the pathway of flow, the local tissue resistance, and the duration of contact. Once the current penetrates the skin, it flows throughout the involved body part, generating heat and damaging tissues. Deep muscle injury may be present even when superficial muscles appear normal or uninjured.

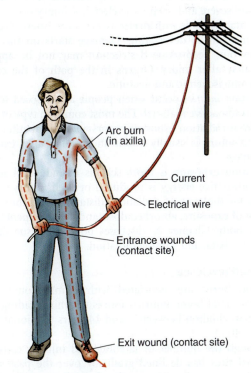

FIG. 26-8 Mechanism of electrical injury: currents passing through the body follow the path of least resistance to the ground.

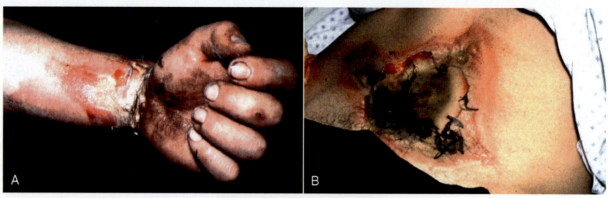

FIG. 26-9 Electrical entrance and exit wounds. **A,** Possible entrance site. **B,** Possible exit site.

The longer the electricity is in contact with the body, the greater the damage. The duration of contact is increased by tetanic contractions of the strong flexor muscles in the forearm, which can prevent the person from releasing the electrical source.

It is difficult to know the exact path a current takes in the body. The course of flow is defined by the locations of the "contact sites," which are the entrance and exit wounds (Fig. 26-9). At first the wounds may not be obvious. The path of the injury may involve many internal organs between the two contact sites.

Burn injuries from electricity can occur as *thermal burns, flash burns,* or *true electrical injury.* Thermal burns occur when clothes ignite from heat or flames produced by electrical sparks. External burn injuries can occur when the electrical current jumps, or "arcs," between two body surfaces. These injuries usually are severe and deep. True electrical injury occurs when direct contact is made with an electrical source. Internal damage results and can be devastating. Damage starts on the inside and goes out; deep-tissue destruction may not be apparent immediately after injury. Organs in the path of the current may become ischemic and necrotic.

Radiation injuries occur when people are exposed to large doses of radioactive material. The most common type of tissue injury from radiation exposure occurs with therapeutic radiation. This injury is usually minor and rarely causes extensive skin damage.

Radiation exposure is more serious in industrial settings where radioactive energy is produced or used. Injury severity depends on the type of radiation, distance from the source, duration of exposure, absorbed dose, and depth of penetration into the body. Chapter 22 discusses potential tissue damage from alpha, beta, and gamma radiation.

Incidence/Prevalence

Fires and burns are associated with unintentional injury deaths and fatal home injuries. Fire is the third leading cause of death in children between 2 and 14 years (National Safety Council, 2017).

Although the number of fatalities and injuries caused by residential fires has declined gradually over the past several decades, many residential fire-related deaths remain preventable and continue to pose a significant public health problem.

An estimated 3280 fire and burn deaths occur each year from all sources of burn injury (Haynes, 2016). Most deaths occur at the scene of the incident or during transport.

The number of deaths from burn injuries decreases with appropriate intervention. Factors that increase the risk for death include age older than 60 years, a burn greater than 40% TBSA, and the presence of an inhalation injury. When a patient has all three of these factors, the risk for death is very high. Better outcomes from burn injuries occur because of vigorous fluid resuscitation, early burn wound excision, improved critical care monitoring, early enteral NUTRITION, antibiotics, and the use of specialized burn centers.

HEALTH PROMOTION AND MAINTENANCE

Minor burns are common, and prevention involves planning and awareness. Teach all people to assess how hot the water is before bathing, showering, or immersing a body part in it. Hot water tanks should be set below 140° F (60° C). Reinforce the use of potholders when taking food from ovens. Stress the importance of never adding a flammable substance (e.g., gasoline, kerosene, alcohol, lighter fluid, charcoal starter) to an open flame. Suggest the use of sunscreen agents and protective clothing to avoid sunburn.

Teach people to reduce the risk for house fires by never smoking in bed, avoiding smoking when drinking alcohol or taking drugs that induce sleep, and keeping matches and lighters out of the reach of children or people who are cognitively impaired. When space heaters are used, stress the importance of keeping clothing, bedding, and other flammable objects away from them. Remind people to keep the screens and doors closed on the fronts of fireplaces and to have chimneys swept each year. Also remind patients using home oxygen not to smoke or have open flames in a room where oxygen is in use.

Leaving a burning building is critical to prevent injury or death. Teach all people to use home smoke detectors and carbon monoxide detectors and to ensure that these are in good working order. The number of detectors needed depends on the size of the home. Recommendations are that each bedroom has a separate smoke detector; there should be at least one detector in the hallway of each story and at least one detector is needed for the kitchen, each stairwell, and each home entrance. Teach everyone to develop a planned escape route with alternatives for when a main route is blocked by fire. Reinforce that no one should ever re-enter a burning building to retrieve belongings.

RESUSCITATION PHASE OF BURN INJURY

Overview

Events within the first hour after injury can make the difference between life and death for the patient with a burn injury. Immediate care focuses on maintaining an open airway, ensuring adequate breathing and circulation, limiting the extent of injury, and maintaining the function of vital organs. Chart 26-1 outlines the emergency management of a burn injury.

The resuscitation phase is the first phase of a burn injury. It begins at the onset of injury and continues for about 24 to 48 hours. During this phase, the injury is evaluated and the immediate problems of fluid imbalance (loss), edema, and reduced blood flow are assessed. The priorities for management during this period are to (1) secure the airway, (2) support circulation and organ PERFUSION by fluid replacement, (3) keep the patient comfortable with analgesics, (4) prevent infection through careful wound care, (5) maintain body temperature, and (6) provide emotional support.

CHART 26-1   Best Practice for Patient Safety & Quality Care QSEN

Emergency Management of Burns

General Management for All Types of Burns
- Assess for airway patency.
- Administer oxygen as needed.
- Cover the patient with a blanket.
- Keep the patient on NPO status.
- Elevate the extremities if no fractures are obvious.
- Obtain vital signs.
- Initiate an IV line and begin fluid replacement.
- Administer tetanus toxoid for prophylaxis.
- Perform a head-to-toe assessment.

Specific Management
Flame Burns
- Smother the flames.
- Remove smoldering clothing and all metal objects.

Chemical Burns
- If dry chemicals are present on skin or clothing, DO NOT WET THEM.
- Brush off any dry chemicals present on the skin or clothing.
- Remove the patient's clothing.
- Ascertain the type of chemical causing the burn.
- Do not attempt to neutralize the chemical unless it has been positively identified and the appropriate neutralizing agent is available.

Electrical Burns
- At the scene, separate the patient from the electrical current.
- Smother any flames that are present.
- Initiate cardiopulmonary resuscitation.
- Obtain an electrocardiogram (ECG).

Radiation Burns
- Remove the patient from the radiation source.
- If the patient has been exposed to radiation from an unsealed source, remove his or her clothing (using tongs or lead protective gloves).
- If the patient has radioactive particles on the skin, send him or her to the nearest designated radiation decontamination center.
- Help the patient bathe or shower.

❖ INTERPROFESSIONAL COLLABORATIVE CARE

Care of the patient with burns may take place in various locations depending on the severity of burn. Patients with very minor burns may be treated in an outpatient setting, whereas patients with more serious burns are likely to be treated initially in an emergency department (ED) and then hospitalized.

◆ Assessment: Noticing

History. Knowledge of circumstances surrounding the burn injury is valuable in planning the management of a burn patient. If possible, obtain information directly from the patient. If this is not possible, ask family members or witnesses to the event. Ask about the circumstances of the injury, the time and place of injury, and the source and cause of injury. Asked detailed questions about how the burn occurred and the events occurring from the time of injury until help arrived. Also obtain demographic data, health history (including pre-existing illness), drug use, any additional injuries, and pain information.

Demographic data include age, weight, and height. The rate of serious complications and death from burn injuries is increased among adults older than 50 years. Chart 26-2 lists the age-related differences in older adults' responses to a burn injury. The patient's preburn weight is used to calculate fluid rates, energy requirements, and drug doses. This weight is the *dry weight*, because it is the patient's weight before edema forms. Calculations based on a weight obtained after fluid replacement is started are not accurate. Height is important in determining total body surface area (TBSA), which is used to calculate NUTRITION needs.

A health history, including any pre-existing illnesses, must be known for appropriate management. Obtain specific information about the patient's history of cardiac or kidney problems, chronic alcoholism, substance abuse, and diabetes mellitus; any of these problems influence fluid resuscitation. The stress of a burn can make a mild disease process worsen. Obtain a drug history that includes allergies, current drugs, and immunization status from the patient or family. Determine the dose and time the last drug was taken. Ask whether the patient smokes or drinks alcohol daily; these factors influence treatment plans and responses.

Other injuries may occur at the time of the burn. Such injuries increase the risk for complications or death. Determine whether additional injuries such as fractures, chest injuries, and abdominal trauma are causing alterations in COMFORT.

Physical Assessment/Signs and Symptoms. Physical assessment findings in the resuscitation phase differ greatly from findings later in the course of the injury. Use a systematic approach to ensure that no problem is missed. Assessment of the respiratory system is most critical to prevent life-threatening complications.

Respiratory Assessment. Patients with major burn injuries and those with inhalation injury, as listed in Table 26-3, are at risk for respiratory problems. *Thus continuous airway assessment is a nursing priority.*

Direct Airway Injury. The degree of inhalation damage depends on the fire source, temperature, environment, and types of toxic gases generated. Ask about the source of the fire, duration of exposure, and whether the fire was in an enclosed space. Inspect the mouth, nose, and pharynx. Burns of the lips, face, ears, neck, eyelids, eyebrows, and eyelashes are strong indicators that an inhalation injury may be present. Burns inside the mouth and

CHART 26-2   Nursing Focus on the Older Adult

Age-Related Changes Increasing Complications from Burn Injury

AGE-RELATED CHANGES	COMPLICATIONS AND NURSING CONSIDERATIONS
Thinner skin, sensory impairment, decreased mobility	Sensory impairment and decreased mobility increase the risk for burn injury. Thinner skin increases the depth of injury even when the exposure to the cause of injury is of shorter duration.
Slower healing time	Longer time with open areas results in a greater risk for infection, metabolic derangements, and loss of function from contracture formation and scar tissue.
More likely to have cardiac impairments	Limits the aggressiveness of fluid resuscitation. Increases the risk for shock and acute kidney injury (AKI).
Reduced inflammatory and immune responses	Increases the risk for infection and sepsis. Patient may not have a fever when infection is present.
Reduced thoracic and pulmonary compliance	Increased risk for atelectasis, hypoxia, and other pulmonary complications.
More likely to have pre-existing medical conditions such as diabetes mellitus, kidney impairment, or pulmonary impairment	Any of these disorders compromise vital organ function and can interfere with fluid resuscitation efforts or other treatments.

TABLE 26-3   Factors Determining Inhalation Injury or Airway Obstruction

- Patients who were injured in a closed space
- Intra-oral charcoal, especially on teeth and gums
- Patients who were unconscious at the time of injury
- Patients with singed scalp hair, nasal hairs, eyelids, or eyelashes
- Patients who are coughing up carbonaceous sputum
- Changes in voice such as hoarseness or brassy cough
- Use of accessory muscles or stridor
- Poor oxygenation or ventilation
- Edema, erythema, and ulceration of airway mucosa
- Wheezing, bronchospasm
- Patients with extensive burns or burns of the face

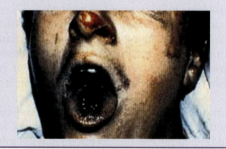

singed nasal hairs also indicate possible inhalation injury. Black particles of carbon in the nose, mouth, and sputum and edema of the nasal septum indicate smoke inhalation, as does a "smoky" smell to the patient's breath.

A change in respiratory pattern may indicate a pulmonary injury. The patient may:

- Become progressively hoarse
- Develop a brassy cough
- Drool or have difficulty swallowing
- Produce sounds on exhalation that include audible wheezes, crowing, and stridor

Any of these changes may mean the patient is about to lose his or her airway.

Upper-airway edema and inhalation injury are most common in the trachea and mainstem bronchi. Auscultation of these areas may reveal wheezes, which indicate partial obstruction.

! NURSING SAFETY PRIORITY (QSEN)

Critical Rescue

Monitor patient's respiratory efforts closely to recognize possible airway involvement. For a burn patient in the resuscitation phase who is hoarse, has a brassy cough, drools or has difficulty swallowing, or produces an audible breath sound on exhalation, respond by immediately applying oxygen and notifying the Rapid Response Team.

Patients with severe inhalation injuries may have such rapid obstruction that, within a short time, they cannot force air through the narrowed airways. As a result, the wheezing sounds disappear. This finding indicates impending airway obstruction and demands immediate intubation. Many patients are intubated when an inhalation injury is first suspected rather than waiting until obstruction makes intubation difficult or impossible.

Carbon Monoxide Poisoning. Carbon monoxide (CO) is one of the leading causes of death from a fire. It is a colorless, odorless, tasteless gas released in the process of combustion. Inhalation injury is a risk for carbon monoxide poisoning (Lafferty et al., 2017).

CO is rapidly transported across the lung membrane and binds tightly to hemoglobin in place of oxygen to form carboxyhemoglobin (COHb), which impairs oxygen unloading at the tissue level. Even though the oxygen-carrying capacity of the hemoglobin is reduced, the blood gas value of partial pressure of arterial oxygen (PaO_2) is normal (Laing, 2013). The vasodilating action of carbon monoxide causes the "cherry red" color (or at least the absence of cyanosis) in these patients. Symptoms vary with the concentration of COHb (Table 26-4).

Thermal (Heat) Injury. Except for steam inhalation, aspiration of scalding liquid, or explosion of flammable gases under pressure, thermal burns to the respiratory tract are usually limited to the upper airway above the glottis (nasopharynx, oropharynx, and larynx).

Inhaled steam can injure the lower respiratory tract down to the major bronchioles. Ulcerations, redness, and edema of the mouth and epiglottis occur first, with rapid swelling leading to upper airway obstruction. Stridor, hoarseness, and shortness of breath result.

TABLE 26-4 Physiologic Effects of Carbon Monoxide Poisoning

CARBON MONOXIDE LEVEL	PHYSIOLOGIC EFFECTS
1%-10% (normal)	Increased threshold to visual stimuli Increased blood flow to vital organs
11%-20% (mild poisoning)	Headache Decreased cerebral function Decreased visual acuity Slight breathlessness
21%-40% (moderate poisoning)	Headache Tinnitus Nausea Drowsiness Vertigo Altered mental state Confusion Stupor Irritability Decreased blood pressure, increased and irregular heart rate Depressed ST segment on ECG and dysrhythmias Pale to reddish-purple skin
41%-60% (severe poisoning)	Coma Convulsions Cardiopulmonary instability
61%-80% (fatal poisoning)	Death

ECG, Electrocardiogram.

? NCLEX EXAMINATION CHALLENGE 26-1

Health Promotion and Maintenance

The client asks about ways to prevent carbon monoxide poisoning. Which teaching will the nurse provide?
A. "You can see black smoke when carbon monoxide is in the air."
B. "If you are experiencing carbon monoxide poisoning, your skin will begin to turn blue."
C. "The only way to get poisoned from carbon monoxide gas is if you are in the presence of a fire."
D. "It is important to have carbon monoxide detectors in your home because this is an odorless gas."

! NURSING SAFETY PRIORITY QSEN

Action Alert

Heat damage of the pharynx is often severe enough to produce edema and upper airway obstruction, especially epiglottitis. The problem can occur any time during resuscitation. In the unresuscitated patient, supraglottic edema may be delayed because of the dehydration that occurs with hypovolemia. However, during fluid resuscitation, the tissues rehydrate and then swell. When it is known that the upper airways were exposed to heat, intubation may be performed as an early intervention before obstruction occurs. When intubation has not been performed in a patient whose upper airways were exposed to heat or toxic gases, continually assess the upper airway for recognition of edema and obstruction.

Smoke Poisoning. Smoke poisoning, or chemical injury from the inhalation of combustion by-products, is a common type of inhalation injury. Toxic by-products are produced when plastics or home furnishings are burned. The products impair respiratory cell function.

Pulmonary Fluid Overload. Pulmonary edema can occur even when the lung tissues have not been damaged directly. Other damaged tissues release such large amounts of inflammatory mediators, causing capillary leak, that even lung capillaries leak fluid into the pulmonary tissue spaces.

Circulatory overload from fluid resuscitation may cause congestive heart failure. This problem creates high pressure within pulmonary blood vessels that pushes fluid into the lung tissue spaces. Excess lung tissue fluid makes GAS EXCHANGE difficult. *The patient is short of breath and has dyspnea in the supine position. Crackles are heard on auscultation.*

! NURSING SAFETY PRIORITY QSEN

Critical Rescue

Monitor patients' respiratory efforts closely to recognize possible development of pulmonary edema. When signs and symptoms of pulmonary edema are present, respond by elevating the head of the bed to at least 45 degrees, applying oxygen, and notifying the burn team or the Rapid Response Team.

External Factors. Patients with burn injuries also may have breathing problems from external factors, such as tight eschar from deep circumferential chest burns. The eschar either restricts chest movement or compresses structures in the neck and throat so airflow is impaired. Inspect the patient's chest hourly for ease of respiration, amount of chest movement, rate of breathing, and effort. If the patient is being mechanically ventilated, increased airway pressures may indicate the need for an escharotomy. Use continuous pulse oximetry to assess breathing effectiveness in maintaining blood oxygen levels.

Cardiovascular Assessment. Changes in the cardiovascular system begin immediately after the burn injury and include shock as a result of disrupted FLUID AND ELECTROLYTE BALANCE. *Hypovolemic shock is a common cause of death in the resuscitation phase in patients with serious injuries.* See Chapter 37 for discussion of shock.

At first, cardiac signs and symptoms are caused by hypovolemia and decreased cardiac output. Monitor the degree of edema and assess cardiac status by measuring central and peripheral pulses, blood pressure, capillary refill, and pulse oximetry. Noninvasive blood pressure readings are inaccurate in patients with large burns of the upper extremities, and invasive blood pressure monitoring may be needed. At first, the patient has tachycardia, decreased blood pressure, and decreased peripheral pulses. Peripheral capillary refill is slow or absent as blood flow decreases. With fluid resuscitation, peripheral edema increases, as does the patient's weight.

Electrocardiographic (ECG) changes can indicate damage to the heart as a result of electrical burn injuries or stress that induces a myocardial infarction. Obtain baseline ECG tracings at the time of admission and continue the ECG monitoring throughout the resuscitation phase. Compare current ECG tracings with the initial tracings to assess whether the patient is experiencing new-onset conduction abnormalities from the burn injury or the fluid resuscitation.

Kidney/Urinary Assessment. Changes in kidney function with burn injury are related to decreased blood flow and cellular debris. During the fluid shift, blood flow to the kidney may not be adequate for filtration. As a result, urine output is greatly decreased compared with IV fluid intake. The urine is very concentrated and has a high specific gravity.

Other substances may be present in the blood that flows through the kidney. Destroyed red blood cells release hemoglobin and potassium. When muscle damage occurs from a major burn or electrical injury, *myoglobin* is released from damaged muscle and circulates to the kidney. Most damaged cells release proteins that form uric acid. All of these large molecules in the blood may precipitate in the kidney tubular system. A "sludge" then forms that blocks kidney blood and urine flow and may cause kidney failure.

Assess kidney function by accurately measuring urine output hourly and comparing this value with fluid intake. Urine output is decreased during the first 24 hours of the resuscitation phase. Fluid resuscitation is provided at the rate needed to maintain urine output at 30 to 50 mL per hour or 0.5 mL/kg/hr. Assess response to fluid resuscitation by measuring urine specific gravity, blood urea nitrogen (BUN), serum creatinine, and serum sodium levels in addition to hourly urine output. Examine the urine for color, odor, and the presence of particles or foam.

Skin Assessment. Assess the skin to determine the size and depth of burn injury. The size of the injury is first estimated in comparison with the *total body surface area (TBSA)*. For example, a burn that involves 40% of the TBSA is a 40% burn. The size of the injury is important not only for diagnosis and prognosis but also for calculating drug doses, fluid replacement volumes, and caloric needs.

Inspect the skin TISSUE INTEGRITY to identify injured areas and changes in color and appearance. Except with electrical burns, this initial size assessment usually can be made accurately with specific assessment tools and charts.

The most rapid method for calculating the size of a burn injury in adult patients whose weights are in normal proportion to their heights is the *rule of nines* (Fig. 26-10). With this method, the body is divided into areas that are multiples of 9%. It is useful at the site of injury, but more accurate evaluations using other methods are made in the burn unit.

Because specific treatments are related to the depth of the burn injury, initial assessment of the skin includes estimations of burn depth. Criteria for depth of injury are based on appearance and associated characteristics (see the Depth of Burn Injury section).

Accurate evaluation of burn depth is performed using thermography, vital dyes, indocyanine green (ICG) video angiography, and laser Doppler imaging (LDI), which provide precise measurement of the amount of PERFUSION of the injured tissue. ICG and LDI are the most accurate of the three methods. LDI is used more frequently because it is relatively accurate, less invasive, and faster than the other methods (Park et al., 2013).

Gastrointestinal Assessment. Although the GI tract usually is not injured directly, changes in function occur in all burn patients. The decreased blood flow and sympathetic stimulation reduce GI motility and promote development of a paralytic ileus. Bowel sounds are usually reduced or absent in a patient with severe burns. Other indications of a paralytic ileus include nausea, vomiting, and abdominal distention. Patients with burns of 25% TBSA or who are intubated generally require a nasogastric (NG) tube inserted to prevent aspiration and remove gastric secretions. Assess the tube for placement and patency after insertion. Examine each stool and vomitus for gross blood or other material that indicates partially digested

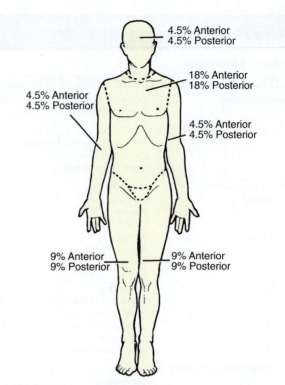

FIG. 26-10 Rule of nines for estimating burn percentage.

4.5% Anterior
4.5% Posterior

18% Anterior
18% Posterior

4.5% Anterior
4.5% Posterior

4.5% Anterior
4.5% Posterior

9% Anterior
9% Posterior

9% Anterior
9% Posterior

blood ("coffee ground"–appearing crumbs). Test for the presence of occult blood on any vomit or stool.

Laboratory Assessment. Certain changes in laboratory test values are found in different phases of postburn recovery and reflect tissue damage or compensatory responses. However, other changes in specific laboratory findings may suggest complications.

During the resuscitation phase and before the start of fluid resuscitation, blood analysis reflects the fluid shift and direct tissue damage. Baseline laboratory test values and early postburn expected changes are listed in Chart 26-3.

Changes in the total white blood cell (WBC) count and differential reflect immune function and inflammatory responses to the burn injury. The burn patient's total WBC count, especially the neutrophil percentage, first rises and then drops rapidly, with a "left shift" (see Chapter 17) as the immune system becomes unable to sustain its defenses. If sepsis occurs, the total WBC count may be as low as 2000 cells/mm^3 (2×10^9/L).

Other laboratory tests that provide useful information about the burn patient's status include urine electrolyte assays, urine cultures, liver enzyme studies, and clotting studies. Drug and alcohol screens are obtained if drug or alcohol intoxication is suspected.

🌐 **CULTURAL/SPIRITUAL CONSIDERATIONS**
Patient-Centered Care **QSEN**

For African-American patients, a sickle cell preparation is performed if sickle status is unknown. The trauma of a burn injury can trigger a sickle cell crisis in patients who have the disease and those who carry the trait.

CHART 26-3 Laboratory Profile

Burn Assessment During the Resuscitation Phase

TEST	NORMAL RANGE FOR ADULTS	NORMAL RANGE FOR ADULTS (🍁)	SIGNIFICANCE OF ABNORMAL FINDINGS
Serum Studies			
Hemoglobin	12-16 g/dL (women) 14-18 g/dL (men)	120-160 g/L (women) 140-180 g/L (men)	Elevated as a result of fluid volume loss
Hematocrit	37%-47% (women) 42%-52% (men)	0.37-0.47 volume fraction (women) 0.42-0.52 volume fraction (men)	Elevated as a result of fluid volume loss
Urea nitrogen	10-20 mg/dL	3.6-7.1 mmol/L (older adult may be slightly higher)	Elevated as a result of fluid volume loss
Glucose	74-106 mg/dL	4.1-5.9 mmol/L	Elevated as a result of the stress response and altered uptake across injured tissues
Electrolytes			
Sodium	136-145 mEq/L (mmol/L)	136-145 mEq/L (mmol/L)	Decreased; sodium is trapped in edema fluid and lost through plasma leakage
Potassium	3.5-5.0 mEq/L (mmol/L)	3.5-5.0 mEq/L (mmol/L)	Elevated as a result of disruption of the sodium-potassium pump, tissue destruction, and red blood cell hemolysis
Chloride	98-106 mEq/L (mmol/L)	98-106 mEq/L (mmol/L)	Elevated as a result of fluid volume loss and reabsorption of chloride in urine
Arterial Blood Gas Studies			
PaO_2	80-100 mm Hg	80-100 mm Hg	Slightly decreased
$PaCO_2$	35-45 mm Hg	35-45 mm Hg	Slightly increased from respiratory injury
pH	7.35-7.45	7.35-7.45	Low as a result of metabolic acidosis
Carboxyhemoglobin (COHb)	0%-10%	No greater than 10%; over 20% is considered critical	Elevated as a result of inhalation of smoke and carbon monoxide
Other			
Total protein	6.4-8.3 g/dL	64-83 g/L	Low; protein exudate is lost through the wound
Albumin	3.5-5.0 g/dL	35-50 g/L	Low; protein is lost through the wound and through vascular membranes because of increased permeability

Data from Pike-MacDonald, S. (Ed.). (2013). *Mosby's Canadian manual of diagnostic and laboratory tests* (1st Canadian ed.). Toronto: Elsevier Canada; and Pagana, K., Pagana, T. J., & Pagana, T. N. (2017). *Mosby's diagnostic and laboratory test reference* (13th ed.). St. Louis: Mosby.

Imaging Assessment. Standard x-rays and scans do not provide direct assessment data about the burn wound. These assessments are not performed unless other trauma is suspected.

Other Diagnostic Assessment. Specific diagnostic studies are performed when deep organ trauma is suspected. Such studies include renal scans, computed tomography (CT), ultrasonography, bronchoscopy, and magnetic resonance imaging (MRI). When burn injuries involve the eye, an ophthalmic evaluation is performed to detect corneal damage (see Chapters 46 and 47 for specific eye and vision evaluation procedures).

◆ *Analysis: Interpreting*

The priority collaborative problems for patients with burn injuries in the resuscitation phase who have sustained a burn injury greater than 25% of the TBSA include:

1. Potential for decreased oxygenation due to upper airway edema, pulmonary edema, airway obstruction, or pneumonia
2. Potential for shock due to increase in capillary permeability, active fluid volume loss, electrolyte imbalance, and inadequate fluid resuscitation
3. Pain (acute and chronic) due to tissue injury, damaged or exposed nerve endings, débridement, dressing changes, invasive procedures, and donor sites

4. Potential for acute respiratory distress syndrome (ARDS) due to inhalation injury

◆ *Planning and Implementation: Responding*

Supporting Oxygenation

Planning: Expected Outcomes. With proper intervention, the patient is expected to maintain a patent airway and have adequate oxygenation. Indicators include that the patient should have either normal or nearly normal oxygen saturation, PaO_2, $PaCO_2$, and arterial pH.

Interventions. Nursing and medical interventions are used to support normal pulmonary function and prevent the pulmonary problems that can result from lung injury or fluid overload and heart failure. (Even young healthy people can develop fluid overload and heart failure.) Specific management plans depend on the cause of the problem and the status of the respiratory tract. *Thus monitoring the patient's respiratory status is a priority nursing intervention.*

Nonsurgical Management. Interventions include airway maintenance, promotion of ventilation, monitoring GAS EXCHANGE, oxygen therapy, drug therapy, positioning, and deep breathing.

Airway maintenance begins at the burn scene in an unconscious patient and may involve only a chin-lift or a head-tilt maneuver. *Remember that upper airway edema becomes*

pronounced 8 to 12 hours after the beginning of fluid resuscitation. Then patients often require nasal or oral intubation if crowing, stridor, or dyspnea is present.

A bronchoscopy is performed to examine the vocal cords and airways of patients at risk for obstruction. Patients with severe smoke inhalation or poisoning may require a bronchoscopy on admission and routinely thereafter for examination of the respiratory tract, deep suctioning of the lungs, and removal of sloughing necrotic tissue. Assess the endotracheal tube hourly to ensure patency and location in intubated patients.

Other causes of airway obstruction are excessive secretions and sloughed tissue from damaged lungs. Suction as indicated based on clinical assessment. Vigorous endotracheal or nasotracheal tube suctioning is performed after chest physiotherapy and aerosol treatments. Patients report that deep endotracheal suctioning is extremely painful. Therefore suctioning the endotracheal tube often requires increased analgesia or sedation.

Promoting ventilation includes ensuring that skeletal muscle movement of the chest is adequate for ventilation. Chest movement can be restricted by eschar and tight dressings that cover the neck, chest, and abdomen. Observe the patient for ease of respiratory movements and loosen tight dressings as needed to assist with ventilation.

Monitor for GAS EXCHANGE by using laboratory tests (e.g., arterial blood gas, carboxyhemoglobin levels) and assessing for cyanosis, disorientation, and increased pulse rate. Additional monitoring may include chest x-ray findings, pulmonary artery catheter pressures, and central venous pressure measurement.

Cyanide poisoning may occur in patients burned in house fires. An elevated plasma lactate level is one indicator of cyanide toxicity even in patients who do not have severe burns.

Oxygen therapy with humidified oxygen by facemask, cannula, or hood is used to manage any breathing impairment in the burn patient. Arterial oxygenation less than 60 mm Hg is an indication for intubation and mechanical ventilation. Keep emergency airway equipment near the bedside. This equipment includes oxygen, masks, cannulas, manual resuscitation bags, laryngoscope, endotracheal tubes, and equipment for tracheostomy. Chapter 32 addresses specific nursing actions for patients during mechanical ventilation.

Drug therapy with antibiotics is used when pneumonia or other pulmonary infections impair breathing. Drug selection is based on known culture and sensitivity reports or on the specific organisms common to that burn unit.

Patients with pulmonary edema and any degree of heart failure may receive beta blockers to improve left ventricular function and prevent or treat pulmonary edema. Diuretics, a mainstay of therapy for pulmonary edema from other causes, may or may not be used in the resuscitation phase, depending on the patient's blood volume and kidney function.

When a patient's activity during mechanical ventilation severely compromises respiratory mechanics, it may be necessary to use a paralytic drug, such as atracurium or vecuronium. Paralytic drugs remove all breathing control from the patient, making mechanical ventilation easier. *These drugs do not prevent the patient from seeing and hearing or from experiencing fear, pain, and loss of control. Any patient receiving neuromuscular blockade drugs must also receive drugs for sedation, analgesia, and antianxiety unless clinically contraindicated.*

> **! NURSING SAFETY PRIORITY** **QSEN**
>
> **Action Alert**
>
> As required by The Joint Commission's National Patient Safety Goals, ensure that all alarms are operative on ventilators. Check patients who are receiving neuromuscular blockage frequently, because they cannot call for help if they become extubated accidentally.

Positioning and deep breathing can improve breathing and GAS EXCHANGE. Turn the patient frequently and assist him or her out of bed to a chair as much as possible. Teach the patient to use coughing and deep-breathing exercises. Urge him or her to use incentive spirometry hourly while awake. Chest physiotherapy may be helpful to mobilize lung secretions.

Surgical Management. A tracheotomy may be needed when long-term intubation is expected. This procedure increases the risk for infection in burn patients even more than in nonburned patients. Emergency tracheotomies are performed when an airway becomes occluded and oral or nasal intubation cannot be achieved.

Other surgical procedures for improving the burn patient's GAS EXCHANGE include inserting chest tubes and performing an escharotomy. Chest tubes are used to re-expand the lung when a pneumothorax or hemothorax has occurred (see Chapter 32). Tight eschar on the neck, chest, or abdomen can restrict respiratory movement. Escharotomies (described in the following Surgical Management section) can relieve this restriction and permit greater respiratory movement.

Preventing Hypovolemic Shock and Inadequate Gas Exchange

Planning: Expected Outcomes. With appropriate intervention, the patient is expected to have blood pressure and tissue oxygenation restored to normal. Indicators include these vital signs and assessment parameters:

- Blood pressure at or near the patient's normal range
- Palpable peripheral pulses (or heard with Doppler) in all extremities
- Oxygen saturation, partial pressure of arterial oxygen (PaO_2), partial pressure of arterial carbon dioxide ($PaCO_2$), and arterial pH at or near the normal ranges

Interventions. Interventions focus on increasing blood fluid volume, supporting compensation, and preventing complications. Nonsurgical management is often sufficient for achieving these aims. Surgical management may be needed for full-thickness burns.

Nonsurgical Management. Fluid volume and tissue blood flow (PERFUSION) are restored through IV fluid therapy and drug therapy. Priority nursing interventions are carrying out fluid resuscitation and monitoring for indications of effectiveness or complications.

Rapid infusion of IV fluids, known as *fluid resuscitation,* is needed to maintain sufficient blood volume for normal cardiac output, mean arterial pressure, and tissue oxygenation. Chart 26-4 lists best practices for fluid resuscitation. There are many formulas for calculating IV fluid needs, but the most commonly used one for adult patients is the Parkland Formula (4 mL/kg/%TBSA burn of crystalloid solution). For example, the calculated fluid needs for a 154-lb man with a 50% TBSA burn would be 4 mL × 70 kg × 50% TBSA = 14,000 mL over the first 24 hours. Although the types and amounts of electrolytes,

◎ **CHART 26-4** **Best Practice for Patient Safety & Quality Care** QSEN

Fluid Resuscitation of the Burn Patient

- Initiate and maintain at least one large-bore IV line in an area of intact skin (if possible).
- Coordinate with physicians to determine the appropriate fluid type and total volume to be infused during the first 24 hours postburn.
- Administer one half of the total 24-hour prescribed volume within the first 8 hours postburn and the remaining volume over the next 16 hours.
- Assess IV access site, infusion rate, and infused volume at least hourly.
- Monitor these vital signs at least hourly:
  - Blood pressure
  - Pulse rate
  - Respiratory rate
  - Breath sounds
  - Voice quality (if not intubated)
  - Oxygen saturation
  - End-tidal carbon dioxide levels
- Assess urine output at least hourly:
  - Volume
  - Color
  - Specific gravity
  - Character
  - Presence of protein
- Assess for fluid overload:
  - Formation of dependent edema
  - Engorged neck veins
  - Rapid, thready pulse
  - Presence of lung crackles or wheezes on auscultation
- Measure additional body fluid output hourly.

crystalloids, and colloids vary, the purpose of any formula is to prevent shock by maintaining blood fluid volume.

Resuscitation for a severe burn requires large fluid loads in a short time to maintain blood flow to vital organs. All common formulas recommend that half of the calculated fluid volume for 24 hours be given in the first 8 hours after injury. The other half is given over the next 16 hours for a total of 24 hours (Culleiton & Simko, 2013a). Fluid boluses are avoided because they increase capillary pressure and worsen edema. In the second 24-hour period after a burn injury, the volume and content of the IV fluids are based on the patient's specific FLUID AND ELECTROLYTE BALANCE needs and his or her response to treatment. This resuscitation involves hourly infusion volumes that are greatly in excess of the 125 mL to 150 mL per hour common infusion rates.

Fluid replacement formulas are calculated from the time of injury and not from the time of arrival at the hospital. For example, if a burn injury occurred at 8 AM but the patient was not admitted to the hospital until 10 AM, the first 8-hour period would be completed at 4 PM (8 hours after the injury). Thus if resuscitation was delayed by 2 hours until admission to the hospital, calculated fluids would need to be given over the next 6-hour period rather than an 8-hour period. Burn resuscitation formulas are guides. The patient's response to therapy determines exact fluid requirements.

The management of extensive burns requires a large-bore central venous catheter so massive fluid loads can be given. Peripheral lines are less useful.

Monitoring patient responses is critical to determine the adequacy of resuscitation for hydration and blood PERFUSION

of the brain, heart, and kidneys. Urine output is the most common and most sensitive noninvasive assessment parameter for cardiac output and tissue PERFUSION. *Regardless of the total amount of fluid calculated as needed for the patient, the amount of fluid given depends on how much IV fluid per hour is needed to maintain the hourly urine output at 0.5 mL/kg (about 30 mL/hr).* Adjustment of the IV fluid rate on the basis of urine output plus serum electrolyte values is known as the *titration* of fluid. In burns larger than 35% TBSA, the use of invasive cardiac and pulmonary function monitoring may be needed in addition to urine output and vital signs to guide resuscitation.

Burn patients can develop severe hypovolemic shock and need invasive cardiac monitoring. Vital parameters such as central venous pressure, pulmonary artery pressures, and cardiac output are obtained on an hourly to continuous basis.

Monitor the ECG activity of patients who have sustained large burns. Compare current ECG findings with those obtained on admission.

❓ **NCLEX EXAMINATION CHALLENGE 26-2**

Safe and Effective Care Environment

Which assessment finding does the nurse interpret as demonstrating a client's fluid resuscitation adequacy?
A. Decreased skin turgor
B. Decreased pulse pressure
C. Decreased core body temperature
D. Decreased urine specific gravity

Drug therapy for shock prevention in burn patients is different from that for the heart failure patient. A common mistake in management is giving diuretics to increase urine output rather than changing the amount and rate of fluid infused. *Diuretics do not increase cardiac output; they actually decrease circulating volume and cardiac output by pulling fluid from the circulating blood volume to enhance diuresis.* This effect reduces blood flow to other vital organs (especially the heart, lungs, and brain) and greatly increases the risk for severe hypovolemic shock. Therefore diuretics are not generally used to improve urine output for burn patients. An exception is the patient with an electrical burn injury. In electrical burns, muscle and deep-tissue damage release the large protein myoglobin, which precipitates in and obstructs the renal tubules. Although the diuretic mannitol (Osmitrol) is often used in this situation, it should always be given after adequate urine output has been established. Hourly urine output should be maintained at 0.5 mL/kg in adults (Rice et al., 2017).

Surgical Management. The surgical procedure for the treatment of inadequate tissue PERFUSION is *escharotomy*. An

🧓 **CONSIDERATIONS FOR OLDER ADULTS**

Patient-Centered Care QSEN

In older patients, especially those with cardiac disease, a complicating factor in fluid resuscitation may be heart failure or myocardial infarction. Drugs that increase cardiac output (e.g., dopamine [Intropin]) or that strengthen the force of myocardial contraction may be used along with fluid therapy. Assess the cardiac status of older adults at least every hour during fluid resuscitation.

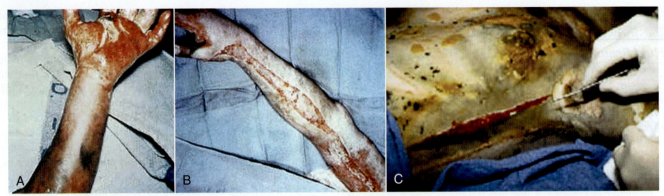

FIG. 26-11 Escharotomy to release circumferential burn eschar and improve circulation to a distal extremity. **A,** Tight circumferential eschar restricting swelling as edema forms in the tissue beneath the eschar. Edema compresses blood vessels, which inhibits blood flow to the distal extremity. **B,** An escharotomy incision allows outward swelling of edematous tissues. The restricted blood flow to the distal extremity is relieved. **C,** An anterior axillary incision is made bilaterally to relieve respiratory distress.

incision through the burn eschar relieves pressure caused by the constricting force of fluid buildup under circumferential burns on the extremity or chest and improves circulation. If the pressure is not relieved, arterial compression can occur with a loss of blood flow to the extremity, leading to ischemia and possible necrosis. Incisions are made along the length of the extremity and extend into the subcutaneous tissue, relieving the tourniquet effect of the eschar (see Fig. 26-5 and Fig. 26-11). If tissue pressure remains elevated after escharotomy, a *fasciotomy* (a deeper incision extending through the fascia) may be needed.

Managing Pain and Alterations in COMFORT. The pain associated with burn injuries is both chronic and acute, with the causes being multifactorial. Accurate assessment of the patient's pain and COMFORT level before and during procedures is an essential part of pain management.

Planning: Expected Outcomes. The patient's pain level is expected to be alleviated or reduced. Indicators that a patient has pain or an alteration in COMFORT include reports of pain, moaning and/or crying, demonstrating facial grimace, and/or loss of appetite. Indicators that the patient's pain level or alteration in comfort has decreased include verbalization of lessened pain, relaxed facial expressions, and interest in activities that are within the patient's current capabilities (e.g., eating, therapy).

Interventions. Pain management is tailored to the patient's tolerance for pain, expectation for COMFORT level, coping mechanisms, and physical status. *The priority nursing actions include continually assessing the patient's pain level, using appropriate pain-reducing strategies, and preventing complications.*

Nonsurgical Management. Interventions for the patient having pain or COMFORT alterations include drug therapy, complementary therapy measures, and environmental manipulation.

Drug therapy for pain usually requires opioid analgesics (e.g., morphine sulfate, hydromorphone [Dilaudid], fentanyl) and nonopioid analgesics. Although these drugs may provide adequate pain relief when no procedures are being performed, they rarely offer more than moderate relief during painful procedures. They may depress respiratory function and reduce intestinal motility. Thus nonpharmacologic interventions also are needed for the burn patient.

During the resuscitation phase, the IV route is used for giving opioid drugs because of problems with absorption from the muscle and stomach (Culleiton & Simko, 2013b). When given IM or subcutaneously, these drugs remain in the tissue spaces and do not relieve pain. When edema is present, all the doses are rapidly absorbed at once when the fluid shift is resolving. This delayed but rapid absorption can result in lethal blood levels of opioids.

> **⚠ NURSING SAFETY PRIORITY** (QSEN)
>
> ***Drug Alert***
>
> Give opioid drugs for pain only by the IV route during the resuscitation phase to prevent delayed rapid absorption leading to lethal blood levels.

Anesthetic agents, such as ketamine (Ketalar) and nitrous oxide, also reduce pain. Use strict protocols when giving these agents to prevent serious complications.

Complementary and integrative therapy measures for pain reduction include relaxation techniques, meditative breathing, guided imagery, music therapy, massage, and healing or therapeutic touch. Hypnosis and autohypnosis can be used by lucid, cooperative patients under the direction of trained therapists. Therapeutic touch, acupuncture, and acupressure are used to a limited extent for burn patients; the results are variable. Active music interventions for distraction have been useful in reducing patients' perceptions of pain and anxiety.

Environmental changes, such as providing a quiet environment, using nonpainful tactile stimulation, and increasing the patient's control, can increase COMFORT. Sleep deprivation increases patients' discomfort. Increasing sleep or rest time in a quiet environment helps reduce the adverse effects of sleep deprivation, replenishes hormone stores, helps prevent critical care unit psychosis, and restores the diurnal effects of endorphins. Coordinate with the interprofessional health care team to ensure that procedures are performed during the patient's waking hours.

Tactile stimulation can reduce pain. Help the patient change positions every 2 hours to reduce pressure on any specific area, improve circulation to painful areas, and ease pain. Massage nonburn areas to reduce pain transmission and stimulate endorphin release. Apply heat and maintain warm room temperatures to prevent shivering.

To reduce anxiety and increase feelings of confidence and independence, encourage the patient to participate in pain control measures. For example, make a contract with the patient that specifies how long a painful procedure will last. This helps patients deal with the pain for that particular period. Patient-controlled analgesia (PCA) also reduces pain. Important issues and techniques for the best use of PCA include giving an initial bolus of 5 to 10 mg of morphine (or equivalent drug), increasing the PCA dose as needed to achieve pain relief, and planning for a change in dosing regimens at night (e.g., giving a bolus dose at bedtime). See Chapter 4 for a detailed discussion of combination drug therapy for pain management.

Surgical Management. Early surgical excision of the burn wound is used in many burn centers (see the Surgical Excision section). Early excision under anesthesia reduces the pain from daily débridement at the bedside or during hydrotherapy.

Preventing Acute Respiratory Distress Syndrome (ARDS)

Planning: Expected Outcomes. The patient with a burn injury is expected to:

- Not experience acute respiratory distress
- Have arterial blood gases (ABGs) within normal limits
- Maintain normal lung compliance

Interventions. Patients who develop acute respiratory distress syndrome (ARDS) from burn injuries require thorough assessments and interventions. Interventions focus on increasing lung compliance and improving partial pressure of arterial oxygen (PaO_2) levels. The priority nursing care actions are coordinating respiratory therapy strategies and monitoring the patient's response to these interventions.

In collaboration with the health care provider and respiratory therapist, give positive end-expiratory pressure (PEEP) to provide a continuous positive pressure in the airways and alveoli. This procedure enhances the diffusion of oxygen across the alveolar-capillary membrane. PEEP can be combined with intermittent mandatory volume (IMV) to enhance its effectiveness.

Assess and document the patient's response so needed ventilator changes can be made. Monitor pulse oximetry and ABG levels to assess changes in respiratory status.

> **! NURSING SAFETY PRIORITY** QSEN
>
> **Critical Rescue**
>
> Recognize indications of respiratory distress or change in respiratory patterns and respond by immediately reporting assessment findings to the burn team and the respiratory therapist.

Neuromuscular blocking drugs (atracurium) can be used in patients receiving mechanical ventilation to reduce oxygen consumption (see the discussion of specific nursing care in the Supporting Gas Exchange section).

◆ Evaluation: Reflecting

Evaluate the care of the patient in the resuscitation phase of burn injury based on the identified priority patient problem. The primary expected outcomes are that the patient will be properly oxygenated without GAS EXCHANGE complications, not experience hypovolemic shock, experience absence of or manageable levels of pain, and avoid Acute Respiratory Distress Syndrome (ARDS).

> **? CLINICAL JUDGMENT CHALLENGE 26-1**
>
> **Patient-Centered Care; Teamwork and Collaboration; Evidence-Based Practice** QSEN
>
> You are caring for a patient who sustained burns that are pink, moist, sensate, and blanching. Vital signs show a heart rate of 150 beats/min and blood pressure of 90/30. The patient's urine output is 15 mL/hr.
>
> 1. Based on the information provided, is the patient experiencing signs of shock?
> 2. Which degree burn does this patient have? Provide rationale.
> 3. How do you anticipate administering pain medication during the acute phase of burn injury?
> 4. With whom will you collaborate to provide the highest quality interprofessional care for this patient?

ACUTE PHASE OF BURN INJURY

Overview

The acute phase of burn injury begins about 36 to 48 hours after injury, when the fluid shift resolves, and lasts until wound closure is complete. During this phase, the nurse coordinates interprofessional care that is directed toward continued assessment and maintenance of the cardiovascular and respiratory systems and toward GI and NUTRITION status, burn wound care, pain control, and psychosocial interventions.

❖ INTERPROFESSIONAL COLLABORATIVE CARE

Patients in the acute phase of a more serious burn injury are most likely to be treated in an emergency department (ED).

◆ Assessment: Noticing

Physical Assessment/Signs and Symptoms

Cardiopulmonary Assessment. *In the acute phase of burn injury, the priority nursing interventions are to assess the cardiovascular and respiratory systems to maintain these systems and to identify or prevent complications.* At this time, the patient may develop pneumonia that can result in respiratory failure requiring mechanical ventilation. Although cardiovascular problems related to the fluid shift should be resolved, the patient is at risk for infection and sepsis, which affect cardiovascular function.

Neuroendocrine Assessment. The increased metabolic demands placed on the body after a severe burn injury can severely deplete NUTRITION stores. Weigh the patient daily without dressings or splints and compare the weight with his or her preburn weight. A 2% loss of body weight indicates a mild deficit. A 10% or more weight loss requires the evaluation and modification of calorie intake. For very accurate calorie requirements, indirect calorimetry may be used. This method assesses energy expenditure by measuring oxygen consumption and carbon dioxide production. Measurements are taken while the patient is at rest—usually at least 30 minutes after the most recent dressing changes or other stressful procedures. Indirect calorimetry may be performed on admission to a burn center and then weekly until the wounds are closed.

Immune Assessment. The patient with a burn injury is at risk for infection because of open wounds and reduced immune function. *Burn wound sepsis is a serious complication of burn injury, and infection is the leading cause of death during the acute phase of recovery.* Continually assess the patient for signs and symptoms of local and systemic infections (Table 26-5), including changes in wound appearance, changes in neurologic and GI function, and subtle changes in vital signs. Monitor for signs and symptoms of gram-positive, gram-negative, and fungal infections (Table 26-6). Enforce meticulous handwashing by all care personnel.

> ! **NURSING SAFETY PRIORITY** QSEN
>
> *Action Alert*
>
> Use aseptic technique in caring for wounds and during invasive monitoring to prevent infection.

Musculoskeletal Assessment. Patients with a burn injury are at risk for musculoskeletal and MOBILITY problems as a result of other injuries, immobility, healing processes, and treatment. The musculoskeletal status is evaluated on admission and throughout the postburn period. Assess active and passive range of motion for all joints, including the neck. Give special attention to joints in the burn area. Ranges and limitations are documented for future reference.

◆ **Analysis: Interpreting**

During the acute phase of the burn injury, the patient may have initial problems that extend into the acute phase and may develop new problems. The priority collaborative problems for patients with burn injuries greater than 25% TBSA in the acute phase of recovery include:

1. Wound care management due to impaired TISSUE INTEGRITY associated with burn injury and skin grafting procedures
2. Potential for infection of open burn wounds due to the presence of multiple invasive catheters, reduced immune function, and poor NUTRITION
3. Weight loss due to increased metabolic rate, reduced calorie intake, and increased urinary nitrogen losses
4. Decreased MOBILITY due to open burn wounds, pain, scars, and contractures
5. Decreased self-esteem due to trauma, changes in physical appearance and lifestyle, and alterations in sensory and motor function

◆ **Planning and Implementation: Responding**

Managing Wound Care

Planning: Expected Outcomes. With appropriate intervention, the burn patient is expected to have no wound extension and have wounds healed. Indicators include that the patient:

- Has presence of granulation, re-epithelialization, and scar tissue formation
- Has decreased wound size
- Has no new wounds

Interventions. Interventions focus on preserving skin TISSUE INTEGRITY, enhancing burn wound healing, and preventing complications.

Nonsurgical Management. Nonsurgical burn wound management involves removing exudates and necrotic tissue, cleaning the area, stimulating granulation and revascularization, and applying dressings. Restoring skin TISSUE INTEGRITY, whether by natural healing or grafting, starts with the removal of eschar and other cellular debris from the burn wound. This removal is called **débridement** and can be performed nonsurgically through mechanical or enzymatic actions that separate eschar over time. The purpose is to prepare the wound for grafting and wound closure by a natural process. *Priority nursing interventions include assessing the wound, providing wound care, and preventing infection and other complications.*

Mechanical Débridement. Burn wounds are débrided and cleaned one or two times each day during **hydrotherapy** (the application of water for treatment). Nurses, unlicensed assistive personnel (UAP), and physical therapists perform hydrotherapy daily to débride and examine the wounds. Hydrotherapy is performed by showering the patient on a special shower table

TABLE 26-5 Local and Systemic Indicators of Infection

Local Indicators	Systemic Indicators
• Conversion of a partial-thickness injury to a full-thickness injury	• Altered level of consciousness
• Ulceration of healthy skin at the burn site	• Changes in vital signs (tachycardia, tachypnea, temperature instability, hypotension)
• Erythematous, nodular lesions in uninvolved skin and vesicular lesions in healed skin	• Increased fluid requirements for maintenance of a normal urine output
• Edema of healthy skin surrounding the burn wound	• Hemodynamic instability
• Excessive burn wound drainage	• Oliguria
• Pale, boggy, dry, or crusted granulation tissue	• GI dysfunction (diarrhea, vomiting, abdominal distention, paralytic ileus)
• Sloughing of grafts	• Hyperglycemia
• Wound breakdown after closure	• Thrombocytopenia
• Odor	• Change in total white blood cell count (above or below normal)
	• Metabolic acidosis
	• Hypoxemia

TABLE 26-6 Indications of Sepsis Caused by Different Organisms

SIGNS AND SYMPTOMS	GRAM-POSITIVE	GRAM-NEGATIVE	FUNGAL
Onset	Insidious, 2-6 days	Rapid, 12-36 hr	Delayed
Cognition	Severe disorientation and lethargy	Mild disorientation	Mild disorientation
Ileus	Severe	Severe	Mild
Diarrhea	Rare	Severe	Occasional
Temperature	Fever	Hypothermia	Fever
Hypotension	Late	Early	Late
White blood cell count	Neutrophilia	Neutropenia	Neutrophilia
Platelets	Normal	Low	Low

or washing only small areas of the wound at the bedside. Showering enhances wound inspection and allows water temperature to be kept constant. Immersion of the patient in a tub or whirlpool is no longer performed because it increases the risk for infection.

Nurses and skilled technicians use forceps and scissors to remove loose, dead tissue during hydrotherapy. At most burn units, small blisters are left intact because they are a protective barrier that promotes wound healing. Larger blisters are opened. Washcloths or gauze sponges are used to débride soft, "cheesy" eschar. Wash burn areas thoroughly and gently with mild soap or detergent and water. Then rinse these areas with room-temperature water.

Enzymatic Débridement. Enzymatic débridement can occur naturally by autolysis or artificially by the application of exogenous agents. Autolysis is the disintegration of tissue by the action of the patient's own cellular enzymes. This process is seldom used alone in North America for larger burns because it is slow and prolongs the hospital stay, increasing the risk for infection.

Topical enzyme agents, such as collagenase (Santyl), are used for rapid wound débridement. When these agents are applied to the burn wound in a once-a-day dressing change, the enzymes digest collagen in necrotic tissues.

Dressing the Burn Wound. After burn wounds are cleaned and débrided, topical antibiotics are reapplied to prevent infection (see the Minimizing Infection section). Some type of dressing is then applied to the burn wound. Burn dressings include standard wound dressings, biologic dressings, synthetic dressings, and artificial skin.

Standard Wound Dressings. Standard dressings are multiple layers of gauze applied over the topical agents on the wound. The number of gauze layers depends on:

- Depth of the injury
- Amount of drainage expected
- Area injured
- Patient's MOBILITY
- Frequency of dressing changes

The gauze layers are held in place with roller-type gauze bandages applied in a distal to proximal direction or with circular net fabrics. Cover gauze dressings on the patient's extremities with elastic wraps, especially if the patient is ambulatory. Dressings are generally changed and reapplied every 12 to 24 hours after thoroughly cleaning the areas.

Biologic Dressings. Biologic dressings are often used for temporary wound coverage and closure. These dressings are skin or membranes obtained from human tissue donors (homograft or allograft) or animals (heterograft or xenograft). When applied over open wounds, a biologic dressing adheres and promotes healing or prepares the wound for permanent skin graft coverage.

Various biologic materials are used in healing partial-thickness and granulating full-thickness wounds that are clean and free of eschar. The type of biologic dressing selected depends on the type of wound to be covered and the availability of the material.

Homografts, also called *allografts,* are human skin obtained from a cadaver and provided through a skin bank. Disadvantages to the use of homografts are the high costs and the risk for transmitting a bloodborne infection.

Heterografts, also called *xenografts,* are skin obtained from another species. Pigskin (porcine) is the most common

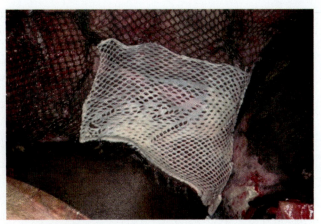

FIG. 26-12 Burn wound covered with a porcine dressing.

heterograft and is compatible with human skin. Pigskin is assessed daily for adherence and need for replacement. Fig. 26-12 shows a small burn covered with a porcine dressing.

Cultured skin can be grown from a small specimen of epidermal cells from an unburned area of the patient's body. The cells are grown in a laboratory to produce cell sheets that can be grafted on the patient to generate a permanent skin surface. The length of time for culturing and growing the skin is long, and the cell sheets are fragile. This process is very costly.

Artificial skin is a substance with two layers—a Silastic epidermis and a porous dermis made from beef collagen and shark cartilage. After the artificial skin is applied to a clean, excised wound surface, fibroblasts move into the collagen part and create a structure similar to normal dermis. The artificial dermis slowly dissolves and is replaced with blood vessels and connective tissue *(neodermis).* The neodermis supports a standard autograft placed over it when the Silastic layer is removed.

Biosynthetic Wound Dressings. Biosynthetic wound dressings are a combination of biosynthetic and synthetic materials. Biobrane is commonly used and effective in the treatment of clean superficial partial-thickness burns such as scalds, as a covering for meshed autografts, and as a donor site dressing. It is made of a nylon fabric that is partially embedded into a silicone film. Collagen is incorporated into both the silicone and the nylon components. The nylon fabric comes into contact with the wound surface and adheres to it until epithelialization has occurred. The porous silicone film allows exudates to pass through.

Synthetic Dressings. Synthetic dressings are made of solid silicone and plastic membranes. They are applied directly to the surface of a prepared wound and remain in place until they fall off or are removed. Many of these dressings are transparent or translucent, and the wound can be inspected without removing the dressing. Pain is reduced at the site because these agents also prevent contact of the wound's nerve endings with air. These dressings also are used to cover donor sites where skin was obtained for autografting.

Transparent film is the dressing commonly used for the care of donor site wounds (Fig. 26-13). This dressing type promotes faster healing with low infection rates, minimal pain, and reduced cost.

Surgical Management. Grafting is used for wound closure when full-thickness injuries cannot close and when natural

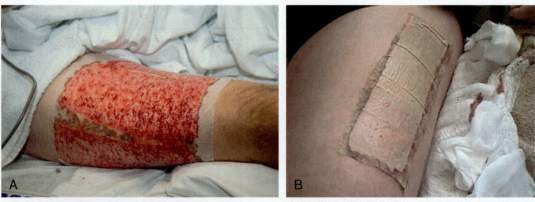

FIG. 26-13 A, Donor site covered with a transparent dressing. **B,** Donor site covered with Xeroform dressing.

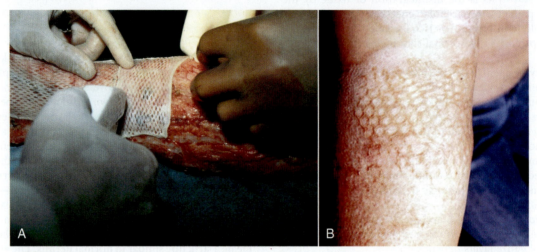

FIG. 26-14 Typical appearance of meshed autografts. **A,** Appearance of meshed autograft at application. **B,** Appearance of meshed autograft after healing.

healing would result in loss of joint function, an unacceptable cosmetic appearance, or a high potential for wound recurrence. Successful skin grafting requires a clean and granulating or freshly excised wound bed. Partial-thickness (split-thickness) or full-thickness strips of skin are removed from the donor area, transferred to the wound, and sutured or stapled in place. Full-thickness free grafts and myocutaneous flaps are used to cover deep, massive ulcers or ulcers in which vital structures, such as bone or tendon, are exposed.

Surgical management of burn wounds involves excision and wound covering. Surgical excision is performed early in the postburn period. Autografting by taking an area of the patient's healthy skin with intact TISSUE INTEGRITY and transplanting it to an excised burn wound may be performed throughout the acute phase when wounds are ready and donor sites are available. Early grafting reduces the time patients are at risk for infection and sepsis.

Surgical Excision. Surgical excision is a common treatment for full-thickness and deep partial-thickness wounds. The patient is taken to the operating room within the first 5 days after injury and again as needed until all wounds are closed permanently.

The surgeon excises the burn wound usually by removing very thin layers of the necrotic burn surface until bleeding tissue is encountered. (Bleeding indicates that a bed of healthy dermis or subcutaneous fat has been reached.) For very deep burns, the surgeon cuts away the wound to the level of superficial fascia. Blood loss is minimal, and grafting is usually successful.

Wound Covering. Permanent skin coverage for large full-thickness injuries occurs by applying an autograft. Skin for an autograft is taken from the patient's body. The surgeon removes a piece of skin from a remote unburned area of the body and transplants it to cover the burn wound. Skin grafts are generally of split thickness, and a partial-thickness injury is formed at the site of surgical removal (the *donor site*). Grafts are placed either on a clean granulated bed or over an area from which dead tissue has just been removed.

Patients with larger burns may have only 5% to 20% of the skin surface available to use for covering the 80% to 95% burned area. Coverage for these wounds may require either repeated skin removal from the same donor site (with time allowed between harvests for healing) or meshing of the split-thickness skin grafts (Fig. 26-14). This technique allows a small graft to be stretched to cover a larger area. Healing time is slower for a meshed graft because the skin must fill in open meshed areas (and attach to the granulation bed).

After surgery, graft sites are immobilized with bulky cotton pressure dressings for 3 to 5 days to allow vascularization, or "take," of the newly grafted skin. Do not disturb the dressing and encourage elevation and complete rest of the grafted area to allow blood vessels to connect the graft with the wound bed. Any activity that might cause movement of the dressing against the body and separation of the graft from the wound is prohibited.

After dressings are removed, monitor the graft for indications of failure to vascularize, nonadherence to the wound, or graft necrosis. A dusky color or sharp line of color change suggests inadequate venous or lymphatic drainage. Other techniques to monitor trends of blood flow in the graft, depending on the graft's location, include pulse oximetry, laser Doppler imaging, ultrasonography, and transcutaneous oxygen determination.

Grafts and donor sites on posterior body surfaces present special problems. For the graft to become fully vascularized or for the donor sites to dry, the patient must be immobilized in a side-lying or prone position for 7 to 10 days.

An alternative to this positioning is the use of special low-pressure or air-fluidized beds, such as the Clinitron bed or KinAir bed, which not only reduces ischemia of the graft while the patient is supine but also helps prevent breakdown of intact skin.

Minimizing Potential for Infection. Burn wound infection occurs through auto-contamination, in which the patient's own normal flora overgrows and invades other body areas; and cross-contamination, in which organisms from other people or environments are transferred to the patient. Signs of infection include foul-smelling discharge, fever, blood culture and/or wound site colonization, and white blood count elevation.

Planning: Expected Outcomes. The patient is expected to remain free from infection and not develop sepsis.

Interventions. Interventions focus on preventing infection and removing infected tissue.

Nonsurgical Management. *Priority nursing interventions include using principles of infection control to prevent transmission, providing a safe environment, and monitoring for early detection of infection.* Drug therapy, isolation therapy, and environmental management are strategies for preventing and managing infection.

Drug Therapy for Infection Prevention. Burn wound conditions promote the growth of *Clostridium tetani*, and all burn patients are at risk for this deadly infection. Tetanus toxoid administration enhances immunity to *C. tetani* and is routinely given on admission. Administration of tetanus immune globulin (human) (Hyper Tet) is recommended when the patient's tetanus immunization status is not known.

Topical antimicrobial drugs are used for infection prevention in burn wounds. Chart 26-5 lists commonly used topical agents. The expected outcome of this therapy is to reduce bacterial

---

Chart 26-5 Common Examples of Drug Therapy

Burn Wounds

TOPICAL DRUG	NURSING IMPLICATIONS
Silver sulfadiazine (Silvadene, Thermazene)	Watch for allergic reaction causing a drop in white blood cell count. Do not use if reaction to sulfonamide has occurred. Use on deep partial-thickness or full-thickness wounds. Monitor wounds for infection.
Collagenase (Santyl) with Polysporin powder	Apply once a day. Use on partial-thickness wounds with eschar. Monitor wounds for infection. May be used with barrier dressing such as Xeroform.
Mafenide acetate (Sulfamylon)	Premedicate for pain before application. Monitor blood gas and serum electrolyte levels. Monitor wounds for infection.
Nitrofurazone (Furacin)	Observe closely for signs of allergic reaction and evidence of superinfection.
Gentamicin sulfate (Garamycin, Gentamar)	Nephrotoxic; monitor kidney function closely, especially changes in serum creatinine and blood urea nitrogen. Ototoxic; monitor hearing weekly.
Polymyxin B-bacitracin (Poly-Bac, Polysporin)	Apply every 2-8 hours to keep area moist.
Acticoat	Do not use with oil-based products or other antimicrobials. Do not use for any patient with a known sensitivity to any of the components of this drug. May dry out and adhere to wound surface; soak off to remove.
PolyMem	Normally leave in place for 7 days. Remove earlier if exudate is visible through outer membrane. Use on partial-thickness wounds and donor sites. Cover with a secondary dressing. Monitor wounds for infection.
Aquacel Ag	Use on partial-thickness wounds and donor sites. Cover with a secondary dressing. Do not use for patients who have allergic reactions to the dressing or any of its components. Moisten with sterile water or normal saline to ease removal. Do not use with oil-based products.
Mepilex Ag	Do not use along with oxidizing agents such as hydrogen peroxide. Cover with secondary dressing. May be used with partial-thickness burns, full-thickness burns, skin grafts, and donor sites.

growth in the wound and prevent sepsis. A variety of agents can be used. Some topicals come in a form of ointments and creams (e.g., silver sulfadiazine, Sulfamylon, bacitracin) and need to be applied once or twice daily. Other products such as Acticoat, Mepilex Ag, and Aquacel Ag contain antimicrobials, which release over a period of several days and can be left on the wound for up to 7 days, thus eliminating the need for daily dressing changes.

Drug Therapy for Treatment of Infection. Systemic antibiotics are used when burn patients have symptoms of an actual infection, including septicemia. Broad-spectrum antibiotics are given until the results of blood cultures and sensitivity status are available. At that time, antibiotics that are effective against the specific organism(s) causing the infection are used. Often burn patients require a higher dose of these drugs to maintain effective blood levels. Peak and trough blood levels may be used to determine treatment effectiveness and risk for toxicity.

Providing a Safe Environment. Providing a safe environment can include isolation therapy, which is used in some burn centers in the belief that it reduces cross-contamination. More often it involves coordinating all members of the health care team in the use of asepsis and monitoring for early recognition of actual infection. Proper and consistent handwashing is the most effective technique for preventing infection transmission.

Use of asepsis requires all health care personnel to wear gloves during all contact with open wounds. The use of sterile versus clean gloves for routine wound care varies by agency and is a matter of debate. Regardless of sterility, change gloves when handling wounds on different areas of the body and between handling old and new dressings.

The equipment on burn units is not shared among patients. Disposable items (e.g., pillows, dishes) are used as much as possible. Assign any equipment used in daily routine care (e.g., blood pressure cuffs, stethoscopes) to each patient for the duration of his or her stay. Daily cleaning of the equipment and general housekeeping are essential for infection control. All other equipment must be cleaned after use on one patient and before use on another. Because *Pseudomonas* has been found in plants, the presence of plants and flowers is prohibited. Some burn units do not permit patients to eat raw foods (e.g., salads, fruit, pepper) to reduce exposure to organisms. Rugs and upholstered articles harbor organisms, and their use is restricted.

Visitors are restricted when the patient is immunosuppressed. Ill people, small children, and other patients should not come into direct contact with the burn patient. Some burn units recommend that all visitors wear protective clothing (gowns, gloves, masks, and shoe and hair covers) in the burn patient's room, but no data support the effectiveness of this approach.

Early detection involves careful monitoring of the burn wounds at each dressing change. Examine all wounds for signs of infection, which include pervasive odor, texture or color changes (especially focal, dark red, or brown discoloration in the eschar), purulent drainage, exudate, sloughing grafts, and/or redness of wound edges extending to the nonburned skin.

Laboratory cultures and biopsies are recommended. Quantitative biopsies of the eschar and granulation tissue are performed routinely to monitor the growth of organisms.

Surgical Management. Infected burn wounds with colony counts at or near 10^5 colonies per gram of tissue may be life threatening, even with antibiotic therapy. Surgical excision of the wound may be needed to control these infections.

NCLEX EXAMINATION CHALLENGE 26-3
Safe and Effective Care Environment

Which nursing intervention(s) decrease(s) the risk for cross-contamination in the client with a severe burn injury? **Select all that apply.**
A. Place client in isolation.
B. Encourage multiple visitors to support client.
C. Ensure that no plants or flowers are in the client's room.
D. Teach family members not to bring fresh fruit and vegetables to the client.
E. Change gloves after cleaning and dressing of one wound area, before cleaning and dressing another.

Minimizing Weight Loss

Planning: Expected Outcomes. The patient is expected to maintain adequate nutrient intake for meeting the body's calorie needs. Indicators include that the patient should have mild or no deviations from the normal ranges for:
- Weight/height ratio
- Food intake
- Hematocrit and hemoglobin
- Serum albumin and prealbumin
- Blood glucose

Interventions. Interventions include calculating the patient's calorie needs and providing an adequate daily source of calories and nutrients that the patient can ingest. Coordinate with a registered dietitian to meet the expected outcomes regarding the patient's NUTRITION status. Therapy begins with calculating the patient's current daily calorie needs. Several formulas and charts are used for this calculation. Nutrition requirements for a patient with a large burn area can exceed 5000 kcal/day. Not meeting this need leads to very rapid weight loss. In addition to a high-calorie intake, a diet high in protein is needed for wound healing. Work with the dietitian and the patient to plan additions to standard nutrition patterns.

Oral diet therapy may be delayed for several days after the injury until the GI tract is motile. Nasoduodenal tube feedings are often started soon after admission. Beginning enteral feedings early helps decrease weight loss, gut atrophy, bacterial translocation, and sepsis. This type of supplement prevents NUTRITION deficits in severely burned patients.

Encourage patients who can eat solid foods to ingest as many calories as possible. Consider the patient's preferences with diet planning and food selection. Encourage patients to request food whenever they feel they can eat, not just according to the hospital's standard meal schedule. Offer frequent high-calorie, high-protein supplemental feedings. Keep an accurate calorie count for foods and beverages that are actually ingested by the patient.

Patients who cannot swallow but who have adequate gastric motility may meet calorie and NUTRITION needs through enteral tube feedings (see Chapter 60). Parenteral nutrition may be used when the GI tract is not functional or when the patient's nutrition needs cannot be met by oral and enteral feeding. This method is used as a last resort because it is invasive and can lead to infectious and metabolic complications.

Maintaining Mobility

Planning: Expected Outcomes. The patient with a burn injury is expected to maintain or regain an optimal MOBILITY.

Indicators include that the patient has minimal limitations in these actions:

- Muscle movement
- Joint MOBILITY
- Walking
- Self-positioning

Interventions. Interventions focus on maintaining or achieving the patient's preburn range of joint motion and MOBILITY and preventing contracture formation.

Nonsurgical Management. Nonsurgical management includes the nursing interventions of positioning, range-of-motion exercises, ambulation, and pressure dressings.

Positioning is critical for patients with burn injuries because the position of COMFORT for the patient is often one of joint flexion, which leads to contracture development. Maintain the patient in a neutral body position with minimal flexion. Best practices for preventing contractures are listed in Chart 26-6. Splints and other devices may be used to maintain good positioning of the hands, elbows, knees, neck, and axillae.

Range-of-motion exercises to maintain MOBILITY are performed actively at least three times a day. If the patient cannot move a joint actively, perform passive range-of-motion exercises. Give burned hands special attention. Urge the patient to perform active range-of-motion exercises for the hand, thumb, and fingers every hour while he or she is awake.

Ambulation is started as soon as possible after the fluid shifts have resolved because it maintains MOBILITY, inhibits bone density loss, strengthens muscles, stimulates immune function, promotes ventilation, and prevents many complications.

? NCLEX EXAMINATION CHALLENGE 26-4

Health Promotion and Maintenance

The nurse is encouraging range-of-motion exercises for the client, who states, "This hurts terribly; I don't want to do this." Identify the appropriate nursing response(s). **Select all that apply.**
A. "You have to do the exercises to get well."
B. "Range of motion helps promote mobility."
C. "Just visualize a beach to get your mind off of the pain."
D. "Let me check when you were last given pain medication."
E. "Which techniques for pain management have you used in the past that were helpful?"
F. "The health care provider has ordered these exercises, and it is important that you do them as instructed."

Patients with attached equipment (IV catheters, nasogastric tubes, ECG leads, extensive dressings) can ambulate with preparation and assistance. This activity is performed two or three times a day and progresses in length each time.

Compression dressings are applied after grafts heal to help prevent contractures and tight hypertrophic scars, which can inhibit MOBILITY. They also inhibit venous stasis and edema in areas with decreased lymph flow. Compression dressings may be elastic wraps or specially designed, custom-fitted, elasticized clothing that provides continuous pressure. Fig. 26-15 shows such a garment. For best effectiveness, pressure garments must be worn at least 23 hours a day, every day, until the scar tissue is mature (12 to 24 months). They can be uncomfortable with itchiness and increased warmth. Reinforce to the patient and

---

◎ CHART 26-6   Best Practice for Patient Safety & Quality Care QSEN

Positioning to Prevent Contractures

AFFECTED BODY PART	POSITION OF FUNCTION	INTERVENTION
Head and neck	Hyperextension	No pillow. Place a towel roll under the patient's neck or shoulder. Neck splint.
Posterior neck	Flexion	Have patient turn the head from side to side.
Upper chest and chest	Shoulder retraction	Place patient in supine position. Place a folded towel under the spine, between the scapulae.
Lateral trunk	Flexion to uninvolved side	Place patient supine with the arm on the affected side up over the head.
Anterior shoulder	Abduction and external rotation	Maintain the upper arm at 90 degrees of abduction from the lateral aspect of the trunk.
Posterior shoulder	Slight flexion and interior rotation	Keep the arm slightly behind the midline.
Axilla	Abduction with 10- to 15-degree forward flexion and external rotation	Support the abducted arm with suspension from IV pole or bedside table. Axilla splint.
Elbow	Extension and supination	Keep the joint in the extended position.
Wrist	30 to 45 degrees of extension	Use a splint.
Fingers		
MP joints	70 to 90 degrees of flexion	Use a splint.
PIP and DIP joints	Extension	Use a splint.
Ankle	90 degrees of dorsiflexion	Use a padded footboard or splint with heels free of pressure.
Legs	15 to 20 degrees of abduction	Place small pillow between legs.
Hip	Extension and neutral rotation	Place patient supine with lower extremity extended. Use trochanter roll. Use foam wedge along lateral aspect of thigh.

DIP, Distal interphalangeal; *MP,* metatarsophalangeal; *PIP,* proximal interphalangeal.

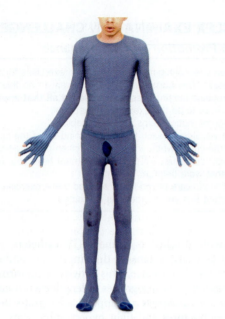

FIG. 26-15 Patient wearing full-body compression garments. (From Herndon, D. N. [2012]. *Total burn care* (4th ed.). Philadelphia: Saunders.)

family that wearing pressure garments is beneficial in saving mobility and reducing scarring.

Surgical Management. Surgical management restores MOBIL-ITY rather than prevents immobility. Surgical release of contractures is commonly performed in the neck, axilla, elbow flexion areas, and hand. Specific surgical procedures vary for each patient.

Nursing responsibilities include interventions to prevent contractures from re-forming and the care of new grafts and suture lines. Constantly reinforce the need for the patient to adhere to exercise and splinting regimens to prevent the recurrence of joint immobility.

Supporting Positive Self-Esteem

Planning: Expected Outcomes. After intervention, the patient with a burn injury is expected to have a positive perception of his or her own appearance, body functions, and self-worth. Indicators include that the patient should consistently demonstrate these behaviors:

- Willingness to touch the affected body part
- Adjustment to changes in body function
- Willingness to use strategies to enhance appearance and function
- Successful progression through the grieving process
- Use of support systems

Interventions. Nonsurgical and surgical interventions can assist patients who have self-image problems as a result of burn injury.

Nonsurgical Management. Understanding the stages of grief is helpful in managing care for the patient with burns. Assess which stage of grief the patient is currently experiencing and help interpret his or her behaviors. The patient often is unaware of or is confused by his or her feelings. Reassure the patient that feelings of grief, loss, anxiety, anger, fear, and guilt are normal. The patient may be grieving the loss of body parts, appearance, role identity, social identity, and family members. Coordinate with other health care team members (e.g., psychologist,

psychiatrist, social worker, case manager, spiritual leader of the patient's choosing) to address these issues.

Accept the physical and psychological features of the patient. Present patients and families with realistic expected outcomes for the patient's functional capacity and physical appearance. Provide information sessions and counseling for the family to identify patterns of support. Facilitate the patient's use of these systems and the development of new support systems. Make referrals to support groups. Evaluate the effectiveness and use of support resources throughout the course of recovery.

Engaging in decision making and independent activities fosters feelings of self-worth. Plan and encourage the patient's active participation in care activities. Assist family members to understand that it is more beneficial for the patient to perform these activities than to have them performed by someone else. Urge families to include the patient in family decision making to the same degree that he or she participated in this process before the injury.

Surgical Management. Reconstructive and cosmetic surgery can be performed many years after the burn injury. Restoring function and improving appearance through surgical techniques often promote the patient's positive self-image and self-worth. Many patients have unrealistic expectations of reconstructive surgery and envision an appearance identical to or equal in quality to the preburn state. Teach the patient and family about expected cosmetic outcomes.

◆ Evaluation: Reflecting

Evaluate the care of the patient in the acute phrase of burn injury on the basis of the identified priority patient problems. The expected outcomes include that the patient will have appropriately managed wound care, remain free from infection, experience minimal weight loss, maintain MOBILITY, and have positive self-esteem.

REHABILITATIVE PHASE OF BURN INJURY

Overview

Although rehabilitation efforts are started at the time of admission, the technical rehabilitative phase begins with wound closure and ends when the patient achieves his or her highest level of functioning. The emphasis is on the psychosocial adjustment of the patient; the prevention of scars and contractures; and the resumption of preburn activity, including resuming work, family, and social roles. This phase may take years or even last a lifetime as patients adjust to life after a burn (Cukor et al., 2015).

❖ INTERPROFESSIONAL COLLABORATIVE CARE

Although attention is placed first on the physical interventions for the burn injury, psychological care is equally important. Continue to provide psychosocial support to the patient and family throughout hospitalization and in the rehabilitative phase.

Obtaining information from the patient and family aids in the assessment and diagnosis of psychological problems and directs management. Explore the patient's feelings about the burn injury. It is extremely difficult for patients to concentrate on the many tasks before them when obstacles such as guilt and grief are in the forefront.

Ask whether there is a history of psychological problems. To assist with a future plan of care, assess and document the type of coping mechanisms the patient has used successfully during times of stress. Also assess the patient's family unit and the history of interaction. Consider cultural, spiritual, and ethnic factors when planning psychosocial interventions.

Throughout the hospitalization, the patient progresses through a variety of stages and exhibits many feelings, including denial, regression, and anger. Assess the patient's feelings at each stage so appropriate plans of care can be implemented.

Care Coordination and Transition Management

Discharge planning for the patient with a burn injury begins at admission to the hospital or burn center. The interdisciplinary team meets regularly to evaluate the progress of each discipline and help the patient reach mutually established discharge outcomes. Table 26-7 lists common discharge needs of the patient with burns.

Psychosocial Preparation. During the recovery period and for some time after discharge, patients with severe burn injuries often have psychological problems that require intervention. Such problems include post-traumatic stress disorder, sexual dysfunction, and severe depression. Assistance is coordinated with the patient, family, and health care team. Psychosocial assistance is best provided by a professional counselor with experience in helping burn patients.

One specific area to address with the patient is the reaction of others to the sight of healing wounds and disfiguring scars. Patients with facial burns are especially subjected to stares and other negative reactions from the public. Visits from friends and short public appearances before discharge may help the patient begin adjusting to this problem. Community reintegration programs can assist the psychosocial and physical recovery of the patient with serious burns.

Home Care Management. The patient with severe burns is discharged from the acute care setting when serious complications are resolved and minimal wound areas remain open.

TABLE 26-7 Needs to Address Before Discharge of the Patient With Burns

- Early patient assessment
- Financial assessment
- Evaluation of family resources
- Weekly discharge planning meeting
- Psychological referral
- Patient and family teaching (home care)
- Designation of principal learners (specific family members or significant others who will help with care)
- Development of teaching plan
- Training for wound care
- Rehabilitation referral
- Home assessment (on-site visit)
- Medical equipment
- Public health nursing referral
- Evaluation of community resources
- Visit to referral agency
- Re-entry programs for school or work environment
- Long-term care placement
- Environmental interventions
- Auditory testing
- Speech therapy
- Prosthetic rehabilitation

During the first weeks at home, the patient usually needs at least daily wound care, physical therapy, NUTRITION support, symptom management, and drug therapy.

Although the patient usually views going home positively, the problems of physical care and the psychological stresses from changes in appearance, role, function, and lifestyle may overwhelm the patient and family. Successful discharge depends on extensive planning and preparation of the patient, family, and home environment through education and the involvement of appropriate support agencies and services.

Preparation for discharge includes assessment of the family and home care situation from physical and social perspectives. Consider the needs of the patient when evaluating the home for cleanliness; access to bathing facilities, electricity, and running water; stairways; number of occupants; temperature control; and safety. If the burn injuries occurred in a house fire, a new residence may need to be established.

Self-Management Education. Education about burn care and living with the consequences of burn injuries begins when the patient is admitted to the hospital or burn center. A weekly plan for patient education is outlined; a positive outcome is progression toward independence for the patient and family. Critical for this outcome is teaching patients and family members to perform such care tasks as dressing changes. Allow patients and family members to first observe dressing changes, then to assist in performing the changes, and then to change the dressings independently under your supervision.

Before discharge, all people who will be involved in the patient's home care participate in discharge planning and teaching sessions. In addition to details about dressing changes, explain signs and symptoms of infection, drug regimens, proper use of prosthetic and positioning devices, correct application and care of pressure garments, COMFORT measures to reduce pruritus, and dates for follow-up appointments.

Health Care Resources. The interprofessional health care team evaluates the family's capacity and willingness to assist in caring for the patient after discharge. A visiting nurse or case manager with extensive experience in providing burn care can help the family with care problems arising at home. This nurse can help the family determine which special equipment, supplies, or services will be needed. The frequency of home visits depends on the patient's condition and the ability of family members to function as care providers. The home care nurse may need a brief visit to the patient while in the hospital and may need to observe burn wound care.

The home care of a patient after a serious burn often involves daily physical therapy and rehabilitation sessions at special centers. Address and resolve transportation problems before the patient is discharged.

When rehabilitation is prolonged, the patient may be discharged to a rehabilitation facility. Consult with the rehabilitation team and provide copies of the care and teaching plans used with the patient.

◆ Evaluation: Reflecting

Evaluate the care of the patient in the rehabilitative phase of burn injury on the basis of the identified priority patient problems. The expected outcomes include that the patient will:
- Maintain adequate GAS EXCHANGE and PERFUSION to all vital organs

❓ CLINICAL JUDGMENT CHALLENGE 26-2

Patient-Centered Care; Teamwork and Collaboration; Evidence-Based Practice QSEN

You are caring for a veteran who was involved in combat where he experienced an explosion near a burn pit that left him with multiple burns. The patient tells you that he has trouble sleeping and is having frequent flashbacks. He can't look at his burns during dressing changes, is asking his family to feed him, and is not participating in occupational and physical therapy.

1. Which interventions would be appropriate for this patient?
2. Which other member of the interprofessional team may you need to contact?
3. What teaching can you provide to the patient's family?
4. Which specific veteran-focused resources may be helpful to your patient?

- Maintain a patent airway
- Have cardiac output restored to normal
- Have pain alleviated or reduced
- Experience no further loss of skin TISSUE INTEGRITY
- Have wounds healed without complications
- Remain free from infection
- Not experience sepsis
- Maintain an adequate NUTRITION for meeting the body's calorie needs
- Regain and maintain an optimal ability to move purposefully
- Have a positive perception of his or her own appearance and body functions

GET READY FOR NCLEX® EXAMINATION!

KEY POINTS

Review these Key Points for each NCLEX Examination Client Needs Category.

Safe and Effective Care Environment

- Use strict aseptic technique when caring for patients who have open burn wounds to prevent infection. **QSEN: Safety**
- Monitor vital signs at least every 8 hours and assess wounds at least daily for signs of wound infection or sepsis. (For patients with greater than 25% TBSA burn, monitor vital signs more frequently.) **QSEN: Safety**
- Administer prescribed opioid analgesics intravenously during the resuscitation phase of burn recovery. **QSEN: Evidence-Based Practice**

Health Promotion and Maintenance

- Encourage adults to have and maintain home smoke and carbon monoxide detectors. **QSEN: Safety**
- Teach patients to not smoke in bed or in rooms where home oxygen is in use and to not smoke when taking substances that induce sedation (drugs or alcohol). **QSEN: Safety**
- Teach patients who have reduced sensation in hands or feet to use a bath thermometer to check water temperature before bathing. **QSEN: Safety**
- Teach patients to avoid exposing burned skin to the sun or to temperature extremes. **QSEN: Safety**
- Instruct adults to set hot water tank temperatures to manufacturer recommendations. **QSEN: Safety**

Psychosocial Integrity

- Allow patients time to grieve over a change in body image and other fire-related loss. **QSEN: Patient-Centered Care**
- Reassure patients that pain will be managed effectively and COMFORT will be promoted. **QSEN: Patient-Centered Care**
- Explain procedures to the patient and family. **Ethics**
- Assess the patient's and family's use of coping strategies related to burn injury, treatment, possible role changes, and possible outcomes. **QSEN: Patient-Centered Care**
- Support the patient and family in coping with permanent changes in appearance and function. **QSEN: Patient-Centered Care**

- Encourage the patient with wounds and scars related to burn injury to participate in self-care. **QSEN: Patient-Centered Care**

Physiological Integrity

- Always prioritize the airway and adequacy of breathing. **QSEN: Safety**
- Keep an endotracheal or tracheostomy kit at the bedside of any patient with facial burns, burns inside the mouth, singed nasal hairs, or a "smoky" smell to the breath. **QSEN: Safety**
- Notify the Rapid Response Team immediately if the patient with an inhalation injury becomes more breathless or audible wheezes disappear. **QSEN: Safety**
- Administer analgesics, sedatives, and antianxiety drugs to patients receiving paralytic drugs during mechanical ventilation. **QSEN: Evidence-Based Practice**
- Administer half of the fluid volume calculated for the first 24 hours after burn injury in the first 8 hours postburn. **QSEN: Evidence-Based Practice**
- Use laboratory and assessment data to determine the effectiveness of fluid resuscitation during the resuscitation phase of burn injury. **QSEN: Evidence-Based Practice**
- Encourage the patient to actively participate in pain control measures. **QSEN: Patient-Centered Care**
- Position patients to promote COMFORT, prevent contractures, and promote joint function. **QSEN: Evidence-Based Practice**
- Assist patients to ambulate several times each day as soon as the fluid shifts have resolved. **QSEN: Evidence-Based Practice**
- Coordinate with the registered dietitian to meet the NUTRITION needs for the patient during the acute phase of burn injury. **QSEN: Teamwork and Collaboration**
- Evaluate wound healing during the acute phase of burn injury. **Clinical Judgment**
- Use appropriate positioning and range-of-motion interventions for prevention of MOBILITY problems. **QSEN: Safety**

SELECTED BIBLIOGRAPHY

Cukor, J., Wyka, K., Leahy, N., & Yurt, R. (2015). The treatment of posttraumatic stress disorder and related psychosocial consequences of burn injury: A pilot study. *Journal of Burn Care & Research*, *36*(1), 184-192.

Culleiton, A., & Simko, L. (2013a). Caring for patients with burn injuries. *Nursing 2013 Critical Care*, *8*(1), 14–22.

Culleiton, A., & Simko, L. (2013b). Managing burn injuries in the ICU. *Nursing 2013 Critical Care*, *8*(2), 22–30.

Haynes, J. (2016). *Fire loss in the United States during 2015*. National Fire Protection Association. http://www.nfpa.org/research/reports-and-statistics/fires-in-the-us/overall-fire-problem/fire-loss-in-the-united-states.

Lafferty, K., et al. (2017). *Smoke inhalation injury*. MedScape. http://emedicine.medscape.com/article/771194-overview.

Laing, C. (2013). Acute carbon monoxide toxicity: Be alert for this easy-to-miss illness. *Nursing2013 Critical Care*, *8*(1), 30–34.

Lewis, C. (2013). Stem cell application in acute burn care and reconstruction. *Journal of Wound Care*, *11*(1), 7–16.

McCance, K., Huether, S., Brashers, V., & Rote, N. (2014). *Pathophysiology: The biologic basis for disease in adults and children* (7th ed.). St. Louis: Mosby.

National Safety Council. (2017). *Fire a leading cause of death for kids*. http://www.nsc.org/learn/safety-knowledge/Pages/safety-at-home-fires-burns.aspx.

Pagana, K., Pagana, T. J., & Pagana, T. N. (2017). *Mosby's diagnostic and laboratory test reference* (13th ed.). St. Louis: Mosby.

Park, Y., Choi, Y., Lee, H., Moon, D., Kim, S., Lee, J., et al. (2013). The impact of laser Doppler imaging on the early decision-making process for surgical intervention in adults with indeterminate burns. *Burns: Journal of the International Society for Burn Injuries*, *39*(4), 655–661.

Pike-MacDonald, S. (Ed.), (2013). *Mosby's Canadian manual of diagnostic and laboratory tests* (1st Canadian ed.). Toronto: Elsevier Canada.

Rice, P., et al. (2017). *Emergency care of moderate and severe thermal burns in adults*. http://www.uptodate.com/contents/emergency-care-of-moderate-and-severe-thermal-burns-in-adults.

Tompkins, R. (2015). Survival from burns in the new millennium: 70 years' experience from a single institution. *Annals of Surgery*, *261*(2), 263–268.

Touhy, T., & Jett, K. (2015). *Ebersole and Hess' gerontological nursing healthy aging* (9th ed.). St. Louis: Mosby.

27 | CHAPTER

Assessment of the Respiratory System

Harry Rees

 http://evolve.elsevier.com/Iggy/

PRIORITY AND INTERRELATED CONCEPTS

The priority concept for this chapter is GAS EXCHANGE.

The interrelated concept for this chapter is PERFUSION.

LEARNING OUTCOMES

Safe and Effective Care Environment

1. Collaborate with the interprofessional team to perform a complete respiratory assessment, including GAS EXCHANGE and PERFUSION.

Health Promotion and Maintenance

2. Explain how physiologic aging changes of the respiratory system affect GAS EXCHANGE, PERFUSION, and the associated care of older adults.
3. Teach all adults measures to take to protect the respiratory system, including the avoidance of tobacco use.

Psychosocial Integrity

4. Implement patient-centered nursing interventions to help patients and families cope with the psychosocial impact caused by a respiratory system problem.

Physiological Integrity

5. Apply knowledge of anatomy and physiology to perform an evidence-based assessment for the patient with a respiratory health problem.
6. Interpret assessment findings for the patient with a respiratory health problem.
7. Teach the patient and caregivers about diagnostic procedures associated with respiratory health problems.

The respiratory system uses ventilation to provide the body with atmospheric oxygen (O_2), which is an essential nutrient for all cells. GAS EXCHANGE is the oxygen transport to the cells and carbon dioxide transport away from cells through ventilation and diffusion. Once ventilation and diffusion exchange these gases in the lungs, blood oxygen is then available to cells by perfusion and diffusion. PERFUSION is the arterial blood flow through the tissues (peripheral perfusion) and blood that is pumped by the heart (central perfusion). See Chapter 2 for overviews of the concepts of gas exchange and perfusion.

The respiratory system includes the upper airways, lungs, lower airways, and alveolar air sacs. Air with oxygen enters the nose and mouth and moves through the airways (trachea, bronchi, bronchioles) and into the air sacs (alveoli) of the

lungs. Once in the air sacs, the oxygen from the air diffuses into the blood so it can be transported to all tissues and organs. Carbon dioxide (CO_2), the waste gas created in the tissues, diffuses from the blood into the lungs so it can be exhaled. All systems depend on adequate GAS EXCHANGE for tissue PERFUSION. Any respiratory problem affects total body health and well-being.

ANATOMY AND PHYSIOLOGY REVIEW

The purpose of breathing is to ensure GAS EXCHANGE. This process has two parts: (1) oxygenation for tissue PERFUSION so cells have enough oxygen to metabolize and generate energy; and (2) removal of carbon dioxide, the waste product of

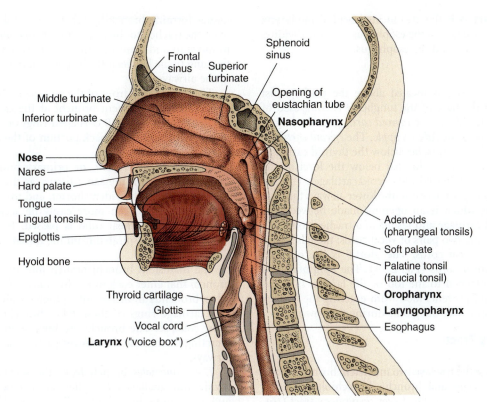

FIG. 27-1 Structures of the upper respiratory tract.

metabolism. The respiratory system also influences acid-base balance, speech, smell, fluid balance, and temperature control.

Upper Respiratory Tract

The upper airways include the nose, the sinuses, the pharynx, and the larynx (Fig. 27-1).

Nose and Sinuses

The nose is the organ of smell, with receptors from cranial nerve I *(olfactory)* located in the upper areas. The nose is rigid with a bony upper portion and a cartilaginous moveable lower portion. The septum divides the nose into two cavities that are lined with mucous membranes and have a rich blood supply. The **anterior nares** are the external openings into the nasal cavities. The posterior nares are openings from the nasal cavity into the throat.

The **turbinates** are three bones that protrude into the nasal cavities from the internal portion of the nose (see Fig. 27-1). Turbinates increase the total surface area for filtering, warming, and humidifying inspired air before it passes into the nasopharynx.

The **paranasal sinuses** are air-filled cavities within the bones that surround the nasal passages (Fig. 27-2). Lined with ciliated membrane, the sinuses provide resonance to speech, decrease the weight of the skull, and act as shock absorbers in the event of facial trauma.

Pharynx

The pharynx (throat) is a passageway for both the respiratory and digestive tracts. It is located behind the oral and nasal cavities. The throat is divided into the nasopharynx, the oropharynx, and the laryngopharynx (see Fig. 27-1).

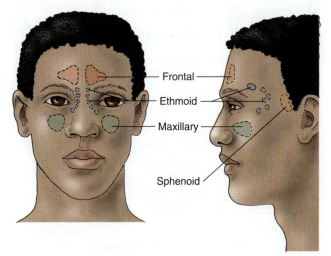

FIG. 27-2 Paranasal sinuses.

The nasopharynx is located behind the nose, above the soft palate. It contains the adenoids and the opening of the eustachian tube. The adenoids trap organisms that enter the nose or mouth. The **eustachian tubes** connect the nasopharynx with the middle ears and open during swallowing to equalize pressure within the middle ear.

The oropharynx is located behind the mouth, below the nasopharynx. It extends from the soft palate to the base of the tongue and is used for breathing and swallowing. The *palatine tonsils,* which are part of the immune system, are located on the sides of the oropharynx and protect against invading organisms.

The laryngopharynx is the area located behind the larynx from the base of the tongue to the esophagus. It is the dividing point between the larynx and the esophagus.

Larynx

The larynx ("voice box") is located above the trachea, just below the throat at the base of the tongue. It is composed of several cartilages (Fig. 27-3). The *thyroid cartilage* is the largest and is commonly called the *Adam's apple*. The *cricoid cartilage*, which contains the vocal cords, lies below the thyroid cartilage. The *cricothyroid membrane* is located below the level of the vocal cords and joins the thyroid and cricoid cartilages. This site is used in an emergency for access to the lower airways through a *cricothyroidotomy*, which is an opening made between the thyroid and cricoid cartilage and results in a tracheostomy.

Inside the larynx are two pairs of vocal cords: the false vocal cords and the true vocal cords. The glottis is the opening between the true vocal cords (Fig. 27-4). The epiglottis is a small, elastic flap attached to the top of the larynx. It opens during breathing and prevents food from entering the trachea (aspiration) by closing over the glottis during swallowing.

Lower Respiratory Tract
Airways

The lower airways are the trachea; two mainstem bronchi; lobar, segmental, and subsegmental bronchi; bronchioles; alveolar ducts; and alveoli (Fig. 27-5). The lower respiratory tract (*tracheobronchial tree*) consists of muscle, cartilage, and elastic tissues forming branching tubes. These tubes decrease in size from the trachea to the respiratory bronchioles and allow gases to move to and from the lungs. GAS EXCHANGE takes place in the lung tissue between the alveoli and the lung capillaries, not in the airways.

The trachea is in front of the esophagus. It branches into the right and left mainstem bronchi at the *carina* junction. The trachea contains 6 to 10 C-shaped rings of cartilage. The open portion of the C is the back portion of the trachea and shares a wall with the esophagus.

The mainstem bronchi, or primary bronchi, begin at the carina and contain the same tissues as the trachea. The right bronchus is slightly wider, shorter, and more vertical than the left bronchus and can more easily be accidentally intubated when an endotracheal tube is passed. In addition, when a foreign object is aspirated from the throat, it usually enters the right bronchus.

The mainstem bronchi branch into the secondary (lobar) bronchi that enter each of the five lobes of the two lungs. Each lobar bronchus branches into progressively smaller divisions. The cartilage rings of these lobar bronchi are complete and resist collapse. The bronchi are lined with a ciliated, mucus-secreting membrane that moves particles away from the lower airways.

The bronchioles branch from the secondary bronchi and divide into smaller and smaller tubes, which are the terminal and respiratory bronchioles (Fig. 27-6). These tubes have a small diameter, have no cartilage, and depend entirely on the elastic recoil of the lung to remain open.

Alveolar ducts branch from the respiratory bronchioles and resemble a bunch of grapes. Alveolar sacs arise from these ducts and contain groups of alveoli, which are the basic units of GAS EXCHANGE (see Fig. 27-6). A pair of healthy adult lungs has about 290 million alveoli, which are surrounded by lung capillaries. These numerous small alveoli normally make a large surface area for GAS EXCHANGE (about the size of a tennis court). Acinus is a term for the structural unit consisting of a respiratory bronchiole, an alveolar duct, and an alveolar sac.

The alveolar walls have cells called *type II pneumocytes* that secrete surfactant, a fatty protein that reduces surface tension in the alveoli. Without surfactant, atelectasis (alveolar collapse) occurs, reducing GAS EXCHANGE because the alveolar surface area is reduced.

Lungs

The lungs are elastic, cone-shaped organs located in the pleural cavity in the chest. The apex (top) of each lung extends above the clavicle; the base (bottom) of each lung lies just above the diaphragm. The lungs are composed of millions of alveoli and their related ducts, bronchioles, and bronchi. The right lung, which is larger and wider than the left, is divided into three lobes: upper, middle, and lower. The left lung is divided into only two lobes. About 60% to 65% of lung function occurs in the right lung. Any problem with the right lung interferes with GAS EXCHANGE and PERFUSION to a greater degree than a problem in the left lung.

The pleura is a continuous smooth membrane with two surfaces that totally enclose the lungs. The parietal pleura lines the inside of the chest cavity and the upper surface of the diaphragm. The visceral pleura covers the lung surfaces. These surfaces are lubricated by a thin fluid that allows the surfaces to glide across each other smoothly during breathing.

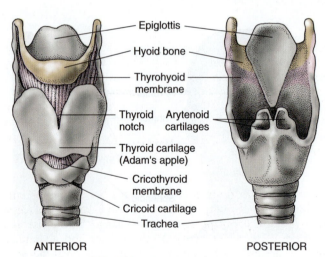

FIG. 27-3 Structures of the larynx.

FIG. 27-4 Detail of the glottis (two vocal folds and the intervening space, the rima glottidis).

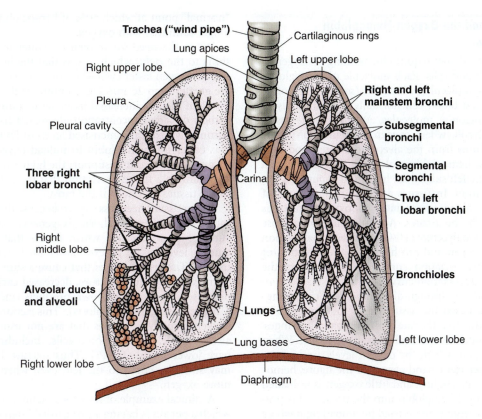

FIG. 27-5 Structures of the lower respiratory tract.

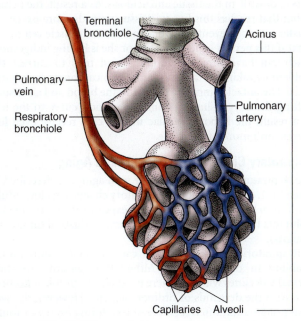

FIG. 27-6 The terminal bronchioles and the acinus.

the heart into the pulmonary artery. This artery eventually branches into arterioles to form capillary networks that are meshed around and through the alveoli—the site of GAS EXCHANGE (see Fig. 27-6). Freshly oxygenated blood travels from the capillaries to the pulmonary veins and then to the left atrium. From the left atrium, oxygenated blood flows into the left ventricle, where it is pumped throughout the systemic circulation.

Accessory Muscles of Respiration

Breathing occurs through changes in the size of and pressure within the chest cavity. Contraction and relaxation of chest muscles (and the diaphragm) cause changes in the size and pressure of the chest cavity. At times, back and abdominal muscles are used in addition to chest muscles when the work of breathing is increased.

? NCLEX EXAMINATION CHALLENGE 27-1

Physiological Integrity

Which description of respiratory physiologic features is correct?
A. The elastic tissues of the tracheobronchial tree are the major structures responsible for gas exchange.
B. The epiglottis closes during speech to divert air movement into and through the vocal cords to produce sound.
C. Any problem with the right lung interferes with gas exchange and perfusion to a greater degree than a problem in the left lung.
D. The left lung is responsible for approximately 60% of gas exchange, and the right lung is responsible for 60% of pulmonary perfusion.

Blood flow in the lungs occurs through two separate systems: bronchial and pulmonary. The bronchial system carries the blood needed to oxygenate lung tissues. These arteries are part of systemic circulation and do not participate in gas exchange.

The pulmonary circulation is a highly vascular capillary network. Oxygen-poor blood travels from the right ventricle of

Oxygen Delivery and the Oxygen-Hemoglobin Dissociation Curve

Oxygen delivery to the tissues requires the binding of oxygen to hemoglobin in red blood cells. Each molecule of hemoglobin can bind four oxygen molecules, which fills (*saturates*) all of its binding sites. Each red blood cell normally has hundreds of thousands of hemoglobin molecules. When blood passes through the lung alveoli, where oxygen concentration is the greatest, oxygen diffuses from the alveoli into red blood cells and binds to all those hemoglobin molecules. This oxygen-rich blood then goes to the left side of the heart and is pumped out into systemic circulation. In tissues away from the source of oxygen, hemoglobin unloads (**dissociates**) the oxygen molecules and delivers them to the tissues. A by-product of glucose metabolism, diphosphoglycerate (DPG) reduces the attraction of hemoglobin for oxygen and can help shift the direction of the oxyhemoglobin dissociation curve. Fig. 27-7 shows the oxygen-hemoglobin dissociation curve.

Tissue oxygen delivery through dissociation or "unloading" from hemoglobin is based on tissues' need for oxygen. The curve in Fig. 27-7 shows that the rate of this unloading changes, depending on how much oxygen is already in the tissues. When blood perfuses tissues in which the oxygen levels are high, as indicated in the upper right-hand corner of the figure, hemoglobin binds oxygen very tightly, and little oxygen is unloaded or dissociated from the hemoglobin into the tissues. This prevents oxygen delivery from being wasted by unloading it where it is not needed. When blood perfuses tissues in which oxygen levels are very low, as indicated in the lower left-hand corner of Fig. 27-7, hemoglobin binds oxygen less tightly and will rapidly and easily unload its remaining oxygen to provide these tissues with needed oxygen. So how rapidly and easily hemoglobin dissociates oxygen to the tissues changes depending on oxygen need. The S-shaped curve indicates that it is harder for oxygen to dissociate from hemoglobin in tissues that are well oxygenated and much easier in tissues that are "starving" for oxygen.

The curve in Fig. 27-7 indicates that, on average, 50% of hemoglobin molecules have completely dissociated their oxygen molecules when blood perfuses tissues that have an oxygen tension (concentration) of 26 mm Hg. This is considered a "normal" point at which 50% of hemoglobin molecules are no longer saturated with oxygen.

When the need for oxygen is greater in tissues, this curve shifts to the *right*, which means that the hemoglobin will dissociate oxygen faster even when the tissue oxygen tension levels are greater than 26 mm Hg. Conditions that shift the curve to the right include increased tissue temperature, increased tissue carbon dioxide concentration, decreased tissue pH (acidosis), chronic hypoxia, and increased levels of DPG. This means that it is easier for hemoglobin to unload oxygen to these tissues because they need it to support the higher metabolism, and the right shift is a tissue protection that increases oxygen delivery to the tissues that need it the most.

When tissues need less oxygen because they are metabolizing more slowly than usual, the oxygen-hemoglobin dissociation curve shifts to the *left*, which means that the tissue oxygen tension level has to be even *lower* for hemoglobin to unload oxygen. Tissue conditions that cause a shift to the left include decreased tissue temperature, decreased carbon dioxide levels, decreased glucose breakdown products (including DPG), and a higher tissue pH (alkalosis). This action prevents wasting oxygen delivery to tissues that are not using the oxygen they already have. Aging blood cells, including banked blood, have lower levels of DPG. Thus massive blood transfusions may shift the curve to the left, even when tissues could use more oxygen.

A clinical example of how these actions are helpful is one in which a person is having a myocardial infarction (heart attack). Blood flow to the area is reduced; and the heart muscle is metabolizing under hypoxic conditions, which creates more carbon dioxide in the tissue and acidosis. As a result, the hemoglobin that reaches this hypoxic tissue unloads more oxygen at a faster rate to prevent ischemia and cardiac muscle cell death. What if this person believes that he or she is having indigestion, which can have similar symptoms, and tries to correct the problem by taking in large amounts of bicarbonate-based antacids? The antacids increase the pH in the blood and all tissues, shifting the oxygen-hemoglobin dissociation curve to the left. As a result, the hypoxic cardiac muscle cells receive even less oxygen, and more of them die.

Respiratory Changes Associated With Aging

The respiratory changes that occur with aging are described in Chart 27-1. Many additional respiratory changes in older adults result from heredity and a lifetime of exposure to environmental pollutants (e.g., cigarette smoke, bacteria, industrial fumes and irritants).

Respiratory disease is a major cause of illness and chronic disability in older patients. Although respiratory function normally declines with age, there is usually no problem keeping pace with the demands of ordinary activity. However, the sedentary older adult often feels breathless during exercise (Touhy & Jett, 2016).

It is difficult to determine which respiratory changes in older adults are related to normal aging and which changes are caused by respiratory disease or exposure to pollutants. Age-related changes in the muscles and the cardiac and vascular system also may cause abnormal breathing, even if the lungs are normal.

Health Promotion and Maintenance

Lung and breathing problems are common causes of death in North America (McCance et al., 2014). Some respiratory

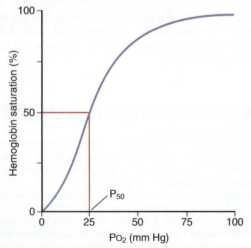

FIG. 27-7 The oxygen-hemoglobin dissociation curve. P_{50}, The partial pressure of O_2 at which hemoglobin is 50% saturated; PO_2, oxygen partial pressure.

CHART 27-1 Nursing Focus on the Older-Adult

Changes in the Respiratory System Related to Aging

PHYSIOLOGIC CHANGE	NURSING INTERVENTIONS	RATIONALES
Alveoli Alveolar surface area decreases. Diffusion capacity decreases. Elastic recoil decreases. Bronchioles and alveolar ducts dilate. Ability to cough decreases. Airways close early.	Encourage vigorous pulmonary hygiene (i.e., encourage patient to turn, cough, and deep breathe) and use of incentive spirometry, especially if he or she is confined to bed or has had surgery. Encourage upright position.	Potential for mechanical or infectious respiratory complications is increased in these situations. The upright position minimizes ventilation-perfusion mismatching.
Lungs Residual volume increases. Vital capacity decreases. Efficiency of oxygen and carbon dioxide exchange decreases. Elasticity decreases.	Include inspection, palpation, percussion, and auscultation in lung assessments. Help patient actively maintain health and fitness. Assess patient's respirations for abnormal breathing patterns. Encourage frequent oral hygiene.	Inspection, palpation, percussion, and auscultation are needed to detect normal age-related changes. Health and fitness help keep losses in respiratory functioning to a minimum. Periodic breathing patterns (e.g., Cheyne-Stokes) can occur. Oral hygiene aids in the removal of secretions.
Pharynx and Larynx Muscles atrophy. Vocal cords become slack. Laryngeal muscles lose elasticity, and airways lose cartilage.	Have face-to-face conversations with patient when possible.	Patient's voice may be soft and difficult to understand.
Pulmonary Vasculature Vascular resistance to blood flow through pulmonary vascular system increases. Pulmonary capillary blood volume decreases. Risk for hypoxia increases.	Assess patient's level of consciousness and cognition.	Patient can become confused during acute respiratory conditions because of reduced oxygen levels in the brain.
Exercise Tolerance Body's response to hypoxia and hypercarbia decreases.	Assess for subtle manifestations of hypoxia.	Early assessment helps prevent complications.
Muscle Strength Respiratory muscle strength, especially the diaphragm and the intercostals, decreases.	Encourage pulmonary hygiene and help patient actively maintain health and fitness.	Regular pulmonary hygiene and overall fitness help maintain maximal functioning of the respiratory system and prevent illness.
Susceptibility to Infection Effectiveness of the cilia decreases. Immunoglobulin A decreases. Alveolar macrophages are altered.	Encourage pulmonary hygiene and help patient actively maintain health and fitness.	Regular pulmonary hygiene and overall fitness help maintain maximal functioning of the respiratory system and prevent illness.
Chest Wall Anteroposterior diameter increases. Thorax becomes shorter. Progressive kyphoscoliosis occurs. Chest wall compliance (elasticity) decreases. Mobility of chest wall may decrease. Osteoporosis is possible, leading to chest wall abnormalities.	Discuss the normal changes of aging. Discuss the need for increased rest periods during exercise. Encourage adequate calcium intake (especially during a woman's premenopause phase).	Patients may be anxious because they must work harder to breathe. Older patients have less tolerance for exercise. Calcium intake helps prevent osteoporosis by building bone in younger patients.

 NCLEX EXAMINATION CHALLENGE 27-2

Physiological Integrity

Which conditions are **most** likely to cause a "left shift" of the oxyhemoglobin dissociation curve? **Select all that apply.**
A. Reduced blood and tissue levels of diphosphoglycerate (DPG)
B. Reduced blood and tissue pH
C. Increased metabolic demands
D. Alkalosis
E. Increased body temperature
F. Reduced blood and tissue levels of oxygen

problems are chronic, and the patient has physical and lifestyle limitations. Many acute health problems, medical therapies, and surgeries adversely affect respiratory function temporarily or permanently. Exposure to inhalation irritants, especially to cigarette smoke, is the most common cause of chronic respiratory problems and physical limitations. In addition, smoking is a modifiable factor that greatly increases the risk for cardiovascular disease, stroke, and many types of cancer. Three compounds in cigarette smoke that have been implicated in the development of these serious diseases are tar, nicotine, and carbon monoxide. In the years after a patient has stopped smoking, his or her risk for respiratory-related disorders decreases significantly. Therefore assessing smoking habits, actively promoting smoking cessation, determining exposure to other inhalation irritants, and teaching adults to protect the respiratory system are important nursing functions. Although cigarette smoking has declined in both countries, about 21% of the United States population continues to smoke cigarettes (Nguyen et al., 2015), and slightly less than 20% of the Canadian population continues to smoke cigarettes (Statistics Canada, 2016).

Assessing smoking habits begins by determining whether the patient is a current smoker or has ever smoked. The smoking history includes the number of cigarettes smoked daily, the duration of the smoking habit, and the age of the patient when smoking started even for patients who are not current smokers. Record the smoking history in **pack-years**, which is the number of packs per day multiplied by the number of years the patient has smoked.

Ask those who do not currently smoke whether and to what extent they are exposed to the smoke of others. Passive smoking has two origins: direct exposure to smoke by being in the same environment with an adult(s) who is actively smoking *(second-hand smoke [SHS])*; and indirect exposure from smoke that clings to hair and clothing *(thirdhand smoke)*. Passive smoking contributes to health problems, especially when chronic exposure occurs in small, confined spaces.

Social smokers are adults who smoke cigarettes only in the presence of others, borrow rather than purchase cigarettes, prefer the company of nonsmokers, and do not smoke for stress relief. Often the social smoker does not consider himself or herself to be a smoker and must be asked specifically, "Do you ever smoke in social situations?" Even intermittent smoking has adverse effects on respiratory and cardiovascular health and may lead to nicotine addiction.

Hookah or water-pipe smoking is increasing in North America, especially among young adults. Many smokers have the false belief that hookah smoking is safer than cigarette smoking. The exposure to inhaled toxins during hookah smoking is as great or greater than with cigarette smoking.

Electronic nicotine delivery systems (ENDS) with either battery-powered electronic cigarettes or a vape pen, also known as *vaping,* are an alternative to traditional cigarettes and sometimes are used as a method of quitting smoking. A vape pen is a larger device with a greater volume of liquid often worn as a pendant or necklace around the neck. An advantage of ENDS is that they do not contain combustion products that affect either the user or bystanders (Antolin & Barkley, 2015). The liquids and the vapors produced contain nicotine; and new evidence indicates that other lung toxins are present in the flavorings, especially diacetyl (Hua & Talbot, 2016). These toxins appear responsible for new-onset bronchiolitis obliterans ("popcorn lung") and for worsening of other existing lung injury conditions. This issue is especially problematic for adults using vape pens because these devices allow almost continuous use and exposure to the liquids. Although previously unregulated, the Food and Drug Administration now has responsibility for assessing health effects of ENDS and setting safety standards (American Lung Association [ALA]), 2016).

Promoting smoking cessation is a sensitive and sometimes uncomfortable issue for nurses and other health care professionals to approach with patients who smoke. However, this opportunity for a "teachable moment" may be the beginning

GENDER HEALTH CONSIDERATIONS
Patient-Centered Care QSEN

Lesbian women, gay men, bisexual men and women, and transgender (LGBT) adults report higher rates of smoking compared with their heterosexual counterparts (ALA, 2015). Therefore screening for smoking and tobacco-related health conditions is especially important when working with LGBT patients.

CULTURAL/SPIRITUAL CONSIDERATIONS
Patient-Centered Care QSEN

The prevalence of smoking is higher among African Americans, blue-collar workers, and less-educated adults than in the overall North American population. It is highest among Native American and Native Canadian Indians. Development of culturally appropriate smoking-cessation programs and research examining barriers to cessation in these populations may help reduce this disparity.

support a patient needs to be successful in this healthful pursuit, especially if the patient is hospitalized for a smoking-related illness (Keating, 2016). Acute care settings have automatic smoking-cessation protocols that attach to the patient's electronic medical record when an active smoking history is recorded. **The Joint Commission requires documentation of screening for tobacco use and that a tobacco treatment program be offered or provided as part of their quality measures.**

Ask about the patient's desire to quit, past attempts to quit, and the methods used. A "yes" response to any of the following questions indicates nicotine dependence. The more "yes" responses, the greater the nicotine dependence. Ask the smoker these questions:

- How soon after you wake up in the morning do you smoke?
- Do you wake up in the middle of your sleep time to smoke?
- Do you find it difficult not to smoke in places where smoking is prohibited?
- Do you smoke when you are ill?

Drug therapies are available over the counter and by prescription to help those addicted to nicotine to modify their behavior and stop smoking. Over-the-counter nicotine replacement therapies (NRTs) include nicotine-releasing transdermal patches, gums, and lozenges. Prescribed NRT products include nasal sprays and inhalers. NRT products have a success rate of smoking cessation of at least 50% (Barnett et al., 2015). They have the highest success rates when used along with a smoking-cessation program. Chart 27-2 lists suggestions for you to use in providing support to the person interested in stopping cigarette smoking.

! NURSING SAFETY PRIORITY QSEN
Drug Alert

Teach adults using drugs for nicotine replacement therapy that smoking while taking these drugs greatly increases circulating nicotine levels and the risk for stroke or heart attack.

CHART 27-2 Patient and Family Education: Preparing for Self-Management

Smoking Cessation

- Make a list of the reasons you want to stop smoking (e.g., your health and the health of those around you, saving money, social reasons).
- Set a date to stop smoking and keep it. Decide whether you are going to begin to cut down on the amount you smoke or are going to stop "cold turkey." Whichever way you decide to do it, keep this important date!
- Ask for help from those around you. Find someone who wants to quit smoking and "buddy up" for support. Look for assistance in your community, such as formal smoking-cessation programs, counselors, and certified acupuncture specialists or hypnotists.
- Consult your health care provider about nicotine replacement therapy (e.g., patch, gum) or other pharmacologic therapy to assist in smoking cessation.
- Remove ashtrays and lighters from your view.
- Talk to yourself! Remind yourself of all the reasons you want to quit.
- Think of a way to reward yourself with the money you save from not smoking for a year.
- Avoid places that might tempt you to smoke. If you are used to having a cigarette after meals, get up from the table as soon as you are finished eating. Think of new things to do at times when you used to smoke (e.g., taking a walk, exercising, calling a friend).
- Find activities that keep your hands busy: needlework, painting, gardening, even holding a pencil.
- Take five deep breaths of clean, fresh air through your nose and out your mouth if you feel the urge to smoke.
- Keep plenty of healthy, low-calorie snacks, such as fruits and vegetables, on hand to nibble on. Try sugarless gum or mints as a substitute for tobacco.
- Drink at least eight glasses of water each day.
- Begin an exercise program with the approval of your primary health care provider. Be aware of the positive, healthy changes in your body since you stopped smoking.
- List the many reasons why you are glad that you quit. Keep the list handy as a reminder of the positive things you are doing for yourself.
- If you have a cigarette, think about the conditions that caused you to light it. Try and think of a strategy to avoid that (or those) conditions.
- Don't beat yourself up for backsliding; just face the next day as a new day.
- Think of each day without tobacco as a major accomplishment. It is!

Additional drug therapy for smoking cessation includes the oral drugs bupropion (Zyban) and varenicline (Chantix). Bupropion decreases cravings and withdrawal symptoms, as well as reduces the depression associated with nicotine-withdrawal symptoms. Varenicline interferes with the nicotine receptors. This promotes smoking cessation by reducing the pleasure derived from nicotine and the symptoms of nicotine withdrawal.

! NURSING SAFETY PRIORITY QSEN

Drug Alert

Both bupropion and varenicline carry a black box warning that use of these drugs can cause manic behavior and hallucinations. These drugs also may unmask serious mental health issues. Teach patients prescribed either of these drugs and their families to report any change in behavior or thought processes to the prescriber immediately.

♥ VETERANS' HEALTH CONSIDERATIONS
Patient-Centered Care QSEN

Cigarette smoking among military veterans is declining more slowly than among the general population, with a 27% smoking rate among veterans compared with a 21% smoking rate among the nonveteran population. Health care costs from cigarette smoking in military veterans is about 7.8% of the total budget for the Veterans' Health Administration (VHA), with costs related to in-patient care as high as 11.4% (Barnett et al., 2015). The slower decline appears to be related to a remaining high smoking prevalence among veterans who have psychiatric and substance use disorders and among female veterans. The VHA has implemented several strategies to promote smoking cessation among veterans, including extending the use of NRT to veterans who are not part of a formal smoking cessation program and eliminating copayments for NRT. Be sure to assess the smoking status of all veterans and inform them of VHA smoking-cessation assistance.

Assessing exposure to inhalation irritants should be part of any health assessment within the demographic history. Include the patient's current and past geographic living area, home conditions, occupation, and hobbies. Areas with high levels of air pollution contribute to respiratory problems. Exposure to dust, particles, chemicals, gases. or toxic fumes can occur in the workplace, making work history information important. Ask about dates of employment and a brief job description. Exposure to industrial dusts of any type or to chemical fumes may cause breathing disorders. Bakers, coalminers, stone masons, cotton handlers, woodworkers, welders, potters, plastic and rubber manufacturers, printers, farm workers, those working in grain elevators or flour mills, and steel foundry workers are at risk for work-related breathing problems.

Ask about the type of heat used at home (e.g., gas heater, wood-burning stove, fireplace, kerosene heater). Determine exposure to irritants (e.g., fumes, chemicals, animals, birds, air pollutants). Ask about hobbies such as painting, ceramics, model airplanes, refinishing furniture, or woodworking, which may expose the patient to harmful chemicals.

Protecting the respiratory system starts with making adults aware of the sources of inhalation irritants. Teach adults who live in areas with high levels of air pollution to remain indoors with windows closed on days when air quality is poor and not to engage in heavy physical activity. Teach adults who have workplace or home exposure to inhalation irritants to wear masks during these exposures and ensure that the area is well ventilated.

ASSESSMENT: NOTICING AND INTERPRETING

Patient History

Accurate patient information is important for identifying the type and severity of breathing problems that may interfere with GAS EXCHANGE. Age, gender, and race can affect the physical and diagnostic findings related to breathing (Jarvis, 2016). Many diagnostic studies for respiratory disorders (e.g., pulmonary function tests) use these data for determining predicted normal values. As described in the Health Promotion and Maintenance section, explore the home, community, and workplace for environmental factors that could cause or worsen lung disease. Use this opportunity to teach patients about measures to protect the respiratory system.

GENDER HEALTH CONSIDERATIONS
Patient-Centered Care QSEN

Women, especially smokers, have greater bronchial responsiveness (i.e., bronchial hyperreactivity) and larger airways than men. This factor increases the risk for a more rapid decline in lung function as a woman ages, especially in women who were or are smokers. Be sure to measure gas exchange adequacy with pulse oximetry when assessing women.

CULTURAL/SPIRITUAL CONSIDERATIONS
Patient-Centered Care QSEN

Compared with white adults, black adults and others with dark skin usually show a lower oxygen saturation (3% to 5% lower) as measured by pulse oximetry; this results from deeper coloration of the nail bed and does not reflect true oxygen status. Use additional respiratory assessment techniques to assess gas exchange adequacy in adults with dark skin.

Ask patients about their respiratory history (Table 27-1), including smoking history, drug use, travel, and area of residence. Document the smoking history in pack-years.

Drug use, both prescribed drugs and illicit drugs, can affect lung function, even when taken systemically. Ask about drugs taken for breathing problems and those taken for other conditions. For example, a cough can be a side effect of some antihypertensive drugs (angiotensin-converting enzyme inhibitors [ACEIs] and angiotensin receptor blockers [ARBs]). Determine which over-the-counter drugs (e.g., cough syrups, antihistamines, decongestants, inhalants) the patient uses. Assess use of complementary and integrative therapies. Ask about past drug use. Some drugs for other conditions can cause permanent changes in lung function. For example, patients may have

---

TABLE 27-1 Important Aspects to Assess in a Respiratory System History

- Smoking history
- Childhood illnesses:
  - Asthma
  - Pneumonia
  - Communicable diseases
  - Hay fever
  - Allergies
  - Eczema
  - Frequent colds
  - Croup
  - Cystic fibrosis
- Adult illnesses:
  - Pneumonia
  - Sinusitis
  - Tuberculosis
  - HIV and AIDS
  - Lung disease such as emphysema and sarcoidosis
  - Diabetes
  - Hypertension
  - Heart disease
  - Influenza, pneumococcal (Pneumovax), and BCG vaccinations

- Surgeries of the upper or lower respiratory system
- Injuries to the upper or lower respiratory system
- Hospitalizations
- Date of last chest x-ray, pulmonary function test, tuberculin test, or other diagnostic tests and results
- Recent weight loss
- Night sweats
- Sleep disturbances
- Lung disease and condition of family members
- Geographic areas of recent travel
- Occupation and leisure activities

AIDS, Acquired immune deficiency syndrome; *BCG,* bacille Calmette-Guérin; *HIV,* human immune deficiency virus.

---

pulmonary fibrosis if they received bleomycin (Blenoxane) as chemotherapy for cancer or amiodarone (Cordarone) for cardiac problems. Marijuana and illicit drugs, such as cocaine, are often inhaled and can affect lung function.

Allergies to foods, dust, molds, pollen, bee stings, trees, grass, animal dander and saliva, or drugs can affect breathing. Ask the patient to describe specific allergic responses. For example, does he or she wheeze, have trouble breathing, cough, sneeze, or have rhinitis after exposure to the allergen? Has he or she ever been treated for an allergic response? If the patient has allergies, ask about the specific cause, treatment, and response to treatment.

! NURSING SAFETY PRIORITY QSEN
Action Alert

Document any known allergies, especially to drugs, and the specific type of allergic response in a prominent place in the patient's medical record.

Travel and geographic area of residence may reveal exposure to certain diseases. For example, *histoplasmosis,* a fungal disease caused by inhalation of contaminated dust, is found in the central parts of the United States and Canada. *Coccidioidomycosis* is found in the western and southwestern parts of the United States, in Mexico, and in parts of Central America, as is *Hantavirus.* With veterans, ask about location of deployments within the past year.

Family History and Genetic Risk

Obtain a family history to assess for respiratory disorders that have a genetic component, such as cystic fibrosis, some lung cancers, and emphysema. Patients with asthma often have a family history of allergy. Ask about a history of infectious disease, such as tuberculosis, because family members may have similar environmental exposures.

Current Health Problems

Whether the breathing problem is acute or chronic, the current health problem usually includes cough, sputum production, chest pain, and shortness of breath at rest or on exertion. Explore the current illness in chronologic order. Ask about the onset of the problem, how long it lasts, the location of the problem, how often it occurs, whether the problem has become worse over time, which symptoms occur with it, which actions or interventions provide relief and which ones make it worse, and which treatments have been used.

Cough is a sign of lung disease. Ask the patient how long the cough has been present and whether it occurs at a specific time of day (e.g., on awakening in the morning) or in relation to any physical activity. Ask whether the cough produces sputum or is dry, tickling, or hacking.

Sputum production is an important symptom associated with coughing. Check the color, consistency, odor, and amount of sputum.

Describe the consistency of sputum as thin, thick, watery, or frothy. Smokers with chronic bronchitis have mucoid sputum. Excessive pink, frothy sputum is common with pulmonary edema. Bacterial pneumonia often produces rust-colored sputum, and a lung abscess may cause foul-smelling sputum. Hemoptysis (blood in the sputum) may be seen in patients with chronic bronchitis or lung cancer. Grossly bloody sputum may occur with tuberculosis, pulmonary infarction, lung cancer, or lung abscess.

Ask the patient to quantify sputum by describing its volume in terms such as teaspoon, tablespoon, and cup. Normally the lungs can produce up to 90 mL of sputum per day.

Chest pain can occur with other health problems in addition to with lung problems. A detailed description of chest pain helps distinguish its cause. Ask whether the pain is continuous or made worse by coughing, deep breathing, or swallowing. Cardiac pain is usually intense and "crushing" and may radiate to the arm, shoulder, or neck. Pulmonary pain varies, depending on the cause, and most often feels like something is "rubbing" inside. Pain may appear only on deep inhalation or be present at the end of inhalation and the end of exhalation. Pulmonary pain is not made worse by touching or pressing over the area.

Dyspnea (difficulty in breathing or breathlessness) is a subjective perception and varies among patients (Baker et al., 2013). A patient's feeling of dyspnea may not be consistent with the severity of the problem. However, patients with chronic lung disease can reliably report dyspnea levels that accurately correspond to the severity of their disease (Croucher, 2014). Determine the type of onset (slow or abrupt), the duration, relieving factors (position changes, drug use, activity cessation), and whether wheezing or stridor occurs with dyspnea.

Try to quantify dyspnea by asking whether this symptom interferes with ADLs and, if so, how severely. For example, does dyspnea occur after walking one block or climbing one flight of stairs? Table 27-2 classifies dyspnea with changes in ADL performance. Because dyspnea can be an independent predictor of life-threatening illness, early assessment provides an opportunity to optimize care, improve symptom management, ensure the appropriate level of intervention and care, and determine best use of resources (Baker et al., 2013).

Ask about orthopnea, which is shortness of breath occurring when lying down and is relieved by sitting up. Assess for paroxysmal nocturnal dyspnea (PND), which awakens the patient from sleep with the feeling of an inability to breathe. PND also occurs while lying flat and is relieved by sitting up. It often occurs with chronic lung disease and left-sided heart failure.

TABLE 27-2 Correlation of Dyspnea Classification With Performance of ADLs

CLASSIFICATION	ADLs KEY
Class I: No significant restrictions in normal activity. Employable. Dyspnea occurs only on more-than-normal or strenuous exertion.	4: No breathlessness, normal.
Class II: Independent in essential ADLs but restricted in some other activities. Dyspneic on climbing stairs or on walking on an incline but not on level walking. Employable only for sedentary job or under special circumstances.	3: Satisfactory, mild breathlessness. Complete performance is possible without pause or assistance but not entirely normal.
Class III: Dyspnea commonly occurs during usual activities such as showering or dressing, but the patient can manage without assistance from others. Not dyspneic at rest; can walk for more than a city block at own pace but cannot keep up with others of own age. May stop to catch breath partway up a flight of stairs. Is not likely to be employed.	2: Fair, moderate breathlessness. Must stop during activity. Complete performance is possible without assistance, but performance may be too debilitating or time consuming.
Class IV: Dyspnea produces dependence on help in some essential ADLs such as dressing and bathing. Not usually dyspneic at rest. Dyspneic on minimal exertion; must pause on climbing one flight, walking more than 100 yards, or dressing. Often restricted to home if lives alone. Has minimal or no activities outside of home.	1: Poor, marked breathlessness. Incomplete performance; assistance is necessary.
Class V: Entirely restricted to home and often limited to bed or chair. Dyspneic at rest. Dependent on help for most needs.	0: Performance not indicated or recommended; too difficult.

ADLs, Activities of daily living.

? NCLEX EXAMINATION CHALLENGE 27-3

Safe and Effective Care Environment

Which assessment findings are **most important** for the nurse to determine when assessing a client with dyspnea? **Select all that apply.**
A. Onset of or when the client first noticed dyspnea
B. Results of most recent pulmonary function test
C. Conditions that relieve the dyspnea sensation
D. Whether or not dyspnea interferes with ADLs
E. Inspection of the external nose and its symmetry
F. Whether stridor is present with dyspnea

Physical Assessment

Assessment of the Nose and Sinuses

Inspect the patient's external nose for deformities or polyps and the nares for symmetry of size and shape. To observe the interior nose, ask the patient to tilt the head back for a penlight examination. The experienced nurse may use a nasal speculum and nasopharyngeal mirror for a more thorough inspection of the nasal cavity.

Inspect for color, swelling, drainage, and bleeding. Nasal mucous membranes normally appear redder than the oral mucosa but are pale, engorged, and bluish-gray in patients with allergic rhinitis. Check the nasal septum for bleeding, perforation, or deviation. Septal deviation is common and appears as an S shape, tilting toward one side or the other. A perforated septum is present if the light shines through the perforation into the opposite side; this condition is often found in cocaine users. Nasal polyps are pale, shiny, gelatinous lumps or "bags" attached to the turbinates. Block one naris at a time to check how well air moves through the unblocked side.

Assessment of the Pharynx, Trachea, and Larynx

Assessment of the pharynx begins with inspection of the mouth. To examine the posterior pharynx, use a tongue depressor to press down one side of the tongue at a time (to avoid stimulating the gag reflex). As the patient says "ah," observe the rise and fall of the soft palate and inspect for color and symmetry, drainage, edema or ulceration, and enlarged tonsils.

Inspect the neck for symmetry, alignment, masses, swelling, bruises, and the use of accessory neck muscles in breathing. Palpate lymph nodes for size, shape, mobility with palpation, consistency, and tenderness.

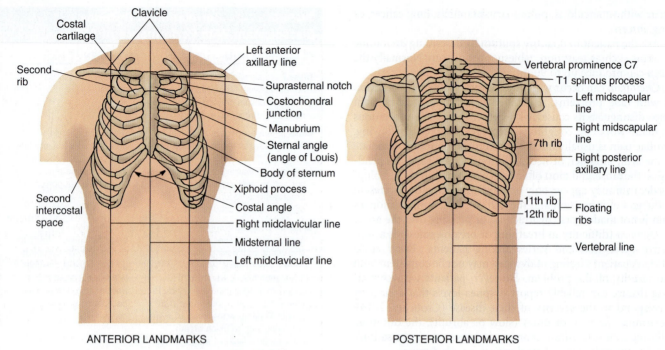

FIG. 27-8 Anterior and posterior chest landmarks.

Gently palpate the trachea for position, mobility, tenderness, and masses. The trachea should be in the midline. Many lung disorders cause the trachea to deviate from the midline. Tension pneumothorax, large pleural effusion, mediastinal mass, and neck tumors push the trachea *away* from the affected area. Pneumonectomy, fibrosis, and atelectasis pull it *toward* the affected area.

The larynx is usually examined by a specialist with a laryngoscope. An abnormal voice, especially hoarseness, may be heard when there are problems of the larynx.

Assessment of the Lungs and Thorax

Inspection. Inspect the front and back of the thorax with the patient sitting up. Normal landmarks of the chest front (anterior) and back (posterior) are shown in Fig. 27-8. The patient should be undressed to the waist. Observe the chest and compare one side with the other. Work from the top (apex) and move downward toward the base, going from side to side, while inspecting for discoloration, scars, lesions, masses, and spinal curvatures. Assessing from side to side allows you to compare the findings for each lung at the same level (Jarvis, 2016).

Observe the rate, rhythm, and depth of inspirations and the symmetry of chest movement. Impaired movement or unequal expansion may indicate disease. Observe the type of breathing (e.g., pursed-lip or diaphragmatic breathing) and the use of accessory muscles.

Examine the shape of the patient's chest, and compare the anteroposterior (AP or front-to-back) diameter with the lateral (side-to-side) diameter. This ratio normally is about 1:1.5, depending on body build. It increases to 1:1 in patients with emphysema, which results in the typical barrel-chest appearance.

Normally the ribs slope downward. Patients with air trapping in the lungs caused by emphysema have ribs that are more horizontal. Observe or palpate the distance between the ribs (*intercostal space*). This distance is usually one finger-breadth (2 cm). It increases in disorders that cause air trapping, such as emphysema. Observe for retraction of muscle between the ribs and at the sternal notch. Retractions are areas that get sucked inward when the patient inhales. This does not occur during normal respiratory effort. Retractions may occur when the patient is working hard to inhale around an obstruction.

Palpation. Palpate the chest after inspection to assess respiratory movement symmetry and observable abnormalities. Palpation also can help identify areas of tenderness and check vocal or tactile **fremitus** (vibration).

Assess chest expansion by placing your thumbs on the patient's spine at the level of the ninth ribs and extending the fingers sideways around the rib cage. As the patient inhales, both sides of the chest should move upward and outward together in one symmetric movement, moving your thumbs apart. On exhalation, the thumbs should come back together as they return to the midline. Unequal expansion may be a result of pain, trauma, or air in the pleural cavity. Respiratory lag or slowed movement on one side indicates a pulmonary problem (Jarvis, 2016).

Palpate any abnormalities found on inspection (e.g., masses, lesions, swelling). Also palpate for tenderness, especially if the patient reports pain. **Crepitus** (air trapped in and under the skin, also known as *subcutaneous emphysema*) is felt as a crackling sensation beneath the fingertips. Document this finding and report it to the primary health care provider when it occurs around a wound site or a tracheostomy site or if a pneumothorax is suspected.

Tactile (vocal) fremitus is felt as a vibration of the chest wall produced when the patient speaks. Fremitus is decreased if sound wave transmission from the larynx to the chest wall is slowed, such as when the pleural space is filled with air (pneumothorax) or fluid (**pleural effusion**) or when the bronchus is obstructed. Fremitus is increased with pneumonia and lung abscesses because the increased density of the chest enhances vibration transmission.

Percussion. Use percussion to assess for pulmonary resonance, the boundaries of organs, and diaphragmatic excursion. Percussion involves tapping the chest wall, which sets the underlying tissues into motion and produces audible sounds (Fig. 27-9). This action produces five different sounds that help determine whether the lung tissue contains air or fluid or is solid (Table 27-3).

Auscultation. Lung auscultation is listening with a stethoscope for normal breath sounds, abnormal (*adventitious*) sounds, and voice sounds. It provides information about the flow of air through the trachea and lungs and helps identify fluid, mucus, or obstruction in the respiratory system.

Begin auscultation with the patient sitting in an upright position. With the stethoscope pressed firmly against the chest wall (clothing can muffle sounds), instruct the patient to breathe slowly and deeply through an open mouth. (Breathing through the nose sets up turbulent sounds that are transmitted to the lungs.) Use a systematic approach, beginning at the lung apices and moving from side to side down through the intercostal spaces to the lung bases (Fig. 27-10). Avoid listening over bony structures. Listen to a full respiratory cycle, noting the quality and intensity of the breath sounds.

Normal breath sounds are produced as air vibrates while moving through the passages from the larynx to the alveoli. Breath sounds are identified by their location, intensity, pitch, and duration within the respiratory cycle (e.g., early or late inspiration and expiration). Normal breath sounds are known as "bronchial" or "tubular" (harsh hollow sounds heard over the trachea and mainstem bronchi), "bronchovesicular" (heard over the branching bronchi), and "vesicular" (soft rustling sounds heard in lung tissue over small bronchioles) (Table 27-4). Describe these sounds as *normal, increased, diminished,* or *absent*.

Bronchial breath sounds heard at the lung edges are abnormal and occur when the bronchial sounds are transmitted to an area of increased density, such as with atelectasis, tumor, or pneumonia. When heard in an abnormal location, bronchovesicular breath sounds may indicate normal aging or an abnormality such as consolidation and chronic airway disease.

Adventitious sounds are additional breath sounds along with normal sounds, and they indicate pathologic changes in the lung. Table 27-5 describes adventitious sounds: crackle, wheeze, rhonchus, and pleural friction rub. These sounds vary in pitch, intensity, and duration and can occur in any phase of the respiratory cycle. Document exactly what you hear on auscultation.

Voice sounds (vocal resonance) through the normally air-filled lung are muffled and unclear because sound vibrations travel poorly through air. These sounds become louder and more distinct when the sound travels through a solid tissue or liquid. The presence of pneumonia, atelectasis, pleural effusion, tumor, or abscess causes increased vocal resonance.

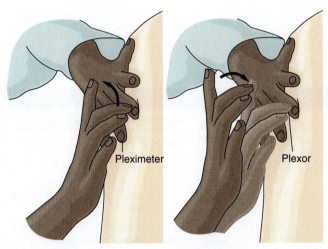

FIG. 27-9 Percussion technique.

❓ NCLEX EXAMINATION CHALLENGE 27-4

Safe and Effective Care Environment

The nurse assessing the respiratory status of a client discovers that tactile fremitus has increased from the assessment performed yesterday. For which possible respiratory problem should the nurse assess further?
A. Pneumothorax
B. Pneumonia
C. Pleural effusion
D. Emphysema

TABLE 27-3	Characteristics of the Five Percussion Notes				
NOTE	**PITCH**	**INTENSITY**	**QUALITY**	**DURATION**	**FINDINGS**
Resonance	Low	Moderate to loud	Hollow	Long	Resonance is characteristic of normal lung tissue.
Hyperresonance	Higher than resonance	Very loud	Booming	Longer than resonance	Hyperresonance indicates the presence of trapped air, so it is commonly heard over an emphysematous or asthmatic lung and occasionally over a pneumothorax.
Flatness	High	Soft	Extreme dullness	Short	An example location is the sternum. Flatness percussed over the lung fields may indicate a massive pleural effusion.
Dullness	Medium	Medium	Thudlike	Medium	Example locations are over the liver and the kidneys. Dullness can be percussed over an atelectatic lung or a consolidated lung.
Tympany	High	Loud	Musical, drumlike	Short	Examples are the cheek filled with air and the abdomen distended with air. Over the lung, a tympanic note usually indicates a large pneumothorax.

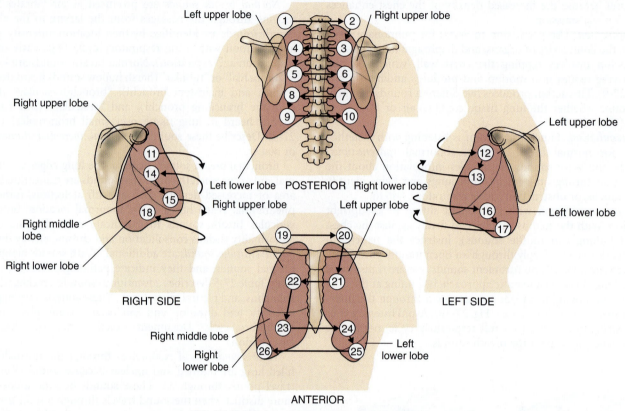

FIG. 27-10 Sequence for percussion and auscultation.

TABLE 27-4	**Characteristics of Normal Breath Sounds**				
	PITCH	**AMPLITUDE**	**DURATION**	**QUALITY**	**NORMAL LOCATION**
Bronchial (tubular, tracheal)	High	Loud	Inspiration < expiration	Harsh, hollow, tubular, blowing	Trachea and larynx
Bronchovesicular	Moderate	Moderate	Inspiration = expiration	Mixed	Over major bronchi where fewer alveoli are located; posterior, between scapulae (especially on right); anterior, around upper sternum in first and second intercostal spaces
Vesicular	Low	Soft	Inspiration > expiration	Rustling, like the sound of the wind in the trees	Over peripheral lung fields where air flows through smaller bronchioles and alveoli

From Jarvis, C. (2016). *Physical examination and health assessment* (7th ed.). St. Louis: Saunders.

Other Indicators of Respiratory Adequacy

Assess other indicators of respiratory adequacy, because GAS EXCHANGE affects all body systems. Some indicators (e.g., cyanosis) reflect immediate gas exchange and PERFUSION problems. Other changes (e.g., clubbing, weight loss) reflect long-term oxygenation problems.

Skin and mucous membrane changes (e.g., pallor, cyanosis) may indicate inadequate GAS EXCHANGE and PERFUSION. Assess the nail beds and the mucous membranes of the oral cavity.

Examine the fingers for clubbing (see Fig. 30-10), which indicates long-term hypoxia.

General appearance includes muscle development and general body build. Long-term respiratory problems lead to weight loss and a loss of general muscle mass. Arms and legs may appear thin or poorly muscled. Neck and chest muscles may be hypertrophied, especially in the patient with chronic obstructive pulmonary disease (COPD) (McCance et al., 2014).

Endurance decreases when breathing is inadequate for GAS EXCHANGE. Observe how easily the patient moves and whether

TABLE 27-5	Characteristics of Adventitious Breath Sounds	
ADVENTITIOUS SOUND	**CHARACTER**	**ASSOCIATION**
Fine crackles Fine rales High-pitched rales	Popping, discontinuous sounds caused by air moving into previously deflated airways; sounds like hair being rolled between fingers near the ear "Velcro" sounds late in inspiration usually associated with restrictive disorders	Asbestosis Atelectasis Interstitial fibrosis Bronchitis Pneumonia Chronic pulmonary diseases
Coarse crackles Low-pitched crackles	Lower-pitched, coarse, rattling sounds caused by fluid or secretions in large airways; likely to change with coughing or suctioning	Bronchitis Pneumonia Tumors Pulmonary edema
Wheeze	Squeaky, musical, continuous sounds associated with air rushing through narrowed airways; may be heard without a stethoscope Arise from the small airways Usually do not clear with coughing	Inflammation Bronchospasm (bronchial asthma) Edema Secretions Pulmonary vessel engorgement (as in cardiac "asthma")
Rhonchus (rhonchi)	Lower-pitched, coarse, continuous snoring sounds Arise from the large airways	Thick, tenacious secretions Sputum production Obstruction by foreign body Tumors
Pleural friction rub	Loud, rough, grating, scratching sounds caused by the inflamed surfaces of the pleura rubbing together; often associated with pain on deep inspirations Heard in lateral lung fields	Pleurisy Tuberculosis Pulmonary infarction Pneumonia Lung cancer

he or she is short of breath while resting or becomes short of breath when walking 10 to 20 steps. Note how often the patient stops for breath between words while speaking.

Psychosocial Assessment

Breathing difficulty often induces anxiety. The patient may be anxious because of reduced oxygen to the brain or because the sensation of not getting enough air is frightening. The thought of having a serious problem, such as lung cancer, can also induce anxiety. Encourage the patient to express his or her feelings and fears about symptoms and their possible meaning.

Assess those aspects of the patient's lifestyle that either can affect respiratory function or are affected by it. Some respiratory problems may become worse with stress. Ask about current life stresses and usual coping mechanisms.

Chronic respiratory disease may cause changes in family roles or relationships, social isolation, financial problems, and unemployment or disability. Discuss coping mechanisms to assess the patient's reaction to these stressors and identify strengths. For example, the patient may react to stress with dependence on family members, withdrawal, or failure to adhere to interventions. Help the patient identify available support systems.

Diagnostic Assessment
Laboratory Assessment

Several laboratory tests (Chart 27-3) are useful in assessing respiratory problems. A red blood cell (RBC) count provides data about oxygen transport. Hemoglobin, found in RBCs, transports oxygen to the tissues. A deficiency of hemoglobin could cause hypoxemia.

Arterial blood gas (ABG) analysis assesses GAS EXCHANGE and PERFUSION as oxygenation (partial pressure of arterial oxygen [Pao$_2$]), alveolar ventilation (partial pressure of arterial carbon dioxide [Paco$_2$]), and acid-base balance. Blood gas studies provide information for monitoring treatment results, adjusting oxygen therapy, and evaluating the patient's responses. See Chapter 12 for more details on blood gas analysis.

Sputum specimens can help identify organisms or abnormal cells. Sputum culture and sensitivity analyses identify bacterial infection and determine which specific antibiotics will be most effective. Cytologic examination can identify cancer cells. Allergic conditions may be identified by cytologic testing.

Imaging Assessment

Chest x-rays with digital images are used for patients with pulmonary problems to evaluate chest status and provide a baseline for comparison with future changes. These chest x-rays are performed from **posteroanterior** (PA; back to front) and left lateral (LL) positions.

Chest x-rays are used to assess lung pathology such as with pneumonia, atelectasis, pneumothorax, and tumor. They also can detect pleural fluid and the placement of an endotracheal tube or other invasive catheters. A computer-enhanced image can be adjusted to emphasize a specific area. However, these images have limitations and may appear normal, even when severe chronic bronchitis, asthma, or emphysema is present.

Sinus and facial x-rays are used to assess fluid levels in the sinus cavities to assist in the diagnosis of acute or chronic sinusitis.

Computed tomography (CT) assesses soft tissues with consecutive cross-sectional views of the entire chest. This type of

CHART 27-3   **Laboratory Profile**

Respiratory Assessment

TEST	NORMAL RANGE FOR ADULTS	SIGNIFICANCE OF ABNORMAL FINDINGS
Blood Studies		
Complete Blood Count		
Red blood cells	*Females:* 4.2-5.4 million/mm³, or 4.2-5.4 × 10¹²/L *Males:* 4.7-6.1 million/mm³, or 4.7-6.1 × 10¹²/L	*Elevated levels* (polycythemia) are often related to the excessive production of erythropoietin in response to a chronic hypoxic state, as in COPD, and from living at a high altitude. *Decreased levels* indicate possible anemia, hemorrhage, or hemolysis.
Hemoglobin, total	*Females:* 12-16 g/dL, or 120-160 g/L *Males:* 14-18 g/dL, or 140-180 g/L	Same as for red blood cells.
Hematocrit	*Females:* 37%-47%, or 0.37-0.47 volume fraction *Males:* 42%-52%, or 0.42-0.52 volume fraction	Same as for red blood cells.
WBC count (leukocyte count, WBC count)	*Total:* 5000-10,000/mm³, or 5-10 × 10⁹/L	*Elevations* indicate possible acute infections or inflammations. *Decreased levels* may indicate an overwhelming infection, an autoimmune disorder, or immunosuppressant therapy.
Differential White Blood Cell (Leukocyte) Count		
Neutrophils	2500-8000/mm³, or 50%-62% of total, or 5-6.2 × 10⁹/L	*Elevations* indicate possible acute bacterial infection (pneumonia), COPD, or inflammatory conditions (smoking). *Decreased levels* indicate possible viral disease (influenza).
Eosinophils	50-500/mm³, or 1%-4% of total, or 0.0-0.3 × 10⁹/L	*Elevations* indicate possible COPD, asthma, or allergies. *Decreased levels* indicate pyogenic infections.
Basophils	15-50/mm³, or 0.5%-1% of total, or 0.02-0.05 × 10⁹/L	*Elevations* indicate possible inflammation; seen in chronic sinusitis, hypersensitivity reactions. *Decreased levels* may be seen in an acute infection.
Lymphocytes	1000-4000/mm³, or 20%-40% of total, or 1.0-4.0 × 10⁹/L	*Elevations* indicate possible viral infection, pertussis, and infectious mononucleosis. *Decreased levels* may be seen during corticosteroid therapy.
Monocytes	100-700/mm³, or 2%-8% of total, or 0.1-0.7 × 10⁹/L	*Elevations:* see Lymphocytes; also may indicate active tuberculosis. *Decreased levels:* see Lymphocytes.
Arterial Blood Gases		
PaO₂	80-100 mm Hg *Older adults:* values may be lower	*Elevations* indicate possible excessive oxygen administration. *Decreased levels* indicate possible COPD, asthma, chronic bronchitis, cancer of the bronchi and lungs, cystic fibrosis, respiratory distress syndrome, anemias, atelectasis, or any other cause of hypoxia.
PaCO₂	35-45 mm Hg	*Elevations* indicate possible COPD, asthma, pneumonia, anesthesia effects, or use of opioids (respiratory acidosis). *Decreased levels* indicate hyperventilation/respiratory alkalosis.
pH	*Up to 60 yr:* 7.35-7.45 *60-90 yr:* 7.31-7.42 *>90 yr:* 7.26-7.43	*Elevations* indicate metabolic or respiratory alkalosis. *Decreased levels* indicate metabolic or respiratory acidosis.
HCO₃⁻	21-28 mEq/L (21-28 mmol/L)	*Elevations* indicate possible respiratory acidosis as compensation for a primary metabolic alkalosis. *Decreased levels* indicate possible respiratory alkalosis as compensation for a primary metabolic acidosis.
SpO₂	95%-100% *Older adults:* values may be slightly lower	*Decreased levels* indicate possible impaired ability of hemoglobin to release oxygen to tissues.

Data from Pagana, K., Pagana, T. J., & Pagana, T. N. (2017). *Mosby's diagnostic and laboratory test reference* (13th ed.). St. Louis: Mosby; and Pagana, K., Pagana, T., & Pike-MacDonald, S. (2013). *Mosby's Canadian manual of diagnostic and laboratory tests.* St. Louis: Mosby.

COPD, Chronic obstructive pulmonary disease; HCO₃, bicarbonate ion; *PaCO₂,* partial pressure of arterial carbon dioxide; *PaO₂,* partial pressure of arterial oxygen; *SpO₂,* peripheral oxygen saturation; *WBC,* white blood cell.

imaging can verify the identity of a suspicious lesion or clot. CT scans may require a contrast agent injected IV to enhance the visibility of tumors, blood vessels, and heart chambers. Your role is to provide information to the patient and determine whether he or she has any sensitivity to the contrast material. Ask the patient whether he or she has a known allergy to iodine or shellfish. In addition, IV contrast medium can be nephrotoxic. Ask about his or her kidney function and whether he or she takes drugs for type 2 diabetes. If the patient usually takes metformin, the drug is stopped at least 24 hours before contrast medium is used and is not restarted until adequate kidney function is confirmed (see Chapter 65).

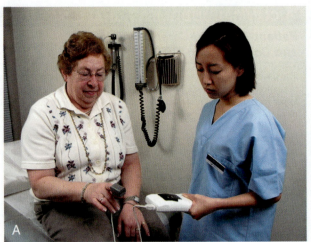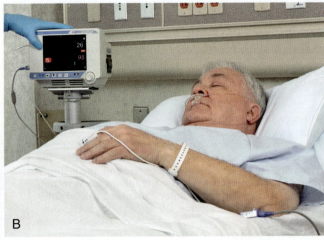

FIG. 27-11 A, A typical pulse oximeter. **B,** Typical capnography equipment without the use of an endotracheal tube. (**A** From Young, A. P., & Proctor, D. [2008]. *Kinn's the medical assistant: An applied learning approach* (10th ed.). St. Louis: Saunders. **B** Copyright ©2016 Medtronic. All rights reserved. Used with the permission of Medtronic.)

Other Noninvasive Diagnostic Assessment

Pulse Oximetry. Pulse oximetry identifies hemoglobin saturation with oxygen. Usually hemoglobin is almost 100% saturated with oxygen in superficial tissues. The pulse oximeter uses a wave of infrared light and a sensor placed on the patient's finger, toe, nose, earlobe, or forehead (Fig. 27-11). Ideal normal pulse oximetry values are 95% to 100%. Normal values are a little lower in older patients and in those with dark skin. To avoid confusion with the PaO_2 values from arterial blood gases, pulse oximetry readings are recorded as the SpO_2 (peripheral arterial oxygen saturation) or SaO_2.

Pulse oximetry can detect desaturation before symptoms (e.g., dusky skin, pale mucosa, pale or blue nail beds) occur. Causes for low readings include patient movement, hypothermia, decreased peripheral blood flow, ambient light (sunlight, infrared lamps), decreased hemoglobin, edema, and fingernail polish. When patients have any degree of impaired peripheral blood flow, the most accurate place to test oxygen saturation is on the forehead. Some brands of inexpensive portable oximeters have been shown to produce unreliable results in acutely ill patients compared with arterial blood sampling for SaO_2 and should not be used in patients who have known abnormal oxygen saturation values (Jones et al., 2015).

Results lower than 91% in an adult who does not have a chronic respiratory problem (and certainly below 86%) are an emergency and require immediate assessment and treatment. When the SpO_2 is below 85%, body tissues have a difficult time becoming oxygenated. An SpO_2 lower than 70% is usually life threatening, but in some cases values below 80% may be life threatening. Pulse oximetry is less accurate at lower values.

Capnometry and Capnography. Capnometry and capnography are methods that measure the amount of carbon dioxide present in exhaled air, which is an indirect measurement of arterial carbon dioxide levels. These noninvasive tests measure the partial pressure of end-tidal carbon dioxide ($PEtCO_2$, also known as $EtCO_2$) levels in both intubated patients and those breathing spontaneously. With capnometry, the exhaled air sample is tested with a sensor that changes the CO_2 level into a color or number for analysis. With capnography, the CO_2 level is graphed as a specific waveform along with a number. These methods provide information about CO_2 production, pulmonary perfusion, alveolar ventilation, respiratory patterns, ventilator effectiveness, and possible rebreathing of exhaled air. Because capnography is a more sensitive indicator of gas exchange adequacy than pulse oximetry, it can be especially useful in early detection of respiratory depression (Carlisle, 2015). See the Quality Improvement box for an example of its use.

The normal value of the partial pressure of end-tidal carbon dioxide ($PEtCO_2$) ranges between 20 and 40 mm Hg. Changes in $PEtCO_2$ reflect changes in breathing effectiveness and GAS EXCHANGE. These changes occur before hypoxia can be detected using pulse oximetry because, even in the presence of diseased lungs, carbon dioxide moves out of the body more easily than oxygen moves into it. The use of both pulse oximetry and $PEtCO_2$ for patients at risk for respiratory problems can provide information to direct early intervention (Carlisle, 2014).

Conditions that increase $PEtCO_2$ above normal levels are those that reflect inadequate GAS EXCHANGE or an increase in cellular metabolism, both of which increase production of carbon dioxide (CO_2). Conditions of inadequate gas exchange include hypoventilation, partial airway obstruction, and rebreathing exhaled air. Conditions that increase cellular metabolism include fever, acidosis, and heavy exercise.

Conditions that decrease $PEtCO_2$ below normal levels are those that reflect poor pulmonary ventilation, such as pulmonary embolism, apnea, total airway obstruction, and malposition of an endotracheal tube. Other causes of low $PEtCO_2$ include hyperventilation not based on oxygen need in which CO_2 is blown off faster than it is generated in the tissues. Cardiopulmonary arrest decreases $PEtCO_2$, and $PEtCO_2$ may be used to determine the effectiveness of CPR and whether there is a spontaneous return of circulation.

Pulmonary Function Tests. Pulmonary function tests (PFTs) assess lung function and breathing problems. These tests measure lung volumes and capacities, flow rates, diffusion capacity, GAS EXCHANGE, airway resistance, and distribution of ventilation. The results are interpreted by comparing the patient's data with expected findings for age, gender, race, height, weight, and smoking status.

QUALITY IMPROVEMENT QSEN

Reducing Cases of Opioid-Induced Respiratory Depression With Increased Use of Capnography

Carlisle, H. (2015). Promoting the use of capnography in acute care settings. An evidence-based practice project. *Journal of PeriAnesthesia Nursing, 30*(3), 201-208.

Opioid-induced respiratory depression (OIRD) is a common yet preventable complication of opioid analgesia. The incidence of this life-threatening problem is on the rise as better pain management with opioid analgesics has increased. **The Joint Commission, the American Society for Pain Management Nursing, the Institute for Safe Medication Practices, and many other groups recommend using capnography to monitor patients at risk for OIRD for the need for early intervention.** Capnography has been proven to be superior for early detection of respiratory changes over the more commonly used pulse oximetry.

This quality improvement project was developed at a large university medical center hospital after two deaths from OIRD had occurred. Because OIRD can be prevented, the hospital examined the number of patients considered to be at risk for OIRD (determined by meeting one or more of the established risk criteria) who actually were being monitored with capnography. Of the patients who qualified as being at risk, only 4.4% were being monitored with capnography. The goal of the project was to increase the number of at-risk patients being monitored using capnography and reducing the overall incidence of OIRD.

The team charged with the improvement project first assessed the barriers to the use of capnography. The major barriers included (1) confusion about whether capnography monitoring required a physician order; (2) inadequate numbers of monitors; and (3) lack of familiarity of this proper use and interpretation of capnography monitoring.

Implementation of the project involved acting on all three barriers. The hospital increased the number of monitors by nearly 50% to a total of 93. A variety of information sessions, videos, and other in-service type education methods were used to increase the registered nurse's understanding of, comfort with, and correct use of capnography monitoring. Over time, an inactive computer-generated standing conditional order for capnography monitoring was developed and designed to open whenever a patient met one or more of the at-risk criteria for OIRD. This order served as a reminder to physicians and nurses and could be activated by either professional. This move empowered nurses to use their clinical judgment in deciding which patients would be best served with capnography monitoring.

A re-evaluation of the use of capnography monitoring in patients at-risk for OIRD a year after the implementation of the project demonstrated an increase in its use from 4.4% to 15%. Although this increase is positive, it is not yet at recommended levels.

Commentary: Implications for Practice and Research

This quality improvement project demonstrated that empowering nurses results in better patient care and earlier intervention for serious complications associated with the widespread use of opioid analgesics, especially in the early postoperative period. Although the use of capnography monitoring increased, so did the quantity and quality of nursing assessments for at-risk patients. The authors of the project warn that, as the use of capnography monitoring increases, it should not ever substitute for close clinical monitoring by knowledgeable registered nurses.

? CLINICAL JUDGMENT CHALLENGE 27-1

Patient-Centered-Care; Teamwork and Collaboration QSEN

The patient is an 82-year-old woman who was admitted from home with pneumonia. Your assessment findings reveal coarse crackles in her right lower lobe and oxygen saturation (SpO$_2$) of 88% without supplemental oxygen. Her temperature is 100.4°F (38°C).

1. Which additional assessment information is it most important for you to obtain now?
2. Which interprofessional team members should be contacted and why?
3. What are some additional diagnostic assessments you should anticipate for this patient?
4. Which additional referrals might be appropriate for this patient?

surgery may identify patients at risk for lung complications after surgery. The most common reason for performing PFTs is to determine the cause of dyspnea. When performed while the patient exercises, PFTs help determine whether dyspnea is caused by lung problems or cardiac problems or by muscle weakness.

Patient Preparation. Explain the purpose of the tests and advise the patient not to smoke for 6 to 8 hours before testing. Depending on the reasons for testing, bronchodilator drugs may be withheld for 4 to 6 hours before the test. The patient with breathing problems often fears further breathlessness and is anxious before these "breathing" tests. Help reduce anxiety by describing what will happen during and after the testing.

Procedure. PFTs can be performed at the bedside or in the respiratory laboratory by a respiratory therapist or respiratory technician. The patient is asked to breathe through the mouth only. A nose clip may be used to prevent air from escaping. The patient performs different breathing maneuvers while measurements are obtained. Table 27-6 describes the most commonly used PFTs and their uses.

Follow-Up Care. Because many breathing maneuvers are performed during PFTs, assess the patient for increased dyspnea or bronchospasm after these studies. Document any drugs given during testing.

Exercise Testing. Exercise increases metabolism and increases gas transport because energy is used. Exercise testing assesses the patient's ability to work and perform ADLs, differentiates reasons for exercise limitation, evaluates disease influence on exercise capacity, and determines whether supplemental oxygen is needed during exercise. These tests are performed on a treadmill or bicycle or by a self-paced 12-minute walking test. Exercise in the patient with normal pulmonary function is limited by circulatory factors, whereas exercise in the pulmonary patient is limited by breathing capacity, GAS EXCHANGE compromise, or both. Explain exercise testing, and assure the patient that he or she will be closely monitored by trained professionals throughout the test.

Other Invasive Diagnostic Assessment

Endoscopic Examinations. Endoscopic studies to assess breathing problems include bronchoscopy, laryngoscopy, and mediastinoscopy. With *laryngoscopy*, a tube for visualization is inserted into the larynx to assess the function of the vocal cords, remove foreign bodies caught in the larynx, or obtain tissue samples for biopsy or culture. A *mediastinoscopy* is the

PFTs are useful in screening patients for lung disease even before the onset of symptoms (Parker, 2014). Repeated testing over time provides data that may be used to guide management (e.g., changes in lung function can support a decision to continue, change, or discontinue a specific therapy). Testing before

TABLE 27-6 Characteristics and Purposes of Pulmonary Function Tests

TEST	PURPOSE
FVC (forced vital capacity) records the maximum amount of air that can be exhaled as quickly as possible after maximum inspiration.	Indicates respiratory muscle strength and ventilatory reserve. Reduced in obstructive and restrictive diseases.
FEV$_1$ (forced expiratory volume in 1 sec) records the maximum amount of air that can be exhaled in the first second of expiration.	Is effort dependent and declines normally with age. It is reduced in certain obstructive and restrictive disorders.
FEV$_1$/FVC is the ratio of expiratory volume in 1 sec to FVC.	Indicates obstruction to airflow. This ratio is the hallmark of obstructive pulmonary disease. It is normal or increased in restrictive disease.
FEF$_{25\%-75\%}$ records the forced expiratory flow over the 25%-75% volume (middle half) of the FVC.	This measure provides a more sensitive index of obstruction in the smaller airways.
FRC (functional residual capacity) is the amount of air remaining in the lungs after normal expiration. FRC test requires use of the helium dilution, nitrogen washout, or body plethysmography technique.	Increased FRC indicates hyperinflation or air trapping, often from obstructive pulmonary disease. FRC is normal or decreased in restrictive pulmonary diseases.
TLC (total lung capacity) is the amount of air in the lungs at the end of maximum inhalation.	Increased TLC indicates air trapping from obstructive pulmonary disease. Decreased TLC indicates restrictive disease.
RV (residual volume) is the amount of air remaining in the lungs at the end of a full, forced exhalation.	RV is increased in obstructive pulmonary disease such as emphysema.
DLCO (diffusion capacity of the lung for carbon monoxide) reflects the surface area of the alveolocapillary membrane. The patient inhales a small amount of CO, holds for 10 sec, and then exhales. The amount inhaled is compared with the amount exhaled.	Is reduced whenever the alveolocapillary membrane is diminished (emphysema, pulmonary hypertension, and pulmonary fibrosis). It is increased with exercise and in conditions such as polycythemia and congestive heart disease.

insertion of a flexible tube through the chest wall just above the sternum into the area between the lungs. It is performed in the operating room with the patient under general anesthesia to examine for the presence of tumors and obtain tissue samples for biopsy or culture. Most complications are related to the anesthetic agents and bleeding. The most common procedure is the bronchoscopy.

A **bronchoscopy** is the insertion of a tube in the airways as far as the secondary bronchi to view airway structures and obtain tissue samples. It is used to diagnose and manage pulmonary diseases. Rigid bronchoscopy usually requires general anesthesia in the operating room. Flexible bronchoscopy can be performed in the ICU or a special endoscopy suite with low-dose sedation. It is used to evaluate the airway and to help with placing or changing an endotracheal tube, collecting specimens, and diagnosing infections. It is often used for lung cancer staging and removal of secretions that are not cleared with normal suctioning. Stents can be placed during bronchoscopy to open up strictures in the trachea and bronchus.

Patient Preparation. Explain the procedure to the patient and verify that consent for the procedure was obtained. Expected outcomes, risks, and benefits of the procedure must be discussed with the patient by the primary health care provider performing the procedure. Document patient allergies. Other tests before the procedure may include a complete blood count, platelet count, prothrombin time, electrolytes, and chest x-ray. The patient should be NPO for 4 to 8 hours before the procedure to reduce the risk for aspiration. Premedication with one of the benzodiazepines may be used to provide both sedation and amnesia. Opioids may also be used.

! NURSING SAFETY PRIORITY **QSEN**

Action Alert

In accordance with The Joint Commission's National Patient Safety Goals, verify the patient's identity with two types of identifiers (name and at least one person-specific number such as birth date, medical record number, or social security number) before a bronchoscopy.

Benzocaine spray as a topical anesthetic to numb the oropharynx is used cautiously, if at all. This agent may induce a condition called **methemoglobinemia**, which is the conversion of normal hemoglobin to methemoglobin (Wesley, 2014). Methemoglobin is an altered iron state that does not carry oxygen, resulting in tissue hypoxia. Other topical anesthetic sprays, such as lidocaine, are less likely to induce this problem.

The normal blood level of methemoglobin is less than 1%. When this level increases, tissue GAS EXCHANGE is reduced. Cyanosis occurs with methemoglobin levels between 10% and 20%, and death can occur when levels reach 50% to 70%. Suspect methemoglobinemia if a patient becomes cyanotic after receiving a topical anesthetic, if he or she does not respond to supplemental oxygen, and if blood is a characteristic chocolate-brown in color. It can be reversed with oxygen and IV injection of 1% methylene blue (1 to 2 mg/kg).

! NURSING SAFETY PRIORITY **QSEN**

Critical Rescue

Assess patients who receive a benzocaine topical anesthetic to the oropharynx to recognize indications of methemoglobinemia. These include cyanosis that is unresponsive to oxygen therapy and chocolate-brown–colored blood. If either of these symptoms is present, respond by notifying the Rapid Response Team.

Procedure. The procedure can be done in a bronchoscopy suite or at the ICU bedside. The bronchoscope is inserted through either the naris or the oropharynx. Maintain IV access and continuously monitor the patient's pulse, blood pressure, respiratory rate, and oxygen saturation. Apply supplemental oxygen.

Follow-Up Care. Monitor the patient until the effects of the sedation have resolved and a gag reflex has returned. Continue to monitor vital signs, including oxygen saturation, and assess breath sounds every 15 minutes for the first 2 hours. Also assess for potential complications, including bleeding, infection, or hypoxemia.

Thoracentesis. Thoracentesis is the needle aspiration of pleural fluid or air from the pleural space for diagnostic or management purposes. Microscopic examination of the pleural fluid helps in making a diagnosis. Pleural fluid may be drained to relieve blood vessel or lung compression and the respiratory distress caused by cancer, empyema, pleurisy, or tuberculosis. Drugs can also be instilled into the pleural space during thoracentesis.

Patient Preparation. Patient preparation is essential before thoracentesis to ensure cooperation during the procedure and prevent complications. Tell the patient to expect a stinging sensation from the local anesthetic agent and a feeling of pressure when the needle is pushed through the posterior chest. Stress the importance of not moving, coughing, or deep breathing during the procedure to avoid puncture of the pleura or lung.

Ask the patient about any allergy to local anesthetic agents. Verify that he or she has signed an informed consent. The entire chest or back is exposed, and the hair on the skin over the aspiration site is clipped if necessary. The site depends on the volume and location of the fluid.

Fig. 27-12 shows the best position for thoracentesis, which widens the spaces between the ribs and permits easy access to the pleural fluid. Properly position and physically support the patient during the procedure. Use pillows to make the patient comfortable and to provide physical support. When the sitting position is used for the procedure, stand in front of the patient to prevent the table from moving and the patient from falling

Procedure. Thoracentesis is often performed at the bedside by a nurse practitioner or a physician, although CT or ultrasound may be used to guide it. The person performing the procedure and any assistants wear goggles and masks to prevent accidental eye or oral splash exposure to the pleural fluid. After the skin is prepped, a local anesthetic is injected into the selected site. Keep the patient informed of the procedure while

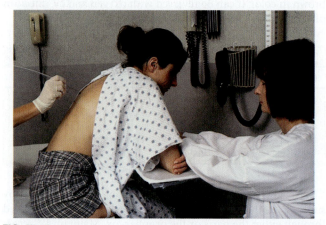

FIG. 27-12 Position for thoracentesis. (From Harkreader, H., Hogan, M. A., & Thobaben, M. [2007]. *Fundamentals of nursing: Caring and clinical judgment* [3rd ed.]. Philadelphia: Saunders.)

observing for shock, pain, nausea, pallor, diaphoresis, cyanosis, tachypnea, and dyspnea.

The short 18- to 25-gauge thoracentesis needle (with an attached syringe) is advanced into the pleural space. Fluid in the pleural space is slowly aspirated with gentle suction. A vacuum collection bottle may be needed to remove larger volumes of fluid. To prevent re-expansion pulmonary edema, usually no more than 1000 mL of fluid is removed at one time. If a biopsy is performed, a second, larger needle with a cutting edge and collection chamber is used. After the needle is withdrawn, pressure is applied to the puncture site, and a sterile dressing is applied. In some cases, pigtail drain catheters may be left in place to a water-seal drainage system, rather than doing a thoracentesis aspiration on a recurring basis.

Follow-Up Care. After thoracentesis, a chest x-ray is performed to rule out possible pneumothorax and mediastinal shift (shift of central thoracic structures toward one side). Monitor vital signs, and listen to the lungs for absent or reduced sounds on the affected side. Check the puncture site and dressing for leakage or bleeding. Assess for complications, such as reaccumulation of fluid in the pleural space, subcutaneous emphysema, infection, and tension pneumothorax. Urge the patient to breathe deeply to promote lung expansion. Document the procedure, including the patient's response; the volume and character of the fluid removed; any specimens sent to the laboratory; the location of the puncture site; and respiratory assessment findings before, during, and after the procedure.

Teach the patient about the symptoms of a pneumothorax (partial or complete collapse of the lung), which can occur within the first 24 hours after a thoracentesis. Symptoms include:

- Pain on the affected side that is worse at the end of inhalation and the end of exhalation
- Rapid heart rate
- Rapid, shallow respirations
- A feeling of air hunger
- Prominence of the affected side that does not move in and out with respiratory effort
- Trachea slanted more to the unaffected side instead of being in the center of the neck
- New onset of "nagging" cough
- Cyanosis

Instruct the patient to go to the nearest emergency department immediately if these symptoms occur.

Lung Biopsy. A lung biopsy is performed to obtain tissue for histologic analysis, culture, or cytologic examination. The samples are used to make a definite diagnosis of inflammation, cancer, infection, or lung disease. There are several types of lung biopsies. The site and extent of the lesion determine which one is used. Transbronchial biopsy (TBB) and transbronchial needle aspiration (TBNA) are performed during bronchoscopy. Transthoracic needle aspiration is performed through the skin (percutaneous) for areas that cannot be reached by bronchoscopy.

Patient Preparation. The patient may worry about the outcome of the biopsy and may associate the term *biopsy* with *cancer*. Explain what to expect before and after the procedure and explore the patient's feelings. An analgesic or sedative may be prescribed before the procedure. Inform the patient undergoing percutaneous biopsy that discomfort is reduced with a local anesthetic agent but that pressure may be felt during needle insertion and tissue aspiration. Open lung biopsy is performed in the operating room with the patient under general anesthesia, and the usual preparations before surgery apply (see Chapter 14).

Procedure. Percutaneous lung biopsy is usually performed in the radiology department after an informed consent has been obtained. Fluoroscopy or CT is used to visualize the area and guide the procedure. The patient is usually placed in the side-lying position, depending on the location of the lesion. The skin is cleansed with an antiseptic agent, and a local anesthetic is given. Under sterile conditions, a spinal-type needle is inserted through the skin into the desired area, and tissue is obtained for microscopic examination. A dressing is applied after the procedure. A CT scan or chest x-ray must follow the biopsy to confirm that there is no pneumothorax.

An open-lung biopsy is performed in the operating room. The patient undergoes a thoracotomy in which lung tissue is exposed and appropriate tissue specimens are taken. A chest tube is placed to remove air and fluid so the lung can re-inflate, and then the chest is closed.

Follow-Up Care. Monitor the patient's vital signs and breath sounds at least every 4 hours for 24 hours and assess for signs of respiratory distress (e.g., dyspnea, pallor, diaphoresis, tachypnea). Pneumothorax is a serious complication of needle biopsy and open-lung biopsy. Report reduced or absent breath sounds immediately. Monitor for hemoptysis (which may be scant and transient) or, in rare cases, for frank bleeding from vascular or lung trauma.

🎯 CLINICAL JUDGMENT CHALLENGE 27-2

Safety; Patient-Centered Care; Teamwork and Collaboration QSEN

Your patient is a 56-year-old man who had an extensive open abdominal surgery yesterday. He has thick secretions and developed a mucus plug. He has just returned from a bronchoscopy.

1. What are your priorities for postprocedure care? Provide a rationale for your choices.
2. The patient is also receiving frequent opioids for pain control after his recent surgery. What, if any, concerns do you have about this therapy?
3. Would you consider using capnography to monitor this patient? Why or why not?
4. Which interprofessional team members would be most important to consider involving in the care of this patient?

GET READY FOR THE NCLEX® EXAMINATION!

KEY POINTS

Review these Key Points for each NCLEX Examination Client Needs Category.

Safe and Effective Care Environment

- Assess any patient's geographic, home, occupational, and recreational exposure to inhalation irritants. **QSEN: Safety**
- Document any known specific allergies that have respiratory symptoms. **QSEN: Safety**
- Assess the patient's respiratory status every 15 minutes for at least the first 2 hours after undergoing an endoscopic test for respiratory disorders. **QSEN: Safety**

Health Promotion and Maintenance

- Teach the older adult about the effects of aging on the respiratory system. **QSEN: Patient-Centered Care**
- Encourage all adults to use masks and adequate ventilation when exposed to inhalation irritants. **QSEN: Evidence-Based Practice**
- Promote smoking cessation for adults who smoke. **QSEN: Patient-Centered Care**
- Support the adult who chooses to stop smoking by helping him or her decide about drug therapy for smoking cessation and finding an appropriate smoking-cessation program. **QSEN: Patient-Centered Care**

Psychosocial Integrity

- Allow the patient the opportunity to express fear or anxiety about tests of respiratory function or about a potential change in respiratory function. **QSEN: Patient-Centered Care**

Physiological Integrity

- Ask the patient about respiratory problems in any other members of the family because some problems have a genetic component. **QSEN: Patient-Centered Care**
- Ask the patient about current and past drug use (prescribed, over-the-counter, and illicit), and evaluate drug use for potential lung damage. **QSEN: Patient-Centered Care**
- Calculate the pack-year smoking history for the patient who smokes or who has ever smoked cigarettes. **QSEN: Patient-Centered Care**
- Distinguish between normal and abnormal (adventitious) breath sounds. **QSEN: Patient-Centered Care**
- Interpret arterial blood gas values to assess the patient's respiratory status. **QSEN: Patient-Centered Care**
- Assess the degree to which breathing problems interfere with the patient's ability to perform ADLs. **QSEN: Patient-Centered Care**
- Assess the airway and breathing effectiveness for any patient who has shortness of breath or any change in mental status. **QSEN: Evidence-Based Practice**
- Teach patients and caregivers about what to expect during tests and procedures to assess respiratory function and respiratory disease. **QSEN: Patient-Centered Care**
- Explain nursing care needs for the patient after bronchoscopy or open lung biopsy. **QSEN: Patient-Centered Care**

SELECTED BIBLIOGRAPHY

American Lung Association (2015). *Disparities in lung health series: Tobacco use in the LBGT community.* http://www.lung.org/our-initiatives/research/lung-health-disparities/tobacco-use-lgbt-community.html.

American Lung Association. (2016). *E-cigarettes and lung health.* www.lung.org/stop-smoking/smoking-facts/e-cigarettes-and-lung-health.html?referrer=https://www.google.com/.

Anatolin, V., & Barkley, T. (2015). Electronic cigarettes: What nurses need to know. *Nursing2015, 45*(11), 60–64.

Baker, K., Barsamian, J., Leone, D., Donovan, B., Williams, D., Carnevale, K., et al. (2013). Routine dyspnea assessment on unit admission. *AJN, 113*(11), 42–49.

Barnett, P., Hamlett-Berry, K., Sung, H.-Y., & Max, W. (2015). Health care expenditures attributable to smoking in military veterans. *Nicotine & Tobacco Research, 17*(5), 586–591.

Carlisle, H. (2014). The case for capnography in patients receiving opioids. *American Nurse Today, 9*(9), 22–26.

Carlisle, H. (2015). Promoting the use of capnography in acute care settings: An evidence-based practice project. *Journal of Perianesthesia Nursing, 30*(3), 201–208.

Croucher, B. (2014). The challenge of diagnosing dyspnea. *AACN Advanced Critical Care, 25*(3), 284–290.

Flott, E. (2015). Smoking cessation strategies for patients with COPD. *Home Healthcare Now, 33*(7), 375–379.

Frederick, D. (2014). Pulmonary issues in the older adult. *Critical Care Nursing Clinics of North America, 26*(1), 91–97.

Genzler, L., Johnson, P., Ghildayal, N., Pangarakis, S., & Sendlebach, S. (2013). End-tidal carbon dioxide as a measure of stress response to clustered nursing interventions in neurologic patients. *American Journal of Critical Care, 22*(3), 239–245.

Haynes, J. (2014). Pulmonary function test quality in the elderly: A comparison with younger adults. *Respiratory Care, 59*(1), 16–21.

Hooley, J. (2015). Decoding the oxyhemoglobin dissociation curve. *American Nurse Today, 10*(1), 18–23.

Hua, M., & Talbot, P. (2016). Potential health effects of electronic cigarettes: A systematic review of case reports. *Preventive Medicine Reports, 4,* 169–178.

Jarvis, C. (2016). *Physical examination & health assessment* (7th ed.). St. Louis: Elsevier Saunders.

Jones, M., Olorvida, E., Monger, K., Yarborough, V., Bennetts, H., Harris, D., et al. (2015). How well do inexpensive, portable pulse oximeter values agree with arterial oxygen saturation in acutely ill patients? *Medsurg Nursing, 24*(6), 391–396.

Keating, S. (2016). Presurgical tobacco cessation counseling. *American Journal of Nursing, 116*(3), 11.

McCance, K., Huether, S., Brashers, V., & Rote, N. (2014). *Pathophysiology: The biologic basis for disease in adults and children* (7th ed.). St. Louis: Mosby.

Nguyen, K., Marshall, L., Hu, S., & Neff, L. (2015). State-specific prevalence of current cigarette smoking and smokeless tobacco use among adults aged > 18 years-United States, 2011-2013. *Morbidity and Mortality Weekly Report, 64*(19), 532–536.

Pagana, K., Pagana, T. J., & Pagana, T. N. (2017). *Mosby's diagnostic and laboratory test reference* (13th ed.). St. Louis: Mosby.

Pagana, K., Pagana, T., & Pike-MacDonald, S. (2013). *Mosby's Canadian manual of diagnostic and laboratory tests.* St. Louis: Mosby.

Parker, M. (2014). Interpreting spirometry: The basics. *Otolaryngologic Clinics of North America, 47*(1), 39–53.

Statistics Canada. (2016). *Report on smoking prevalence in Canada.* www.statcan.gc.ca/eng/subjects/Health?text=cigarette+smoking.

Touhy, T., & Jett, K. (2016). *Ebersole and Hess' toward healthy aging: Human needs & nursing response* (9th ed.). St. Louis: Mosby.

Wesley, C. (2014). Understanding acquired methemoglobinemia. *Nursing2014, 44*(2), 67.

CHAPTER 28

Care of Patients Requiring Oxygen Therapy or Tracheostomy

Harry Rees

http://evolve.elsevier.com/Iggy/

PRIORITY AND INTERRELATED CONCEPTS

The priority concept for this chapter is GAS EXCHANGE.

❋ The GAS EXCHANGE concept exemplar for this chapter is Tracheostomy, p. 537.

The interrelated concept for this chapter is TISSUE INTEGRITY.

LEARNING OUTCOMES

Safe and Effective Care Environment

1. Collaborate with the interprofessional team to coordinate high-quality care and promote GAS EXCHANGE in patients requiring oxygen therapy or tracheostomy.
2. Teach the patient receiving oxygen or who has a tracheostomy and caregiver(s) about home safety affected by oxygen therapy or tracheostomy.
3. Prioritize evidence-based care for patients requiring oxygen therapy or tracheostomy for problems affecting GAS EXCHANGE.

Health Promotion and Maintenance

4. Identify community resources for patients requiring oxygen therapy or tracheostomy.

Psychosocial Integrity

5. Implement nursing interventions to decrease the psychosocial impact caused by requiring oxygen therapy or tracheostomy.

Physiological Integrity

6. Apply knowledge of anatomy and physiology to assess patients with respiratory problems affecting GAS EXCHANGE who require oxygen therapy or tracheostomy.
7. Explain appropriate techniques to administer prescribed oxygen therapy and provide tracheostomy care.

GAS EXCHANGE with oxygenation and tissue perfusion are impaired as a result of many problems with the respiratory system. Oxygen therapy through various delivery systems, including tracheostomy, can help improve gas exchange and tissue perfusion.

OXYGEN THERAPY

Overview

In addition to being an essential body nutrient, oxygen (O_2) is a gas used as a drug for relief of **hypoxemia** (low levels of oxygen in the blood) and **hypoxia** (decreased tissue oxygenation). The oxygen content of atmospheric air is about 21%. Oxygen therapy is prescribed for both acute and chronic breathing problems when the patient's oxygen needs cannot be met by atmospheric ("room") air alone. Indications for use include decreased partial pressure of arterial oxygen (Pao_2) levels or decreased arterial oxygen saturation (Sao_2). Nonrespiratory conditions, such as heart failure, sepsis, fever, and decreased hemoglobin levels or poor hemoglobin quality, can affect GAS EXCHANGE and also are indications for oxygen therapy. These conditions increase oxygen demand, decrease the oxygen-carrying capability of the blood, or decrease cardiac output.

The purpose of oxygen therapy is to use the lowest *fraction of inspired oxygen (Fio₂)* to have an acceptable blood oxygen level without causing harmful side effects. *Although oxygen improves the Pao₂ level, it does not cure the problem or stop the disease process.* Most patients with hypoxia require an oxygen flow of 2 to 4 L/min via nasal cannula or up to 40% via Venturi mask to achieve an oxygen saturation of at least 95%. For a patient who is hypoxemic and has chronic **hypercarbia** (increased partial pressure of arterial carbon dioxide [$Paco_2$] levels), the Fio_2 delivered should be titrated to correct the hypoxemia and achieve generally acceptable oxygen saturations in the range of 88% to 92%.

❖ INTERPROFESSIONAL COLLABORATIVE CARE

Oxygen therapy may be used in any setting. Most patients are prescribed oxygen therapy through their primary health care provider without first having been hospitalized.

◆ *Assessment: Noticing*

Arterial blood gas (ABG) analysis is the best measure to determine the need for oxygen therapy and evaluate its effects. Oxygen need is also determined by noninvasive monitoring such as pulse oximetry and capnography (Carlisle, 2014).

◆ *Interventions: Responding*

Before starting oxygen therapy and while caring for a patient receiving oxygen therapy, you must be knowledgeable about oxygen hazards and complications. Know the rationale and the expected outcome related to oxygen therapy for each patient receiving oxygen. Chart 28-1 lists best practices for patients using oxygen therapy.

Hazards and Complications of Oxygen Therapy

Combustion. Oxygen does not burn, but it enhances combustion so fire burns better in its presence. For example, when the oxygen content of the air around a lighted cigarette is nearly 50%, the entire cigarette flames up and can catch items nearby on fire. Open fires, even small ones such as candles or cigarettes, should not be in the same room during oxygen therapy. Take precautions during oxygen delivery, including posting a sign on the door of the patient's room. Smoking is prohibited in the patient's room, including at home, when oxygen is in use.

All electrical equipment in rooms where oxygen is in use must have grounded plugs and be plugged into grounded outlets to prevent fires from electrical arcing sparks. Frayed cords are not used because they can spark and ignite a flame. Flammable solutions (containing high concentrations of alcohol or oil) are not used in rooms in which oxygen is in use. (This does not include alcohol-based hand rubs.)

Oxygen-Induced Hypoventilation. For many years oxygen was thought to induce hypoventilation in the patient with chronic lung disease who also had carbon dioxide retention (**hypercarbia**). As a result, nurses and physicians were reluctant to administer oxygen to these hypoxic patients, leading to serious problems and even deaths related to inadequate GAS EXCHANGE. Research disproves the hypoxic drive theory and has found that patients with chronic lung disease are at risk for oxygen-induced hypercapnia but not for severely reduced respiratory effort (Makic et al., 2013). Therefore oxygen therapy is prescribed at the lowest liter flow needed to manage hypoxemia. A system that delivers more precise oxygen levels (e.g., a Venturi mask) is preferred. Monitor the patient's response to therapy closely to ensure adequate gas exchange and correction of hypoxemia. Responses to monitor include the level of consciousness, respiratory pattern and rate, and pulse oximetry. *Untreated or inadequately treated hypoxemia is a threat to life for any person with a breathing problem.*

Oxygen Toxicity. Oxygen toxicity is related to the concentration of oxygen delivered, duration of oxygen therapy, and degree of lung disease present. A continuous oxygen level greater than 50% for more than 24 to 48 hours may injure the TISSUE INTEGRITY of the lungs.

The causes and indications of lung injury from oxygen toxicity are the same as those for acute respiratory distress syndrome (ARDS) (see Chapter 32). Initial problems include dyspnea, nonproductive cough, chest pain beneath the sternum, GI upset, and crackles on auscultation. As exposure to high levels of oxygen continues, the problems become more severe, with decreased vital capacity, decreased compliance, and hypoxemia. With prolonged exposure to high oxygen levels, atelectasis, pulmonary edema, hemorrhage, and hyaline membrane formation may result. Surviving this critical condition depends on correcting the underlying disease process and decreasing the oxygen amount delivered.

The toxic effects of oxygen are difficult to manage, making prevention a priority. The lowest level of oxygen needed to maintain GAS EXCHANGE and prevent oxygen toxicity is prescribed. Monitor arterial blood gases (ABGs) during oxygen therapy and notify the primary health care provider when Pao_2 levels become greater than 90 mm Hg. Also monitor the prescribed oxygen level and length of therapy to identify patients at risk. High oxygen levels are avoided unless absolutely necessary. The use of noninvasive positive airway pressure techniques with oxygen or the use of mechanical ventilation (see Chapter 32) may reduce the amount of oxygen needed. As soon as the patient's condition allows, the prescribed amount of oxygen is decreased.

Absorptive Atelectasis. Normally nitrogen in the air maintains patent airways and alveoli. Making up 79% of room air, nitrogen prevents alveolar collapse. When high oxygen levels are delivered, nitrogen is diluted, oxygen diffuses from the alveoli into the blood, and the alveoli collapse. Collapsed alveoli cause atelectasis (called *absorptive atelectasis*), which is detected as crackles and decreased breath sounds on auscultation.

Drying of the Mucous Membranes. When the prescribed oxygen flow rate is higher than 4 L/min, humidify the delivery system to prevent damage to TISSUE INTEGRITY (Fig. 28-1). Ensure that oxygen bubbles through the water in the humidifier.

◎ CHART 28-1 Best Practice for Patient Safety & Quality Care QSEN

Oxygen Therapy

- Check the health care provider's prescription with the type of delivery system and liter flow or percentage of oxygen actually in use.
- Obtain a prescription for humidification if oxygen is being delivered at 4 L/min or more.
- Be sure that the oxygen and humidification equipment are functioning properly.
- Check the skin around the patient's ears, back of the neck, and face every 4 to 8 hours for pressure points, signs of irritation, and loss of TISSUE INTEGRITY.
- Ensure that mouth care is provided every 8 hours and as needed; assess nasal and oral mucous membranes for cracks or other signs of dryness or impaired tissue integrity.
- Pad the elastic band and change its position frequently to prevent skin breakdown.
- Pad tubing in areas that put pressure on the skin.
- Cleanse the cannula or mask by rinsing with clear, warm water every 4 to 8 hours or as needed.
- Cleanse skin under the tubing, straps, and mask every 4 to 8 hours or as needed.
- Lubricate the patient's nostrils, face, and lips with nonpetroleum cream to relieve the drying effects of oxygen.
- Position the tubing so it does not pull on the patient's face, nose, or artificial airway.
- Ensure that there is no smoking and that no candles or matches are lit in the immediate area.
- Assess and document the patient's response to oxygen therapy.
- Ensure that the patient has an adequate oxygen source during any periods of transport.
- Provide the patient with ongoing teaching and reassurance to enhance his or her adherence to oxygen therapy.

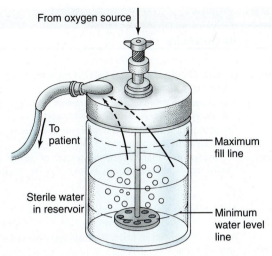

From oxygen source

To patient

Maximum fill line

Sterile water in reservoir

Minimum water level line

FIG. 28-1 Bubble humidifier bottle used with oxygen therapy

! **NURSING SAFETY PRIORITY** (QSEN)

Action Alert

Monitor the patient receiving high levels of oxygen closely to recognize indications of absorptive atelectasis (new onset of crackles and decreased breath sounds) every 1 to 2 hours when oxygen therapy is started and as often as needed thereafter.

Oxygen can also be humidified via a large-volume jet nebulizer in mist form (aerosol). A heated nebulizer raises the humidity even more and is used for oxygen delivery through an artificial airway. Usually the upper airway passages warm the air during breathing, but these passages are bypassed with an artificial airway, such as an endotracheal tube.

For the patient to receive humidified oxygen, the humidifier or nebulizer must have a sufficient amount of sterile water, and the flow rate must be adequate. Condensation often forms in the tubing. Remove this condensation as it collects by disconnecting the tubing and emptying the water. Minimize the time the tubing is disconnected because the patient does not receive oxygen during this period. Some humidifiers and nebulizers have a water trap that hangs from the tubing so the condensation can be drained without disconnecting. Check the water level and change the humidifier as needed.

! **NURSING SAFETY PRIORITY** (QSEN)

Action Alert

Assess the tubing system used for oxygen delivery to recognize buildup of condensation. Respond by draining condensation. To prevent bacterial contamination of the oxygen delivery system, never drain the fluid from the water trap back into the humidifier or nebulizer.

Infection. The humidifier or nebulizer may be a source of bacteria, especially if it is heated. Oxygen delivery equipment such as cannulas and masks can also harbor organisms. Change equipment per agency policy, which ranges from every 24 hours for humidification systems to every 7 days or whenever necessary for cannulas and masks.

? **NCLEX EXAMINATION CHALLENGE 28-1**

Safe and Effective Care Environment

The nurse notes that a client with a history of chronic obstructive pulmonary disease (COPD) who is receiving oxygen therapy at 2 L/min and had an oxygen saturation of 88% 1 hour ago now has dyspnea and an oxygen saturation of 80%. Should the nurse increase the FiO_2?
A. No; increasing the FiO_2 will severely depress the respiratory rate by blunting the hypoxic drive.
B. No; an oxygen saturation of 80% is acceptable for a client with COPD.
C. Yes; hypoxia must be treated despite the risk for oxygen-induced hypercapnia.
D. Yes; the expected outcome for any client with hypoxia is to achieve a saturation of at least 97%.

Oxygen Delivery Systems. Oxygen can be delivered by many systems. Regardless of the type of delivery system used, it is important to understand its indications, advantages, and disadvantages. Use the equipment properly and ensure appropriate equipment maintenance. Provide interprofessional collaboration by consulting a respiratory therapist whenever there is a question or concern about an oxygen delivery system.

The type of delivery system used depends on:
- Oxygen concentration required by the patient
- Oxygen concentration achieved by a delivery system
- Importance of accuracy and control of the oxygen concentration
- Patient comfort
- Importance of humidity
- Patient mobility

Oxygen delivery systems are classified by the rate of oxygen delivery as either low-flow or high-flow systems. Low-flow systems have a low fraction of inspired oxygen (FiO_2) and do not provide enough oxygen to meet the patient's total oxygen and air volume needs. Thus part of the tidal volume is supplied by the patient as he or she breathes room air. The total level of oxygen inspired depends on the respiratory rate and tidal volume. High-flow systems have a flow rate that meets the entire oxygen need and tidal volume, regardless of the patient's breathing pattern. These systems are used for critically ill patients and when delivery of precise levels of oxygen is needed.

If the patient needs a mask but is able to eat, request a prescription for a nasal cannula to be used at mealtimes only. Reapply the mask after the meal is completed. To increase mobility, up to 50 feet of connecting tubing can be used with connecting pieces, although the longer tubing can be a safety issue for patients who are unsteady while ambulating.

Low-Flow Oxygen Delivery Systems. Low-flow systems include the nasal cannula, simple facemask, partial rebreather mask, and nonrebreather mask (Table 28-1). These systems are easy to use and fairly comfortable, but the amount of oxygen delivered varies and depends on the patient's breathing pattern. The oxygen is diluted with room air (21% oxygen), which lowers the amount actually inspired.

Nasal Cannula. The nasal cannula (prongs) (Fig. 28-2) is used at flow rates of 1 to 6 L/min. Oxygen concentrations of 24% (at 1 L/min) to 44% (at 6 L/min) can be achieved. Flow rates greater than 6 L/min do not increase GAS EXCHANGE

TABLE 28-1   Comparison of Low-Flow Oxygen Delivery Systems

FiO₂ DELIVERED	NURSING INTERVENTIONS	RATIONALES
Nasal Cannula		
24%-40% FiO₂ at 1-6 L/min	Ensure that prongs are in the nares properly.	A poorly fitting nasal cannula leads to hypoxemia and skin breakdown with loss of TISSUE INTEGRITY.
≈ 24% at 1 L/min		
≈ 28% at 2 L/min	Apply water-soluble jelly to nares PRN.	This substance prevents mucosal irritation related to the drying effect of oxygen; promotes comfort.
≈ 32% at 3 L/min		
≈ 36% at 4 L/min	Assess the patency of the nostrils.	Congestion or a deviated septum prevents effective delivery of oxygen through the nares.
≈ 40% at 5 L/min		
≈ 44% at 6 L/min	Assess the patient for changes in respiratory rate and depth.	The respiratory pattern affects the amount of oxygen delivered. A different delivery system may be needed.
Simple Facemask		
40%-60% FiO₂ at 5-8 L/min; flow rate must be set at least at 5 L/min to flush mask of carbon dioxide	Be sure that mask fits securely over nose and mouth.	A poorly fitting mask reduces the FiO₂ delivered.
≈ 40% at 5 L/min	Assess skin and provide skin care to the area covered by the mask.	Pressure and moisture under the mask may cause loss of TISSUE INTEGRITY.
≈ 45%-50% at 6 L/min	Monitor the patient closely for risk for aspiration.	The mask limits the patient's ability to clear the mouth, especially if vomiting occurs.
≈ 55%-60% at 8 L/min	Provide emotional support to the patient who feels claustrophobic.	Emotional support decreases anxiety, which contributes to a claustrophobic feeling.
	Suggest to the primary health care provider to switch the patient from a mask to the nasal cannula during eating.	Use of the cannula promotes GAS EXCHANGE during eating.
Partial Rebreather Mask		
60%-75% at 6-11 L/min, a liter flow rate high enough to maintain reservoir bag two-thirds full during inspiration and expiration	Make sure that the reservoir does not twist or kink, which results in a deflated bag.	Deflation results in decreased oxygen delivered and increases the rebreathing of exhaled air.
	Adjust the flow rate to keep the reservoir bag inflated.	The flow rate is adjusted to meet the pattern of the patient.
Nonrebreather Mask		
80%-95% FiO₂ at a liter flow high enough to maintain reservoir bag two-thirds full	Interventions as for partial rebreather mask; this patient requires close monitoring.	Rationales as for partial rebreather mask. Monitoring ensures proper functioning and prevents harm.
	Make sure that valves and rubber flaps are patent, functional, and not stuck. Remove mucus or saliva.	Valves should open during expiration and close during inhalation to prevent dramatic decrease in FiO₂. Suffocation can occur if the reservoir bag kinks or if the oxygen source disconnects.
	Closely assess the patient on increased FiO₂ via nonrebreather mask. Intubation is the only way to provide more precise FiO₂.	The patient may require intubation.

FiO₂, Fraction of inspired oxygen.

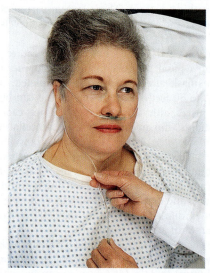

FIG. 28-2 Nasal cannula (prongs). (From Perry, A. G., Potter, P. A., & Ostendorf, W. R. [2017]. *Clinical nursing skills and techniques* [9th ed.]. St. Louis: Mosby.)

because the **anatomic dead space** (places where air flows but the structures are too thick for gas exchange) is full. High flow rates also increase mucosal irritation and damage to TISSUE INTEGRITY.

The nasal cannula is often used for chronic lung disease and for any patient needing long-term oxygen therapy. Place the nasal prongs in the nostrils, with the openings facing the patient, following the natural anatomic curve of the nares.

Facemasks. Facemasks can deliver a wide range of oxygen flow rates and concentrations.

Simple facemasks are used to deliver oxygen concentrations of 40% to 60% for short-term oxygen therapy or in an emergency (Fig. 28-3). A minimum flow rate of 5 L/min is needed to prevent rebreathing of exhaled air. Ensure that the mask fits well to maintain inspired oxygen levels. Care for the skin under the mask and strap to prevent breakdown (Ambutas et al., 2014).

Partial rebreather masks provide oxygen concentrations of 60% to 75% with flow rates of 6 to 11 L/min. These masks have a reservoir bag but no flaps (Fig. 28-4). With each breath, the patient rebreathes one third of the exhaled tidal volume, which

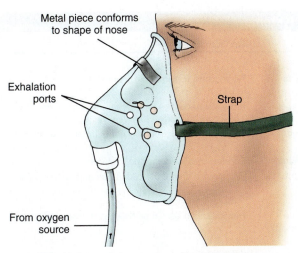

FIG. 28-3 Simple facemask used to deliver oxygen.

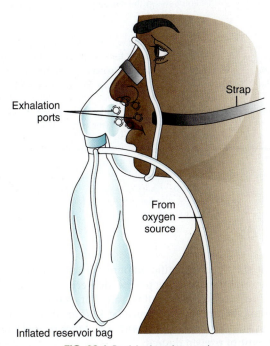

FIG. 28-4 Partial rebreather mask.

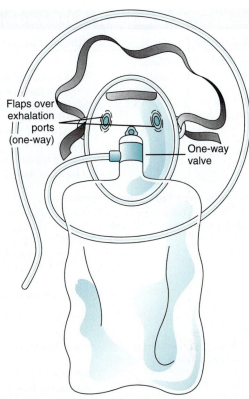

FIG. 28-5 Nonrebreather mask.

valve prevents exhaled air from re-entering the reservoir bag. The flow rate is kept high (10 to 15 L/min) to keep the bag inflated during inhalation. Assess for this safety feature at least hourly.

> ! **NURSING SAFETY PRIORITY** QSEN
>
> *Critical Rescue*
>
> Ensure that the valve and flaps on a nonrebreather mask are intact and functional during each breath. If the oxygen source should fail or be depleted when both flaps are in place, the patient would not be able to inhale room air.

is high in oxygen and increases the fraction of inspired oxygen (FiO_2). For best oxygen delivery, be sure that the bag remains slightly inflated at the end of inspiration. If needed, call the respiratory therapist for assistance.

Nonrebreather masks provide the highest oxygen level of the low-flow systems and can deliver an FiO_2 greater than 90%, depending on the patient's breathing pattern. This mask is often used with patients whose respiratory status is unstable and who may require intubation.

The nonrebreather mask has a one-way valve between the mask and the reservoir and usually has two flaps over the exhalation ports (Fig. 28-5). The valve allows the patient to draw all needed oxygen from the reservoir bag, and the flaps prevent room air from entering through the exhalation ports (which would dilute the oxygen concentration). During exhalation, air leaves through these exhalation ports while the one-way

High-Flow Oxygen Delivery Systems. High-flow systems (Table 28-2) include the Venturi mask, aerosol mask, face tent, Vapotherm high-flow nasal cannula, tracheostomy collar, and T-piece. These devices deliver an accurate oxygen level when properly fitted, with oxygen concentrations from 24% to 100% at 8 to 15 L/min. More recently, high-flow nasal cannulas (HFNCs) such as Vapotherm are more widely used for precise temperature and oxygen control along with humidification. With use of these devices at liter flows of 40 to 60 L/min, an FiO_2 approaching that of a nonrebreather system can be achieved.

Venturi masks (Venti masks) deliver the most accurate oxygen concentration without intubation. They work by pulling in a proportional amount of room air for each liter flow of oxygen. An adaptor is located between the bottom of the mask and the oxygen source (Fig. 28-6). Adaptors with holes of

TABLE 28-2 **Comparison of High-Flow Oxygen Delivery Systems**

Fio₂ DELIVERED	NURSING INTERVENTIONS	RATIONALES
Venturi Mask (Venti Mask)		
24%-50% Fio₂ with flow rates as recommended by the manufacturer, usually 4-10 L/min; provides high humidity	Perform constant surveillance to ensure an accurate flow rate for the specific Fio₂.	An accurate flow rate ensures Fio₂ delivery.
	Keep the orifice for the Venturi adaptor open and uncovered.	If the Venturi orifice is covered, the adaptor does not function, and oxygen delivery varies.
	Provide a mask that fits snugly and tubing that is free of kinks.	Fio₂ is altered if kinking occurs or if the mask fits poorly.
	Assess the patient for dry mucous membranes.	Comfort measures may be indicated.
	Change to a nasal cannula during mealtime.	Oxygen is a drug that needs to be given continuously.
Aerosol Mask, Face Tent, Tracheostomy Collar		
24%-100% Fio₂ with flow rates of at least 10 L/min; provides high humidity	Assess that aerosol mist escapes from the vents of the delivery system during inspiration and expiration.	Humidification should be delivered to the patient.
	Empty condensation from the tubing.	Emptying prevents the patient from being lavaged with water, promotes an adequate flow rate, and ensures a continued prescribed Fio₂.
	Change the aerosol water container as needed.	Adequate humidification is ensured only when there is sufficient water in the canister.
T-Piece		
24%-100% Fio₂ with flow rates of at least 10 L/min; provides high humidity	Empty condensation from the tubing.	Condensation interferes with flow rate delivery of Fio₂ and may drain into the tracheostomy if not emptied.
	Keep the exhalation port open and uncovered.	If the port is occluded, the patient can suffocate.
	Position the T-piece so it does not pull on the tracheostomy or endotracheal tube.	The weight of the T-piece pulls on the tracheostomy and causes pain or erosion of skin at the insertion site.
	Make sure the humidifier creates enough mist. A mist should be seen during inspiration and expiration.	An adequate flow rate is needed to meet the inspiration effort of the patient. If not, the patient will be "air-hungry."

Fio₂, Fraction of inspired oxygen.

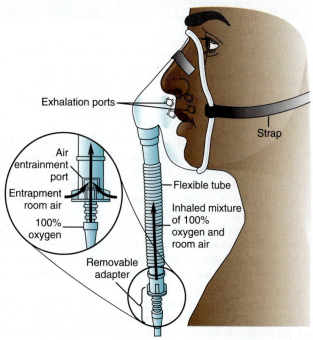

Exhalation ports

Strap

Air entrainment port

Entrapment room air

100% oxygen

Flexible tube

Inhaled mixture of 100% oxygen and room air

Removable adapter

FIG. 28-6 Venturi mask for precise oxygen delivery.

different sizes allow specific amounts of air to mix with the oxygen, resulting in more precise delivery of oxygen. Each adaptor requires a different flow rate. For example, to deliver 24% of oxygen, the flow rate must be 4 L/min. Another type of Venturi mask has one adaptor with a dial that is used to select the amount of oxygen desired.

Other high-flow systems include the face tent, aerosol mask, tracheostomy collar, and T-piece. They are often used to provide high humidity with oxygen delivery. A dial on the humidity source regulates the delivered oxygen level. A face tent fits over the chin, with the top extending halfway across the face. Although the oxygen level delivered varies, the face tent is useful for patients who have facial trauma or burns. An aerosol mask is used when high humidity is needed. The tracheostomy collar is used to deliver high humidity and the desired oxygen to the patient with a tracheostomy. A special adaptor, called the *T-piece,* is used to deliver any desired Fio₂ to the patient with a tracheostomy, laryngectomy, or endotracheal tube (Fig. 28-7). Adjust the flow rate so the aerosol appears on the exhalation side of the T-piece. The high-flow nasal cannula (HFNC) is increasing in use for adults. Some systems require heated humidification, and some use blenders to more accurately adjust Fio₂. The Fio₂ and flow rates can be adjusted independently and may achieve an actual Fio₂ close to the predicted

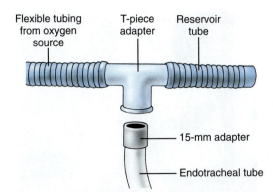

FIG. 28-7 T-piece apparatus for attachment to an endotracheal or tracheostomy tube.

Fio₂. The use of pulse oximetry is recommended to titrate the HFNC to patient response.

Noninvasive Positive-Pressure Ventilation. Noninvasive positive-pressure ventilation (NPPV) is a type of noninvasive ventilation (NIV). This technique uses positive pressure to keep alveoli open and improve GAS EXCHANGE without the need for and dangers of intubation (Bajaj et al., 2015). It is used to manage dyspnea, hypercarbia and acute exacerbations of chronic obstructive pulmonary disease (COPD), cardiogenic pulmonary edema, and acute asthma attacks (see the Evidence-Based Practice box). Although NPPV prevents the complications associated with intubation, including ventilator-associated pneumonia (VAP), risks and complications are associated with it. Masks must fit tightly to form a proper seal, which can lead to loss of TISSUE INTEGRITY with skin breakdown over the nose or face. Full facemasks cause fewer skin problems than do nasal-oral masks (Schallom et al., 2015). Leaks can cause uncomfortable pressure around the eyes, and gastric insufflation can lead to vomiting and the potential for aspiration. Thus NPPV should be used only on alert patients who have the ability to protect their airway, although a nasogastric (NG) tube may still be required for safety.

NPPV can deliver oxygen or may use just room air. A nasal mask, nasal pillows, or full-facemask delivery system allows mechanical delivery. The three most common modes of delivery for NPPV are (1) continuous positive airway pressure (CPAP), which delivers a set positive airway pressure throughout each cycle of inhalation and exhalation; (2) volume-limited or flow-limited, which delivers a set tidal volume with the patient's inspiratory effort; and (3) pressure-limited, which includes pressure support, pressure control, and bi-level positive airway pressure (BiPAP), which cycles different pressures at inspiration and expiration.

For BiPAP, a cycling machine delivers a set inspiratory positive airway pressure each time the patient begins to inspire. As he or she begins to exhale, the machine delivers a lower set end-expiratory pressure. Together, these two pressures improve tidal volume, can reduce respiratory rate, and may relieve dyspnea.

For CPAP the effect is to open collapsed alveoli. Patients who may benefit from this form of oxygen or air delivery include those with atelectasis after surgery or cardiac-induced pulmonary edema or those with COPD. It is not helpful for patients with respiratory failure following extubation. However, both

EVIDENCE-BASED PRACTICE QSEN

When Is Noninvasive Ventilation (NIV) Most Effective?

Bajaj, A., Rathor, P., Sehgal, V., & Shetty, A. (2015). Efficacy of noninvasive ventilation after planned extubation: A systematic review and meta-analysis of randomized controlled trials. *Heart & Lung, 44*(2), 150-157.

Extubation failure with subsequent reintubation places patients at continuing risk for complications and the possibility of permanent intubation. Therefore the use of methods that reduce intubation failure have great clinical importance. The objective of this meta-analysis was to update the evidence on the efficacy of noninvasive ventilation (NIV) compared with conventional oxygen therapy after planned extubation. The method used was a systematic literature review of PubMed, EMBASE, and Cochrane for randomized controlled trials (RCTs) comparing NIV with conventional oxygen therapy after planned extubation. The results of this large analysis showed that NIV decreased reintubation rate significantly compared to conventional oxygen therapy in chronic obstructive pulmonary disease (COPD) and patients at high risk for extubation failure. However, in a mixed medical ICU population, there was no statistical difference of reintubation rate between the two groups. These results indicate that use of NIV after planned extubation significantly decreases the reintubation rate in COPD patients and patients at high risk for extubation failure.

Level of Evidence: 1
The study was a meta-analysis of nine large, multi-site RCTs. In addition, the study added a separate analysis of three different subgroups to determine if NIV was more effective with a particular group of patients.

Commentary: Implications for Practice and Research
The use of NIV immediately after planned extubation among patients with COPD or other identified high risk for extubation failure decreased the rate of reintubation, ICU mortality, hospital mortality, and ICU length of stay when compared with conventional oxygen therapy. This therapy is relatively low cost for actual expenses and those caused by increased lengths of stay or more invasive interventions. Reduction of patient risks and increased comfort are also benefits. Nurses should consider requesting this type of respiratory support after planned extubation for patients with COPD and those at high risk for extubation failure. Nursing research assessing patient and family tolerance and perceptions of NIV may provide results that further promote its use.

CPAP and BiPAP are used after extubation to prevent respiratory failure and the need for re-intubation. NPPV is used in palliative care to relieve dyspnea, including for those patients with "do-not-intubate" orders. However, this practice is controversial. The Society of Critical Care Medicine recommends discussing goals and expected outcomes with the patient and family before initiating therapy.

NPPV is used for sleep apnea. The effect is to hold open the upper airways (Fig. 28-8). Patients using CPAP or BiPAP at home for sleep apnea often bring their home equipment to the hospital. They feel more comfortable using their own equipment. The reasons for using NPPV remain when the patient enters the hospital, and the need continues while hospitalized.

The number of patients using NPPV therapy is increasing in every setting. Nurses caring for the patient with NPPV must be knowledgeable about the equipment, technique, and potential complications. Respiratory therapy support can help safely manage a patient receiving NPPV.

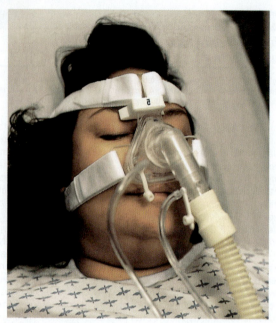

FIG. 28-8 Nasal continuous positive airway pressure (CPAP). (From Perry, A. G., Potter, P. A., & Ostendorf, W. R. [2017]. *Clinical nursing skills and techniques* [9th ed.]. St. Louis: Mosby.)

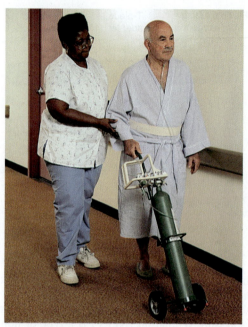

FIG. 28-9 Small E-size oxygen tank (cylinder) for portability. (From Perry, A. G., Potter, P. A., & Ostendorf, W. R. [2017]. *Clinical nursing skills and techniques* [9th ed.]. St. Louis: Mosby.)

Transtracheal Oxygen Therapy. Transtracheal oxygen (TTO) is a long-term method of delivering oxygen directly into the lungs. A small, flexible catheter is passed into the trachea through a small incision with the patient under local anesthesia. TTO avoids damage to TISSUE INTEGRITY from nasal prongs and is less visible. A TTO team provides patient education, including the purpose of TTO and care of the catheter. Different flow rates are prescribed for rest and activity. A flow rate also is prescribed for the nasal cannula, which is used when the TTO catheter is being cleaned.

⍰ CLINICAL JUDGMENT CHALLENGE 28-1

Patient-Centered Care; Teamwork and Collaboration; Evidence-Based Practice QSEN

Your patient is a 56-year-old woman who just had laparoscopic surgery. She is morbidly obese, has COPD, and is a current smoker. She does not use oxygen at home. During this early postoperative period, she is prescribed oxygen.

1. Which type of oxygen delivery device do you believe will deliver the most precise FiO₂ for this patient?
2. For which potential complication of a higher FiO₂ would this patient be at risk, and how could this be avoided?
3. The PACU report indicates that the patient had frequent episodes of snoring with decreased oxygen saturation while sleeping. Should you request a referral and to whom?
4. Your patient continues to require oxygen to maintain a saturation of 88%. It appears that she will need home oxygen. With whom should you consult for this possibility?

Care Coordination and Transition Management

Home Care Management. The patient must be stable before home oxygen is considered. For Medicare to cover the cost of home oxygen therapy, the patient must have severe hypoxemia defined as a partial pressure of arterial oxygen (PaO_2) level of less than 55 mm Hg or arterial oxygen saturation (SpO_2) of less

than 88% on room air and at rest. The criteria vary when hypoxemia is caused by nonpulmonary problems or when oxygen is needed only at night or with exercise.

Self-Management Education. When home oxygen therapy is prescribed, begin a teaching plan about it. The nurse or respiratory therapist teaches the patient about the equipment needed for home oxygen therapy and the safety aspects of using and maintaining the equipment. Equipment may include oxygen source, delivery devices, and humidity sources. Work with the discharge planner to help the patient select a durable medical equipment (DME) company to deliver oxygen equipment and select a community health nursing agency for follow-up care in the home. Re-evaluation of the need for oxygen therapy occurs on a periodic basis.

While providing discharge planning and teaching, be sensitive to the patient's emotional adjustment to oxygen therapy. Encourage the patient to share feelings and concerns. He or she may be concerned about social acceptance. Help him or her realize that adherence to oxygen therapy is important for being able to participate in ADLs and other events that bring enjoyment.

Home Care Preparation. Home oxygen therapy is provided in one of three ways: compressed gas in a tank or a cylinder, liquid oxygen in a reservoir, or an oxygen concentrator. Compressed gas in an oxygen tank (green) is the most often used oxygen source. The large H cylinder may be used as a stationary source, and the smaller E tank is available for transporting the patient (Fig. 28-9). Even smaller cylinders are available for the patient to carry. Teach the patient and family to check the gauge daily to assess the amount of oxygen left in the tank. As a safety precaution, the tanks must always be in a stand or rack. A tank that is accidentally knocked over could suddenly decompress and move around in an uncontrolled manner.

Liquid oxygen for home use is oxygen gas that has been liquefied. A concentrated amount of oxygen is available in a lightweight and easy-to-carry container similar to a Thermos

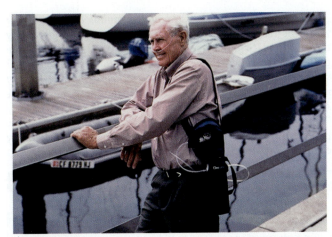

FIG. 28-10 Portable liquid oxygen. (Courtesy Chad Therapeutics, Chatsworth, CA.)

bottle (Fig. 28-10). This portable tank is filled from a large stationary liquid vessel. Liquid oxygen lasts longer than gaseous oxygen but is more expensive.

The oxygen concentrator or *oxygen extractor* is a machine that removes nitrogen from room air, increasing oxygen levels to more than 90%. This device is the least expensive system and does not need to be filled. It is often used in the home as a stationary system. A smaller version that can plug into DC electrical outlets can be rented for longer car or boat trips.

Regardless of the type of oxygen delivery system used, review safety issues with the patient and all family members.

! **NURSING SAFETY PRIORITY** QSEN

Action Alert

Assess the patient's and caregivers' knowledge of oxygen therapy to recognize any deficiencies. Respond by providing safety information and stressing the importance of not smoking when he or she is using oxygen. Teach the patient and all family members that smoking materials, candles, gas burners, and fireplaces (and other open flames) are not to be used in the same room that oxygen is being used.

💡 **NCLEX EXAMINATION CHALLENGE 28-2**

Health Promotion and Maintenance

What must the nurse include for discharge education for a client who is newly prescribed to use oxygen therapy at home? **Select all that apply.**
A. The consequences of smoking while using oxygen
B. The need to limit potted plants in the home
C. The types of oxygen delivery devices available for home use
D. The use of oxygen when performing ADLs
E. The need to travel only in specially designated cars
F. Performing proper skin care under the device and its straps

---

✳ **GAS EXCHANGE CONCEPT EXEMPLAR**
Tracheostomy

Overview

Tracheotomy is the surgical incision into the trachea to create an airway to help maintain GAS EXCHANGE. Tracheostomy is the tracheal *stoma* (opening) that results from the tracheotomy. A tracheotomy can be an emergency procedure or a scheduled surgery. Tracheostomies can be temporary or permanent. Indications for tracheostomy include acute airway obstruction, the need for airway protection, laryngeal or facial trauma or burns, and airway involvement during head or neck surgery. They also are used for prolonged unconsciousness, paralysis, or the inability to be weaned from mechanical ventilation. With temporary tracheostomies, the nurse is key in evaluating patient readiness for progression toward decannulation (removal of the tracheostomy tube) (Morris et al., 2014).

❖ INTERPROFESSIONAL COLLABORATIVE CARE

Although the initial tracheotomy to form a tracheostomy is usually performed in an acute care setting, care of the patient who has a tracheostomy often occurs in the community. Care for the patient requiring long-term tracheostomy is best when a team approach is used. In addition to the nurse, interprofessional team members often include the primary health care provider, respiratory therapist, registered dietitian, discharge planner, and social worker.

◆ Analysis: Interpreting

The priority collaborative problems for patients requiring tracheostomy include:
1. Decreased GAS EXCHANGE due to weak chest muscles, obstruction, or other physical problems that interfere with ventilation and diffusion of gases
2. Inadequate communication due to tracheostomy or intubation
3. Potential for weight loss due to inadequate nutrition from presence of endotracheal tube
4. Potential for infection due to invasive procedures or problems with the normal protective mechanisms of the respiratory tract
5. Potential for loss of tracheal TISSUE INTEGRITY due to pressure and trauma from tracheostomy tubes

◆ Interventions: Responding

Preoperative Care. The care for the patient having a tracheotomy is similar to that for a laryngectomy (see Chapter 29). Focus on his or her knowledge deficits through teaching and discuss tracheostomy care, communication, and speech.

Operative Procedures. Initially the neck is extended, and an endotracheal (ET) tube is placed by the anesthesia provider to maintain the airway. Incisions are made through the neck and the tracheal rings to enter the trachea (Fig. 28-11).

After the trachea is entered, the ET tube is removed while the tracheostomy tube is inserted. The tracheostomy tube is secured in place with sutures and tracheostomy ties or Velcro tube holders. A chest x-ray determines proper placement of the tube.

Postoperative Care. Immediately after surgery, focus care on ensuring a patent airway. Confirm the presence of bilateral breath sounds. Perform a respiratory assessment at least hourly. Assess the patient for complications from the procedure.

Complications. Major complications can arise after surgery. Table 28-3 lists symptoms, management, and prevention of complications of tracheostomy.

Tube obstruction can occur as a result of secretions or by cuff displacement. Indicators are difficulty breathing; noisy respirations; difficulty inserting a suction catheter; thick, dry secretions; and high peak pressures (if a mechanical ventilator is used). Assess the patient at least hourly for tube patency. Prevent obstruction by helping the patient cough and deep breathe, providing inner cannula care, humidifying oxygen, and suctioning. If tube obstruction results from cuff prolapse over the end of the tube, the primary health care provider repositions or replaces the tube.

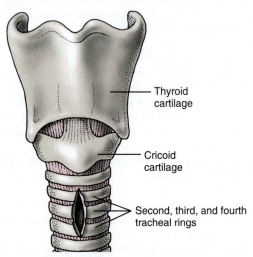

Thyroid cartilage

Cricoid cartilage

Second, third, and fourth tracheal rings

FIG. 28-11 Vertical tracheal incision for a tracheostomy.

Tube dislodgment and accidental decannulation can occur when the tube is not secure. Prevent this problem by securing the tube in place to reduce movement and traction or accidental pulling by the patient. *Tube dislodgment in the first 72 hours after surgery is an emergency because the tracheostomy tract has not matured and replacement is difficult. The tube may end up in the subcutaneous tissue instead of in the trachea (also referred to as "false passage"). The patient will not be able to be ventilated.* Obese patients or those with short, large necks may be particularly difficult to recannulate if the tracheostomy tube is dislodged.

> ! **NURSING SAFETY PRIORITY** **QSEN**
>
> ***Critical Rescue***
>
> Monitor the patient for tube placement. When you recognize that the tube is dislodged on an immature tracheostomy, respond by ventilating the patient using a manual resuscitation bag and facemask while another nurse calls the Rapid Response Team.

For safety, ensure that a tracheostomy tube of the same type (including an obturator) and size (or one size smaller) is at the bedside at all times, along with a tracheostomy insertion tray. If decannulation occurs after 72 hours, extend the patient's neck and open the tissues of the stoma with a curved Kelly clamp to secure the airway. With the obturator inserted into the

TABLE 28-3	**Complications of Tracheostomy**		
COMPLICATIONS AND DESCRIPTION	**MANIFESTATIONS**	**MANAGEMENT**	**PREVENTION**
Tracheomalacia: Constant pressure exerted by the cuff causes tracheal dilation and erosion of cartilage, leading to loss of tissue integrity.	An increased amount of air is required in the cuff to maintain the seal. A larger tracheostomy tube is required to prevent an air leak at the stoma. Food particles are seen in tracheal secretions. The patient does not receive the set tidal volume on the ventilator.	No special management is needed unless bleeding occurs.	Use an uncuffed tube as soon as possible. Monitor cuff pressure and air volumes closely and detect changes.
Tracheal stenosis: Narrowed tracheal lumen is caused by scar formation from irritation of tracheal mucosa and impaired tissue integrity by the cuff.	Stenosis is usually seen after the cuff is deflated or the tracheostomy tube is removed. The patient has increased coughing, inability to expectorate secretions, or difficulty breathing or talking.	Tracheal dilation or surgical intervention is used.	Prevent pulling of and traction on the tracheostomy tube. Properly secure the tube in the midline position. Maintain proper cuff pressure. Minimize oronasal intubation time.
Tracheoesophageal fistula (TEF): Excessive cuff pressure causes erosion of the posterior wall of the trachea and loss of TISSUE INTEGRITY. A hole is created between the trachea and the anterior esophagus. The patient at highest risk also has a nasogastric tube present.	Similar to tracheomalacia: Food particles are seen in tracheal secretions. Increased air in cuff is needed to achieve a seal. The patient has increased coughing and choking while eating. The patient does not receive the set tidal volume on the ventilator.	Manually administer oxygen by mask to prevent hypoxemia. Use a small, soft feeding tube instead of a nasogastric tube for tube feedings. A gastrostomy or jejunostomy may be performed by the physician. Monitor the patient with a nasogastric tube closely; assess for TEF and aspiration.	Maintain cuff pressure. Monitor the amount of air needed for inflation and detect changes. Progress to a deflated cuff or cuffless tube as soon as possible.
Trachea—innominate artery fistula: A malpositioned tube causes its distal tip to push against the lateral wall of the tracheostomy. Continued pressure causes necrosis and erosion of the innominate artery. **This is a medical emergency.**	The tracheostomy tube pulsates in synchrony with the heartbeat. There is heavy bleeding from the stoma. This is a life-threatening complication.	Remove the tracheostomy tube immediately. Apply direct pressure to the innominate artery at the stoma site. Prepare the patient for immediate surgical repair.	Correct the tube size, length, and midline position. Prevent pulling or tugging on the tracheostomy tube. Immediately notify the physician of the pulsating tube.

tracheostomy tube, quickly and gently replace the tube and remove the obturator. Check for airflow through the tube and for bilateral breath sounds. *If you cannot secure the airway, notify a more experienced nurse, respiratory therapist, or physician for assistance. Ventilate with a bag-valve-mask. If the patient is in distress, call the Rapid Response Team for help.* To reduce tube dislodgment problems, many institutions have a "difficult airway" cart for high-risk patients.

Pneumothorax (air in the chest cavity) can develop during the tracheotomy procedure if the chest cavity is entered. Chest x-rays after placement are used to assess for pneumothorax.

Subcutaneous emphysema occurs when there is an opening or tear in the trachea and air escapes into the fresh tissue planes of the neck. Air can progress throughout the chest and other tissues into the face. Inspect and palpate for air under the skin around the new tracheostomy.

> ### ! NURSING SAFETY PRIORITY (QSEN)
> #### Critical Rescue
> Assess the skin around a new tracheostomy to recognize subcutaneous emphysema. If it is puffy and you can feel a crackling sensation when pressing on this skin, respond by notifying the physician immediately.

Bleeding in small amounts from the tracheotomy incision is expected for the first few days, but constant oozing is abnormal. Wrap gauze around the tube and pack gauze gently into the wound to apply pressure to the bleeding sites. Bleeding can occur in the trachea itself or in the tissues surrounding the incision. If hemorrhage occurs, the site may need surgical exploration or ligation of blood vessels.

Infection can occur at any time. In the hospital, use sterile technique to prevent infection during suctioning and tracheostomy care. Assess the stoma site at least once every 8 hours for purulent drainage, redness, pain, swelling, or loss of TISSUE INTEGRITY. Tracheostomy dressings may be used to keep the stoma clean and dry. These dressings resemble a 4 × 4 gauze pad with an area removed to fit around the tube. If tracheostomy dressings are not available, fold standard sterile 4 × 4s to fit around the tube. *Do not cut the dressing because small bits of gauze could then be aspirated through the tube.* Change these dressings often because moist dressings provide a medium for bacterial growth. Careful wound care prevents most local infections.

Tracheostomy Tubes. Many types of tracheostomy tubes are available (Fig. 28-12). The one chosen depends on patient needs. Tubes are available in many sizes and are made of plastic or metal. Most tubes are disposable. A tracheostomy tube may have a cuff and an inner cannula. A cuffed tube is used for patients receiving mechanical ventilation. The cuff is a small balloon surrounding the outside of the tracheostomy tube (see Figure 28-12). When inflated to the proper size and pressure, the cuff comes into contact with the trachea and seals it off so that all air movement occurs within the tracheostomy tube, not around it. Usually the cuff is inflated through the use of a pilot balloon, which remains on the outside of the body where it can be accessed. As shown in Figure 28-12, the pilot balloon is a small balloon with a valve on one end and a thin long tube on the other end. The thin tube is connected to the cuff. To inflate the cuff, an air-filled syringe is attached to the pilot balloon valve. As the syringe is pressed, air first enters the pilot balloon and then moves through the thin tube to inflate the cuff. In addition to the function of inflating the cuff, the pilot balloon can determine whether any air is in the cuff because the pilot remains inflated when the cuff is inflated. It does not indicate air volume or pressure in the cuff.

For tubes with a reusable inner cannula, inspect, suction, and clean the inner cannula. During the first 24 hours after surgery, perform cannula care as often as needed, perhaps hourly. Thereafter care is determined by the patient's needs and agency policy. In planning for self-care, teach the patient to remove the inner cannula and check for cleanliness. Instruct him or her about suctioning and tracheostomy cleaning.

Because breathing and swallowing move the tube, even a cuffed tube does not protect against aspiration. Having a cuffed tube inflated may give a false sense of security that aspiration cannot occur during feeding or mouth care. In addition, the pilot balloon does not reflect whether the correct amount of air is present in the cuff.

A fenestrated tube functions in many different ways. When the inner cannula is in place, the fenestration is closed, and this tube works like a double-lumen tube. With the inner cannula removed and the plug or stopper locked in place, air can pass through the fenestration, around the tube, and up through the natural airway so the patient can cough and speak. If the patient has trouble with these actions, he or she should be evaluated for proper tube placement, patency, size, and fenestration. *Do not cap the tube until the problem is identified and corrected.*

A fenestrated tube may or may not have a cuff. With a cuff, some air flows through the natural airway when the patient is not being mechanically ventilated.

> ### ! NURSING SAFETY PRIORITY (QSEN)
> #### Action Alert
> Always deflate the cuff before capping the tube with the decannulation cap; otherwise the patient has no airway.

Patients with metal tracheostomy tubes scheduled for MRI need to change to a plastic tube. Metal tubes could be dislodged or heat up with exposure to the magnetic field during the scan.

Care Issues for the Patient With a Tracheostomy

Preventing Tissue Damage. Loss of TISSUE INTEGRITY can occur at the point where the inflated cuff presses against the tracheal mucosa. Mucosal ischemia occurs when the pressure exerted by the cuff on the mucosa exceeds the capillary perfusion pressure. To reduce the risk for tracheal damage, keep the cuff pressure between 14 and 20 mm Hg or 20 and 30 cm H_2O (ideally, 25 cm H_2O or less).

Most cuffs use a high volume of air while keeping low pressure on the tracheal mucosa. Inflate the cuff to form a seal between the trachea and the cuff with the least amount of pressure. If the cuff cannot be inflated to seal well enough, a larger-diameter tube may be needed. A pressure cuff inflator can be used to inflate the cuff to a specified pressure or to check the cuff pressure (Fig. 28-13).

Check the cuff pressure at least once during each shift using either a pressure cuff inflator or the minimal leak technique. When using an inflator, keep the pressure at 14 to 20 mm Hg or 20 to 30 cm H_2O. In rare situations, the cuff pressure is increased to maintain ventilator volumes when peak pressures are greater than 50 mm Hg (65 cm H_2O) and positive end-expiratory pressure (PEEP) is greater than 10 mm Hg (14 cm

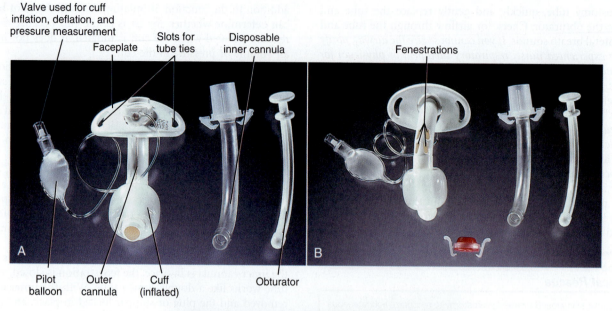

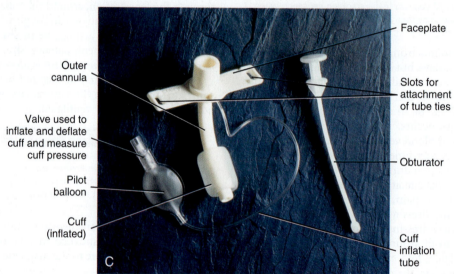

FIG. 28-12 Tracheostomy tubes. **A,** Dual-lumen cuffed tracheostomy tube with disposable inner cannula. **B,** Single-lumen cannula cuffed tracheostomy tube. **C,** Dual-lumen cuffed fenestrated tracheostomy tube. (Courtesy Mallinckrodt, Inc., Shiley Tracheostomy Products, St. Louis, MO.)

H_2O). High PEEP values can deflate the cuff over time, and more air may need to be added to maintain a proper seal. Manufacturers have guidelines for the specific volumes for each cuff size. Most cuffs are adequately inflated with less than 10 mL of air.

When using the minimal leak technique to ensure adequate cuff pressure and reduce the risk for pressure injury, a pressure cuff inflator is not used. Instead, after completing tracheostomy care and suctioning the airway above the cuff, attach a 10-mL Luer-Lok syringe to the valve in the pilot balloon. Place a stethoscope on the side of the patient's neck near the tracheostomy tube and slowly deflate the cuff with the syringe while listening for a loud, gurgling air rush as the seal is broken and air bypasses the tracheostomy tube on inhalation. Then while re-injecting the air in the syringe, continue to listen for air passing the cuff. When air is no longer heard passing the cuff,

the airway is sealed. At this point, remove 1 mL of air from the cuff. This ensures that the airway is sealed sufficiently to allow adequate ventilation and keep the tube fitting just loose enough to prevent tracheal injury.

Although a high cuff pressure alone can injure tracheal TISSUE INTEGRITY, other factors contribute to the risk for damage (Makic et al., 2013). The patient who is malnourished, dehydrated, hypoxic, older, or receiving corticosteroids is at risk for greater tissue damage. Tube friction and movement damage the mucosa and lead to tracheal stenosis. Reduce local airway damage by maintaining proper cuff pressures, stabilizing the tube, suctioning only when needed, and preventing malnutrition, dehydration, and hypoxia.

Ensuring Air Warming and Humidification. The tracheostomy tube bypasses the nose and mouth, which normally humidify and warm the inspired air. If humidification and

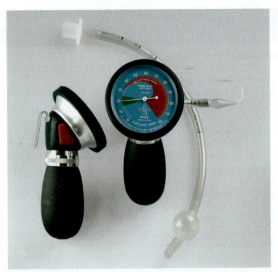

FIG. 28-13 Aneroid pressure manometer for cuff inflation and measuring cuff pressures. (Courtesy J. T. Posey Company, Arcadia, CA.)

warming are not adequate, tracheal damage can occur. Inadequate humidity promotes thick, dried secretions that can occlude the airways.

To prevent these complications, humidify the air as prescribed. Continually assess for a fine mist emerging from the tracheostomy collar or T-piece during ventilation. To increase the amount of humidity delivered, a warming device can be attached to the water source with a temperature probe in the tubing circuit. Monitor the circuit temperature hourly by feeling the tubing and by checking the probe. Ensure adequate hydration, which also helps liquefy secretions. Increasing the flow rate at the flow meter increases the amount of delivered humidity.

! **NURSING SAFETY PRIORITY** QSEN

Action Alert

Keep the temperature of the air entering a tracheostomy between 98.6° and 100.4° F (37° and 38° C) and never exceed 104° F (40° C).

Suctioning. Suctioning maintains a patent airway and promotes GAS EXCHANGE by removing secretions when the patient cannot cough adequately. Chart 28-2 lists best practices for suctioning. Assess the patient's need for suctioning (e.g., audible or noisy secretions; crackles or wheezes heard on auscultation; restlessness, increased pulse or respiratory rates, or mucus present in the artificial airway) (Morris et al., 2013). Other indications include patient requests for suctioning or an increase in the peak airway pressure on the ventilator.

Deep endotracheal suctioning is painful. Unconscious patients may still feel pain, and this should be kept in mind during the suctioning procedure. At the very least, provide verbal acknowledgment of the discomfort and reassurance of when the procedure will end.

Suctioning is often performed through an artificial airway, but the nose or mouth also can be used. Suctioning of both routes is routine for the patient with retained secretions.

Suctioning through the nose has complications and can be painful. Selecting a small suction catheter and coating it with a water-soluble lubricant helps minimize trauma and increase

---

⊚ **CHART 28-2** **Best Practice for Patient Safety & Quality Care** QSEN

Suctioning the Artificial Airway

- Assess the need for suctioning (routine unnecessary suctioning causes mucosal damage, bleeding, and bronchospasm).
- Wash hands. Don protective eyewear. Maintain Standard Precautions.
- Explain to the patient that sensations such as shortness of breath and coughing are to be expected but that any discomfort will be very brief.
- Check the suction source. Occlude the suction source and adjust the pressure dial to between 80 and 120 mm Hg to prevent hypoxemia and trauma to the mucosa.
- Set up a sterile field.
- Preoxygenate the patient with 100% oxygen for 30 seconds to 3 minutes (at least three hyperinflations) to prevent hypoxemia. Keep hyperinflations synchronized with inhalation.
- Quickly insert the suction catheter until resistance is met. *Do not apply suction during insertion.*
- Withdraw the catheter 0.4 to 0.8 inch (1 to 2 cm) and begin to apply suction. Apply continuous suction and use a twirling motion of the catheter during withdrawal to avoid injury to TISSUE INTEGRITY. *Never suction longer than 10 to 15 seconds.*
- Hyperoxygenate for 1 to 5 minutes or until the patient's baseline heart rate and oxygen saturation are within normal limits.
- Repeat as needed for up to three total suction passes.
- Suction mouth as needed and provide mouth care.
- Remove gloves and wash hands.
- Describe secretions and document patient's responses.

---

comfort. Slow, careful placement of the catheter following the nasopharyngeal anatomy reduces pain and prevents injuring TISSUE INTEGRITY. Placing a nasopharyngeal airway and suctioning through it can prevent trauma to the nasal mucosa. Advance the catheter through the nasopharynx and into the laryngopharynx while the patient receives oxygen by mask or nasal cannula. Once the catheter enters the larynx, the patient may cough. On inhalation, insert the catheter into the trachea. If needed, disconnect the catheter from suction and attach it to an oxygen source so the patient receives oxygen via the catheter.

Suctioning can cause hypoxia, injury to mucosal TISSUE INTEGRITY, trauma, infection, vagal stimulation, bronchospasm, and cardiac dysrhythmias.

Hypoxia can be caused by these factors in the patient with a tracheostomy:

- Ineffective oxygenation before, during, and after suctioning
- Use of a catheter that is too large for the artificial airway
- Prolonged suctioning time
- Excessive suction pressure
- Too frequent suctioning

Prevent hypoxia by hyperoxygenating the patient with 100% oxygen using a manual resuscitation bag attached to an oxygen source. Instruct the patient to take deep breaths 3 or 4 times with the existing oxygen delivery system before suctioning. Monitor the heart rate or use a pulse oximeter while suctioning to assess tolerance of the procedure. Assess for hypoxia (e.g., increased heart rate and blood pressure, oxygen desaturation, cyanosis, restlessness, anxiety, dysrhythmias). Oxygen saturation below 90% by pulse oximetry indicates hypoxemia. If hypoxia occurs, stop the suctioning procedure. Using the 100%

oxygen delivery system, reoxygenate the patient until baseline parameters return.

Use a correct-size catheter to reduce the risk for hypoxia and still remove secretions effectively. The size should not exceed half of the size of the tracheal lumen. The standard catheter size for an adult is 12 Fr or 14 Fr.

Loss of TISSUE INTEGRITY by trauma results from frequent suctioning, prolonged suctioning, excessive suction pressure, and nonrotation of the catheter. Prevent trauma to the mucosa by suctioning only when needed and lubricating the catheter with sterile water or saline before insertion. *Apply continuous suction only during catheter withdrawal because intermittent suction does not protect the mucosa and can lead to "dropping" of secretions in the airway.* Use a twirling motion during withdrawal to prevent grabbing of the mucosa.

Apply suction for only 10 to 15 seconds. Estimate this time frame by holding your own breath and counting to 10 or 15 while suctioning. Longer suctioning can cause alveolar collapse.

Infection is possible because each catheter pass introduces bacteria into the trachea. In the hospital, use sterile technique for suctioning and for all suctioning equipment (e.g., suction catheters, gloves, saline or water). Suction the mouth or nose *after* suctioning the artificial airway. Clean technique is used at home because the number of virulent organisms in the home environment is lower than in the hospital.

! NURSING SAFETY PRIORITY QSEN

Action Alert

Never use oral suction equipment for suctioning an artificial airway because this can introduce oral bacteria into the lungs.

Vagal stimulation and bronchospasm are possible during suctioning. Vagal stimulation results in bradycardia, hypotension, heart block, ventricular tachycardia, or other dysrhythmias. *If vagal stimulation occurs, stop suctioning immediately and oxygenate the patient manually with 100% oxygen.* Bronchospasm may occur when the catheter passes into the airway. The patient may need a bronchodilator to relieve bronchospasm and respiratory distress. The hypoxia caused by suctioning can stimulate a variety of cardiac dysrhythmias. If the patient has cardiac monitoring in place, check the monitor during suctioning.

? NCLEX EXAMINATION CHALLENGE 28-3

Safe and Effective Care Environment

For which possible complication of tracheostomy tube dislodgment does the nurse remain alert in a client during the first 72 hours after placement?
A. Oxygen toxicity
B. Increased secretions
C. Movement of the tube into a "false passage"
D. Increased risk for aspiration during swallowing

Providing Tracheostomy Care. Tracheostomy care keeps the tube free of secretions, maintains a patent airway, and provides wound care (Schreiber, 2015). It is performed whether or not the patient can clear secretions. Perform tracheostomy care according to agency policy, usually every 8 hours and as needed. Chart 28-3 outlines best practices for tracheostomy care.

◎ CHART 28-3 Best Practice for Patient Safety & Quality Care QSEN

Tracheostomy Care

- Assemble the necessary equipment.
- Wash hands. Maintain Standard Precautions.
- Suction the tracheostomy tube if necessary.
- Remove old dressings and excess secretions.
- Set up a sterile field.
- Remove and clean the inner cannula. Use half-strength hydrogen peroxide to clean the cannula and sterile saline to rinse it. If the inner cannula is disposable, remove the cannula and replace it with a new one.
- Clean the stoma site and then the tracheostomy plate with half-strength hydrogen peroxide followed by sterile saline. Ensure that none of the solutions enters the tracheostomy.
- Change tracheostomy ties if they are soiled. Secure new ties in place before removing soiled ones to prevent accidental decannulation. If a knot is needed, tie a square knot that is visible on the side of the neck. Only one finger should be able to be placed between the tie tape and the neck.
- Wash hands.
- Document the type and amount of secretions and the general condition of the stoma and surrounding skin tissue integrity. Document the patient's response to the procedure and any teaching or learning that occurred.

📋 CHART 28-4 Focused Assessment

The Patient With a Tracheostomy

- Note the quality, pattern, and rate of breathing:
  - Within patient's baseline?
  - Tachypnea can indicate hypoxia.
  - Dyspnea can indicate secretions in the airway.
- Assess for any cyanosis, especially around the lips, which could indicate hypoxia.
- Check the patient's pulse oximetry reading.
- If oxygen is prescribed, is the patient receiving the correct amount, with the correct equipment and humidification?
- Assess the tracheostomy site:
  - Note the color, consistency, and amount of secretions in the tube or externally.
  - If the tracheostomy is sutured in place, is there any redness, swelling, or drainage from suture sites?
  - If the tracheostomy is secured with ties, what is the condition of the ties? Are they moist with secretions or perspiration? Are the secretions dried on the ties? Is the tie secure?
  - Assess the condition of the skin around the tracheostomy and neck for tissue integrity. Be sure to check underneath the neck for secretions that may have drained to the back. Check for any skin breakdown related to pressure from the ties or related to excess secretions.
  - Assess behind the faceplate for the size of the space between the outer cannula and the patient's tissue. Are any secretions collected in this area?
- If the tube is cuffed, check cuff pressure.
- Auscultate the lungs.
- Are a second (emergency) tracheostomy tube and obturator available?

Before tracheostomy care, assess the patient as described in Chart 28-4. The need for suctioning and tracheostomy care is determined by the secretions, the specific disorder, the ability of the patient to cough, the need for mechanical ventilation, and wound care. Using a penlight, inspect the inner lumen of a single-lumen tube to assess for secretions.

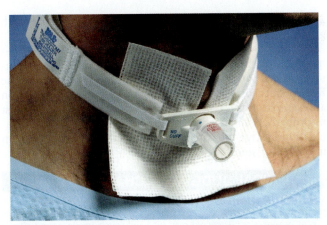

FIG. 28-14 Placement of tracheostomy gauze dressing and Velcro tracheostomy tube holder. (Courtesy Dale Medical Products, Inc., Plainville, MA.)

Secure tracheostomy tubes in place using either twill tape ties or commercial tube holders. Both methods have advantages and disadvantages over the other, and both are acceptable (Smith, 2016). These devices require changing when soiled or at least daily to keep them clean, to prevent infection, and to assess TISSUE INTEGRITY under the ties. Whenever possible, use the assistance of a coworker to stabilize the tube and prevent decannulation while changing the ties or tube holder (Schreiber, 2015). A properly secured tie or holder allows space for only one finger to be placed between the tie or holder and the neck (Morris et al., 2013). Tube movement causes irritation and coughing and may lead to decannulation. Keeping the tube secure while changing the ties or holder to prevent accidental decannulation is critical. Include the patient in tracheostomy care as a step toward self-care. Fig. 28-14 shows correct placement of a tracheostomy dressing.

! NURSING SAFETY PRIORITY OSEN

Critical Rescue

Prevent decannulation during tracheostomy care by keeping the old ties or holder on the tube while applying new ties or holder or by keeping a hand on the tube until it is securely stable. (This is best performed with the assistance of a coworker.)

Providing Bronchial and Oral Hygiene. Bronchial hygiene promotes a patent airway and prevents infection. Turn and reposition the patient every 1 to 2 hours, support out-of-bed activities, and encourage ambulation to promote lung expansion and GAS EXCHANGE and help remove secretions. Coughing and deep breathing, combined with the chest percussion, vibration, and postural drainage, promote pulmonary hygiene (see Chapter 30).

Good oral hygiene keeps the airway patent, prevents bacterial overgrowth, and promotes comfort. Avoid using glycerin swabs or mouthwash that contains alcohol for oral care because these products dry the mouth, change its pH, and promote bacterial growth. Instead use a sponge tooth cleaner or soft-bristle toothbrush moistened in water for mouth care. Diluted hydrogen peroxide solutions can help remove crusted matter but may break down healing tissue and should be used only if prescribed. Help the patient rinse the mouth with normal saline every 4 hours while awake or as often as he or she desires.

◎ CHART 28-5 Best Practice for Patient Safety & Quality Care OSEN

Preventing Aspiration During Swallowing

- Avoid serving meals when the patient is tired.
- Provide smaller and more frequent meals.
- Provide adequate time; do not "hurry" the patient.
- Provide close supervision if the patient is self-feeding.
- Keep emergency suctioning equipment close at hand and turned on.
- Avoid water and other "thin" liquids.
- Thicken all liquids, including water.
- Avoid foods that generate thin liquids during the chewing process such as fruit.
- Position the patient in the most upright position possible.
- When possible, completely (or at least partially) deflate the tube cuff during meals.
- Suction after initial cuff deflation to clear the airway and allow maximum comfort during the meal.
- Feed each bite or encourage the patient to take each bite slowly.
- Encourage the patient to "dry swallow" after each bite to clear residue from the throat.
- Avoid consecutive swallows of liquids.
- Provide controlled small volumes of liquids, using a spoon.
- Encourage the patient to "tuck" his or her chin down and move the forehead forward while swallowing.
- Allow the patient to indicate when he or she is ready for the next bite.
- If the patient coughs, stop the feeding until he or she indicates that the airway has been cleared.
- Continuously monitor tolerance to oral food intake by assessing respiratory rate, ease, pulse.

Examine the mouth for changes in TISSUE INTEGRITY. Ulcers and infections are treated medically. Apply lip balm or water-soluble jelly to prevent cracked lips and promote comfort. Mouth care promotes oral health and comfort. Offering an opportunity for the patient or family member to perform mouth care allows participation in care and increases self-esteem.

Oral secretions can move down the trachea and collect above the inflated cuff of the endotracheal tube. When the cuff is deflated, the secretions can move into the lungs. Some endotracheal tubes have an extra lumen open to the area above the cuff, which allows suctioning of the airway above the cuff before deflating and reduces the risk for aspiration.

Ensuring Nutrition. Swallowing can be a major problem for the patient with a tracheostomy tube in place. In a normal swallow, the larynx lifts and moves forward to prevent food and saliva from entering. The tracheostomy tube sometimes tethers the larynx in place, making it unable to move effectively. The result is difficulty in swallowing. In addition, when the tracheostomy tube cuff is inflated, it can balloon backward and interfere with food passage in the esophagus because the wall separating the trachea from the esophagus is thin.

Instruct the patient to keep the head of the bed elevated for at least 30 minutes after eating. Chart 28-5 outlines best practices to prevent aspiration during swallowing.

Maintaining Communication. The patient can speak when there is a cuffless tube, when a fenestrated tracheostomy tube is in place, and when the fenestrated tube is capped or covered. Until natural speech is feasible, teach him or her and the family about other communication means. A writing tablet, a board with pictures and letters, communication "flash cards" on a ring, hand signals, and smartphones, as well as a call light within reach, are used to promote communication and decrease frustration from not being able to speak or be understood. Concerns about infection control have been raised with techniques that involve shared equipment, such as communication boards and flash cards. Studies exploring the patient's use of his or her own smartphones for text messaging are ongoing (Bell, 2016). Phrase questions for "yes" or "no" answers to help the patient respond easily. Mark the central call light system to indicate that he or she cannot speak. For any patient with a communication problem, including a speech-language pathologist as part of the interprofessional team promotes better outcomes (Vento-Wilson et al., 2015).

The inability to talk is a stressor for the patient. Helping communication is an important nursing action and is required by The Joint Commission's National Patient Safety Goals (NPSGs). When the patient can tolerate cuff deflation, he or she places a finger over the tracheostomy tube on exhalation, forcing air up through the larynx and mouth for speech.

A device to facilitate speech for the patient with a tracheostomy is a one-way valve that fits over the tube and replaces the need for finger occlusion. The valve allows him or her to breathe in through the tracheostomy tube. On exhalation, the valve closes so air is forced through the vocal cords, allowing speech. For this valve to assist in speech, the patient must not be connected to a ventilator, must have the cuff deflated, and must be able to breathe around the tube. Some valves have a port for supplemental oxygen without impairing the ability to speak.

Supporting Psychosocial Needs and Self-Concept. Addressing psychological concerns is an important aspect of nursing care for patients recovering from a tracheostomy. Always keep in mind the emotional impact of an artificial airway. Acknowledge the patient's frustration with communication and allow sufficient time for communication. When speaking to him or her, use a normal tone of voice because hearing and understanding are not altered by the presence of a tube.

The patient may have a change in self-image because of the presence of a stoma or artificial airway, speech changes, a change in the method of eating, or difficulty with speech. Help him or her set realistic goals, starting with involvement in self-care.

Work with the caregivers to ease the patient into a more normal social environment. Provide encouragement and positive reinforcement while demonstrating acceptance and caring behaviors. Assess the caregiver(s) for the need for counseling.

After surgery the patient may feel shy and socially isolated. He or she can wear loose-fitting shirts, decorative collars, or scarves to cover the tracheostomy tube.

Weaning. Weaning the patient from a tracheostomy tube entails a gradual decrease in the tube size and ultimate removal of the tube. Carefully monitor this process, especially after each change. The physician or advanced practice nurse performs the steps in the process.

First, the cuff is deflated as soon as the patient can manage secretions and does not need mechanical ventilation. This change allows him or her to breathe through the tube and through the upper airway. Next, the tube is changed to an uncuffed tube. If this is tolerated, the size of the tube is gradually decreased. When a small fenestrated tube is placed, the tube is capped so all air passes through the upper airway and the fenestra, with none passing through the tube. Assess the patient to ensure adequate airflow around the tube when it is capped. The tube may be removed after he or she tolerates more than

24 hours of capping. Place a dry dressing over the stoma (which gradually heals on its own).

Another device used for the transition from tracheostomy to natural breathing is a *tracheostomy button*. The button maintains stoma patency and assists spontaneous breathing. The Kistner tracheostomy tube and Olympic tracheostomy button are examples of this type of device. To function, the button must fit properly. A disadvantage is the possibility of covert decannulation (i.e., the tube can dislodge from the trachea but remain in the neck tissues).

❓ CLINICAL JUDGMENT CHALLENGE 28-2
Safety; Patient-Centered Care QSEN

Your patient is a 59-year-old man who requires a tracheostomy after being unable to wean from the ventilator. He no longer requires mechanical ventilation and has a tracheostomy collar with an FiO_2 of 40%.
1. Which supplies should you maintain at the bedside? Explain your choices.
2. What precautions should you take to help this patient eat with a tracheostomy tube?
3. What can you do to minimize tracheal damage?
4. The patient is concerned about communicating. What are his options at this time?

Care Coordination and Transition Management

Self-Management Education. By the time of discharge, the patient should be able to provide self-care, including tracheostomy care, nutrition care, suctioning, and communication. Although education begins before surgery, most self-care is taught in the hospital. Teach the patient and caregiver how to care for the tracheostomy tube. Review airway care, including cleaning and signs of infection or loss of TISSUE INTEGRITY. Teach clean suction technique and review the plan of care.

Instruct the patient to use a shower shield over the tracheostomy tube when bathing to prevent water from entering the airway. Teach him or her to cover the airway loosely with a small cotton cloth to protect it during the day. Covering the opening filters the air entering the stoma, keeps humidity in the airway, and enhances appearance. Attractive coverings are available as cotton scarves, decorative collars, and jewelry.

Home Care Management. Teach the patient to increase humidity in the home. Tell him or her to wear a medical alert bracelet that identifies the inability to speak.

Health Care Resources. The interprofessional health care team assesses specific discharge needs and makes referrals to home care agencies and durable medical equipment companies (for suction equipment and tracheostomy supplies). Follow-up visits occur early after discharge. The home care nurse initiates and coordinates the services of dietitians, nurses, speech and language pathologists, and social workers and identifies appropriate community resources.

👤 CONSIDERATIONS FOR OLDER ADULTS
Patient-Centered Care QSEN

Self-managing tracheostomy care and oxygen therapy can be difficult for the older patient who has vision problems or difficulty with upper arm movement. Teach him or her to use magnifying lenses or glasses to ensure the proper setting on the oxygen gauge. Assess his or her ability to reach and manipulate the tracheostomy. If possible, work with a family member who can provide assistance during tracheostomy care.

◆ *Evaluation: Reflecting*

Evaluate the care of the patient with a tracheostomy based on the identified priority patient problems. The expected outcomes of care are that the patient should:

- Attain and maintain GAS EXCHANGE at a level within his or her chronic baseline values
- Communicate effectively
- Achieve and maintain a body weight within 10% of his or her ideal weight
- Avoid serious respiratory infections
- Maintain TISSUE INTEGRITY of the airway mucosa and skin surrounding the tracheostomy.

GET READY FOR THE NCLEX® EXAMINATION!

KEY POINTS

Review the following key points for each NCLEX Examination Client Needs Category.

Safe and Effective Care Environment

- Never allow water condensation in an oxygen delivery system to drain back into the system. **QSEN: Safety**
- Use sterile technique when performing endotracheal or tracheal suctioning. **QSEN: Safety**
- Assess TISSUE INTEGRITY of the oral mucous membranes for injury each shift for anyone who has an endotracheal tube. **QSEN: Safety**
- Keep a tracheostomy tube (and obturator) and tracheostomy insertion tray at the bedside for the first 72 hours after a tracheostomy has been created. **QSEN: Safety**
- Never use oral suctioning equipment to suction an artificial airway. **QSEN: Safety**
- Use Aspiration Precautions for any patient with an altered level of consciousness or who has an endotracheal tube (see Chart 28-5). **QSEN: Safety**
- Verify safe use of appropriate oxygen delivery systems and tracheostomy equipment. **QSEN: Safety**
- Keep the tracheal cuff pressure between 14 and 20 mm Hg to prevent injury to the TISSUE INTEGRITY. **QSEN: Safety**
- Teach the patient and caregivers about home management of oxygen therapy, including the avoidance of smoking or open flames in rooms in which oxygen is being used. **QSEN: Safety**
- Teach the patient and caregivers how to perform tracheostomy care (see Chart 28-3). **QSEN: Safety**

Health Promotion and Maintenance

- Ensure that the patient and caregiver(s) know whom to contact about needed supplies and durable medical equipment. **QSEN: Patient-Centered Care**

Psychosocial Integrity

- Provide opportunity for the patient and caregivers to express concerns about a change in breathing status or the possibility of intubation and mechanical ventilation. **QSEN: Patient-Centered Care**
- Teach caregivers and family members ways to communicate with a patient who is intubated or being mechanically ventilated. **QSEN: Patient-Centered Care**
- Reassure patients who are intubated that the loss of speech is temporary. **QSEN: Patient-Centered Care**
- Encourage patients with permanent tracheostomies to become involved in self-care. **QSEN: Patient-Centered Care**

Physiological Integrity

- Apply oxygen to anyone who is hypoxemic. **QSEN: Evidence-Based Practice**
- Ensure that oxygen therapy delivered to the patient is humidified appropriately. **QSEN: Evidence-Based Practice**
- Monitor arterial blood gases (ABGs) and oxygen saturation of all patients receiving oxygen therapy. **QSEN: Evidence-Based Practice**
- Assess the skin under the mask and under the plastic tubing every shift for patients receiving oxygen by mask. **QSEN: Patient-Centered Care**
- Assess the TISSUE INTEGRITY of the nares and under the elastic band every shift for patients receiving oxygen by nasal cannula. **QSEN: Patient-Centered Care**
- Observe any patient receiving oxygen at greater than a 50% concentration for early signs and symptoms of oxygen toxicity (i.e., dyspnea, nonproductive cough, chest pain, GI upset). **QSEN: Patient-Centered Care**
- Use a manual resuscitation bag to ventilate the patient if the tracheostomy tube has dislodged or become decannulated. **QSEN: Safety**
- Assess the new tracheostomy stoma site at least once per shift for purulent drainage, redness, pain, and swelling as indicators of infection or loss of TISSUE INTEGRITY. **QSEN: Evidence-Based Practice**

SELECTED BIBLIOGRAPHY

Ambutas, S., Staffileno, B., & Fogg, L. (2014). Reducing nasal pressure ulcers with an alternative taping device. *Medsurg Nursing, 23*(2), 96–100.

Bajaj, A., Rathor, P., Sehgal, V., & Shetty, A. (2015). Efficacy of noninvasive ventilation after planned extubation: A systematic review and meta-analysis of randomized controlled trials.

Heart and Lung: The Journal of Critical Care, 44(2), 150–157.

Bell, L. (2016). Caring for patients who are unable to speak. *American Journal of Critical Care, 25*(2), 109.

Bull, A. (2014). Primary care of chronic dyspnea in adults. *The Nurse Practitioner, 39*(8), 34–40.

Carlisle, H. (2014). The case for capnography in patients receiving opioids. *American Nurse Today, 9*(9), 22–26.

Makic, M. B., Martin, S., Burns, S., Philbrick, D., & Rauen, C. (2013). Putting evidence into nursing practice: Four traditional practices not supported by the evidence. *Critical Care Nurse, 33*(2), 28–42.

McCance, K., Huether, S., Brashers, V., & Rote, N. (2014). *Pathophysiology: The biologic basis for disease in adults and children* (7th ed.). St. Louis: Mosby.

Morris, L., McIntosh, E., & Whitmer, A. (2014). The importance of tracheostomy progression in the intensive care unit. *Critical Care Nurse, 34*(1), 40–48.

Morris, L., Whitmer, A., & McIntosh, E. (2013). Tracheostomy care and complications in the intensive care unit. *Critical Care Nurse, 33*(5), 18–30.

Nishimura, M. (2015). High-flow nasal cannula oxygen therapy in adults. *J Intensive Care, 15*, 1–8. http://www.ncbi.nlm.nih.gov/pmc/articles/PMC4393594/.

Schallom, M., Cracchiolo, L., Falker, A., Foster, J., Hager, J., Morehouse, T., et al. (2015). Pressure ulcer incidence in patients wearing nasal-oral versus full-face noninvasive ventilation masks. *American Journal of Critical Care, 24*(4), 349–357.

Schreiber, M. (2015). Tracheostomy: Site care, suctioning, and readiness. *Medsurg Nursing, 24*(2), 121–124.

Seckel, M. (2014). Oxygen and oxygenation. *Critical Care Nurse, 34*(5), 73–74.

Smith, S. (2016). Best method for securing an endotracheal tube. *Critical Care Nurse, 36*(2), 78–79.

Vento-Wilson, M., McGuire, A., & Ostergren, J. (2015). Role of the speech-language pathologist. *Dimensions of Critical Care Nursing, 34*(2), 112–119.

CHAPTER 29

Care of Patients With Noninfectious Upper Respiratory Problems

M. Linda Workman

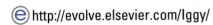
http://evolve.elsevier.com/Iggy/

PRIORITY AND INTERRELATED CONCEPTS

The priority concepts for this chapter are:
- CELLULAR REGULATION
- GAS EXCHANGE

❊ The CELLULAR REGULATION concept exemplar for this chapter is Head and Neck Cancer, below.

The interrelated concepts for this chapter are:
- NUTRITION
- TISSUE INTEGRITY

LEARNING OUTCOMES

Safe and Effective Care Environment

1. Collaborate with the interprofessional team to coordinate high-quality care and promote GAS EXCHANGE for patients who have upper respiratory problems.
2. Protect patients with upper respiratory problems from hypoxia, injury, infection, and reduced GAS EXCHANGE.
3. Prioritize evidence-based care for critically ill patients with respiratory problems that decrease GAS EXCHANGE.
4. Teach the patient and family how to manage a chronic upper respiratory disorder and avoid injury and complications in the home.

Health Promotion and Maintenance

5. Teach all adults measures to take to protect the upper respiratory system from damage and cancer (loss of CELLULAR REGULATION), including the avoidance of known environmental causative agents.

6. Identify community resources for patients requiring assistance with long-term complications of upper respiratory problems.

Psychosocial Integrity

7. Implement nursing interventions to help the patient and family cope with the psychosocial impact caused by upper respiratory problems.

Physiological Integrity

8. Apply knowledge of anatomy and physiology to assess patients with upper respiratory problems affecting GAS EXCHANGE.
9. Teach the patient and caregiver(s) about common drugs and other management strategies used for upper respiratory problems.
10. Prioritize the nursing care needs of the patient and family experiencing head and neck cancer.

The upper airway structures are the nose, sinuses, oropharynx, larynx, and trachea. These structures contribute to GAS EXCHANGE by providing the entrance site for air. Any problem of the upper airways can interfere with airflow and gas exchange. The nursing priority for patients with disorders of the upper respiratory tract is to promote gas exchange by ensuring a patent airway.

❊ CELLULAR REGULATION CONCEPT EXEMPLAR
Head and Neck Cancer

❖ PATHOPHYSIOLOGY

Head and neck cancer can disrupt breathing (GAS EXCHANGE), eating, facial appearance, self-image, speech, and communica-

tion. This form of cancer can be devastating, even when cured. The care needs for patients with these problems are complex, requiring a coordinated interprofessional team approach. Common team members include an oncologist, surgeon, nurse, registered dietitian, speech and language pathologist, dentist, respiratory therapist, social worker, wound care specialist, clergy, occupational and physical therapists, and psychosocial counselors.

Head and neck cancers are usually squamous cell carcinomas. These slow-growing tumors are curable when diagnosed and treated at an early stage. The prognosis for those who have more advanced disease at diagnosis depends on the extent and location of the tumors. Untreated, these cancers are often fatal within 2 years of diagnosis (American Cancer Society [ACS], 2017).

The cancer begins as a loss of CELLULAR REGULATION when the mucosa is chronically irritated and becomes tougher and thicker (*squamous metaplasia*). At the same time, genes controlling cell growth are damaged, allowing excessive growth of these abnormal cells, which eventually become malignant. These lesions may then be seen as white, patchy lesions (leukoplakia) or red, velvety patches (erythroplakia).

Head and neck cancer first spreads (metastasizes) into local lymph nodes, muscle, and bone. Later spread is systemic to distant sites, usually to the lungs or liver.

The cancer type and stage are determined by cellular analysis. Earlier-stage cancers are described as *carcinoma in situ* and *well differentiated*. Without treatment, cancers progress to be *moderately differentiated* and, finally, *poorly differentiated*. Most head and neck cancers arise from the mucous membrane and skin, but they also can start from salivary glands, the thyroid, tonsils, or other structures. Treatment is based on tumor cell type and degree of spread at diagnosis.

Etiology

The two most important risk factors for head and neck cancer are tobacco and alcohol use, especially in combination. Other risk factors include voice abuse, chronic laryngitis, exposure to chemicals or dusts, poor oral hygiene, long-term gastroesophageal reflux disease, and oral infection with the human papillomavirus (HPV) (ACS, 2017; McKiernan & Thom, 2016; Rettig & D'Souza, 2015).

Incidence and Prevalence

The frequency of head and neck carcinoma is increasing in North America. About 67,200 new cases of oral, pharyngeal, and laryngeal cancers are diagnosed each year and account for more than 14,000 deaths per year (ACS, 2017; Canadian Cancer Society, 2016). They affect men twice as often as women and are most common in adults older than 60 years.

❖ INTERPROFESSIONAL COLLABORATIVE CARE

Adults with head and neck cancer may be treated on an outpatient basis with radiation for early-stage disease. When surgery is needed, care starts in an acute care environment and can involve a stay of 5 days or more. Chemotherapy is usually performed in an outpatient setting.

◆ Assessment: Noticing

History. The patient may have difficulty speaking because of hoarseness, shortness of breath, tumor bulk, and pain. Pace the interview to avoid tiring the patient.

Ask about tobacco and alcohol use, history of acute or chronic laryngitis or pharyngitis, oral sores, swallowing difficulty, and lumps in the neck. Calculate the patient's pack-years of smoking history (see Chapter 27). Ask about alcohol intake (how many drinks per day and for how many years). Also ask about oral exposure to the human papilloma virus (Schiech, 2016).

Assess problems related to risk factors. For example, NUTRITION may be poor because of alcohol intake, impaired liver function, and difficulty swallowing. Assess dietary habits and any weight loss. Ask about chronic lung disease, which also may have an impact on GAS EXCHANGE.

Physical Assessment/Signs and Symptoms. Table 29-1 lists the warning signs of head and neck cancer. With laryngeal cancer, painless hoarseness may occur because of tumor size

TABLE 29-1	Warning Signs of Head and Neck Cancer
• Pain
• Lump in the mouth, throat, or neck
• Difficulty swallowing
• Color changes in the mouth or tongue to red, white, gray, dark brown, or black
• Oral lesion or sore that does not heal in 2 weeks
• Persistent or unexplained oral bleeding
• Numbness of the mouth, lips, or face
• Change in the fit of dentures
• Burning sensation when drinking citrus juices or hot liquids
• Persistent, unilateral ear pain
• Hoarseness or change in voice quality
• Persistent or recurrent sore throat
• Shortness of breath
• Anorexia and weight loss

and an inability of the vocal cords to come together for normal speech. Vocal cord lesions form early in laryngeal cancer. Any adult who has a history of hoarseness, mouth sores, or a lump in the neck for 3 to 4 weeks should be evaluated for laryngeal cancer.

Inspect the head and neck for symmetry and the presence of lumps or lesions. An advanced practice nurse or physician may perform a laryngeal examination using a laryngeal mirror or fiberoptic laryngoscope. The neck is palpated to assess for enlarged lymph nodes.

Psychosocial Assessment. Often the patient with head and neck cancer has a long-standing history of tobacco or alcohol use or both. Assess the adequacy of support systems and coping mechanisms. Document social and family support because the patient needs extensive assistance at home after treatment. A social worker should be a member of the patient's interprofessional team. Assess the level of education or literacy of the patient and family to plan teaching before and after surgery.

Document any family history of cancer and the patient's age, gender, occupation, and ability to perform ADLs. Ask the patient whether his or her occupation requires continual oral communication. Job retraining may be needed if treatment affects speech.

Laboratory Assessment. Diagnostic tests include a complete blood cell count, bleeding times, urinalysis, and blood chemistries. The patient with chronic alcoholism may have low protein and albumin levels from poor NUTRITION. Liver and kidney function tests are performed to rule out cancer spread and to evaluate the patient's ability to metabolize drugs and chemotherapy agents. A blood test for the presence of human papilloma virus (HPV) is often performed.

Imaging Assessment. Many types of imaging studies, including x-rays of the skull, sinuses, neck, and chest, are useful in diagnosing cancer spread, other tumors, and the extent of tumor invasion. CT with contrast medium helps evaluate the tumor's exact location. MRI can help differentiate normal from diseased tissue.

The brain, bone, and liver are evaluated with nuclear imaging, bone scans, single-photon emission computerized tomography (SPECT) scans, and positron emission tomography CT (PET-CT) scans (National Comprehensive Cancer Network [NCCN], 2016). These tests locate additional tumor sites.

Other Diagnostic Assessment. Other helpful tests include direct and indirect laryngoscopy, tumor mapping, and biopsy. *Panendoscopy* (laryngoscopy, nasopharyngoscopy, esophagoscopy, and bronchoscopy) is performed with general anesthesia to define the extent of the tumor. Tumor-mapping biopsies are performed to identify tumor location. Biopsy tissues taken at the time of the panendoscopy confirm the diagnosis, tumor type, cell features, location, and stage (see Chapter 21).

◆ *Analysis: Interpreting*

The priority collaborative problems for patients with head and neck cancer include:

1. Potential for airway obstruction due to edema and presence of tumor
2. Potential for aspiration due to edema, anatomic changes, or altered protective reflexes
3. Anxiety due to threat of death, change in role status, or change in economic status
4. Decreased self-esteem due to cancer and cancer treatment side effects

◆ *Planning and Implementation: Responding*

Preventing Airway Obstruction. Without treatment, head and neck cancers grow, obstruct the airway, and prevent GAS EXCHANGE. Airway obstruction also can occur as a complication of treatment modalities.

Planning: Expected Outcomes. The patient with head and neck cancer is expected to attain and maintain adequate GAS EXCHANGE and tissue oxygenation. Indicators include:

- Arterial blood gas values within the normal range
- Rate and depth of respiration within the normal range
- Pulse oximetry within the normal range

Interventions. The focus of treatment is to remove or eradicate the cancer while preserving as much function as possible. The oncologist presents the available treatment options. Surgery, radiation, chemotherapy, or biotherapy may be used alone or in combination, depending on the stage of the disease and the patient's general health. Considerations for treatment options include the patient's physical condition, NUTRITION status, and age; the effects of the tumor on body function; and the patient's personal choice. Treatment for laryngeal cancer may range from radiation therapy (for a small specific area or tumor) to total laryngopharyngectomy with bilateral neck dissections followed by radiation therapy, depending on the extent and location of the lesion. Voice-conservation procedures are used only if they do not risk incomplete removal of the tumor. Nursing care focuses on preoperative preparation, optimal in-hospital care, discharge planning and teaching, and extensive outpatient rehabilitation.

Nonsurgical Management. Monitor GAS EXCHANGE and the respiratory system by assessing respiratory rate, breath sounds, pulse oximetry, and arterial blood gas values. Airway obstruction can occur from tumor growth, edema, or both. Teach the patient to use the Fowler's and semi-Fowler's positions for best gas exchange. Sitting upright in a reclining chair may promote more comfortable breathing. Chapters 4 and 7 provide additional information on palliation and pain control for patients who elect not to have therapy and for those whose therapy has not been effective.

Radiation therapy for treatment of small cancers in specific locations has a cure rate of at least 80%. Standard therapy uses 5000 to 7500 rad (radiation absorbed dose), usually over 6 weeks and in daily or twice-daily doses. Intensity-modulated

radiotherapy (IMRT) is recommended to provide higher doses directly to the tumor with less damage to surrounding normal tissues (NCCN, 2016). Radiation may be used alone or in combination with surgery and chemotherapy (see Chapter 22). It can be performed before or after surgery. Most patients have hoarseness, dysphagia, skin problems, impaired taste, and dry mouth for a few weeks after radiation therapy (McLaughlin & Mahon, 2014a).

Hoarseness may become worse during therapy. Reassure the patient that voice improves within 4 to 6 weeks after completion of radiation therapy. Urge him or her to use voice rest and alternative means of communication until the effects of radiation therapy have passed. Collaborate with the speech and language pathologist to help the patient communicate.

Most patients have a sore throat and difficulty swallowing during radiation therapy to the neck. Gargling with saline or sucking ice may decrease discomfort. Mouthwashes and throat sprays containing a local anesthetic agent such as lidocaine or diphenhydramine can provide temporary relief. Analgesic drugs may be prescribed.

The skin at the site of irradiation becomes red and tender and may peel during therapy. Instruct the patient to avoid exposing this area to sun, heat, cold, and abrasive actions such as shaving. Teach the patient to wear protective clothing made of soft cotton and to wash this area gently daily with a mild soap such as Dove. Using appropriate skin care products (approved by the radiation-oncology department) can reduce the intensity of skin reactions.

If the salivary glands are in the irradiation path, the mouth becomes dry (xerostomia). This effect is long term and may be permanent, and a dental consultation is needed. Some of the problems from reduced saliva include increased risk for dental caries, increased risk for oral infections, bad breath, and taste changes. Fluoride gel trays and nightly fluoride treatments can reduce the incidence of tooth deterioration. The trays can be worn during radiation therapy to prevent radiation scatter from the beam deflecting off existing metal inside the mouth. Although there is no cure for xerostomia, interventions can help reduce the discomfort. Heavy fluid intake, particularly water, and humidification can help ease the discomfort. Some patients benefit from the use of artificial saliva such as Salivart, moisturizing sprays or gels such as Mouth Kote, or saliva stimulants such as Salagen and cevimeline (cholinergic drugs).

Chemotherapy can be used alone or in addition to surgery or radiation for head and neck cancer. Often chemotherapy and radiation therapy *(chemoradiation)* are used at the same time. Although the exact drugs used may vary, depending on cancer cell features, most chemotherapy regimens for head and neck cancers include cisplatin (or another platinum-based drug) in combination with 5FU (NCCN, 2016). The oral cavity effects of radiation are intensified with concurrent chemotherapy. These can be uncomfortable, and patients often request breaks in the treatment regimen. However, these breaks in treatment do affect treatment outcome and should be avoided. Intense patient education before and support during treatment can improve patient adherence to the treatment plan (Mason et al., 2013). Chapter 22 discusses the general care needs of patients receiving chemotherapy.

Biotherapy (targeted therapy) with an epidermal growth-factor receptor inhibitor (EGFRI) such as cetuximab (Erbitux) (NCCN, 2016) is used for patients whose tumors overexpress the receptor. Although it is a targeted therapy, this drug blocks

EGFRs in normal tissues, as well as those in the tumor. As a result, severe skin reactions are common and difficult for the patient.

❓ NCLEX EXAMINATION CHALLENGE 29-1

Health Promotion and Maintenance

A client about to undergo radiation therapy for head and neck cancer (pharyngeal) asks what side effects are expected from this therapy. Which side effects does the nurse teach the client to expect? **Select all that apply.**
A. Scalp and eyebrow alopecia
B. Taste sensation loss or changes
C. Increased risk for sinus infections
D. Increased risk for skin breakdown
E. Moderate weight gain
F. Increased risk for cavities

Surgical Management. Tumor size, node number, and metastasis location (TNM classification) determine the type of surgery needed for the specific head and neck cancer (see Chapter 21). Very small, early-stage tumors may be removed by laser therapy or photodynamic therapy; however, few head and neck tumors are found at this stage, and most require extensive traditional surgery. Reconstruction is determined by the tumor size and amount of tissue to be resected and reconstructed. Surgical procedures for head and neck cancers include laryngectomy (total and partial), tracheotomy, and oropharyngeal cancer resections. The major types of surgery for laryngeal cancer include cord stripping, removal of a vocal cord (**cordectomy**), partial laryngectomy, and total laryngectomy. If cancer is in the lymph nodes in the neck, the surgeon performs a nodal neck dissection along with removal of the primary tumor ("radical neck").

Preoperative Care. Teach the patient and family about the tumor. The surgeon explains the surgical procedure and obtains informed consent. Discuss and interpret the implications of such consent with the patient and family. Chapter 14 describes general preoperative assessment and education needs.

Explain about self-management of the airway, suctioning, pain-control methods, the critical care environment (including ventilators and critical care routines), NUTRITION support, feeding tubes, and plans for discharge. The patient will need to learn new methods of speech, at least during the time that mechanical ventilation is used and, depending on surgery type, perhaps forever. Along with the speech and language pathologist, help the patient prepare for this change before surgery and practice the use of the selected form of communication (see Chart 29-1 and the discussion of Maintaining Communication in Chapter 28). Determine the communication method preferred by the patient.

Operative Procedures. Table 29-2 lists specific information about the various surgical procedures for laryngeal cancer. Hemilaryngectomy (vertical or horizontal) and supraglottic laryngectomy are types of partial voice-conservation laryngectomies.

To protect the airway, a tracheostomy is needed. With a partial laryngectomy, the tracheostomy is usually temporary. With a total laryngectomy, the upper airway is separated from the throat and esophagus, and a permanent laryngectomy stoma in the neck is created.

Neck dissection includes the removal of lymph nodes, the sternocleidomastoid muscle, the jugular vein, the 11th cranial

◎ CHART 29-1   Best Practice for Patient Safety & Quality Care QSEN

Communicating With a Patient Who Is Unable To Speak

- Assess the patient's reading skills and cognition.
- Determine in what language (languages) the patient is most fluent.
- Collaborate with a speech and language pathologist.
- If the patient requires vision-enhancing or hearing-enhancing devices, be sure these are available and in use.
- Provide the patient with a variety of techniques to practice before verbal skills are lost to determine with which one(s) the patient feels most comfortable. These may include:
  - Alphabet board
  - Picture board
  - Paper and pencil
  - Magic Slate
  - Hand signals/gestures
  - Computer with e-triloquist program
  - Programmable speech-generating devices (text-to-speech communication aid)
- Reinforce to the patient the technique for esophageal speech presented by the speech and language pathologist and provide the time for practice.
- Use a normal tone of voice to talk with the patient (unless hearing is a pre-existing problem, a change in the ability to speak does not interfere with the patient's ability to hear).
- Ensure that the call-light board at the nurses' station indicates a nonspeaking patient.
- Teach the patient to make noise to indicate that immediate attention is needed at the bedside when he or she signals by call light. Such noises can include tapping the side rail with a spoon, making clicking noises with the tongue, using a bell, or working a noisemaker. Be sure that whatever method is selected is listed on the call-light board.
- When face-to-face with the patient:
  - Phrase questions in a "yes" or "no" format.
  - Watch the patient's face for indications of understanding or the lack of it.
  - Listen attentively to any sound the patient makes.
- If writing is selected as the method to communicate, assess whether the patient is right handed or left handed and ensure appropriate writing materials are within reach. Use the other arm for IV placement.
  - Ensure that the preferred method of communication is documented in the patient record and is communicated to all care providers.
  - Encourage the family to work with the patient in the use of the selected method.
  - Provide praise and encouragement.
  - Do not avoid talking with the patient.
  - Allow the patient to set the pace for communication.

nerve, and surrounding soft tissue. Shoulder drop is expected after extensive surgery. Physical therapy can help the patient ease the shoulder drop by using other muscle groups.

Postoperative Care. Head and neck surgery often lasts 8 hours or longer, and the patient spends the immediate period after surgery in an ICU environment. Monitor airway patency, vital signs, hemodynamic status, and comfort level. Monitor for hemorrhage and other general complications of anesthesia and surgery (see Chapter 16). Take vital signs hourly for the first 24 hours and then according to agency policy until the patient is stable. After the patient is transferred from the ICU, vital signs are monitored according to agency policy.

Complications after surgery include airway obstruction, hemorrhage, wound breakdown, and tumor recurrence. *The first priorities after head and neck surgery are airway maintenance*

TABLE 29-2 Surgical Procedures for Laryngeal Cancer and Their Effect on Voice Quality

PROCEDURE	DESCRIPTION	RESULTING VOICE QUALITY
Laser surgery	Tumor reduced or destroyed by laser beam through laryngoscope	Normal/hoarse
Transoral cordectomy	Tumor (early lesion) resected through laryngoscope	Normal/hoarse (high cure rate)
Laryngofissure	No cord removed (early lesion)	Normal (high cure rate)
Supraglottic partial laryngectomy	Hyoid bone, false cords, and epiglottis removed Neck dissection on affected side performed if nodes involved	Normal/hoarse
Hemilaryngectomy or vertical laryngectomy	One true cord, one false cord, and one half of thyroid cartilage removed	Hoarse
Total laryngectomy	Entire larynx, hyoid bone, strap muscles, one or two tracheal rings removed Nodal neck dissection if nodes involved	No natural voice

and GAS EXCHANGE. Other priorities are wound, flap, and reconstructive tissue care; pain management; NUTRITION; and psychological adjustment, including speech and language therapy.

Airway Maintenance and Gas Exchange. Immediately after surgery, the patient may need ventilatory assistance. Most patients wean easily from the ventilator after this type of surgery because the thoracic and abdominal cavities are not entered. During weaning, the patient usually uses a tracheostomy collar (over the artificial airway or open stoma) with oxygen and humidity to help move mucus secretions. Secretions may remain blood tinged for 1 to 2 days. Use Standard Precautions and report any increase in bleeding to the surgeon. Humidity helps remove crusts and prevents obstruction of the tube with secretions. A laryngectomy tube is used for patients who have undergone a *total laryngectomy* and need an appliance to prevent scar tissue shrinkage of the skin-tracheal border. This tube is similar to a tracheostomy tube but is shorter and wider with a larger lumen. Laryngectomy tube care is similar to tracheostomy tube care (see Chapter 28), except that the patient can change the laryngectomy tube daily or as needed. A laryngectomy button is similar to a laryngectomy tube but is softer, has a single lumen, and is very short. A button is comfortable for the patient, is easily removed for cleaning, and is available in various sizes for a custom fit. Provide alternative communication techniques because the patient cannot speak.

Coughing and deep breathing are usually effective in clearing secretions. Instruct the patient how to cough and deep breathe to clear secretions.

Oral secretions can be suctioned by the alert patient using a Yankauer or tonsillar suction or a soft flexible catheter. Teach the patient to suction *away* from the surgical side to prevent opening the wound. Using a table mirror helps the patient see the area more clearly. Provide a clean environment for the catheter.

Stoma care after a total laryngectomy is a combination of wound care and airway care. Inspect the stoma with a flashlight. Clean the suture line with sterile saline (or a prescribed solution) to prevent secretions from forming crusts and obstructing the airway. Perform suture line care every 1 to 2 hours during the first few days after surgery and then every 4 hours. The mucosa of the stoma and trachea should be bright and shiny and without crusts, similar to the appearance of the oral mucosa.

Wound, Flap, and Reconstructive Tissue Care. Tissue "flaps" may be used to close the wound and improve appearance. Flaps are skin, subcutaneous tissue, and sometimes muscle, taken from other body areas used for reconstruction after head and neck resection. After neck dissection, the surgeon places a split-thickness skin graft (STSG) over the exposed carotid artery before covering it with skin flaps or reconstructive flaps.

The first 24 hours after surgery are critical. Evaluate all grafts and flaps hourly for the first 72 hours. Monitor capillary refill, color, drainage, and Doppler activity of the major blood vessel to the area. Report changes to the surgeon immediately because surgical intervention may be needed. Position the patient so the surgical flaps are not dependent.

Hemorrhage. Hemorrhage is a possible complication after any surgery, but it is uncommon with laryngectomy. The surgeon often places a closed surgical drain in the neck area to collect blood and drainage for about 72 hours after surgery. The drain also helps maintain the position of the reconstructed skin flaps. Any drain obstruction or equipment malfunction may cause a buildup of blood or fluid under the flaps that can impair blood flow and result in flap failure. A sudden stoppage of drainage may indicate drain obstruction by a clot. Monitor and record the amount and character of drainage. Check the patency and functioning of the drainage system. Report any drain malfunction or change in flap appearance to the surgeon. Depending on the surgeon's preference and the agency's policy, you may need to empty the drainage container or "milk" the drain (but avoid creasing or "stripping" the tubing).

Wound Breakdown. Wound breakdown with loss of TISSUE INTEGRITY is a complication caused by poor NUTRITION, a long smoking history, alcohol use, wound contamination, and radiation therapy before surgery. Manage wound breakdown with packing and local care as prescribed to keep the wound clean and stimulate the growth of healthy granulation tissue. Wounds may be extensive, and the carotid artery may be exposed. Split-thickness skin grafts often are placed over the carotid artery for protection in the event of wound dehiscence. As the wound heals, granulation tissue covers the artery and prevents rupture. If granulation is slow and the carotid artery is at risk, another surgical flap may be made to cover the artery and close the wound.

When the carotid artery ruptures, large amounts of bright red blood spurt quickly. It is also possible for the carotid artery to have a small leak, with continuous oozing of bright red blood. Usually a small leak leads to a complete rupture within a short time.

Pain Management. Pain is caused by the surgical cutting or manipulation of tissue and by nerve compression. Pain should

! **NURSING SAFETY PRIORITY** QSEN

Critical Rescue

Assess the patient hourly for the first several days after head and neck surgery to recognize a carotid artery leak. If you suspect a leak, respond by calling the Rapid Response Team and **do not touch the area because additional pressure could cause an immediate rupture.** If the carotid artery actually ruptures because of drying or infection, immediately place constant pressure over the site and secure the airway. Maintain direct manual, continuous pressure on the carotid artery and immediately transport the patient to the operating room for carotid resection. Do not leave the patient. Carotid artery rupture has a high risk for stroke and death.

be controlled, and the patient should still be able to participate in his or her care. Morphine (Duramorph, Statex ✦) often is given IV by a patient-controlled analgesia (PCA) pump for the first 1 to 2 days after surgery. As the patient progresses, liquid opioid analgesics can be given by feeding tube. Oral drugs for pain and discomfort are started only after the patient can tolerate oral intake. After discharge, the patient still requires pain management, especially if he or she is receiving radiation therapy. An adjunct to the pain regimen may be liquid NSAIDs along with opioid analgesics. Tricyclic antidepressants may also be used for the lancinating pain of nerve-root involvement.

Nutrition. Many patients with head and neck cancer have taste changes and some degree of inadequate NUTRITION (malnutrition) before cancer treatment begins (McLaughlin & Mahon, 2014b). All patients are at risk for malnutrition during treatment for head and neck cancer. A nasogastric, gastrostomy, or jejunostomy tube is placed during surgery for nutrition support while the head and neck heal. After the intestinal tract is motile, nutrients can be given via the feeding tube. The dietitian assesses the patient before surgery and is available for consultation after surgery. Replacement for calorie, protein, and water losses is calculated carefully for each patient (Ardilio, 2011).

The feeding tube usually remains in place for 7 to 10 days after surgery. Before removing the tube, assess the patient's ability to swallow if NUTRITION is to be given by mouth. Aspiration *cannot* occur after a total laryngectomy because the airway is completely separated from the esophagus. Stay with the patient during the first few swallowing attempts. Swallowing may be uncomfortable at first, and analgesics may be needed. If difficulty persists, a swallowing study may be needed.

Speech and Language Rehabilitation. The patient's voice quality and speech are altered after surgery. Although this problem has enormous effects on the patient's ability to maintain social interactions, continue employment, and maintain a desired quality of life, it is often poorly addressed while he or she is hospitalized. Working with him or her and the family toward developing an acceptable communication method during the inpatient period is essential for a satisfactory outcome.

Together with the speech and language pathologist (SLP), discuss the principles of speech therapy with the patient and family early in the course of the treatment plan (see Chart 29-1). Voice and speech differences depend on the type of surgical resection (see Table 29-2). Speech production varies with patient practice, amount of tissue removed, and radiation effects but can be very understandable. Patients have reported ongoing difficulties with speech and communication to be the most distressing problem for months to years after head and neck cancer therapy.

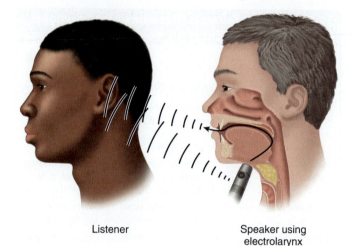

Listener   Speaker using electrolarynx

FIG. 29-1 An electrolarynx to generate speech after a laryngectomy.

The speech rehabilitation plan for patients who have a total laryngectomy at first consists of writing, using a picture board, or using a computer. The patient then uses an artificial larynx and may eventually learn esophageal speech. For success, the patient needs encouragement and support from the SLP, hospital team, and family while relearning to speak. This process is time consuming and requires concentration each time the patient speaks. Having a **laryngectomee** (an adult who has had a laryngectomy) from one of the local self-help organizations visit the patient and family is often beneficial. The International Association of Laryngectomees is very supportive, as is the ACS Visitor Program.

Esophageal speech is attempted by most patients who have a total laryngectomy. Sound can be produced this way by "burping" the air swallowed or injected into the esophageal pharynx and shaping the words in the mouth. The voice produced is a monotone; it cannot be raised or lowered and carries no pitch. If patients do not have adequate hearing, esophageal speech will be difficult because they need to use their mouth to shape the words as they hear them. Hearing-impaired patients may need hearing aids.

Mechanical devices, called *electrolarynges,* may be used for communication. Most are battery-powered devices placed against the side of the neck or cheek (Fig. 29-1). The air inside the mouth and throat is vibrated, and the patient moves his or her lips and tongue as usual. The quality of speech generated with mechanical devices is robotlike.

Tracheoesophageal puncture (TEP) may be used if esophageal speech is ineffective and if the patient meets strict criteria. A small surgical puncture is created between the trachea and the esophagus using a special catheter. After the puncture heals, a silicone prosthesis (e.g., the Blom-Singer prosthesis or the Panje Voice Button) is inserted in place of the catheter. The patient covers the stoma and the opening of the prosthesis with a finger or with a special valve to divert air from the lungs, through the trachea, into the esophagus, and out of the mouth where lip and tongue movement produces speech.

Surgical Procedures for Other Head and Neck Cancers. The surgeries for other head and neck cancers are called *composite resections.* These resections are a combination of surgical procedures, including partial or total glossectomies (tongue removal), partial mandibulectomies (jaw removal) and, if needed, nodal neck dissections. Tracheostomy may be planned to provide an adequate airway. (See Chapter 53 for more information about oral cancer.)

Tracheotomy. A tracheotomy is a surgical incision into the trachea for the purpose of establishing an airway (tracheostomy). It can be performed as an emergency procedure or as a scheduled surgical procedure. A tracheostomy can be temporary or permanent. Chapter 28 discusses the nursing care of a patient with a tracheostomy.

Preventing Aspiration

Planning: Expected Outcomes. The patient with head and neck cancer is expected to not aspirate food, gastric contents, or oral secretions into the lungs. Indicators include that the patient often or consistently demonstrates these behaviors:

- Positions self upright for eating or drinking
- Selects foods according to swallowing ability
- Chooses liquids and foods of proper consistency

Interventions. The surgical changes in the upper respiratory tract and altered swallowing mechanisms increase the patient's risk for aspiration. Aspiration can result in pneumonia, weight loss, and prolonged hospitalization. Chart 28-5 lists actions for aspiration prevention.

A nasogastric (NG) feeding tube increases the risk for aspiration because it keeps the lower esophageal sphincter partially open. The one exception is the patient who has undergone a total laryngectomy. In these cases, the airway is separated from the esophagus, making aspiration impossible; and the patient is *not* at risk. Most patients who need enteral feeding supplementation have a percutaneous endoscopic gastrostomy (PEG) tube placed rather than an NG tube. See Chapter 60 for care of patients receiving enteral NUTRITION by NG or PEG tube.

A dynamic swallow study, such as a barium swallow under fluoroscopy, evaluates a patient's ability to protect the airway from aspiration and helps determine the appropriate method of swallow rehabilitation (Balusik, 2014). In many cases, enteral feedings are used because of either the patient's inability to swallow or continued aspiration risk.

Swallowing can be a problem for the patient who has a tracheostomy tube. It can be normal if the cranial nerves and anatomic structures are intact. In a normal swallow, the larynx rises and moves forward to protect itself from the passing stream of food and saliva. The tracheostomy tube may fix the larynx in place, resulting in difficulty swallowing.

An inflated tracheostomy tube cuff can balloon backward into the esophagus and interfere with the passage of food. The wall between the posterior trachea and the esophagus is very thin, which allows this pushing action. The patient who is cognitively intact may adapt to eating normal food when the tracheostomy tube is small and the cuff is not inflated.

The patient who has had a partial vertical or supraglottic laryngectomy *must* be observed for aspiration. It is critical to teach the patient to use alternate methods of swallowing without aspirating. The "supraglottic" method of swallowing is especially effective after a partial laryngectomy or base-of-tongue resection (Chart 29-2). To reinforce teaching and learning, place a chart in the patient's room detailing the steps. A dynamic swallow study is performed to guide rehabilitation for swallowing and to evaluate the patient's ability to protect the airway.

Minimizing Anxiety

Planning: Expected Outcomes. The patient with head and neck cancer is expected to have decreased anxiety. Indicators include that the patient often or consistently demonstrates:

> **CHART 29-2** Patient and Family Education: Preparing for Self-Management
>
> **The Supraglottic Method of Swallowing**
>
> 1. Place yourself in an upright, preferably out-of-bed, position.
> 2. Clear your throat.
> 3. Take a deep breath.
> 4. Place ½ to 1 teaspoon of food into your mouth.
> 5. Hold your breath or "bear down" (Valsalva maneuver).
> 6. Swallow twice.
> 7. Release your breath and clear your throat.
> 8. Swallow twice again.
> 9. Breathe normally.
>
> This method exaggerates the normal protective mechanisms of cessation of respiration during the swallow. The double swallow attempts to clear food that may be pooling in the pharynx, vallecula, and piriform sinuses. This method is used only after a dynamic radiographic swallow study has demonstrated that it is appropriate and safe for the patient.

- Verbalization of reduced anxiety
- Absence of distress, irritability, and facial tension
- Effective use of coping strategies

Interventions. Conferences with all members of the interprofessional care team and the general nursing staff may be beneficial. Explore the reason for anxiety (e.g., fear of the unknown, lack of teaching, fear of pain, fear of death, loss of control, uncertainty). The patient and family often benefit from further information. Before the patient is scheduled for surgery (and while still at home), home care nurses or community-sponsored programs, such as the ACS, may be able to decrease fears about the disease process and surgical interventions.

Give prescribed antianxiety drugs, such as diazepam (Valium), with caution because of the risk for respiratory depression and because some of these drugs are eliminated slowly. Shorter-duration drugs, such as lorazepam (Ativan), may have fewer respiratory side effects. The location of the tumor and the presence of other lung disease may cause some degree of airway obstruction. For anxiety in these patients, drug therapy may include lorazepam (Ativan, Novo-Lorazem ✦) rather than a sedating agent.

Supporting Self-Esteem

Planning: Expected Outcomes. The patient with head and neck cancer is expected to accept body image changes. Indicators include that the patient often or consistently demonstrates:

- Willingness to touch and care for the affected body part
- Willingness to use strategies to enhance appearance
- Interaction with visitors, staff, and family members

Interventions. The patient with head and neck cancer usually has a change in self-concept and self-image resulting from issues such as the presence of a stoma or artificial airway, speech changes, and a change in the method of eating. Psychosocial issues may include guilt, regret, and uncertainty. He or she may not be able to speak at all or may have permanent speech deficits. Help the patient set realistic goals, starting with involvement in self-care. Teach the patient alternative communication methods so he or she can communicate in the hospital and after discharge.

Teach the family to ease the patient into a normal social environment. Use positive reinforcement and encouragement while demonstrating acceptance and caring behaviors. The family also may benefit from counseling sessions while the patient is still in the hospital.

After surgery, the patient may feel socially isolated because of the change in voice and facial appearance. Loose-fitting, high-collar shirts or sweaters, scarves, and jewelry can be worn to cover the laryngectomy stoma, tracheostomy tube, and other changes related to surgery. Cosmetics may aid in covering disfigurement. Most surgeons try to place the incisions in the natural skinfold lines if doing so does not pose a risk for cancer recurrence.

Care Coordination and Transition Management

If no complications occur, the patient is usually discharged home or to an extended-care facility within 2 weeks. At the time of discharge, he or she or a family member should be able to perform tracheostomy or stoma care and participate in NUTRITION, wound care, and communication methods.

The patient and family may feel more secure about discharge with a referral to support groups or a community health agency familiar with the care of patients recovering from head and neck cancer. Coordinate the efforts of the interprofessional team in assessing the specific discharge needs and making the appropriate referrals to home care agencies. Coordinate the scheduling for chemotherapy or radiation therapy with the patient and family.

Home Care Management. Extensive home care preparation is needed after a laryngectomy for cancer. The convalescent period is long, and airway management is complicated. The patient or family must be able to take an active role in care.

General cleanliness of the home is assessed by the home care nurse or case manager. For the patient with severe respiratory problems, home changes to allow for one-floor living may be needed. Increased humidity is needed. A humidifier add-on to a forced-air furnace can be obtained, or a room humidifier or vaporizer may be used. Be sure to stress that meticulous cleaning of these items is needed to prevent spread of mold or other sources of infection.

A home care nurse is often an important resource for the patient and family. This nurse assesses the patient and home situation for problems in self-care, complications, adjustment, and adherence to the medical regimen. Chart 29-3 lists assessment areas for the patient in the home after a laryngectomy. This nurse reinforces health care teaching, self-care teaching, and smoking-cessation regimens.

Self-Management Education. Education begins before surgery, and most self-care is taught in the hospital. Teach the patient and family how to care for the stoma or tracheostomy or laryngectomy tube, depending on the type of surgery performed. Review incision and airway care, including cleaning and inspecting for signs of infection. Chart 29-4 lists self-care actions for the patient after laryngeal cancer surgery. Many of these actions also apply to any surgery for head and neck cancer.

Stoma care teaching is focused on protection, which is needed as a result of the anatomic changes resulting from surgery. Instruct the patient to use a shower shield over the tube or stoma when bathing to prevent water from entering the airway. Teach men who use electric shavers to cover the stoma while shaving to keep hair from falling into it. Suggest that the patient wear a protective cover or stoma guard to protect the stoma during the day. Covering the opening has two benefits: (1) to

CHART 29-3 Home Care Assessment

Patients After Laryngectomy

Assess respiratory status and effectiveness of GAS EXCHANGE:
- Observe rate and depth of respiration.
- Auscultate lungs.
- Check patency of airway.
- Examine the tracheostomy drainage for amount, color, and character.
- Examine nail beds and mucous membranes for evidence of cyanosis.
- Obtain a pulse oximetry reading.

Assess condition of wound and TISSUE INTEGRITY:
- Remove dressings (noting condition of dressings).
- Cleanse the wound.
- Compare with previous notations of wound condition:
  - Presence, amount, and nature of exudate
  - Presence/absence of cellulitis
  - Presence/absence of odor

Assess patient's psychosocial status:
- Ask the patient about passing the time, visitors, and trips outside the house.
- Observe whether the patient communicates responses directly or whether a family member speaks for him or her.
- Observe patient and family member interactions.
- Determine which method of communication the patient has selected and observe the patient's skill with it.
- Observe whether the patient is wearing pajamas or is dressed in street clothes.
- Take the patient's temperature at each home care visit.

Assess the patient's understanding of illness and adherence to treatment:
- Manifestations to report to the health care provider
- Medication plan (correct timing and dose)
- Ambulation or positioning schedule
- Dressing changes/skin care
- Diet modifications (24-hour diet recall)
- Skill in tracheostomy or dressing care

Assess patient's NUTRITION status:
- Change in muscle mass
- Lackluster nails/sparse hair
- Recent weight loss greater than 10% of usual weight
- Impaired oral intake
- Difficulty swallowing
- Generalized edema

CHART 29-4 Patient and Family Education: Preparing for Self-Management

Home Laryngectomy Care

- Avoid swimming and use care when showering or shaving.
- Lean slightly forward and cover the stoma when coughing or sneezing.
- Wear a stoma guard or loose clothing to cover the stoma.
- Clean the stoma with mild soap and water. Lubricate the stoma with a non–oil-based ointment as needed.
- Increase humidity by using saline in the stoma as instructed, a bedside humidifier, pans of water, and houseplants.
- Obtain and wear a MedicAlert bracelet and emergency care card for life-threatening situations.

filter the air entering the stoma while keeping humidity in the airway; and (2) to enhance aesthetic appearance. Attractive coverings are available in the form of scarves, crocheted collars, and jewelry.

The skill level needed to be competent at tracheostomy care can be frightening to the patient and to the caregiver. Most adults are not familiar with sterile technique and suctioning, and cleaning the tube to prevent serious consequences can be daunting (Loerzel et al., 2014). The Quality Improvement box describes the development and implementation of a pilot project designed to increase the confidence and competence of patients and caregivers in the performance of this important care in the home.

Instruct the patient how to increase humidity in the home. Stress the importance of keeping well hydrated to prevent secretions from thickening.

Communication involves having the patient continue the selected communication method that began in the hospital. Instruct him or her to wear a medical alert (MedicAlert) bracelet and carry a special identification card. For patients with a laryngectomy, this card is available from the local chapters of the International Association of Laryngectomees. The card instructs the reader about providing an emergency airway or resuscitating someone who has a stoma.

Smoking cessation is a difficult but important issue after head and neck cancer surgery. Stress that smoking cessation can reduce the risk for developing other cancers and can increase the rate of healing from surgery. See Chapter 27 for details about smoking cessation.

Psychosocial Preparation. The many changes resulting from a laryngectomy influence physical, social, and emotional functioning for both the patient and his or her significant other (Sterba et al., 2016). Patients may perceive changes in their quality of life. Begin preparing the patient and family by scheduling a visit from an adult who has adjusted to these changes.

The patient with a permanent stoma, tracheostomy tube, NG or PEG tube, and wounds has an altered body image. Stress the importance of returning to as normal a lifestyle as possible. Most patients can resume many of their usual activities within 4 to 6 weeks after surgery. A longer time is needed after a combination of radiation therapy and surgery and for patients who also have other chronic diseases. The patient may be frustrated at times while trying to adjust to the many changes resulting from treatment of head and neck cancer.

The patient with a total laryngectomy cannot produce sounds during laughing and crying. Mucus secretions may appear unexpectedly when these emotions arise or when coughing or sneezing occurs. The mucus can be embarrassing, and the patient needs to be prepared to cover the stoma with a handkerchief or gauze. The patient who has undergone composite resections has difficulty with speech *and* swallowing. He or she may need to deal with tracheostomy and feeding tubes in public places.

Health Care Resources. Inform the patient and family of community organizations (e.g., ACS) and local laryngectomee clubs, which can offer support, information, and friendships. When the patient has problems paying for health care services, equipment, and prescriptions, a visiting nurse agency and social worker may be helpful in locating available resources.

In many areas, the local unit of the ACS or Canadian Cancer Society can help provide dressing materials and NUTRITION supplements to patients in need. These organizations may also provide transportation to and from follow-up visits or radiation therapy.

QUALITY IMPROVEMENT QSEN

Support and Education Reduce Caregiver Anxiety for Patients With Tracheostomies

Loerzel, V., Crosby, W., Reising, E., & Sole, M. (2014). Developing the tracheostomy care anxiety relief through education and support (T-CARES) program. *Clinical Journal of Oncology Nursing, 18*(5), 522-527.

Permanent tracheostomies are a common method of breathing for patients who have surgery for later-stage head and neck cancer. Both the patient and the caregiver must learn proper tracheostomy care for best function and to prevent complications. The care is considered complicated by non–health care adults and creates anxiety for the patient and the caregiver; a problem with the care of the tracheostomy at home is a common reason for hospital readmission.

A group of oncology nursing experts identified one cause of anxiety to be a lack of "hands on" practice with time for education and feedback for patients with tracheostomies and their caregivers. This group developed the pilot project T-CARES program of "Tracheostomy Care Anxiety Relief through Education and Support." The program consisted of an hour-long teaching session for tracheostomy care with an 18-minute video demonstration, group discussion with return demonstration, and assessment of 14 procedure-related skills. Instruction included basic airway anatomy, tube function description, and demonstrations of suctioning, tube cleaning and maintenance, emergency decannulation and reinsertion procedures, and equipment/supply use. The program also used hands-on practice performance of the techniques of gloving, suctioning, and other tracheostomy care using an anatomic training dummy. After completion of the 1-hour program, participants were permitted to continue the hands-on practice.

Both state and trait anxiety levels of the participants were measured before and after completion of the program. State anxiety decreased from a preprogram score of 50.5 to a postprogram score of 34.3, which reached statistical significance. After the program, all participants demonstrated acceptable competence on at least 9 of the 14 skills assessed.

Commentary: Implications for Practice and Research

Reducing anxiety in adults performing a new skill can improve competence and confidence for both the adult performing the skill and the adult who has the tracheostomy. This pilot project did not have a control group for comparison purposes. In addition, the article explaining the project did not indicate whether the participants were provided with a copy of the video to allow reinforcement of the information presented. Further research using a control group and a retest of participants 6 weeks after the initial program could help determine the utility of the T-CARES program. Another outcome to assess for program effectiveness is a comparison of the readmission rate between program participants and a control group who only receive "standard home-going instructions."

◆ Evaluation: Reflecting

Evaluate the care of the patient with head and neck cancer based on the identified priority patient problems. The expected outcomes are that the patient:

- Maintains a patent airway
- Performs self-care of the artificial airway and wound
- Performs ADLs independently or with minimal assistance
- Attains or maintains adequate NUTRITION
- Does not aspirate gastric contents or food
- Engages in desired social interactions

CLINICAL JUDGMENT CHALLENGE 29-1

Patient-Centered Care; Teamwork and Collaboration; Evidence-Based Practice QSEN

A 68-year-old man is diagnosed with stage 3 cancer of the larynx. He exercises daily, has never smoked, is a healthy weight, and serves as a deacon in his church. His only other health problem is asthma, which is well controlled with daily preventive drugs. He describes himself as a "social drinker" of no more than three martinis a day. His older brother died of lung cancer 3 years ago. He is very angry and states that all of his healthy living was a "waste." He is also concerned about his ability to keep on serving as a deacon, which requires public speaking. He asks whether you think God is angry with him. He is scheduled for hemilaryngectomy surgery.

1. Which, if any, risk factors does he have for cancer of the larynx?
2. Is his concern about public speaking valid? Why or why not?
3. How will you answer his question about God?
4. Which members of the interprofessional team could be most helpful with his current concerns?

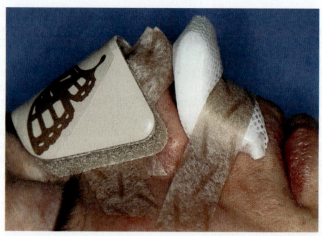

FIG. 29-2 Immediate postoperative appearance of a patient who has undergone rhinoplasty. Note the splint and gauze drip pad (moustache dressing). (From Tardy, M. E. [1997]. *Rhinoplasty: The art and science.* Philadelphia: Saunders. Used with permission.)

CANCER OF THE NOSE AND SINUSES

Tumors of the nasal cavities and sinuses result from the loss of CELLULAR REGULATION. Malignant tumors are rare and are more common among adults with chronic exposure to wood dusts, dusts from textiles, leather dusts, flour, nickel and chromium dust, mustard gas, and radium. Cigarette smoking along with these exposures increases the risk (ACS, 2017).

The onset of sinus cancer is slow, and symptoms resemble sinusitis. These include persistent nasal obstruction, drainage, bloody discharge, and pain that persists after treatment of sinusitis. Lymph node enlargement often occurs on the side with tumor mass. Tumor location is identified with x-ray, CT, or MRI imaging. A biopsy is performed to confirm the diagnosis.

Surgical removal of all or part of the tumor is the main treatment for nasopharyngeal cancers. It is usually combined with radiation therapy, especially intensity-modulated radiation therapy (IMRT) (see Chapter 22). Chemotherapy may be used in conjunction with surgery and radiation for some tumors. Problems after surgery include a change in body image or speech and altered NUTRITION, especially when the maxilla and floor of the nose are involved in the surgery. Patients often also have changes in taste and smell.

Provide general postoperative care (see Chapter 16), including maintaining a patent airway, monitoring for hemorrhage, providing wound care, assessing nutrition status, and performing tracheostomy care (if needed). (See Chapter 28 for tracheostomy care.) Perform careful mouth and sinus cavity care with saline irrigations using an electronic irrigation system (e.g., Water-Pik, Sonicare) or a syringe. Assess the patient for pain and infection. Collaborate with the dietitian to help the patient make food selections that promote healing.

FRACTURES OF THE NOSE

❖ PATHOPHYSIOLOGY

Nasal fractures often result from injury and can interfere with GAS EXCHANGE. If the bone or cartilage is not displaced and no complications are present, treatment may not be needed. However, displacement of either the bone or cartilage can cause

airway obstruction or cosmetic deformity and is a potential source of infection.

❖ INTERPROFESSIONAL COLLABORATIVE CARE

◆ Assessment: Noticing

Document any nasal problem, including deviation, malaligned nasal bridge, a change in nasal breathing, crackling of the skin *(crepitus)* on palpation, bruising, and pain. Blood or clear fluid (cerebrospinal fluid [CSF]) rarely drains from one or both nares as a result of a simple nasal fracture and, if present, indicates a serious injury (e.g., skull fracture). CSF can be differentiated from normal nasal secretions because CSF contains glucose that will test positive with a dipstick test for glucose. When CSF dries on a piece of filter paper, a yellow "halo" appears as a ring at the dried edge of the fluid.

◆ Interventions: Responding

The primary health care provider performs a simple **closed reduction** (moving the bones by palpation to realign them) of the nasal fracture using local or general anesthesia within the first 24 hours after injury. After 24 hours the fracture is more difficult to reduce because of edema and scar formation. Then reduction may be delayed for several days until edema is gone. Simple closed fractures may not need surgical intervention. Management focuses on pain relief and cold compresses to decrease swelling.

Rhinoplasty. Reduction and surgery may be needed for severe fractures or for those that do not heal properly. **Rhinoplasty** is a surgical reconstruction of the nose. It can be performed to repair a fractured nose and also to change the shape of the nose. The patient returns from surgery with packing in both nostrils, which prevents bleeding and provides support for the reconstructed nose. As long as the packing is in place, the patient cannot breathe through the nose. A "moustache" dressing (or drip pad), often a folded 2 × 2 gauze pad, is usually placed under the nose (Fig. 29-2). A splint or cast may cover the nose for better alignment and protection. Change or teach the patient to change the drip pad as necessary.

After surgery observe for edema and bleeding. Check vital signs every 4 hours until the patient is discharged. The patient with uncomplicated rhinoplasty is discharged the day of surgery. Instruct him or her and the family about the routine care described in the following paragraphs.

! NURSING SAFETY PRIORITY (QSEN)

Action Alert

Assessing how often the patient swallows after nasal surgery is a priority because repeated swallowing may indicate posterior nasal bleeding. Use a penlight to examine the throat for bleeding and notify the surgeon if bleeding is present.

Instruct the patient to stay in a semi-Fowler's position and to move slowly. Suggest that he or she rests and uses cool compresses on the nose, eyes, and face to help reduce swelling and bruising. If a general anesthetic was used, soft foods can be eaten once the patient is alert and the gag reflex has returned. Urge the patient to drink at least 2500 mL/day.

To prevent bleeding, teach the patient to limit Valsalva maneuvers (e.g., forceful coughing or straining during a bowel movement), not to sniff upward or blow the nose, and not to sneeze with the mouth closed for the first few days after the packing is removed. Instruct the patient to avoid aspirin and other NSAIDs to prevent bleeding. Antibiotics may be prescribed to prevent infection. Recommend the use of a humidifier to prevent mucosal drying. Explain that edema lasts for weeks and that the final surgical result will be evident in 6 to 12 months.

Nasoseptoplasty. Nasoseptoplasty, or **submucous resection** (SMR), may be needed to straighten a deviated septum when chronic symptoms or discomfort occurs. Slight nasal septum deviation causes no symptoms. Major deviations may obstruct the nasal passages or interfere with airflow and sinus drainage. The deviated section of cartilage and bone is removed or reshaped as an ambulatory surgical procedure. Nursing care is similar to that for a rhinoplasty.

? NCLEX EXAMINATION CHALLENGE 29-2

Health Promotion and Maintenance

Which interventions are **most appropriate** for the nurse to teach a client with a nasal fracture to reduce bleeding from the injury? **Select all that apply.**
A. "Avoid blowing or picking the nose."
B. "Drink at least 2000 mL of fluid daily."
C. "Take the antibiotics for as long as they are prescribed."
D. "Take in only liquids and eat no solid food for at least a week."
E. "Change the drip (moustache) dressing as soon as it becomes wet."
F. "Use acetaminophen for pain rather than aspirin or other NSAIDS."

EPISTAXIS

❖ PATHOPHYSIOLOGY

Epistaxis (nosebleed) is a common problem because of the many capillaries within the nose. Nosebleeds occur as a result of trauma, hypertension, blood dyscrasia (e.g., leukemia), inflammation, tumor, decreased humidity, nose blowing, nose picking, chronic cocaine use, and procedures such as nasogastric suctioning. Older adults tend to bleed most often from the posterior portion of the nose.

◎ CHART 29-5 Best Practice for Patient Safety & Quality Care (QSEN)

Emergency Care of a Patient With an Anterior Nosebleed

- Maintain Standard Precautions or Body Substance Precautions.
- Position the patient upright and leaning forward to prevent blood from entering the stomach and possible aspiration.
- Reassure the patient and attempt to keep him or her quiet to reduce anxiety and blood pressure.
- Apply direct lateral pressure to the nose for 10 minutes and apply ice or cool compresses to the nose and face if possible.
- If nasal packing is necessary, loosely pack both nares with gauze or nasal tampons.
- To prevent rebleeding from dislodging clots, instruct the patient to not blow the nose for 24 hours after the bleeding stops.
- Seek medical assistance if these measures are ineffective or if the bleeding occurs frequently.

❖ INTERPROFESSIONAL COLLABORATIVE CARE

The patient often reports that the bleeding started after sneezing or blowing the nose. Document the amount and color of the blood and take vital signs. Ask about the number, duration, and causes of previous bleeding episodes.

Chart 29-5 lists the best practices for emergency care of the patient with a nosebleed. An additional intervention for use at home or in the emergency department is a special nasal plug that contains an agent to promote blood clotting (sold by HemCon). The plug expands on contact with blood and compresses mucosal blood vessels.

Medical attention is needed if the nosebleed does not respond to these interventions. In such cases, the affected capillaries may be cauterized with silver nitrate or electrocautery, and the nose packed. Anterior packing controls bleeding from the anterior nasal cavity.

Posterior nasal bleeding is an emergency because it cannot be easily reached and the patient may lose a lot of blood quickly (Vacca & Poirier, 2013). Posterior packing, epistaxis catheters (nasal pressure tubes), or gel tampons are used to stop bleeding that originates in the posterior nasal region. With packing, the primary health care provider positions a large gauze pack in the posterior nasal cavity above the throat, threads the attached string through the nose, and tapes it to the patient's cheek to prevent pack movement. Epistaxis catheters look like very short (about 6 inches) urinary catheters (Fig. 29-3A). These tubes have an exterior balloon along the tube length in addition to an anchoring balloon on the end. Placement of posterior packing or pressure tubes is uncomfortable; and the airway may be obstructed with reduced GAS EXCHANGE if the pack slips. Fig. 29-3B shows a patient with tubes in place for a posterior nasal bleed.

Observe the patient for respiratory distress and tolerance of the packing or tubes. Humidity, oxygen, bedrest, and antibiotics may be prescribed. Opioid drugs may be prescribed for pain. Assess patients receiving opioids at least hourly for gag and cough reflexes. Use pulse oximetry to monitor for hypoxemia. The tubes or packing is usually removed after 1 to 3 days.

For posterior bleeds that do not respond to packing or tubes, additional options include cauterizing the blood vessels, ligating the vessels, or performing an embolization of the bleeding artery with interventional radiology. Potential complications of

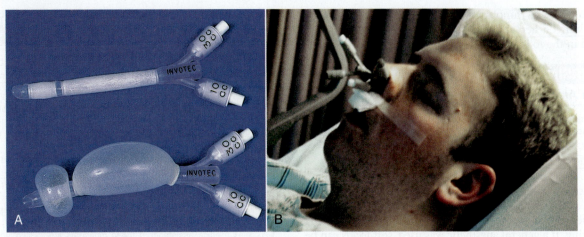

FIG. 29-3 A, Ultra-Stat epistaxis catheter. **B,** Patient with epistaxis catheters in place to control a posterior nasal bleed. (**A** courtesy Invotec International, Jacksonville, FL.)

embolization include facial pain, necrosis of skin or nasal mucosa, facial nerve paralysis, and blindness (Poetker, 2013).

After the tubes or packing is removed, teach the patient and family these interventions to use at home for comfort and safety:

- Petroleum jelly can be applied sparingly to the nares for lubrication and comfort. (Excessive application could cause inhalation of the jelly into the lungs and increase the risk for pneumonia.)
- Nasal saline sprays and humidification add moisture and prevent rebleeding.
- Avoid vigorous nose blowing, the use of aspirin or other NSAIDs, and strenuous activities such as heavy lifting for at least 1 month.

FACIAL TRAUMA

❖ PATHOPHYSIOLOGY

Facial trauma is described by the specific bones (e.g., mandibular, maxillary, orbital, nasal fractures) and the side of the face involved. Mandibular (lower jaw) fractures are the most common. *Le Fort I* is a nasoethmoid complex fracture. *Le Fort II* is a maxillary *and* nasoethmoid complex fracture. *Le Fort III* combines I and II plus an orbital-zygoma fracture, called *craniofacial disjunction* because the midface has no connection to the skull. The rich facial blood supply results in extensive bleeding and bruising.

❖ INTERPROFESSIONAL COLLABORATIVE CARE
◆ Assessment: Noticing

The priority action when caring for a patient with facial trauma is airway assessment for GAS EXCHANGE. Signs of airway obstruction are stridor, shortness of breath, dyspnea, anxiety, restlessness, hypoxia, hypercarbia (elevated blood levels of carbon dioxide), decreased oxygen saturation, cyanosis, and loss of consciousness. After establishing the airway, assess the trauma site for bleeding and obvious fractures. Check for soft-tissue edema, facial asymmetry, pain, or leakage of spinal fluid through the ears or nose, indicating a skull fracture. Assess vision and eye movement because orbital and maxillary fractures can entrap the eye nerves and muscles. Check behind the ears (mastoid area) for extensive bruising, known as the "battle sign," which is often associated with skull fracture and brain

trauma. Because facial trauma can occur with spinal trauma and skull fractures, cranial CT, facial series, and cervical spine x-rays are obtained.

◆ Interventions: Responding

The priority action is to establish and maintain an airway for adequate GAS EXCHANGE. Anticipate the need for emergency intubation, *tracheotomy,* or *cricothyroidotomy* (creation of a temporary airway by making a small opening in the throat between the thyroid cartilage and the cricoid cartilage). Care at first focuses on establishing an airway to ensure GAS EXCHANGE, controlling hemorrhage, and assessing for the extent of injury. If shock is present, fluid resuscitation and identification of bleeding sites are started immediately.

Time is critical in stabilizing the patient who has head and neck trauma. Early response and treatment by special interprofessional services (e.g., trauma team, maxillofacial surgeon, general surgeon, otolaryngologist, plastic surgeon, dentist) optimize the patient's recovery.

Stabilizing the fractured jaw allows the teeth to heal in proper alignment and involves *fixed occlusion* (wiring the jaws together with the mouth in a closed position). The patient remains in fixed occlusion for 6 to 10 weeks. Treatment delay, tooth infection, or poor oral care may cause jaw bone infection. This condition may then require surgical removal of dead tissue, IV antibiotic therapy, and a longer period with the jaws in a fixed position.

Extensive jaw fractures may require open reduction with internal fixation (ORIF) procedures. Compression plates and reconstruction plates with screws may be applied. Plates may be made of stainless steel, titanium, or Vitallium. If the mandibular fracture is repaired with titanium plates, the plates are permanent and do not interfere with MRI studies.

Facial fractures may be repaired with microplating surgical systems that involve bone substitutes or commercial bone graft. Shaping plates hold the bone fragments in place until new bone growth occurs. Bone cells grow into the bone substitute and re-matrix into a stable bone support. The plates may remain in place permanently or may be removed after healing.

With inner maxillary fixation (IMF), the bones are realigned and then wired in place with the bite closed. Nondisplaced aligned fractures can be repaired in a clinic or office using local dental anesthesia. General anesthesia is used to repair displaced or complex fractures or fractures that occur with other facial bone fractures.

After surgery, teach the patient about oral care with an irrigating device such as a Water-Pik or Sonicare. If the patient has inner maxillary fixation, teach self-management with wires in place, including a dental liquid diet. If the patient vomits, watch for aspiration because of the patient's inability to open the jaws to allow ejection of the emesis. Teach him or her how to cut the wires if vomiting occurs to maintain GAS EXCHANGE. If the wires are cut, instruct the patient to return to the surgeon for rewiring as soon as possible to reinstitute fixation.

> **! NURSING SAFETY PRIORITY** QSEN
>
> **Action Alert**
>
> Instruct the patient to keep wire cutters with him or her at all times to prevent aspiration if vomiting occurs.

NUTRITION is important and difficult for a patient with fractures because of oral fixation, pain, and surgery. Collaborate with the dietitian for patient teaching and support.

OBSTRUCTIVE SLEEP APNEA

❖ PATHOPHYSIOLOGY

Obstructive sleep apnea (OSA) is a breathing disruption during sleep that lasts at least 10 seconds and occurs a minimum of five times in an hour. The most common cause is upper airway obstruction by the soft palate or tongue. Factors that contribute to OSA include obesity, a large uvula, a short neck, smoking, enlarged tonsils or adenoids, and oropharyngeal edema.

During sleep the muscles relax, and the tongue and neck structures are displaced. As a result, the upper airway is obstructed, but chest movement is unimpaired. The apnea decreases GAS EXCHANGE, increases blood carbon dioxide levels, and decreases the pH. These blood gas changes stimulate neural centers. The sleeper awakens after 10 seconds or longer of apnea and corrects the obstruction, and respiration resumes. After he or she goes back to sleep, the cycle begins again, sometimes as often as every 5 minutes.

This cyclic pattern of disrupted sleep prevents the deep sleep needed for best rest, and the adult may have excessive daytime sleepiness, an inability to concentrate, and irritability. Long-term effects of chronic OSA include increased risk for hypertension, stroke, cognitive deficits, weight gain, diabetes, and pulmonary and cardiovascular disease (Veenstra & Untalan, 2014).

❖ INTERPROFESSIONAL COLLABORATIVE CARE

◆ Assessment: Noticing

Patients are often unaware that they have sleep apnea. The disorder should be suspected for any adult who has persistent daytime sleepiness or reports "waking up tired," particularly if he or she also snores heavily. Other symptoms include irritability and personality changes. Sleep apnea may be verified by family members who observe the problem when the adult sleeps. A complete assessment is performed when excessive daytime sleepiness is a problem.

A beginning assessment includes having the patient complete the STOP-Bang Sleep Apnea Questionnaire (Nations & Mayo, 2016). The patient is asked to answer yes or no to eight items (*S*noring, *T*iredness, *O*bserved as stopped breathing during sleep, *P*-treatment for high blood pressure, *B*ody mass index >35, *A*ge >50, *N*eck circumference >40 cm, and *G*ender-male). A yes score to fewer than three items indicates a low risk for OSA. A yes score to higher than three items indicates a high risk for OSA. This questionnaire is easy to administer and interpret and has both high reliability and validity. The results correlate well to overnight sleep study results and have some predictive value for both difficult intubations and postoperative respiratory complications (Nations & Mayo, 2016).

The most accurate test for sleep apnea is an overnight sleep study. The patient is directly observed while wearing a variety of monitoring equipment to evaluate depth of sleep, type of sleep, respiratory effort, oxygen saturation, and muscle movement. Monitoring devices include an electroencephalograph (EEG), an electrocardiograph (ECG), a pulse oximeter, and an electromyograph (EMG).

◆ Interventions: Responding

Changes in sleeping position or weight loss may correct mild sleep apnea and improve GAS EXCHANGE. Position-fixing devices may prevent subluxation of the tongue and reduce obstruction. Severe OSA requires additional methods to prevent obstruction.

A common method to prevent airway collapse is the use of noninvasive positive-pressure ventilation (NPPV) to hold open the upper airways. A nasal mask or full-facemask delivery system allows mechanical delivery of either bi-level positive airway pressure (BiPAP), autotitrating positive airway pressure (APAP), or nasal continuous positive airway pressure (CPAP). With BiPAP, a machine delivers a set inspiratory positive airway pressure at the beginning of each breath. As the patient begins to exhale, the machine delivers a lower end-expiratory pressure. These two pressures hold open the upper airways. With APAP, the machine adjusts continuously, resetting the pressure throughout the breathing cycle to meet the patient's needs. Nasal CPAP delivers a set positive airway pressure continuously during each cycle of inhalation and exhalation. For any positive-pressure ventilation delivered through a facemask during sleep, a small electric compressor is required. Proper fit of the mask over the nose and mouth or just over the nose is key to successful treatment (see Fig. 28-8). Although noisy, these methods are accepted by most patients after an adjustment period.

One drug has been approved to help manage the daytime sleepiness associated with OSA (modafinil [Attenace, Provigil]) and may help patients who have *narcolepsy* (uncontrolled daytime sleep) by promoting daytime wakefulness. This drug does *not* treat the cause of OSA. Sleep-inducing sedatives also are not considered first-line therapy.

Surgical intervention may involve a simple adenoidectomy, uvulectomy, or remodeling of the entire posterior oropharynx (uvulopalatopharyngoplasty [UPP]). Both conventional and laser surgeries are used for this purpose. A tracheostomy may be needed for very severe sleep apnea that is not relieved by more moderate interventions.

LARYNGEAL TRAUMA

Laryngeal trauma and damage occur with a crushing or direct-blow injury, fracture, or prolonged endotracheal intubation. Symptoms include difficulty breathing (dyspnea), inability to

? NCLEX EXAMINATION CHALLENGE 29-3

Safe and Effective Care Environment

With which client does the nurse anticipate complications from obstructive sleep apnea following abdominal surgery?
A. 28-year-old who is 80 lbs (36.4 kg) overweight and has a short neck
B. 48-year-old who has type 1 diabetes and chronic sinusitis
C. 58-year-old who has had gastroesophageal reflux disease for 10 years
D. 78-year-old who wears upper and lower dentures and has asthma

produce sound *(aphonia)*, hoarseness, and **subcutaneous emphysema** (air present in the subcutaneous tissue). Bleeding from the airway (**hemoptysis**) may occur, depending on the location of the trauma. The primary health care provider performs a direct visual examination of the larynx by laryngoscopy or fiberoptic laryngoscopy to determine the extent of the injury.

Management of patients with laryngeal injuries consists of assessing the effectiveness of GAS EXCHANGE and monitoring vital signs (including respiratory status and pulse oximetry) every 15 to 30 minutes. *Maintaining a patent airway is a priority.* Apply oxygen and humidification as prescribed to maintain adequate oxygen saturation. Signs of respiratory difficulty include tachypnea, nasal flaring, anxiety, sternal retraction, shortness of breath, restlessness, decreased oxygen saturation, decreased level of consciousness, and stridor.

! NURSING SAFETY PRIORITY **QSEN**

Critical Rescue

Assess the patient to recognize signs of respiratory difficulty (tachypnea, nasal flaring, anxiety, sternal retraction, shortness of breath, restlessness, decreased oxygen saturation, decreased level of consciousness, stridor). If any signs are present, respond by staying with the patient and instructing other trauma team members or the Rapid Response Team to prepare for an emergency intubation or tracheotomy.

Surgical intervention is needed for lacerations of the mucous membranes, cartilage exposure, and cord paralysis. Laryngeal repair is performed as soon as possible to prevent laryngeal stenosis and to cover any exposed cartilage. An artificial airway may be needed.

UPPER AIRWAY OBSTRUCTION

❖ PATHOPHYSIOLOGY

Upper airway obstruction is the interruption of airflow through nose, mouth, pharynx, or larynx. When GAS EXCHANGE is impaired, obstruction can be a life-threatening condition. Early recognition is essential to prevent complications, including respiratory arrest. Causes of upper airway obstruction include:
- Tongue edema (surgery, trauma, angioedema as an allergic response to a drug)
- Tongue occlusion (e.g., loss of gag reflex, loss of muscle tone, unconsciousness, coma)
- Laryngeal edema
- Peritonsillar and pharyngeal abscess
- Head and neck cancer
- Thick secretions
- Stroke and cerebral edema

- Smoke inhalation edema
- Facial, tracheal, or laryngeal trauma
- Foreign-body aspiration
- Burns of the head or neck area
- Anaphylaxis

One preventable cause of airway obstruction leading to asphyxiation is *inspissated* (thickly crusted) oral and nasopharyngeal secretions. In this condition, poor oral hygiene leads to thickening and hardening of secretions that can completely block the airway and lead to death. Proper nursing care can eliminate this cause of airway obstruction. Patients at highest risk are those who have an altered mental status and level of consciousness, are dehydrated, are unable to communicate, are unable to cough effectively, or are at risk for aspiration.

! NURSING SAFETY PRIORITY **QSEN**

Action Alert

Assess the oral care needs of the patient with risk factors for inspissated (thickly crusted) secretions daily. Ensure that whoever provides oral care understands the importance and the correct techniques for preventing secretion buildup and airway obstruction.

❖ INTERPROFESSIONAL COLLABORATIVE CARE

An acute airway obstruction from a foreign body may be managed in the community or emergency department. When chronic problems cause airway obstruction, more intensive interventions may be needed in an acute care setting.

◆ Assessment: Noticing

Airway obstruction is frightening, and prompt care is essential to prevent a partial obstruction from progressing to a complete obstruction. Partial obstruction produces general symptoms such as diaphoresis, tachycardia, and elevated blood pressure. Persistent or unexplained symptoms must be evaluated even though vague. Diagnostic procedures include chest or neck x-rays, laryngoscopic examination, and CT.

Observe for hypoxia and hypercarbia, restlessness, increasing anxiety, sternal retractions, a "seesawing" chest, abdominal movements, or a feeling of impending doom from air hunger. Use pulse oximetry or end-tidal carbon dioxide ($ETCO_2$ or $PETCO_2$) for ongoing monitoring of GAS EXCHANGE. Continually assess for stridor, cyanosis, and changes in level of consciousness.

◆ Interventions: Responding

Assess for the cause of the obstruction. When the obstruction is caused by the tongue falling back or excessive secretions, slightly extend the patient's head and neck and insert a nasal or an oral airway. Suction to remove any obstructing secretions. If the obstruction is caused by a foreign body, perform abdominal thrusts (Fig. 29-4).

Upper airway obstruction may require emergency procedures such as cricothyroidotomy, endotracheal intubation, or tracheotomy to improve GAS EXCHANGE. Laryngoscopy may be performed to determine the cause of obstruction or to remove foreign bodies.

Cricothyroidotomy is an emergency procedure performed by emergency medical personnel as a stab wound at the cricothyroid membrane between the thyroid cartilage and the cricoid cartilage (see Fig. 27-3). Any hollow tube—but preferably a

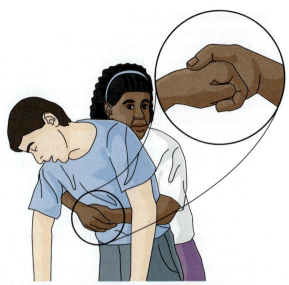

With the conscious victim standing or sitting, place your fist between the victim's lower rib cage and navel. Wrap the palm of your hand around your fist. A quick inward, upward thrust expels the air remaining in the victim's lungs, and with it the foreign body. If the first thrust is unsuccessful, repeat several thrusts in rapid succession until the foreign body is expelled or until the victim loses consciousness.

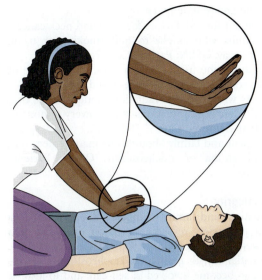

With the unconscious victim lying supine, straddle the victim's thighs. Place one hand on top of the other as shown, with the heel of the bottom hand just above the victim's navel. Quickly thrust inward and upward, toward the victim's head.

FIG. 29-4 Abdominal thrust maneuver (formerly known as the *Heimlich maneuver*) for relief of upper airway obstruction caused by a foreign body.

tracheostomy tube—can be placed through the opening to hold this airway open until a tracheotomy can be performed. This procedure is used when it is the *only* way to secure an airway. Another emergency procedure to bypass an obstruction is the insertion of a 14-gauge needle or a very small endotracheal tube directly into the cricoid space to allow airflow into and out of the lungs.

Endotracheal intubation is performed by inserting a tube into the trachea via the nose *(nasotracheal)* or mouth *(orotracheal)* by a physician, anesthesia provider, or other specially trained personnel.

Tracheotomy is a surgical procedure and takes about 5 to 10 minutes to perform. It is best performed in the operating room (OR) with the patient under local or general anesthesia but can be performed at the bedside. Local anesthesia is used if there is concern that the airway will be lost during the induction of anesthesia. A tracheotomy is reserved for the patient who cannot be easily intubated with an endotracheal tube. An emergency tracheotomy can establish an airway in less than 2 minutes. See Chapter 28 for a discussion of care of the patient with a tracheotomy.

Patients receiving mechanical ventilation for upper airway obstruction or respiratory failure may require a tracheostomy after 7 or more days of continuous intubation. In such cases, a tracheotomy is performed to prevent laryngeal injury by the endotracheal tube.

GET READY FOR THE NCLEX® EXAMINATION!

KEY POINTS

Review these Key Points for each NCLEX Examination Client Needs Category.

Safe and Effective Care Environment

- Use sterile technique when performing endotracheal or tracheal suctioning. **QSEN: Safety**
- Use Standard Precautions when caring for a patient with epistaxis. **QSEN: Safety**
- Supervise care delegated to licensed practical nurses/licensed vocational nurses (LPNs/LVNs) or nursing assistants to patients who have risk factors for airway obstruction. **QSEN: Safety**

- Use Aspiration Precautions for any patient with an altered level of consciousness or who has an endotracheal tube (see Chart 28-5). **QSEN: Safety**
- Apply knowledge of anatomy to prevent aspiration in a patient with a tracheostomy. **QSEN: Safety**
- Use correct technique to suction via a tracheostomy or laryngectomy tube. **QSEN: Safety**
- Teach the patient and family how to perform tracheostomy care (see Chart 28-3). **QSEN: Safety**
- Teach family members ways to communicate with a patient who cannot speak after surgery for head and neck cancer. **QSEN: Patient-Centered Care**

Health Promotion and Maintenance

- Assess the patient for risk factors for head and neck cancer.
- Encourage adults who smoke to quit smoking or using tobacco in any way. **QSEN: Patient-Centered Care**
- Encourage adults who use alcohol to reduce their intake of alcoholic beverages. **QSEN: Evidence-Based Practice**
- Teach patients who have had radiation therapy to the oral cavity to have dental examinations at least every 6 months. **QSEN: Patient-Centered Care**
- Teach the patient and family about home management of a laryngectomy stoma or tracheostomy. **QSEN: Patient-Centered Care**

Psychosocial Integrity

- Allow the patient and family members the opportunity to express fear or anxiety regarding a cancer diagnosis or a change in breathing status. **QSEN: Patient-Centered Care**
- Encourage patients with permanent tracheostomies or laryngectomies to become involved in self-care and to look at the wound and touch the affected area. **QSEN: Patient-Centered Care**
- Allow the patient and family to grieve the loss of function and change in body image. **QSEN: Patient-Centered Care**
- Allow time to communicate with the patient who has voice loss. **QSEN: Patient-Centered Care**
- Refer patients and families to local chapters of the ACS or the Canadian Cancer Society after surgery for head and neck cancer. **QSEN: Patient-Centered Care**

Physiological Integrity

- Assess the airway patency of any patient who experiences facial or nasal trauma. **QSEN: Safety**
- Perform a focused upper respiratory assessment and re-assessment to determine adequacy of GAS EXCHANGE and tissue perfusion. **QSEN: Patient-Centered Care**
- Notify the Rapid Response Team when a patient experiences a posterior nasal bleed. **QSEN: Safety**
- Check the airway and packing at least every hour for a patient who has posterior nasal packing placed after nasal surgery or posterior epistaxis. **QSEN: Evidence-Based Practice**
- Instruct patients who have had mandibular immobilization or fixation after a mandibular fracture to keep wire cutters with them at all times. **QSEN: Safety**
- Apply oxygen to any patient who develops stridor. **QSEN: Safety**
- Use a manual resuscitation bag to ventilate the patient if the tracheostomy tube has dislodged or been decannulated. **QSEN: Safety**
- Assess the new tracheostomy stoma site at least once per shift for purulent drainage, redness, pain, and swelling as indicators of infection. **QSEN: Safety**
- Keep the tracheal cuff pressure between 14 and 20 mm Hg to prevent tissue injury. **QSEN: Evidence-Based Practice**

SELECTED BIBLIOGRAPHY

Asterisk indicates a classic or definitive work on this subject.

American Cancer Society (ACS). (2017). *Cancer facts and figures, 2017.* 01-300M–No. 500817. Atlanta: Author.

*Ardilio, S. (2011). Calculating nutrition needs for a patient with head and neck cancer. *Clinical Journal of Oncology Nursing, 15*(5), 457–459.

Balusik, B. (2014). Management of dysphagia in patients with head and neck cancer. *Clinical Journal of Oncology Nursing, 18*(2), 149–150.

Canadian Cancer Society, & Statistics Canada. (2016). *Canadian cancer statistics, 2016.* Toronto, ON: Canadian Cancer Society. www.cancer.ca/~/media/cancer.ca/CW/cancer%20information/cancer%20101/Canadian%20cancer%20statistics/Canadian-Cancer-Statistics-2016-EN.pdf?la=en.

Fronczek, A. (2015). A phenomenologic study of family caregivers of patients with head and neck cancers. *Oncology Nursing Forum, 42*(6), 593–600.

Loerzel, V., Crosby, W., Reising, E., & Sole, M. (2014). Developing the tracheostomy care anxiety relief through education and support (T-CARES) program. *Clinical Journal of Oncology Nursing, 18*(5), 522–527.

Mason, H., DeRubeis, M., Foster, J., Taylor, J., & Worden, F. (2013). Outcomes evaluation of a weekly nurse practitioner-managed symptom management clinic for patients with head and neck cancer treated with chemotherapy. *Oncology Nursing Forum, 40*(6), 581–586.

McCance, K., Huether, S., Brashers, V., & Rote, N. (2014). *Pathophysiology: The biologic basis for disease in adults and children* (7th ed.). St. Louis: Mosby.

McKiernan, J., & Thom, B. (2016). Human papillomavirus-related oropharyngeal cancer: A review of nursing considerations. *The American Journal of Nursing, 116*(8), 34–43.

McLaughlin, L., & Mahon, S. (2014a). A meta-analysis of the relationship among impaired taste and treatment, treatment type, and tumor site in head and neck cancer treatment survivors. *Oncology Nursing Forum, 41*(3), E194–E202.

McLaughlin, L., & Mahon, S. (2014b). Taste dysfunction and eating behaviors in survivors of head and neck cancer treatment. *Medsurg Nursing, 230*(3), 165–170.

National Comprehensive Cancer Network (NCCN). (2016). NCCN Clinical practice guidelines in oncology: Head and neck cancers *(version 1.2015).* www.nccn.org/professionals/physician_gls/pdf/head-and-neck.pdf.

Nations, R., & Mayo, A. (2016). Critique of the STOP-Bang sleep apnea questionnaire. *Clinical Nurse Specialist CNS, 30*(1), 11–14.

Poetker, D. (2013). Adults with epistaxis. *Patient management perspectives in otolaryngology, 42*(6), 1–26.

Rettig, E., & D'Souza, G. (2015). Epidemiology of head and neck cancer. *Surgical Oncology Clinics of North America, 24*(3), 379–396.

Schiech, L. (2016). Tonsillar cancer: What nurses need to know. *Nursing, 46*(7), 36–44.

Sterba, K., Zapka, J., Cranos, C., Laursen, A., & Day, T. (2016). Quality of life in head and neck patient-caregiver dyads. *Cancer Nursing, 39*(3), 238–250.

Vacca, V., & Poirier, W. (2013). Action STAT: Posterior epistaxis. *Nursing, 43*(1), 72.

Veenstra, A., & Untalan, E. (2014). Implications and interventions related to obstructive sleep apnea. *Critical Care Nursing Clinics of North America, 26*, 499–509.

CHAPTER 30

Care of Patients With Noninfectious Lower Respiratory Problems

M. Linda Workman

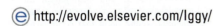
http://evolve.elsevier.com/Iggy/

PRIORITY AND INTERRELATED CONCEPTS

The priority concept for this chapter is GAS EXCHANGE.

❋ The GAS EXCHANGE concept exemplar for this chapter is Chronic Obstructive Pulmonary Disease, p. 572.

The interrelated concepts for this chapter are:
- PERFUSION
- CELLULAR REGULATION

LEARNING OUTCOMES

Safe and Effective Care Environment

1. Collaborate with the interprofessional team to coordinate high-quality care and promote GAS EXCHANGE in patients with chronic lower respiratory problems.
2. Protect patients with lower respiratory problems from injury or infection.
3. Teach the patient and family how to manage a chronic lower respiratory disorder and avoid injury and complications in the home.

Health Promotion and Maintenance

4. Teach all adults measures to take to protect the respiratory system from damage and cancer, including the avoidance of known environmental causative agents.
5. Identify community resources for patients requiring assistance with long-term GAS EXCHANGE issues related to chronic lower airway problems.

Psychosocial Integrity

6. Implement nursing interventions to help the patient and family cope with the psychosocial impact of living with a chronic lower respiratory problem.

Physiological Integrity

7. Apply knowledge of anatomy, physiology, and pathophysiology to assess critically ill patients with respiratory problems affecting GAS EXCHANGE or PERFUSION.
8. Teach the patient and caregiver(s) about common drugs and other management strategies used for acute or chronic lower respiratory problems.
9. Use assessment information to identify adults at increased genetic risk for a respiratory disease that affects GAS EXCHANGE or PERFUSION.
10. Prioritize nursing care for the patient with chest tubes.

Airflow through the entire respiratory tubular system is needed for oxygen to reach the alveolar ducts and alveoli for GAS EXCHANGE to occur. When the function of any of these structures is reduced, both gas exchange and systemic PERFUSION are impaired. Many noninfectious lower airway problems, whether they affect airflow or gas exchange, are chronic and progressive, requiring changes in lifestyle, especially for older adults (Touhy & Jett, 2016). Chart 30-1 lists nursing issues for the older patient with a respiratory problem.

ASTHMA

❖ PATHOPHYSIOLOGY

Asthma is a chronic disease in which reversible airway obstruction occurs intermittently, reducing airflow (Fig. 30-1). Airway obstruction occurs by both inflammation and airway tissue

sensitivity (hyperresponsiveness) with bronchoconstriction. Inflammation obstructs the airway lumens (i.e., the insides) (Fig. 30-2). Airway hyperresponsiveness and constriction of bronchial smooth muscle narrow the tubular structure of the airways. Airway inflammation and sensitivity can trigger bronchiolar constriction, and many adults with asthma have both problems. Severe airway obstruction reduces GAS EXCHANGE and can be fatal. At least 3630 deaths from acute asthma occur in the United States each year (Centers for Disease Control and Prevention [CDC], 2015). The risk for death from asthma is higher among older adults (Arjona, 2015).

Etiology and Genetic Risk

Although asthma is classified into types based on what triggers the attacks, the effect on GAS EXCHANGE is the same. Inflammation of the mucous membranes lining the airways is a key event

CHART 30-1   Nursing Focus on the Older-Adult

Chronic Respiratory Disorder

- Provide rest periods between activities such as bathing, meals, and ambulation.
- Place the patient in an upright position for meals to prevent aspiration.
- Encourage nutritional fluid intake after the meal to promote increased calorie intake.
- Schedule drugs around routine activities to increase adherence to drug therapy.
- Arrange chairs in strategic locations to allow the patient with dyspnea to stop and rest while walking.
- Urge the patient to notify the primary health care provider promptly for any symptoms of infection.
- Encourage the patient to receive the pneumococcal vaccine and to have an annual influenza vaccination.
- For patients who are prescribed home oxygen, keep tubing coiled when walking to reduce the risk for tripping.

in triggering an asthma attack. It occurs in response to the presence of specific allergens; general irritants such as cold air, dry air, or fine airborne particles; microorganisms; and aspirin and other NSAIDs. Increased airway sensitivity (hyperresponsiveness) can occur with exercise or upper respiratory illness and for unknown reasons.

GENETIC/GENOMIC CONSIDERATIONS

Patient-Centered Care QSEN

Genetic studies indicate that more than 50 gene variations are associated with asthma, although asthma is a disorder with both genetic and environmental input needed for expression (Online Mendelian Inheritance in Man [OMIM], 2015). Variation in the gene that controls the activity of beta-adrenergic receptors also has an impact on drug therapy for asthma. Adults with this mutation do not respond as expected to beta agonist drugs. Teaching these adults about why their drug therapies are different from standard recommendations is a nursing responsibility that can assist with therapy adherence.

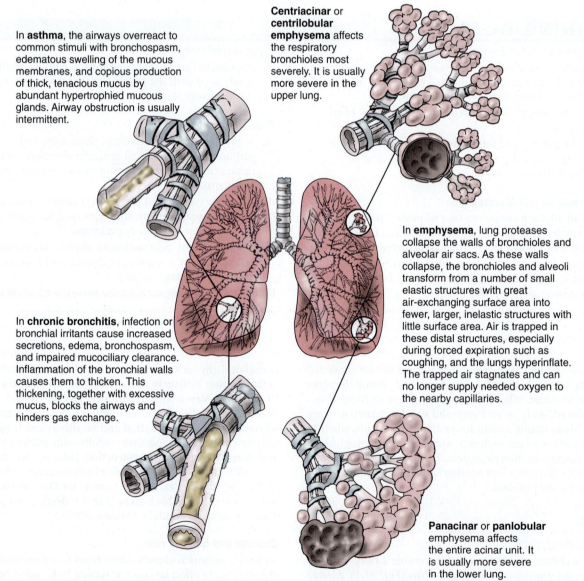

In **asthma**, the airways overreact to common stimuli with bronchospasm, edematous swelling of the mucous membranes, and copious production of thick, tenacious mucus by abundant hypertrophied mucous glands. Airway obstruction is usually intermittent.

Centriacinar or **centrilobular emphysema** affects the respiratory bronchioles most severely. It is usually more severe in the upper lung.

In **chronic bronchitis**, infection or bronchial irritants cause increased secretions, edema, bronchospasm, and impaired mucociliary clearance. Inflammation of the bronchial walls causes them to thicken. This thickening, together with excessive mucus, blocks the airways and hinders gas exchange.

In **emphysema**, lung proteases collapse the walls of bronchioles and alveolar air sacs. As these walls collapse, the bronchioles and alveoli transform from a number of small elastic structures with great air-exchanging surface area into fewer, larger, inelastic structures with little surface area. Air is trapped in these distal structures, especially during forced expiration such as coughing, and the lungs hyperinflate. The trapped air stagnates and can no longer supply needed oxygen to the nearby capillaries.

Panacinar or **panlobular** emphysema affects the entire acinar unit. It is usually more severe in the lower lung.

FIG. 30-1 Pathophysiology of chronic airflow limitation (CAL).

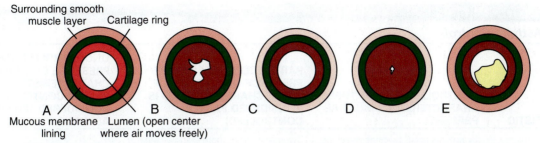

FIG. 30-2 Causes of narrowed airways. **A,** Cross-section of a small airway showing the tissue layers. **B,** Mucosal swelling. **C,** Constriction of smooth muscle. **D,** Mucosal swelling and constriction of smooth muscle. **E,** Mucus plug.

When asthma is well controlled, airway changes are temporary and reversible. With poor control, chronic inflammation leads to airway damage and altered CELLULAR REGULATION with enlargement of the bronchial epithelial cells, including mucus-secreting cells, and changes in the bronchial smooth muscle (Lynn & Kushto-Reese, 2015). With frequent asthma attacks, even exposure to low levels of the triggering agent or event may stimulate an attack.

Inflammation triggers asthma for some adults when allergens bind to specific antibodies (especially immunoglobulin E [IgE]). These antibodies are attached to tissue *mast cells* and white blood cells (WBCs) called *basophils,* which are filled with chemicals that can start local inflammatory responses (see Chapters 17 and 20). Some chemicals, such as histamine, start an immediate inflammatory response, which can be blocked by drugs such as diphenhydramine (Benadryl). Others, such as leukotriene and eotaxin, are slower and cause later, prolonged inflammatory responses, which can be blocked by drugs such as montelukast (Singulair), zafirlukast (Accolate), and zileuton (Zyflo). Chemicals also attract more WBCs to the area, which then continue the responses of blood vessel dilation and capillary leak, causing mucous membrane swelling and increased mucus production (McCance et al., 2014). These responses narrow the lumens even more, which then interferes with airflow and GAS EXCHANGE. Inflammation can also occur through general irritation rather than allergic responses.

Bronchospasm is narrowing of the bronchial tubes by constriction of the smooth muscle around and within the bronchial walls. It can occur when small amounts of pollutants or respiratory viruses stimulate nerve fibers, causing constriction of bronchial smooth muscle. If an inflammatory response is stimulated at the same time, the chemicals released during inflammation also trigger constriction. Severe bronchospasm alone, especially in smaller bronchioles, can profoundly limit airflow to the alveoli and greatly reduce GAS EXCHANGE.

Aspirin and other NSAIDs can trigger asthma in some adults, although this response is not a true allergy. It results from increased production of leukotriene when aspirin or NSAIDs suppress other inflammatory pathways.

Gastroesophageal reflux disease (GERD) can trigger asthma in some adults and causes asthma symptoms at night (Global Initiative for Asthma [GINA], 2017). With GERD, highly acidic stomach contents enter the airway and make pre-existing tissue sensitivity worse.

Incidence and Prevalence

Asthma can occur at any age. About half of adults with asthma also had the disease in childhood. Asthma affects nearly 21 million adults in the United States and Canada (18.5 million in the United States and 2.5 million in Canada) (CDC, 2015; Statistics Canada, 2016a). It is more common in urban settings than in rural settings.

CONSIDERATIONS FOR OLDER ADULTS
Patient-Centered Care QSEN

Asthma occurs as a new disorder in about 3% of adults older than 55 years, and another 3% of adults older than 60 years have asthma as a continuing chronic disorder (Arjona, 2015). Lung and airway changes as a part of aging make breathing problems more serious in the older adult. One problem related to aging is a decrease in the sensitivity of beta-adrenergic receptors. When stimulated, these receptors relax smooth muscle and cause bronchodilation. As these receptors become less sensitive, they no longer respond as quickly or as strongly to agonists (epinephrine, dopamine) and beta-adrenergic drugs, which are often used as rescue therapy during an acute asthma attack. Thus teaching older patients how to avoid asthma attacks and how to correctly use preventive drug therapy is a nursing priority.

❖ INTERPROFESSIONAL COLLABORATIVE CARE

As a treatable chronic disorder, asthma is generally managed in the community with health care oversight (Keep et al., 2016). Acute exacerbations may require management in emergency departments or ICUs. Because asthma is a common disorder, adults admitted to the hospital for other health problems or surgery may also have asthma. For asthma control, the management plan must continue, regardless of setting.

◆ Assessment: Noticing

Asthma is classified on the basis of how well controlled the symptoms are and on the patient's response to asthma drugs. These classes are the basis for current asthma therapy (Charts 30-2 and 30-3).

History. The patient with asthma usually has a pattern of intermittent episodes of dyspnea (shortness of breath), chest tightness, coughing, wheezing, and increased mucus production. Ask whether the symptoms occur continuously, seasonally, in association with specific activities or exposures, at work, or more frequently at night. Some patients have symptoms for 4 to 8 weeks after a cold or other upper respiratory infection. The patient with atopic (allergic) asthma also may have other allergic problems. Ask whether any family members have asthma or respiratory problems. Ask about current or previous smoking habits. If the patient smokes, use this opportunity to teach him or her about smoking cessation (see Chart 27-2). Wheezing in nonsmokers is important in the diagnosis of asthma.

⟩⟩ **CHART 30-2   Key Features**

Levels of Asthma Control

CHARACTERISTIC	CONTROLLED (ALL OF THESE CHARACTERISTICS MUST BE PRESENT)	PARTLY CONTROLLED (THE PRESENCE OF ANY ONE OF THESE CHARACTERISTICS IS CONSIDERED PARTLY CONTROLLED)	UNCONTROLLED (THE PRESENCE OF THREE OR MORE CHARACTERISTICS FROM THE PARTLY CONTROLLED LIST IS CONSIDERED UNCONTROLLED ASTHMA)
Daytime symptoms	Symptoms occur twice per week or less	Symptoms occur more than twice per week	
Activity limitations	None	Any	
Nighttime symptoms	None	Any	
Reliever drug use	Reliever used twice per week or less	Reliever used more than twice per week	
PEF or FEV₁	Normal	Less than 80% of predicted or established personal best	
Treatment action	Find and maintain lowest step level that controls symptoms	Increase step until symptoms are controlled on a regular basis and then reduce step to the lowest step level that consistently controls symptoms	Increase step (step up) until control is reached and maintained

FEV₁, Forced expiratory volume in the first second; *PEF*, peak expiratory flow.

⟩⟩ **CHART 30-3   Key Features**

The Step System for Medication Use in Asthma Control

STEP 1	STEP 2	STEP 3	STEP 4	STEP 5
As-needed rapid-acting beta₂ agonist (relief inhaler)	As-needed rapid-acting beta₂ agonist (relief inhaler)	As-needed rapid-acting beta₂ agonist (relief inhaler)	As-needed rapid-acting beta₂ agonist (relief inhaler)	As-needed rapid-acting beta₂ agonist (relief inhaler)
No daily drugs needed	Daily treatment involves the use of *one* of these two options:	Daily treatment involves the use of *one* of these four options:	Daily treatment involves the use of the Step 3 option that provided the best degree of control and was well tolerated along with one or more of these two options:	Daily treatment involves the use of the Step 4 option(s) that provided the best degree of control and was well tolerated along with either of these two options:
	Low-dose ICS	Low-dose ICS *and* long-acting beta₂ agonist	Medium-dose or high-dose ICS *and* long-acting beta₂ agonist	Oral glucocorticosteroid (lowest dose)
	Leukotriene modifier*	Medium-dose or high-dose ICS Low-dose ICS and leukotriene modifier Low-dose ICS and sustained-release theophylline	Leukotriene modifier and sustained-release theophylline	Anti-IgE† treatment

Data compiled from Global Initiative for Asthma (GINA). (2017). *Pocket guide for asthma management and prevention.* http://ginasthma.org/2017-pocket-guide-for-asthma -management-and-prevention/.
ICS, Inhaled corticosteroid.
*Leukotriene modifier = Leukotriene receptor antagonist or leukotriene synthesis inhibitor.
†IgE = Immunoglobulin E.

Physical Assessment/Signs and Symptoms. The patient with mild-to-moderate asthma may have no symptoms between asthma attacks. During an acute episode, common symptoms are an audible wheeze and increased respiratory rate. At first the wheeze is louder on exhalation. When inflammation occurs with asthma, coughing may increase.

The patient may use accessory muscles to help breathe during an attack. Observe for muscle retraction at the sternum and the suprasternal notch and between the ribs. The patient with long-standing, severe asthma may have a "barrel chest," caused by air trapping (Fig. 30-3). The anteroposterior (AP) diameter (diameter between the front and the back of the chest)

increases with air trapping, giving the chest a rounded rather than an oval shape. The normal chest is about 1.5 times as wide as it is deep. In severe, chronic asthma, the AP diameter may equal or exceed the lateral diameter (Jarvis, 2016). Compare the chest AP diameter with the lateral diameter. Chronic air trapping also flattens the diaphragm and increases the space between the ribs.

Along with an audible wheeze, the breathing cycle is longer, with prolonged exhalation, and requires more effort. The patient may be unable to speak more than a few words between breaths. Hypoxia occurs with severe attacks. Pulse oximetry shows **hypoxemia** (poor blood oxygen levels). Examine the oral

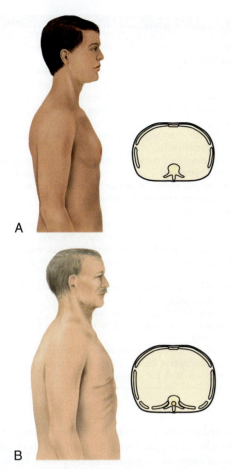

FIG. 30-3 A, Normal adult. The thorax has an oval shape with an antero-posterior-to-transverse diameter of 1 : 1.5 or 5 : 7. **B,** Barrel chest. Note equal anteroposterior-to-transverse diameter and that ribs are horizontal instead of the normal downward slope. This is associated with chronic obstructive pulmonary disease and severe asthma as a result of hyperinflation of the lungs. (From Jarvis, C. [2016]. *Physical examination and health assessment* [7th ed.]. Philadelphia: Saunders.)

mucosa and nail beds for cyanosis. Other indicators of hypoxemia include changes in the level of cognition or consciousness and tachycardia.

Laboratory Assessment. Laboratory tests can determine asthma type and the degree of breathing impairment. Arterial blood gas (ABG) levels show the effectiveness of GAS EXCHANGE (see Chapter 12 for discussion of ABGs). The arterial oxygen level (Pao$_2$) may decrease during an asthma attack. Early in the attack, the arterial carbon dioxide level (Paco$_2$) may be decreased as the patient increases the breathing rate and depth. Later in an asthma episode, Paco$_2$ rises, indicating carbon dioxide retention. Allergic asthma often occurs with elevated serum eosinophil counts and immunoglobulin E (IgE) levels. The sputum may contain eosinophils and mucus plugs with shed epithelial cells (Curschmann's spirals).

Pulmonary Function Tests. The most accurate tests for measuring airflow in asthma are the pulmonary function tests (PFTs) using spirometry. Baseline PFTs are obtained for all patients diagnosed with asthma. The most important PFTs for a patient with asthma are the forced vital capacity (FVC), the forced expiratory volume in the first second (FEV$_1$), and the peak expiratory flow (PEF), sometimes called *peak expiratory rate flow (PERF)* (Lynn & Kushto-Reese, 2015). Definitions of

PFTs are listed in Chapter 27. A decrease in either the FEV$_1$ or the PEF (PERF) of 15% to 20% below the expected value for age, gender, and size is common for the patient with asthma. Asthma is diagnosed when these values increase by 12% or more after treatment with bronchodilators. Airway responsiveness is tested by measuring the PEF and FEV$_1$ before and after the patient inhales the drug *methacholine*, which induces bronchospasm in susceptible adults.

◆ Interventions: Responding

The purposes of asthma therapy are to control and prevent episodes, improve airflow and GAS EXCHANGE, and relieve symptoms. Asthma is best controlled when the patient is an active partner in the management plan. Priority nursing actions focus on patient education about using his or her personal asthma action plan, which includes drug therapy and lifestyle management strategies to help him or her understand the disease and its management (GINA, 2017).

Self-Management Education. Asthma often has intermittent overt symptoms. With guided self-care, patients can co-manage this disease, increasing symptom-free periods and decreasing the number and severity of attacks. Good management decreases hospital admissions and increases participation in patient-chosen work and leisure activities. Self-care requires extensive education for the patient to be able to self-assess respiratory status, self-manage (by adjusting the frequency and dosage of prescribed drugs), and know when to consult the primary health care provider (Keep et al., 2016).

Ideally a personal asthma action plan is developed by the health care provider and the patient. The plan is tailored to meet the patient's personal triggers, asthma symptoms, and drug responses. It includes:

- The prescribed daily controller drug(s) schedule and prescribed reliever drug directions
- Patient-specific daily asthma control assessment questions
- Directions for adjusting the daily controller drug schedule
- When to contact the primary health care provider (in addition to regularly scheduled visits)
- Emergency actions to take when asthma is not responding to controller and reliever drugs

Teach the patient to assess asthma severity at least daily with a peak flow meter (Fig. 30-4) and to adjust drugs according to his or her personal asthma action plan to prevent or relieve symptoms. Chart 30-4 describes the correct method for using the peak flow meter. The patient first establishes a baseline or "personal best" peak expiratory flow (PEF) by measuring his or her PEF twice daily for 2 to 3 weeks when asthma is well controlled and recording the results. This way, the patient will know when his or her peak flow is reduced to the point that more drugs are needed or that emergency assistance is needed. When the patient has established a "personal best," all other readings are compared with this value. Some meters are color coded to help the patient interpret the results. Green zone readings are at least 80% of or above the "personal best." This is the ideal range for asthma control and indicates that no increases in drug therapy are needed. Yellow is a range between 50% and 80% of personal best. When a patient has a reading in this range, he or she needs to use the prescribed reliever drug. Within a few minutes after using the reliever drug, another PEF reading should be made to determine whether it is working. *Frequent*

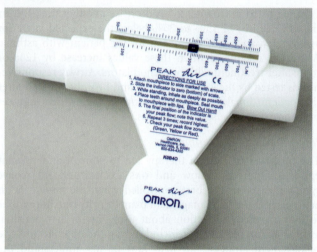

FIG. 30-4 Typical peak flow meter. This model will show faster exhalation rates in *green,* reduced exhalation rates in *yellow,* and seriously reduced exhalation rates in *red.* (From Aehlert, B. [2011]. *Paramedic practice today: Above and beyond.* St. Louis: Mosby.)

CHART 30-4 Patient and Family Education: Preparing for Self-Management

Using a Peak Flow Meter

- Set the peak flow meter at zero.
- Use a standing position, without leaning or supporting yourself on anything, if possible.
- Take as deep a breath as you can.
- Place the mouthpiece of the meter in your mouth, taking care to wrap your lips tightly around it.
- Blow your breath out through the mouthpiece as hard and as fast as you are able. (If you cough, sneeze, or have any type of interruption while you exhale, reset the meter and perform the test again.)
- Reset and perform the test two additional times.
- The highest reading of the three is your current peak flow rate.
- Keep a record or graph of your peak flow rates and examine these for trends.

readings in the yellow zone or increasing use of reliever drugs indicates the need to reassess the asthma plan for the need to change controller drugs. Red is a range below 50% of the patient's personal best, indicating serious respiratory obstruction.

⚠ NURSING SAFETY PRIORITY **QSEN**

Action Alert

Teach the patient that, if a red zone reading occurs when using the peak flow meter, to immediately use the reliever drugs and seek emergency help.

Teach the patient to keep a symptom and intervention diary to learn specific triggers of asthma, early cues for impending attacks, and personal response to drugs. Stress the importance of proper use of his or her personal asthma action plan for any severity of asthma. Chart 30-5 lists areas to emphasize when teaching the patient with asthma.

Drug Therapy. Pharmacologic management of adults with asthma is based on the step category for severity and treatment (see Charts 30-2 and 30-3) (GINA, 2017). **Control therapy drugs**

CHART 30-5 Patient and Family Education: Preparing for Self-Management

Asthma Management

- Avoid potential environmental asthma triggers, such as smoke, fireplaces, dust, mold, and weather changes of warm to cold.
- Avoid drugs that trigger your asthma (e.g., aspirin, NSAIDs, beta blockers).
- Avoid food that has been prepared with monosodium glutamate (MSG) or metabisulfite.
- If you have exercise-induced asthma, use your bronchodilator inhaler 30 minutes before exercise to prevent or reduce bronchospasm.
- Be sure that you know the proper technique and correct sequence when you use metered dose inhalers.
- Get adequate rest and sleep.
- Reduce stress and anxiety; learn relaxation techniques; adopt coping mechanisms that have worked for you in the past.
- Wash all bedding with hot water to destroy dust mites.
- Monitor your peak expiratory flow rates with a flow meter at least twice daily.
- Seek immediate emergency care if you experience any of these:
  - Gray or blue fingertips or lips
  - Difficulty breathing, walking, or talking
  - Retractions of the neck, chest, or ribs
  - Nasal flaring
  - Failure of drugs to control worsening symptoms
  - Peak expiratory rate flow (PERF) declining steadily after treatment, or a flow rate 50% below your usual flow rate

are used to reduce airway sensitivity (responsiveness) to prevent asthma attacks from occurring to maintain GAS EXCHANGE. *They are used every day, regardless of symptoms.* **Reliever drugs** (also called *rescue drugs*) are used to actually stop an attack once it has started. Some patients may need drug therapy only during an asthma episode. For others, daily drugs are needed to keep asthma episodic rather than a more frequent problem. Therapy involves the use of bronchodilators and various drug types to reduce inflammation. Some drugs reduce the asthma response, and other drugs actually prevent it. Combination drugs are two agents from different classes combined together for better response. Chart 30-6 lists the most common preferred drugs in each class for control and relief therapy of asthma. The actions and interventions for most drugs within a single class are similar. Be sure to consult a drug handbook for information on a specific drug.

Bronchodilators. Bronchodilators cause bronchiolar smooth muscle relaxation but have no effect on inflammation. Thus, for patients who have airflow obstruction by both bronchospasm and inflammation, at least two types of drug therapy are needed. Bronchodilators include beta$_2$ agonists and cholinergic antagonists.

Beta$_2$ agonists bind to and stimulate the beta$_2$-adrenergic receptors in the same way that epinephrine and norepinephrine do. This causes an increase in smooth muscle relaxation. Short-acting beta$_2$ agonists (SABAs) provide rapid but short-term relief. These inhaled drugs are most useful when an attack begins (as relief) or as premedication when the patient is about to begin an activity that is likely to induce an attack (GINA, 2017). Such agents include albuterol (ProAir, Proventil, Ventolin), levalbuterol (Xopenex), and terbutaline (Brethaire). Teach the patient the correct technique for using an inhaled drug with a metered dose inhaler (MDI) (Chart 30-7). Fig. 30-5 shows a patient using a "spacer" with an MDI. Spacer use increases the

CHART 30-6 Common Examples of Drug Therapy

Asthma Prevention and Treatment

DRUG	NURSING IMPLICATIONS
Bronchodilators—Cause bronchodilation through relaxing bronchiolar smooth muscle by binding to and activating pulmonary beta$_2$ receptors.	
Short-Acting Beta$_2$ Agonist (SABA)—Primary use is a fast-acting reliever (rescue) drug to be used either during an asthma attack or just before engaging in activity that usually triggers an attack.	
Albuterol (ProAir, Proventil, Ventolin) (inhaled drug) Levalbuterol (Xopenex)	Teach patients to carry drug with them at all times *because it can stop or reduce life-threatening bronchoconstriction.* Teach patient to monitor heart rate *because excessive use causes tachycardia and other systemic symptoms.* When taking any of these drugs with other inhaled drugs, teach patient to use it at least 5 minutes before the other inhaled drugs *to allow the bronchodilation effect to increase the penetration of the other inhaled drugs.* Teach patient the correct technique for using the MDI or *DPI to ensure that the drug reaches the site of action.*
Long-Acting Beta$_2$ Agonist (LABA)—Causes bronchodilation through relaxing bronchiolar smooth muscle by binding to and activating pulmonary beta$_2$ receptors. Onset of action is slow with a long duration. Primary use is prevention of an asthma attack.	
Salmeterol (Serevent) (inhaled drug) Indacaterol (Arcapta Neohaler) (COPD only) (inhaled drug) Formoterol (Perforomist) Arformoterol (Brovana) (COPD only)	Teach patient to not use these drugs as reliever drugs *because they have a slow onset of action and do not relieve acute symptoms.* Teach patient the correct technique for using the MDI or DPI *to ensure that the drug reaches the site of action.*
Cholinergic Antagonist—Causes bronchodilation by inhibiting the parasympathetic nervous system, allowing the sympathetic system to dominate, releasing norepinephrine that activates beta$_2$ receptors. Purpose is to both relieve and prevent asthma and improve GAS EXCHANGE.	
Ipratropium (Atrovent, Apo-Ipravent ✦) (inhaled drug) Tiotropium (Spiriva)	If patient is to use any of these as a reliever drug, teach him or her to carry it at all times *because it can stop or reduce life-threatening bronchoconstriction.* Teach patient to shake MDI well before using *because the drugs separate easily.* Teach patient to increase daily fluid intake *because the drugs cause mouth dryness.* Teach patient to observe for and report blurred vision, eye pain, headache, nausea, palpitations, tremors, inability to sleep *as these are systemic symptoms of overdose and require intervention.* Teach patient the correct technique for using the MDI or DPI *to ensure that the drug reaches the site of action.*
Anti-Inflammatories—All of these drugs help improve bronchiolar airflow and increase GAS EXCHANGE by decreasing the inflammatory response of the mucous membranes in the airways. *They do not cause bronchodilation.*	
Corticosteroids—Disrupt production pathways of inflammatory mediators. The main purpose is to prevent an asthma attack caused by inflammation or allergies (controller drug).	
Fluticasone (Ellipta) (MDI inhaled drug) Beclomethasone (Qvar) (MDI inhaled drug) Budesonide (Pulmicort) (MDI inhaled drug)	Teach patient to use the drug daily, *even when no symptoms are present, because maximum effectiveness requires continued use for 48-72 hr and depends on regular use.* Teach patient to use good mouth care and to check mouth daily for lesions or drainage *because these drugs reduce local immunity and increase the risk for local infections, especially* Candida albicans *(yeast).* Teach patient to not use these drugs as reliever drugs *because they have a slow onset of action and do not relieve acute symptoms.* Teach patient the correct technique for using the MDI *to ensure that the drug reaches the site of action.*
Prednisone (oral drug)	Teach patient about expected side effects *because knowing which side effects to expect may reduce anxiety when they appear.* Teach patient to avoid anyone who has an upper respiratory infection *because the drug reduces all protective inflammatory responses, increasing the risk for infection.* Teach patient to avoid activities that lead to injury *because blood vessels become more fragile, leading to bruising and petechiae.* Teach patient to take drug with food *to help reduce the side effect of GI ulceration.* Teach patient not to suddenly stop taking the drug for any reason *because the drug suppresses adrenal production of corticosteroids, which are essential for life.*

Continued

CHART 30-6   Common Examples of Drug Therapy—cont'd

Asthma Prevention and Treatment

DRUG	NURSING IMPLICATIONS
Cromone—Stabilizes the membranes of mast cells and prevents the release of inflammatory mediators. Purpose is to prevent asthma attack triggered by inflammation or allergens.	
Nedocromil (Tilade) (inhaled drug)	Teach patient to use the drug daily, *even when no symptoms are present, because maximum effectiveness requires continued use for 48-72 hr and depends on regular use.* Teach patient to not use this drug as a reliever drug *because it has a slow onset of action and does not relieve acute symptoms.* Teach patient the correct technique for using the MDI *to ensure that the drug reaches the site of action.*
Leukotriene Modifier—Blocks the leukotriene receptor, preventing the inflammatory mediator from stimulating inflammation. Purpose is to prevent asthma attack triggered by inflammation or allergens.	
Montelukast (Singulair) (oral drug)	Teach patient to use the drug daily, *even when no symptoms are present, because maximum effectiveness requires continued use for 48-72 hr and depends on regular use.* Teach patient not to decrease the dose of or stop taking any other asthma drugs unless instructed by the health care professional *because this drug is for long-term asthma control and does not replace other drugs, especially corticosteroids and reliever (rescue) drugs.*

Data from Global Initiative for Asthma (GINA). (2017). *Pocket guide for asthma management and prevention.* http://ginasthma.org/2017-pocket-guide-for-asthma-management-and-prevention/; and Global Initiative for Chronic Obstructive Lung Disease (GOLD). (2017). *Global strategy for the diagnosis, management, and prevention of chronic obstructive pulmonary disease.* http://goldcopd.org/wp-content/uploads/2016/12/wms-GOLD-2017-Pocket-Guide.pdf.
COPD, Chronic obstructive pulmonary disease; *DPI,* dry powder inhaler; *MDI,* metered dose inhaler.

CHART 30-7   Patient and Family Education: Preparing for Self-Management

How to Use an Inhaler Correctly

With a Spacer (Preferred Technique)

1. Before each use, remove the caps from the inhaler and the spacer.
2. Insert the mouthpiece of the inhaler into the nonmouthpiece end of the spacer.
3. Shake the whole unit vigorously three or four times.
4. Fully exhale and then place the mouthpiece into your mouth, over your tongue, and seal your lips tightly around it.
5. Press down firmly on the canister of the inhaler to release one dose of medication into the spacer.
6. Breathe in slowly and deeply. If the spacer makes a whistling sound, you are breathing in too rapidly.
7. Remove the mouthpiece from your mouth; and, keeping your lips closed, hold your breath for at least 10 seconds and then breathe out slowly.
8. Wait at least 1 minute between puffs.
9. Replace the caps on the inhaler and the spacer.
10. At least once a day, clean the plastic case and cap of the inhaler by thoroughly rinsing in warm, running tap water; at least once a week, clean the spacer in the same manner.

Without a Spacer

1. Before each use, remove the cap and shake the inhaler according to the instructions in the package insert.
2. Tilt your head back slightly and breathe out fully.
3. Open your mouth and place the mouthpiece 1 to 2 inches away.
4. As you begin to breathe in deeply through your mouth, press down firmly on the canister of the inhaler to release one dose of medication.
5. Continue to breathe in slowly and deeply (usually over 5-7 sec).
6. Hold your breath for at least 10 seconds to allow the medication to reach deep into the lungs and then breathe out slowly.
7. Wait at least 1 minute between puffs.
8. Replace the cap on the inhaler.
9. At least once a day, remove the canister and clean the plastic case and cap of the inhaler by thoroughly rinsing in warm, running tap water.
10. Avoid spraying in the direction of the eyes.

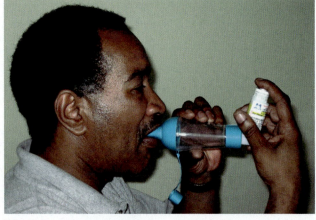

FIG. 30-5 Patient using an aerosol metered dose inhaler with a spacer.

⚠ NURSING SAFETY PRIORITY (QSEN)

Action Alert

Teach the patient with asthma to always carry the relief drug inhaler with him or her and to ensure that enough drug remains in the inhaler to provide a quick dose when needed.

amount of drug that is delivered to the lungs. Chart 30-8 describes the care and use of a dry powder inhaler (DPI).

Dry powder inhalers indicate the amount of remaining drug. Most aerosol inhalers (MDIs) now have meters that indicate the number of doses left in the canister, but some do not. It is recommended that the patient count the number of doses as they are used; however, many patients have difficulty keeping the dose count accurate.

Long-acting beta$_2$ agonists (LABAs) are also delivered by inhaler directly to the site of action—the bronchioles. Proper use of the long-acting agonists decreases the need to use reliever

CHART 30-8 Patient and Family Education: Preparing for Self-Management

How to Use a Dry Powder Inhaler (DPI)

For Inhalers Requiring Loading
- First load the drug by:
  - Turning the device to the next dose of drug, _or_
  - Inserting the capsule into the device, _or_
  - Inserting the disk or compartment into the device

After Loading the Drug and for Inhalers That Do Not Require Drug Loading
- Read your doctor's instructions for how fast you should breathe for your particular inhaler.
- Exhale fully away from the inhaler.
- Place your lips over the mouthpiece and breathe in forcefully (there is no propellant in the inhaler; only your breath pulls the drug in).
- Remove the inhaler from your mouth as soon as you have breathed in.
- _Never exhale (breathe out) into your inhaler._ Your breath will moisten the powder, causing it to clump and not be delivered accurately.
- _Never wash or place the inhaler in water._
- _Never shake your inhaler._
- Keep your inhaler in a dry place at room temperature.
- If the inhaler is preloaded, discard it after it is empty.
- Because the drug is a dry powder and there is no propellant, you may not feel, smell, or taste it as you inhale.

drugs as often. Unlike short-acting agonists, long-acting drugs need time to build up an effect, but the effects are longer lasting. These drugs are useful in _preventing_ an asthma attack but cannot stop an acute attack. Therefore teach patients not to use LABAs alone to relieve symptoms of an attack or when wheezing is getting worse but, instead, to use a SABA. Examples of LABAs include formoterol (Perforomist, Zenhale ✦) and salmeterol (Serevent). Both drugs are associated with increased asthma deaths, especially when used as the only therapy for asthma, and have a black box warning from the Food and Drug Administration (FDA).

! NURSING SAFETY PRIORITY QSEN
Drug Alert

LABAs should never be prescribed as the _only_ drug therapy for asthma and are not to be used during an acute asthma attack or bronchospasm. Teach the patient to use these control drugs daily as prescribed, even when no symptoms are present, and to use a SABA to relieve acute symptoms. Any patient using these drugs must be monitored closely.

Cholinergic antagonists, also called _anticholinergic drugs_ or _long-acting muscarinic antagonists (LAMAs),_ are similar to atropine and block the parasympathetic nervous system. This action increases bronchodilation and decreases secretions. The main drug in this class is ipratropium (Apo-Ipravent ✦, Atrovent), which is used as an inhalant. Most cholinergic antagonists are short acting and are used several times a day. Long-acting agents such as tiotropium (Spiriva) are used once a day.

Xanthines such as theophylline and aminophylline are used rarely, only when other types of management are ineffective. These drugs are given systemically, and the dosage that is effective is close to the dosage that produces many dangerous side

effects. Blood levels must be monitored closely to ensure that the drug level is within the therapeutic range.

Anti-Inflammatory Agents. Anti-inflammatory agents decrease airway inflammation. The inhaled forms have fewer systemic side effects than those taken systemically. _All of the anti-inflammatory drugs, whether inhaled or taken orally, are controller drugs only._

! NURSING SAFETY PRIORITY QSEN
Drug Alert

Anti-inflammatory drug therapy for asthma is for prevention or control of asthma. They are _not_ effective in reversing symptoms during an asthma attack and should not be used alone as reliever drugs. Teach patients to take anti-inflammatory asthma drugs on a scheduled basis, even when no symptoms are present.

Corticosteroids decrease inflammation mainly by reducing the production of inflammatory chemicals. Inhaled corticosteroids (ICSs) can be helpful in controlling asthma symptoms. High-potency steroid inhalers, such as fluticasone (Flovent), budesonide (Pulmicort), and mometasone (Asmanex), may be used once per day for maintenance. Newer approved drugs for asthma control include those that are combinations of an inhaled corticosteroid and an inhaled beta$_2$ agonist, such as Breo Elipta (fluticasone and vilanterol). This combination comes in different strengths and is used once daily.

Systemic corticosteroids, because of severe side effects, are avoided for mild-to-moderate intermittent asthma and are used on a short-term basis for moderate asthma. For some patients with severe asthma, daily oral corticosteroids may be needed.

Cromones, either inhaled or taken orally, are useful as _controller_ asthma therapy when taken on a scheduled basis. These agents reduce airway inflammation by either inhibiting the release of inflammatory chemicals (nedocromil [Tilade]) or preventing mast cell membranes from opening when an allergen binds to IgE (cromolyn sodium [Intal]).

Leukotriene modifiers are oral drugs that work in several ways to control asthma when taken on a scheduled basis. Montelukast (Singulair) and zafirlukast (Accolate) block the leukotriene receptor. Zileuton (Zyflo) prevents leukotriene synthesis.

Exercise and Activity. Regular exercise is a recommended part of asthma therapy to maintain cardiac health, strengthen muscles, and promote GAS EXCHANGE and PERFUSION. Teach patients to examine the conditions that trigger an attack and adjust the exercise routine as needed. Some may need to use an inhaled SABA before beginning activity. For others, adjusting the environment may be needed (e.g., changing from outdoor ice-skating in cold, dry air to indoor ice-skating).

Oxygen Therapy. Supplemental oxygen by mask or nasal cannula is often used during an acute asthma attack. High-flow delivery may be needed when bronchospasms are severe and limit flow of oxygen through the bronchiole tubes (see Chapter 28 for high-flow delivery systems).

! NURSING SAFETY PRIORITY QSEN
Action Alert

Ensure that no open flames (e.g., cigarette smoking, fireplaces, burning candles) or other combustion hazards are in rooms where oxygen is in use.

Status Asthmaticus. Status asthmaticus is a severe, life-threatening acute episode of airway obstruction that intensifies once it begins and often does not respond to usual therapy. The patient arrives in the emergency department with extremely labored breathing and wheezing. Use of accessory muscles for breathing and distention of neck veins are observed. *If the condition is not reversed, the patient may develop pneumothorax and cardiac or respiratory arrest.* IV fluids, potent systemic bronchodilators, steroids, epinephrine, and oxygen are given immediately to reverse the condition. Magnesium sulfate also may be used. Prepare for emergency intubation. Sudden absence of wheezing indicates complete airway obstruction and requires a tracheotomy. When breathing improves, management is similar to that for any patient with asthma.

❓ NCLEX EXAMINATION CHALLENGE 30-1

Health Promotion and Maintenance

A client newly diagnosed with moderate asthma asks whether he can just take salmeterol instead of salmeterol and albuterol, because he has read that they are both beta agonists. What is the nurse's **best** advice?

A. Yes; both of these drugs have the same action, and you only need one.

B. Yes, because they both need to be used daily whether you are having symptoms or not; just take a little more of the salmeterol and don't take any of the albuterol.

C. No; albuterol is used to relieve the symptoms during an actual asthma attack, and salmeterol is used to prevent an attack. Both are needed."

D. No; albuterol is taken through the use of an aerosol inhaler, and salmeterol is an oral drug (tablet) that is activated in the stomach. Both are needed."

✳ GAS EXCHANGE CONCEPT EXEMPLAR
Chronic Obstructive Pulmonary Disease

❖ *PATHOPHYSIOLOGY*

Chronic obstructive pulmonary diseases (COPD) interfere with airflow and GAS EXCHANGE. These disorders include emphysema and chronic bronchitis. Although these are separate disorders with different pathologic processes, many patients with emphysema also have chronic bronchitis (Fig. 30-6).

Emphysema

The two major changes that occur with emphysema are loss of lung elasticity and hyperinflation of the lung (see Fig. 30-1).

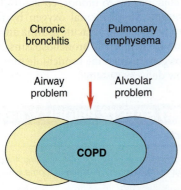

FIG. 30-6 The interaction of chronic bronchitis and emphysema in chronic obstructive pulmonary disease (COPD).

These changes result in dyspnea, reduced GAS EXCHANGE, and the need for an increased respiratory rate.

In the healthy lung, enzymes called *proteases* are present to destroy and eliminate particulates inhaled during breathing. Cigarette smoking triggers increased synthesis of these enzymes. When these proteases are present in higher-than-normal levels, they damage the alveoli and the small airways by breaking down elastin. Over time, alveolar sacs lose their elasticity, and the small airways collapse or narrow. Some alveoli are destroyed, and others become large and flabby, with less area for GAS EXCHANGE.

An increased amount of air is trapped in the lungs. Causes of air trapping are loss of elastic recoil in the alveolar walls, overstretching and enlargement of the alveoli into air-filled spaces called *bullae*, and collapse of small bronchioles. These changes greatly increase the work of breathing and interfere with airflow to the lungs. The hyperinflated lung flattens the diaphragm (Fig. 30-7), weakening the effectiveness of this muscle. As a result, the patient with emphysema needs to use accessory muscles in the neck, chest wall, and abdomen to inhale and exhale. This increased effort increases the need for oxygen, making the patient have an "air hunger" sensation. Inhalation starts before exhalation is completed, resulting in an uncoordinated breathing pattern.

GAS EXCHANGE is affected by the increased work of breathing and the loss of alveolar tissue. Although some alveoli enlarge, the curves of alveolar walls decrease, and less surface area is available for gas exchange. Often the patient adjusts

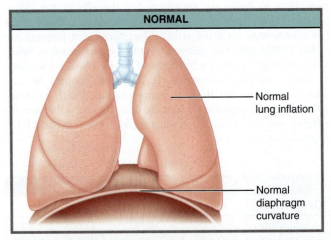

NORMAL

— Normal lung inflation

— Normal diaphragm curvature

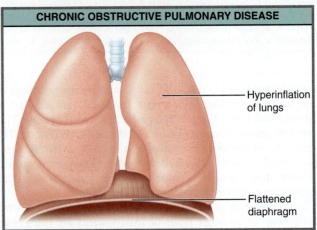

CHRONIC OBSTRUCTIVE PULMONARY DISEASE

— Hyperinflation of lungs

— Flattened diaphragm

FIG. 30-7 Diaphragm shape and lung inflation in the normal patient and in the patient with chronic airflow limitation (CAL), especially chronic obstructive pulmonary disease (COPD).

by increasing the respiratory rate, so arterial blood gas (ABG) values may not show gas exchange problems until the patient has advanced disease. Then carbon dioxide is produced faster than it can be eliminated, resulting in carbon dioxide retention and chronic respiratory acidosis (see Chapter 12). The patient with late-stage emphysema also has a low arterial oxygen (PaO_2) level because it is difficult for oxygen to move from diseased alveoli into the blood.

Emphysema is classified as *panlobular, centrilobular,* or *paraseptal,* depending on the pattern of destruction and dilation of the gas-exchanging units (acini) (see Fig. 30-1). Each type can occur alone or in combination in the same lung. Most are associated with smoking or chronic exposure to other inhaled particles such as wood smoke and biomass fuels (Global Initiative for Chronic Obstructive Lung Disease [GOLD], 2017).

Chronic Bronchitis

Bronchitis is an inflammation of the bronchi and bronchioles caused by exposure to irritants, especially cigarette smoke. The irritant triggers inflammation, vasodilation, mucosal edema, congestion, and bronchospasm. Bronchitis affects only the airways, not the alveoli.

Chronic inflammation increases the number and size of mucus-secreting glands, which produce large amounts of thick mucus. The bronchial walls thicken and impair airflow. This thickening, along with excessive mucus, blocks some of the smaller airways and narrows larger ones. The increased mucus provides a breeding ground for organisms and leads to chronic infection.

Chronic bronchitis impairs airflow and GAS EXCHANGE because mucus plugs and infection narrow the airways. As a result, the PaO_2 level decreases (hypoxemia), and the arterial carbon dioxide ($PaCO_2$) level increases (respiratory acidosis).

Etiology and Genetic Risk

Cigarette smoking is the greatest risk factor for COPD. The patient with a 20–pack-year history or longer often has early-stage COPD with changes in pulmonary function tests (PFTs).

The inhaled smoke triggers the release of excessive proteases in the lungs. These enzymes break down elastin, the major component of alveoli. By impairing the action of cilia, smoking also inhibits the cilia from clearing the bronchi of mucus, cellular debris, and fluid.

Alpha₁-antitrypsin deficiency is a less common but important risk factor for COPD, although it is often underrecognized (Kessenich & Bacher, 2015). The enzyme alpha$_1$-antitrypsin (AAT) is normally present in the lungs. AAT inhibits excessive protease activity so the proteases only break down inhaled pollutants and organisms and do not damage lung structures.

The production of normal amounts of AAT depends on the inheritance of a pair of normal gene alleles for this protein. The AAT gene is recessive. Thus if one of the pair of alleles is faulty and the other allele is normal, the adult makes enough AAT to prevent COPD unless there is significant exposure to cigarette smoke or other inhalation irritants. However, this adult is a carrier for AAT deficiency. When both alleles are faulty, COPD develops at a fairly young age even when the person is not exposed to cigarette smoke or other irritants.

About 100,000 Americans have severe AAT deficiency, and many more have mild-to-moderate deficiencies. Although an AAT deficiency also can cause problems in the skin and liver, lung diseases are more common (Kessenich & Bacher, 2014).

TABLE 30-1 Characteristics Associated With the Most Common Alpha$_1$-Antitrypsin Gene Mutations

MUTATION GENOTYPE	LEVEL OF SERUM ALPHA$_1$-ANTITRYPSIN (% OF NORMAL)	DISEASE SEVERITY
M/S	80%	No detectable disease
S/S	50%-60%	Minimal to no disease expression
M/Z	50%-55%	Minimal to no disease expression
S/Z	30%-35%	Pulmonary disease, early age
Z/Z	10%-15%	Severe COPD, extrapulmonary involvement

COPD, Chronic obstructive pulmonary disease.

⚕ GENETIC/GENOMIC CONSIDERATIONS

Patient-Centered Care QSEN

The gene for AAT has many known variations, and some increase the risk for emphysema. Different variations result in different levels of AAT deficiency, which is why the disease is more severe for some adults than for others (OMIM, 2016b). The most serious variation for emphysema risk is the Z mutation, although others also increase the risk but to a lesser degree. Table 30-1 shows the most common AAT mutations increasing the risk for emphysema. Urge patients who have any AAT deficiency to avoid smoking and other environmental pollutants.

In addition to genetic and environmental factors, asthma also appears to be a risk factor for COPD. The incidence of COPD is reported to be 12 times greater among adults with asthma than among adults without asthma after adjusting for smoking history (GOLD, 2017).

Incidence and Prevalence

The prevalence of chronic bronchitis and emphysema in the United States has been estimated at about 15.8 million and 800,000 in Canada (CDC, 2016; Statistics Canada, 2016b). More than 10% of nursing home residents have COPD. COPD is the fourth leading cause of morbidity and mortality in the United States (GOLD, 2017).

Complications

COPD affects GAS EXCHANGE and the oxygenation of all tissues. Complications include hypoxemia, acidosis, respiratory infection, cardiac failure, dysrhythmias, and respiratory failure.

Hypoxemia and acidosis occur because the patient with COPD has reduced gas exchange, leading to decreased oxygenation and increased carbon dioxide levels. These problems reduce cellular function.

Respiratory infection risk increases because of the increased mucus and poor GAS EXCHANGE. Bacterial infections are common and make COPD symptoms worse by increasing inflammation and mucus production and inducing more bronchospasm. Airflow becomes even more limited, the work of breathing increases, and dyspnea results.

Cardiac failure, especially cor pulmonale (right-sided heart failure caused by pulmonary disease), occurs with bronchitis or

> ### CHART 30-9 Key Features
> #### Cor Pulmonale
>
> - Hypoxia and hypoxemia
> - Increasing dyspnea
> - Fatigue
> - Enlarged and tender liver
> - Warm, cyanotic hands and feet, with bounding pulses
> - Cyanotic lips
> - Distended neck veins
> - Right ventricular enlargement (hypertrophy)
> - Visible pulsations below the sternum
> - GI disturbances such as nausea or anorexia
> - Dependent edema
> - Metabolic and respiratory acidosis
> - Pulmonary hypertension

emphysema. Air trapping, airway collapse, and stiff alveolar walls increase the lung tissue pressure and narrow lung blood vessels, making blood flow more difficult. The increased pressure creates a heavy workload on the right side of the heart, which pumps blood into the lungs. To pump blood through the narrowed vessels, the right side of the heart generates high pressures. In response to this heavy workload, the right chambers of the heart enlarge and thicken, causing right-sided heart failure with backup of blood into the general venous system. Chart 30-9 lists key features of cor pulmonale.

Cardiac dysrhythmias are common in patients with COPD. They result from hypoxemia (from decreased oxygen to the heart muscle), other cardiac disease, drug effects, or acidosis.

Health Promotion and Maintenance

The incidence and severity of COPD would be greatly reduced by smoking cessation. Urge all adults who smoke to quit smoking. Chart 27-2 provides tips to teach adults about smoking cessation. In addition, as described in Chapter 27, teach all adults specific actions to take to avoid exposure to other inhalation irritants.

❖ INTERPROFESSIONAL COLLABORATIVE CARE

Although COPD is a life-limiting chronic disorder, most patients live decades in the community, although management is continuous. Acute infections and other complications often require hospital stays. Adults with COPD may be admitted to the hospital for other health problems or surgery and require continued COPD management.

COPD can affect every aspect of a patient's life, and care is best provided by an interprofessional team. In addition to primary health care providers and nurses, other professionals important to ensuring optimal management include registered dietitians, pharmacists, respiratory therapists, occupational therapists, physical therapists, social workers, patient navigators, community health workers, and mental health practitioners (Bracken, 2016). Like many chronic disorders, COPD management is most effective when the patient and family are full partners with the health care team.

The Concept Map addresses interprofessional care issues related to COPD.

◆ Assessment: Noticing

History. Ask about risk factors such as age, gender, and occupational history. COPD is seen more often in older men. Some types of emphysema occur in families, especially those with alpha₁-antitrypsin (AAT) deficiency.

Obtain a thorough smoking history, because tobacco use is a major risk factor. Ask about the length of time the patient has smoked and the number of packs smoked daily. Use these data to determine the pack-year smoking history.

Ask the patient to describe the breathing problems and assess whether he or she has any difficulty breathing while talking. Does he or she speak in complete sentences, or is it necessary to take a breath between every one or two words? Ask about the presence, duration, or worsening of wheezing, coughing, and shortness of breath. Determine which activities trigger these problems. Assess any cough, and ask whether sputum is clear or colored and how much is produced each day. Ask about the time of day when sputum production is greatest. Smokers often have a productive cough when they get up in the morning; nonsmokers generally do not.

Ask the patient to compare the activity level and shortness of breath now with those of a month ago and a year ago. Ask about any difficulty with eating and sleeping. Many patients sleep in a semi-sitting position because breathlessness is worse when lying down (**orthopnea**). Ask about any difficulty with ADLs or sexual activity. Document this assessment to personalize the intervention plan.

Weigh the patient and compare this weight with previous weights. Unplanned weight loss is likely when COPD severity increases, because the work of breathing increases metabolic needs. Dyspnea and mucus production often result in poor food intake and inadequate nutrition. Ask the patient to recall a typical day's meals and fluid intake. When heart failure is present with COPD, general edema with weight gain may occur.

Physical Assessment/Signs and Symptoms. *General appearance* can provide clues about respiratory status and energy level. Observe weight in proportion to height, posture, mobility, muscle mass, and overall hygiene. The patient with increasingly severe COPD is thin, with loss of muscle mass in the extremities, although the neck muscles may be enlarged. He or she tends to be slow moving and slightly stooped. The patient often sits in a forward-bending posture with the arms held forward, a position known as the *orthopneic* or *tripod position* (Fig. 30-8). When dyspnea becomes severe, activity intolerance may be so great that bathing and general grooming are neglected.

Respiratory changes occur as a result of obstruction, changes in chest size, and fatigue. Inspect the chest and assess the breathing rate and pattern. The patient with respiratory muscle fatigue breathes with rapid, shallow respirations and may have an abnormal breathing pattern in which the abdominal wall is sucked in during inspiration or may use accessory muscles in the abdomen or neck. During an acute exacerbation, the respiratory rate could be as high as 40 to 50 breaths/min and requires immediate medical attention. As respiratory muscles become fatigued, respiratory movement is jerky and appears uncoordinated.

Check the patient's chest for retractions and asymmetric chest expansion. The patient with emphysema has limited diaphragmatic movement (excursion) because the diaphragm is flattened and below its usual resting state. Chest vibration (fremitus) is often decreased, and the chest sounds hyperresonant on percussion because of trapped air (Jarvis, 2016).

Auscultate the chest to assess the depth of inspiration and any abnormal breath sounds. Wheezes and other abnormal sounds often occur on inspiration and expiration, although crackles are usually not present. Reduced breath sounds are common, especially with emphysema. Note the pitch and location of the sound and the point in the respiratory cycle at which the sound

CONCEPT MAP

PERFUSION   CELLULAR REGULATION

Chronic Obstructive Pulmonary Disease (COPD)

GAS EXCHANGE

Concept Map by Deanne A. Blach, MSN, RN

INTERVENTIONS—RESPONDING

1 — History Assessment—Noticing

- Assess ability to perform ADLs. *Good management maintains adequate GAS EXCHANGE and improves overall health.*
- Trend and monitor weight. *Monitors for unplanned weight loss when work of breathing increases metabolic needs.*
- Ask patient to recall a typical day's meals and fluid intake. *Evaluates for inadequate nutrition.*

2 — Physical Assessment—Noticing

- Observe weight/height proportion, posture, mobility, muscle mass, and overall hygiene. *Provides clues about GAS EXCHANGE and energy level.*
- Inspect chest size and shape; assess breath sounds, respiratory rate, pattern, depth of inspiration, presence of retractions, asymmetry of chest expansion, cyanosis and sputum production. *Determines state of respiratory distress and whether chronic symptoms are present.*
- Assess degree of dyspnea using VADS, cyanosis, delayed capillary refill, and finger clubbing. *Indicates decreased arterial oxygen levels and poor GAS EXCHANGE.*
- Assess heart rate & rhythm, dependent edema or other signs and symptoms of right heart failure. *Indicates cardiac changes related to COPD-associated anatomic changes.*
- Examine nail beds and oral mucous membranes. *Indicates adequacy of GAS EXCHANGE and oxygenation of all tissues.*

3 — Nursing Priority - Improving GAS EXCHANGE

- Teach patient to participate in COPD management: airway maintenance, breathing techniques, positioning, effective coughing, oxygen therapy, exercise conditioning, suctioning, hydration, use of a vibratory positive pressure device, and adhering to prescribed drug therapy. *Promotes airway maintenance to improve GAS EXCHANGE.*
- Consult with registered dietitian for nutritional assessment. Monitor weight and serum prealbumin levels. *Prevents loss of muscle mass and strength, lung elasticity, and alveolar-capillary surface area, which reduce GAS EXCHANGE.*
- Assist patient with strategies to manage anxiety. *Keeps patient calm during acute dyspneic episodes.*
- Assist with ADLs. Encourage patient to self-pace activities, note skin color changes, pulse rate and regularity, O_2 saturation and work of breathing, supplemental low-dose O_2 for high energy activities. *Helps to manage chronic fatigue.*
- Teach patient to avoid crowds and get pneumonia and influenza vaccines. *Prevents risk for respiratory tract infections.*

4 — Interpreting Laboratory Assessment

- Review ABG values and monitor pulse oximetry. *Assesses changes in respiratory status and gauges treatment response to identify abnormal GAS EXCHANGE.*
- Obtain sputum samples for culture & sensitivity and white blood cell count. *Evaluates for infections and helps identify necessary treatment.*
- Review hemoglobin & hematocrit. Assess electrolytes. *Assesses for polycythemia. Evaluates for acidosis. Low electrolyte levels reduce muscle strength.*

5 — Drug Therapy

- Teach patient about drug management and correct techniques for inhaler use. *Helps ensure patient receives full dose of inhaled medication and ensures correct sequence is done.*

6 — Psychosocial Assessment

- Assess patient's home environment, interests, hobbies, and potential factors that contribute to respiratory infections. *Helps prevent isolation due to fatigue or embarrassment from coughing and excessive sputum production.*
- Explore economic impact of disease on patient. *Evaluates patient ability to purchase and take drugs correctly.*
- Encourage the expression of concerns about lifestyle, disease progression, and use of support groups. *Urges patient to participate in a full life, and reduces anxiety and fear from feelings of breathlessness.*

EXPECTED OUTCOMES

- Attain and maintain GAS EXCHANGE at usual baseline level: SpO_2 at least 88%, no cyanosis, maintain cognitive orientation, cough and clear secretions effectively, and maintain respiratory rate and rhythm appropriate to activity level.
- Achieve and maintain body weight within 10% of ideal: maintain appropriate weight/height ratio, maintain serum albumin or prealbumin within normal range.
- Have decreased anxiety, identify contributory factors, and perform activities to decrease or eliminate anxiety.
- Increase activity to an acceptable level: maintain baseline SpO_2 with activity, perform ADLs with no or minimal assistance, perform selected activities with minimal dyspnea or tachycardia, participate in family, work, or social activities as desired.
- Avoid serious respiratory infection: describe signs and symptoms, monitoring procedures, preventive strategies, and seek medical assistance when signs of respiratory infection appear.

Planning

PATIENT PROBLEMS

- Hypoxemia with hypercapnia
- Weight loss related to dyspnea, excessive secretions, anorexia, and fatigue
- Anxiety related to dyspnea, a change in health status, and situational crisis
- Activity Intolerance
- Potential for pneumonia or other respiratory infections

Interpreting the Data

NOTICE IN THE HISTORY

Nick Williams, age 66, is a long-time smoker admitted with an exacerbation of COPD. He reports shortness of breath and a productive cough with thick yellow sputum.

NOTICING— Physical Assessment

ABGs—pH 7.31; PaO_2 66; $PaCO_2$ 59; HCO_3^- 26. Bilateral wheezing, dyspnea and tachypnea 28/min, O_2 sat 86%, T 100.6° F, HR 104; BP 140/88; use of accessory muscles; productive cough; thick yellow sputum; digital clubbing; barrel-shaped chest; skin cool and dry. No peripheral edema.

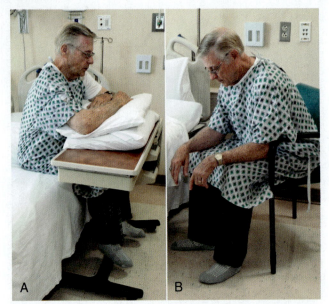

FIG. 30-8 Orthopnea positions that patients with chronic obstructive pulmonary disease (COPD) often assume to ease the work of breathing.

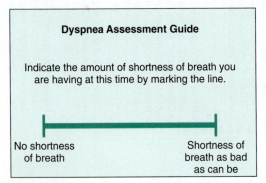

Dyspnea Assessment Guide

Indicate the amount of shortness of breath you are having at this time by marking the line.

No shortness of breath ——— Shortness of breath as bad as can be

FIG. 30-9 Visual analog scale to assess dyspnea. (Modified from Gift, A. [1989]. A dyspnea assessment guide. *Critical Care Nurse, 9*[8], 79. Used with permission.)

is heard. A silent chest may indicate serious airflow obstruction or pneumothorax.

Assess the degree of dyspnea using a visual analog dyspnea scale (VADS), which is a straight line with verbal anchors at the beginning and end of a 100-mm line (Fig. 30-9). Ask the patient to place a mark on the line to indicate his or her breathing difficulty. Document and use this scale to determine the therapy effectiveness and pace the patient's activities.

Examine the patient's chest for the presence of a "barrel chest" (see Fig. 30-3). With a barrel chest, the ratio between the anteroposterior (AP) diameter of the chest and its lateral diameter is 1:1 rather than the normal ratio of 1:1.5, as a result of lung overinflation and diaphragm flattening (Jarvis, 2016).

The patient with chronic bronchitis often has a cyanotic, or blue-tinged, dusky appearance and has excessive sputum production. Assess for cyanosis, delayed capillary refill, and finger clubbing (Fig. 30-10), which indicate chronically decreased arterial oxygen levels and poor GAS EXCHANGE.

Cardiac changes occur as a result of the anatomic changes associated with COPD. Assess the patient's heart rate and rhythm. Check for swelling of the feet and ankles (dependent edema) or other signs of right-sided heart failure. Examine nail beds and oral mucous membranes. In late-stage emphysema the patient may have pallor or cyanosis and is usually underweight.

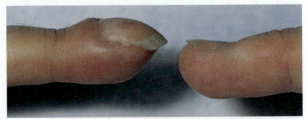

FIG. 30-10 Late digital clubbing *(on left)* compared with a normal digit *(on right)*. (From Swartz, M. H. (2009). *Textbook of physical diagnosis: History and examination* [6th ed.]. Philadelphia: Saunders.)

Psychosocial Assessment. COPD affects all aspects of a patient's life. He or she may be isolated because dyspnea causes fatigue or because of embarrassment from coughing and excessive sputum production.

Ask the patient about interests and hobbies to assess whether socialization has decreased or whether hobbies cause exposure to irritants. Ask about home conditions for exposure to smoke or crowded living conditions that promote transmission of respiratory infections.

Economic status may be affected by the disease through changes in income and health insurance coverage. Drugs, especially the metered dose inhalers (MDIs) and dry powder inhalers (DPIs), are expensive, and many patients with limited incomes may use them only during exacerbations and not as prescribed on a scheduled basis.

Anxiety and fear from feelings of breathlessness may reduce the patient's ability to participate in a full life. Work, family, social, and sexual roles can be affected. Encourage the patient and family to express their feelings about the limitations on lifestyle and disease progression. Assess their use of support groups and community services.

Laboratory Assessment. Arterial blood gas (ABG) values identify abnormal GAS EXCHANGE, oxygenation, ventilation, and acid-base status. Compare repeated ABG values to assess changes in respiratory status. Once baseline ABG values are obtained, pulse oximetry can gauge treatment response. As COPD worsens, the amount of oxygen in the blood decreases (hypoxemia), and the amount of carbon dioxide increases (hypercarbia). Chronic respiratory acidosis (increased arterial carbon dioxide [$Paco_2$]) then results; metabolic alkalosis (increased arterial bicarbonate) occurs as compensation by kidney retention of bicarbonate. This change is seen on ABGs as an elevation of HCO_3^- although pH remains lower than normal. Not all patients with COPD are CO_2 retainers, even when hypoxemia is present, because CO_2 diffuses more easily across lung membranes than does oxygen. Hypercarbia is a problem in advanced emphysema (because the alveoli are affected) rather than in bronchitis (in which the airways are affected).

Sputum samples are obtained for culture from hospitalized patients with an acute respiratory infection. The infection is treated on the basis of symptoms and the common bacterial organisms in the local community. A WBC count helps confirm the presence of infection.

Other blood tests include hemoglobin and hematocrit to determine *polycythemia* (a compensatory increase in red blood cells [RBCs] and iron in the chronically hypoxic patient). Serum electrolyte levels are examined because acidosis can change electrolyte values. Low phosphate, potassium, calcium, and magnesium levels reduce muscle strength. In patients with a family history of COPD, serum AAT levels may be drawn.

TABLE 30-2	Gold Classification of COPD Severity	
CLASS	**PULMONARY FUNCTION TEST RESULTS**
GOLD 1: Mild	FEV_1 ≥80% of predicted
GOLD 2: Moderate	FEV_1 50% to 79% of predicted
GOLD 3: Severe	FEV_1 30% to 49% of predicted
GOLD 4: Very severe	FEV_1 <30% of predicted

Data from Global Initiative for Chronic Obstructive Lung Disease (GOLD). (2017). *Global strategy for the diagnosis, management, and prevention of chronic obstructive pulmonary disease.* http://goldcopd.org/wp-content/uploads/2016/12/wms-GOLD-2017-Pocket-Guide.pdf.
COPD, Chronic obstructive pulmonary disease; *FEV₁,* volume of air blown out as hard and fast as possible during the first second of the most forceful exhalation after the greatest full inhalation; *FVC,* functional vital capacity.

Imaging Assessment. Chest x-rays are used to rule out other lung diseases and to check the progress of patients with respiratory infections or chronic disease. With advanced emphysema, chest x-rays show hyperinflation and a flattened diaphragm.

Other Diagnostic Assessments. COPD is classified from mild to very severe on the basis of symptoms and pulmonary function test (PFT) changes (Table 30-2; see Table 27-6). Airflow rates and lung volume measurements help distinguish airway disease (obstructive diseases) from interstitial lung disease (restrictive diseases). PFTs determine lung volumes, flow volume curves, and diffusion capacity. Each test is performed before and after the patient inhales a bronchodilator agent. Encourage the patient to express his or her feelings about testing and the potential impact of the results. Explain the preparations for the procedures (if any), whether pain or discomfort will be involved, and any needed follow-up care.

Although the severity classification in Table 30-2 can help clinicians determine overall disease severity, it does not predict how well the patient can manage his or her activity on a daily basis and how likely an acute exacerbation could occur. So this classification was modified in 2017 to include the severity indications based on symptom scores obtained with the patient responses to the COPD Assessment Test (CAT) (GOLD, 2017). This 8-item test requires the patient to rate his or her specific symptoms on a 0 (no symptom) to a 5 (worst symptom) scale. Scores can range from 0 to 40, with lower scores indicating less severe problems. As a result, each of the GOLD classes also can contain an ABCD designation for actual symptom severity as an indicator of risk for exacerbation. An *A* designation indicates a low risk for exacerbation, even when the patient has a GOLD class of 4 (very severe disease), whereas a *D* designation indicates a high risk for exacerbation (and need for hospitalization), even if the patient meets PFT results associated with a GOLD class of 1 (mild disease). It is hoped that use of the new classification can help clinicians better recognize when interventions are needed to prevent an acute exacerbation.

The lung volumes measured for COPD are vital capacity (VC), residual volume (RV), forced expiratory volume (FEV), and total lung capacity (TLC). Although all volumes and capacities change to some degree in COPD, the RV is most affected, with increases reflecting the trapped, stale air remaining in the lungs that interferes with GAS EXCHANGE.

A diagnosis of COPD is based mostly on the FEV_1 (the FEV in the first second of exhalation). FEV_1 can also be expressed as a percentage of the forced vital capacity (FVC). As the disease progresses, the ratio of FEV_1 to FVC becomes smaller.

The diffusion test measures how well a test gas (carbon monoxide) diffuses across the alveolar-capillary membrane and combines with hemoglobin. In emphysema, alveolar wall destruction decreases the large surface area for diffusion of gas into the blood, leading to a decreased diffusion capacity. In bronchitis alone, the diffusion capacity is usually normal.

The patient with COPD has decreased oxygen saturation, often much lower than 90%. Changes in SpO_2 below the patient's usual saturation require medical attention. Patients who have been managing COPD for a long time often are aware of their usual SpO_2 values.

Peak expiratory flow meters are used to monitor the effectiveness of drug therapy to relieve obstruction. Peak flow rates increase as obstruction resolves. Teach the patient to self-monitor the peak expiratory flow rates at home and adjust drugs as needed.

◆ *Analysis: Interpreting*

The priority collaborative problems for patients with chronic obstructive pulmonary disease (COPD) include:

1. Decreased GAS EXCHANGE due to alveolar-capillary membrane changes, reduced airway size, ventilatory muscle fatigue, excessive mucus production, airway obstruction, diaphragm flattening, fatigue, and decreased energy
2. Weight loss due to dyspnea, excessive secretions, anorexia, and fatigue
3. Anxiety due to a change in health status, and situational crisis
4. Decreased endurance due to fatigue, dyspnea, and an imbalance between oxygen supply and demand
5. Potential for pneumonia or other respiratory infections due to presence of thick secretions and the immunosuppressive effects of some drugs

◆ *Planning and Implementation: Responding*
 Improving Gas Exchange and Reducing Carbon Dioxide Retention

Planning: Expected Outcomes. The patient with COPD is expected to attain and maintain GAS EXCHANGE at his or her usual baseline level. Indicators include that the patient:

- Maintains SpO_2 of at least 88%
- Remains free from cyanosis
- Maintains cognitive orientation
- Coughs and clears secretions effectively
- Maintains a respiratory rate and rhythm appropriate to his or her activity level

Interventions. Most patients with COPD use nonsurgical management to improve or maintain GAS EXCHANGE. Surgical management requires that the patient meet strict criteria.

Nonsurgical Management. Nursing management for patients with COPD focuses on airway maintenance, monitoring, breathing techniques, positioning, effective coughing, oxygen therapy, exercise conditioning, suctioning, hydration, and use of a vibratory positive-pressure device. A nursing priority is to teach the patient how to be a partner in COPD management by participating in therapies to improve GAS EXCHANGE and by adhering to prescribed drug therapy.

Before any intervention, assess the breathing rate, rhythm, depth, and use of accessory muscles. The accessory muscles are less efficient than the diaphragm, and the work of breathing increases. Determine whether any factors are contributing to the increased work of breathing, such as respiratory infection. *Airway maintenance is the most important focus of interventions to improve GAS EXCHANGE.*

Monitoring. Monitoring for changes in respiratory status is key to providing prompt interventions to reduce complications. Assess the hospitalized patient with COPD at least every 2 hours, even when the purpose of hospitalization is not COPD management. Apply prescribed oxygen, assess the patient's response to therapy, and prevent complications.

If the patient's condition worsens, more aggressive therapy is needed. Noninvasive ventilation (NIV) may be useful for patients with stable, very severe COPD and daytime hypercapnia (GOLD, 2017). Intubation and mechanical ventilation may be needed for patients in respiratory failure.

Breathing Techniques. Diaphragmatic or abdominal and pursed-lip breathing may be helpful for managing dyspneic episodes. Teach the patient to use these techniques, shown in Chart 30-10, during all activities to reduce the amount of stale air in the lungs and manage dyspnea. Teach these techniques when the patient has less dyspnea.

In diaphragmatic breathing, the patient consciously increases movement of the diaphragm. Lying on the back allows the abdomen to relax. Breathing through pursed lips creates mild resistance, which prolongs exhalation and increases airway pressure. This technique delays airway compression and reduces air trapping.

Positioning. Placing the patient in an upright position with the head of the bed elevated can help alleviate dyspnea by increasing chest expansion and keeping the diaphragm in the proper position to contract. This position conserves energy by supporting the patient's arms and upper body. Help the patient who can tolerate sitting in a chair to get out of bed for 1-hour periods two to three times a day.

Effective Coughing. Coughing effectively can improve GAS EXCHANGE by helping increase airflow in the larger airways. The patient with COPD has difficulty removing secretions, which results in poor gas exchange. Excessive mucus increases the risk for infections.

Controlled coughing is helpful in removing excessive mucus. Teach the patient to cough on arising in the morning to eliminate mucus that collected during the night. Coughing to clear mucus before mealtimes may make meals more pleasant. Coughing before bedtime may help clear lungs for a less interrupted night's sleep.

For effective coughing, teach the patient to sit in a chair or on the side of a bed with feet placed firmly on the floor. Instruct him or her to turn the shoulders inward and to bend the head slightly downward, hugging a pillow against the stomach. The patient then takes a few breaths, attempting to exhale more fully. After the third to fifth breath (in through the nose, out through pursed lips), instruct him or her to take a deeper breath and bend forward slowly while coughing two or three times ("mini" coughs) from the same breath. On return to a sitting position, the patient takes a comfortably deep breath. The entire coughing procedure is repeated at least twice.

Oxygen Therapy. Oxygen is prescribed for relief of hypoxemia and hypoxia. The need for oxygen therapy and its effectiveness can be determined by arterial blood gas (ABG) values and oxygen saturation. The patient with COPD may need an oxygen flow of 2 to 4 L/min via nasal cannula or up to 40% via Venturi mask. Ensure that there are no open flames in rooms in which oxygen is in use. See Chapter 28 for information on oxygen therapy.

In the past, the patient with COPD was thought to be at risk for extreme hypoventilation with oxygen therapy because of a decreased drive to breathe as blood oxygen levels rose. However,

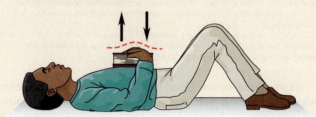

CHART 30-10 Patient and Family Education: Preparing for Self-Management

Breathing Exercises

Diaphragmatic or Abdominal Breathing
- If you can do so comfortably, lie on your back with your knees bent. If you cannot lie comfortably, perform this exercise while sitting in a chair.
- Place your hands or a book on your abdomen to create resistance.
- Begin breathing from your abdomen while keeping your chest still. You can tell if you are breathing correctly if your hands or the book rises and falls accordingly.

Pursed-Lip Breathing
- Close your mouth and breathe in through your nose.
- Purse your lips as you would to whistle. Breathe out slowly through your mouth, without puffing your cheeks. Spend at least twice the amount of time it took you to breathe in.
- Use your abdominal muscles to squeeze out every bit of air you can.
- Remember to use pursed-lip breathing during any physical activity. Always inhale before beginning the activity and exhale while performing it. Never hold your breath.

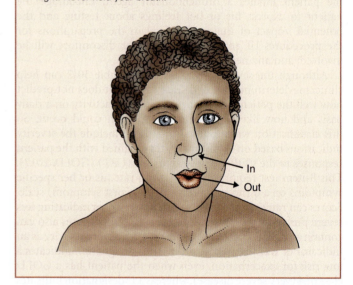

this concern has not been shown to be evidence based and has been responsible for ineffective management of hypoxia in patients with COPD. All hypoxic patients, even those with COPD and hypercarbia, should receive oxygen therapy at rates appropriate to reduce hypoxia and bring Spo$_2$ levels up between 88% and 92% (Burt & Corbridge, 2013; Makic et al., 2013).

Drug Therapy. Drugs used to manage COPD are the same drugs as for asthma and include beta-adrenergic agents, cholinergic antagonists, xanthines, corticosteroids, and cromones (see Chart 30-6). The focus is on long-term control therapy with longer-acting drugs, such as arformoterol (Brovana); indacaterol (Arcapta Neohaler); tiotropium (Spiriva); aclidinium bromide (Tudorza Pressair); olodaterol (Striverdi); and the combination drugs, such as fluticasone/vilanterol (BREO ELLIPTA), olodaterol/tiotropium (STIOLTO RESPIMAT), and vilanterol/umeclidinium (ANORO ELLIPTA). The patient with COPD is more likely to be taking systemic agents in addition to inhaled drugs. Another drug class for COPD is the mucolytics, which thin the thick secretions, making them easier to cough up and expel. Nebulizer treatments with normal saline or a mucolytic agent such as acetylcysteine (Mucosil, Mucomyst ✦) or dornase alfa (Pulmozyme) and normal saline help thin secretions. Guaifenesin (Organidin, Naldecon Senior EX) is a systemic mucolytic that is taken orally. A combination of guaifenesin and dextromethorphan (Mucinex DM) also raises the cough threshold.

Stepped therapy, which adds drugs as COPD progresses, is recommended for patients with chronic bronchitis or emphysema, although the patient's response to drug therapy is the best indicator of when drugs or their dosages need changing. Ideally the patient notices changes and participates in management strategies. Teach patients and family members the correct techniques for using inhalers and to care for them properly.

Many inhalers for COPD drug therapy are dry powder inhalers (DPIs). These often require having the patient "load in" each dose. The steps for this process involve opening the inhaler's capsule chamber, removing the dry powder capsule from a separate blister pack, placing the capsule in the chamber, closing the inhaler until it clicks and punctures the capsule, and then using the inhaler. Often the patient with severe COPD is older, has muscle weakness, has poor manual dexterity, and may have some problems with cognition. All of these issues can be barriers to proper use of a DPI inhaler for COPD management.

Exercise Conditioning. Exercise for conditioning and pulmonary rehabilitation can improve function and endurance in patients with COPD. Patients often respond to the dyspnea of COPD by limiting their activity, even basic ADLs. Over time, the muscles used in breathing weaken, resulting in increased dyspnea with lower activity levels.

Pulmonary rehabilitation involves education and exercise training to prevent muscle deconditioning. Each patient's exercise program is personalized to his or her current limitations and planned outcomes. The simplest plan is having the patient walk (indoors or outdoors) daily at a self-paced rate until symptoms limit further walking, followed by a rest period, and then continue walking until 20 minutes of actual walking has been accomplished. As the time during rest periods decreases, the patient can add 5 more minutes of walking time. Teach patients whose symptoms are severe to modify the exercise by using a walker with wheels or, if needed, to use oxygen while exercising. Exercise needs to be performed at least two or three times weekly for best improvement. Formal pulmonary rehabilitation programs can be beneficial even for patients who are severely impaired. Additional exercise techniques to retrain ventilatory muscles include isocapneic hyperventilation and resistive breathing. Isocapneic hyperventilation, in which the patient hyperventilates into a machine that controls the levels of oxygen and carbon dioxide, increases endurance. In resistive breathing the patient breathes against a set resistance. Resistive breathing increases respiratory muscle strength and endurance.

Suctioning. Perform suctioning only when needed—not routinely. Nasotracheal suction is used only for patients with a weak cough, weak pulmonary muscles, and inability to expectorate effectively. Assess for dyspnea, tachycardia, and dysrhythmias during the procedure. Assess for improved breath sounds after suctioning. Suctioning is discussed in detail in Chapter 28.

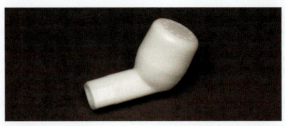

FIG. 30-11 The FLUTTER® valve mucus clearance device, a type of vibratory positive-pressure device. (Courtesy Axcan Pharma, Mont-Saint-Hilaire, Quebec, Canada.)

Hydration. Maintaining hydration may thin the thick, tenacious (sticky) secretions, making them easier to remove by coughing. Unless hydration needs to be avoided for other health problems, teach the patient with COPD to drink at least 2 L/day. Humidifiers may be useful for those living in a dry climate or those who use dry heat during the winter.

Vibratory Positive Expiratory Pressure Device. The use of a vibratory positive expiratory pressure device can help patients remove airway secretions. The device is a small, handheld plastic pipe with a short, fat stem and a perforated lid over the bowl (Fig. 30-11). A movable steel ball is inside the bowl. The patient inhales deeply and then exhales through the device, causing the ball to move and set up vibrations that are transmitted to the chest and airways. The vibrations loosen secretions and allow them to be coughed out more easily.

Surgical Management. Lung transplantation and lung reduction surgery can improve GAS EXCHANGE in the patient with COPD. Transplantation is a relatively rare procedure because of cost and the scarce availability of donor lungs. The more common surgical procedure for patients with emphysema is lung reduction surgery.

The purpose of lung reduction surgery is to improve GAS EXCHANGE through removal of hyperinflated lung tissues that are filled with stagnant air containing little, if any, oxygen. The level of carbon dioxide is the same as that in the capillary, and no gas exchange occurs. Successful lung reduction results in increased forced expiratory volume and decreased total lung capacity and residual volume. Activity tolerance increases, and oxygen therapy may no longer be needed.

Preoperative Care. Patients who are selected for this procedure have end-stage emphysema, minimal chronic bronchitis, and stable cardiac function. They also must be ambulatory; not ventilator dependent; free of pulmonary fibrosis, asthma, or cancer; and not have smoked for at least 6 months. The patient must be rehabilitated to the stage that he or she is able to walk, without stopping, for 30 minutes at 1 mile/hr and maintain a 90% or better oxygen saturation level.

In addition to standard preoperative testing, tests to determine the location of greatest lung hyperinflation and poorest lung blood flow are performed. These tests include pulmonary plethysmography, gas dilution, and PERFUSION scans.

Operative Procedures. Usually lung reduction is performed on both lungs, most often by the minimally invasive surgical technique of video-assisted thoracoscopic surgery (VATS) (GOLD, 2016). Each lung is examined for areas of hyperinflation. The surgeon removes as much of the hyperinflated tissue as possible.

Postoperative Care. After lung reduction surgery, the patient needs close monitoring for continuing respiratory problems and usual postoperative complications. Bronchodilator and mucolytic therapies are maintained. Pulmonary hygiene includes incentive spirometry 10 times per hour while awake, chest physiotherapy starting on the first day after surgery, and hourly pulmonary assessment.

Preventing Weight Loss

Planning: Expected Outcomes. The patient with COPD is expected to achieve and maintain a body weight within 10% of ideal. Indicators include that the patient:

- Maintains an appropriate weight/height ratio
- Maintains serum albumin or prealbumin within the normal range

Interventions. The patient with COPD often has nausea, *early satiety* (feeling too "full" to eat), poor appetite, and meal-related dyspnea. The work of breathing raises calorie and protein needs, which can lead to protein-calorie malnutrition. Malnourished patients lose muscle mass and strength, lung elasticity, and alveolar-capillary surface area, all of which reduce GAS EXCHANGE and PERFUSION.

Identify patients at risk for or who have this complication and collaborate with a registered dietitian to perform a nutrition assessment. Monitor weight and other indicators of nutrition, such as serum prealbumin levels.

Dyspnea management is needed because shortness of breath interferes with eating. Teach the patient to plan the biggest meal of the day for the time when he or she is most hungry and well rested. Four to six small meals a day may be preferred to three larger ones. Remind patients to use pursed-lip and abdominal breathing and to use the prescribed bronchodilator 30 minutes before the meal to reduce bronchospasm.

Food selection can help prevent weight loss. Abdominal bloating and a feeling of fullness often prevent the patient from eating a complete meal. Collaborate with the dietitian to teach about foods that are easy to chew and not gas-forming. Advise the patient to avoid dry foods that stimulate coughing and caffeine-containing drinks that increase urine output and may lead to dehydration.

Urge the patient to eat high-calorie, high-protein foods. Supplements such as Pulmocare provide nutrition with reduced carbon dioxide production. If early satiety is a problem, advise him or her to avoid drinking fluids before and during the meal and to eat smaller, more frequent meals.

❓ NCLEX EXAMINATION CHALLENGE 30-2

Health Promotion and Maintenance

Which interventions are important for the nurse to teach a client with severe chronic obstructive pulmonary disease (COPD) to help ensure adequate nutrition? **Select all that apply.**
A. Avoid eating gas-producing foods.
B. Cough to clear mucus right before eating.
C. Drink plenty of fluid with every meal.
D. Eat smaller meals more frequently.
E. Rest immediately following a meal.
F. Eat more raw fruits and vegetables.
G. Use your bronchodilator about 30 minutes before each meal.

Minimizing Anxiety

Planning: Expected Outcomes. The patient with COPD is expected to have decreased anxiety. Indicators include that the patient consistently demonstrates these behaviors:

- Identifies factors that contribute to anxiety
- Identifies activities to decrease anxiety
- States that anxiety is reduced or absent

Interventions. Patients with COPD become anxious during acute dyspneic episodes, especially when excessive secretions are present. Anxiety also may cause dyspnea.

Help the patient understand that anxiety can increase dyspnea and have a plan for dealing with anxiety. Together with the patient, develop a written plan that states exactly what he or she should do if symptoms flare. Having a plan provides confidence and control in knowing what to do, which often helps reduce anxiety. Stress the use of pursed-lip and diaphragmatic breathing techniques during periods of anxiety or panic.

Family, friends, and support groups can be helpful. Recommend professional counseling, if needed, as a positive suggestion. Stress that talking with a counselor can help identify techniques to maintain control over dyspnea and panic.

Explore other approaches to help the patient manage dyspneic episodes and panic attacks, such as progressive relaxation, hypnosis therapy, and biofeedback. For some patients, antianxiety drug therapy may be needed for severe anxiety.

Improving Endurance

Planning: Expected Outcomes. The patient with COPD is expected to increase activity to a level acceptable to him or her. Indicators include that the patient:

- Maintains his or her baseline Spo$_2$ with activity
- Performs ADLs with no or minimal assistance
- Participates in family, work, or social activities as desired

Interventions. The patient with COPD often has chronic fatigue. During acute exacerbations, he or she may need extensive help with the ADLs of eating, bathing, and grooming. As the acute problem resolves, encourage the patient to pace activities and perform as much self-care as possible. Teach him or her to not rush through morning activities, because rushing increases dyspnea, fatigue, and hypoxemia. As activity gradually increases, assess the patient's response by noting skin color changes, pulse rate and regularity, oxygen saturation, and work of breathing. Suggest the use of oxygen during periods of high energy use such as bathing or walking.

Energy conservation is the planning and pacing of activities for best tolerance and minimum discomfort. Ask the patient to describe a typical daily schedule. Help him or her divide each activity into its smaller parts to determine whether that task can be performed in a different way or at a different time. Teach about planning and pacing daily activities with rest periods between activities. Help the patient develop a chart outlining the day's activities and planned rest periods.

Encourage the patient to avoid working with the arms raised. Activities involving the arms decrease exercise tolerance because the accessory muscles are used to stabilize the arms and shoulders rather than to assist breathing. Many activities involving the arms can be done sitting at a table leaning on the elbows. Teach the patient to adjust work heights to reduce back strain and fatigue. Remind him or her to keep arm motions smooth and flowing to prevent jerky motions that waste energy. Work with the occupational therapist to teach about the use of adaptive tools for housework, such as long-handled dustpans, sponges, and dusters, to reduce bending and reaching.

Suggest organizing work spaces so items used most often are within easy reach. Measures such as dividing laundry or groceries into small parcels that can be handled easily, using disposable plates to save washing time, and letting dishes dry in the rack also conserve energy. Teach the patient to not talk when engaged in other activities that require energy, such as walking. In addition, teach him or her to avoid breath holding while performing any activity.

Preventing Respiratory Infection

Planning: Expected Outcomes. The patient with COPD is expected to avoid serious respiratory infection. Indicators include that the patient consistently demonstrates these behaviors:

- Describes signs and symptoms of respiratory infection
- Describes respiratory infection-monitoring procedures
- Uses prevention activities such as pneumonia and influenza vaccination and crowd avoidance
- Seeks medical assistance when signs of respiratory infection first appear

Interventions. Pneumonia is a common complication of COPD, especially among older adults. Patients who have excessive secretions are at increased risk for respiratory tract infections. Teach patients to avoid crowds and stress the importance of receiving a pneumonia vaccination and a yearly influenza vaccine.

Care Coordination and Transition Management

Home Care Management. Most patients with COPD are managed in the ambulatory care setting and cared for at home. When pneumonia or a severe exacerbation develops, the patient often returns home after hospitalization. For those with advanced disease, 24-hour care may be needed for ADLs and for monitoring. If home care is not possible, placement in a long-term care setting may be needed.

Patients with hypoxemia may use oxygen at home either as needed or continually. Continuous, long-term oxygen therapy can reverse tissue hypoxia and improve cognition and well-being. For more information on home oxygen therapy, see Chapter 28.

Collaborate with the case manager to obtain the equipment needed for care at home. Patient needs may include oxygen therapy, a hospital-type bed, a nebulizer, a tub transfer bench or shower chair, and scheduled visits from a home care nurse for monitoring and evaluation.

The patient with COPD faces a lifelong disease with remissions and exacerbations. Explain to the patient and family that he or she may have periods of anxiety, depression, and ineffective coping. The patient who was a smoker may also have self-directed anger.

Self-Management Education. Patients with COPD need to know as much about the disease as possible so they can better manage it and themselves. Patients and families should be able to discuss drug therapy, signs of infection, avoidance of respiratory irritants, the nutrition therapy regimen, and activity progression. Instruct them to identify and avoid stressors that can worsen the disease.

Reinforce the techniques of pursed-lip breathing, diaphragmatic breathing, positioning, relaxation therapy, energy conservation, and coughing and deep breathing. Teaching about all of the needed topics may require coordination with the home care or clinic staff.

Health Care Resources. Provide appropriate referrals as needed. Home care visits may be needed, especially when home oxygen therapy is first prescribed. Chart 30-11 lists assessment areas for the patient with COPD at home. Referral to assistance programs, such as Meals on Wheels, can be helpful. Provide a list of support groups and Better Breather clubs sponsored by the American Lung Association. If the patient wants to quit smoking, make the appropriate referrals.

◆ Evaluation: Reflecting

Evaluate the care of the patient with COPD based on the identified priority patient problems. The expected outcomes of care are that the patient will:

🏠 **CHART 30-11** **Home Care Assessment**

The Patient With Chronic Obstructive Pulmonary Disease

Assess respiratory status and adequacy of GAS EXCHANGE.
- Measure rate, depth, and rhythm of respirations.
- Examine mucous membranes and nail beds for evidence of hypoxia.
- Determine use of accessory muscles.
- Examine chest and abdomen for paradoxical breathing.
- Count number of words patient can speak between breaths.
- Determine need and use of supplemental oxygen. (How many liters per minute is the patient using?)
- Determine level of consciousness and presence/absence of confusion.
- Auscultate lungs for abnormal breath sounds.
- Measure oxygen saturation by pulse oximetry.
- Determine sputum production, color, and amount.
- Ask about activity level.
- Observe general hygiene.
- Measure body temperature.

Assess cardiac status for adequate PERFUSION.
- Measure rate, quality, and rhythm of pulse.
- Check dependent areas for edema.
- Check neck veins for distention with the patient in a sitting position.
- Measure capillary refill.

Assess nutritional status.
- Check weight maintenance, loss, or gain.
- Determine food and fluid intake.
- Determine use of nutritional supplements.
- Observe general condition of the skin.

Assess patient's and caregiver's adherence and understanding of illness and treatment, including:
- Correct use of supplemental oxygen
- Correct use of inhalers
- Drug schedule and side effects
- Symptoms to report to the primary health care provider indicating the need for acute care
- Increasing severity of resting dyspnea
- Increasing severity of usual symptoms
- Development of new symptoms associated with poor GAS EXCHANGE
- Respiratory infection
- Failure to obtain the usual degree of relief with prescribed therapies
- Unusual change in condition
- Use of pursed-lip and diaphragmatic breathing techniques
- Scheduling of rest periods and priority activities
- Participation in rehabilitation activities

- Attain and maintain GAS EXCHANGE at a level within his or her chronic baseline values
- Achieve an effective breathing pattern that decreases the work of breathing
- Maintain a patent airway
- Achieve and maintain a body weight within 10% of his or her ideal weight
- Have decreased anxiety
- Increase activity to a level acceptable to him or her
- Avoid serious respiratory infections

CYSTIC FIBROSIS

❖ PATHOPHYSIOLOGY

Cystic fibrosis (CF) is a genetic disease that affects many organs and lethally impairs lung function. Although CF is present from birth and usually is first seen in early childhood, almost half of

---

? **CLINICAL JUDGMENT CHALLENGE 30-1**

Patient-Centered Care; Teamwork and Collaboration QSEN

A 60-year-old patient has recently been diagnosed with GOLD 2 class COPD. He is a current smoker and has only had COPD symptoms for the past year. He and his wife, a retired registered nurse, are attending a class on COPD management. Before the class starts, he complains to you that his wife is pressuring him to make some big changes. First she wants him to stop smoking, which he has agreed to do and has started on pharmacologic therapy to assist in this process. She wants to sell their current home (where they have lived for 25 years) and move to a one-story house. She has started mowing the lawn, which has always been his job, and which he wants to continue to do. She also has asked him to stop his hobby of refinishing furniture to avoid the fumes. He says, "I'm not dying yet, and I don't want to give up any of these things." She says, "I'm just thinking of your best interests and am planning ahead." She then asks you to support her suggestions (demands).

1. How should you respond to her request to support her suggestions? What do you think her motive(s) is (are)?
2. Is there justification for any or all of these suggested changes? Provide a rationale for your responses.
3. Should you continue this conversation with both of them together or separately? Provide a rationale for your choice.
4. Which members of the interprofessional team for COPD management would be helpful in this situation? Provide a rationale for your choices.

---

patients with CF in the United States are adults (Cystic Fibrosis Foundation [CFF], 2015).

The underlying problem of CF is blocked chloride transport in the cell membranes. Poor chloride transport causes the formation of mucus that has little water content and is thick. The thick, sticky mucus causes problems in the lungs, pancreas, liver, salivary glands, and testes. The mucus plugs up the airways in the lungs and the glandular tissues in nonpulmonary organs, causing atrophy and organ dysfunction. Nonpulmonary problems include pancreatic insufficiency, malnutrition, intestinal obstruction, poor growth, male sterility, and cirrhosis of the liver. Additional problems of CF in young adults include osteoporosis and diabetes mellitus. Respiratory failure is the main cause of death. Improved management has increased life expectancy, even among those with severe disease, to about 40 years (CFF, 2015).

The pulmonary problems of CF result from the constant presence of thick, sticky mucus and are the most serious complications of the disease. The mucus narrows airways, reducing airflow and interfering with GAS EXCHANGE. The constant presence of mucus results in chronic respiratory tract infections, chronic bronchitis, and dilation of the bronchioles (bronchiectasis). Lung abscesses are common. Over time, the bronchioles distend, and mucus-producing cells have increased numbers (hyperplasia) and increased size (hypertrophy). Complications include pneumothorax, arterial erosion and hemorrhage, and respiratory failure.

CF is most common among whites, and about 4% are carriers (CFF, 2015). It is rare among African Americans and Asians. Males and females are affected equally.

❖ **INTERPROFESSIONAL COLLABORATIVE CARE**
◆ *Assessment: Noticing*
Usually, but not always, CF is diagnosed in childhood. The major diagnostic test is sweat chloride analysis (Pagana et al.,

---

🧬 **GENETIC/GENOMIC CONSIDERATION**

Patient-Centered Care QSEN

CF is an autosomal-recessive disorder in which both gene alleles must be mutated for the disease to be expressed. The CF gene *(CTFR)* produces a protein that controls chloride movement across cell membranes. The severity of CF varies; however, life expectancy is always reduced, with an average of 40 years. Adults with one mutated allele are carriers and have few or no symptoms of CF but can pass the abnormal allele on to their children. More than 1700 different mutations have been identified, which is responsible for variation in disease severity (OMIM, 2016c). Help patients understand why their symptoms may be more or less severe than others with the disease.

2017). The sweat chloride test is positive for CF when the chloride level in the sweat ranges between 60 and 200 mEq/L (mmol/L), compared with the normal value of less than 40 mEq/L (mmol/L) (CFF, 2015). Values of 40 to 59 mEq/L (mmol/L) are considered borderline. Genetic testing can be performed to determine which specific mutation an adult may have. Different mutations result in different degrees of disease severity.

Nonpulmonary symptoms include abdominal distention, gastroesophageal reflux, rectal prolapse, foul-smelling stools, and **steatorrhea** (excessive fat in stools). The patient is often malnourished and has many vitamin deficiencies, especially of the fat-soluble vitamins (e.g., vitamins A, D, E, K). As pancreatic function decreases, diabetes mellitus develops with loss of insulin production. The adult with severe CF is usually smaller and thinner than average. Another problem seen in adults with CF is the early onset of osteoporosis and osteopenia, with a greatly increased risk for bone fracture (CFF, 2015).

Pulmonary symptoms caused by CF are progressive. Respiratory infections are frequent or chronic with exacerbations. Patients usually have chest congestion, limited exercise tolerance, cough, sputum production, use of accessory muscles, and decreased pulmonary function (especially forced vital capacity [FVC] and forced expiratory volume in the first second of exhalation [FEV_1]). Chest x-rays show infiltrate and an increased anteroposterior (AP) diameter.

During an acute exacerbation or when the disease progresses to end stage, the patient has increased chest congestion, reduced activity tolerance, increased crackles, increased cough, increased sputum production (often with hemoptysis), and severe dyspnea with fatigue. Arterial blood gas (ABG) studies show acidosis (low pH), greatly reduced arterial oxygen (Pao_2) levels, increased arterial carbon dioxide ($Paco_2$) levels, and increased bicarbonate levels.

With infection, the patient has fever, an elevated white blood cell count, and decreased oxygen saturation. Other symptoms of infection include tachypnea, tachycardia, intercostal retractions, weight loss, and increased fatigue.

◆ *Interventions: Responding*
The patient with CF needs daily therapy to slow disease progress and enhance GAS EXCHANGE. There is no cure for CF.

Nonsurgical Management. The management of the patient with CF is complex and lifelong. Nutrition management focuses on weight maintenance, vitamin supplementation, diabetes management, and pancreatic enzyme replacement. Pulmonary management focuses on preventive maintenance and management of exacerbations. Priority nursing interventions focus on

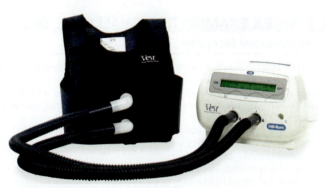

FIG. 30-12 Inflatable chest physiotherapy vest for high-frequency chest wall oscillation (HFCWO). (Modified ©2015 Hill-Rom Services, Inc. Reprinted with permission—all rights reserved.)

teaching about drug therapy, infection prevention, pulmonary hygiene, nutrition, and vitamin supplementation.

Preventive/maintenance therapy involves the use of positive expiratory pressure, active cycle of breathing technique, and an individualized exercise program. Daily chest physiotherapy with postural drainage is beneficial for the patient with CF. This therapy uses chest percussion, chest vibration, and dependent drainage to loosen secretions and promote drainage. Increasingly the use of a chest physiotherapy (CPT) vest is recommended (Fig. 30-12). This system uses an inflatable vest that rapidly fills and deflates, gently compressing and releasing the chest wall up to 25 times per second, a process called high-frequency chest wall oscillation (HFCWO). The action creates mini-coughs that dislodge mucus from the bronchial walls, increase mobilization, and move it toward central airways where it can be removed by coughing or suctioning. HFCWO also thins secretions, making them easier to clear. Pulmonary function tests are monitored regularly. Daily drugs include bronchodilators, anti-inflammatories, mucolytics, and antibiotics.

Exacerbation therapy is needed when the patient with CF has increased chest congestion, reduced activity tolerance, increased or new-onset crackles, and a 10% decrease in FEV_1. Other symptoms include increased sputum production with bloody or purulent sputum, increased coughing, decreased appetite, weight loss, fatigue, decreased SpO_2, and chest muscle retractions. Often infection is present, with fever, increased lung infiltrate on x-ray, and an elevated white blood cell count.

Every attempt is made to avoid mechanical ventilation for the patient with CF. Bi-level positive airway pressure (BiPAP) may be a part of daily therapy for the patient with advanced disease (see Chapter 28 for information on BiPAP). Management focuses on airway clearance, increased GAS EXCHANGE, and antibiotic therapy. Supplemental oxygen is prescribed on the basis of SpO_2 levels. The respiratory therapist initiates airway clearance techniques four times a day. Bronchodilator and mucolytic therapies are intensified. Steroidal agents are started or increased.

Depending on the severity of the exacerbation, a 14- to 21-day course of oral antibiotics may be prescribed. Antibiotic choice is based on which bacteria are found in the patient's sputum. If antibiotics are not effective or if the exacerbation is very severe, IV antibiotics are used, usually an aminoglycoside such as tobramycin and colistin, or meropenem (Merrem).

A serious bacterial infection for patients with CF is *Burkholderia cepacia*. The organism lives in the respiratory tracts of patients with CF and is often resistant to antibiotic therapy. It is spread by casual contact from one CF patient to another.

It is possible for *B. cepacia* to be transmitted to a CF patient during clinic and hospital visits; thus special infection control measures that limit close contact between adults with CF are needed. These measures include separating infected CF patients from noninfected CF patients on hospital units and seeing them in the clinic on different days. Strict CFF-approved procedures are used to clean clinic rooms and respiratory therapy equipment. Drug therapy for this infection usually includes co-trimoxazole (a combination of trimethoprim and sulfamethoxazole [Bactrim, Septra]) along with the usual drugs used for exacerbation therapy.

Teach patients about protecting themselves by not routinely shaking hands or kissing in social settings. Handwashing is critical because the organism also can be acquired indirectly from contaminated surfaces such as sinks and tissues.

As life span increases for patients with CF, other problems, such as bronchiole bleeding from lung arteries, may develop. Interventional radiology may be needed to embolize the bleeding arterial branches. Patients with CF may undergo this procedure repeatedly to control hemoptysis. See Chapter 36 for information on interventional radiology vascular procedures.

Other problems that occur with CF over time include severe gastroesophageal reflux disease (GERD), osteoporosis, and sensory hearing loss. Osteoporosis increases the risk for bone fractures.

Gene therapy for CF is available for use in patients with specific gene mutations (Nakano & Tluczek, 2014). The drug ivacaftor (Kalydeco) has been found to be of value to patients with CF who have any one of the following specific mutations in the *CFTR* gene: G551D, G1244E, G1349D, G178R, G551S, S1251N, S1255P, S549N, or S549R. A newly approved combination drug, lumacaftor/ivacaftor (Orkambi), is effective for patients whose CF is caused by the F508del mutation, the most common mutation involved in CF. For patients with the involved mutations, the oral drugs specifically target and potentiate the CFTR channel opening so this transporter can move chloride ions across the cell membrane. This action reduces sodium and fluid absorption so mucus is less thick and sticky. These drugs have no effect in patients whose *CFTR* gene does not have the specific mutations described.

Surgical Management. The surgical management of the patient with CF is lung transplantation. The patient has greatly reduced symptoms but is at continuing risk for lethal pulmonary infections, especially with anti-rejection drug therapy. The nonpulmonary problems are not helped by this treatment. Transplantation extends life for 1 to 15 years with an average of 7 years; but the transplant rejection rate is high, possibly caused by poor GI absorption of anti-rejection drugs (CFF, 2015).

Fewer lung transplants are performed compared with transplantation of other solid organs because of the scarcity of available lungs. In addition, many patients who could benefit from lung transplantation have serious problems in other organs that make the procedure even more dangerous.

Lung transplant procedures include two lobes or single-lung transplantation, as well as double-lung transplantation. The type of procedure is determined by the patient's overall condition and the life expectancy after transplantation. Usually the patient with CF has a bilateral lobe transplant from either a cadaver donor or a living-related donor.

Preoperative Care. Many factors are considered before lung transplantation surgery. Recipient and donor criteria vary from one program to another, but some criteria are universal.

Recipient criteria for the patient with CF include that he or she must have severe, irreversible lung damage and still be well enough to survive the surgery. Common exclusion criteria include a cancer diagnosis, systemic infection, HIV/AIDS, and irreversible heart, kidney, or liver disease.

Donor criteria, regardless of whether the lung tissue is obtained from a cadaver or from a living-related donor, include that the donor be infection free and cancer free, have healthy lung tissue, be a close tissue match with the recipient, and have the same blood type as the recipient. When the donor is a living relative, additional criteria include an age restriction and that he or she has healthy organs and has not had previous chest surgery.

The two nursing priorities before surgery are teaching the patient the expected regimen of pulmonary hygiene to be used in the period immediately after surgery and assisting him or her in a pulmonary muscle strengthening/conditioning regimen.

Operative Procedures. The patient may or may not need to be placed on cardiopulmonary bypass, depending on the exact procedure. Those having single-lung or lobe transplantation usually do not need bypass; those having double-lung transplantation usually do.

The most common incision used for lung transplantation is a transverse thoracotomy ("clamshell"). The diseased lung or lungs are removed. The new lobes, lung, or lungs are placed in the chest cavity with proper connections made to the trachea, bronchi, and blood vessels. Usually lung transplantation surgery is completed within 4 to 6 hours.

Postoperative Care. The patient is intubated for at least 48 hours, and chest tubes and arterial lines are in place. The care needed is the same as that for any thoracic surgery.

Major problems after lung transplantation are bleeding, infection, and transplant rejection. The patient usually remains in the ICU for several days after transplantation. Postoperative chest physiotherapy often is performed with high-frequency chest wall oscillation (HFCWO) at this time.

Anti-rejection drug regimens are started immediately after surgery, which increases the risk for infection. Combination therapy with the anti-rejection drugs, described in Chapter 17, is used for the rest of the patient's life. Corticosteroids are avoided in the first 10 to 14 days after surgery because of their negative impact on the healing process.

After transplantation, patients have more energy and usually feel very good. The drug regimen for nonpulmonary CF problems is continued for the rest of the patient's life or until after a pancreatic transplant is performed. Exercise is gradually increased; and some patients even participate in intense activities, such as jogging, running, skiing, skating, and swimming.

PULMONARY ARTERIAL HYPERTENSION

❖ PATHOPHYSIOLOGY

General pulmonary hypertension can occur as a complication of other lung disorders. Primary pulmonary arterial hypertension (PAH) (also known as *idiopathic pulmonary hypertension*) occurs in the absence of other lung disorders, and its cause is unknown; however, exposure to some drugs, such as fenfluramine/phentermine (Pondimin or "Fen-Phen") or dasatinib (Sprycel), increase the risk. The disorder is rare and occurs mostly in women between the ages of 20 and 40 years (McCance et al., 2014). The familial PAH form appears to be transmitted in an autosomal-dominant pattern with reduced penetrance (OMIM, 2016d).

? NCLEX EXAMINATION CHALLENGE 30-3
Psychosocial Integrity

A client with CF who is 2 months postoperative from a bilateral lung transplant wants to begin riding his bicycle again, as his pulmonary specialist has said he can do, but his wife is concerned that this will "wear out" his new lungs faster. How will the nurse advise this couple?
A. Remind the wife that activity does not damage or "wear out" the lungs and that exercise will reduce the risk for other health complications.
B. Tell the wife that, because the client has a reduced life expectancy, she should allow him to do whatever he wants.
C. Remind the client that this is the "honeymoon phase" of recovery and that he will not feel well for very long.
D. Advise the client to protect his lungs at all cost.

The pathologic problem in PAH is blood vessel constriction with increasing vascular resistance in the lung. Pulmonary blood pressure rises, and blood flow decreases through the lungs, leading to poor PERFUSION and GAS EXCHANGE with hypoxemia. Eventually the right side of the heart fails (*cor pulmonale*) from the continuous workload of pumping against the high pulmonary pressures. Without treatment, death usually occurs within 2 years after diagnosis.

🧬 GENETIC/GENOMIC CONSIDERATIONS
Patient-Centered Care QSEN

About 50% of patients with pulmonary arterial hypertension have a genetic mutation in the BMPR2 gene, which codes for a growth factor receptor. Excessive activation of this receptor allows increased growth of arterial smooth muscle in the lungs, making these arteries thicker. Many more adults have mutations in this gene than have PAH. It is thought that these mutations increase the susceptibility to PAH when other, often unknown, environmental factors also are present. Mutations in other genes, such as the PPH1 gene and the SMAD9 gene, are also associated with thickening of lung arteries and increased risk for PAH (OMIM, 2016d).

Often PAH is not diagnosed until late in the disease process when the lungs and heart have already been damaged significantly. Teach adults, especially women, who have a first-degree relative (parent or sibling) with PAH to have regular health checks and to consult a primary health care provider whenever pulmonary problems are present.

❖ INTERPROFESSIONAL COLLABORATIVE CARE

◆ Assessment: Noticing

The most common early symptoms are dyspnea and fatigue in an otherwise healthy adult. Some patients also have angina-like chest pain. Table 30-3 lists the classification of PAH.

Diagnosis is made from the results of right-sided heart catheterization showing elevated pulmonary pressures. Other test results suggesting PAH include abnormal ventilation-perfusion scans, pulmonary function tests (PFTs) showing reduced functional pulmonary volumes with reduced diffusion capacity, and an abnormal appearance on CT.

◆ Interventions: Responding

Drug therapy can reduce pulmonary pressures and slow the development of cor pulmonale by dilating pulmonary vessels

TABLE 30-3 Severity Classification for Primary Pulmonary Arterial Hypertension

CLASS	SYMPTOMS
I	Pulmonary hypertension diagnosed by pulmonary function tests and right-sided cardiac catheterization No limitation of physical activity Moderate physical activity does not induce dyspnea, fatigue, chest pain, or light-headedness
II	No symptoms at rest Mild-to-moderate physical activity induces dyspnea, fatigue, chest pain, or light-headedness
III	No or slight symptoms at rest Mild (less than ordinary) activity induces dyspnea, fatigue, chest pain, or light-headedness
IV	Dyspnea and fatigue present at rest Unable to carry out any level of physical activity without symptoms Symptoms of right-sided heart failure apparent (dependent edema, engorged neck veins, enlarged liver)

and preventing clot formation. Warfarin (Coumadin) is taken daily to achieve an international normalized ratio (INR) of 1.5 to 2.0. Calcium channel blockers have been used to dilate blood vessels. The three classes of drugs that have been shown to be most effective in the treatment of PAH are the endothelin-receptor antagonists, prostacyclin agents, and guanylate cyclase stimulators.

Endothelin-receptor agonists, such as bosentan (Tracleer), induce blood vessel relaxation and decrease pulmonary arterial pressure. However, these agents cause general vessel dilation and some degree of hypotension. Another endothelin receptor antagonist drug, macitentan (Opsumit), is an oral agent taken once daily. Teach patients to take the drug with a glass of water; and teach them not to break, chew, or crush the tablet.

Because macitentan can cause birth defects, its use is contraindicated for women who are pregnant or breast-feeding. Instruct women who are sexually active and within childbearing age to use two reliable methods of contraception while taking this drug. In addition, the drug can harm the liver, and patients should avoid drinking alcoholic beverages while taking it.

Natural and synthetic prostacyclin agents provide the best specific dilation of pulmonary blood vessels. Continuous infusion of epoprostenol (Flolan, Veletri) or treprostinil (Remodulin) through a small IV pump reduces pulmonary pressures and increases lung blood flow. Treprostinil also can be delivered by continuous subcutaneous infusion. These continuous infusions of prostacyclin drugs can be performed by the patient at home and in other settings. These drugs also are continued when the patient is hospitalized for any reason. The unusual continuous infusion, the need to keep an IV line dedicated strictly to prostacyclin infusion, and the varied dosages of the different brands of prostacyclins contribute to a high drug error rate when infusing this drug.

The prostacyclin agents iloprost (Ilomedin, Ventavis, Ventavis) and treprostinil (Tyvaso) can be delivered by inhalation. A new oral prostacyclin agonist is selexipag (Uptravi) (Aschenbrenner, 2016). A drug given along with prostacyclins is oral or IV sildenafil (Revatio, Viagra).

Guanylate cyclase stimulators increase the amount an intracellular substance (cGMP) in endothelial cells that induces relaxation and vasodilation. The oral agent in this class is

riociguat (Adempas). It is usually used in combination with other classes of drugs for PAH. Riociguat is known to cause birth defects.

Although most patients with PAH need to stay on prostacyclin drugs until lung transplantation or disease progression to death, a small percentage have been successfully weaned off prostacyclin drug therapy. These patients are maintained on oral bosetan, sildenafil, and warfarin therapy (Demerouti et al., 2013).

❗ NURSING SAFETY PRIORITY (QSEN)

Action Alert

A critical nursing priority for a patient undergoing therapy with IV prostacyclin agents is to ensure that the drug therapy is never interrupted. Deaths have been reported if the drug delivery is interrupted even for a matter of minutes. Teach the patient to always have backup drug cassettes and battery packs. If these are not available or if the line is disrupted, the patient should go to the emergency department immediately.

Another critical priority is helping the patient receiving IV prostacyclin agents prevent sepsis. The central line IV setup provides an access for organisms to enter the bloodstream directly. Teach the patient to use strict aseptic technique for all aspects of the drug delivery system. Also teach him or her to notify the pulmonologist at the first sign of any infection.

When the heart has undergone hypertrophy and cardiac output has fallen, the patient may be started on a regimen of digoxin (Lanoxin) and diuretics. Oxygen therapy is used when dyspnea is uncomfortable. This therapy improves function and reduces symptoms but does not cure PAH.

Surgical management of PAH involves lung transplantation. When cor pulmonale also is present, the patient may need combined heart-lung transplantation. It is not known whether the process of pulmonary vasoconstriction can begin again in the transplanted lungs.

❓ NCLEX EXAMINATION CHALLENGE 30-4

Safe and Effective Care Environment

A client with pulmonary artery hypertension on a continuous IV epoprostenol infusion is in the emergency department with symptoms of possible sepsis. The primary health care provider prescribes a broad-spectrum antibiotic to be administered IV immediately. What is the nurse's **best** action?

A. Request a prescription for an oral antibiotic.

B. Start a peripheral IV line and administer the antibiotic.

C. Administer the IV antibiotic through the continuous infusion's side port.

D. Stop the epoprostenol infusion for 15 minutes to administer the IV antibiotic.

IDIOPATHIC PULMONARY FIBROSIS

❖ PATHOPHYSIOLOGY

Idiopathic pulmonary fibrosis is a common restrictive lung disease. The patient usually is an older adult with a history of cigarette smoking, chronic exposure to inhalation irritants, or exposure to the drugs amiodarone (Cordarone) or ambrisentan (Letairis, Volibris). Most patients have progressive disease with few remission periods. Even with proper treatment, most patients usually survive less than 5 years after diagnosis.

Pulmonary fibrosis is an example of excessive wound healing with loss of CELLULAR REGULATION. Once lung injury occurs, inflammation begins tissue repair. The inflammation continues beyond normal healing time, causing fibrosis and scarring. These changes thicken alveolar tissues, making GAS EXCHANGE difficult.

❖ INTERPROFESSIONAL COLLABORATIVE CARE

The onset is slow, with early symptoms of mild dyspnea on exertion. Pulmonary function tests show decreased forced vital capacity (FVC). High-resolution computed tomography (HRCT) shows a "honeycomb" pattern in affected lung tissue. As the fibrosis progresses, the patient becomes more dyspneic, and hypoxemia becomes severe. Eventually he or she needs high levels of oxygen and often is still hypoxemic. Respirations are rapid and shallow.

Therapy focuses on slowing the fibrotic process and managing dyspnea. Corticosteroids and other immunosuppressants are the mainstays of therapy. Immunosuppressant drugs include cytotoxic drugs such as cyclophosphamide (Cytoxan, Neosar, Procytox ❖), azathioprine (Imuran), chlorambucil (Leukeran), or methotrexate (Folex). These drugs have many side effects, including increased infection risk, nausea, and lung and liver damage and have shown limited benefit. Studies using the combination therapy of corticosteroids, azathiaprine, interferon gamma 1b, and N-acetylcysteine show promise of slowing disease progression. Newer approved drugs include nintedanib (Ofev), a tyrosine kinase inhibitor, and pirfenidone (Esbriet), an antifibrotic agent. Both drugs help improve CELLULAR REGULATION of fibrous cell growth.

Starting any drug therapy early is critical, even though not all patients respond to therapy. Even among those who have a response to therapy, the disease eventually continues to progress and leads to death by respiratory failure. Lung transplantation is a curative therapy; however, the selection criteria, cost, and availability of organs make this option unlikely for most patients.

The patient and family need support and help with community resources. Nursing care focuses on helping the patient and family understand the disease process and maintaining hope for fibrosis control. It is important to prevent respiratory infections. Teach the patient and family about the symptoms of infection and to avoid respiratory irritants, crowds, and people who are ill.

Home oxygen is needed by the time the patient has dyspnea because significant fibrosis has already occurred and GAS EXCHANGE is reduced. Teach about oxygen use as a continuous therapy. Fatigue is a major problem. Teach the patient and family about energy conservation measures (see the discussion of activity intolerance in the Chronic Obstructive Pulmonary Disease section). These measures and rest help reduce the work of breathing and oxygen consumption. Encourage the patient to pace activities and accept assistance as needed.

In the later stages of the disease, the focus is to reduce the sensation of dyspnea. This is often accomplished with the use of oral, parenteral, or nebulized morphine. Provide information about hospice, which supports and coordinates resources to meet the needs of the patient and family when the prognosis for survival is less than 6 months (see Chapter 7).

LUNG CANCER

❖ PATHOPHYSIOLOGY

Lung cancer is a leading cause of cancer-related deaths worldwide. In North America, more deaths from lung cancer occur each year than from prostate cancer, breast cancer, and colon cancer combined. In the United States, more than 243,000 new cases are diagnosed each year, and more than 160,000 deaths occur from lung cancer annually (American Cancer Society [ACS], 2017). In Canada, more than 26,600 new cases are diagnosed each year, and more than 20,900 deaths from lung cancer occur annually (Canadian Cancer Society, 2016). The overall 5-year survival for all patients with lung cancer is only 16%. This poor long-term survival is because most lung cancers are diagnosed at a late stage, when metastasis is present. Only 15% of patients have small tumors and localized disease at the time of diagnosis. The 5-year survival rate for this population is 52% (ACS, 2017).

The prognosis for advanced lung cancer remains poor. Treatment often focuses on relieving symptoms or increasing survival time (**palliation**) rather than cure.

Most primary lung cancers arise as a result of failure of CELLULAR REGULATION in the bronchial epithelium. These cancers are collectively called *bronchogenic carcinomas*. Lung cancers are classified as small cell lung cancer (SCLC) and non–small cell lung cancer (NSCLC). Chapter 21 discusses the general mechanisms and processes of cancer development.

Metastasis (spread) of lung cancer occurs by direct extension, through the blood, and by invading lymph glands and vessels. Tumors in the bronchial tubes can grow and obstruct the bronchus partially or completely. Tumors in other areas of lung tissue can grow so large that they can compress and obstruct the airway. Compression of the alveoli, nerves, blood vessels, and lymph vessels can occur and also interfere with GAS EXCHANGE. Lung cancer can spread to the lung lymph nodes; distant lymph nodes; and other tissues, including bone, liver, brain, and adrenal glands.

Additional symptoms, known as *paraneoplastic syndromes,* complicate certain lung cancers. The paraneoplastic syndromes are caused by hormones secreted by tumor cells and occur most commonly with SCLC. Table 30-4 lists the endocrine paraneoplastic syndromes that may occur.

Staging of lung cancer is performed to assess the size and extent of the disease. These factors are related to survival. Lung cancer staging is based on the TNM system (T, primary tumor;

TABLE 30-4 Endocrine Paraneoplastic Syndromes Associated With Lung Cancer

ECTOPIC HORMONE	SYMPTOMS
Adrenocorticotropic hormone (ACTH)	Cushing's syndrome
Antidiuretic hormone	Syndrome of inappropriate antidiuretic hormone (SIADH) Weight gain General edema Dilution of serum electrolytes
Follicle-stimulating hormone (FSH)	Gynecomastia
Parathyroid hormone	Hypercalcemia
Ectopic insulin	Hypoglycemia

N, number of regional lymph **n**odes; M, distant **m**etastasis). See Table 21-5 for a cancer staging system. Higher numbers represent later stages and less chance for cure or long-term survival.

Incidence and Prevalence

Lung cancers occur as a result of repeated exposure to inhaled substances that cause chronic tissue irritation or inflammation interfering with CELLULAR REGULATION of cell growth. Cigarette smoking is the major risk factor and is responsible for 85% of all lung cancer deaths (ACS, 2017). The risk for lung cancer is directly related to the total exposure to cigarette smoke as determined by the number of years of smoking and number of packs of cigarettes smoked per day (pack-years). Pipe and cigar smoking also increase risk.

Etiology and Genetic Risk

Nonsmokers exposed to "secondhand" or "thirdhand" smoke also have a greater risk for lung cancer than do nonsmokers who are minimally exposed to cigarette smoke (Sherry, 2017). See Chapter 27 for a discussion of passive smoking risks.

Other lung cancer risk factors include chronic exposure to asbestos, beryllium, chromium, coal distillates, cobalt, iron oxide, mustard gas, petroleum distillates, radiation, tar, nickel, and uranium (Held-Warmkessel & Schiech, 2014). Air pollution with benzopyrenes and hydrocarbons also increases the risk for lung cancer.

GENETIC/GENOMIC CONSIDERATIONS

Patient-Centered Care (QSEN)

Lung cancer development varies among adults with similar smoking histories, suggesting that genetic factors can influence susceptibility. Genome-wide association studies have found specific variations in a variety of genes that increase the susceptibility to lung cancer development (OMIM, 2016a). Differences in a gene that regulates cell division, the Tp53 gene, may be the most important genetic susceptibility link for lung cancer development. Mutations in the alleles of this gene are known to increase the susceptibility to a wide variety of cancers both with and without exposure to environmental risks, including lung cancer development among smokers and nonsmokers. Help patients understand that lung cancer susceptibility varies by both genetic issues and exposure to carcinogens.

Health Promotion and Maintenance

Primary prevention for lung cancer is directed at reducing tobacco smoking. Chapter 27 discusses strategies for helping adults reduce smoking and ways to protect lungs from other exposures to inhalation irritants linked to lung cancer development.

Secondary prevention by early detection involves screening adults at high risk for lung cancer development. Annual CT scans can detect cancers at stage I, when cure is probable and long-term survival (longer than 5 years) is very likely (ACS, 2016; Qiu et al., 2016).

❖ INTERPROFESSIONAL COLLABORATIVE CARE

◆ Assessment: Noticing

History. Ask the patient about risk factors, including smoking, hazards in the workplace, and warning signals (Table 30-5). Calculate the pack-year smoking history as described in Chapter 27.

TABLE 30-5	**Warning Signals Associated With Lung Cancer**

- Hoarseness
- Change in respiratory pattern
- Persistent cough or change in cough
- Blood-streaked sputum
- Rust-colored or purulent sputum
- Frank hemoptysis
- Chest pain or chest tightness
- Shoulder, arm, or chest wall pain
- Recurring episodes of pleural effusion, pneumonia, or bronchitis
- Dyspnea
- Fever associated with one or two other signs
- Wheezing
- Weight loss
- Clubbing of the fingers

Ask about the presence of lung cancer symptoms, such as hoarseness, cough, sputum production, hemoptysis, shortness of breath, or change in endurance. Assessing for and documenting these symptoms provide information about the extent of nursing care and teaching the patient needs now and can be used later to determine therapy effectiveness. Symptoms often have been present for years. Ask the patient to describe any recent symptom changes or if position affects them.

Assess for chest pain or discomfort, which can occur at any stage of tumor development. Chest pain may be localized or on just one side and can range from mild to severe. Ask about any sensation of fullness, tightness, or pressure in the chest, which may suggest obstruction. A piercing chest pain or pleuritic pain may occur on inspiration. Pain radiating to the arm results from tumor invasion of nerve plexuses in advanced disease.

Physical Assessment/Signs and Symptoms—Pulmonary. Symptoms of lung cancer are often nonspecific and appear late in the disease. Specific symptoms depend on tumor location. Chills, fever, and cough may be related to pneumonitis or bronchitis that occurs with obstruction. Assess sputum quantity and character. Blood-tinged sputum may occur with bleeding from a tumor. Hemoptysis is a later finding in the course of the disease. If infection or necrosis is present, sputum may be purulent and copious.

Breathing may be labored or painful. Obstructive breathing may occur as prolonged exhalation alternating with periods of shallow breathing. Rapid, shallow breathing occurs with pleuritic chest pain and an elevated diaphragm. Look for and document abnormal retractions, the use of accessory muscles, flared nares, stridor, and asymmetric diaphragmatic movement on inspiration. Dyspnea and wheezing may be present with airway obstruction. Ask about dyspnea severity at rest, with activity, and in the supine position. Assess how much the dyspnea interferes with the patient's participation in ADLs, work, recreational activities, and family responsibilities. Ask him or her to compare participation in activities during the past week with that of a month ago and a year ago.

Areas of tenderness or masses may be felt when palpating the chest wall. Increased vibrations felt on the chest wall (**fremitus**) indicate areas of the lung where air spaces are replaced with tumor or fluid. Fremitus is decreased or absent when the bronchus is obstructed. The trachea may be displaced from midline if a mass is present in the area.

Lung areas with masses sound dull or flat rather than hollow or resonant on chest percussion. Breath sounds may change with the presence of a tumor. Wheezes indicate partial obstruction of airflow in passages narrowed by tumors. Decreased or absent breath sounds indicate complete obstruction of an airway by a tumor or fluid. Increased loudness or sound intensity of the voice while listening to breath sounds indicates increased density of lung tissue from tumor compression. A pleural friction rub may be heard when inflammation is present.

Physical Assessment/Signs and Symptoms—Nonpulmonary.
Many other systems can be affected by lung cancer and have changes at the time of diagnosis. Heart sounds may be muffled by a tumor or fluid around the heart (*cardiac tamponade*). Dysrhythmias may occur as a result of hypoxemia or direct pressure of the tumor on the heart. Cyanosis of the lips and fingertips or clubbing of the fingers may be present (see Fig. 30-10).

Bones lose density with tumor invasion and break easily. The patient may have bone pain or pathologic fractures. Handle him or her carefully. Thin bones can fracture with little pressure and without trauma. Even heavy coughing can break a rib.

Late symptoms of lung cancer usually include fatigue, weight loss, anorexia, dysphagia, and nausea and vomiting. *Superior vena cava syndrome may result from tumor pressure in or around the vena cava. This syndrome is an emergency (see Chapter 22) and requires immediate intervention.* The patient may have confusion or personality changes from brain metastasis. Bowel and bladder tone or function may be affected by tumor spread to the spine and spinal cord, which can change gait.

Psychosocial Assessment.
The poor prognosis for lung cancer has made it a much-feared disease. Dyspnea and pain add to the patient's fear and anxiety. The patient with a history of cigarette smoking may feel guilt and shame. Convey acceptance and interact with the patient in a nonjudgmental way. Encourage the patient and family to express their feelings about the possible diagnosis of lung cancer.

Diagnostic Assessment.
The diagnosis of lung cancer is made by examination of cancer cells. Cytologic testing of early-morning sputum specimens may identify tumor cells; however, cancer cells may not be present in the sputum. When pleural effusion is present, fluid is obtained by thoracentesis for cytology.

Most commonly, lung lesions are first identified on chest x-rays. CT scans are then used to identify the lesions more clearly and guide biopsy procedures.

A thoracoscopy to directly view lung tissue may be performed through a video-assisted thoracoscope entering the chest cavity via small incisions through the chest wall. Spread to mediastinal lymph nodes is assessed with a mediastinoscopy through a small chest incision.

Other diagnostic studies may be needed to determine how widely the cancer has spread. Such tests include needle biopsy of lymph nodes, direct surgical biopsy, and thoracentesis with pleural biopsy. MRI and radionuclide scans of the liver, spleen, brain, and bone help determine the location of metastatic tumors. Pulmonary function tests (PFTs) and arterial blood gas (ABG) analysis help determine the overall respiratory status. Positron emission tomography (PET) scanning is becoming the most thorough way to locate metastases. These tests help determine the extent of the cancer and the best methods to treat it.

◆ Interventions: Responding

Interventions for Cure.
Interventions for the patient with lung cancer can have the purposes of curing the disease, increasing survival time, and enhancing quality of life through palliation. Both nonsurgical and surgical interventions are used to achieve these purposes. Some patients with lung cancer may undergo interventions for all three purposes at different stages in the disease process. Cure is most likely for patients who undergo treatment for stage I or II disease. Cure is rare for patients who undergo treatment for stage III or IV disease, although survival time is increasing.

Nonsurgical Management. *Chemotherapy* is often the treatment of choice for lung cancers, especially small cell lung cancer (SCLC). It may be used alone or as adjuvant therapy in combination with surgery for non–small cell lung cancer (NSCLC). The combination of drugs used depends on tumor response and the overall health of the patient; however, most include platinum-based agents.

Side effects that occur with chemotherapy for lung cancer include chemotherapy-induced nausea and vomiting (CINV), **alopecia** (hair loss), open sores on mucous membranes (**mucositis**), immunosuppression with neutropenia, anemia, **thrombocytopenia** (decreased numbers of platelets), and peripheral neuropathy. Consult Chapter 22 for a thorough discussion of the nursing care needs for patients who have these side effects.

Immunosuppression with neutropenia, which greatly increases the risk for infection, is the major dose-limiting side effect of chemotherapy for lung cancer. It can be managed by the use of growth factors to stimulate bone marrow production of immune system cells. Teach the patient and family about precautions to take to reduce the patient's risk for infection (see Chart 22-4). (See Chapter 22 for information about chemotherapy and associated nursing care.)

Targeted therapy is common in the treatment of non–small cell lung cancer (NSCLC). These agents take advantage of one or more differences in cancer cell growth or metabolism that is either not present or only slightly present in normal cells. Agents used as targeted therapies work to disrupt cancer cell division in one of several ways. However, these agents only work when the cancer cell has the particular target or specific genetic mutation. Therefore testing of the cancer cells is needed before therapy begins, and not all cancers of the same type express the target. Some of these drugs are used alone for metastatic NSCLC, and others are used in combination with chemotherapy. These agents are increasing survival time for patients with NSCLC but do not lead to a cure. Table 30-6 lists targeted agents and indications. Chapter 22 describes general issues with targeted therapy agents.

Radiation therapy can be an effective treatment for locally advanced lung cancers confined to the chest. Best results are seen when radiation is used in addition to surgery or chemotherapy. Radiation may be performed before surgery to shrink the tumor and make resection easier.

Usually radiation therapy for lung cancer is performed daily for a 5- to 6-week period. Only the areas thought to have cancer are positioned in the radiation path. The immediate side effects of this treatment are skin irritation and peeling, fatigue, nausea, and taste changes. Some patients have esophagitis during therapy, making nutrition more difficult. Collaborate with a dietitian to teach patients to eat foods that are soft, bland, and high in calories. Suggest that the patient drink liquid nutrition

TABLE 30-6 Targeted Agents for Non–Small Cell Lung Cancer (NSCLC)

AGENT AND ROUTE OF ADMINISTRATION	SPECIFIC INDICATIONS OR TARGETS
afatinib (Gilotrif) Oral	First-line therapy for metastatic NSCLC that is positive for a mutation in the EGFR gene of either exon 19 deletion or exon 21 L858R substitution mutations
alectinib (Alcensa) Oral	Second-line therapy for metastatic NSCLC that has progressed after initial treatment and is ALK-positive
bevacizumab (Avastin) IV	First-line treatment of unresectable, locally advanced, recurrent, or metastatic nonsquamous NSCLC in combination with carboplatin and paclitaxel
crizotinib (Xalkori) Oral	First-line treatment of metastatic NSCLC that is ALK-positive
erlotinib (Tarceva) Oral	First-line treatment of metastatic NSCLC with EGFR exon 19 deletions or exon 21 (L858R) substitution mutations
necitamumab (Portrazza) IV	First-line treatment of metastatic squamous NSCLC in combination with gemcitabine and cisplatin
nivolumab (Opdivo) IV	Second-line treatment of metastatic NSCLC, with progression on or after platinum-based chemotherapy and after progression on EGFR- or ALK-targeted therapy
ramucirumab (Cyramza) IV	Second-line treatment of metastatic NSCLC in combination with docetaxel, with disease progression on or after platinum-based chemotherapy

ALK, Anaplastic lymphoma kinase *EGFR,* epidermal growth factor receptor.

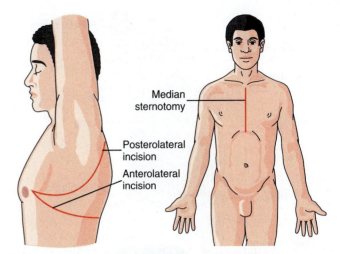

FIG. 30-13 Common incision locations for partial or total pneumonectomy.

supplements between meals to maintain weight and energy levels.

Skin care in the radiation-treated area can be difficult, and consultation with a wound care specialist may be needed. Because skin in the radiation path is more sensitive to sun damage, advise patients to avoid direct skin exposure to the sun during treatment and for at least 1 year after radiation is completed. See Chapter 22 for other nursing care issues associated with radiation therapy.

Photodynamic therapy (PDT) may be used to remove small bronchial tumors when they are accessible by bronchoscopy. The patient is first injected with an agent that sensitizes cells to light. This drug enters all cells but leaves normal cells more rapidly than cancer cells. Usually, within 48 to 72 hours, most of the drug has collected in high concentrations in cancer cells. At this time, the patient goes to the operating room where, under anesthesia and intubation, a laser light is focused on the tumor. The light activates a reaction that causes irreversible damage to the cells retaining the sensitizing drug. Some cells die and slough immediately; others continue to slough for several days.

With PDT, the patient may require a stay in the ICU for airway management. Sloughing tissue and airway edema from inflammation can block the airways. The patient is at risk for bronchial hemorrhage, fistula formation, and hemoptysis.

Surgical Management. Surgery is the main treatment for stage I and stage II NSCLC. Total tumor removal may result in a cure. If complete resection is not possible, the surgeon removes the bulk of the tumor. The specific surgery depends on the stage of the cancer and the patient's overall health. Lung cancer surgery may involve removal of the tumor only, removal of a lung segment, removal of a lobe (**lobectomy**), or removal of the entire lung (**pneumonectomy**). These procedures can be performed by open thoracotomy or by minimally invasive surgery in select patients.

Preoperative Care. The focus of nursing care before surgery is to relieve anxiety and promote the patient's participation (see Chapter 14 for routine preoperative care). Encourage the patient to express fears and concerns, reinforce the surgeon's explanation of the procedure, and provide education related to what is expected after surgery. Teach about the probable location of the surgical incision or thoracoscopy openings, shoulder exercises, and the chest tube and drainage system (except after pneumonectomy).

Operative Procedures. Three types of incisions can be made, depending on the location of the cancer: posterolateral, anterolateral, and median sternotomy (Fig. 30-13). The incisions are large and are held open with retractors during surgery, contributing to pain after surgery.

Surgery may consist of a lobectomy, pneumonectomy, segmental resection, or wedge resection. A segmental resection is a lung resection that includes the bronchus, pulmonary artery and vein, and tissue of the involved lung segment or segments of a lobe. A **wedge resection** is removal of the peripheral portion of small, localized areas of disease.

A lobe or entire lung can be removed through video-assisted thoracoscopic surgery (VATS), which is minimally invasive, in select patients. The procedure involves making three small incisions in the chest for placement of the instruments. These same openings are used later for placement of drains and chest tubes. The lung section, lobe, or lung then is isolated from its airway, which is surgically closed. The lobe or the lung is closed off from the rest of the lung using a double-stapling technique. The tissue is sealed in a bag to prevent leakage of tumor tissue and possible seeding of the cancer. The bagged lung is then removed whole through one of the small incisions.

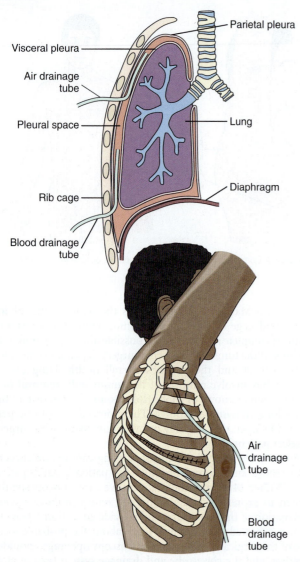

FIG. 30-14 Chest tube placement.

Labels for the figure:
- Visceral pleura
- Parietal pleura
- Air drainage tube
- Pleural space
- Lung
- Rib cage
- Diaphragm
- Blood drainage tube
- Air drainage tube
- Blood drainage tube

Postoperative Care. Care after surgery for patients who have undergone thoracotomy (except for pneumonectomy) requires closed-chest drainage to drain air and blood that collect in the pleural space. A **chest tube**, a drain placed in the pleural space, allows lung re-expansion (Fig. 30-14). The chest tube also prevents air and fluid from returning to the chest. The drainage system consists of one or more chest tubes or drains, a collection container placed below the chest level, and a water seal to keep air from entering the chest. The drainage system may be a stationary, disposable, self-contained system (Fig. 30-15); or a smaller, portable, disposable, self-contained system that requires no connection to a vacuum source (Fig. 30-16). The nursing care priorities for the patient with a chest tube are to ensure the integrity of the system, promote comfort, ensure chest tube patency, and prevent complications.

Chest Tube Placement and Care. The tip of the tube used to drain air is placed near the front lung apex (see Fig. 30-14). The tube that drains liquid is placed on the side near the base of the lung. After lung surgery, two tubes, anterior and posterior, are used. The wounds are covered with airtight dressings.

The chest tube is connected by about 6 feet of tubing to a collection device placed below the chest, which allows gravity to drain the pleural space. The tubing allows the patient to turn and move without pulling on the chest tube. When two chest tubes are inserted, they are joined by a Y-connector near the patient's body; the 6 feet of tubing is attached to the Y-connector.

Stationary chest tube drainage systems use a water-seal mechanism that acts as a one-way valve to prevent air or liquid from moving back into the chest cavity. The Pleur-evac system is a common device using a one-piece disposable plastic unit with three chambers. The three chambers are connected to one another. The tube(s) from the patient is (are) connected to the first chamber in the series of three. This chamber is the drainage collection container. The second chamber is the water seal to prevent air from moving back up the tubing system and into the chest. The third chamber, when suction is applied, is the suction regulator.

In setting up the system, chamber one (nearest to the patient) does not at first have fluid in it. The tubing from the patient penetrates shallowly into this chamber, as does the tube connecting chamber one with chamber two.

Chamber one collects the fluid draining from the patient. This fluid is measured hourly during the first 24 hours. *The fluid in chamber one must never fill to the point that it comes into contact with any tubes! If the tubing from the patient enters the fluid, drainage stops and can lead to a tension pneumothorax.*

Chamber two is the water seal that prevents air from re-entering the patient's pleural space. As the trapped air leaves the pleural space, it will pass through chamber one (drainage collection chamber) before entering chamber two (the water-seal chamber), which should always contain at least 2 cm of water to prevent air from returning to the patient. As trapped air from the patient's pleural space passes through the water seal, which serves as a one-way valve, the water will bubble. Once all the air has been evacuated from the pleural space, bubbling of the water seal stops.

> **! NURSING SAFETY PRIORITY** (QSEN)
> **Action Alert**
>
> For a water-seal chest tube drainage system, 2 cm of water is the minimum needed in the water seal to prevent air from flowing backward into the patient. Check the water level every shift and add sterile water to this chamber to the level marked on the indicator (specified by the manufacturer of the drainage system).

The bubbling of the water in the water-seal chamber indicates air drainage from the patient. Bubbling is seen when intrathoracic pressure is greater than atmospheric pressure, such as when the patient exhales, coughs, or sneezes. When the air in the pleural space has been removed, bubbling stops. A blocked or kinked chest tube also can cause bubbling to stop (Muzzy & Butler, 2015). Excessive bubbling in the water-seal chamber (chamber two) may indicate an air leak. The water in the narrow column of the water-seal chamber normally rises 2 to 4 inches during inhalation and falls during exhalation, a process called *tidaling.* An absence of fluctuation may mean that the lung has fully re-expanded or that there is an obstruction in the chest tube.

Chamber three is the suction control of the system. There are different types of suction, most commonly wet or dry. With wet suction, the fluid level in chamber three is prescribed by the primary health care provider (usually −20 cm water). The

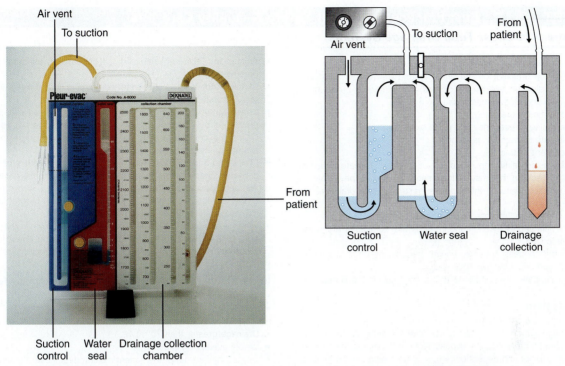

FIG. 30-15 **A,** Pleur-evac drainage system, a commercial three-chamber chest drainage device. **B,** Schematic of the drainage device.

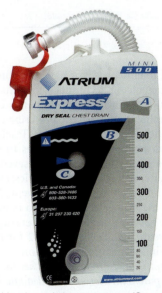

FIG. 30-16 Portable chest drainage system. (Courtesy Atrium Medical Corporation, Hudson, NH.)

chamber is connected to wall suction, which is turned up until there is gentle bubbling in the chamber. With dry suction, the primary health care provider prescribes the suction level to be dialed in on the device. When connected to wall suction, the regulator is set to the amount indicated by the device's manufacturer. For either type of suction, the amount of suction in the system is determined not by the wall suction unit but by the chest tube drainage device.

Chart 30-12 summarizes best safety practices when caring for a patient with a water-seal chest tube drainage system. Check hourly to ensure the sterility and patency of the drainage

system. Tape tubing junctions to prevent accidental disconnections and keep an occlusive dressing at the chest tube insertion site. Keep sterile gauze at the bedside to cover the insertion site immediately if the chest tube becomes dislodged. Also keep padded clamps at the bedside for use if the drainage system is interrupted. Position the drainage tubing to prevent kinks and large loops of tubing, which can block drainage and prevent lung re-expansion.

If any tube manipulation is needed, gentle hand-over-hand "milking" of the tube, stopping between each handhold, is used to move blood clots and prevent obstruction. Follow surgeon prescriptions and agency policies and guidelines on this action.

> ## ! NURSING SAFETY PRIORITY QSEN
> ### Action Alert
> Manipulation of the chest tube should be kept to a minimum. Do not vigorously "strip" the chest tube because this can create up to −400 cm of water negative pressure and damage lung tissue.

Assess the respiratory status and document the amount and type of drainage hourly on the collection chamber. Notify the surgeon if more than 70 mL/hr of drainage occurs. After the first 24 hours, assess drainage at least every 8 hours. Usually the drainage in chamber one is not emptied unless it is so full that the fluid is in danger of coming into contact with the chest drainage tube.

Check the water-seal chamber for unexpected bubbling created by an air leak in the system. Bubbling is normal during forceful expiration or coughing because air in the chest is being expelled. Continuous bubbling indicates an air leak (Muzzy & Butler, 2015). Notify the primary health care provider if

CHART 30-12 Best Practice for Patient Safety & Quality Care QSEN

Management of Chest Tube Drainage Systems

Patient

- Ensure that the dressing on the chest around the tube is tight and intact. Depending on agency policy and the surgeon's preference, reinforce or change loose dressings.
- Assess for difficulty breathing.
- Assess breathing effectiveness by pulse oximetry.
- Listen to breath sounds for each lung.
- Check alignment of trachea.
- Check tube insertion site for condition of the skin. Palpate area for puffiness or crackling that may indicate subcutaneous emphysema.
- Observe site for signs of infection (redness, purulent drainage) or excessive bleeding.
- Check to see if tube "eyelets" are visible.
- Assess for pain and its location and intensity and administer drugs for pain as prescribed.
- Assist patient to deep breathe, cough, perform maximal sustained inhalations, and use incentive spirometry.
- Reposition the patient who reports a "burning" pain in the chest.

Drainage System

- Do not "strip" the chest tube.
- Keep drainage system lower than the level of the patient's chest.
- Keep the chest tube as straight as possible from the bed to the suction unit, avoiding kinks and dependent loops. Extra tubing can be loosely coiled on the bed.
- Ensure that the chest tube is securely taped to the connector and that the connector is taped to the tubing going into the collection chamber.
- Assess bubbling in the water-seal chamber; should be gentle bubbling on patient's exhalation, forceful cough, position changes.

- Assess for "tidaling" (rise and fall of water in chamber three with breathing).
- Check water level in the water-seal chamber and keep at the level recommended by the manufacturer.
- Check water level in the suction control chamber and keep at the level prescribed by the surgeon (unless dry suction system is used).
- Clamp the chest tube only for brief periods to change the drainage system or when checking for air leaks.
- Check and document amount, color, and characteristics of fluid in the collection chamber as often as needed according to the patient's condition and agency policy.
- Empty collection chamber or change the system before the drainage makes contact with the bottom of the tube.
- When a sample of drainage is needed for culture or other laboratory test, obtain it from the chest tube; after cleaning chest tube, use a 20-gauge (or smaller) needle and draw up specimen into a syringe.

Immediately Notify Physician or Rapid Response Team for:

- Tracheal deviation
- Sudden onset or increased intensity of dyspnea
- Oxygen saturation less than 90%
- Drainage greater than 70 mL/hr
- Visible eyelets on chest tube
- Chest tube falls out of the patient's chest (first, cover the area with dry, sterile gauze)
- Chest tube disconnects from the drainage system (first, put end of tube in a container of sterile water and keep below the level of the patient's chest)
- Drainage in tube stops (in the first 24 hours)

---

bubbling occurs continuously in the water-seal chamber. With a prescription, gently apply a padded clamp briefly on the drainage tubing close to the occlusive dressing. If the bubbling stops, the air leak may be at the chest tube insertion site or within the chest, requiring physician intervention. Bubbling that does not stop when a padded clamp is applied indicates that the air leak is between the clamp and the drainage system. Release the clamp as soon as this assessment is made.

Mobile or portable chest tube drainage systems are "dry" chest drainage systems without a water seal to prevent air from re-entering the patient's lung through the chest tube. Instead, these lightweight devices use a dynamic control "flutter" valve that prevents backflow of air. When the patient exhales, air is forced from the chest cavity into the chest tube under pressure. This pressure forces the soft flutter valve open, and air moves into the harder surrounding tube shell (which has a vent for air). Portable units allow the patient to ambulate and go home with chest tubes still in place.

Chest tube removal is performed when drainage is minimal and lung expansion is stable, as confirmed by x-ray. Usually the primary health care provider removes the chest tube at the bedside. Most patients find chest tube removal painful during the actual procedure. After removal, the site is dressed and sealed with an occlusive dressing and observed for drainage. Assess the patient hourly for respiratory distress for the first few hours after chest tube removal. Respiratory distress may signal lung collapse and the need for chest tube reinsertion.

Pain Management. Most patients have intense pain after an open thoracotomy. Pain is considerably less for the patient after surgery using minimally invasive techniques. However, pain control is needed in either case for patient comfort and to help him or her participate in techniques to reduce the risk for complications, such as incentive spirometry, coughing, deep breathing, and ambulating. Give the prescribed drugs for pain and assess the patient's responses to them. Teach patients using patient-controlled analgesia (PCA) devices to self-administer the drug before pain intensity becomes too severe. Monitor vital signs before and after giving opioid analgesics, especially for the patient who is not being mechanically ventilated. Plan care activities around the timing of analgesia to reduce pain.

Respiratory Management. Immediately after surgery the patient is mechanically ventilated. See Chapter 32 for nursing care of the patient receiving mechanical ventilation.

Once the patient is breathing on his or her own, the priorities are to maintain a patent airway, ensure adequate ventilation, and prevent complications. Assess the patient at least every 2 hours for adequacy of ventilation and GAS EXCHANGE. Check the alignment of the trachea. Assess oxygen saturation and the rate and depth of respiration. Listen to breath sounds in all lobes on the nonoperative side, particularly noting the presence of crackles. Assess the oral mucous membranes for cyanosis and the nail beds for rate of capillary refill. Perform oral suctioning as necessary.

Usually the patient receives oxygen by mask or nasal cannula for the first 2 days after surgery. Warm and humidify the oxygen. Assist the patient to a semi-Fowler's position or up in a chair as soon as possible. Encourage him or her to use the incentive spirometer every hour while awake. If coughing is permitted, help him or her cough by splinting any incision and ensuring that the chest tube does not pull with movement. Ensuring that pain is well managed increases the patient's ability to cough and deep breathe effectively.

❓ **NCLEX EXAMINATION CHALLENGE 30-5**

Safe and Effective Care Environment

The chest tube of a client who is 12 hours postoperative from a lobectomy separates from the drainage system. What is the nurse's best **first** action?
A. Immediately call the surgeon or rapid response team.
B. Notify respiratory therapy to set up a new drainage system.
C. Cover the insertion site with a sterile occlusive dressing and tape down on three sides.
D. Place the end of the disconnected tube into a container of sterile water positioned below the chest.

Pneumonectomy Care. After pneumonectomy, the pleural cavity on the affected side is an empty space. The surgeon sometimes inserts a clamped chest tube for only a day. Serous fluid collection in the empty space creates adhesions that help reduce mediastinal shift toward the affected side. Closed-chest drainage is not usually used.

Complications of a pneumonectomy include *empyema* (purulent material in the pleural space) and development of a bronchopleural *fistula* (an abnormal duct that develops between the bronchial tree and the pleura). Positioning of the patient after pneumonectomy varies according to surgeon preference and the patient's comfort. Some surgeons want the patient placed on the nonoperative side immediately after a pneumonectomy to reduce stress on the bronchial stump incision. Others prefer to place the patient on the operative side to allow fluids to fill in the now empty space.

Interventions for Palliation. *Oxygen therapy* is prescribed when the patient is hypoxemic. Even if the hypoxemia is not severe, humidified oxygen may be prescribed to relieve dyspnea and anxiety. (See Chapter 28 for issues related to home oxygen therapy.)

Drug therapy with bronchodilators and corticosteroids is prescribed for the patient with bronchospasm to decrease bronchospasm, inflammation, and edema. Mucolytics may help ease removal of thick mucus and sputum. Bacterial infections are treated with antibiotic therapy.

Radiation therapy can help relieve hemoptysis, obstruction of the bronchi and great veins (superior vena cava syndrome), difficulty swallowing from esophageal compression, and pain from bone metastasis. Radiation for palliation uses higher doses for shorter periods. Skin care issues and fatigue are the same as those occurring with radiation therapy for cure.

Thoracentesis is performed when pleural effusion is a problem for the patient with lung cancer. The excess fluid increases dyspnea, discomfort, and the risk for infection. The purpose of treatment is to remove pleural fluid and prevent its formation. Thoracentesis is fluid removal by suction after the placement of a large needle or catheter into the intrapleural space. Fluid removal temporarily relieves hypoxia; however, the fluid can rapidly re-form in the pleural space. When fluid development is continuous and uncomfortable, a continuously draining catheter may be placed into the intrapleural space to collect the fluid.

Dyspnea management is needed because the patient with lung cancer tires easily and is often most comfortable resting in a semi-Fowler's position. Dyspnea is reduced with oxygen, use of a continuous morphine infusion, and positioning for comfort. The severely dyspneic patient may be most comfortable sitting in a lounge chair or reclining chair.

Pain management may be needed to help the patient be as pain free and comfortable as possible. Pain may be present in the chest or in almost any area when bone metastasis occurs. Perform a complete pain assessment with attention to onset, intensity, quality, duration, and the patient's description of the pain.

Pharmacologic management with opioid drugs as oral, parenteral, or transdermal preparations is needed. Analgesics are most effective when given around the clock. Additional PRN analgesics are used for breakthrough pain. Ongoing evaluation of pain control effectiveness is a primary nursing responsibility.

Hospice care can be beneficial for the patient in the terminal phase of lung cancer. Hospice programs provide support to the terminally ill patient and the family, meet physical and psychosocial needs, adjust the palliative care regimen as needed, make home visits, and provide volunteers for errands and respite care. (See Chapter 7 for a more complete discussion of end-of-life issues.) Family and significant others who are caregivers also have many needs and require support during this time. The American Cancer Society or the Canadian Cancer Society may provide assistance through support groups for patients and families or through the use of equipment such as a hospital bed or bedside commode.

GET READY FOR THE NCLEX® EXAMINATION!

▎KEY POINTS

Review these Key Points for each NCLEX Examination Client Needs Category.

Safe and Effective Care Environment
- Ensure there are no open flames or combustion hazards in rooms where oxygen is in use. **QSEN: Safety**
- Ensure that oxygen therapy delivered to the patient is humidified. **QSEN: Safety**
- Protect the patient with cystic fibrosis from hospital-acquired pulmonary infections. **QSEN: Safety**
- Ensure proper function of chest tube drainage equipment. **QSEN: Safety**

Health Promotion and Maintenance
- Teach patients who come into contact with inhalation irritants in their workplaces or leisure-time activities to use a mask to avoid respiratory contact with these substances. **QSEN: Safety**
- Teach adults who smoke that smoking increases the risk for development of many pulmonary problems. **QSEN: Evidence-Based Practice**

- Teach patients with asthma to develop a management plan based on their identified personal best on peak expiratory rate flow testing. **QSEN: Patient-Centered Care**
- Encourage all patients older than 50 years and anyone with a respiratory problem to receive a yearly influenza vaccination. **QSEN: Patient-Centered Care**
- Teach all patients who smoke the warning signs of lung cancer. **QSEN: Evidence-Based Practice**
- Help patients and families contact community support agencies such as the American Cancer Society and the Canadian Cancer Society. **QSEN: Patient-Centered Care**

Psychosocial Integrity
- Encourage the patient and family to express their feelings regarding the diagnosis of a chronic respiratory disease or cancer and about management/treatment regimens. **QSEN: Patient-Centered Care**
- Explain all diagnostic procedures, restrictions, and follow-up care to the patient scheduled for tests. **QSEN: Patient-Centered Care**
- Help patients use strategies to improve their appearance when alopecia occurs. **QSEN: Patient-Centered Care**

Physiological Integrity
- Assess the airway and effectiveness of GAS EXCHANGE for any patient who experiences shortness of breath or any change in mental status. **QSEN: Evidence-Based Practice**

- Assess the degree to which breathing problems interfere with the patient's ability to perform ADLs, work, and leisure-time activities. **QSEN: Patient-Centered Care**
- Apply oxygen to anyone who is hypoxemic. **QSEN: Evidence-Based Practice**
- Monitor arterial blood gases and oxygen saturation of all patients receiving oxygen therapy. **QSEN: Evidence-Based Practice**
- Teach patients receiving radiation therapy how to care for the skin in the radiation path (see Chart 22-2). **QSEN: Patient-Centered Care**
- Collaborate with respiratory therapists, registered dietitians, and social workers to meet the hospital and home care needs of patients with chronic lower respiratory problems. **QSEN: Teamwork and Collaboration**
- Remind patients with lung cancer that targeted therapies can be used only for tumors that express the targets and cancer cell testing is needed to identify these. **QSEN: Patient-Centered Care**
- Instruct patients with asthma or COPD who are prescribed to use inhalers how to use and care for them properly. **QSEN: Patient-Centered Care**
- Instruct patients with asthma to carry a reliever inhaler with them at all times. **QSEN: Safety**
- Teach patients receiving chemotherapy for lung cancer the signs and symptoms of infection. **QSEN: Patient-Centered Care**

SELECTED BIBLIOGRAPHY

Adams, B., & Ferguson, K. (2014). Pharmacologic management of pulmonary artery hypertension. *AACN Advanced Critical Care, 25*(4), 309–316.

American Cancer Society (ACS). (2017). *Cancer facts and figures—2017.* No. 01-300M–No. 500817. Atlanta: Author.

Ari, A. (2015). Patient education and adherence to aerosol therapy. *Respiratory Care, 60*(6), 941–958.

Arjona, N. (2015). Near-fatal asthma in the elderly. *Dimensions of Critical Care Nursing, 34*(1), 26–31.

Aschenbrenner, D. (2015). Drug watch: Asthma medication receives new warning. *The American Journal of Nursing, 115*(1), 22–23.

Aschenbrenner, D. (2016). Drug watch: A new treatment for pulmonary artery hypertension. *The American Journal of Nursing, 116*(4), 21.

Bracken, N. (2016). Reducing readmissions in COPD patients. *American Nurse Today, 11*(7), 24–28.

Burchum, J., & Rosenthal, L. (2015). *Lehne's pharmacology for nursing care* (9th ed.). St. Louis: Elsevier.

Burt, L., & Corbridge, S. (2013). COPD exacerbations: Evidence-based guidelines for identification, assessment, and management. *The American Journal of Nursing, 113*(2), 34–43.

Canadian Cancer Society, Statistics Canada. (2016). *Canadian Cancer Statistics, 2016.* Toronto, ON: Canadian Cancer Society. www.cancer.ca/~/media/cancer.ca/CW/cancer%20information/cancer%20101/Canadian%20cancer%20statistics/Canadian-Cancer-Statistics-2016-EN.pdf?la=en.

Centers for Disease Control and Prevention (CDC). (2016). *FastStats—Chronic obstructive pulmonary disease (COPD).* www.cdc.gov/nchs/fastats/copd.htm.

Centers for Disease Control and Prevention (CDC). (2015). *FastStats—Asthma.* www.cdc.gov/nchs/fastats/asthma.htm.

Cystic Fibrosis Foundation (CFF). (2015). *About cystic fibrosis.* http://www.jointcommision.org/certification/inpatient_diabetes.aspx.

Demerouti, E., Manginas, A., Athanassopoulis, G., Karatasakis, G., Leontiadis, E., & Pavlides, G. (2013). Successful epoprostenol

withdrawal in pulmonary arterial hypertension: Case report and literature review. *Respiratory Care, 58*(2), e1–e5.

Duquette, S. (2015). A patient with pulmonary hypertension on a medical-surgical unit. *Medsurg Nursing, 24*(2), 83–88.

Global Initiative for Asthma (GINA). (2017). *Pocket guide for asthma management and prevention.* http://ginasthma.org/2017-pocket-guide-for-asthma-management-and-prevention/.

Global Initiative for Chronic Obstructive Lung Disease (GOLD). (2017). *Global strategy for the diagnosis, management, and prevention of chronic obstructive pulmonary disease.* http://goldcopd.org/wp-content/uploads/2016/12/wms-GOLD-2017-Pocket-Guide.pdf.

Held-Warmkessel, J., & Schiech, L. (2014). Non–small cell lung cancer: Recent advances. *Nursing, 44*(2), 32–42.

Jarvis, C. (2016). *Physical examination & health assessment* (7th ed.). St. Louis: Elsevier.

Keep, S., Reiffer, A., & Bahl, T. (2016). Supporting self-management of asthma care. *Home Healthcare Now, 34*(3), 126–134.

Kessenich, C., & Bacher, K. (2014). Alpha-1 antitrypsin deficiency. *The Nurse Practitioner, 39*(7), 12–14.

Kessenich, C., & Bacher, K. (2015). Alpha-1 antitrypsin deficiency: An under-recognized inherited disorder. *Nursing Critical Care, 10*(3), 11–13.

Lynn, S., & Kushto-Reese, K. (2015). Understanding asthma pathophysiology, diagnosis, and management. *American Nurse Today, 10*(7), 49–51.

Makic, M. B., Martin, S., Burns, S., Philbrick, D., & Rauen, C. (2013). Putting evidence into practice: Four traditional practices not supported by the evidence. *Critical Care Nurse, 33*(2), 28–42.

Mazurek, J., & White, G. (2015). Work-related asthma-22 states, 2012. *MMWR. Morbidity and Mortality Weekly Report, 64*(13), 343–346.

McCance, K., Huether, S., Brashers, V., & Rote, N. (2014). *Pathophysiology: The biologic basis for disease in adults and children* (7th ed.). St. Louis: Mosby.

Miller, S., Owens, L., & Silverman, E. (2015). Physical examination of the adult patient with chronic respiratory disease. *Medsurg Nursing, 24*(3), 195–198.

Muzzy, A., & Butler, A. (2015). Managing chest tubes: Air leaks and unplanned tube removal. *American Nurse Today, 10*(5), 10–13.

Nakano, S., & Tluczek, A. (2014). Genomic breakthroughs in the diagnosis and treatment of cystic fibrosis. *The American Journal of Nursing, 114*(6), 36–43.

Online Mendelian Inheritance in Man (OMIM). (2015). *Asthma, susceptibility to.* www.omim.org/entry/600807.

Online Mendelian Inheritance in Man (OMIM). (2016a). *Adenocarcinoma of the lung.* www.omim.org/entry/211980.

Online Mendelian Inheritance in Man (OMIM). (2016b). *Alpha-1-antitrypsin deficiency.* www.omim.org/entry/613490.

Online Mendelian Inheritance in Man (OMIM). (2016c). *Cystic fibrosis; CF.* www.omim.org/entry/219700.

Online Mendelian Inheritance in Man (OMIM). (2016d). *Pulmonary hypertension, primary.* www.omim.org/entry/178600.

Pagana, K., Pagana, T. J., & Pagana, T. N. (2017). *Mosby's diagnostic and laboratory test reference* (13th ed.). St. Louis: Mosby.

Pagana, K., Pagana, T., & Pike-MacDonald, S. (2013). *Mosby's Canadian Manual of Diagnostic and Laboratory Tests.* St. Louis: Mosby.

Qiu, R., Copeland, A., Sercy, E., Porter, N., McDonnell, K., & Eberth, J. (2016). Planning and implementation of low-dose computed tomography lung cancer screening programs in the United States. *Clinical Journal of Oncology Nursing, 20*(1), 52–58.

Sherry, V. (2017). Lung cancer: Not just a smoker's disease. *American Nurse Today, 12*(2), 16–20.

Smith, C., York, N., Kane, C., & Weitendorf, F. (2015). Care of the patient with pulmonary artery hypertension. *Dimensions of Critical Care Nursing, 34*(6), 340–347.

Statistics Canada. (2016a). *Asthma, by age group and sex.* http://www.statcan.gc.ca/tables-tableaux/sum-som/l01/cst01/health49a-eng.htm.

Statistics Canada. (2016b). *Chronic obstructive pulmonary disease by age group and sex.* http://www.statcan.gc.ca/tables-tableaux/sum-som/l01/cst01/health104a-eng.htm.

Touhy, T., & Jett, K. (2016). *Ebersole and Hess' toward healthy aging: human needs & nursing response* (9th ed.). St. Louis: Mosby.

Care of Patients With Infectious Respiratory Problems

Meg Blair

 http://evolve.elsevier.com/Iggy/

PRIORITY AND INTERRELATED CONCEPTS

The priority concepts for this chapter are:
- GAS EXCHANGE
- IMMUNITY

✳ The GAS EXCHANGE concept exemplar for this chapter is Pneumonia, p. 598.

✳ The IMMUNITY concept exemplar for this chapter is Pulmonary Tuberculosis, p. 605.

The interrelated concept for this chapter is COGNITION.

LEARNING OUTCOMES

Safe and Effective Care Environment
1. Collaborate with the interprofessional team to coordinate high-quality care and promote GAS EXCHANGE in patients with infectious respiratory problems.
2. Teach the patient and caregiver(s) about home safety affected by infectious respiratory problems.
3. Prioritize evidence-based care for patients with common infectious respiratory problems affecting GAS EXCHANGE.

Health Promotion and Maintenance
4. Identify community resources for patients with infectious respiratory problems.
5. Teach adults how to decrease the risk for respiratory infections.

Psychosocial Integrity
6. Implement nursing interventions to help the patient and family cope with the psychosocial impact caused by respiratory infection.

Physiological Integrity
7. Apply knowledge of pathophysiology to assess patients with common respiratory infections that impair GAS EXCHANGE.
8. Teach the patient and caregiver(s) about common drugs used for pneumonia, tuberculosis, and other respiratory infections.

SEASONAL INFLUENZA

❖ PATHOPHYSIOLOGY

Seasonal influenza, or "flu," is a highly contagious acute viral respiratory infection that can occur at any age. Epidemics are common and lead to complications of pneumonia or death, especially in older adults or immunocompromised patients. Between 5% and 20% of the U.S. population get influenza each year, and up to 49,000 deaths in a single year have been caused by the flu (Centers for Disease Control and Prevention [CDC], 2015k). Most patients are treated at home, but hospitalization may be needed when symptoms are severe or the patient develops complications such as pneumonia. Influenza may be caused by one of several virus families, referred to as A, B, and C.

The patient with influenza often has a rapid onset of severe headache, muscle aches, fever, chills, fatigue, and weakness. Adults are contagious from 24 hours before symptoms occur and up to 5 days after they begin. Sore throat, cough, and watery nasal discharge can also occur. Infection with influenza strain B can lead to nausea, vomiting, and diarrhea. Most patients feel fatigued for 1 to 2 weeks after the acute episode has resolved.

Health Promotion and Maintenance

Vaccinations for the prevention of influenza are widely available and are recommended for adults by The Joint Commission's National Patient Safety Goals (NPSGs). The vaccine is changed every year based on which specific viral strains are most likely to cause illness during the influenza season (i.e., late fall and winter in the Northern Hemisphere). Usually the vaccines contain antigens for the three or four expected viral strains. The recommended influenza vaccination for all adults is an IM injection (Fluvirin, Fluzone). The intranasal vaccine was found to be ineffective and is no longer available (CDC, 2016). An annual vaccination is especially important for those older than 50 years, adults with chronic illness or immune compromise, those living in institutions, adults living with or caring for adults with health problems that put them at risk for severe complications of influenza, and health care personnel providing direct care to patients (CDC, 2015f). Nurses have an opportunity to urge vaccination in the community and can show support for this action by receiving annual vaccinations themselves (Wiley, 2015).

Teach the patient who is sick to reduce the risk for spreading the flu by thoroughly washing hands, especially after nose blowing, sneezing, coughing, rubbing the eyes, or touching the face. Other precautions include staying home from work, school, or crowded places; covering the mouth and nose with a tissue when sneezing or coughing; disposing properly of used tissues immediately; and avoiding close contact with other people (Wiley, 2015). Although handwashing is a good way to prevent transmitting the virus, many people cannot wash their hands immediately after sneezing. The technique recommended by the CDC for controlling flu spread is to sneeze or cough into the upper sleeve rather than into the hand (CDC, 2015c). (Respiratory droplets on the hands can contaminate surfaces and be transmitted to others.)

❖ INTERPROFESSIONAL COLLABORATIVE CARE

Tests for influenza are available; however, in a community that has already seen the disease, the diagnosis is usually based on the patient's reported symptoms. The rapid influenza diagnostic test (RIDT) is common but has high false-negative rates, and the patient should be treated if influenza is suspected even if the RIDT is negative. Other tests, including cultures, are usually recommended only in specific situations.

Viral infections do not respond to antibiotic therapy. Antiviral agents such as oseltamivir (Tamiflu), zanamivir (Relenza), and peramivir (Rapivab) have been effective in the prevention and treatment of some strains of influenza A and B. They can be given to adults at high risk for complications who have been exposed to influenza but have not yet been vaccinated. These drugs also shorten the duration of influenza. The drugs prevent viral spread in the respiratory tract by inhibiting a viral enzyme that allows the virus to penetrate respiratory cells. To be effective as treatment, they must be taken within 24 to 48 hours after symptoms begin. Zanamivir should be used with caution in patients who have chronic obstructive pulmonary disease (COPD) or asthma and in older adults. Peramivir is available only as an IV drug. Patients older than 65 years should be treated with antiviral drugs as soon as possible to reduce their risks for hospitalization, complications, and disability (CDC, 2015d).

The patient should rest for several days and increase fluid intake unless another problem requires fluid restriction. Saline gargles may ease sore throat pain. Antihistamines may reduce the rhinorrhea. Other supportive measures are the same as those for acute rhinitis.

PANDEMIC INFLUENZA

❖ PATHOPHYSIOLOGY

Many viral infections in animals and birds are not usually transmitted to humans. A few historic exceptions have occurred when these animal and bird viruses mutated and became highly infectious to humans. These infections are termed **pandemic** because they have the potential to spread globally and because the virus is new to humans who have no IMMUNITY to it. Such

? NCLEX EXAMINATION CHALLENGE 31-1
Health Promotion and Maintenance

A nurse is providing community education on seasonal influenza. What information will the nurse include in this presentation? **Select all that apply.**
A. Adults older than 65 years should get the Prevnar-13 vaccination annually.
B. All adults older than 49 years should receive a Fluzone immunization annually.
C. Sneeze into a disposable tissue or into your sleeve instead of your hand.
D. Avoid large crowds during spring and summer to limit the chance for getting the flu.
E. Wash your hands frequently and after blowing your nose, coughing, or sneezing.
F. Call your primary health care provider for an antiviral prescription within 3 days of getting symptoms.

pandemics include the 1918 "Spanish" influenza that resulted in 40 million to 100 million deaths worldwide. This virus, the H1N1 strain, also known as *swine flu,* mutated and became highly infectious to humans. Most recently it caused a pandemic in 2009, spreading to 215 countries. In the United States, the number of people infected during the pandemic was estimated at 61 million with more than 12,000 deaths (CDC, 2015e). A vaccine was developed in 2009 and was administered separately from the seasonal influenza vaccine. Now the seasonal influenza vaccine contains the H1N1 antigen.

A new avian virus is the H5N1 strain, known as "avian influenza" or "bird flu." This virus has infected millions of birds, especially in Asia, and now has started to spread by human-to-human contact. World health officials are concerned that this strain could become a pandemic and spread worldwide, leading to very high mortality rates. Another avian strain, H7N9, has appeared in China, resulting in several deaths. This virus seems to be able to spread from person to person in limited situations. Travelers have brought the virus outside of China, but there are no cases originating outside of that country (CDC, 2015e).

Health Promotion and Maintenance

The prevention of a worldwide influenza pandemic of any virus is the responsibility of everyone. Health officials have been monitoring human outbreaks and testing both wild and domestic bird species throughout the world. A vaccine (Vepacel) is available in case of H5N1 outbreaks, but it is stockpiled and not part of general influenza vaccination. The recommended approach for any potential pandemic is early recognition of cases and implementing community and personal quarantine. Social-distancing behaviors also will help to reduce viral exposure.

Plans to prevent and contain pandemic flu in North America have been developed with the cooperation of the United States and Canadian governments. When a cluster of cases is discovered in an area, the stockpiled vaccine will be made available for immunization. Vepacel requires two injections 28 days apart.

The antiviral drugs oseltamivir (Tamiflu) and zanamivir (Relenza) should be widely distributed. These drugs may reduce the severity of the infection and the mortality rate. Infected patients must be cared for in strict isolation. All nonessential public activities in the area should be stopped, including public gatherings of any type, attendance at schools, religious services, shopping, and many types of employment. Adults should stay home and use the food, water, and drugs they have stock-piled to last at least 2 weeks per person (see Chapter 10). Travel to and from this area should be stopped.

Urge all adults to pay attention to public health announcements and early warning systems for disease outbreaks. Teach them the importance of starting prevention behaviors as soon as an outbreak is announced. They should also have a battery-powered radio (and batteries) to keep informed of updates. See Chapter 10 for more information on items to have ready in the home for disaster preparedness. *An influenza pandemic is a disaster, and containing it requires the cooperation of all adults.*

❖ INTERPROFESSIONAL COLLABORATIVE CARE

The care priorities for the patient with avian or any pandemic influenza are supporting the patient and preventing spread of the disease. Both are equally important. The initial signs and symptoms of avian influenza are similar to those of other respiratory infections—cough, fever, and sore throat. These progress rapidly to shortness of breath and pneumonia. In addition, diarrhea, vomiting, abdominal pain, and bleeding from the nose and gums can occur. *Ask any patient with these symptoms if he or she has recently (within the past 10 days) traveled to areas of the world affected by H5N1. If such travel has occurred, coordinate with the health care team to place the patient in an airborne isolation room with negative air pressure. These precautions remain until the diagnosis of H5N1 is ruled out or the threat of contagion is over.* Diagnosis is made based on signs and symptoms and positive testing. Rapid influenza diagnostic testing is available along with other measures such as cultures.

When caring for the patient with avian influenza, personal protective equipment is essential. Anyone entering the patient's room for any reason needs to wear a fit-tested respirator. Use other Airborne, Droplet, and Contact Precautions as described in Chapter 23. Teach others to monitor themselves for illness, especially respiratory infection, for at least a week after the last contact with the patient. Use the antiviral drug *oseltamivir* (Tamiflu) or *zanamivir* (Relenza) within 48 hours of contact with the infected patient. All health care personnel working with patients suspected of having avian influenza should receive the vaccine in the recommended two-step process.

No effective treatment for this infection currently exists. Interventions are supportive to allow the patient's own immune system to fight the infection. Oxygen is given when hypoxia, breathlessness, or a sudden change in COGNITION is present. Respiratory treatments to dilate the bronchioles and move respiratory secretions are used. If hypoxemia is not improved with oxygen therapy, intubation and mechanical ventilation may be needed. Antibiotics are used to treat a bacterial pneumonia that may occur with H5N1.

In addition to the need for respiratory support, the patient with H5N1 may have severe diarrhea and need fluid therapy. Transmission Precautions may prevent using a scale to weigh the patient. Monitor his or her hydration status, and carefully measure intake and output. The type of fluid therapy varies with the patient's cardiovascular status and blood osmolarity. Two important areas to monitor during rehydration are pulse rate and quality and urine output.

MIDDLE EAST RESPIRATORY SYNDROME (MERS)

Middle East respiratory syndrome (MERS) is another example of a disease that could cause a pandemic. MERS is caused by a "novel" or new virus from the large family of coronaviruses. Viruses from this family cause many respiratory illnesses such as the common cold. They also can cause critical infections such as severe acute respiratory syndrome (SARS). There have been 1611 confirmed cases of MERS since 2012 and 575 deaths. MERS was first identified in Saudi Arabia and has now been reported in 26 countries. The most recent outbreak started in 2015 in the Republic of Korea ("South Korea"). Only two cases of MERS have been confirmed in North America, and both patients were health care workers who lived in Saudi Arabia and traveled to North America (WHO, 2015b).

Patients with MERS typically report respiratory symptoms (cough and shortness of breath) along with fever. Pneumonia is common. GI problems, such as diarrhea, have also been reported. Symptoms may be mild or progress rapidly to multisystem organ failure, sepsis, and death. With severe distress, arterial blood gas analysis is performed to determine the need for oxygen therapy and possible ventilation support.

The only tests available for MERS are through the CDC. To be tested, patients must have symptoms of MERS and have either traveled to areas where MERS has been reported or have had close contact with someone who was confirmed to have MERS. Other patients considered for testing may be part of a cluster of cases of severe, unknown respiratory disease that is being investigated. The CDC test uses the reverse-transcriptase polymerase chain reaction assay (rRT-PCR). It is also possible to test a patient for a prior infection by assessing for MERS antibodies.

There is no specific treatment for MERS. Supportive care is used to manage and prevent complications. The patient may need mechanical ventilation and fluids. If kidney function is severely reduced, dialysis is performed. Hemorrhage from disseminated intravascular coagulation is managed with blood products. (See Chapter 37 for management of septic shock.) "Convalescent serum," which is the serum taken from a patient who has recovered from the disease, is a potential treatment but requires that the patient have the same blood type as the convalescent patient. This therapy was used successfully with a few patients during the 2014 Ebola outbreak. Patients being treated for MERS must be maintained in Contact and Airborne Precautions (CDC, 2015g).

❗ NURSING SAFETY PRIORITY **QSEN**

Action Alert

When performing procedures for the patient with a pandemic influenza that normally induce coughing or promote aerosolization of particles (e.g., suctioning, using a positive-pressure facemask, obtaining a sputum culture, or giving aerosolized treatments), protect yourself and other health care workers. Wear a disposable particulate mask respirator and protective eyewear during the procedures. Keep the door to the patient's room closed. Avoid touching your face with contaminated gloves. Wash your hands after you remove the gown, gloves, eyewear, and face shield and whenever you leave the patient's room. Wear gloves when disinfecting contaminated surfaces or equipment.

✳ GAS EXCHANGE CONCEPT EXEMPLAR Pneumonia

❖ PATHOPHYSIOLOGY

Pneumonia is excess fluid in the lungs from an inflammatory process. This disease can seriously reduce gas exchange. GAS EXCHANGE is oxygen transport to the cells and carbon dioxide

---

💡 NCLEX EXAMINATION CHALLENGE 31-2

Physiological Integrity

A nurse is caring for a client who suddenly developed acute respiratory distress after returning home from an extended business trip in a foreign country. Which actions by the nurse are **most appropriate** before the cause of the problem is identified? **Select all that apply.**

A. Ask the client where the travel specifically occurred and whether he or she was exposed to anyone who was ill.

B. Use Contact Precautions with this client and use gloves and gown for care.

C. Prepare to administer isoniazid (INH) as soon as the first dose is available.

D. Monitor the results of the client's blood urea nitrogen (BUN), creatinine, and liver function studies.

E. Collaborate with the interprofessional team to obtain arterial blood gases and prepare to intubate the client.

F. Assist with obtaining sputum cultures for acid-fast bacilli to send to the laboratory for analysis.

TABLE 31-1   Risk Factors for Pneumonia

Community-Acquired Pneumonia
- Is an older adult
- Has never received the pneumococcal vaccination or received it more than 5 years ago
- Did not receive the influenza vaccine in the previous year
- Has a chronic health problem or other coexisting condition that reduces IMMUNITY
- Has recently been exposed to respiratory viral or influenza infections
- Uses tobacco or alcohol or is exposed to high amounts of secondhand smoke

Health Care–Acquired Pneumonia
- Is an older adult
- Has a chronic lung disease
- Has presence of gram-negative colonization of the mouth, throat, and stomach
- Has an altered level of consciousness
- Has had a recent aspiration event
- Has presence of endotracheal, tracheostomy, or nasogastric tube
- Has poor nutritional status
- Has reduced IMMUNITY (from disease or drug therapy)
- Uses drugs that increase gastric pH (histamine [H_2] blockers, antacids) or alkaline tube feedings
- Is currently receiving mechanical ventilation (ventilator-associated pneumonia [VAP])

---

transport away from cells through ventilation and diffusion. See Chapter 2 for a discussion that summarizes the concept of gas exchange.

Inflammation causing pneumonia can be triggered by infectious organisms and by inhaling irritating agents. Inflammation occurs in the interstitial spaces, the alveoli, and often the bronchioles. The process begins when organisms penetrate the airway mucosa and multiply in the alveolar spaces. White blood cells (WBCs) migrate to the area of infection, causing local capillary leak, edema, and exudate. These fluids collect in and around the alveoli, and the alveolar walls thicken. Both events seriously reduce GAS EXCHANGE by interfering with diffusion in the lungs. This leads to hypoxemia, which has the potential to cause death. Red blood cells (RBCs) and fibrin move into the alveoli, and capillary leak spreads the infection to other areas of the lung. If the organisms move into the bloodstream, septicemia results; if the infection extends into the pleural cavity, empyema (a collection of pus in the pleural cavity) results.

The fibrin and edema stiffen the lung, reducing compliance and decreasing the vital capacity. Alveolar collapse (atelectasis) reduces GAS EXCHANGE even more. As a result, arterial oxygen levels fall, causing hypoxemia.

Pneumonia may occur as *lobar pneumonia* with consolidation (solidification, lack of air spaces) in a segment or an entire lobe of the lung or as *bronchopneumonia* with diffusely scattered patches around the bronchi. The extent of lung involvement depends on the host defenses. Bacteria multiply quickly in a person whose immune system is compromised. Tissue necrosis results when an abscess forms and perforates the bronchial wall.

Etiology

Pneumonia develops when a patient's IMMUNITY cannot overcome the invading organisms (Arsbad et al., 2016). Organisms from the environment (especially after natural disasters), from invasive devices, equipment and supplies, or other people can invade the body. Risk factors are listed in Table 31-1. Pneumonia can be caused by bacteria, viruses, mycoplasmas, fungi, rickettsiae, protozoa, and helminths (worms). Noninfectious causes of pneumonia include inhalation of toxic gases, chemical fumes, and smoke and aspiration of water, food, fluid (including saliva), and vomitus. Pneumonia can be categorized as community-acquired (CAP), hospital-acquired (HAP), health

care–acquired (HCAP) or ventilator-associated (VAP) (see Table 31-2).

Incidence and Prevalence

In the United States 2 to 5 million cases of pneumonia occur annually. About 1 million people are hospitalized for treatment, and more than 50,000 deaths result from the disease (CDC, 2015k). In Canada, influenza and pneumonia incidence and deaths are reported together; and both disorders are common, accounting for about 6000 deaths annually (Statistics Canada, 2015). The rate of pneumonia is higher among older adults, nursing home residents, hospitalized patients, patients with neurological problems or difficulty swallowing, and those being mechanically ventilated. CAP is more common than HAP and occurs most often in late fall and winter, frequently as a complication of influenza.

Health Promotion and Maintenance

Patient education about vaccination is important in the prevention of pneumonia (Chart 31-1). The Joint Commission National Patient Safety Goals [NPSGs] recommend that nurses especially encourage adults older than 65 years and those with a chronic health problem to receive immunization against pneumonia. There are two pneumonia vaccines: pneumococcal polysaccharide vaccine (PPSV 23), known as *Pneumovax*; and pneumococcal conjugate vaccine (PCV-13), known as *Prevnar 13*. The CDC recommends that adults older than 65 years be vaccinated with both, first with Prevnar 13 followed by Pneumovax about 6 to 12 months later. Adults who have already received the Pneumovax should have Prevnar 13 about a year or more later. These recommendations also apply to adults between 19 and 64 years of age who have specific risk factors such as chronic illnesses (CDC, 2015j). Because pneumonia often follows influenza, especially among older adults, urge all adults to receive the seasonal vaccination annually.

TABLE 31-2   Differentiation of Types of Pneumonia

TYPE OF PNEUMONIA	DEFINITION	MANAGEMENT CONSIDERATIONS
Community-acquired	Contracted outside a health care setting; acquired in the community	Most common bacterial agents: *Streptococcus pneumoniae, Haemophilus influenzae* Most common viral agents: influenza, respiratory syncytial virus (RSV) Antibiotics are often empirical based on multiple patient and environmental factors Treatment length: minimum of 5 days Prompt initiation of antibiotics required; in ED setting, first dose given before patient leaves unit for inpatient bed or within 6 hours of presentation to the ED
Health care–associated	Onset/diagnosis of pneumonia occurs <48 hours after admission in patient with specific risk factors: • In hospital for >48 hours in the past 90 days • Living in nursing home or assisted-living facility • Received IV therapy, wound care, antibiotics, chemotherapy in the past 30 days • Seen at a hospital or dialysis clinic within the past 30 days	May have multidrug-resistant organisms Hand hygiene critical
Hospital-acquired	Onset/diagnosis of pneumonia >48 hours after admission to hospital	Encourage pulmonary hygiene and progressive ambulation Provide adequate hydration Assess risk for aspiration using an evidence-based tool Monitor for early signs of sepsis Hand hygiene is critical Provide vigorous oral care

Ventilator-associated	Onset/diagnosis of pneumonia within 48-72 hours after endotracheal intubation	Presence of ET tube increases risk for pneumonia by bypassing protective airway mechanisms and allowing aspiration of secretions from the oropharynx and stomach; dental plaque also increases risk
		Initiate ventilator bundle order set, including:
		  Elevate HOB at least 30 degrees
		  Daily sedation "vacation" and weaning assessment
		  DVT prophylaxis
		  Oral care regimen
		  Stress ulcer prophylaxis
		  Suctioning, either as needed or continuous subglottal suction
		Hand hygiene is critical

Data from Sopena, N., Heras, E., Casas, I., Bechini, J., Gausch, I., Pedro-Botet, et al. (2014). Risk factors of hospital-acquired pneumonia outside the intensive care unit. *American Journal of Infection Control, 42*, 38-42; Peyrani, P. (2013). A three-step critical pathway for community-acquired pneumonia reduces duration of hospital stay and intravenous antibiotic use by 2 days. *Evidence-Based Nursing, 16* (2), 48-49; Driver, C., (2014). The common causes of community-acquired pneumonia. *Nursing in Residential Care, 16*(4), 202-205; Quinn, B., & Baker, D.L. (2015). Comprehensive oral care helps prevent hospital non-ventilator acquired pneumonia. *American Nurse Today, 10*(3), 18-23; Gianakis, A., McNett, M., Belle, J., Moran, C., & Grimm, D. (2015). Risk factors for ventilator-associated pneumonia. *Journal of Trauma Nursing, 22*(3), 125-113; Liao, Yu-Mei, Tsai, Jung-Rung; & Chou, Fan-Hao. (2015). The effectiveness of an oral health program for preventing ventilator-associated pneumonia. *Nursing in Critical Care, 10*(2), 89-97. *DVT,* Deep vein thrombosis; *ED,* emergency department; *ET,* endotracheal; *HOB,* head of bed.

CHART 31-1   Patient and Family Education: Preparing for Self-Management

Preventing Pneumonia

- Know whether you are at risk for pneumonia (older than 65 years, have a chronic health problem [especially a respiratory problem], or have limited mobility and are confined to a bed or chair during your waking hours).
- Have the annual influenza vaccine after discussing appropriate timing of the vaccination with your primary health care provider.
- Discuss the pneumococcal vaccine with your primary health care provider and have the vaccination as recommended.
- Avoid crowded public areas during flu and holiday seasons.
- If you have a mobility problem, cough, turn, move about as much as possible, and perform deep-breathing exercises.

- If you are using respiratory equipment at home, clean the equipment as you have been taught.
- Avoid indoor pollutants, such as dust, secondhand (passive) smoke, and aerosols.
- If you do not smoke, do not start.
- If you smoke, seek professional help on how to stop (or at least decrease) your habit.
- Be sure to get enough rest and sleep on a daily basis.
- Eat a healthy, balanced diet.
- Drink at least 3 L (quarts) of nonalcoholic fluids each day (unless fluid restrictions are needed because of another health problem).

QUALITY IMPROVEMENT QSEN

Enhancing Interprofessional Collaboration Toward Reaching a Core Measure

Michaels, K., & Sidone, L. (2014). Adhering to The Joint Commission's pneumonia core measure. *Nursing, 44*(2), 20-22.

Because of the high morbidity and mortality associated with community-acquired pneumonia, one of The Joint Commission's core measures for hospitalized patients is pneumonia, with vaccination receipt as the outcome measure. This Quality Improvement project was an interprofessional process improvement project at Suburban Hospital in Maryland to meet this core measure.

Before the project, Suburban hospital's nurse-driven pneumonia vaccination program gave nurses the authority to screen patients and implement standing orders for the pneumonia vaccine based on patient eligibility. The patients were screened and then vaccinated on the day of discharge. On audit, the compliance rate for this activity was only 47%.

After a thorough investigation into the practice by a multidisciplinary team, it was determined that vaccination on the day of discharge was the probable barrier. Reasons for this included patients being in a hurry to leave and not wanting to wait or having other concerns and questions during the discharge process.

The team established a pilot program in which nurses screened patients for vaccine eligibility when they were admitted and a pharmacist administered the vaccination on the second or third day of the hospital stay. The pharmacist was responsible for obtaining a prescription from the provider and securing the vaccine, which had been removed from the medication dispensing units on the floors.

The program included educating nurses and pharmacists about the changes, generating new reports that contained vaccination information for each patient, collaborating with other members of the health care team (social workers, unit managers, and staff educators), and a protocol for determining vaccine status from patients admitted from long-term care facilities.

After the program was implemented, Suburban Hospital's program demonstrated compliance rates of 95% to 99% for vaccination.

Commentary: Implications for Practice and Research

This Quality Improvement project demonstrates the value of creative, out-of-the-box thinking and interprofessional collaboration. Identification of a probable barrier to consistently attaining 100% compliance was found to be short (<24 hour) hospital admissions. The team is implementing a new process in which the reports on vaccine eligibility are reviewed twice a day.

Vaccination for pneumonia is now available at the hospital for patients admitted for any other condition. **The Joint Commission's NPSGs include that all inpatients should have their pneumonia vaccination status checked and, if needed, be vaccinated while on in-patient status.** Although this is now a Core Measure, compliance has remained less than desirable. See the Quality Improvement box to learn about one hospital's program to increase the compliance with this core measure.

Other prevention techniques include strict handwashing to avoid spreading organisms and avoiding crowds during cold and flu season. Teach the patient who has a cold or the flu to see his or her primary health care provider if fever lasts more than 24 hours, if the problem lasts longer than 1 week, or if symptoms worsen.

Respiratory therapy equipment must be well maintained and decontaminated or changed as recommended. Use sterile water rather than tap water in GI tubes and institute Aspiration Precautions as indicated, including screening patients for aspiration risk.

VAP is on the rise, but the risk can be reduced with conscientious assessment and meticulous nursing care. The preventive care for VAP is discussed in detail in Chapter 32.

! NURSING SAFETY PRIORITY QSEN

Action Alert

Because pneumonia is a frequent cause of sepsis, use a sepsis screening tool to monitor patients who have pneumonia. For patients with pneumonia, always check oxygen saturation with vital signs.

❖ *INTERPROFESSIONAL COLLABORATIVE CARE*

Depending on the patient's overall health status, the specific cause of the pneumonia, and the severity of hypoxemia, patients may be cared for in the home or other residential setting or may need acute hospital care. The Concept Map addresses assessment and nursing care issues related to patients who have pneumonia. Signs and symptoms of pneumonia differ in older patients compared with younger patients.

◆ *Assessment: Noticing*

History. Assess for the risk factors for infection (see Table 31-1). Document age; living, work, or school environment; diet, exercise, and sleep routines; swallowing problems; presence of a nasogastric tube; tobacco and alcohol use; and past and current use of or addiction to "street" drugs. Remember that often aspiration is "silent" with no signs or symptoms. Ask about past respiratory illnesses and whether the patient has been exposed to influenza or pneumonia or has had a recent viral infection.

If the patient has chronic respiratory problems, ask whether respiratory equipment is used in the home. Assess whether the patient's home cleaning routine is adequate to prevent infection. Ask when he or she received the last influenza or pneumococcal vaccine. Ask family members whether they have noticed a change in the patient's COGNITION.

Physical Assessment/Signs and Symptoms. Observe the general appearance. Many patients with pneumonia have flushed cheeks and an anxious expression. The patient may have chest pain or discomfort, myalgia, headache, chills, fever, cough, tachycardia, dyspnea, tachypnea, hemoptysis, and sputum production. Severe chest muscle weakness also may be present from sustained coughing.

Observe the patient's breathing pattern, position, and use of accessory muscles. The patient with hypoxia and reduced GAS EXCHANGE may be uncomfortable in a lying position and will sit upright, balancing with the hands ("tripod position"). Assess the cough and the amount, color, consistency, and odor of sputum produced.

Crackles are heard with auscultation when fluid is in interstitial and alveolar areas, and breath sounds may be diminished. Wheezing may be heard if inflammation or exudate narrows the airways. Bronchial breath sounds are heard over areas of density or consolidation. Fremitus is increased over areas of pneumonia, and percussion is dulled. Chest expansion may be diminished or unequal on inspiration.

In evaluating vital signs, compare the results with baseline values. The patient with pneumonia, especially the older adult, is often hypotensive with orthostatic changes because of vasodilation and dehydration. A rapid, weak pulse may indicate

CONCEPT MAP

IMMUNITY

COMMUNITY-ACQUIRED PNEUMONIA (CAP)

GAS EXCHANGE

INTERVENTIONS—RESPONDING

1 Nursing Priority – Improving GAS EXCHANGE, Eliminating Infection
- Deliver oxygen therapy; assist with bronchial hygiene. *Promotes GAS EXCHANGE and oxygenation.*
- Administer antibiotics for 5-7 days; reinforce, clarify, and provide information regarding drug therapy. *Helps to rid body of infection and encourages drug compliance.*

2 Providing Safe and Effective Care
- Apply principles of infection control (e.g., hand hygiene, Isolation or Airborne Precautions). *Protects client and health care providers from infection transmission.*

3 Respiratory Assessment: Pattern of Responses—Noticing
- Perform focused respiratory assessment and re-assessment; observe breathing pattern, position, and use of accessory muscles. *Assesses for respiratory distress.*
- Assess cough and amount, color, consistency, odor produced by sputum. *Assesses for infection and inadequate GAS EXCHANGE.*
- Assess for breath sounds and document wheezes, rhonchi, crackles, and evidence of decreased breath sounds. *Crackles indicate fluid in interstitial and alveolar areas; wheezing indicates inflammation or exudate in airways; bronchial breath sounds indicate areas of density or consolidation.*

4 Interpreting Vital Signs Assessment
- Evaluate oxygen saturation and vital sign trends, effectiveness of antibiotics, fluids, and antipyretics. *Monitors for signs of sepsis, hypotension with orthostatic changes; rapid, weak pulse; and dysrhythmias.*

5 Promoting Breathing
- Assist with coughing, deep breathing, and incentive spirometry at least every 2 hours. Encourage alert patient to drink at least 2 L of fluid daily, unless contraindicated. *Promotes removal of secretions, hydration, and ensures adequate GAS EXCHANGE and oxygenation.*
- Monitor intake & output, especially when fever and tachypnea are present. *Monitors for signs of dehydration.*

6 Interpreting Diagnostic Tests
- Obtain complete blood count with differential, sputum and blood cultures. *Determines whether organisms have invaded the blood and caused sepsis.*
- Determine oxygenation status by arterial blood gas values and pulse oximetry. *Determines baseline PaO₂ and PaCO₂ and helps identify need for supplemental oxygen.*
- Assess electrolytes, blood urea nitrogen (BUN), and creatinine levels. *Checks for dehydration and kidney function.*
- Review chest x-rays. *Provides early diagnosis in older adults because pneumonia symptoms are often vague.*

7 Responding to Psychosocial Issues—Minimizing Anxiety
- Assess expressions and general tenseness of facial and shoulder muscles. Listen using calm, slow approach. *Encourages calmness because pain, fatigue, and dyspnea promote anxiety.*

8 Nursing Safety Priority: Action Alert!
Teach the importance of completing the entire course of antibiotic therapy even when symptoms improve or subside. *Helps eradicate organisms and prevents drug resistance.*

Concept Map by Deanne A. Blach, MSN, RN

EXPECTED OUTCOMES

Adequate GAS EXCHANGE:
- Maintains patent airway; SaO₂ of at least 95% or in patient's normal range
- Maintains cognitive orientation
- Effective cough with absence of chest pain, crackles, or hemoptysis
- Absence of tachycardia or tachypnea, breathing discomfort with speaking, or cyanosis
- Returns to pre-pneumonia health status

INFLAMMATION:
- Absence of wheezing

INFECTION:
- Free from invading organisms in blood and sputum
- WBC and differential within normal limits
- Afebrile

Data Synthesis →

PATIENT PROBLEMS
- Impaired GAS EXCHANGE related to decreased diffusion at the alveolar-capillary membrane
- Potential for airway obstruction related to excessive tracheobronchial secretions, fatigue, chest discomfort, muscle weakness
- Potential for sepsis related to the presence of microorganisms in a very vascular area and decreased IMMUNITY.

Planning and implementation: Responding

Noticing Older Adult Differences

Most common sign/symptom is acute confusion from hypoxia. Other signs/symptoms: weakness, fatigue, lethargy, poor appetite. Fever and cough may be absent. White blood cells may not be elevated until infection is severe. Greatly increased risk for sepsis and death.

NOTICE IN THE HISTORY

60-year-old Diane Owens is admitted with CAP. She says, "My chest hurts from coughing so much." She is coughing up thick, green and rust-colored sputum. She is becoming confused and has lost her appetite.

NOTICING— Physical Assessment →

- Confused.
- T 99.1° F; HR 128, pulse weak; RR 24; BP 96/58 mm Hg
- Cheeks are flushed; fatigued, weak, lethargic; pain present; dyspneic; anxious
- Bilateral crackles and wheezing; fremitus over RLL; dulled percussion; unequal chest expansion on inspiration

TABLE 31-3 Pathophysiology of Common Signs and Symptoms of Pneumonia

SIGN OR SYMPTOM	PATHOPHYSIOLOGY
Increased respiratory rate/dyspnea	Stimulation of chemoreceptors Increased work of breathing as a result of decreased lung compliance Stimulation of J receptors Anxiety Pain
Hypoxemia	Alveolar consolidation Pulmonary capillary shunting
Cough	Fluid accumulation in the receptors of the trachea, bronchi, and bronchioles
Purulent, blood-tinged, or rust-colored sputum	A result of the inflammatory process in which fluid from the pulmonary capillaries and red blood cells moves into the alveoli
Fever	Phagocytes release pyrogens that cause the hypothalamus to increase body temperature
Pleuritic chest discomfort	Inflammation of the parietal pleura causes pain on inspiration

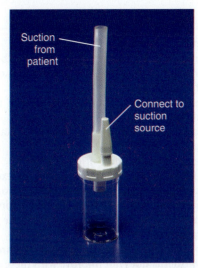

FIG. 31-1 Lukens tube for collection of sterile sputum/mucus specimens. (Courtesy Covidien, AG, Switzerland.)

hypoxemia, dehydration, or impending sepsis and shock. Dysrhythmias may occur from cardiac tissue hypoxia. Common pneumonia signs and symptoms and their causes are listed in Table 31-3.

Use an evidence-based pneumonia severity scale to help determine where the patient should be managed. Two such tools are the Pneumonia Severity Index (PSI) and the CURB-65. The PSI uses four risk categories (demographics, comorbid conditions, physical examination, and selected laboratory values) to determine a score that shows the severity of the patient's pneumonia. The CURB-65 relies on laboratory values (blood urea nitrogen [BUN], age, respiration, blood pressure, and presence of confusion).

CONSIDERATIONS FOR OLDER ADULTS
Patient-Centered Care [QSEN]

The older adult with pneumonia has weakness, fatigue (which can lead to falls), lethargy, confusion, and poor appetite. Fever and cough may be absent, but hypoxemia is often present. The most common symptom of pneumonia in the older-adult patient is a change in COGNITION with acute confusion from hypoxia. The WBC count may not be elevated until the infection is severe. Waiting to treat the disease until more typical symptoms appear greatly increases the risk for sepsis and death (Touhy & Jett, 2016).

Psychosocial Assessment. The patient with pneumonia often has pain, fatigue, and dyspnea, all of which promote anxiety. Assess anxiety by looking at his or her facial expression and general tenseness of facial and shoulder muscles. Listen to the patient carefully, and use a calm approach. Because of airway obstruction and muscle fatigue, the patient with dyspnea speaks in broken sentences. Keep the interview short if severe dyspnea or breathing discomfort is present.

Laboratory Assessment. Sputum is obtained and examined by Gram stain, culture, and sensitivity testing; however, the

responsible organism often is not identified. A sputum sample is easily obtained from the patient who can cough into a specimen container. Extremely ill patients may need suctioning to obtain a sputum specimen. In these situations, a specimen is obtained by sputum trap (Fig. 31-1) during suctioning. A complete blood count (CBC) is obtained to assess for an elevated WBC count, which is a common finding except in older adults. Blood cultures may be performed to determine whether the organism has entered the bloodstream.

In severely ill patients, arterial blood gases (ABGs) may be assessed to determine baseline arterial oxygen and carbon dioxide levels and to help identify a need for supplemental oxygen. Serum electrolyte, blood urea nitrogen (BUN), and creatinine levels also are assessed. A high BUN level may occur as a result of dehydration. Hypernatremia (high blood sodium levels) occurs with dehydration. A lactate level may be ordered to help assess for sepsis.

Imaging Assessment. Chest x-ray is the most common diagnostic test for pneumonia but may not show changes until 2 or more days after symptoms are present. It usually appears on chest x-ray as an area of increased density. It may involve a lung segment, a lobe, one lung, or both lungs. *In the older adult, the chest x-ray is essential for early diagnosis because pneumonia symptoms are often vague* (Touhy & Jett, 2016).

Other Diagnostic Assessments. Pulse oximetry is used to assess for hypoxemia. Thoracentesis is used in patients who have an accompanying pleural effusion.

◆ **Analysis: Interpreting**

The priority collaborative problems for patients with pneumonia include:

1. Decreased GAS EXCHANGE due to decreased diffusion at the alveolar-capillary membrane
2. Potential for airway obstruction due to excessive pulmonary secretions, fatigue, muscle weakness
3. Potential for sepsis due to the presence of microorganisms in a very vascular area and decreased IMMUNITY.
4. Potential for pulmonary empyema due to spread of infectious organisms from the lung into the pleural space.

◆ *Planning and Implementation: Responding*

Improving Gas Exchange

Planning: Expected Outcomes. The patient with pneumonia is expected to have adequate GAS EXCHANGE and oxygenation. Indicators of adequacy are:

- Maintenance of Sao_2 of at least 95% or in the patient's normal range
- Absence of crackles and wheezes on auscultation
- Absence of cyanosis
- Maintenance of cognitive orientation

Interventions. Interventions to improve GAS EXCHANGE are similar to those for the patient with asthma or chronic obstructive pulmonary disease (see Chapter 30). Nursing priorities include delivery of oxygen therapy and assisting the patient with bronchial hygiene.

Oxygen therapy is usually delivered by nasal cannula or mask unless the hypoxemia does not improve with these devices. The patient who is confused may not tolerate a facemask. Check the skin under the device and under the elastic band, especially around the ears, for areas of redness or skin breakdown. Actions for oxygen therapy are listed in Chart 28-1.

Incentive spirometry is used to improve inspiratory muscle action and prevent or reverse atelectasis (alveolar collapse). Instruct the patient to sit up if possible; exhale fully; place the mouthpiece in his or her mouth; take a long, slow, deep breath, raising the piston as high as possible; and then hold the breath for 2 to 4 seconds before slowly exhaling. Evaluate technique and record the volume of air inspired. Teach the patient to perform 5 to 10 breaths per session every hour while awake.

Preventing Airway Obstruction

Planning: Expected Outcomes. The patient with pneumonia is expected to maintain a patent airway. Indicators are:

- Effective cough
- Absence of pallor or cyanosis
- Pulse oximetry at or above 95%

Interventions. Interventions to improve GAS EXCHANGE by avoiding airway obstruction in pneumonia are similar to those for chronic obstructive pulmonary disease (COPD) or asthma. Because of fatigue, muscle weakness, chest discomfort, and excessive secretions, the patient often has difficulty clearing secretions. Help him or her cough and deep breathe at least every 2 hours. The alert patient may use an incentive spirometer to facilitate deep breathing and stimulate coughing. Encourage the alert patient to drink at least 2 L of fluid daily to prevent dehydration and to thin secretions unless another health problem requires fluid restriction. Monitor intake and output; oral mucus membranes; and skin turgor to assess hydration status, especially when fever and tachypnea are present.

Bronchodilators, especially beta$_2$ agonists (see Chart 30-6), are prescribed when bronchospasm is present. They can be given by nebulizer or metered-dose inhaler. Inhaled or IV steroids are used with acute pneumonia when airway swelling is present. Expectorants such as guaifenesin (Mucinex) may be used.

Preventing Sepsis

Planning: Expected Outcomes. The patient with pneumonia is expected to be free of the invading organism and to return to a pre-pneumonia health status. Indicators are:

- Absence of fever
- Absence of pathogens in blood and sputum cultures
- WBC count and differential within normal limits

Interventions. Eliminating the infecting organism is key to treating pneumonia and preventing sepsis. When sepsis occurs with pneumonia, the risk for death is high. Anti-infectives are given for all types of pneumonias except those caused by viruses. Which drugs and the route of delivery prescribed are based on how the pneumonia was acquired (i.e., CAP, HAP, or HCAP), how ill the patient is, which organism is involved, and whether the patient has conditions that increase the risk for complications, especially reduced IMMUNITY. The primary health care provider must consider drug resistance in the specific geographic area and in that hospital setting. Drug resistance is becoming increasingly common, especially for infections with *Streptococcus pneumoniae* (drug-resistant *S. pneumoniae* [DRSP]). Usually anti-infectives are used for 5 to 7 days for a patient with uncomplicated CAP and up to 21 days for a patient with severely impaired immunity or one with HAP.

For pneumonia caused by aspiration of food or stomach contents, interventions focus on preventing lung damage and treating the infection. Aspiration of acidic stomach contents can cause widespread inflammation, leading to acute respiratory distress syndrome (ARDS) and permanent lung damage. See Chapter 32 for a discussion of ARDS.

Managing Empyema. When pulmonary empyema occurs as a result of pneumonia, further interventions are needed. Pulmonary empyema is a collection of pus in the pleural space most commonly caused by pulmonary infection. When empyema is present, GAS EXCHANGE can be impaired by both reduced lung diffusion and reduced effective ventilation.

Empyema is suspected when chest wall motion is reduced, fremitus is reduced or absent, percussion is flat, and breath sounds are decreased. Abnormal breath sounds, including bronchial breath sounds, egophony, and whispered pectoriloquy, also may be present. Diagnosis is made by chest x-ray or CT scan and a sample of the pleural fluid (obtained via thoracentesis). Empyema fluid is thick, opaque, exudative, and foul smelling.

Treatment includes draining the empyema cavity, re-expanding the lung, and controlling the infection. Appropriate antibiotics are prescribed. A chest tube(s) to closed-chest drainage is used to promote lung expansion and drainage. The tube is removed when the lung is fully expanded and the infection is under control. Chest surgery may be needed for thick pus or excessive pleural thickening. Nursing interventions are similar to those for patients with a pleural effusion, pneumothorax, or infection. Chapters 30 and 32 discuss these interventions in more detail.

❓ NCLEX EXAMINATION CHALLENGE 31-3

Safe and Effective Care Environment

When reviewing the laboratory values for a client admitted with pneumonia, which result will cause the nurse to collaborate quickly with the primary health care provider?

A. White blood cell (WBC) count of 14,526 mm^3
B. PaO$_2$ 68 mm Hg
C. PaCO$_2$ 46 mm Hg
D. Blood glucose 146 mg/dL

Care Coordination and Transition Management

The patient needs to continue the anti-infective drugs as prescribed. An important nursing role is to reinforce, clarify, and provide information to the patient and family as needed.

CHART 31-2 Focused Assessment

The Patient Recovering from Pneumonia

Ask whether the patient has had any of these:
- New-onset confusion
- Chills
- Fever
- Persistent cough
- Dyspnea
- Wheezing
- Hemoptysis
- Increased sputum production
- Chest discomfort
- Increasing fatigue
- Any other symptoms that have failed to resolve

Assess the patient for:
- Fever
- Diaphoresis
- Cyanosis, especially around the mouth or conjunctiva
- Dyspnea, tachypnea, or tachycardia
- Adventitious or abnormal breath sounds
- Weakness

Home Care Management. No special changes are needed in the home. If the home has a second story, the patient may prefer to stay on one floor for a few weeks, because stair climbing can be tiring. Toileting needs may be met by using a bedside commode if a bathroom is not located on the level the patient is using. Home care needs depend on the patient's level of fatigue, dyspnea, and family and social support.

The long recovery phase, especially in the older adult, can be frustrating. Fatigue, weakness, and a residual cough can last for weeks. Some patients fear they will never return to a "normal" level of functioning. Prepare them for the disease course and offer reassurance that complete recovery will occur. After discharge a home nursing assessment may be helpful. Chart 31-2 details the assessment of a patient recovering from pneumonia.

Self-Management Education. Review all drugs with the patient and family and emphasize the importance of completing anti-infective therapy. Teach the patient to notify the primary health care provider if chills, fever, persistent cough, dyspnea, wheezing, hemoptysis, increased sputum production, chest discomfort, or increasing fatigue returns or fails to go away completely. Instruct him or her to get plenty of rest and increase activity gradually.

An important aspect of education for the patient and family is avoiding upper respiratory tract infections and viruses. Teach him or her to avoid crowds (especially in the fall and winter when viruses are prevalent), people who have a cold or flu, and exposure to irritants such as smoke. A balanced diet and adequate fluid intake are essential.

Health Care Resources. Inform patients who smoke that smoking is a risk factor for pneumonia. **Provide them with information on local smoking-cessation classes and nicotine replacement options as recommended by The Joint Commission's NPSGs** (see Chapter 27). Teach about pneumonia and urge the patient who has not already been vaccinated against influenza or pneumonia to get these vaccinations after the pneumonia has resolved. Vaccinations will boost IMMUNITY to these diseases.

! NURSING SAFETY PRIORITY QSEN

Drug Alert

Warn the patient using nicotine patches or supplements of the danger of myocardial infarction if smoking is continued while using other forms of nicotine.

◆ *Evaluation: Reflecting*

Evaluate the care of the patient with pneumonia based on the identified priority patient problems. The expected outcomes are that he or she:
- Attains or maintains adequate GAS EXCHANGE
- Maintains patent airways
- Is free of the invading organism
- Avoids empyema
- Returns to his or her pre-pneumonia health status

✳ **IMMUNITY CONCEPT EXEMPLAR**
Pulmonary Tuberculosis

❖ *PATHOPHYSIOLOGY*

Tuberculosis (TB) is a highly communicable disease caused by *Mycobacterium tuberculosis*. It is one of the most common bacterial infections worldwide. The organism is transmitted via aerosolization (i.e., an airborne route) (Fig. 31-2). When a person with active TB coughs, laughs, sneezes, whistles, or sings, infected respiratory droplets become airborne and may be inhaled by others. Far more adults are infected with the bacillus than actually develop active TB. This is because the normal protection of IMMUNITY prevents full development of TB in the healthy person. Immunity is the body's physiologic defense mechanisms that protect from illness or disease. See Chapter 2 for a discussion that summarizes the concept of immunity.

The bacillus multiplies freely when it reaches a susceptible site (bronchi or alveoli). An exudative response occurs, causing pneumonitis. With the development of acquired IMMUNITY to TB, further growth of bacilli is controlled in most cases. The lesions usually resolve and leave little or no residual bacilli. Only a small percentage of adults infected with the bacillus ever develop active TB.

Cell-mediated IMMUNITY against TB develops 2 to 10 weeks after infection and is manifested by a positive reaction to a tuberculin test. The primary infection may be so small that it does not appear on a chest x-ray. The process of infection occurs in this order:

1. The granulomatous inflammation created by the TB bacillus in the lung becomes surrounded by collagen, fibroblasts, and lymphocytes.
2. Caseation necrosis, which is necrotic tissue being turned into a granular mass, occurs in the center of the lesion. If this area shows on x-ray, it is the *primary* lesion.

Areas of caseation then undergo resorption, degeneration, and fibrosis. These necrotic areas may calcify (*calcification*) or liquefy (*liquefaction*). If liquefaction occurs, this material then empties into a bronchus, and the emptied area becomes a cavity (*cavitation*). Bacilli continue to grow in the necrotic cavity wall and spread through the lymph channels into new areas of the lung.

A lesion also may grow by direct extension if bacilli multiply rapidly during inflammation. The lesions can extend through the pleura, resulting in pleural or pericardial effusion. Miliary

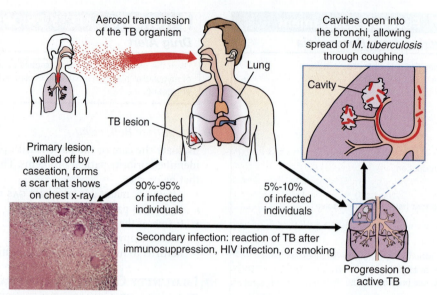

FIG. 31-2 Primary TB infection with progression to secondary infection and active disease. *HIV,* Human immune deficiency virus; *M. tuberculosis, Mycobacterium tuberculosis; TB,* tuberculosis. (Illustration from Workman, M. L., & LaCharity, L. (2016). *Understanding pharmacology* (2nd ed.). St. Louis: Saunders; photo from Kumar, V., Abbas, A., & Aster, J. (2015). *Robbins and Cotran pathologic basis for disease* [9th ed.]. Philadelphia: Saunders.)

or **hematogenous TB** is the spread of TB throughout the body when a large number of organisms enter the blood. Many tiny nodules scattered throughout the lung are seen on chest x-ray. Other body areas can become infected as a result of this spread.

Initial infection is seen more often in the middle or lower lobes of the lung. The local lymph nodes are infected and enlarged. An asymptomatic period usually follows the primary infection and can last for years or decades before clinical symptoms develop. This is called *latent TB. An infected person is not contagious to others until symptoms of disease occur.*

Secondary TB is a reactivation of the disease in a previously infected person. It is more likely when defenses are lowered and IMMUNITY is reduced. This is seen in older adults, those with chronic diseases, and especially those with HIV disease. The upper lobes are common sites of reactivation.

Etiology

M. tuberculosis is a slow-growing, acid-fast rod transmitted via the airborne route. Adults most often infected are those having repeated close contact with an infectious person who has not yet been diagnosed with TB. The risk for transmission is reduced after the infectious person has received proper drug therapy for 2 to 3 weeks, clinical improvement occurs, and acid-fast bacilli (AFB) in the sputum are reduced.

Incidence and Prevalence

Worldwide, 9.5 million people were diagnosed, and an additional 1.45 million people died from TB in 2012 (WHO, 2016). About one-third of the entire world population has latent TB (WHO, 2015a). In the United States, there were over 9000 new cases of TB in 2014 (CDC, 2015m). The incidence of TB has been steadily decreasing in North America, although increases in incidence are seen in many other countries (WHO, 2015a). In North America, the adults who are at greatest risk for development of TB are:

- Those in constant, frequent contact with an untreated person

- Those who have reduced IMMUNITY or HIV
- Adults who live in crowded areas such as long-term care facilities, prisons, homeless shelters, and mental health facilities
- Older homeless adults
- Abusers of injection drugs or alcohol
- Lower socioeconomic groups
- Foreign immigrants (WHO, 2015a)

Health Promotion and Maintenance

Many adults who acquire TB have risk factors such as homelessness, living in very crowded conditions, or substance abuse with malnutrition. These risk factors are best managed on a societal level. Communities need to work toward providing adequate housing, substance-abuse programs that are accessible, and feeding centers or food banks for those in need. On a personal level, many health conditions make it more likely to contract TB if exposed. Adults with these health conditions should avoid people who are ill, stay well nourished, and practice good handwashing. Any adult who works with people at high risk of having TB should be screened annually.

❖ INTERPROFESSIONAL COLLABORATIVE CARE
◆ Assessment: Noticing

Early detection of TB depends on subjective patient reports rather than observable signs or symptoms. TB has a slow onset, and patients are not aware of problems until the disease is advanced. *TB should be considered for any patient with a persistent cough or other symptoms of TB, such as unintended weight loss, anorexia, night sweats, hemoptysis, shortness of breath, fever, or chills.*

History. Assess the patient's past exposure to TB. Ask about his or her country of origin and travel to foreign countries where incidence of TB is high. It is important to ask about the results of any previous tests for TB. Also ask whether the patient has had bacille Calmette-Guérin (BCG) vaccine (often given in childhood overseas), which contains attenuated tubercle bacilli.

Anyone who has received BCG vaccine within the previous 10 years will have a positive skin test that can complicate interpretation. Usually the size of the skin response decreases each year after BCG vaccination. These patients should be evaluated for TB with a chest x-ray or the QuantiFERON-TB Gold test (CDC, 2015l).

Physical Assessment/Signs and Symptoms. The patient with TB has progressive fatigue, lethargy, nausea, anorexia, weight loss, irregular menses, and a low-grade fever. Symptoms may have been present for weeks or months. Night sweats may occur with the fever. A cough with mucopurulent sputum, which may be streaked with blood, is present. Chest tightness and a dull, aching chest pain occur with the cough. Ask about, assess for, and document the presence of any of these symptoms to help with diagnosis, establish a baseline, and plan nursing interventions.

When assessing the patient, you may note dullness with percussion over the involved lung fields, bronchial breath sounds, crackles, and increased transmission of spoken or whispered sounds. Partial obstruction of a bronchus from the disease or compression by lymph nodes may produce localized wheezing.

Psychosocial Assessment. Tuberculosis is a frightening diagnosis. Explain the disease thoroughly, including the need to maintain good hygiene and avoid infecting others. The patient may feel isolated and shunned. Take time to listen to him or her and help to resolve any concerns. The family and friends of the patient may have similar concerns as well. Often close contacts will be afraid they have contracted the illness. Encourage all close contacts to get tested. Help the patient notify his or her employer if needed about required time off. Directly observed therapy may feel threatening. Explain how this helps improve adherence to the long treatment schedule.

Diagnostic Assessment. There are several methods to test for TB. In addition to chest x-ray, sputum cultures of blood or respiratory secretions can be tested. The most accurate and rapid test for TB is the fully automated nucleic acid amplification test (NAAT) used on respiratory secretions. Results are available in less than 2 hours.

Sputum culture confirms the diagnosis. Enhanced TB cultures take up to 4 weeks for a valid result. After drug therapy is started, sputum samples are obtained at intervals to determine therapy effectiveness. Cultures are usually negative after 3 months of effective treatment (CDC, 2015l).

Blood analysis can be done with interferon-gamma release assays, or IGRAs. The two available tests are the QuantiFERON-TB Gold In-Tube test and the T-SPOT TB test. Both tests show how the patient's immune system responds to the TB bacterium. A positive result means that the person is infected with TB but does not indicate whether the infection is latent or active. Another blood test, the Xpert MTB/RIF can detect drug-resistant strains of TB and is also recommended for testing people with HIV infection. A new test (GeneXpert Omni) will be available in the future for point-of-care testing (WHO, 2015a).

The tuberculin test (Mantoux test) is the most commonly used reliable screening test for TB. A small amount (0.1 mL) of purified protein derivative (PPD) is placed intradermally in the forearm. The test is "read" in 48 to 72 hours. An area of induration (localized swelling with hardness of soft tissue), not just redness, measuring 10 mm or greater in diameter, indicates exposure to and possible infection with TB (Fig. 31-3). In certain adults, such as those with decreased IMMUNITY, induration of

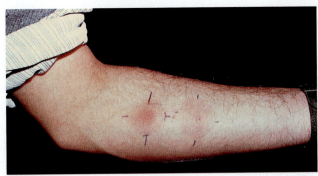

FIG. 31-3 Positive tuberculin skin test with induration. (From Zitelli, B. J., McIntire, S. C., & Nowalk, A. J. (2012). *Zitelli and Davis' atlas of pediatric physical diagnosis* (6th ed.). Philadelphia: Saunders; courtesy Kenneth Schuitt, MD.)

5 mm is a positive result. If possible, the site is re-evaluated after 72 hours because false-negative readings occur more often after only 48 hours (CDC, 2015l). *A positive reaction indicates exposure to TB or the presence of inactive (dormant) disease, not active disease. A reduced skin reaction or a negative skin test does not rule out TB disease or infection of the very old or anyone who has severely reduced IMMUNITY.* Failure to have a skin response because of reduced immunity when infection is present is called anergy.

Annual screening is needed for anyone who comes into contact with people who may be infected with TB, including some health care workers. Screening is very important for foreign-born people and migrant workers. Participation in screening programs is higher when programs are delivered in a culturally sensitive and nonthreatening manner. Urge anyone who is considered high risk to have an annual TB screening test.

Imaging Assessment. Once a person's skin test is positive for TB, a chest x-ray is used to detect active TB or old, healed lesions. Caseation and inflammation may be seen on the x-ray if the disease is active. The chest x-rays of HIV-infected patients may be normal or may show infiltrates in any lung zone and lymph node enlargement.

◆ **Analysis: Interpreting**

The priority collaborative problems for patients with tuberculosis include:

1. Potential for airway obstruction due to thick secretions and weak cough effort
2. Potential for development of drug-resistant disease and spread of infection due to inadequate adherence to therapy regimen
3. Anxiety due to diagnosis
4. Weight loss due to inadequate intake and nausea from therapy regimen
5. Fatigue due to lengthy illness, poor GAS EXCHANGE, and increased energy demands

◆ **Planning and Implementation: Responding**

Promoting Airway Clearance

Planning: Expected Outcomes. The patient with TB is expected to maintain a patent and adequate airway. Indicators of adequacy are:

• Effective cough
• Able to expectorate secretions

- Adequate GAS EXCHANGE
- Absence of cyanosis

Interventions. Interventions to maintain a patent airway are similar to those for pneumonia and COPD. Instruct the patient to drink plenty of fluids unless another condition requires restriction. Teach him or her to take a deep breath before coughing. An incentive spirometer may facilitate effective coughing.

Decreasing Drug Resistance and Infection Spread

Planning: Expected Outcomes. The patient with TB is expected to become free of active disease and not spread the disease to others.

Interventions. Interventions to help the patient become disease free include antimicrobial therapy.

Combination drug therapy is the most effective method of treating TB and preventing transmission. Active TB is treated with a combination of drugs to which the organism is sensitive. Therapy continues until the disease is under control. Multiple-drug regimens destroy organisms as quickly as possible and reduce the emergence of drug-resistant organisms. First-line therapy uses isoniazid (INH, Nidrazid), rifampin (Rifadin), pyrazinamide, and ethambutol (Myambutol) for the first 8 weeks, which is called *the initial phase of treatment.* The continuation phase lasts another 18 weeks, and the patient takes INH and rifampin either daily or twice a week (CDC, 2015l) (Chart 31-3). These drugs are now available in two- or three-drug combinations. One example is Rifater, which combines isoniazid, pyrazinamide, and rifampin. Variations of the first-line drugs along with other drug types are used when the patient does not tolerate the standard first-line therapy. Nursing interventions focus on patient teaching for drug therapy adherence and infection control.

CHART 31-3 Common Examples of Drug Therapy

First-Line Treatment for Tuberculosis

DRUG	NURSING IMPLICATIONS
Isoniazid (INH, Hydrazide, PDP-Isoniazid ◆) Kills actively growing mycobacteria outside the cell and inhibits the growth of dormant bacteria inside macrophages and caseating granulomas	Instruct the patient to avoid antacids and to take the drug on an empty stomach (1 hour before or 2 hours after meals) *to prevent slowing of drug absorption in the GI tract.* Teach the patient to take a daily multiple vitamin that contains the B-complex vitamins while on this drug *because the drug can deplete the body of this vitamin.* Remind the patient to avoid drinking alcoholic beverages while on this drug *because the liver-damaging effects of this drug are potentiated by drinking alcohol.* Tell the patient to report darkening of the urine, a yellow appearance to the skin or whites of the eyes, and an increased tendency to bruise or bleed, *which are signs and symptoms of liver toxicity or failure.*
Rifampin (RIF, Rifadin, Rimactane, Rofact ◆) Kills slower-growing organisms, even those that reside inside macrophages and caseating granulomas	Warn patients to expect an orange-reddish staining of the skin and urine, and all other secretions to have a reddish-orange tinge; also, soft contact lenses will become permanently stained *because knowing the expected side effects decreases anxiety when they appear.* Instruct sexually active women using oral contraceptives to use an additional method of contraception while taking this drug and for 1 month after stopping it *because this drug reduces the effectiveness of oral contraceptives.* Remind the patient to avoid drinking alcoholic beverages while on this drug *because the liver-damaging effects of this drug are potentiated by drinking alcohol.* Tell the patient to report darkening of the urine, a yellow appearance to the skin or whites of the eyes, and an increased tendency to bruise or bleed, *which are signs and symptoms of liver toxicity or failure.* Ask the patient about all other drugs in use *because this drug interacts with many other drugs.*
Pyrazinamide (PZA) Can effectively kill organisms residing within the very acidic environment of macrophages (which is where the tuberculosis bacillus sequesters) Available only in combination with other anti-TB drugs	Ask whether the patient has ever had gout *because the drug increases uric acid formation and will make gout worse.* Instruct patients to drink at least 8 ounces of water when taking this tablet and to increase fluid intake *to prevent uric acid from precipitating, making gout or kidney problems worse.* Teach the patient to wear protective clothing, a hat, and sunscreen when going outdoors in the sunlight *because the drug causes photosensitivity and greatly increases the risk for sunburn.* Remind the patient to avoid drinking alcoholic beverages while on this drug *because the liver-damaging effects of this drug are potentiated by drinking alcohol.* Tell the patient to report darkening of the urine, a yellow appearance to the skin or whites of the eyes, and an increased tendency to bruise or bleed, *which are signs and symptoms of liver toxicity or failure.*
Ethambutol (EMB, Etibi ◆, Myambutol) Inhibits bacterial RNA synthesis, thus suppressing bacterial growth Slow acting and bacteriostatic rather than bactericidal; thus it must be used in combination with other anti-TB drugs	Instruct patients to report any changes in vision, such as reduced color vision, blurred vision, or reduced visual fields, immediately to his or her primary health care provider *because the drug can cause optic neuritis, especially at high doses, and can lead to blindness.* Minor eye problems are usually reversed when the drug is stopped. Remind the patient to avoid drinking alcoholic beverages while on this drug *because the drug induces severe nausea and vomiting when alcohol is ingested.* (At one time ethambutol was used as drug therapy to help alcoholic patients stop drinking because of the drug's side effects in association with alcohol.) Ask whether the patient has ever had gout because *the drug increases uric acid formation and will make gout worse.* Instruct patients to drink at least 8 ounces of water when taking this drug and to increase fluid intake *to prevent uric acid from precipitating, making gout or kidney problems worse.*

Bedaquiline fumarate (Sirturo) is specifically targeted to multidrug-resistant TB. Side effects of this drug can be life threatening, so it is not used when other drugs will work. It should be given through directly observed therapy. Several other drugs for multidrug-resistant TB are in different phases of clinical trials.

Strict adherence to the prescribed drug regimen is crucial for suppressing the disease. Adherence is difficult because of the long duration of treatment. (Duration of therapy is often 26 weeks but can be as long as 2 years for multidrug-resistant [MDR] TB.) Thus your major role is teaching the patient about drug therapy and stressing the importance of taking each drug regularly, exactly as prescribed, for as long as it is prescribed. Provide accurate information in multiple formats, such as pamphlets, videos, and drug-schedule worksheets. To determine whether the patient understands how to take the drugs, ask him or her to describe the treatment regimen, side effects, and when to call the health care agency and physician.

! NURSING SAFETY PRIORITY QSEN

Drug Alert

The first-line drugs used as therapy for TB all can damage the liver. Warn the patient to not drink any alcoholic beverages for the entire duration of TB therapy. Bedaquiline fumarate can prolong the QT interval, cause ventricular dysrhythmias, and lead to sudden death. Patients on this drug need to have regular electrocardiograms (ECGs) and serum electrolyte evaluations.

The patient with TB often has concerns about the disease prognosis. Offer a positive outlook for the patient who adheres to the drug regimen. *However, with current resistant strains of TB, emphasize that not taking the drugs as prescribed could lead to an infection that is drug resistant.*

Some *multidrug-resistant TB* (MDR TB) strains are emerging as extensively drug-resistant (XDR TB). MDR TB is an infection that resists INH and rifampin. XDR TB is resistant not only to the first-line anti-tuberculosis drugs but also to the second-line antibiotics, including the fluoroquinolones and at least one of the aminoglycosides. The WHO estimates that 3.5% of all TB cases are drug resistant. The most common cause of MDR TB and XDR TB is mismanagement of drug therapy, either from inappropriate selection or use of antibiotics. Patients with acquired immune deficiency syndrome (AIDS) also often have MDR TB (WHO, 2015a). Drug therapy for MDR TB and XDR TB is more limited than standard first-line therapy and requires higher doses for longer periods. Patients who contract TB from a person with a resistant strain will also have a resistant strain of TB. So teaching patients to adhere to their drug regimens will also help them prevent the spread of the disease in both forms.

! NURSING SAFETY PRIORITY QSEN

Action Alert

Warn patients with extensively drug-resistant TB that absolute adherence to therapy is critical for survival and cure of the disease. These patients should receive directly observed therapy (DOT) (described under the "Self-Management Education" section).

The hospitalized patient with active TB is placed on Airborne Precautions (see Chapter 23) in a well-ventilated room that has at least six exchanges of fresh air per minute. All health care workers must use a personal respirator when caring for the patient. Use Standard Precautions with appropriate protection as with all patients. **In accordance with The Joint Commission's NPSGs, perform handwashing before and after patient care.** Precautions are discontinued when the patient is no longer contagious.

Other care issues for the patient with TB include teaching about infection prevention and what to expect about disease monitoring and participating in activities. TB is often treated outside the acute care setting, with the patient convalescing at home. Airborne Precautions are not necessary in this setting because family members have already been exposed; however, all members of the household need to undergo TB testing. Teach the patient to cover the mouth and nose with a tissue when coughing or sneezing, to place used tissues in plastic bags, and to wear a mask when in contact with crowds until the drugs suppress infection.

Tell the patient that sputum specimens are needed usually every 2 to 4 weeks once drug therapy is initiated. When the results of three consecutive sputum cultures are negative, the patient is no longer infectious (contagious) and may return to former activities. Remind him or her to avoid exposure to any inhalation irritants because these can cause further lung damage.

? NCLEX EXAMINATION CHALLENGE 31-4

Health Promotion and Maintenance

Which information is **most important** for a nurse to include when teaching a client with tuberculosis about the prescribed first-line drug therapy?
A. "Report darkening or reddening of the urine while taking Rifampin."
B. "Do not drink alcohol in any quantity while taking Isoniazid."
C. "Restrict fluid intake to 2 quarts of liquid a day on pyrazinamide."
D. "Temporary visual changes while taking ethambutol are not serious."

Managing Anxiety

Planning: Expected Outcomes. The patient with TB is expected to have adequate knowledge about the disease and report decreased anxiety. Indicators of decreased anxiety include:

- Patient report of reduced anxiety
- Relaxed facial features and muscles
- Ability to listen and retain information

Interventions. The nurse can provide many interventions to decrease anxiety if present. First assess the patient for subjective reports of anxiety and work with him or her to determine the source. Most patients will need education regarding the disease. When teaching the patient and family with either MDR TB or XDR TB, stress that it is the organism, not the patient, that is drug resistant because that can sometimes be misunderstood. Patients may be anxious about isolation if hospitalized or about spreading the disease to housemates or visitors. They may also be concerned about contacting an employer. Provide education and support. Refer the patient to social services if he or she does not have sick leave and will lose pay during the time off work.

Improving Nutrition

Planning: Expected Outcomes. The patient with TB is expected to have improved nutrition. Indicators of improved nutrition include:

- Weight gain
- Improvement in laboratory values indicating nutritional status
- Improved stamina
- Reports eating a healthy, balanced diet

Interventions. The patient with TB often has a long-standing history of malnutrition. Conduct a nutrition assessment using an evidence-based tool. Determine patient likes/dislikes, the ability to buy healthy food, condition of teeth or dentures, weight and body mass index, and history of substance abuse. When inadequate nutrition is a problem, be sure to include a registered dietitian as part of the interprofessional team.

Drugs to treat TB often cause nausea. If this happens, instruct the patient to take once-a-day drugs at night. Antiemetics can also be prescribed. If food doesn't interfere with the drug absorption (check the label), taking pills with a small snack of simple carbohydrates may help. Refer the patient to Meals on Wheels or other meal-delivery service. Instruct him or her about good oral hygiene, which makes food taste better. Weigh the patient once a week at the primary health care provider's office or, if he or she is receiving home health care services, have the agency weigh the patient and report the results to the provider.

For best healing, the patient should eat a diet with quality protein; iron; vitamins A, B, C, and E; and abundant fresh produce. Educate him or her about nutrition in consultation with a registered dietitian. Tell the patient to avoid alcohol. Alcohol can cause liver damage, and so can most of the antituberculosis drugs. Alcohol is also a source of "empty calories," and adults who abuse alcohol often are malnourished. An adult who gets a large number of calories from alcohol will not feel hungry. A special problem for this group of patients is lack of phosphorus, which is part of the cellular energy compound ATP. With low phosphorus, the patient will lack energy. Refer the patient to support groups if alcoholism or other substance abuse is present. Improved nutrition will improve IMMUNITY.

Managing Fatigue

Planning: Expected Outcomes. The patient with TB is expected to have improved stamina and less fatigue. Indicators of improved fatigue include:

- Patient report of increased energy
- Increased activity and activity tolerance
- Increased ability to concentrate

Interventions. Many of the interventions for fatigue will be the same as those for improving nutrition. Poor nutrition can lead directly to fatigue. Encourage the patient to resume activities slowly and get plenty of rest. Reassure him or her that the fatigue will improve as therapy progresses. Assess the patient's sleep-wake habits and encourage a full night's sleep with short day-time naps. Help him or her develop a healthy bed-time ritual if needed. Mental stamina may be decreased as a result of the lengthy convalescence. Reassure the patient that, by taking drugs as directed, the disease will be cured and energy levels will increase.

Care Coordination and Transition Management

Home Care Management. Most patients with TB are managed outside the hospital; however, patients may be diagnosed with TB while in the hospital for another problem. Discharge may be delayed if the living situation is high risk or if nonadherence is likely. Ensure collaboration with other members of the interprofessional team, including the case manager or social service worker in the hospital or the community health nursing agency, to ensure that the patient is discharged to the appropriate environment with continued supervision.

Self-Management Education. Teach the patient to follow the drug regimen exactly as prescribed and always to have a supply on hand. Teach about side effects and ways of reducing them to promote adherence. Remind him or her that the disease is usually no longer contagious after drugs have been taken for 2 to 3 consecutive weeks and clinical improvement is seen; however, *he or she must continue with the prescribed drugs for 6 months or longer as prescribed.* Directly observed therapy (DOT), in which a health care professional watches the patient swallow the drugs, may be indicated in some situations. This practice leads to more treatment successes, fewer relapses, and less drug resistance.

The patient who has weight loss and severe lethargy should gradually resume usual activities. Proper nutrition is needed to prevent infection recurrence.

Provide the patient with information about how TB can be spread to others. A key to preventing transmission is identifying those in close contact with the infected person so they can be tested and treated if needed. Identified contacts are assessed with a TB test and possibly a chest x-ray to determine infection status. Multidrug therapy may be indicated to prevent TB in heavily exposed individuals or for those who have other health problems that reduce IMMUNITY.

Health Care Resources. Teach the patient to receive follow-up care by a primary health care provider for at least 1 year after active treatment. The American Lung Association (ALA) can provide free information to the patient about the disease and its treatment. In addition, Alcoholics Anonymous (AA) and other health care resources for patients with alcoholism are available if needed. Assist the patient who uses illicit drugs to locate a drug-treatment program. **In accordance with The Joint Commission's NPSGs, urge smokers to quit and help them find an appropriate smoking-cessation program** (see Chapter 27).

◆ Evaluation: Reflecting

Evaluate the care of the patient with TB based on the identified priority patient problems. The expected outcomes are that he or she:

- Effectively clears his or her airways
- Is free of the invading organism and does not spread the infection
- Has reduced anxiety
- Demonstrates improved nutrition
- Reports decreased fatigue and increased energy
- Returns to his or her pre-tuberculosis health status

RHINOSINUSITIS

❖ PATHOPHYSIOLOGY

Rhinosinusitis is an inflammation of the mucous membranes of one or more of the sinuses and is usually seen with rhinitis, especially the common cold (coryza). Anything that interferes with sinus drainage (e.g., deviated nasal septum, nasal polyps or tumors, inhaled air pollutants or cocaine, allergies, facial trauma, and dental infection) can lead to rhinosinusitis. Even when the problem starts with a noninfectious cause such as seasonal allergies, swelling usually blocks the flow of secretions from the sinuses, which may then become infected.

Most episodes of rhinosinusitis are caused by viruses and usually develop in the maxillary and frontal sinuses, although bacterial infections also can occur. Complications include cellulitis, abscess, and meningitis.

Diagnosis is made based on the patient's history and symptoms, but other tests in complicated cases include endoscopic examination and CT scans. Plain x-rays are not helpful in viewing sinuses and are not recommended. Purulent drainage, fever, and lack of response to decongestants can indicate a bacterial infection. Cultures are not usually necessary but may be useful in patients who do not respond to therapy or who develop complications.

❖ INTERPROFESSIONAL COLLABORATIVE CARE

Overwhelmingly rhinosinusitis is managed as an outpatient problem. Even when sinus surgery is needed, it usually takes place in an ambulatory surgical setting.

Assess for signs and symptoms of rhinosinusitis. Common symptoms include pain over the cheek radiating to the teeth, tenderness to percussion over the sinuses, referred pain to the temple or back of the head, and general facial pain that is worse when bending forward. Additional symptoms in bacterial infection include purulent nasal drainage with postnasal drip, sore throat, fever, erythema, swelling, fatigue, dental pain, and ear pressure.

Management focuses on symptom relief and patient education. Teach him or her about correct use of the drug therapy prescribed.

Drug therapy commonly includes decongestants and intranasal steroid spray. *Antihistamines, leukotriene inhibitors,* and *mast cell stabilizers* block or reduce the amount of chemical mediators in nasal and sinus tissues and prevent local edema and itching. *Decongestants* constrict blood vessels and decrease edema. *Antipyretics* are given if fever is present, and analgesics may be given for pain.

🧓 CONSIDERATIONS FOR OLDER ADULTS
Patient-Centered Care QSEN

First-generation antihistamines are potentially inappropriate drugs for use in older adults. In this population, problems with these drugs include reduced drug clearance, higher risk for confusion, and anticholinergic effects such as dry mouth and constipation. Common drugs in this category include chlorpheniramine (Chlor-Trimeton), diphenhydramine (Aller-Aid ✦, Allerdryl ✦, Benadryl), and hydroxyzine (Vistaril). Educate older adults that they should not take these drugs.

Treatment for bacterial rhinosinusitis includes broad-spectrum antibiotics (e.g., amoxicillin [Amoxil, Novamoxin ✦]), decongestants (e.g., phenylephrine [Neo-Synephrine]), and antipyretics. In some cases, nasal steroids or systemic steroids may be prescribed. If no improvement is seen within 48 hours, the patient may need further evaluation. Endoscopic sinus surgery to relieve obstruction and promote sinus drainage may be needed if nonsurgical management fails to provide relief.

Supportive therapy such as humidification, nasal irrigation, and applying hot wet packs over the sinus area can increase the patient's comfort and help prevent spread of the infection.

❗ NURSING SAFETY PRIORITY QSEN
Action Alert

Teach patients with any bacterial infection the importance of completing the entire antibiotic prescription, even when symptoms improve or subside. This will help eradicate the organism and prevents development of resistant bacterial strains.

Instruct the patient about the importance of rest (8 to 10 hours a day) and fluid intake of at least 2000 mL/day unless other health problems require fluid restriction. Humidifying the air helps relieve congestion. Humidity can be increased with a room humidifier or by breathing steamy air in the bathroom after running hot shower water. Nasal saline irrigation is an inexpensive treatment with few side effects. Sleeping with the head of the bed elevated and avoiding cigarette smoke may reduce discomfort. If the condition is caused by allergies, limiting exposure to the offending agent is helpful (see Chapter 20).

Teach patients to reduce the risk for spreading infections by thoroughly washing hands, especially after nose blowing, sneezing, coughing, rubbing the eyes, or touching the face. Other precautions include staying home from work, school, or other crowded places; covering the mouth and nose with a tissue when sneezing or coughing; disposing properly of used tissues immediately; and avoiding close contact with others.

PERITONSILLAR ABSCESS

Peritonsillar abscess (PTA) is a rare complication of acute tonsillitis. The infection spreads from the tonsil to the surrounding tissue and forms an abscess. The most common cause of PTA is group A beta-hemolytic *Streptococcus,* although the abscess often contains multiple organisms (Shah, 2014).

Signs and symptoms include a collection of pus behind the tonsil causing swelling on one side of the throat, pushing the uvula toward the unaffected side. The patient may have severe throat pain radiating to the ear or teeth, a muffled voice, fever, and difficulty swallowing. He or she may also have a tonic contraction of the muscles of chewing (trismus) and difficulty breathing. Bad breath is present, and lymph nodes on the affected side are swollen. Diagnosis is usually made based on the patient's symptoms, but needle aspiration and culture of pus collected is the preferred test.

Most patients can be treated as outpatients with antibiotics. However, antibiotics alone are often ineffective. The patient may need steroids to reduce the swelling, and some may need drainage of the abscess. Pain control is important; drugs may include topical anesthetics, over-the-counter analgesics, and opioids. The patient may need liquid drugs because of swallowing difficulty. *Stress the importance of completing the antibiotic regimen and coming to the emergency department quickly if symptoms of obstruction (drooling and stridor) appear.* Hospitalization is needed when the airway is endangered or when the infection does not respond to antibiotic therapy. A tonsillectomy may be performed to prevent recurrence.

INHALATION ANTHRAX
❖ PATHOPHYSIOLOGY

Inhalation anthrax (respiratory anthrax) is a bacterial infection caused by the gram-positive organism *Bacillus anthracis.* This organism lives as a spore in soil where grass-eating animals live and graze. Most cases of anthrax are on the skin (cutaneous). Inhalation anthrax accounts for only about 5% of cases, and GI anthrax accounts for about 1% of cases of the disease. When infection occurs through the lungs, the disease is nearly 100% fatal without treatment (CDC, 2015b). Inhalation anthrax is rare in North America and is not spread by person-to-person contact. It is an occupational hazard of veterinarians; farmers; taxidermists; and others who frequently contact animal wool, hides, bone meal, and skin (CDC, 2015a).

> ! **NURSING SAFETY PRIORITY** **QSEN**
> **Action Alert**
>
> Because inhalation anthrax is so rare, any occurrence in a person who does not have an occupational risk is considered an intentional act of bioterrorism. Report the presence of symptoms consistent with inhalation anthrax to hospital authorities immediately.

This organism first forms a spore (i.e., an encapsulated organism that is inactive). Spores can live for years, even decades. When many spores are inhaled deeply into the lungs, macrophages engulf them. Once inside the macrophage, the organism leaves its capsule and replicates. The active bacteria produce several toxins that are released into the infected tissues and the blood that make the infection worse. Massive edema occurs along with hemorrhage and destruction of lung cells. Infected macrophages carry the organisms to the lymph nodes; and the organisms spread rapidly, causing bacteremia, sepsis and meningitis. Lethal toxins produced by the bacteria are the most common cause of death (CDC, 2015b).

❖ INTERPROFESSIONAL COLLABORATIVE CARE

Inhalation anthrax has two stages: prodromal (or incubation period) and fulminant (with active disease). Symptoms take up to 8 weeks to develop after exposure (Chart 31-4).

The prodromal stage is early and difficult to distinguish from influenza or pneumonia. Symptoms include low-grade fever, fatigue, mild chest pain, and a dry, harsh cough. *A special feature of inhalation anthrax is that it is* **not** *accompanied by upper respiratory symptoms of sore throat or rhinitis.* Usually the patient starts to feel better and symptoms improve in 2 to 4 days.

> ⫸ **CHART 31-4** **Key Features**
> **Inhalation Anthrax**
>
> | PRODROMAL STAGE (EARLY) | FULMINANT STAGE (LATE) |
> | --- | --- |
> | • Fever | • Sudden onset of breathlessness |
> | • Fatigue | • Dyspnea |
> | • Mild chest pain | • Diaphoresis |
> | • Dry cough | • Stridor on inhalation and exhalation |
> | • No signs or symptoms of upper respiratory infection | • Hypoxia |
> | • Mediastinal "widening" on chest x-ray | • High fever |
> | | • Mediastinitis |
> | | • Pleural effusion |
> | | • Hypotension |
> | | • Septic shock |

If the patient begins appropriate antibiotic therapy at this stage, the likelihood of survival is high. Diagnosis can be made with a Gram stain of blood or a chest x-ray. After several days, blood cultures may be positive for the organism. Genetic material of the bacteria may be found with polymerase chain reaction (PCR) done on serum. Positive results may not be evident until the disease has progressed to the fulminant stage.

The fulminant stage begins after the patient feels a little better. Usually there is a sudden onset of severe illness, including respiratory distress, hematemesis (bloody vomit), dyspnea, diaphoresis, stridor, chest pain, and cyanosis. The patient has a high fever. Hemorrhagic mediastinitis and pleural effusions develop. The patient may have a decreased level of consciousness or frank shock. The disease spreads through the blood, causing septic shock and hemorrhagic meningitis. Death often occurs within 24 to 36 hours even if antibiotics are started in this stage (CDC, 2015b).

The organism found naturally in the environment is sensitive to common antibiotics; however, organisms grown for bioterrorism may have been altered to be resistant to these antibiotics. Therefore the antibiotics used for suspected or diagnosed inhalation anthrax include a combination of drugs (Chart 31-5). The same drugs are used to prevent illness when adults have been exposed to inhalation anthrax but do not yet have symptoms. A new monoclonal antibody drug has been approved to neutralize the toxins produced by the organisms.

A vaccine is available to be used *before* exposure occurs, but distribution is limited to specific at-risk adults. The CDC also recommends that it be considered for patients after exposure and before symptoms appear, but this requires special approval. A new vaccine is currently being tested for postexposure use.

Teach patients with any type of lower respiratory infection to be especially vigilant for changes after they think they are getting well. They need to seek medical attention immediately on having a setback that starts with breathlessness.

> 💊 **CHART 31-5** **Common Examples of Drug Therapy**
> **Prophylaxis and Treatment of Inhalation Anthrax**
>
> | PROPHYLAXIS | TREATMENT |
> | --- | --- |
> | Ciprofloxacin (Cipro) 500 mg orally twice daily | Ciprofloxacin (Cipro IV) 400 mg IV every 12 hr |
> | *or* | *or* |
> | Doxycycline (Vibramycin) 100 mg orally twice daily | Doxycycline (Doxy 100) 100 mg IV every 12 hr |
> | *or (if organism is proven susceptible to penicillin)* | **Plus** *one or two of the following secondary agents (parenteral form (IV); dosage based on patient's weight and age):* |
> | Amoxicillin (Amoxil, Trimox) 500 mg orally every 8 hr or 875 mg orally twice daily | Rifampin (RIF) Clindamycin (Cleocin) Vancomycin (Vancocin, Vancoled) |
> | **Prophylaxis must continue for 60 days (or longer if exposure was heavy).** | **Treatment with IV drugs continues for at least 7 days. When the response is good and the patient improves, IV drugs are changed to oral agents and continued for at least 60 days.** |

PERTUSSIS

Pertussis is a respiratory infection caused by the bacterium *Bordetella pertussis*. It is highly contagious and spreads easily from person to person via respiratory droplets. Once considered a childhood disease, is it making a comeback in adults, perhaps because of decreasing IMMUNITY from childhood vaccinations over time (Masseria & Krishnarajah, 2015). In 1976 there were only 1010 reported cases. In 2014 that number jumped to 32,971 (CDC, 2015h; CDC, 2015i).

The disease has three distinct phases. During the first (*catarrhal*) phase, the patient has symptoms resembling the common cold, including a mild cough. After 1 to 2 weeks, the *paroxysmal* stage begins, and the patient has severe coughing "fits" lasting several minutes. During the coughing spasms the patient may turn red and/or vomit. He or she is frequently exhausted by the coughing. The distinct "whooping" sound common in children at the end of a cough may not be present in adults. There is a bloody, purulent, thick exudate in the small airways that can lead to atelectasis and pneumonia. This stage can last up to 10 weeks. The recovery (*convalescent*) stage lasts for months.

The diagnosis of pertussis can be made based on the patient's reported symptoms, but sputum cultures (obtained by deep suctioning) and PCR laboratory testing are also available. Blood cultures are negative. The CDC recommends testing for anyone who has a cough lasting longer than 3 weeks.

COCCIDIOIDOMYCOSIS

Coccidioidomycosis is a fungal infection caused by the *Coccidioides* organism common in the desert southwest regions of the United States, Mexico, and Central and South America. It is also known as *valley fever* and is becoming more prevalent. The organism is present in the soil as inactive and nonreproducing microfilaments. When the soil is disturbed by excavation or dust storms, the microfilaments become airborne. When the microfilaments are inhaled, they change into the reproductively active spore form of the organism. This can lead to development of an actual pulmonary infection within 1 to 4 weeks after exposure (Buhrow, 2013).

Symptoms of coccidioiomycosis resemble other respiratory infections with fever, cough, headache, muscle aches, chest pain, and night sweats. Bone and joint pain indicates more severe infection. Often the disorder is misdiagnosed and mistreated as influenza or pneumonia. Neither antibacterial drugs nor antiviral drugs are effective therapy. The disease can become widespread and cause symptoms of hemoptysis, meningitis, and involvement of the skin, adrenal glands, liver, and spleen. It also can become chronic and debilitating.

Depending on the health and IMMUNITY of the infected person and the number of spores present in the respiratory tract, the resulting infection can be mild, moderate, severe, or widely disseminated. Most younger healthy adults recover from the infection without treatment. For moderate infection, oral therapy with antifungal agents such as fluconazole (Diflucan), ketoconazole (Nizoral), voriconazole (Vfend) is needed. For those with severe disease or women who are pregnant, IV amphotericin B may be needed. Because the infection is not spread from person to person, Isolation Precautions are not required.

In endemic areas, adults at highest risk are those who work in or around soil, such as farm workers or construction workers. Older adults, anyone who has reduced IMMUNITY, and pregnant women also are at increased risk for developing more severe disease. Because the areas that naturally harbor this organism are often winter vacation destinations, always ask anyone with respiratory infection symptoms whether they have visited endemic regions so the possibility of coccidioidomycosis is considered.

CLINICAL JUDGMENT CHALLENGE 31-1

Patient-Centered Care, Evidence-Based Practice QSEN

A patient has been admitted with an obvious problem with GAS EXCHANGE. The patient's room air ABGs are: pH 7.12, Po_2 62 mm Hg, Pco_2 66 mm Hg, HCO_3 22 mm Hg. The patient's oxygen saturation is 84%, and you assess coarse lung sounds with some wheezing in all fields. The patient is anxious and reports feeling very short of breath. The patient is febrile at 102.3°F (39°C); pulse is 148 beats/min, respirations 38 breaths/min, and blood pressure is 98/52 mm Hg.

1. Which immediate care actions do you anticipate?
2. After addressing the patient's GAS EXCHANGE needs, which care priorities should you focus on next?
3. The primary health care provider leaves the following prescriptions for the patient. In what order should you accomplish them?
   a. Start gentamycin (Garamycin) 500 mg IVPB now
   b. Obtain sputum and blood cultures
   c. Insert indwelling urinary catheter
   d. Administer acetaminophen 1000 mg orally once for rib pain
   e. Increase rate of IV infusion to 150 mL/hr
4. Which member(s) of the interprofessional team would be most helpful in this situation and why?
5. Which other assessments should you perform?

GET READY FOR THE NCLEX® EXAMINATION!

KEY POINTS

Review these Key Points for each NCLEX Examination Client Needs Category.

Safe and Effective Care Environment

- Limit transmission of respiratory infections by washing hands after blowing the nose or using a tissue. **QSEN: Safety**

- Receive a yearly influenza vaccination because you are more likely to care for infected people and because you could spread influenza to adults who have reduced IMMUNITY. **QSEN: Safety**
- Use Airborne Precautions and Isolation Precautions for any patient who has tuberculosis (TB) symptoms until proven otherwise. **QSEN: Safety**

- If possible, place the patient with a respiratory infection in a private room. **QSEN: Safety**
- Keep the door to the room of any patient with a respiratory infection closed until the cause of the infection is identified. **QSEN: Safety**
- Teach adults living with patients who have TB to ensure good ventilation of the home with open windows whenever possible. **QSEN: Safety**
- Administer humidified oxygen therapy to patients with inadequate GAS EXCHANGE and hypoxemia. **QSEN: Evidence-Based Practice**
- Assess the skin under and around a facemask or nasal cannula for evidence of skin breakdown at least every 8 hours. **QSEN: Patient-Centered Care**
- Identify patients who may require a directly observed therapy (DOT) program in which they must be directly observed by a health care professional while swallowing the drug. **QSEN: Safety**

Health Promotion and Maintenance

- Teach everyone the "etiquette" of sneezing or coughing into the upper sleeve rather than the hand when a tissue is not available. **QSEN: Evidence-Based Practice**
- Urge all adults older than 50 years, anyone who has a chronic respiratory problem, anyone who has reduced IMMUNITY, and anyone who lives with a person who is older or immunocompromised or has a chronic respiratory disease to receive the pneumonia vaccine and yearly influenza vaccinations. **QSEN: Evidence-Based Practice**
- Urge all adults to quit smoking or using tobacco in any form. **QSEN: Patient-Centered Care**
- Teach all adults to be prepared for an emergency or disaster by having sufficient food, water, and prescribed drugs for at least 2 weeks (see Chapter 10). **QSEN: Patient-Centered Care**
- Teach all adults to follow community infection containment procedures if there is a possible outbreak of any pandemic influenza virus. **QSEN: Patient-Centered Care**

Psychosocial Integrity

- Assess older patients with acute confusion for pneumonia (cough and fever may not be present). **QSEN: Evidence-Based Practice**

- Assure the family of an older-adult patient with pneumonia who is confused that the new-onset confusion is temporary. **QSEN: Patient-Centered Care**
- Teach adults who may be afraid of contracting inhalational anthrax that this disease is not transmitted by person-to-person contact. **QSEN: Patient-Centered Care**
- Inform patients who have a positive TB test that far more adults are infected with the bacillus than have active TB disease. **QSEN: Patient-Centered Care**

Physiological Integrity

- Assess the respiratory status of any adult suspected of having a respiratory infection by taking vital signs, noting color of nail beds and mucous membranes, measuring oxygen saturation, determining ease of ventilation, determining cognition, and auscultating lung fields. **QSEN: Evidence-Based Practice**
- Ask any patient with a respiratory infection if he or she is from a foreign country or has recently visited a foreign country. **QSEN: Patient-Centered Care**
- Ask patients from other countries whether they have had BCG as a vaccination against TB. For patients who have had BCG, the PPD skin test is a less reliable indicator of TB. **QSEN: Safety**
- Educate the family and the patient with tuberculosis who lives at home about the side effects of anti-TB therapy and when to notify the primary health care provider. **QSEN: Patient-Centered Care**
- Urge patients to complete the anti-infective drug therapy course for any respiratory infection. **QSEN: Patient-Centered Care**
- Assess the patient receiving first-line drug therapy for TB for any symptoms of liver impairment (dark urine, clay-colored stools, anorexia, jaundiced sclera or hard palate). **QSEN: Patient-Centered Care**
- Teach sexually active women taking rifampin or rifapentine as drug therapy for TB that these drugs reduce the effectiveness of oral contraceptives and an additional form of birth control should be used while on this therapy. **QSEN: Patient-Centered Care**

SELECTED BIBLIOGRAPHY

American Lung Association (ALA). (2013). *Trends in tuberculosis morbidity and mortality.* http://www.lung.org/assets/documents/research/tb-trend-report.pdf.

American Lung Association (ALA). (2015). *Trends in pneumonia and influenza morbidity and mortality.* http://www.lung.org/search.jsp?query=pneumonia+trends.

American Lung Association (ALA). (2016). *Tuberculosis.* http://www.lung.org/lung-health-and-diseases/lung-disease-lookup/tuberculosis/?referrer=.

Arsbad, H., Fasanya, A., Cheema, T., & Singh, A. (2016). Acute pneumonia. *Critical Care Nursing Quarterly, 39*(2), 148–160.

Buhrow, S. (2013). Coccidioidomycosis: A differential diagnosis for visitors to the southwest. *The American Journal of Nursing, 113*(11), 52–55.

Burchum, J., & Rosenthal, L. (2016). *Lehne's pharmacology for nursing care* (9th ed.). St. Louis, MO: Elsevier.

Centers for Disease Control and Prevention (CDC). (2015a). *Anthrax prevention.* http://www.cdc.gov/anthrax/medical-care/prevention.html.

Centers for Disease Control and Prevention (CDC). (2015b). *Anthrax treatment.* http://www.cdc.gov/anthrax/medical-care/treatment.html.

Centers for Disease Control and Prevention (CDC). (2015c). *Cover your cough.* www.cdc.gov/flu/protect/covercough.htm.

Centers for Disease Control and Prevention (CDC). (2015d). *Early flu treatment reduces hospitalization time, disability risk in older people.* http://www.cdc.gov/media/releases/2015/p0902-early-flu-treatment.html.

Centers for Disease Control and Prevention (CDC). (2015e). *Information on avian influenza.* www.cdc.gov/flu/avianflu/.

Centers for Disease Control and Prevention (CDC). (2015f). *Key facts about seasonal flu vaccine.* www.cdc.gov/flu/protect/keyfacts.htm.

Centers for Disease Control and Prevention (CDC). (2015g). *Middle East respiratory syndrome (MERS)*. http://www.cdc.gov/CORONA-VIRUS/MERS/INDEX.HTML.

Centers for Disease Control and Prevention (CDC). (2015h). *Pertussis outbreak trends*. http://www.cdc.gov/pertussis/outbreaks/trends.html.

Centers for Disease Control and Prevention (CDC). (2015i). *Pertussis surveillance and reporting*. http://www.cdc.gov/pertussis/surv-reporting/cases-by-year.html.

Centers for Disease Control and Prevention (CDC). (2015j). *Pneumococcal vaccine: Who needs it?* http://www.cdc.gov/vaccines/vpd-vac/pneumo/vacc-in-short.htm.

Centers for Disease Control and Prevention (CDC). (2015k). *Seasonal influenza Q&A*. http://www.cdc.gov/flu/about/qa/disease.htm.

Centers for Disease Control and Prevention (CDC). (2015l). *Testing and diagnosis for TB*. http://www.cdc.gov/tb/topic/testing/default.htm.

Centers for Disease Control and Prevention (CDC). (2015m). *Treatment for TB disease*. http://www.cdc.gov/tb/topic/treatment/tbdisease.html.

Centers for Disease Control and Prevention (CDC). (2016). *New flu information for 2016-2017*. https://www.cdc.gpv/flu/about/season/flu-season-2016-2017.htm.

Jarvis, C. (2016). *Physical examination & health assessment* (7th ed.). St. Louis: Elsevier.

Masseria, C., & Krishnarajah, G. (2015). The estimated incidence of pertussis in people aged 50 years old in the United States, 2006-2010. *BMC Infectious Diseases, 15*, 1–8. doi:10.1186/s12879-015-1269-1.

McCance, K., Huether, S., Brashers, V., & Rote, N. (2014). *Pathophysiology: The biologic basis for disease in adults and children* (7th ed.). St. Louis: Mosby.

Pagana, K., Pagana, T. J., & Pagana, T. N. (2017). *Mosby's diagnostic and laboratory test reference* (13th ed.). St. Louis: Mosby.

Shah, U. K. (2014). Tonsillitis and peritonsillar abscess. *Medscape Reference*. http://emedicine.medscape.com/article/871977-overview.

Statistics Canada. (2015). *Deaths and mortality rate, by selected grouped causes and sex, Canada, provinces and territories*. http://www5.statcan.gc.ca/cansim/a26?Lang=eng&retrLang=eng&id=1020552&paSer=&pattern=&stByVal=1&p1=1&p2=-1&tabMode=dataTable&csid=.

Touhy, T., & Jett, K. (2016). *Ebersole and Hess' toward healthy aging: Human needs & nursing response* (9th ed.). St. Louis: Mosby.

Wiley, S. (2015). Encourage patients to roll up their sleeves for influenza vaccination. *Nursing, 45*(11), 50–54.

World Health Organization (WHO). (2015a). *Global tuberculosis report 2015: Executive summary*. http://www.who.int/tb/publications/global_report/en/.

World Health Organization (WHO). (2015b). *Middle East respiratory syndrome coronavirus (MERS-CoV)*. www.who.int/mediacentre/factsheets/mers-cov/en/.

World Health Organization (WHO). (2016). *Tuberculosis fact sheet*. http://www.who.int/mediacentre/factsheets/fs104/en/.

Care of Critically Ill Patients With Respiratory Problems

Harry Rees

e http://evolve.elsevier.com/Iggy/

PRIORITY AND INTERRELATED CONCEPTS

The priority concept for this chapter is GAS EXCHANGE.

❋ The GAS EXCHANGE concept exemplar for this chapter is Pulmonary Embolism, below.

The interrelated concepts for this chapter are:
• PERFUSION
• CLOTTING

LEARNING OUTCOMES

Safe and Effective Care Environment

1. Collaborate with the interprofessional team to coordinate high-quality care and promote GAS EXCHANGE in critically ill patients with respiratory problems.
2. Teach the patient and caregiver(s) about how decreased GAS EXCHANGE and impaired PERFUSION affect home safety.
3. Prioritize evidence-based care for critically ill patients with respiratory problems that decrease GAS EXCHANGE.

Health Promotion and Maintenance

4. Identify community resources for patients requiring assistance with long-term complications of severe respiratory problems.
5. Teach adults how to decrease the risk for severe respiratory damage or disease.

Psychosocial Integrity

6. Implement nursing interventions to help the patient and family cope with the psychosocial impact caused by severe respiratory problems.

Physiological Integrity

7. Apply knowledge of anatomy, physiology, and pathophysiology to assess critically ill patients with respiratory problems affecting GAS EXCHANGE or PERFUSION.
8. Teach the patient and caregiver(s) about common drugs and other management strategies used for respiratory problems.
9. Implement evidence-based nursing interventions to prevent complications of pulmonary embolism, mechanical ventilation, or any other critical respiratory problem.

Although chronic respiratory problems are more common, acute problems do arise that can interfere with GAS EXCHANGE and tissue PERFUSION to such a degree that death can occur quickly. These problems tax the cardiac system by forcing the heart to work harder to compensate for lung-related impairment of gas exchange (Fig. 32-1). *Thus prompt recognition and interventions are needed to prevent serious complications and death.* Such emergencies include pulmonary embolism, acute respiratory failure, acute respiratory distress syndrome, and chest trauma. The emergent nature of these problems and the potential for fatal outcomes present challenges in caring for these critically ill patients.

❋ GAS EXCHANGE CONCEPT EXEMPLAR
Pulmonary Embolism

❖ PATHOPHYSIOLOGY

A **pulmonary embolism (PE)** is a collection of particulate matter (solids, liquids, or air) that enters venous circulation and lodges in the pulmonary vessels. Large emboli obstruct pulmonary blood flow, leading to reduced GAS EXCHANGE, reduced oxygenation, pulmonary tissue hypoxia, decreased PERFUSION, and potential death. Any substance can cause an embolism, but a blood clot is the most common (McCance et al., 2014; Rali

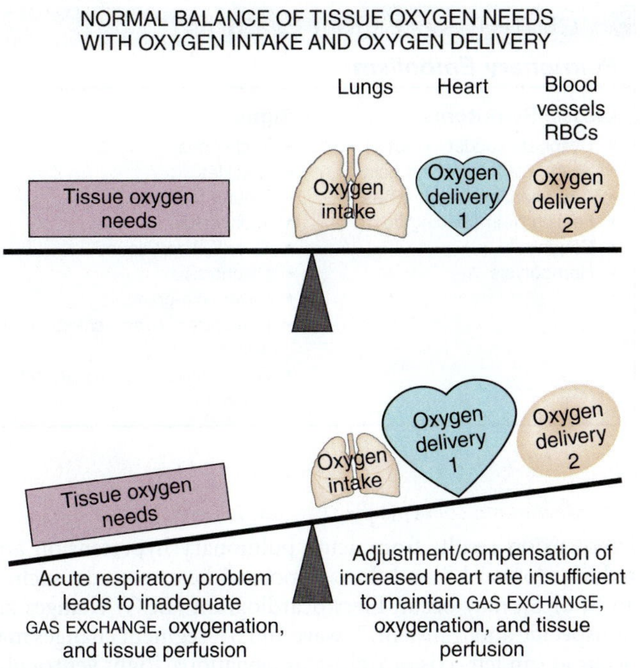

NORMAL BALANCE OF TISSUE OXYGEN NEEDS
WITH OXYGEN INTAKE AND OXYGEN DELIVERY

FIG. 32-1 Rapid-onset acute respiratory problems overwhelm the ability of the cardiac oxygen delivery system to adapt and restore balance. The red blood cell (RBC) oxygen delivery system cannot begin to adapt to the acute respiratory problem.

CHART 32-1 Best Practice for Patient Safety & Quality Care QSEN

Prevention of Pulmonary Embolism

- Start passive and active range-of-motion exercises for the extremities of immobilized and postoperative patients.
- Ambulate patients soon after surgery.
- Use anti-embolism and pneumatic compression stockings and devices after surgery.
- Evaluate patient for criteria indicating the need for anticoagulant therapy.
- Avoid the use of tight garters, girdles, and constricting clothing.
- Prevent pressure under the popliteal space (e.g., do not place a pillow under the knee; instead, use alternating pressure mattress).
- Perform a comprehensive assessment of peripheral circulation.
- Elevate the affected limb 20 degrees or more above the level of the heart to improve venous return, as appropriate.
- Change patient position every 2 hours or ambulate as tolerated.
- Prevent injury to the vessel lumen by preventing local pressure, trauma, infection, or sepsis.
- Refrain from massaging leg muscles.
- Instruct patient not to cross legs.
- Administer prescribed prophylactic low-dose anticoagulant and anti-platelet drugs.
- Teach the patient to avoid activities that result in the Valsalva maneuver (e.g., breath-holding, bearing down for bowel movements, coughing).
- Administer prescribed drugs, such as stool softeners, that will prevent episodes of the Valsalva maneuver.
- Teach the patient and family about precautions.
- Encourage smoking cessation.

et al., 2016). PE is common and may account for as many as 100,000 deaths each year in the United States (Centers for Disease Control and Prevention [CDC], 2015). It may be the most common preventable death in hospitalized patients but is often misdiagnosed, and patients at risk may not be provided the appropriate preventive measures.

Most often, a PE occurs when inappropriate blood CLOT-TING forms a venous thromboembolism (VTE) (also known as a deep vein thrombosis [DVT]) in a vein in the legs or the pelvis and a clot breaks off and travels through the vena cava into the right side of the heart. The clot then lodges in the pulmonary artery or within one or more of its branches. Platelets collect on the embolus, triggering the release of substances that cause blood vessel constriction. Widespread pulmonary vessel constriction and pulmonary hypertension impair GAS EXCHANGE and tissue PERFUSION. Deoxygenated blood moves into arterial circulation, causing hypoxemia (low arterial blood oxygen level), although some patients with PE do *not* have hypoxemia.

Major risk factors for VTE leading to PE are:

- Prolonged immobility
- Central venous catheters
- Surgery
- Obesity
- Advancing age
- Conditions that increase blood CLOTTING
- History of thromboembolism

Smoking, pregnancy, estrogen therapy, heart failure, stroke, cancer (particularly lung or prostate), and trauma increase the risk for VTE and PE (McCance et al., 2014).

Fat, oil, air, tumor cells, amniotic fluid and fetal debris, foreign objects (e.g., broken IV catheters), injected particles, and infected clots can enter a vein and cause PE. Fat emboli can occur with fracture of the femur, and oil emboli can occur from diagnostic procedures. These have a mortality rate of about 10% (Moore, 2016). Fat emboli do not impede lung blood flow; instead, they injure blood vessels and cause acute respiratory distress syndrome (ARDS) (discussed as a disorder later in this chapter). Septic clots often arise from a pelvic abscess, an infected IV catheter, and injections of illegal drugs. The effects of sepsis are more serious than the venous blockage.

Health Promotion and Maintenance

Although pulmonary embolism (PE) can occur in healthy people without warning, certain conditions increase the risk for occurrence. Thus prevention of conditions that lead to PE is a major nursing concern. Preventive actions for PE are those that also prevent venous stasis and VTE. Best nursing practices for PE prevention are outlined in Chart 32-1. Also see Chapter 14 for more information about core measures during the surgical experience for VTE prevention.

Lifestyle changes can help reduce the risk for PE. Tobacco use narrows blood vessels and increases the risk for clot formation. Hormone-based contraceptives also increase blood CLOTTING. Urge patients to stop smoking cigarettes, especially women who use hormone-based contraceptives. Reducing weight and becoming more physically active can reduce risk for PE. Teach patients who are traveling for long periods to drink plenty of water, change positions often, avoid crossing their legs, and get up from the sitting position at least 5 minutes out of every hour to prevent stasis and clot formation.

For patients known to be at risk for PE, small doses of heparin or low-molecular-weight heparin (enoxaparin

[Lovenox]), an indirect thrombin inhibitor, may be prescribed every 8 to 12 hours. Oral direct thrombin inhibitors may be used instead of heparin for VTE prevention in patients who have nonvalvular atrial fibrillation.

For adults who have an ongoing risk for VTE and PE, prevention may include preoperative placement of a retrievable inferior vena cava (IVC) filter. This placement occurs before any surgery in which the patient is expected to be confined to bed for more than just a few days and is retrieved when the patient is fully ambulatory.

❖ INTERPROFESSIONAL COLLABORATIVE CARE

The patient who has a pulmonary embolism (PE) is critically ill and at risk for life-threatening complications. Initial management occurs in an acute care environment, most often an ICU. In addition to medical and nursing care providers, pharmacists and respiratory therapists are key interprofessional team members.

Some patients have ongoing issues or residual problems that impair GAS EXCHANGE and PERFUSION after the acute problems have resolved. These changes may be permanent. Then continuing care occurs in the home or residential setting.

The interprofessional team for ongoing issues includes a variety of specialists for optimal patient function. A pulmonary health care provider in addition to a primary health care provider is needed for continual assessment and management of any reduced lung function. Respiratory therapists assist with prescribed oxygen therapy and delivery needs. Physical therapists can help the patient maintain muscle conditioning. Occupational therapists provide information and home set-up suggestions to help patients conserve energy when endurance is affected. Registered dietitians assess patients' caloric and protein needs and plan personalized interventions to meet these needs. Pastoral care workers and clergy may help patients who experience spiritual distress with this life-altering condition. Social workers together with home care nurses determine which types of home modifications and durable supplies would be most helpful in maintaining functional ability for self-management of ADLs. When significant lifestyle changes are needed, mental health professionals can help the patient and family cope with adjustments.

◆ Assessment: Noticing

Signs and symptoms range from vague, nonspecific discomforts to hemodynamic collapse and death. *It is important to remember that many patients with PE do not have the "classic" symptoms.* This variability in symptoms often leads to PEs being overlooked.

Physical Assessment/Signs and Symptoms. Respiratory symptoms are outlined in Chart 32-2 and are mostly related to decreased GAS EXCHANGE. Assess the patient for difficulty breathing (dyspnea) and pleuritic chest pain (sharp, stabbing-type pain on inspiration) (Wilbeck & Evans, 2015). Other symptoms vary depending on the size and type of embolism. Breath sounds may be normal or include crackles, wheezes, or a pleural friction rub. A dry or productive cough may be present; hemoptysis (bloody sputum) may result from pulmonary infarction.

Cardiac symptoms related to decreased tissue PERFUSION include tachycardia, distended neck veins, syncope (fainting or loss of consciousness), cyanosis, and hypotension. Systemic

---

►► CHART 32-2 Key Features
Pulmonary Embolism

Classic Symptoms	Signs
• Dyspnea, sudden onset • Sharp, stabbing chest pain • Apprehension, restlessness • Feeling of impending doom • Cough • Hemoptysis	• Tachypnea • Crackles • Pleural friction rub • Tachycardia • S_3 or S_4 heart sound • Diaphoresis • Fever, low-grade • Petechiae over chest and axillae • Decreased arterial oxygen saturation (SaO_2)

---

hypotension results from acute pulmonary hypertension and reduced forward blood flow. Abnormal heart sounds, such as an S_3 or S_4, may occur. Electrocardiogram (ECG) changes are nonspecific and transient. T-wave and ST-segment changes may occur as can left-axis or right-axis deviations. Right ventricular dysfunction and failure are extreme complications. The patient may have cardiac arrest or frank shock.

❗ NURSING SAFETY PRIORITY QSEN
Critical Rescue

Monitor patients at risk to recognize signs and symptoms of PE (e.g., shortness of breath, chest pain, and/or hypotension without an obvious cause). If such symptoms are present, respond by notifying the Rapid Response Team. If PE is strongly suspected, prompt categorization and management strategies are started before diagnostic studies have been completed.

Psychosocial Assessment. Symptoms of PE often occur abruptly, and the patient is anxious. Hypoxemia may stimulate a sense of impending doom and cause increased restlessness. The life-threatening nature of PE and admission to an ICU increase the patient's anxiety and fear.

Laboratory Assessment. The hyperventilation triggered by hypoxia and pain first leads to respiratory alkalosis, indicated by low partial pressure of arterial carbon dioxide ($PaCO_2$) on arterial blood gas (ABG) analysis. The PaO_2-FiO_2 (fraction of inspired oxygen) ratio falls as a result of "shunting" of blood from the right side of the heart to the left without picking up oxygen from the lungs. Shunting causes the $PaCO_2$ level to rise, resulting in respiratory acidosis (McCance et al., 2014). Later, metabolic acidosis results from buildup of lactic acid caused by tissue hypoxia. (See Chapter 12 for a more detailed discussion of acidosis.)

Even if ABG studies and pulse oximetry show hypoxemia, these results alone are not sufficient for the diagnosis of PE (McCance et al., 2014). A patient with a small embolus may not be hypoxemic, and PE is not the only cause of hypoxemia.

Other laboratory studies performed when PE is suspected include a general metabolic panel, troponin, brain natriuretic peptide (BNP), and a D-dimer. The D-dimer, a fibrin split product, rises with fibrinolysis. When the value is normal or low, it can rule out a PE. However, even if the value is high, other diagnostic testing is needed to determine whether a PE has occurred (Pagana et al., 2017).

⚕ GENETIC/GENOMIC CONSIDERATIONS
Patient-Centered Care (QSEN)

Factor V Leiden (also known as activated protein C resistance) is an inherited abnormal tendency to develop blood clots. In this disorder, the gene coding for blood clotting factor V (the *F5* gene) has a mutation that changes the nature of the factor V produced. With this genetic alteration, factor V functions normally but is more slowly degraded; and clotting activity continues longer than usual, which increases the risk for developing abnormal blood clots (Lee, 2014). People can inherit either one or both abnormal gene alleles. The risk for developing clots is three to eight times greater in those who inherit only one abnormal allele and up to 80 times greater with two abnormal alleles (United States National Library of Medicine, 2016). The risk for developing DVT, PE, or thrombotic strokes increases greatly when both abnormal gene alleles are present, especially in smokers and those who use hormone-based contraceptives. Testing for factor V Leiden is recommended for people who develop a VTE without a precipitating event and for those who have a first-degree relative with the disorder (Online Mendelian Inheritance in Man [OMIM], 2015).

Imaging Assessment. Pulmonary angiography is the "gold standard" diagnostic test but is not available in all settings. Computed tomography pulmonary angiography (CT-PA) or helical CT may also be used, which has the added advantage of diagnosing other pulmonary abnormalities causing the patient's symptoms. Ventilation-perfusion ($\dot{V}/\dot{Q}$) scans are not as widely used anymore but may be considered in certain circumstances (e.g., allergy to contrast dye). A chest x-ray may diagnose other conditions that mimic acute PE. Doppler ultrasound may be used to document the presence of VTE and to support a diagnosis of PE (York et al., 2015).

◆ Analysis: Interpreting

The priority collaborative problems for patients with PE include:
1. Hypoxemia due to mismatch of lung PERFUSION and alveolar GAS EXCHANGE with oxygenation
2. Hypotension due to inadequate circulation to the left ventricle
3. Potential for excessive bleeding due to anticoagulation or fibrinolytic therapy causing inadequate CLOTTING
4. Anxiety due to hypoxemia and life-threatening illness

◆ Planning and Implementation: Responding

Managing Hypoxemia. When a patient has a sudden onset of dyspnea and chest pain, immediately notify the Rapid Response Team. Reassure the patient and elevate the head of the bed. Prepare for oxygen therapy and blood gas analysis while continuing to monitor and assess for other changes.

Planning: Expected Outcomes. The patient with PE is expected to have adequate tissue PERFUSION in all major organs. Indicators of adequate PERFUSION are that the patient has:
- ABGs within normal limits
- Pulse oximetry above 92%
- Cognitive status unimpaired compared with baseline
- Absence of pallor and cyanosis

◎ CHART 32-3 Best Practice for Patient Safety & Quality Care (QSEN)
Care of the Patient With a Pulmonary Embolism

- Apply oxygen by nasal cannula or mask.
- Reassure patient that the correct measures are being taken.
- Place patient in high-Fowler's position.
- Apply telemetry monitoring equipment.
- Obtain an adequate venous access.
- Assess oxygenation continuously with pulse oximetry.
- Assess respiratory status at least every 30 minutes by:
  - Listening to lung sounds.
  - Measuring the rate, rhythm, and ease of respirations.
  - Checking skin color and capillary refill.
  - Checking position of trachea.
- Assess cardiac status by:
  - Comparing blood pressures in right and left arms.
  - Checking pulse for quality.
  - Checking cardiac monitor for dysrhythmias.
  - Checking for distention of neck veins.
- Ensure that prescribed chest imaging and laboratory tests are obtained immediately (may include complete blood count with differential, platelet count, prothrombin time, partial thromboplastin time, D-dimer level, arterial blood gases).
- Examine the thorax for presence of petechiae.
- Administer prescribed anticoagulants.
- Assess for bleeding.
- Handle patient gently.
- Institute Bleeding Precautions.

Interventions. Nonsurgical management of PE is most common. In some cases invasive procedures also may be needed. Best care practices for the patient with PE are listed in Chart 32-3. Rapid categorization of PE severity and prompt management are required (Table 32-1).

Nonsurgical Management. Management activities for PE focus on increasing GAS EXCHANGE and oxygenation, improving lung PERFUSION, reducing risk for further clot formation, and preventing complications. Priority nursing interventions include implementing oxygen therapy, administering anticoagulation or fibrinolytic therapy to improve tissue perfusion, monitoring the patient's responses to the interventions, and providing psychosocial support (York et al., 2015).

Oxygen therapy is critical for the patient with PE. The severely hypoxemic patient may need mechanical ventilation and close monitoring with ABG studies. In less severe cases oxygen may be applied by nasal cannula or mask. Use pulse oximetry to monitor oxygen saturation and hypoxemia.

Monitor the patient continually for any changes in status. Check vital signs, lung sounds, and cardiac and respiratory status at least every 1 to 2 hours. Document increasing dyspnea, dysrhythmias, distended neck veins, and pedal or sacral edema. Assess for crackles and other abnormal lung sounds along with cyanosis of the lips, conjunctiva, oral mucosa, and nail beds.

Drug therapy begins immediately with anticoagulants to prevent embolus enlargement and more CLOTTING. Unfractionated heparin, low-molecular-weight heparin (enoxaparin [Lovenox]), or fondaparinux (Arixtra) is used unless the PE is massive or occurs with hemodynamic instability. Review the patient's partial thromboplastin time (PTT)—also called

TABLE 32-1	Pulmonary Embolism (PE) Severity and Management Options	
CATEGORY	**POSSIBLE SYMPTOMS**	**MANAGEMENT OPTIONS**
Massive PE Mortality may be as high as 65%	Severe hypotension (SBP <90 mm Hg for at least 15 minutes) Cardiac arrest/cardiopulmonary collapse Severe bradycardia Shock Severe dyspnea/respiratory distress	CPR Inotropic and/or vasopressor support; fluids Fibrinolytic therapy Tissue plasminogen activator (tPA) Alteplase (Activase) Unfractionated heparin initial treatment
Submassive PE	Normotension RV dysfunction on echocardiography RV dilation on echocardiography or CT Right bundle branch block ST elevation or depression T-wave inversion Elevated BNP or troponin	Treatment is controversial; some agents not approved for this group Must weigh benefits of thrombolytic therapy against risk for bleeding Thrombolytics may be preferred if patient appears to be decompensating or if there is RV dysfunction (hypokinesis) or elevation in BNP or troponin LMWH preferred agent Fondaparinux (Arixtra) Unfractionated heparin
Low-risk PE Mortality ranges from 1% to 8%	Normotension No RV dysfunction No elevation in BNP or troponin	Thrombolytics not warranted because of risk for bleeding LMWH Rivaroxaban (Xarelto)

Adapted from Jaff, M. R., McMurtry, M. S., & Archer, S. L. (2011). The use of fibrinolytics in patients with acute pulmonary embolism. *Circulation*, *123*, 1788-1830.
BNP, Brain natriuretic peptide; *CPR*, cardiopulmonary resuscitation; *CT*, computed tomography; *LMWH*, low-molecular-weight heparin; *RV*, right ventricle; *SBP*, systolic blood pressure.

activated partial thromboplastin time (aPTT)—before therapy is started and thereafter according to facility policy. Therapeutic PTT values usually range between 1.5 and 2.5 times the control value for this health problem. Factor anti-Xa levels may be used instead of PTT or aPTT.

Fibrinolytic drugs, such as alteplase (Activase, tPA), are used for treatment of PE when specific criteria are met such as shock, hemodynamic collapse, or instability. Fibrinolytic drugs are used to break up the existing clot. (See Chapter 38 for a discussion of fibrinolytic therapy.)

Both heparin and fibrinolytic drugs are *high-alert drugs*. These drugs have an increased risk to cause harm if given at too high a dose, at too low a dose, or to the wrong patient. Because of the high risk for bleeding, patients receiving fibrinolytic therapy are monitored in an ICU setting.

! NURSING SAFETY PRIORITY QSEN

Drug Alert

Heparin comes in a variety of concentrations in vials that have differing amounts, which contributes to possible medication errors. **In accordance with The Joint Commission's National Patient Safety Goals (NPSGs), check the prescribed dose carefully and ensure that the correct concentration is being used to prevent overdosing or underdosing.**

Heparin therapy usually continues for 5 to 10 days. Most patients are started on an oral anticoagulant, such as warfarin (Coumadin, Jantoven, Warfilone ♣), on day one or two of heparin therapy. Therapy with both heparin and warfarin continues until the international normalized ratio (INR) reaches 2.0 to 3.0. Heparin is usually infused for at least 5 days and continues for 24 hours after the INR is greater than 2. Monitor the platelet count and INR during this time. A low-molecular-weight heparin (e.g., dalteparin [Fragmin], enoxaparin [Lovenox]) or a direct thrombin inhibitor (e.g., rivaroxaban [Xarelto]) is often used instead of warfarin. Oral anticoagulant use continues for 3 to 6

weeks, but some patients may take it indefinitely. Charts 32-4 and 32-5 list common drugs used and the laboratory tests to monitor in a patient with PE. These drugs and the associated nursing care are discussed in Chapters 36, 38, and 39.

🧬 GENETIC/GENOMIC CONSIDERATIONS

Patient-Centered Care QSEN

Many agencies perform genetic tests before starting warfarin therapy to check for variation in two specific genes. One gene, *VKORC1*, produces an enzyme that alters vitamin K so it can help activate the vitamin K–dependent clotting factors. Warfarin interferes with the activity of this enzyme. Patients who have a variation in the enzyme are resistant to the effects of warfarin, and much higher doses are needed to achieve coagulation. On the other hand, the gene *CYP2C19* produces an enzyme that metabolizes warfarin and prepares it for elimination. Patients who have a variation in this gene do not metabolize warfarin well, so higher blood levels remain and more severe side effects are possible. The dosage of warfarin needs to be much lower in patients with this gene variation. When a patient's CLOTTING response to warfarin is either greater than expected or much less than expected, consider the possibility of a gene mutation.

Anticoagulation and fibrinolytic therapy can lead to excessive bleeding. *The antidote for heparin is protamine sulfate; the antidote for warfarin is vitamin K1, which is available as an injectable drug, phytonadione (AquaMEPHYTON, Mephyton). Antidotes for fibrinolytic therapy include clotting factors, fresh frozen plasma, and aminocaproic acid (Amicar).* Antidotes to anticoagulant drugs and fibrinolytic drugs should be readily available either on the unit, from the pharmacy, or from the blood bank for patients undergoing these therapies. Based on hospital policy, blood banks may require that a blood type and screen be completed every 72 hours. This action minimizes delays if a transfusion is indicated.

Surgical Management. Two surgical procedures for the management of PE are embolectomy and inferior vena cava filtration.

CHART 32-4 Common Examples of Drug Therapy
Pulmonary Embolism

DRUG	NURSING IMPLICATIONS
Heparins and Heparinoids—These drugs are used to begin anticoagulation to minimize growth of existing clots and prevent the development of additional clots. They bind to and increase the activity of antithrombin III (AT III). By activating AT III, coagulation factor Xa (thrombin) is indirectly inhibited.	
Heparin sodium (Hepalean) Enoxaparin (Lovenox)	Monitor PTT (or factor anti-Xa) and know expected therapeutic PTT range for each patient *to detect side effects and prevent complications.* Monitor patient for bleeding or bruising, *which are indications of a prolonged PTT and a harbinger of excessive bleeding.* Have *protamine sulfate* available *because it is an antidote to heparin and can prevent hemorrhage when anticoagulation is too great.* Avoid puncturing the skin and apply pressure to venipuncture and IM injection sites *to prevent excessive bruising and bleeding.* Monitor platelet counts *to assess for the complication of heparin-induced thrombocytopenia (HIT).*
Vitamin K Antagonists (VKAs)—These drugs decrease the synthesis of vitamin K in the intestinal tract, which then reduces the production of vitamin K–dependent CLOTTING factors II, VII, IX, and X, along with the anticoagulant proteins C and S. When the clotting factors are reduced, anticoagulation results. It is used for long-term anticoagulation in at-risk patients to prevent the development of future clots.	
Warfarin sodium (Coumadin, Jantoven, Warfilone ✦)	Monitor INR and know expected therapeutic INR range for each patient *to ensure drug effectiveness and identify drug overdose.* Consult the pharmacist about potential drug interactions *because this drug affects the activity of many other drugs.* Teach patients to check with a pharmacist before taking any other prescribed or over-the-counter drug *because this drug affects the activity of many other drugs.* Have *vitamin K (phytonadione)* available *because it is the antidote to be used in case of warfarin overdose.* Avoid puncturing the skin and apply pressure to venipuncture and IM injection sites *to prevent excessive bruising and bleeding.* Teach patients which foods are sources of vitamin K (e.g., leafy dark green vegetables, herbs, spring onions, Brussels sprouts, broccoli, cabbage, asparagus), *because they will reduce the effectiveness of warfarin if eaten in excess.*
Fibrinolytics—These drugs selectively break down fibrin threads present in formed blood clots by activating tissue protein *plasminogen* to its active form, *plasmin,* which then directly attacks and degrades the fibrin molecule. Fibrinolytics are used to promote lysis of large pulmonary emboli in patients who are hemodynamically unstable.	
Alteplase (tissue plasminogen activator, recombinant; tPA; Activase)	Assess hourly for internal and external bleeding while the patient is receiving the drug and for 8 hours after *because hemorrhage is the most common complication.* To administer, reconstitute with sterile water that contains no preservative immediately before use *to ensure drug stability.* Administer with caution to patients who have been receiving aspirin, dipyridamole, heparin, or other anticoagulants *because these drugs also increase the risk for bleeding.*

INR, International normalized ratio; *PTT,* partial thromboplastin time.

NCLEX EXAMINATION CHALLENGE 32-1
Safe and Effective Care Environment

Which laboratory values are **most important** for a nurse to monitor for a client who is receiving a heparin infusion for treatment of a pulmonary embolism when warfarin is added to the drug therapy? **Select all that apply.**
A. Activated partial thromboplastin time
B. Albumin levels
C. Factor V levels
D. Hepatic function tests
E. International normalized ratio
F. Platelet count
G. Serum osmolarity

Embolectomy is the surgical or percutaneous removal of the embolus. It may be performed when fibrinolytic therapy cannot be used for a patient who has massive or multiple large pulmonary emboli with shock or bleeding complications.

Inferior vena cava filtration with placement of a retrievable vena cava filter prevents further emboli from reaching the lungs in patients with ongoing risk for PE. Patients for whom filter placement is considered less risky than drug therapy include those with recurrent or major bleeding while receiving anticoagulants, those with septic PE, and those undergoing pulmonary embolectomy. Placement of a vena cava filter is detailed in Chapter 36.

Managing Hypotension
Planning: Expected Outcomes. The patient with PE is expected to have adequate circulation and tissue PERFUSION. Indicators of adequate circulation are:
- Maintenance of pulse rate and blood pressure within the normal ranges
- Maintenance of a urine output of at least 0.5 to 1 mL/kg/hr
- Absence of cyanosis

Interventions. In addition to the interventions used for hypoxemia, IV fluid therapy and drug therapy are used to increase cardiac output and maintain blood pressure.

IV fluid therapy involves giving crystalloid solutions to restore plasma volume and prevent shock (see Chapter 37). Continuously monitor the ECG and pulmonary artery and central venous/right atrial pressures of the patient receiving IV fluids because increased fluids can worsen pulmonary hypertension and lead to right-sided heart failure. Also

CHART 32-5 Laboratory Profile

Blood Tests Used to Monitor Anticoagulation Therapy

TEST	NORMAL RANGE	SIGNIFICANCE OF ABNORMAL FINDINGS
Partial thromboplastin time (PTT, aPTT [APTT])	Normal values for each local laboratory may vary. When activator reagents are used by the laboratory, the normal CLOTTING time is shortened. Common normal ranges are 20-30 sec in some laboratories and 30-40 sec in others. Therapeutic range for PE is 1.5-2.5 times the normal value (e.g., if normal is 20-30 sec, therapeutic range is 40-75 sec).	*Subtherapeutic times* may signify that the patient is not receiving enough heparin to prevent extension of the blood clot. An increase in the dosage or rate of infusion is usually indicated. *Therapeutic times* mean that the clotting time is increased from normal but this increase is indicated in the case of PE. *Prolonged times* in patients with PE (i.e., >75 sec) indicate that the patient is at risk for serious spontaneous bleeding. Heparin is usually held or decreased until the PTT drops back into the therapeutic range.
Prothrombin time (pro time, PT)	Common normal range is 11-12.5 sec. Therapeutic range for anticoagulant therapy in PE is 1.5-2.0 times the normal or control value in seconds. Control values can vary day to day because reagents used may vary.	*Subtherapeutic values* may signify that the patient is not receiving enough warfarin. An increase in the dosage is usually indicated. *Therapeutic values* mean that the pro time is increased from normal but this increase is indicated in the case of PE. *Prolonged values* in the treatment of PE indicate that the patient is at risk for reduced CLOTTING and increased bleeding. The warfarin dose is usually decreased or held, the patient is instructed to eat foods high in vitamin K, or an injection of vitamin K may be given.
International normalized ratio (INR)	The common normal range is 0.8-1.1. The therapeutic range for PE is 2.5-3.0, or 3.0-4.5 for recurrent PE.	*Subtherapeutic values* may signify that the patient is not receiving enough warfarin. An increase in the dosage is usually indicated. *Therapeutic values* mean that the INR is increased from normal but this increase is indicated in the case of PE. *Prolonged values* (higher than 4.5) in the treatment of PE indicate that the patient is at risk for bleeding. The warfarin dose is usually decreased or held, the patient is instructed to eat foods high in vitamin K, or an injection of vitamin K may be given.

Data from Pagana, K., Pagana, T. J., & Pagana, T. N. (2017). *Mosby's diagnostic and laboratory test reference* (13th ed.). St. Louis: Mosby; and Pagana, K., Pagana, T., & Pike-MacDonald, S. (2013). *Mosby's Canadian manual of diagnostic and laboratory tests*. St. Louis: Mosby.
aPTT or *APTT*, Activated partial thromboplastin time; *INR*, international normalized ratio; *PE*, pulmonary embolism.

monitor indicators of fluid adequacy, including urine output, skin turgor, and moisture of mucous membranes.

Drug therapy with vasopressors is used when hypotension persists despite fluid resuscitation. Commonly used agents include norepinephrine (Levophed), epinephrine (adrenalin), or dopamine (Intropin). Agents that increase myocardial contractility (**positive inotropic agents**), including milrinone (Primacor) and dobutamine (Dobutrex), may be considered. Vasodilators, such as nitroprusside (Nipride, Nitropress), may be used to decrease pulmonary artery pressure if it is impeding cardiac contractility. Assess the patient's cardiac status hourly during therapy with any of these drugs.

Minimizing Bleeding

Planning: Expected Outcomes. The patient with PE is expected to have appropriate CLOTTING and remain free from bleeding. Indicators include that the patient:

- Does not have bruising or petechiae
- Maintains hematocrit, hemoglobin, and platelet count within the normal range

Interventions. Drug therapy that disrupts clots or prevents their formation impairs the patient's ability to start and continue the blood-CLOTTING cascade when injured, increasing the risk for bleeding. Priority nursing actions are ensuring that appropriate antidotes are present on the nursing unit, protecting the patient from situations that could lead to bleeding, ensuring correct drug therapy, assessing laboratory values, and monitoring the amount of bleeding that occurs.

Assess for evidence of bleeding (e.g., oozing, bruises that cluster, petechiae, or purpura) at least every 2 hours. Examine all stools, urine, drainage, and vomitus for gross blood; and test for occult blood. Measure any blood loss as accurately as possible. Measure the patient's abdominal girth every 8 hours (increasing girth can indicate internal bleeding). Best practices to prevent bleeding are listed in Chart 32-6.

Monitor laboratory values daily. Review the complete blood count (CBC) results to determine the risk for impaired CLOTTING and whether actual blood loss has occurred. If the patient has severe blood loss, packed red blood cells may be prescribed (see Transfusion Therapy in Chapter 40). Monitor the platelet count. A decreasing count may indicate ongoing CLOTTING or heparin-induced thrombocytopenia (HIT) caused by the formation of anti-heparin antibodies.

Minimizing Anxiety

Planning: Expected Outcomes. The patient with PE is usually anxious and fearful as a result of the life-threatening nature of the problem. He or she is expected to have anxiety reduced to an acceptable level. Indicators include that he or she consistently demonstrates these behaviors:

- States that anxiety is reduced
- Has no distress, irritability, or facial tension
- Uses coping strategies effectively

Interventions. The patient with PE is anxious and fearful and often has pain. Interventions for reducing anxiety in those with PE include oxygen therapy (see Interventions

CHART 32-6 Best Practice for Patient Safety & Quality Care QSEN

Prevention of Injury for the Patient Receiving Anticoagulant, Fibrinolytic, or Antiplatelet Therapy

- Handle the patient gently.
- Use and teach UAP to use a lift sheet when moving and positioning the patient in bed.
- Avoid IM injections and venipunctures.
- When injections or venipunctures are necessary, use the smallest-gauge needle for the task.
- Apply firm pressure to the needlestick site for 10 minutes or until the site no longer oozes blood.
- Apply ice to areas of trauma.
- Test all urine, vomitus, and stool for occult blood.
- Assess IV sites at least every 4 hours for bleeding.
- Instruct alert patients to notify nursing personnel immediately if any trauma occurs and if bleeding or bruising is noticed.
- Avoid trauma to rectal tissues:
  - Do not administer enemas.
  - If suppositories are prescribed, lubricate liberally and administer with caution.
- Instruct the patient and UAP to use an electric shaver rather than a razor.
- When providing mouth care or supervising others in providing mouth care:
  - Use a soft-bristled toothbrush or tooth sponges.
  - Do not use floss.
  - Check to make certain that dentures fit and do not rub.
- Instruct the patient not to blow the nose forcefully or insert objects into the nose.
- Ensure that the patient wears shoes with firm soles whenever he or she is ambulating.
- Ensure that antidotes to anticoagulation therapy are on the unit.

UAP, Unlicensed assistive personnel.

CHART 32-7 Patient and Family Education: Preparing for Self-Management

Preventing Injury and Bleeding

During the time you are taking anticoagulants:
- Use an electric shaver.
- Use a soft-bristled toothbrush and do not floss.
- Do not have dental work performed without consulting your health care provider.
- Do not take aspirin or any aspirin-containing products. Read the label to be sure that the product does not contain aspirin or salicylates.
- Do not participate in contact sports or any activity likely to result in your being bumped, scratched, or scraped.
- If you are bumped, apply ice to the site for at least 1 hour.
- Avoid hard foods that would scrape the inside of your mouth.
- Eat warm, cool, or cold foods to avoid burning your mouth.
- Check your skin and mouth daily for bruises, swelling, or areas with small, reddish-purple marks that may indicate bleeding.
- Notify your health care provider if you:
  - Are injured and persistent bleeding results
  - Have excessive menstrual bleeding
  - See blood in your urine or bowel movement
- Avoid anal intercourse.
- Take a stool softener to prevent straining during a bowel movement.
- Do not use enemas or rectal suppositories.
- Do not wear clothing or shoes that are tight or that rub.
- Avoid blowing your nose forcefully or placing objects in your nose. If you must blow your nose, do so gently without blocking either nasal passage.
- Avoid playing musical instruments that raise the pressure inside your head, such as brass wind instruments and woodwinds or reed instruments.
- Keep all appointments for laboratory tests.

---

discussion in the Managing Hypoxemia section), communication, and drug therapy.

Communication is critical in allaying anxiety. Acknowledge the anxiety and the patient's perception of a life-threatening situation. Stay with him or her and speak calmly and clearly, providing assurances that appropriate measures are being taken. Explain the rationale and share information when giving drugs, changing position, taking vital signs, or assessing the patient. Coordinate with pastoral care to help provide spiritual comfort.

Drug therapy with an antianxiety drug may be prescribed if the patient's anxiety interferes with diagnostic testing, management, or adequate rest. Unless he or she is mechanically ventilated, sedating agents are avoided to reduce the risk for hypoventilation. Pharmacologic therapy is used for pain management. Care is taken to avoid suppressing the respiratory response.

Care Coordination and Transition Management

The patient with a PE is discharged when hypoxemia and hemodynamic instability are resolved and adequate anticoagulation has been achieved. Anticoagulation therapy usually continues after discharge.

Home Care Management. Some patients are discharged to home with minimal risk for recurrence and no permanent physiologic changes. Others have heart or lung damage that requires home and lifestyle modification.

Patients with extensive lung damage may have activity intolerance from reduced GAS EXCHANGE and become fatigued easily. The living arrangements may need to be modified so patients can spend most of the time on one floor and avoid climbing stairs. Depending on the degree of impairment, patients may require varying amounts of assistance with ADLs. Coordinate with members of the interprofessional team as described earlier in the Interprofessional Collaborative Care section to ensure optimal patient function.

Self-Management Education. The patient with a PE may continue anticoagulation therapy for weeks, months, or years after discharge, depending on the risks for PE, and have impaired CLOTTING. Teach him or her and the family about Bleeding Precautions, activities to reduce the risk for venous thromboembolism (VTE) and recurrence of PE, complications, and the need for follow-up care (Chart 32-7).

Health Care Resources. Patients using anticoagulation therapy with warfarin are usually seen in a clinic or primary health care provider's office frequently for blood tests. Those who are homebound may have a visit from a home care nurse to perform these tests. Enoxaparin (Lovenox) and newer anticoagulation agents (dabigatran [Pradaxa], rivaroxaban [Xarelto], and apixaban [Eliquis]) do not require laboratory monitoring. Patients with severe dyspnea may need home oxygen therapy. Respiratory therapy treatments can be performed in the home. The nurse or case manager coordinates arrangements for oxygen and other respiratory therapy equipment to

CHART 32-8 Home Care Assessment
The Patient After Pulmonary Embolism

Assess respiratory status:
- Observe rate and depth of ventilation.
- Auscultate lungs.
- Examine nail beds and mucous membranes for evidence of cyanosis, indicating reduced GAS EXCHANGE.
- Take a pulse oximetry reading.
- Ask the patient if chest pain or shortness of breath is experienced in any position.
- Ask the patient about the presence of sputum and its color and character.

Assess cardiovascular status:
- Take vital signs, including apical pulse, pulse pressure; assess for presence or absence of orthostatic hypotension and quality and rhythm of peripheral pulses.
- Note presence or absence of peripheral edema.
- Examine hand vein filling in the dependent position.
- Examine neck vein filling in the recumbent and sitting positions.

Assess lower extremities for deep vein thrombosis:
- Examine lower legs and compare with each other for:
  - General edema
  - Calf swelling
  - Surface temperature
  - Presence of red streaks or cordlike, palpable structure
- Measure calf circumference.

Assess for evidence of bleeding:
- Examine the mouth and gums for oozing or frank bleeding.
- Examine all skin areas, especially old puncture sites and wounds, for bleeding, bruising, or petechiae.
- If the patient voids during the visit, test the urine for occult blood.

Assess cognition and mental status:
- Check level of consciousness.
- Check orientation to time, place, and person.
- Can the patient accurately read a seven-word sentence containing no words with more than three syllables?

Assess the patient's understanding of illness and adherence to treatment:
- Symptoms to report to health care provider
- Drug therapy plan (correct timing and dose)
- Bleeding Precautions
- Prevention of venous thromboembolism

CLINICAL JUDGMENT CHALLENGE 32-1
Patient-Centered Care; Safety; Teamwork and Collaboration QSEN

The patient is a 53-year-old woman who had major abdominal surgery for a bowel resection 2 days ago. She is a current smoker with a 40 pack-year smoking history. She also has chronic obstructive pulmonary disease and had a right upper lobe lung removal in the past. The nursing assistant calls you to the patient's room because her pulse oximeter is alarming and indicates an SpO2 of 50%. The patient reports mild shortness of breath, and her blood pressure is 76/42.

1. What should be your first actions? Provide a rationale for your choice(s).
2. The primary health care provider asks you to send a D-dimer laboratory test. Is this test diagnostic for a PE? Why or why not?
3. The primary health care provider believes that the patient has a PE and wants to start anticoagulation before a CT scan is performed for confirmation. Is this an appropriate intervention action? Why or why not?
4. Which other interprofessional team members now would be helpful to involve in this patient's care and why?
5. Your patient does have a PE and has completed her inpatient therapy. She is to be discharged to home on warfarin therapy. Which important issues should be included in the discharge plan?

---

be available if needed at home. See Chart 32-8 for a home care assessment guide.

◆ Evaluation: Reflecting

Evaluate the care of the patient with PE on the basis of the identified priority patient problems. The expected outcomes are that he or she:
- Attains and maintains adequate GAS EXCHANGE and oxygenation
- Does not experience hypovolemia and shock
- Remains free from bleeding episodes
- States that the level of anxiety is reduced
- Uses effective coping strategies

ACUTE RESPIRATORY FAILURE

❖ PATHOPHYSIOLOGY

A near match in the lungs between air movement or ventilation ($\dot{V}$) and blood flow or PERFUSION ($\dot{Q}$) is needed for adequate pulmonary GAS EXCHANGE. When either ventilation or perfusion is mismatched with the other in a lung or lung area, gas exchange is reduced, and respiratory failure can result (Lamba et al., 2016).

Acute respiratory failure (ARF) can be *ventilatory failure, oxygenation (GAS EXCHANGE) failure,* or a *combination of both ventilatory and oxygenation failure* and is classified by abnormal blood gas values. The critical values are:
- Partial pressure of arterial oxygen (Pao_2) less than 60 mm Hg (hypoxemic/oxygenation failure)
- *or* Partial pressure of arterial carbon dioxide ($Paco_2$) more than 45 mm Hg occurring with acidemia (pH <7.35) (hypercapnic/ventilatory failure)
- *and* Arterial oxygen saturation (Sao_2) less than 90% in both cases

Whatever the underlying problem, the patient in acute respiratory failure is always **hypoxemic** (has low arterial blood oxygen levels).

Ventilatory Failure

Ventilatory failure is a problem in oxygen intake (air movement or ventilation) and blood flow (PERFUSION) that causes a ventilation-perfusion ($\dot{V}/\dot{Q}$) mismatch in which blood flow (perfusion) is normal but air movement (ventilation) is inadequate. It occurs when the chest pressure does not change enough to permit air movement into and out of the lungs. As a result, too little oxygen reaches the alveoli, and carbon dioxide is retained. Perfusion is wasted in this area of no air movement from either inadequate oxygen intake or excessive carbon dioxide retention, leading to poor GAS EXCHANGE and hypoxemia.

Ventilatory failure usually results from any of these problems: a physical problem of the lungs or chest wall; a defect in the respiratory control center in the brain; or poor function of the respiratory muscles, especially the diaphragm. The problem is defined by a $Paco_2$ level above 45 mm Hg plus acidemia (pH < 7.35) in patients who have otherwise healthy lungs.

TABLE 32-2	Common Causes of Ventilatory Failure

Extrapulmonary Causes	Intrapulmonary Causes
• Neuromuscular disorders: • Myasthenia gravis • Guillain-Barré syndrome • Poliomyelitis • Spinal cord injuries affecting nerves to intercostal muscles • Central nervous system dysfunction: • Stroke • Increased intracranial pressure • Meningitis • Chemical depression: • Opioid analgesics, sedatives, anesthetics • Kyphoscoliosis • Massive obesity • Sleep apnea • External obstruction/constriction	• Airway disease: • Chronic obstructive pulmonary disease (COPD), asthma • Ventilation-perfusion ($\dot{V}/\dot{Q}$) mismatch: • Pulmonary embolism • Pneumothorax • Acute respiratory distress syndrome (ARDS) • Amyloidosis • Pulmonary edema • Interstitial fibrosis

TABLE 32-3	Common Causes of Oxygenation Failure

- Low atmospheric oxygen concentration:
  - High altitudes, closed spaces, smoke inhalation, carbon monoxide poisoning
- Pneumonia
- Congestive heart failure with pulmonary edema
- Pulmonary embolism (PE)
- Acute respiratory distress syndrome (ARDS)
- Interstitial pneumonitis-fibrosis
- Abnormal hemoglobin
- Hypovolemic shock
- Hypoventilation
- Complications of nitroprusside therapy:
  - Thiocyanate toxicity, methemoglobinemia

Many disorders can result in ventilatory failure. Causes are either extrapulmonary (involving nonpulmonary tissues but affecting respiratory function) or intrapulmonary (disorders of the respiratory tract). Table 32-2 lists causes of ventilatory failure.

Oxygenation (Gas Exchange) Failure

In oxygenation (GAS EXCHANGE) failure, chest pressure changes are normal, and air moves in and out without difficulty but does not oxygenate the pulmonary blood sufficiently. It occurs in the type of $\dot{V}/\dot{Q}$ mismatch in which air movement and oxygen intake (ventilation) are normal but lung blood flow (PERFUSION) is decreased.

Many lung disorders can cause oxygenation failure. Problems include impaired diffusion of oxygen at the alveolar level, right-to-left shunting of blood in the pulmonary vessels, $\dot{V}/\dot{Q}$ mismatch, breathing air with a low oxygen level, and abnormal hemoglobin that fails to bind oxygen. In one type of $\dot{V}/\dot{Q}$ mismatch, areas of the lungs still have PERFUSION, but GAS EXCHANGE does not occur, which leads to hypoxemia. An extreme example of $\dot{V}/\dot{Q}$ mismatch is when systemic venous blood (oxygen-poor) passes through the lungs without being oxygenated and is "shunted" to the left side of the heart and into the systemic arterial system. Normally less than 5% of cardiac output contains venous blood that has bypassed oxygenation. With poor oxygenation in the lungs or a shunt that allows venous blood to bypass the lungs, even more arterial blood is not oxygenated, and applying 100% oxygen does not correct the problem. A classic cause of such a $\dot{V}/\dot{Q}$ mismatch is acute respiratory distress syndrome (ARDS). Table 32-3 lists specific causes of oxygenation failure.

Combined Ventilatory and Oxygenation Failure

Combined ventilatory and oxygenation failure involves hypoventilation (poor respiratory movements). Impaired GAS EXCHANGE at the alveolar-capillary membrane results in poor diffusion of oxygen into arterial blood and carbon dioxide retention. The condition may or may not include poor lung perfusion. When lung PERFUSION is not adequate, $\dot{V}/\dot{Q}$ mismatch

occurs, and both ventilation and perfusion are inadequate. This type of respiratory failure leads to a more profound hypoxemia than either ventilatory failure or oxygenation failure alone.

A combination of ventilatory failure and oxygenation (GAS EXCHANGE) failure occurs in patients who have abnormal lungs, such as those who have any form of chronic bronchitis, emphysema, or cystic fibrosis or are having an asthma attack. The bronchioles and alveoli are diseased (causing oxygenation failure), and the work of breathing increases until the respiratory muscles cannot function effectively, causing ventilatory failure leading to acute respiratory failure (ARF). ARF can also occur in patients who have cardiac failure along with ventilatory failure and is made worse because the cardiac system cannot adapt to the hypoxia by increasing the cardiac output.

❖ INTERPROFESSIONAL COLLABORATIVE CARE

◆ Assessment: Noticing

The symptoms of ARF are related to the systemic effects of hypoxia, hypercapnia, and acidosis. Assess for dyspnea (perceived difficulty breathing)—the hallmark of respiratory failure. Evaluate dyspnea on the basis of how breathless the patient becomes while performing common tasks. Depending on the nature of the underlying problem, the patient might not be aware of changes in the work of breathing.

Dyspnea is more intense when it develops rapidly. Slowly progressive respiratory failure may first be noticed as dyspnea on exertion (DOE) or when lying down. The patient may have orthopnea, finding it easier to breathe in an upright position (Bull, 2014). With chronic respiratory problems, a minor increase in dyspnea may represent severe GAS EXCHANGE problems.

Assess for a change in the patient's respiratory rate or pattern and changes in lung sounds. Pulse oximetry (SpO_2) may show decreased oxygen saturation, but end-tidal CO_2 ($ETCO_2$ or $PETCO_2$) monitoring may be more valuable for monitoring the patient with ARF (Carlisle, 2014). His or her pulse oximetry may show adequate oxygen saturation but, because of increased $ETCO_2$, the patient may be close to respiratory failure. Arterial blood gas (ABG) studies are reviewed to most accurately identify the degree of hypoxia and hypercarbia.

Other symptoms of hypoxic respiratory failure include restlessness, irritability or agitation, confusion, and tachycardia. Symptoms of hypercapnic failure may include decreased level of consciousness (LOC), headache, drowsiness, lethargy, and seizures. The effects of acidosis may lead to decreased LOC, drowsiness, confusion, hypotension, bradycardia, and weak peripheral pulses.

◆ Interventions: Responding

Oxygen therapy is appropriate for any patient with acute hypoxemia. It is used in acute respiratory failure to keep the arterial oxygen (Pao_2) level above 60 mm Hg while treating the cause of the respiratory failure. Oxygen therapy is discussed in detail in Chapter 28. If oxygen therapy does not maintain acceptable Pao_2 levels, indicating adequate GAS EXCHANGE, mechanical ventilation (invasive or noninvasive) may be needed.

Drugs given systemically, by nebulizer, or by metered dose inhaler (MDI) may be prescribed to dilate the bronchioles and decrease inflammation to promote GAS EXCHANGE. Corticosteroids may be used, but their benefit has not been demonstrated conclusively. Analgesics are needed if the patient has pain. If the patient requires mechanical ventilation, he or she may need neuromuscular blockade drugs for optimal ventilator effect. Other management strategies depend on the underlying condition(s) that predisposed the patient to ARF development, which may include diuretic therapy or antibiotic therapy.

Help the patient find a position of comfort that allows easier breathing (i.e., usually a more upright position). To decrease the anxiety occurring with dyspnea, help him or her use relaxation, diversion, and guided imagery. Start energy-conserving measures, such as minimal self-care and no unnecessary procedures. Encourage deep breathing and other breathing exercises.

ACUTE RESPIRATORY DISTRESS SYNDROME

❖ PATHOPHYSIOLOGY

Acute respiratory distress syndrome (ARDS) is acute respiratory failure with these features:
- Hypoxemia that persists even when 100% oxygen is given (**refractory hypoxemia**, a cardinal feature)
- Decreased pulmonary compliance
- Dyspnea
- Noncardiac-associated bilateral pulmonary edema
- Dense pulmonary infiltrates on x-ray (ground-glass appearance)

Often ARDS occurs after an *acute lung injury (ALI)* in people who have no pulmonary disease as a result of other conditions such as sepsis, burns, pancreatitis, trauma, and transfusion. Other terms for ARDS include *adult respiratory distress syndrome* and *shock lung*.

Despite different causes of ALI in ARDS, the trigger is a systemic inflammatory response. As a result, ARDS symptoms are similar regardless of the cause. The main site of injury in the lung is the alveolar-capillary membrane, which normally is permeable only to small molecules. It can be injured during sepsis, pulmonary embolism, shock, aspiration, or inhalation injury. When injured, this membrane becomes more permeable to large molecules, which allows debris, proteins, and fluid into the alveoli. Lung tissue normally remains relatively dry, but in patients with ARDS lung fluid increases and contains more proteins.

Other changes occur in the alveoli and respiratory bronchioles. Normally the type II pneumocytes produce surfactant, a substance that increases lung **compliance** (elasticity) and

prevents alveolar collapse. Surfactant activity is reduced in ARDS because type II pneumocytes are damaged and because the surfactant is diluted by excess lung fluids. As a result, the alveoli become unstable and tend to collapse unless they are filled with fluid. These fluid-filled and collapsed alveoli cannot participate in GAS EXCHANGE. Edema then forms around terminal airways, which are compressed and closed and can be destroyed. Lung volume and compliance are further reduced. As fluid continues to leak in more lung areas, fluid, protein, and blood cells collect in the alveoli and in the spaces between the alveoli. Lymph channels are compressed, and more fluid collects. Poorly inflated alveoli receive blood but cannot oxygenate it, increasing the shunt. Hypoxemia and ventilation-perfusion $\dot{V}/\dot{Q}$ mismatch result.

Transfusion-related acute lung injury (TRALI) is the sudden onset (within 6 hours of a transfusion) of hypoxemic lung disease along with infiltrates on x-ray without cardiac problems. TRALI is associated with the activation of the inflammatory response caused by a recent transfusion of plasma-containing blood products such as packed red blood cells (PRBCs), platelets, and fresh frozen plasma. Other lung complications of transfusion include transfusion-associated circulatory overload (TACO) and transfusion-related immunomodulation (TRIM).

Etiology and Genetic Risk

ALI leading to ARDS has many causes (Table 32-4). Some causes result in direct injury to lung tissue; other causes do not directly involve the lungs. As a result of sepsis, pancreatitis, trauma, and other conditions, inflammatory mediators spread to the lungs, causing damage (McCance et al., 2014).

ARDS also can occur from direct lung injury. Aspiration of acidic gastric contents, pneumonia, drowning, or inhaling toxic fumes are examples of conditions causing direct lung injury. With such events, surfactant production is impaired, and the remaining surfactant is diluted. This situation leads to atelectasis, decreased lung compliance, and shunting (movement of blood in the lungs without GAS EXCHANGE and oxygenation) (McCance et al., 2014).

Incidence and Prevalence

The actual incidence of ARDS is unknown because it is part of other health problems and is not systematically reported as a separate disorder. According to the ARDS Foundation, about 150,000 cases of ARDS occur yearly in North America, although many health care professionals believe this estimate to be low. The mortality rate is estimated at 42% (ARDS Foundation, 2016).

TABLE 32-4 Common Causes of Acute Lung Injury	
• Shock	• Pulmonary aspiration (especially of stomach contents)
• Trauma	
• Serious nervous system injury	• Drug ingestion (e.g., heroin, opioids, aspirin)
• Pancreatitis	• Hemolytic disorders
• Fat and amniotic fluid emboli	• Multiple blood transfusions
• Pulmonary infections	• Cardiopulmonary bypass
• Sepsis	• Submersion in water with water aspiration (especially in fresh water)
• Inhalation of toxic gases (smoke, oxygen)	

🧬 **GENETIC/GENOMIC CONSIDERATIONS**
Patient-Centered Care QSEN

An increased genetic risk is suspected in the development and progression of ARDS. Variations in the genes responsible for surfactant production appear to increase the predisposition to developing ARDS, as does variation in the genes responsible for cytokine production during inflammatory events associated with sepsis. Ask about the patient's previous responses to infection or injury. If the patient has consistently had greater-than-expected inflammatory responses, he or she may be at increased risk for ARDS after ALI and should be monitored for symptoms of the disorder.

Health Promotion and Maintenance

The nursing priority in the prevention of ARDS is early recognition of patients at high risk for the syndrome. Because patients who aspirate gastric contents are at great risk, closely assess and monitor those receiving tube feedings (because the tube keeps the gastric sphincter open) and those with problems that impair swallowing and gag reflexes. **As required by The Joint Commission's NPSGs to prevent ARDS, follow meticulous infection control guidelines, including handwashing, invasive catheter and wound care, and Contact Precautions.** Teach unlicensed assistive personnel (UAP) the importance of always adhering to infection control guidelines. Carefully observe patients who are being treated for any health problem associated with ARDS.

❖ INTERPROFESSIONAL COLLABORATIVE CARE

ARDS is a life-threatening health problem that may result in permanent impairment of lung function requiring major changes in lifestyle. For optimum patient function, a comprehensive interprofessional team approach is needed. Essential team members are the same as those described for pulmonary embolism (see the exemplar earlier in this chapter).

◆ Assessment: Noticing

Physical Assessment/Signs and Symptoms. Assess the breathing of any patient at increased risk for ARDS. Determine whether increased work of breathing is present, as indicated by hyperpnea, noisy respiration, cyanosis, pallor, and retraction intercostally (between the ribs) or substernally (below the ribs). Document sweating, respiratory effort, and any change in mental status. *Abnormal lung sounds are **not** heard on auscultation because the edema occurs first in the interstitial spaces and not in the airways.* Assess vital signs at least hourly for hypotension, tachycardia, and dysrhythmias.

Many patients with ARDS have an altered core body temperature on admission. Those with a temperature elevation early in the course of ARDS appear to have a better outcome with lower mortality than do those who have hypothermia (Schell-Chaple et al., 2015).

Diagnostic Assessment. The diagnosis of ARDS is established by a lowered partial pressure of arterial oxygen (PaO_2) value (decreased GAS EXCHANGE and oxygenation), determined by arterial blood gas (ABG) measurements. Because a widening alveolar oxygen gradient (i.e., increased fraction of inspired oxygen [FiO_2] does not lead to increased PaO_2 levels) develops with increased shunting of blood, the patient has a progressive need for higher levels of oxygen. He or she develops refractory

hypoxemia and often needs intubation and mechanical ventilation. Sputum cultures obtained by bronchoscopy and transtracheal aspiration are used to determine if a lung infection also is present.

The chest x-ray may show diffuse haziness or a "whited-out" (ground-glass) appearance of the lung. An ECG rules out cardiac problems and usually shows no specific changes. Although hemodynamic monitoring with a pulmonary artery catheter has been used in the past to help diagnose ARDS, such invasive monitoring has not shown any benefit and is no longer recommended.

◆ Interventions: Responding

Management Overview. General management of the patient with ARDS focuses on the three phases of ARDS. Timing of the phases varies from patient to patient.

Exudative phase. This phase includes early changes of dyspnea and tachypnea resulting from the alveoli becoming fluid filled and from pulmonary shunting and atelectasis. Early interventions focus on supporting the patient and providing oxygen.

Fibroproliferative phase. Increased lung injury leads to pulmonary hypertension and fibrosis. The body attempts to repair the damage, and increasing lung involvement reduces GAS EXCHANGE and oxygenation. Multiple organ dysfunction syndrome (MODS) can occur. Interventions focus on delivering adequate oxygen, preventing complications, and supporting the lungs.

Resolution phase. Usually occurring after 14 days, resolution of the injury can occur; if not the patient either dies or has chronic disease. Fibrosis may or may not occur. Patients surviving ARDS often have neuropsychological deficits.

Specific Management. The patient with ARDS often needs intubation and mechanical ventilation with positive end-expiratory pressure (PEEP) or continuous positive airway pressure (CPAP). Best practice involves using "open lung" and lung protective ventilation strategies. Low tidal volumes (6 mL/kg of body weight) have been shown to prevent lung injury. PEEP is started at 5 cm H_2O and increased to keep oxygen saturation adequate. PEEP levels may need to be high. Pressure-controlled ventilation is preferred over volume-controlled ventilation to promote the nonfunctional alveoli to participate in GAS EXCHANGE. Because one of the side effects of PEEP is tension pneumothorax, assess lung sounds hourly and suction as often as needed to maintain a patent airway.

Airway pressure-release ventilation (APRV) and high-frequency oscillatory ventilation (HFOV) are alternative modes of mechanical ventilation that improve GAS EXCHANGE with oxygenation and ventilation in patients with moderate-to-severe ARDS. The airway pressure for both APRV and HFOV are significantly higher than for conventional mechanical ventilation. Sedation and paralysis may be needed for adequate ventilation and to reduce tissue oxygen needs, especially with HFOV. Sedation and paralysis are not required with APRV but may be needed to prevent patient disruption of mechanical ventilation. APRV does not allow for spontaneous breathing between mandatory breaths (see the Modes of Ventilation section).

Positioning may be important in promoting GAS EXCHANGE, but the exact position is controversial. Some patients do better in the prone position, especially if it is started early in the disease course (Drahnak & Custer, 2015; Senecal, 2015). Prone positioning may be achieved using a mechanical turning device, although the turning equipment is awkward and care in the prone position is more difficult. Automated kinetic beds are available to assist with turning. Manually turning the patient every 2 hours has been shown to improve PERFUSION; however, this intervention often is not performed as frequently as needed. Early progressive mobility also has demonstrated benefit in reducing ventilator needs, days on the ventilator, and mortality. Automatic turning appears to have a slight advantage of decreasing some pulmonary complications but has not yet shown secondary benefits such as decreased lengths of stay, reduced ICU mortality, or decreased ventilator days.

For severe ARDS, extracorporeal membrane oxygenation (ECMO) using heart-lung bypass equipment has been a successful life support technique when the patient does not improve with more traditional management (Schulman et al., 2014). However, the proper timing of ECMO and standardization of this therapy for best outcomes have not been established.

Drug and Fluid Therapy. Antibiotics are used to treat infections when organisms are identified. Other drugs are used to manage any underlying cause. Currently no treatments reverse the pathologic changes in the lungs, although many interventions that modify the inflammatory responses and reduce oxidative stress are under investigation. These agents include vitamins C and E, *N*-acetylcysteine, nitric oxide, and surfactant replacement (Chudow et al., 2015; Howe et al., 2015).

Research shows that patients with ARDS who receive conservative fluid therapy have improved lung function and a shorter duration of mechanical ventilation and ICU length of stay compared with those who receive more liberal fluid therapy. Conservative fluid therapy involves infusing smaller amounts of IV fluid and using diuretics to maintain fluid balance, whereas liberal fluid therapy often results in an increasingly positive fluid balance and more edema.

Nutrition Therapy. The patient with ARDS is at risk for malnutrition, which further reduces respiratory muscle function and the immune response. The interprofessional team should include a registered dietitian, and enteral nutrition (tube feeding) or parenteral nutrition is started as soon as possible.

⚑ CLINICAL JUDGMENT CHALLENGE 32-2

Safety; Teamwork and Collaboration; Evidence-Based Practice (QSEN)

The patient is a 26-year-old who was admitted to the surgical floor 2 days ago after a motor vehicle crash. His injuries include a thoracic fracture, for which he must remain flat, and some chest bruising. He was started on enteral feeding yesterday. His IV fluid rate is 150 mL/hr, and he is receiving IV morphine every 2 hours for pain. At change of shift, your assessment findings include that the patient is dyspneic and slightly confused. Lung sounds are diminished in the right base, and he is febrile to 101.5° F (38.6° C). Pulse is 120 beats/min; respirations are 36 breaths/min and shallow. Blood pressure is 88/56 mm Hg, pulse oximetry shows an SpO$_2$ of 88%, and capnography shows an end-tidal CO$_2$ (ETCO$_2$) of 48.

1. Is this patient experiencing ventilatory failure, oxygen failure, or a combination of ventilatory and oxygenation failure? Explain your answer.
2. What are some possible causes of the patient's distress?
3. Which interprofessional team members should you contact now and why?
4. Which diagnostic tests should you anticipate?

THE PATIENT REQUIRING INTUBATION AND VENTILATION

❖ PATHOPHYSIOLOGY

With mechanical ventilation, the patient who has severe problems of GAS EXCHANGE may be supported until the underlying problem improves or resolves. Usually mechanical ventilation is a temporary life-support technique. The need for this support may be lifelong for those with severe restrictive lung disease or chronic progressive neuromuscular disease that reduces ventilation.

Mechanical ventilation is most often used for patients with hypoxemia and progressive alveolar hypoventilation with respiratory acidosis. The hypoxemia is usually caused by pulmonary shunting of blood when other methods of oxygen delivery do not provide a sufficiently high fraction of inspired oxygen (FIO$_2$). Mechanical ventilation may be used for patients who need temporary ventilatory support after surgery, those who expend too much energy with breathing and barely maintain adequate GAS EXCHANGE, or those who have general anesthesia or heavy sedation.

❖ INTERPROFESSIONAL COLLABORATIVE CARE

Assess the patient to be intubated in the same way as for other breathing problems. Once mechanical ventilation has been started, assess the respiratory system on an ongoing basis. Monitor and assess for problems related to the artificial airway or ventilator.

Endotracheal Intubation

The patient who needs mechanical ventilation must have an artificial airway. The most common type of airway for a short-term basis is the endotracheal (ET) tube. To reduce tracheal and vocal cord damage, a tracheostomy is considered if an artificial airway is needed for longer than 10 to 14 days (see Chapter 28). The expectations of intubation are to maintain a patent airway, provide a means to remove secretions, and provide ventilation and oxygen.

Endotracheal Tube. An ET tube is a long polyvinyl chloride tube that is passed through the mouth or nose and into the trachea (Fig. 32-2). When properly positioned, the tip of the ET tube rests about 2 cm above the carina (the point at which the trachea divides into the right and left mainstem bronchi). Oral intubation is a fast and easy way to establish an airway and is often performed as an emergency procedure. The nasal route is used for oral surgeries and when oral intubation is not possible. This route is avoided with midface trauma or possible basilar skull fracture. This route is not used if the patient has a blood CLOTTING problem. An anesthesiologist, nurse anesthetist, or respiratory therapist usually performs the intubation.

The shaft of the tube has a radiopaque line running the length of the tube. This line shows on x-ray and is used to determine correct tube placement. Short horizontal lines (depth markings) are used to place the tube correctly at the naris or mouth (at the incisor tooth) and to identify how far the tube has been inserted.

The cuff at the distal end of the tube is inflated after placement and creates a seal between the trachea and the cuff. The seal ensures delivery of a set tidal volume when mechanical ventilation is used. The cuff is inflated using a minimal-leak technique: when the cuff is inflated to an adequate sealing

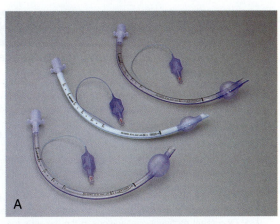 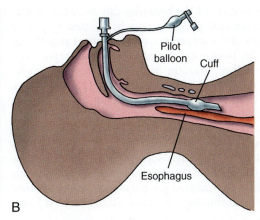

FIG. 32-2 A, Endotracheal tubes. **B,** Correct placement of an oral endotracheal tube. (**A** Courtesy Sims Porter, Inc.)

volume, a minimal amount of air can pass around it to the vocal cords, nose, or mouth. The patient cannot talk when the cuff is inflated.

The pilot balloon with a one-way valve permits air to be inserted into the cuff and prevents air from escaping. This balloon is a guide for determining whether air is present in the cuff, but it does not show how much or how little air is present.

The adaptor connects the ET tube to ventilator tubing or an oxygen delivery system. The ET tube size is listed on the shaft of the tube. Adult tube sizes range from 7 to 9 mm. Tube size selected is based on the size of the patient.

Preparing for Intubation. Know the proper procedure for summoning intubation personnel in the facility to the bedside in an emergency situation. Explain the procedure to the patient as clearly as possible. *Basic life support measures, such as obtaining a patent airway and delivering 100% oxygen by a manual resuscitation bag with a facemask, are crucial to survival until help arrives.*

! **NURSING SAFETY PRIORITY** QSEN

Critical Rescue

Monitor patients at risk for airway obstruction and impaired ventilation. When you recognize the need for emergency intubation and ventilation, respond by bringing the code (or "crash") cart, airway equipment box, and suction equipment (often already on the code cart) to the bedside. Maintain a patent airway through positioning (head-tilt, chin-lift) and the insertion of an oral or nasopharyngeal airway until the patient is intubated. Delivering manual breaths with a bag-valve-mask may also be required.

During intubation, the nurse coordinates the rescue response and continuously monitors the patient for changes in vital signs, signs of hypoxia or hypoxemia, dysrhythmias, and aspiration. Ensure that each intubation attempt lasts no longer than 30 seconds, preferably less than 15 seconds. After 30 seconds, provide oxygen by means of a mask and manual resuscitation bag to prevent hypoxia and cardiac arrest. Suction as necessary.

Verifying Tube Placement. Immediately after an ET tube is inserted, placement should be verified. The most accurate ways to verify placement are by checking end-tidal carbon dioxide levels and by chest x-ray. Assess for breath sounds bilaterally,

sounds over the gastric area, symmetric chest movement, and air emerging from the ET tube. If breath sounds and chest wall movement are absent on the left side, the tube may be in the right mainstem bronchus. The person intubating the patient should be able to reposition the tube without repeating the entire intubation procedure.

If the tube is in the stomach, the abdomen may be distended and must be decompressed with a nasogastric (NG) tube after the ET tube is replaced. Monitor chest wall movement and breath sounds until tube placement is verified by chest x-ray.

Stabilizing the Tube. The nurse, respiratory therapist, or anesthesia provider stabilizes the ET tube at the mouth or nose. The tube is marked at the level where it touches the incisor tooth or naris. Two people working together use a head halter technique to secure the tube. An oral airway also may be inserted, or a commercial bite block placed to keep the patient from biting an oral ET tube. One person stabilizes the tube at the correct position and prevents head movement while a second person applies the tube holding device. Commercial tube holders are preferred over securing the tube with tape. After the procedure is completed, verify and document the presence of bilateral and equal breath sounds and the level of the tube.

Nursing Care. The priority nursing action when caring for an intubated patient is maintaining a patent airway. Assess tube placement, cuff leak, breath sounds, indications of adequate GAS EXCHANGE and oxygenation, and chest wall movement regularly.

! **NURSING SAFETY PRIORITY** QSEN

Critical Rescue

Assess intubated patients to recognize indications of decreased GAS EXCHANGE. When these indications are present, respond by checking for DOPE: *d*isplaced tube, *o*bstructed tube (most often with secretions), *p*neumothorax, and *e*quipment problems.

Prevent the patient from pulling or tugging on the tube to avoid tube dislodgment and check the pilot balloon to ensure that the cuff is inflated. Monitor the pressure within the cuff to ensure that it is maintained between 20 to 30 cm H_2O to stabilize the tube without causing tracheal injury. Suctioning, coughing, and speaking can cause dislodgment. Neck flexion, neck extension, and rotation of the head also can cause the tube to move. In addition, cuff pressures may be affected by patient position changes and may require more frequent monitoring (Lizy et al., 2014). Tongue movement also can change the tube's position. When other measures fail, obtain a prescription for soft wrist restraints and apply these for the patient who is pulling on the tube. *Restraints are used as a last resort to prevent accidental extubation.* To remain in compliance with The Joint Commission's National Patient Safety Goals (NPSG), reassess the need for restraint use daily. If the need continues, a new prescription is needed daily. Adequate sedation (chemical restraint) may be needed to decrease agitation or prevent extubation. Obtain permission for restraints from the patient or family. More information on airway management is found in Chapter 28.

Complications of an ET or nasotracheal tube can occur during placement, while in place, during extubation, or after extubation (either early or late). Common complications include tube obstruction, dislodgment, pneumothorax, tracheal tears, bleeding, and infection. Trauma and other problems can occur to the face; eye; nasal and paranasal areas; oral, pharyngeal, bronchial, tracheal, and pulmonary areas; esophageal and gastric areas; and cardiovascular, musculoskeletal, and neurologic systems.

NCLEX EXAMINATION CHALLENGE 32-2

Safe and Effective Care Environment

The client from Clinical Judgment Challenge 32-2 continues to deteriorate clinically and is to be intubated. What are the **most important** actions for the nurse to implement? **Select all that apply.**
A. Obtain a cervical x-ray.
B. Discontinue the IV fluids.
C. Immediately page anesthesia or the Rapid Response Team (depending on institution policy).
D. Confirm that suction is at the bedside and functioning properly.
E. Have the crash cart available.
F. Place client on nasal cannula oxygen.
G. Have manual resuscitation bag with facemask at bedside.
H. Verify bilateral breath sounds postintubation.

Mechanical Ventilation

Mechanical ventilation to support and maintain GAS EXCHANGE is used in many settings, not just in critical care units. The nurse plays a pivotal role in the coordination of care and prevention of problems. Chart 32-9 lists best practices for patient care during mechanical ventilation.

The purposes of mechanical ventilation are to improve GAS EXCHANGE and decrease the work needed for effective breathing. It is used to support the patient until lung function is adequate or until the acute episode has passed. *A ventilator does not cure diseased lungs; it provides ventilation until the patient can resume the process of breathing on his or her own.* Remember *why* the patient is using the ventilator so your management efforts also can focus on correcting the causes of the respiratory failure. If normal gas exchange with oxygenation, ventilation, and respiratory muscle strength is achieved, mechanical ventilation can be discontinued.

CHART 32-9 Best Practice for Patient Safety & Quality Care QSEN

Care of the Patient Receiving Mechanical Ventilation

- Assess the patient's respiratory status and GAS EXCHANGE at least every 4 hours for the first 24 hours and then as needed:
  - Take vital signs at least every 4 hours.
  - Assess the patient's color (especially lips and nail beds).
  - Observe the patient's chest for bilateral expansion.
  - Assess the placement of the nasotracheal or endotracheal tube.
  - Obtain pulse oximetry reading.
  - Evaluate ABGs as available.
  - Maintain head of the bed more than 30 degrees when patient is supine to prevent aspiration and ventilator-associated pneumonia.
- Document pertinent observations in the patient's medical record.
- Check at least every 8 hours to be sure that the ventilator setting is as prescribed.
- Check to be sure that alarms are set (especially low-pressure and low-exhaled volume).
- If the patient is on PEEP, observe the peak airway pressure dial to determine the proper level of PEEP.
- Check the exhaled volume digital display to be sure that the patient is receiving the prescribed tidal volume.
- Empty ventilator tubings when moisture collects. Never empty fluid in the tubing back into the cascade.
- Ensure humidity by keeping delivered air temperature maintained at body temperature.
- Be sure the tracheostomy cuff (or endotracheal cuff) is adequately inflated to ensure tidal volume.
- Auscultate the lungs for crackles, wheezes, equal breath sounds, and decreased or absent breath sounds.
- Check the patient's need for tracheal, oral, or nasal suctioning every 2 hours and suction as needed.
- Assess the patient's mouth around the ET tube for pressure injuries.
- Perform mouth care every 2 hours.
- Change tracheostomy tube holder or tape or ET tube holder or tape as needed:
  - Carefully move the oral ET tube to the opposite side of the mouth once daily to prevent ulcers.
  - Provide tracheostomy care every 8 hours.
- Assess ventilated patients for GI distress (diarrhea, constipation, tarry stools).
- Maintain accurate intake and output records to monitor fluid balance.
- Turn the patient at least every 2 hours and get the patient out of bed as prescribed to promote pulmonary hygiene and prevent complications of immobility.
- Schedule treatments and nursing care at intervals for rest.
- Monitor the patient's progress on current ventilator settings and make appropriate changes as indicated.
- Monitor the patient for the effectiveness of mechanical ventilation in terms of his or her physiologic and psychological status.
- Monitor for adverse effects of mechanical ventilation: infection, barotrauma, reduced cardiac output.
- Position the patient to facilitate ventilation-perfusion ($\dot{V}/\dot{Q}$) matching ("good lung down"), as appropriate.
- Monitor the effects of ventilator changes on GAS EXCHANGE and the patient's subjective response.
- Monitor readiness to wean.
- Explain all procedures and treatments; provide access to a call light; visit the patient frequently.
- Provide a method of communication. Request consultation with a speech-language pathologist for assistance, if necessary.
- Initiate relaxation techniques, as appropriate.
- Administer muscle-paralyzing agents, sedatives, and narcotic analgesics, as prescribed.
- Include the patient and family whenever possible (especially during suctioning and tracheostomy care).

ABGs, Arterial blood gases; *ET,* endotracheal; *PEEP,* positive end-expiratory pressure.

Types of Ventilators. Many types of ventilators are available. The ventilator selected depends on the severity of the breathing problem and the length of time ventilator support is needed. Most ventilators are positive-pressure ventilators. During inspiration, pressure is generated that pushes air into the lungs and expands the chest. Usually an endotracheal (ET) tube or tracheostomy is needed. Positive-pressure ventilators are classified by the mechanism that ends inspiration and starts expiration. Inspiration is cycled in three major ways: pressure-cycled, time-cycled, or volume-cycled.

Pressure-cycled ventilators push air into the lungs until a preset airway pressure is reached. Tidal volumes and inspiratory time vary. These ventilators are used for short periods, such as just after surgery and for respiratory therapy. Bi-level positive airway pressure (Bi-PAP) ventilators are a newer form of pressure-cycled ventilators in which the ventilator provides a preset inspiratory pressure and an expiratory pressure similar to positive end-expiratory pressure (PEEP).

Time-cycled ventilators push air into the lungs until a preset time has elapsed. Tidal volume and pressure vary, depending on the needs of the patient and the type of ventilator.

Volume-cycled ventilators push air into the lungs until a preset volume is delivered. A constant tidal volume is delivered, regardless of the pressure needed to deliver the tidal volume. However, a set pressure limit prevents excessive pressure from being exerted on the lungs. The advantage of this type of ventilator is that a constant tidal volume is delivered, regardless of changes in lung or chest wall compliance or airway resistance.

Microprocessor ventilators are computer-managed positive-pressure ventilators. A computer is built into the ventilator to allow ongoing monitoring of ventilatory functions, alarms, and patient conditions. It often has components of volume-, time-, and pressure-cycled ventilators. This type of ventilator is more responsive to patients who have severe lung disease and those who need prolonged weaning trials. Examples include the Dräger Evita XL (Fig. 32-3) and Puritan-Bennett 840.

Modes of Ventilation. The mode of ventilation is the way in which the patient receives breaths from the ventilator. The most common modes are assist-control ventilation, synchronized intermittent mandatory ventilation, and bi-level positive airway pressure (BiPAP) ventilation.

Assist-control (AC) ventilation is the mode used most often as a resting mode. The ventilator takes over the work of breathing for the patient. The tidal volume and ventilatory rate are preset. If the patient does not trigger spontaneous breaths, a ventilatory pattern is established by the ventilator. It is programmed to respond to the patient's inspiratory effort if he or she begins a breath. In this case, the ventilator delivers the preset tidal volume while allowing the patient to control the rate of breathing.

A disadvantage of the AC mode is that the ventilator continues to deliver a preset tidal volume even when the patient's spontaneous breathing rate increases. This can cause hyperventilation and respiratory alkalosis. Investigate and correct causes of hyperventilation, such as pain, anxiety, or acid-base imbalances.

Synchronized intermittent mandatory ventilation (SIMV) is similar to AC ventilation in that tidal volume and ventilatory rate are preset. If the patient does not breathe, a ventilatory pattern is established by the ventilator. Unlike the AC mode, SIMV allows spontaneous breathing at the patient's own rate and tidal volume between the ventilator breaths. It can be used as a main ventilatory mode or as a weaning mode. When used for weaning, the number of mechanical breaths (SIMV breaths) is gradually decreased (e.g., from 12 to 2) as the patient resumes spontaneous breathing. The mandatory ventilator breaths are delivered when the patient is ready to inspire. This action coordinates breathing between the ventilator and the patient.

Bi-level positive airway pressure (BiPAP) provides noninvasive pressure support ventilation by nasal mask or facemask. It is most often used for patients with sleep apnea but also may be used for patients with respiratory muscle fatigue or impending respiratory failure to avoid more invasive ventilation methods.

Other modes of ventilation, such as pressure support and continuous flow (flow-by), are part of most microprocessor ventilators. Both types decrease the work of breathing and are used for weaning patients from mechanical ventilation. Other modes are maximum mandatory ventilation (MMV), inverse inspiration-expiration (I/E) ratio, permissive hypercarbia, airway pressure–release ventilation (APRV), proportional assist ventilation, and high-frequency oscillation. Most modes use special ventilators, tubing, or airways.

Ventilator Controls and Settings. The volume-cycled ventilator is the most widely used type in the acute care setting. Regardless of the type of volume-cycled ventilator used, the controls and types of settings are universal (see Fig. 32-3). The pulmonologist or primary health care provider prescribes the ventilator settings, and usually the ventilator is readied or set up by the respiratory therapy department. The nurse assists in connecting the patient to the ventilator and monitors the ventilator settings in conjunction with respiratory therapy.

Tidal volume (V_T) is the volume of air the patient receives with each breath, as measured on either inspiration or expiration. The average prescribed V_T ranges between 6 and 8 mL/kg of body weight. Adding a zero to a patient's weight in kilograms gives an estimate of tidal volume.

Rate, or breaths/min, is the number of ventilator breaths delivered per minute. The rate is usually set between 10 and 14 breaths/min.

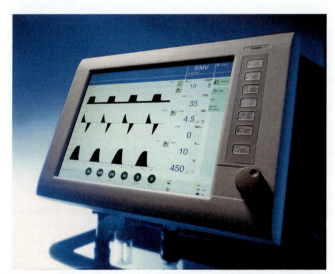

FIG. 32-3 Display signals, alarms, and control panel of a typical volume-cycled ventilator. (© Dräger Medical AG & Co. KG, Lübeck, Germany. All rights reserved. No portion hereof may be reproduced, saved or stored in a data processing system, electronically or mechanically copied or otherwise recorded by any other means without express prior written permission.)

Fraction of inspired oxygen (FiO$_2$) is the oxygen level delivered to the patient. The prescribed FiO$_2$ is based on the ABG values and the patient's condition. The range is 21% to 100% oxygen.

The oxygen delivered to the patient is warmed to body temperature (98.6° F [37° C]) and humidified to 100%. This is needed because upper air passages of the respiratory tree, which normally warm and humidify air, are bypassed. Humidifying and warming prevent mucosal damage.

Peak airway (inspiratory) pressure (PIP) is the pressure used by the ventilator to deliver a set tidal volume at a given lung compliance. The PIP value appears on the display of the ventilator. It is the highest pressure reached during inspiration. Trends in PIP reflect changes in resistance of the lungs and resistance in the ventilator. An increased PIP reading means increased airway resistance in the patient or the ventilator tubing (bronchospasm or pinched tubing, patient biting the ET tube), increased secretions, pulmonary edema, or decreased pulmonary compliance (the lungs or chest wall is "stiffer" and harder to inflate) (Covert & Niu, 2014). An upper pressure limit is set to prevent barotrauma. When the limit is reached, the high-pressure alarm sounds, and the remaining volume is not given.

Continuous positive airway pressure (CPAP) applies positive airway pressure throughout the entire respiratory cycle for spontaneously breathing patients. Sedating drugs are given lightly or not at all when the patient is receiving CPAP so respiratory effort is not suppressed. CPAP keeps the alveoli open during inspiration and prevents alveolar collapse during expiration. This process increases functional residual capacity (FRC) and improves GAS EXCHANGE and oxygenation.

CPAP is commonly used to help in the weaning process. During CPAP, no ventilator breaths are delivered. The ventilator just delivers oxygen and provides monitoring and an alarm system. The respiratory pattern is determined by the patient's efforts. Normal levels of CPAP are 5 to 15 cm H$_2$O to promote adequate GAS EXCHANGE and oxygenation. If no pressure is set, the patient receives no positive pressure. The patient is then using the ventilator as a T-piece with alarms. Modifications of CPAP include nasal CPAP and BiPAP, which are used on a temporary basis for select problems.

Positive end-expiratory pressure (PEEP) is positive pressure exerted during expiration. PEEP improves oxygenation by enhancing GAS EXCHANGE and preventing atelectasis. It is used to treat persistent hypoxemia that does not improve with an acceptable oxygen delivery level. It may be added when the arterial oxygen pressure (PaO$_2$) remains low with an FiO$_2$ of 50% to 70% or greater.

The need for PEEP indicates a severe GAS EXCHANGE problem. *It is important to lower the FiO$_2$ delivered whenever possible because prolonged use of a high FiO$_2$ can damage lungs from the toxic effects of oxygen.* PEEP prevents alveoli from collapsing because the lungs are kept partially inflated so alveolar-capillary gas exchange is promoted throughout the ventilatory cycle. The effect should be an increase in arterial blood oxygenation so the FiO$_2$ can be decreased.

PEEP is "dialed in" on the control panel. The amount of PEEP is usually 5 to 15 cm H$_2$O (although higher PEEP can be used) and is monitored on the peak airway pressure dial, the same dial used to read the PIP. When PEEP is added, the dial does not return to zero at the end of exhalation; rather, it returns to a baseline that is increased from zero by the amount of PEEP applied.

Flow rate is how fast each breath is delivered and is usually set at 40 L/min. *If a patient is agitated or restless, has a widely fluctuating inspiratory pressure reading, or has other signs of air hunger, the flow may be set too low. Increasing the flow should be tried before using chemical restraints.*

Other settings may be used, depending on the type of ventilator and mode of ventilation. Examples include inspiratory and expiratory cycle, waveform, expiratory resistance, and plateau.

Nursing Management. The use of mechanical ventilation involves a collaborative and complex decision-making process for the patient, family, and interprofessional care team. Address the physical and psychological concerns of the patient and family because the mechanical ventilator often causes them anxiety. Explain the purpose of the ventilator and acknowledge the patient's and family's feelings. Encourage the patient and family to express their concerns. Act as the coach to help and support them through this experience. Patients undergoing mechanical ventilation in ICUs often experience delirium, or "ICU psychosis." These patients need frequent, repeated explanations and reassurance.

When caring for a ventilated patient, be concerned with the patient first and the ventilator second. If the ventilator alarm sounds, examine the patient for breathing, color, and oxygen saturation before assessing the ventilator. It is vital to understand *why* mechanical ventilation is needed. Some problems requiring ventilation, such as excessive secretions, sepsis, and trauma, require different interventions to successfully wean from the ventilator. Chronic health problems (e.g., chronic obstructive pulmonary disease, left-sided heart failure, anemia, malnutrition) may slow weaning from mechanical ventilation and require close monitoring and intervention.

> **! NURSING SAFETY PRIORITY** **QSEN**
> *Action Alert*
>
> The nursing priorities in caring for the patient during mechanical ventilation are monitoring and evaluating patient responses, managing the ventilator system safely, and preventing complications.

Monitoring the Patient's Response. Monitor, evaluate, and document the patient's response to the ventilator. Assess vital signs and listen to breath sounds every 30 to 60 minutes at first. Monitor respiratory parameters (e.g., capnography, pulse oximetry) and check ABG values (Carlisle, 2014). Monitoring provides information to guide the patient's activities, such as weaning, physical or occupational therapy, and self-care. Pace activities to ensure effective ventilation with adequate GAS EXCHANGE and oxygenation. Interpret ABG values to evaluate the effectiveness of ventilation and determine whether ventilator settings need to be changed.

Assess the breathing pattern in relation to the ventilatory cycle to determine whether the patient is tolerating or fighting the ventilator. Patient asynchrony with mechanical ventilation has many causes and reduces the effectiveness of GAS EXCHANGE (Mellott et al., 2014). Assess and record breath sounds, including bilateral equal breath sounds, to ensure proper endotracheal (ET) tube placement. Determine the need for suctioning by observing secretions for type, color, and amount. The most common indicator of the need for suctioning is the presence of coarse crackles over the trachea (Sole et al., 2015). Assess the area around the ET tube or tracheostomy site at least every 4 hours for color, tenderness, skin irritation, and drainage, and document the findings.

The nurse spends the most time with the patient and is most likely to be the first person to recognize changes in vital signs or ABG values, fatigue, or distress. If the patient's condition does not respond to current intervention, promptly coordinate with the pulmonary health care provider and respiratory therapist. The pulmonary health care provider may change the prescribed management plan to prevent the patient's condition from deteriorating. The respiratory therapist can most accurately assess the function of the ventilation equipment and make appropriate adjustments or replacements.

> ### ! NURSING SAFETY PRIORITY QSEN
> #### Critical Rescue
>
> Always assess patients being mechanically ventilated for indications of respiratory distress and poor GAS EXCHANGE. When symptoms of respiratory distress develop during mechanical ventilation, respond by immediately removing the ventilator and providing ventilation with a bag-valve-mask device. This action allows quick determination of whether the problem is with the ventilator or the patient.

Serve as a resource for the psychological needs of the patient and family. Anxiety can reduce tolerance for mechanical ventilation. Skilled and sensitive nursing care promotes emotional well-being and synchrony with the ventilator. The patient cannot speak, and communication can be frustrating and anxiety-producing. The patient and family may panic because they believe that the voice has been lost. Reassure them that the ET tube prevents speech only temporarily.

Plan methods of communication to meet the patient's needs, such as a picture board, pen and paper, alphabet board, electronic tablet computer, or programmable speech-generating device. Finding a successful means for communication is important because the patient often feels isolated by the inability to speak (see Chart 29-1). Anticipate his or her needs and provide easy access to frequently used belongings. The observation of facial expressions in noncommunicative patients may indicate pain, especially during suctioning (Darwish et al., 2016; Rahu et al., 2015). Visits from family, friends, and pets and keeping a call light within reach are some ways of giving patients a sense of control over the environment. Urge them to participate in self-care.

Managing the Ventilator System. Ventilator settings are prescribed by the pulmonary health care provider in conjunction with the respiratory therapist. Settings include tidal volume, respiratory rate, fraction of inspired oxygen (Fio$_2$), and mode of ventilation (assist-control [AC] ventilation, synchronized intermittent mandatory ventilation [SIMV], and adjunctive modes such as positive end-expiratory pressure [PEEP], pressure support, or continuous flow).

Perform and document ventilator checks according to the standards of the unit or facility (in many facilities this function is performed by respiratory therapists). Respond promptly to alarms. During a ventilator check, compare the prescribed ventilator settings with the actual settings and confirm these findings with the respiratory therapist. Check the level of water in the humidifier and the temperature of the humidifying system to ensure that they are not too high. Temperature extremes damage the airway mucosa. Remove any condensation

in the ventilator tubing by draining water into drainage collection receptacles and empty them every shift.

> ### ! NURSING SAFETY PRIORITY QSEN
> #### Action Alert
>
> To prevent bacterial contamination, do not allow moisture and water in the ventilator tubing to enter the humidifier.

Mechanical ventilators have alarm systems that warn of a problem with either the patient or the ventilator. **As required by The Joint Commission's NPSGs, alarm systems must be activated and functional at all times. If the cause of the alarm cannot be determined, ventilate the patient manually with a resuscitation bag until the problem is corrected by another health care professional.** Alarms should never be turned off or ignored during mechanical ventilation (Lukasewicz & Mattox, 2015). The major alarms on a ventilator indicate either a high pressure or a low exhaled volume. Table 32-5 lists interventions for causes of ventilator alarms.

Assess and care for the ET or tracheostomy tube. Maintain a patent airway by suctioning when any of these conditions are present:

- Secretions
- Increased peak airway (inspiratory) pressure (PIP)
- Rhonchi
- Decreased breath sounds

Proper care of the ET or tracheostomy tube also ensures a patent airway. *Assess tube position at least every 2 hours, especially when the airway is attached to heavy ventilator tubing that may pull on the tube. Position the ventilator tubing so the patient can move without pulling on the ET or tracheostomy tube, possibly dislodging it.* To detect changes in tube position, mark it where the tube touches the patient's teeth or nose. Give oral care per facility policy. Standardized oral care has been shown to reduce ventilator-associated pneumonia (VAP), specifically using chlorhexidine oral rinses twice daily (Kiyoshi-Teo et al., 2014).

Special attention is needed for the patient being transported while receiving mechanical ventilation. Monitor Spo$_2$ during transport to assess adequacy of GAS EXCHANGE. Assess lung sounds each time the patient is moved, transferred, or turned.

> ### ? NCLEX EXAMINATION CHALLENGE 32-3
> #### Safe and Effective Care Environment
>
> The nurse is trouble-shooting multiple ventilator alarms sounding for a client who is intubated and being mechanically ventilated. The alarms persist despite suctioning, repositioning the client, and ensuring that the ventilator tubing is unobstructed. Which actions will the nurse perform next? **Select all that apply.**
> A. Turn off all ventilator alarms until a cause is found to prevent scaring the client.
> B. Page the primary health care provider to request additional sedation.
> C. Ensure that the endotracheal tube marking is at the client's incisor.
> D. Increase the PEEP to improve GAS EXCHANGE.
> E. Disconnect the client from the ventilator and use the manual resuscitation bag.
> F. Change all ventilator tubing.
> G. Stat page the respiratory therapist.
> H. Determine when the client received the last dose of the paralytic agent.

TABLE 32-5 **Nursing Interventions for Various Causes of Ventilator Alarms**

CAUSE	NURSING INTERVENTIONS
High-Pressure Alarm (sounds when peak inspiratory pressure reaches the set alarm limit [usually set 10-20 mm Hg above the patient's baseline PIP])	
An increased amount of secretions or a mucus plug is in the airways.	Suction as needed.
The patient coughs, gags, or bites on the oral ET tube.	Insert oral airway to prevent biting on the ET tube.
The patient is anxious or fights the ventilator.	Provide emotional support to decrease anxiety. Increase the flow rate. Explain all procedures to the patient. Provide sedation or paralyzing agent as prescribed.
Airway size decreases related to wheezing or bronchospasm.	Auscultate breath sounds. Collaborate with respiratory therapy to provide prescribed bronchodilators.
Pneumothorax occurs.	Alert the pulmonary health care provider or Rapid Response Team about a new onset of decreased breath sounds or unequal chest excursion, which may be caused by pneumothorax. Auscultate breath sounds.
The artificial airway is displaced; the ET tube may have slipped into the right mainstem bronchus.	Assess the chest for unequal breath sounds and chest excursion. Obtain a chest x-ray as prescribed to evaluate the position of the ET tube. After the proper position is verified, secure the tube in place.
Obstruction in tubing occurs because the patient is lying on the tubing or there is water or a kink in the tubing.	Assess the system, beginning with the artificial airway and moving toward the ventilator.
There is increased PIP associated with deliverance of a sigh.	Empty water from the ventilator tubing and remove any kinks. Coordinate with respiratory therapist or pulmonary health care provider to adjust the pressure alarm.
Decreased compliance of the lungs is noted; a trend of gradually increasing PIP is noted over several hours or a day.	Evaluate the reasons for the decreased compliance of the lungs. Increased PIP occurs in ARDS, pneumonia, or any worsening of pulmonary disease.
Low–Exhaled Volume (or Low-Pressure) Alarm (sounds when there is a disconnection or leak in the ventilator circuit or a leak in the patient's artificial airway cuff)	
A leak in the ventilator circuit prevents breath from being delivered.	Assess all connections and all ventilator tubing for disconnection.
The patient stops spontaneous breathing in the SIMV or CPAP mode or on pressure support ventilation.	Evaluate the patient's tolerance of the mode.
A cuff leak occurs in the ET or tracheostomy tube.	Evaluate the patient for a cuff leak. A cuff leak is suspected when the patient can talk (air escapes from the mouth) or when the pilot balloon on the artificial airway is flat (see Tracheostomy Tubes section in Chapter 28).

ARDS, Acute respiratory distress syndrome; *CPAP,* continuous positive airway pressure; *ET,* endotracheal; *PIP,* peak inspiratory pressure; *SIMV,* synchronized intermittent mandatory ventilation.

Preventing Complications. A wide variety of complications, now known as **ventilator-associated events (VAEs),** are defined as "conditions that result in a significant and sustained deterioration in oxygenation (greater than 20% increase in the daily minimum fraction of inspired oxygen or an increase of at least 3 cm H_2O in the daily minimum positive end-expiratory pressure [PEEP] to maintain oxygenation)" (Raoof & Baumann, 2014). Table 32-6 lists the tiers of VAEs. Other complications affecting many body systems are related to positive pressure from the ventilator.

Cardiac problems from mechanical ventilation include hypotension and fluid retention. Hypotension is caused by positive pressure that increases chest pressure and inhibits blood return to the heart. The decreased blood return reduces cardiac output, causing hypotension, especially in patients who are dehydrated or need high PIP for ventilation. Teach the patient to avoid a **Valsalva maneuver** (bearing down while holding the breath).

Fluid is retained because of decreased cardiac output. The kidneys receive less blood flow, which stimulates the renin-angiotensin-aldosterone system to retain fluid. Humidified air

TABLE 32-6 **Tiers of Ventilator-Associated Events**

TIER	CHARACTERISTICS
1. Ventilator-Associated Condition (VAC)	Patient develops hypoxemia for a sustained period of more than 2 days, regardless of its etiology.
2. Infection-Related Ventilator-Associated Complication (IVAC)	Hypoxemia develops in the setting of generalized infection or inflammation, and antibiotics are instituted for a minimum of 4 days.
3. Ventilator-Associated Pneumonia (VAP)	There is additional laboratory evidence of white blood cells or Gram stain of material from a respiratory secretion specimen of acceptable quality and/or presence of respiratory pathogens on quantitative cultures from patients with IVAC.

Adapted from Raoof, S., & Baumann, M. (2014). Ventilator-associated events: The new definition. *American Journal of Critical Care, 23*(1), 7-9.

in the ventilator system contributes to fluid retention. Monitor the patient's fluid intake and output, weight, hydration status, and indications of hypovolemia.

Lung problems from mechanical ventilation include:

- Barotrauma (damage to the lungs by positive pressure)
- Volutrauma (damage to the lung by excess volume delivered to one lung over the other)
- Atelectrauma (shear injury to alveoli from opening and closing)
- Biotrauma (inflammatory response-mediated damage to alveoli)
- Ventilator-associated lung injury/ventilator-induced lung injury (VALI/VILI) (damage from prolonged ventilation causing loss of surfactant, increased inflammation, fluid leakage, and noncardiac pulmonary edema)
- Acid-base imbalance

Barotrauma includes pneumothorax, subcutaneous emphysema, and pneumomediastinum. Patients at highest risk for barotrauma have chronic airflow limitation (CAL), have blebs or bullae, are on PEEP, have dynamic hyperinflation, or require high pressures to ventilate the lungs (because of "stiff" lungs, as seen in acute respiratory distress syndrome [ARDS]). Ventilator-induced lung injury can be prevented by using low tidal volumes combined with moderate levels of PEEP, especially in patients with acute lung injury (ALI) or ARDS. Blood gas problems can be corrected by ventilator changes and adjustment of fluid and electrolyte imbalances.

GI and nutrition problems result from the stress of mechanical ventilation. Stress ulcers occur in many patients receiving mechanical ventilation. These ulcers complicate the nutrition status and, because the mucosa is not intact, increase the risk for systemic infection. Antacids, sucralfate (Carafate, Sulcrate ✦), and histamine blockers such as ranitidine (Zantac) or proton-pump inhibitors such as esomeprazole (Nexium) may be prescribed as soon as the patient is intubated. Because many other acute or life-threatening events occur at the same time, nutrition is often neglected. Malnutrition is an extreme problem for these patients and is a cause of failing to wean from the ventilator. In malnutrition, the respiratory muscles lose mass and strength. The diaphragm, the major muscle of inspiration, is affected early. When it and other respiratory muscles are weak, ineffective breathing results, fatigue occurs, and the patient cannot be weaned.

Balanced nutrition, whether by diet, enteral feedings, or parenteral feeding, is essential during ventilation and is often started within 48 hours of intubation. In addition, nutrition for the patient with chronic obstructive pulmonary disease (COPD) requires a reduction of dietary carbohydrates. During metabolism, carbohydrates are broken down to glucose, which then produces energy, carbon dioxide, and water. Excessive carbohydrate loads increase carbon dioxide production, which the patient with COPD may be unable to exhale. Hypercarbic respiratory failure results. Nutrition formulas with a higher fat content (e.g., Pulmocare, Nutri-Vent, Intralipid) are calorie sources to combat this problem.

Electrolyte replacement is also important because electrolytes influence muscle function. Monitor potassium, calcium, magnesium, and phosphate levels and replace them as prescribed.

Infections are part of two tiers of ventilator-associated events (VAEs) and are a threat for the patient using a ventilator, especially ventilator-associated pneumonia (VAP). The ET or tracheostomy tube bypasses the body's filtering process and provides a direct access for bacteria to enter the lower respiratory system. The artificial airway is colonized with bacteria within 48 hours, which promotes pneumonia development and increases morbidity. Aspiration of colonized fluid from the mouth or stomach can be a source of infection. *Infection prevention through strict adherence to infection control, especially handwashing during suctioning and care of the tracheostomy or ET tube, is essential (Kiyoshi-Teo et al., 2014).*

To prevent VAP, implement "ventilator bundle" sets, which typically include these actions (Munro & Ruggiero, 2014):

- Keeping the head of the bed elevated at least 30 degrees
- Performing oral care per agency policy (usually brushing teeth every 8 hours and antimicrobial rinse [chlorhexidine] every 2 hours)
- Ulcer prophylaxis
- Preventing aspiration
- Pulmonary hygiene, including chest physiotherapy, postural drainage, and turning and positioning

Using the ventilator bundle has greatly reduced the overall incidence of VAP. Vigilant oral care is a key component of the VAP prevention strategy, although actual practice varies regarding timing, products used, and specific application methods (Kiyoshi-Teo et al., 2014; Wong et al., 2016). Additional information on pneumonia can be found in Chapter 31.

Muscle deconditioning and weakness can occur because of immobility. Getting the patient out of bed and having him or her ambulate with help and perform exercises not only improve muscle strength but also boost morale, enhance GAS EXCHANGE, and promote oxygen delivery to all muscles. Early progressive mobility decreases ventilator days and ICU stays. Early passive exercise also may be beneficial (Amidei & Sole, 2013).

Ventilator dependence is the inability to wean off the ventilator and can have both a physiologic and a psychological basis. The longer a patient uses a ventilator, the more difficult the weaning process is because the respiratory muscles fatigue and cannot assume breathing. The health care team uses every method of weaning before a patient is declared "unweanable."

Collaborate with the pulmonologist, social worker or psychologist, and a member of the clergy to discuss with the patient and family the patient's quality of life, goals, and values. As a result of this discussion, arrange for home ventilation, nursing home placement, or withdrawal of life support (in terminal cases). Special units and facilities can maximize the rehabilitation and weaning of ventilator-dependent patients.

Weaning. Weaning is the process of going from ventilatory dependence to spontaneous breathing. The process is prolonged by complications. Many problems can be avoided with appropriate nursing care. For example, turning and positioning the patient not only promote comfort and prevent skin breakdown but also improve GAS EXCHANGE and prevent pneumonia and atelectasis. Table 32-7 lists various weaning techniques.

Extubation. Extubation is the removal of the endotracheal (ET) tube. The tube is removed when the need for intubation has been resolved. Before removal, explain the procedure. Set up the prescribed oxygen delivery system at the bedside and bring in the equipment for emergency reintubation. Hyperoxygenate the patient and thoroughly suction both the ET tube and the oral cavity. Then rapidly deflate the cuff of the ET tube and remove the tube at peak inspiration. Immediately instruct the patient to cough. It is normal for large amounts of oral secretions to collect. Give oxygen by facemask or nasal cannula. The

TABLE 32-7 Weaning Methods

Synchronous Intermittent Mandatory Ventilation

- The patient breathes between the machine's preset breaths/min rate.
- The machine is initially set on an SIMV rate of 12, meaning that the patient receives a minimum of 12 breaths/min by the ventilator.
- The patient's respiratory rate will be a combination of ventilator breaths and spontaneous breaths.
- As the weaning process ensues, the pulmonary health care provider prescribes gradual decreases in the SIMV rate, usually at a decrease of 1 to 2 breaths/min.

T-Piece Technique

- The patient is taken off the ventilator for short periods (initially 5 to 10 minutes) and allowed to breathe spontaneously.
- The ventilator is replaced with a T-piece (see Chapter 28) or CPAP, which delivers humidified oxygen.
- The prescribed FiO_2 may be higher for the patient on the T-piece than on the ventilator.
- Weaning progresses as the patient can tolerate progressively longer periods off the ventilator.
- Nighttime weaning is not usually attempted until the patient can maintain spontaneous respirations most of the day.

Pressure Support Ventilation

- PSV allows the patient's respiratory effort to be augmented by a predetermined pressure assist from the ventilator.
- As the weaning process ensues, the amount of pressure applied to inspiration is gradually decreased.
- Another method of weaning with PSV is to maintain the pressure but gradually decrease the ventilator's preset breaths/min rate.

CPAP, Continuous positive airway pressure; *FiO₂,* fraction of inspired oxygen; *PSV,* pressure support ventilation; *SIMV,* synchronized intermittent mandatory ventilation.

CONSIDERATIONS FOR OLDER ADULTS
Patient-Centered Care QSEN

The older patient, especially one who has smoked or who has a chronic lung problem such as COPD, is at risk for ventilator dependence and failure to wean. Age-related changes, such as chest wall stiffness, reduced ventilatory muscle strength, and decreased lung elasticity, reduce the likelihood of weaning. The usual symptoms of ventilatory failure—hypoxemia and hypercarbia—may be less obvious in the older adult. Use other clinical measures of GAS EXCHANGE and oxygenation, such as a change in mental status, to determine breathing effectiveness (Touhy & Jett, 2016).

fraction of inspired oxygen (FiO_2) is usually prescribed at 10% higher than the level used while the ET tube was in place.

Monitor vital signs after extubation every 5 minutes at first and assess the ventilatory pattern for signs of respiratory distress. It is common for patients to be hoarse and have a sore throat for a few days after extubation. Teach the patient to sit in a semi-Fowler's position, take deep breaths every half-hour, use an incentive spirometer every 2 hours, and limit speaking. These measures help improve GAS EXCHANGE, decrease laryngeal edema, and reduce vocal cord irritation. Observe closely for respiratory fatigue and airway obstruction.

Early symptoms of obstruction are mild dyspnea, coughing, and the inability to expectorate secretions. Stridor is a high-pitched, crowing noise during inspiration caused by laryngospasm or edema around the glottis. It is a late sign of a narrowed airway and requires prompt attention. Racemic epinephrine, a topical aerosol vasoconstrictor, is given, and reintubation may be needed.

⚠ NURSING SAFETY PRIORITY QSEN
Critical Rescue

Monitor the patient frequently to recognize symptoms of obstruction. When stridor or other symptoms of obstruction occur after extubation, respond by immediately calling the Rapid Response Team *before* the airway becomes completely obstructed.

CHEST TRAUMA

Chest injuries are responsible for or contribute to many traumatic deaths in the United States each year. Many of the injured die before arriving at the hospital. Few types of chest injury require thoracotomy. Most can be treated with basic resuscitation, intubation, or chest tube placement. *The first emergency approach to all chest injuries is ABC (airway, breathing, circulation), a rapid assessment and treatment of life-threatening conditions.* See Chapter 8 for more information on care of the trauma patient.

PULMONARY CONTUSION

Pulmonary contusion, a potentially lethal injury, is a common chest injury and occurs most often by rapid deceleration during car crashes. After a contusion, respiratory failure can develop immediately or over time. Hemorrhage and edema occur in and between the alveoli, reducing both lung movement and the area available for GAS EXCHANGE. Localized inflammation can cause further damage. The patient becomes hypoxemic and dyspneic.

Patients may be asymptomatic at first and can later develop various degrees of respiratory failure and possibly pneumonia (Landeen & Smith, 2014). These patients often have decreased breath sounds or crackles and wheezes over the affected area. Other symptoms include bruising over the injury, dry cough, tachycardia, tachypnea, and dullness to percussion. At first the chest x-ray may show no abnormalities. A hazy opacity in the lobes or parenchyma may develop over several days. If there is no disruption of the parenchyma, bruise resorption often occurs without treatment.

Management includes maintenance of ventilation and GAS EXCHANGE. Provide oxygen, give IV fluids as prescribed, and place the patient in a moderate-Fowler's position. If a high FiO_2 is needed, oxygen may be administered using a high-flow nasal cannula (HFNC). When side-lying, the "good lung down" position may be helpful. The patient in obvious respiratory distress may need noninvasive positive-pressure ventilation (NPPV) or mechanical ventilation with positive end-expiratory pressure (PEEP) to inflate the lungs.

A vicious cycle occurs in which more muscle effort is needed for ventilating a lung with a contusion and the patient becomes progressively hypoxemic. This situation causes him or her to tire easily, have reduced GAS EXCHANGE, and become more fatigued and hypoxemic. This condition often leads to acute respiratory distress syndrome (ARDS).

RIB FRACTURE

Rib fractures are a common injury to the chest wall, often resulting from direct blunt trauma to the chest. The force applied to the ribs fractures them and drives the bone ends into the chest. Thus there is a risk for deep chest injury such as pulmonary contusion, pneumothorax, and hemothorax.

The patient has pain on movement and splints the chest defensively. Splinting reduces breathing depth and clearance of secretions. If the patient has pre-existing lung disease, the risk for atelectasis and pneumonia increases. Those with injuries to the first or second ribs, flail chest, seven or more fractured ribs, or expired volumes of less than 15 mL/kg often have a deep chest injury and a poor prognosis.

Management of uncomplicated rib fractures is simple because the fractured ribs reunite spontaneously. The chest is usually not splinted by tape or other materials. The main focus is to decrease pain so adequate GAS EXCHANGE is maintained. An intercostal nerve block may be used if pain is severe. Analgesics that cause respiratory depression are avoided.

FLAIL CHEST

Flail chest is the result of fractures of at least two neighboring ribs in two or more places causing **paradoxical chest wall movement** (inward movement of the thorax during inspiration, with outward movement during expiration) (Fig. 32-4). It usually involves one side of the chest and results from blunt chest trauma—often high-speed car crashes. Because the force required to produce a flail chest is great, it is important to assess for other possible underlying injuries (Poirier & Vacca, 2013).

Flail chest can also occur from bilateral separations of the ribs from their cartilage connections to each other anteriorly, without an actual rib fracture. This condition can occur as a complication of cardiopulmonary resuscitation. Other injuries to the lung tissue under the flail segment may be present. GAS EXCHANGE, coughing, and clearance of secretions are impaired. Splinting further reduces the patient's ability to

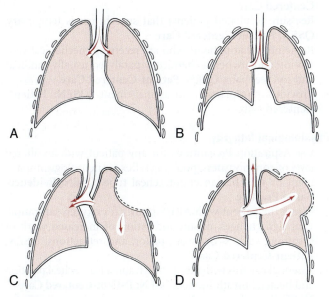

FIG. 32-4 Flail chest. Normal respiration: **A,** Inspiration; **B,** Expiration. Paradoxical motion; **C,** Inspiration—area of the lung underlying unstable chest wall sucks in on inspiration; **D,** Expiration—unstable area balloons out. Note movement of mediastinum toward opposite lung during inspiration. (From McCance, K. L., Huether S. E., Brashers, V. L., & Rote, N. S. (2014). *Pathophysiology: The biologic basis for disease in adults and children* (7th ed.). St. Louis: Mosby.)

exert the extra effort to breathe and may contribute later to failure to wean.

Assess the patient with a flail chest for paradoxical chest movement, dyspnea, cyanosis, tachycardia, and hypotension. The patient is often anxious, short of breath, and in pain. Work of breathing is increased from the paradoxical movement of the involved segment of the chest wall.

Interventions include humidified oxygen, pain management, promotion of lung expansion through deep breathing and positioning, and secretion clearance by coughing and tracheal suction.

The patient with a flail chest may be managed with vigilant respiratory care. Mechanical ventilation is needed if respiratory failure or shock occurs. Monitor ABG values and vital capacity closely. With severe hypoxemia and hypercarbia, the patient is intubated and mechanically ventilated with PEEP. With lung contusion or an underlying pulmonary disease, the risk for respiratory failure increases. Usually flail chest is stabilized by positive-pressure ventilation. Surgical stabilization is used only in extreme cases of flail chest (Messing et al., 2014).

Monitor the patient's vital signs and fluid and electrolyte balance closely so hypovolemia or shock can be managed immediately. If he or she has a lung contusion, provide oxygen as needed and give IV fluids as prescribed. Assess for and relieve pain with prescribed analgesic drugs by IV, epidural, or nerve block route. Give psychosocial support to the anxious patient by explaining all procedures, talking slowly, and allowing time for expression of feelings and concerns.

PNEUMOTHORAX AND HEMOTHORAX

❖ *PATHOPHYSIOLOGY*

A **pneumothorax** is air in the pleural space causing a loss of negative pressure in chest cavity, a rise in chest pressure, and a reduction in vital capacity, which can lead to a lung collapse (Arsbad et al., 2016). It is often caused by blunt chest trauma and may occur with some degree of **hemothorax**, which is bleeding into the chest cavity. It can also occur as a complication of medical procedures. (A *simple* hemothorax is a blood loss of less than 1000 mL into the chest cavity; a *massive* hemothorax is a blood loss of more than 1000 mL.) The pneumothorax can be *open* (pleural cavity is exposed to outside air, as through an open wound in the chest wall) or *closed* (such as when a patient with chronic obstructive pulmonary disease has a spontaneous pneumothorax).

A **tension pneumothorax** is a life-threatening complication of pneumothorax in which air continues to enter the pleural space during inspiration and does not exit during expiration (Loftus, 2014). As a result, air collects under pressure, completely collapsing the lung and compressing blood vessels, which limits blood return. This process leads to decreased filling of the heart and reduced cardiac output. *If not promptly detected and treated, tension pneumothorax is quickly fatal.*

❖ *INTERPROFESSIONAL COLLABORATIVE CARE*
◆ *Assessment: Noticing*

Assessment findings for any type of pneumothorax commonly include:

- Reduced (or absent) breath sounds of the affected side on auscultation
- Hyperresonance on percussion

- Prominence of the involved side of the chest, which moves poorly with respirations
- When severe, deviation of the trachea *away* from the midline and side of injury toward the *unaffected* side (indicating pushing of tissues to the unaffected side [a *mediastinal shift*] from increasing pressure within the injured side)

For tension pneumothorax, additional assessment findings also may include:

- Extreme respiratory distress and cyanosis
- Distended neck veins
- Hemodynamic instability

With a hemothorax, percussion on the involved side produces a dull sound.

In addition to symptoms, chest x-rays, CT scans, or ultrasonography may be used for diagnosis of any type of pneumothorax or hemothorax.

◆ Interventions: Responding

For a stable patient with a small pneumothorax who has mild symptoms and no continuing air leak, no treatment may be needed. For more severe pneumothorax, tension pneumothorax, and hemothorax, chest tube therapy is essential. Chest tube management is discussed in detail in Chapter 30.

Initial management of a tension pneumothorax is an immediate needle thoracostomy, with a large-bore needle inserted by the primary health care provider into the second intercostal space in the midclavicular line of the affected side. A chest tube then is placed into the fourth intercostal space, and the other end is attached to a water-seal drainage system until the lung re-inflates. Interventions for hemothorax include chest tube placement to remove the blood in the pleural space to normalize breathing and prevent infection.

Closely monitor the chest tube drainage. Serial chest x-rays are used to determine treatment effectiveness. Other care includes pain control, pulmonary hygiene, and continued assessment for respiratory failure.

An open thoracotomy is needed when there is initial blood loss of 1000 mL from the chest or persistent bleeding at the rate of 150 to 200 mL/hr over 3 to 4 hours. Monitor the vital signs, blood loss, and intake and output. Assess the patient's response to the chest tubes and infuse IV fluids and blood as prescribed. The blood lost through chest drainage can be infused back into the patient after processing if needed.

GET READY FOR THE NCLEX® EXAMINATION!

■ KEY POINTS

Review these Key Points for each NCLEX Examination Client Needs Category.

Safe and Effective Care Environment

- Use aseptic technique when caring for a patient requiring pulmonary suctioning. **QSEN: Safety**
- Identify patients in your setting who are at risk for developing a pulmonary embolism. **QSEN: Safety**
- Use Bleeding Precautions for patients receiving anti-clotting therapy (see Chart 32-6). **QSEN: Safety**
- Keep antidotes available when patients are receiving heparin (antidote is protamine) or warfarin (antidote is phytonadione). **QSEN: Safety**
- Inspect the mouth and perform oral care every 2 hours for anyone who has an endotracheal tube or is being mechanically ventilated. **QSEN: Safety**
- Check and document ventilator settings hourly. **QSEN: Safety**
- Ensure that alarm systems on mechanical ventilators are activated and functional at all times. **QSEN: Safety**
- Ensure that bag-valve-mask device and suction equipment are at the bedside at all times. **QSEN: Safety**
- Evaluate the need for chemical restraint or soft wrist restraints. **QSEN: Patient-Centered Care**

Health Promotion and Maintenance

- Teach patients ways to promote venous return and avoid venous thromboembolism (VTE), especially when traveling long distances (see Chart 32-1). **QSEN: Patient-Centered Care**
- Teach patients ways to prevent injury when taking drugs that reduce CLOTTING (see Chart 32-7). **QSEN: Patient-Centered Care**

Psychosocial Integrity

- Allow the patient and family members the opportunity to express feelings and concerns about a change in breathing status or the possibility of intubation and mechanical ventilation. **QSEN: Patient-Centered Care**
- Use alternate ways to communicate with a patient who is intubated or being mechanically ventilated. **QSEN: Patient-Centered Care**
- Reassure intubated patients that speech loss is temporary. **QSEN: Patient-Centered Care**
- Remember that patients who are receiving mechanical ventilation and are being chemically paralyzed usually can hear and can feel pain. **QSEN: Patient-Centered Care**
- Provide appropriate pain management. **QSEN: Patient-Centered Care**

Physiological Integrity

- Use Aspiration Precautions for any patient with an altered level of consciousness, poor gag reflex, or neurologic impairment or who has an endotracheal tube. **QSEN: Evidence-Based Practice**
- Check the patient with ARDS hourly for oxygen saturation, vital sign changes, or any indication of increased work of breathing such as cyanosis, pallor, and retractions. **QSEN: Patient-Centered Care**
- Assess all patients with blunt chest trauma for tracheal position and bilateral breath sounds. **QSEN: Patient-Centered Care**
- Notify the pulmonary health care provider immediately for any patient who develops sudden-onset respiratory difficulty. **QSEN: Safety**
- Check GAS EXCHANGE by pulse oximetry for any patient who has trouble breathing or who develops acute confusion. **QSEN: Patient-Centered Care**

- Evaluate ABG values to assess the severity of hypoxia and the patient's response to therapy. **QSEN: Patient-Centered Care**
- Apply oxygen to anyone who is hypoxemic. **QSEN: Evidence-Based Practice**
- Ensure that oxygen therapy delivered to the patient is humidified. **QSEN: Evidence-Based Practice**
- Assess lung sounds bilaterally each hour for patients who are receiving PEEP. **QSEN: Patient-Centered Care**
- Check all ventilator settings against the prescription at least once per shift. **QSEN: Safety**

- Administer drugs for pain to patients who have rib fractures and encourage deep breaths. **QSEN: Patient-Centered Care**
- Evaluate nutrition status and collaborate with the dietitian to meet the patient's nutrition needs. **QSEN: Teamwork and Collaboration**
- If a patient experiences respiratory distress during mechanical ventilation, remove him or her from the ventilator and provide ventilation by bag-valve-mask device. **QSEN: Safety**

SELECTED BIBLIOGRAPHY

Ambutas, S., Staffileno, B., & Fogg, L. (2014). Reducing nasal pressure ulcers with an alternative taping device. *Medsurg Nursing, 23*(2), 96–100.

Amidei, C., & Sole, M. (2013). Physiological responses to passive exercise in adults receiving mechanical ventilation. *American Journal of Critical Care, 22*(4), 337–348.

ARDS Foundation. (2016). *Acute Respiratory Distress Syndrome.* http://www.ardsfoundationil.com/acute-respiratory-distress-syndrome.htm.

Arsbad, H., Young, M., Adyrty, R., & Singh, A. (2016). Acute pneumothorax. *Critical Care Nursing Quarterly, 39*(2), 176–189.

Aust, M. (2014). Compact clinical guide to mechanical ventilation: Foundations of practice for critical care nurses. *Critical Care Nurse, 34*(2), 80.

Bull, A. (2014). Primary care of chronic dyspnea in adults. *The Nurse Practitioner, 39*(8), 34–40.

Burchum, J., & Rosenthal, L. (2016). *Lehne's pharmacology for nursing care* (9th ed.). St. Louis: Elsevier.

Carlisle, H. (2014). The case for capnography in patients receiving opioids. *American Nurse Today, 9*(9), 22–26.

Centers for Disease Control and Prevention (CDC). (2015). *Venous thromboembolism (blood clots): Data & statistics.* http://www.cdc.gov/ncbddd/dvt/data.html.

Chowdhury, M., Moza, A., Siddiqui, N., Bonnell, M., & Cooper, C. (2015). Emergent echocardiography and extracorporeal membrane oxygenation: Lifesaving in massive pulmonary embolism. *Heart and Lung: The Journal of Critical Care, 44*(4), 344–346.

Chudow, M., Carter, M., & Rumbak, M. (2015). Pharmacological treatments for acute respiratory distress syndrome. *AACN Advanced Critical Care, 26*(3), 185–191.

Covert, T., & Niu, N. (2014). Differential diagnosis of high peak airway pressures. *Dimensions of Critical Care Nursing, 34*(1), 19–23.

Darwish, Z., Hamdi, R., & Fallatah, S. (2016). Evaluation of pain assessment tools in patients receiving mechanical ventilation. *AACN Advanced Critical Care, 27*(2), 162–172.

Drahnak, D., & Custer, N. (2015). Prone positioning of patients with acute respiratory distress syndrome. *Critical Care Nurse, 35*(6), 29–36.

Happ, M., Seaman, J., Nilsen, M., Sciulli, A., Tate, J., Saul, M., et al. (2015). The number of mechanically ventilated ICU patients meeting communication criteria. *Heart and Lung: The Journal of Critical Care, 44*(1), 45–49.

Howe, K., Clochesy, J., Goldstein, L., & Owen, H. (2015). Mechanical ventilation antioxidant trial. *American Journal of Critical Care, 24*(5), 440–445.

Kiyoshi-Teo, H., Cabana, M. O., Froelicher, E. S., & Blegen, M. A. (2014). Adherence to institution-specific ventilator-associated pneumonia prevention guidelines. *American Journal of Critical Care, 23*(3), 201–215.

Lacoske, J. (2015). Sedation options for intubated intensive care unit patients. *Critical Care Nursing Clinics of North America, 27*, 131–145.

Lamba, T., Sharara, R., Singh, A., & Balaan, M. (2016). Pathophysiology and classification of respiratory failure. *Critical Care Nursing Quarterly, 39*(2), 85–93.

Landeen, C., & Smith, H. L. (2014). Examination of pneumonia risks and risk levels in trauma patients with pulmonary contusion. *Journal of Trauma Nursing, 21*(2), 41–49.

Lee, A. (2014). Factor V Leiden. *Nursing, 44*(6), 10–12.

Lizy, C., Swinnen, W., Labeau, S., Poelaert, J., Vogelaers, D., Vandewoude, K., et al. (2014). Cuff pressure of endotracheal tubes after changes in body position in critically ill patients treated with mechanical ventilation. *American Journal of Critical Care, 23*(1), e1–e8.

Loftus, T. (2014). Touch and go for a patient with a pneumothorax. *American Nurse Today, 9*(3), 11.

Lukasewicz, C., & Mattox, E. (2015). Understanding clinical alarm safety. *Critical Care Nurse, 35*(4), 45–57.

McCance, K., Huether, S., Brashers, V., & Rote, N. (2014). *Pathophysiology: The biologic basis for disease in adults and children* (7th ed.). St. Louis: Mosby.

Mellott, K. G., Grap, M., Munro, C. L., Sessler, C. N., Wetzel, P. A., Nilsestuen, J. O., et al. (2014). Patient ventilator asynchrony in critically ill adults: Frequency and types. *Heart and Lung: The Journal of Critical Care, 43*(3), 231–243.

Messing, J. A., Gail, V., & Sarani, B. (2014). Successful management of severe flail chest via early operative intervention. *Journal of Trauma Nursing, 21*(2), 83–85.

Moore, D. (2016). Fat embolism threatens a patient's life. *American Nurse Today, 11*(5), 26.

Munro, N., & Ruggiero, M. (2014). Ventilator-associated pneumonia bundle. *AACN Advanced Critical Care, 25*(2), 163–178.

Online Mendelian Inheritance in Man (OMIM). (2015). *Coagulation factor V; F5.* www.omim.org/entry/612309.

Pagana, K., Pagana, T. J., & Pagana, T. N. (2017). *Mosby's diagnostic and laboratory test reference* (13th ed.). St. Louis: Mosby.

Poirier, W., & Vacca, V. (2013). Flail chest. *Nursing, 43*(12), 10–11.

Rahu, M., Grap, M., Furgusin, P., Joseph, P., Sherman, S., & Elswick, R. (2015). Validity and sensitivity of 6 pain scales in critically ill intubated adults. *American Journal of Critical Care, 24*(6), 514–524.

Rali, P., Gandhi, V., & Malik, K. (2016). Pulmonary embolism. *Critical Care Nursing Quarterly, 39*(2), 131–138.

Raoof, S., & Baumann, M. (2014). Ventilator-associated events: The new definition. *American Journal of Critical Care, 23*(1), 7–9.

Schell-Chaple, H., Puntillo, K., Matthay, M., Liu, K., & the National Heart, Lung, and Blood Institute Acute Respiratory Distress Syndrome Network. (2015). Body temperature and mortality in patients with acute respiratory distress syndrome. *American Journal of Critical Care, 24*(1), 15–23.

Schulman, C., Bibro, C., Downey, D., & Lasich, C. (2014). Transferring patients with refractory hypoxemia to a regional extracorporeal membrane oxygenation center. *AACN Advanced Critical Care, 25*(4), 351–364.

Senecal, P. (2015). Prone position for acute respiratory distress syndrome. *Critical Care Nurse, 35*(4), 72–74.

Sole, M., Bennett, M., & Ashworth, S. (2015). Clinical indicators for endotracheal suctioning in adult patients receiving mechanical ventilation. *American Journal of Critical Care, 24*(4), 318–325.

Touhy, T., & Jett, K. (2016). *Ebersole and Hess' toward healthy aging: Human needs & nursing response* (9th ed.). St. Louis: Mosby.

United States National Library of Medicine. (2016). *Genetics Home Reference: Factor V Leiden thrombophilia.* http://ghr.nlm.nih.gov/condition/factor-v-leiden-thrombophilia.

Wilbeck, J., & Evans, D. (2015). Acute chest pain and pulmonary embolism. *The Nurse Practitioner, 40*(1), 43–45.

Wong, T., Schlichting, A., Stoltze, A., Fuller, B., Peacock, A., Harland, K., et al. (2016). No decrease in early ventilator-associated pneumonia after early use of chlorhexidine. *American Journal of Critical Care, 25*(2), 173–177.

York, N., Kane, C., Smith, C., & Minton, L. (2015). Care of the patient with an acute pulmonary embolism. *Dimensions of Critical Care Nursing, 34*(1), 3–9.

A

abdominal acute compartment syndrome (AACS) A complication after abdominal trauma that occurs when the intraabdominal pressure is sustained at greater than 200 mm Hg.

abdominoperineal (AP) resection The surgical removal of the sigmoid colon, rectum, and anus through combined abdominal and perineal incisions. This resection is performed when rectal tumors are present.

ablative The process or act of removing.

abscess A localized collection of pus caused by an inflammatory response to bacteria in tissues or organs.

absolute neutrophil count (ANC) The percentage and actual number of mature circulating neutrophils; used to measure a patient's risk for infection. The higher the numbers, the greater the resistance to infection.

absorption The uptake from the intestinal lumen of nutrients produced by digestion.

acalculia Difficulty with math calculations; caused by brain injury or disease.

acalculous cholecystitis Inflammation of the gallbladder occurring in the absence of gallstones; typically associated with biliary stasis caused by any condition that affects the regular filling or emptying of the gallbladder.

acceleration-deceleration Types of forces that involve rapid or sudden movement forward and then backward.

acclimatization The process of adapting to a high altitude; involves physiologic changes that help the body compensate for less available oxygen in the atmosphere.

accommodation The process of maintaining a clear visual image when the gaze is shifted from a distant object to a near object. The eye adjusts its focus by changing the curvature of the lens.

achlorhydria The absence of hydrochloric acid from gastric secretions.

acid A substance that releases hydrogen ions when dissolved in water. The strength of an acid is measured by how easily it releases hydrogen ions in solution.

acid-base balance The maintenance of arterial blood pH between 7.35 and 7.45 through control of hydrogen ion production and elimination.

acidosis An acid-base imbalance in which blood pH is below normal.

acinus The structural unit of the lower respiratory tract consisting of a respiratory bronchiole, an alveolar duct, and an alveolar sac.

Acorn cardiac support device A polyester mesh jacket that is placed over the ventricles to provide support and to avoid overstretching the myocardial muscle in the patient with heart failure; reduces heart muscle hypertrophy and assists with improvement of ejection fraction.

acoustic neuroma A benign tumor of cranial nerve VIII; symptoms include damage to hearing, facial movements, and sensation. The tumor can enlarge into the brain, damaging structures in the cerebellum.

active euthanasia Purposeful action that directly causes death; not supported by most professional organizations, including the American Nurses Association.

active immunity Resistance to infection that occurs when the body responds to an invading antigen by making specific antibodies against the antigen. Immunity lasts for years and is natural by infection or artificial by stimulation (e.g., vaccine) of the body's immune defenses.

active surveillance (AS) Observation for cancer without immediate active treatment.

activities of daily living (ADLs) The activities performed in the course of a normal day, such as bathing, dressing, feeding, and ambulating.

activity therapist See *recreational therapist.*

acute Having relatively greater intensity; marked by a sudden onset and short duration.

acute adrenal insufficiency A life-threatening event in which the need for cortisol and aldosterone is greater than the available supply. Also called *addisonian crisis.*

acute arterial occlusion The sudden blockage of an artery, typically in the lower extremity, in the patient with chronic peripheral arterial disease.

acute compartment syndrome (ACS) A complication of a fracture characterized by increased pressure within one or more compartments and causing massive compromise of circulation to the area. Compartments are sheaths of inelastic fascia that support and partition muscles, blood vessels, and nerves in the body.

acute coronary syndrome (ACS) A disorder, including unstable angina and myocardial infarction, that results from obstruction of the coronary artery by ruptured atherosclerotic plaque and leads to platelet aggregation, thrombus formation, and vasoconstriction.

acute gastritis Inflammation of the gastric mucosa or submucosa after exposure to local irritants. Various degrees of mucosal necrosis and inflammatory reaction occur in acute disease. Complete regeneration and healing usually occur within a few days.

acute glomerulonephritis Inflammation of the glomerulus that develops suddenly from an excess immunity response within the kidney tissues.

acute hematogenous infection An infection resulting from bacteremia, disease, or nonpenetrating trauma that is disseminated by the blood through the circulation.

acute kidney injury (AKI) A rapid decrease in kidney function, leading to the collection of metabolic wastes in the body; formerly called *acute renal failure (ARF).*

acute pain The unpleasant sensory and emotional experience associated with tissue damage that results from acute injury, disease, or surgery.

acute pancreatitis A serious inflammation of the pancreas characterized by a sudden onset of abdominal pain, nausea, and vomiting. It is caused by premature activation of pancreatic enzymes that destroy ductal tissue and pancreatic cells and results in autodigestion and fibrosis of the pancreas.

acute paronychia Inflammation of the skin around the nail, which usually occurs with a torn cuticle or an ingrown toenail.

acute pericarditis An inflammation or alteration of the pericardium, the membranous sac that encloses the heart; may be fibrous, serous, hemorrhagic, purulent, or neoplastic.

acute pyelonephritis Active bacterial infection in the kidney.

acute respiratory distress syndrome (ARDS) Respiratory failure marked by hypoxemia that persists even when 100% oxygen is given, as well as decreased pulmonary compliance, dyspnea, noncardiac-associated bilateral pulmonary edema, and dense pulmonary infiltrates on x-ray.

acute sialadenitis Inflammation of a salivary gland; can be caused by infectious agents, irradiation, or immunologic disorders.

acute-on-chronic kidney disease A condition in which acute kidney injury occurs in addition to chronic kidney disease.

adaptive immunity The immunity that a person's body makes (or can receive) as an adaptive response to invasion by organisms or foreign proteins; occurs either naturally or artificially through lymphocyte responses and can be either active or passive.

addisonian crisis Acute adrenal insufficiency; a life-threatening event in which the need for cortisol and aldosterone is greater than the available supply.

adenocarcinoma Tumor that arises from the glandular epithelial tissue.

adenohypophysis The anterior lobe of the pituitary gland, which makes up about 70% of the gland.

adiponectin An anti-inflammatory and insulin-sensitizing hormone.

adipose Fatty.

adjuvant therapy Chemotherapy that is used along with surgery or radiation.

adjuvant A substance that aids another substance, such as a cancer treatment that uses chemotherapy in addition to surgery.

adrenal crisis Acute adrenocortical insufficiency, which can be life threatening.

adrenal Cushing's disease An excess of glucocorticoids caused by a problem in the adrenal cortex, usually a benign tumor (adrenal adenoma). This usually occurs in only one adrenal gland.

advance directive (AD) A written document prepared by a competent person to specify what, if any, extraordinary actions he or she would want when no longer able to make decisions about personal health care.

adverse drug event (ADE) An unintended harmful reaction to an administered drug.

adverse events Variations in the standard of care that are usually below the standard.

aerosolization Transmission via fine airborne droplets.

aesthetic plastic surgery Plastic surgery that is cosmetic and aims to alter a person's physical appearance.

afferent arteriole The smallest, most distal portion of the renal arterial system that supplies blood to the nephron. From the afferent arteriole, blood flows into the glomerulus, a series of specialized capillary loops.

after-drop A continued decrease in core body temperature after a victim is removed from a cold environment; results from equilibration of core and peripheral blood temperature and countercurrent cooling of the blood perfusing cold tissue.

afterload The pressure or resistance that the ventricles must overcome to eject blood through the semilunar valves and into the peripheral blood vessels; the amount of resistance is directly related to arterial blood pressure and blood vessel diameter.

agglutination A clumping action that results during the antibody-binding process when antibodies link antigens together to form large and small immune complexes.

agnosia A general term for a loss of sensory comprehension; may include an inability to write, comprehend reading material, or use an object correctly.

agraphia Loss of the ability to write; caused by brain injury or disease.

Airborne Precautions Infection control guidelines from the U.S. Centers for Disease Control and Prevention; used for patients with infections spread by the airborne transmission route, such as tuberculosis. Negative airflow rooms are required to prevent the airborne spread of microbes.

akinesia Slow or no movement, as seen in a patient with Parkinson disease. Also called *bradykinesia.*

albuminuria The presence of albumin in the urine.

alcoholic hepatitis Liver inflammation caused by the toxic effect of alcohol on hepatocytes. The liver becomes enlarged, with cellular degeneration and infiltration by fat, leukocytes, and lymphocytes.

aldosterone The chief mineralocorticoid produced by the adrenal cortex. Aldosterone increases kidney reabsorption of sodium and water, thus restoring blood pressure, blood volume, and blood sodium levels. Aldosterone secretion is regulated by the renin-angiotensin system, serum potassium ion concentration, and adrenocorticotropic hormone.

alert Awake, engaged, and responsive.

alexia Complete inability to understand written language; caused by brain injury or disease.

alkaline reflux gastropathy A complication of gastric surgery in which the pylorus is bypassed or removed. Endoscopic examination reveals regurgitated bile in the stomach and mucosal hyperemia. Symptoms include early satiety, abdominal discomfort, and vomiting. Also called *bile reflux gastropathy.*

alkalosis An acid-base imbalance in which blood pH is above normal.

allele An alternate form (or variation) of a gene.

allergen A foreign protein that is capable of causing a hypersensitivity response, or allergy, that ranges from uncomfortable (itchy, watery eyes or sneezing) to life threatening (allergic asthma, anaphylaxis, bronchoconstriction, or circulatory collapse); causes a release of natural chemicals, such as histamine, in the body.

allergy An increased or excessive response to the presence of a foreign protein or allergen (antigen) to which the patient has been previously exposed.

allogeneic bone marrow transplantation The transplantation of bone marrow from a sibling.

allograft A graft of tissue or bone between individuals of the same species but a different genotype; the donor may be a cadaver or a living person, either related or unrelated. Also called *homograft.*

alopecia Hair loss.

alveolitis Inflammation of the alveoli.

amaurosis fugax A transient, brief episode of blindness in one eye.

ambulatory aid Assistive device such as a cane or a walker.

ambulatory pump Infusion therapy pump generally used with a home care patient to allow a return to his or her usual activities while receiving infusion therapy.

ambulatory A term that refers to a patient who goes to the hospital or physician's office for treatment and returns home on the same day.

amenorrhea The absence of menstrual periods in women.

amnesia Loss of memory.

amputation The removal of a limb or other appendage of the body.

amylase An enzyme that converts starch and glycogen into simple sugars; found most commonly in saliva and pancreatic fluids.

amyotrophic lateral sclerosis (ALS) A progressive and degenerative disease of the motor system that is characterized by atrophy of the hands, forearms, and legs and that results in paralysis and death. There is no known cause, no cure, no specific treatment, no standard pattern of progression, and no method of prevention. Also called *Lou Gehrig's disease.*

anaerobic cellular metabolism Metabolism without oxygen.

anaerobic Lacking adequate oxygen.

anal fissure A painful ulcer at the margin of the anus.

analgesia Pain relief or pain suppression.

anaphylaxis The widespread reaction that occurs in response to contact with a substance to which the person has a severe allergy (antigen); characterized by blood vessel and bronchiolar smooth muscle involvement causing widespread blood vessel dilation, decreased cardiac output, and bronchoconstriction; results in cell damage and the release of large amounts of histamine, severe hypovolemia, vascular collapse, decreased cardiac contraction, and dysrhythmias, and causes extreme whole-body hypoxia.

anasarca Generalized edema.

anastomosis Surgical reattachment. Also a general term meaning "a connection."

anatomic dead space Places in which air flows but the structures are too thick for gas exchange.

anemia A clinical sign of some abnormal condition related to a reduction in one of the following: number of red blood cells, amount of hemoglobin, or hematocrit (percentage of packed red blood cells per deciliter of blood).

anergy The inability to mount an immune response to an antigen.

anesthesia An induced state of partial or total loss of sensation with or without loss of consciousness.

aneuploid (aneuploidy) An abnormal karyotype with more or fewer than 23 pairs of chromosomes.

aneurysm A permanent localized dilation of an artery (to at least 2 times its normal diameter) that forms when the middle layer (media) of the artery is weakened, stretching the inner (intima) and outer (adventitia) layers. As the artery widens, tension in the wall increases and further widening occurs, thus enlarging the aneurysm.

aneurysmectomy A surgical procedure performed to excise an aneurysm.

angina pectoris Literally, "strangling of the chest"; a temporary imbalance between the ability of the coronary arteries to supply oxygen and the demand for oxygen by the cardiac muscle. As a result, the patient experiences chest discomfort.

angioedema Diffuse swelling resulting from a vascular reaction in the deep tissues; can occur in a patient having an anaphylactic reaction.

anion Ion that has a negative charge.

anisocoria A difference in the size of the pupils.

ankle-brachial index (ABI) A ratio derived by dividing the ankle blood pressure by the brachial blood pressure; this calculation is used to assess the vascular status of the lower extremities. To obtain the ABI, a blood pressure cuff is applied to the lower extremities just above the malleoli. The systolic pressure is measured by Doppler ultrasound at both the dorsalis pedis and posterior tibial pulses. The higher of these two pressures is then divided by the higher of the two brachial pulses.

anomia Inability to find words.

anorectal abscess A localized induration and fluctuance that is caused by inflammation of the soft tissue near the rectum or anus and is most often the result of obstruction of the ducts of glands in the anorectal region by feces, foreign bodies, or trauma.

anorectic drugs Drugs that suppress appetite, which reduces food intake and, over time, may result in weight loss; may be prescribed for obese patients in a comprehensive weight reduction program.

anorexia nervosa An eating disorder of self-induced starvation resulting from a fear of fatness, even though the patient is underweight.

anorexia The loss of appetite for food.

anorexin Neuropeptide that decreases appetite.

anoxic Completely lacking oxygen.

antalgic (gait) A term that refers to an abnormality in the stance phase of gait. When part of one leg is painful, the person shortens the stance phase on the affected side.

anterior colporrhaphy Surgery for severe symptoms of cystocele in which the pelvic muscles are tightened for better bladder support.

anterior nares The nostrils or external openings into the nasal cavities.

antibody-mediated immunity (AMI) or antibody-mediated immune system The defense response that produces antibodies directed against certain pathogens. The antibodies inactivate the pathogens and protect against future infection from that microorganism.

antidepressants A group of drugs that help manage clinical depression.

antiepileptic drugs (AEDs) A class of drugs used to control seizures. Also called *anticonvulsants*.

antigen A foreign protein or allergen that is capable of causing an immune response; protein on the surface of a cell.

anuria Complete lack of urine output; usually defined as less than 100 mL/24 hr.

aortic regurgitation The flow of blood from the aorta back into the left ventricle during diastole; occurs when the aortic valve leaflets do not close properly during diastole and the annulus (the valve ring that attaches to the leaflets) is dilated or deformed.

aortic stenosis Narrowing of the aortic valve orifice and obstruction of left ventricular outflow during systole.

aphasia Inability to use or comprehend spoken or written language due to brain injury or disease.

apheresis A procedure in which whole blood is withdrawn from the patient, a blood component (e.g., stem cells) is filtered out, and the plasma is returned to the patient.

aphonia Inability to produce sound; complete but temporary loss of the voice.

aphthous stomatitis Noninfectious stomatitis.

apical impulse The pulse located at the left fifth intercostal space in the midclavicular line in the mitral area (the apex of the heart). Also called the *point of maximal impulse*.

apolipoprotein E One of several regulators of lipoprotein metabolism.

appendectomy Surgical removal of the inflamed appendix.

appendicitis Acute inflammation of the vermiform appendix, which is the blind pouch attached to the cecum of the colon, usually located in the right iliac region just below the ileocecal valve.

approximated In a clean laceration or a surgical incision to be closed with sutures or staples, the act of bringing together the wound edges with the skin layers lined up in correct anatomic position so they can be held in place until healing is complete.

apraxia The loss of the ability to carry out a purposeful motor activity.

aqueous humor The clear, watery fluid that is continually produced by the ciliary processes and fills the anterior and posterior chambers of the eye. This fluid drains through the canal of Schlemm into the blood to maintain balanced intraocular pressure (pressure within the eye).

arcus senilis An opaque ring within the outer edge of the cornea caused by fat deposits. Its presence does not affect vision.

areflexic bladder Urinary retention and overflow (dribbling) caused by injuries to the lower motor neuron at the spinal cord level of S2 to S4 (e.g., multiple sclerosis and spinal cord injury below

T12). Bladder emptying may be achieved by performing a Valsalva maneuver or tightening the abdominal muscles. The effectiveness of these maneuvers should be ascertained by catheterizing the patient for residual urine after voiding. Also called *flaccid bladder*.

arrhythmogenic right ventricular cardiomyopathy (dysplasia) A form of cardiomyopathy that results from the replacement of myocardial tissue with fibrous and fatty tissue.

arterial revascularization The surgical procedure most commonly used to increase arterial blood flow in the affected limb of a patient with peripheral arterial disease.

arterial ulcers A painful complication in the patient with peripheral arterial disease. Typically, the ulcer is small and round, with a "punched out" appearance and well-defined borders. Ulcers develop on the toes (often the great toe), between the toes, or on the upper aspect of the foot. With prolonged occlusion, the toes can become gangrenous.

arteriography Angiography of the arterial vessels; this invasive diagnostic procedure involves fluoroscopy and the use of a contrast medium and is performed when an arterial obstruction, narrowing, or aneurysm is suspected.

arteriosclerosis A thickening, or hardening, of the arterial wall.

arteriotomy A surgical opening into an artery.

arteriovenous malformation (AVM) An abnormality that occurs during embryonic development, resulting in a tangled mass of malformed, thin-walled, dilated vessels. The congenital absence of a capillary network in these vessels forms an abnormal communication between the arterial and venous systems and increases the risk that the vessels may rupture, causing bleeding, such as into the subarachnoid space or into the intracerebral tissue with brain AVMs. In the absence of the capillary network, the thin-walled veins are subjected to arterial pressure.

arthralgia Pain in a joint.

arthritis Inflammation of one or more joints.

arthrodesis The surgical fusion of a joint.

arthrogram An x-ray study of a joint after contrast medium (air or solution) has been injected to enhance its visualization.

arthroscopy Procedure in which a fiberoptic tube is inserted into a joint for direct visualization of the ligaments, menisci, and articular surfaces of the joint.

articulations Joint surfaces.

artifact In the electrocardiogram, interference that is seen on the monitor or rhythm strip and may look like a wandering or fuzzy baseline; can be caused by patient movement, loose or defective electrodes, improper grounding, or faulty equipment.

ASA Physical Status Classification System From the American Society of Anesthesiologists (ASA), a system that assesses the fitness of patients for surgery.

ascending tracts Groups of nerves that originate in the spinal cord and end in the brain.

ascites The accumulation of free fluid within the peritoneal cavity. Increased hydrostatic pressure

from portal hypertension causes this fluid to leak into the peritoneal cavity.

assistive technology Electronic equipment that increases the ability of disabled patients to care for themselves.

assistive/adaptive device Any item that enables the patient to perform all or part of an activity independently.

asterixis A coarse tremor characterized by rapid, nonrhythmic extensions and flexions in the wrists and fingers; a motor disturbance seen in portal-systemic encephalopathy. Also called a *liver flap* or *flapping tremor*.

asthma A chronic respiratory condition in which reversible airway obstruction occurs intermittently, reducing airflow.

asthma A chronic respiratory condition in which reversible airflow obstruction in the airways occurs intermittently.

astigmatism A refractive error caused by unevenly curved surfaces on or in the eye (especially of the cornea) that distort vision.

ataxia Gait disturbance or loss of balance.

atelectasis Collapse of alveoli.

atelectrauma Shear injury to alveoli from opening and closing.

atherectomy An invasive nonsurgical technique in which a high-speed, rotating metal burr uses fine abrasive bits to scrape plaque from inside an artery while minimizing damage to the vessel surface.

atherosclerosis A type of arteriosclerosis that involves the formation of plaque within the arterial wall; the leading contributor to coronary artery and cerebrovascular disease.

atrial fibrillation (AF) A cardiac dysrhythmia in which multiple rapid impulses from many atrial foci, at a rate of 350 to 600 times per minute, depolarize the atria in a totally disorganized manner, with no P waves, no atrial contractions, a loss of the atrial kick, and an irregular ventricular response.

atrial gallop An abnormal fourth heart sound that occurs as blood enters the ventricles during the active filling phase at the end of ventricular diastole; may be heard in patients with hypertension, anemia, ventricular hypertrophy, myocardial infarction, aortic or pulmonic stenosis, and pulmonary emboli.

atrioventricular (AV) junction In the cardiac conduction system, the area consisting of a transitional cell zone, the atrioventricular (AV) node itself, and the bundle of His. The AV node lies just beneath the right atrial endocardium, between the tricuspid valve and the ostium of the coronary sinus.

atrophic gastritis A type of gastritis that involves all layers of the stomach and includes diffuse inflammation and destruction of deeply located glands.

attenuated The quality of making a substance weaker; for example, antigens that are used to make vaccines are specially processed to make them less likely to grow in the body.

atypical angina Angina that manifests itself as indigestion, pain between the shoulders, an aching jaw, or a choking sensation that occurs with exertion. Many women experience atypical angina.

atypical migraine The least common of the three types of migraine headaches, after migraines with aura and migraines without aura; the atypical category includes menstrual and cluster migraines.

aura A sensation that signals the onset of a headache or seizure; the patient may experience visual changes, flashing lights, or double vision.

autoamputation of the distal digits A condition in which the tips of the digits fall off spontaneously; can occur in severe cases of Raynaud's phenomenon.

autoantibodies Antibodies directed against self tissues of cells.

autocontamination The occurrence of infection in which the patient's own normal flora overgrows and penetrates the internal environment.

autodigestion Self-digestion. Specifically, the process of the stomach digesting itself if there is a break in its protective mucosal barrier.

autogenous Belonging to the person, such as a person's vein being moved from one part of the body to another.

autoimmune pancreatitis A chronic inflammatory form of pancreatitis that can also affect the bile ducts, kidneys, and other major connective tissues.

autologous blood transfusion Reinfusing the patient's own blood during surgery.

autologous bone marrow transplantation A type of bone marrow transplant in which patients receive their own stem cells, which were collected before high-dose chemotherapy.

autologous donation The donation of a patient's own blood before scheduled surgery for use, if needed, during the surgery to eliminate transfusion reactions and reduce the risk of bloodborne disease.

autolysis The spontaneous disintegration of tissue by the action of the patient's own cellular enzymes.

automaticity The ability of a cell to initiate an impulse spontaneously and repetitively; in cardiac electrophysiology, the ability of primary pacemaker cells (SA node, AV junction) to generate an electrical impulse.

autonomic dysreflexia (AD) A syndrome that affects the patient with an upper spinal cord injury; characterized by severe hypertension and headache, bradycardia, nasal stuffiness, and flushing; caused by a noxious stimulus, usually a distended bladder or constipation. This is a neurologic emergency and must be promptly treated to prevent a hypertensive brain attack.

autonomic nervous system (ANS) The part of the nervous system that is not under conscious control; consists of the sympathetic nervous system and the parasympathetic nervous system.

autonomy Ethical principle that implies a person's self-determination and self-management.

autosome Any of the 22 pairs of human chromosomes containing genes that code for all the structures and regulatory proteins needed for normal function but do not code for the sexual differentiation of a person.

axial loading A mechanism of injury that involves vertical compression. An example is a diving accident, in which the blow to the top of the head causes the vertebrae to shatter and pieces of bone enter the spinal canal and damage the cord.

azoospermia The absence of living sperm in the semen.

azotemia An excess of nitrogenous wastes (urea) in the blood.

B

Babinski's sign Dorsiflexion of the great toe and fanning of the other toes, which is an abnormal reflex in response to testing the plantar reflex with a pointed (but not sharp) object; indicates the presence of central nervous system disease. The normal response is plantar flexion of all toes.

bacteremia The presence of bacteria in the bloodstream.

bacteriuria Bacteria in the urine.

bad death A death embodied by pain, not having one's wishes followed at the end of one's life, isolation, abandonment, and constant agonizing about losses associated with death.

Baker's cyst Enlarged popliteal bursa.

banding See *endoscopic variceal ligation*.

barbiturate coma The use of drugs such as pentobarbital sodium or sodium thiopental at dosages to maintain complete unresponsiveness; used for patients whose increased intracranial pressure cannot be controlled by other means. These drugs decrease the metabolic demands of the brain and cerebral blood flow, stabilize cell membranes, decrease the formation of vasogenic edema, and produce a more uniform blood supply. The patient in a barbiturate coma requires mechanical ventilation, sophisticated hemodynamic monitoring, and intracranial pressure monitoring.

bariatrics Branch of medicine that manages obesity and its related diseases.

baroreceptors Sensory receptors in the arch of the aorta and at the origin of the internal carotid arteries that are stimulated when the arterial walls are stretched by an increased blood pressure.

barotrauma Damage to the lungs by positive pressure.

Barrett's epithelium Columnar epithelium (instead of the normal squamous cell epithelium) that develops in the lower esophagus during the process of healing from gastroesophageal reflux disease. It is considered premalignant and is associated with an increased risk of cancer in patients with prolonged disease.

Barrett's esophagus Ulceration of the lower esophagus caused by exposure to acid and pepsin, leading to the replacement of normal distal squamous mucosa with columnar epithelium as a response to tissue injury.

base A substance that binds (reduces) free hydrogen ions in solution. Strong bases bind hydrogen ions easily; weak bases bind less readily.

Basic Cardiac Life Support (BCLS) Procedure that involves ventilating the patient who has stopped breathing, as well as giving chest compressions in the absence of a carotid pulse. Also known as *cardiopulmonary resuscitation (CPR)*.

Bell's palsy Acute paralysis of cranial nerve VII; characterized by a drawing sensation and paralysis of all facial muscles on the affected side. The patient cannot close the eye, wrinkle the forehead, smile, whistle, or grimace. The face appears masklike and sags. Also called *facial paralysis*.

beneficence The ethical principle of preventing harm and ensuring the patient's well-being.

benign tumor cells Normal cells growing in the wrong place or at the wrong time.

benign Altered cell growth that is harmless and does not require intervention.

bereavement Grief and mourning experienced by the survivor before and after a death.

bicaval technique Surgical technique in heart transplantation in which the intact right atrium of the donor heart is preserved by anastomoses at the recipient's superior and inferior vena cavae.

bifurcation The point of division of a single structure into two branches.

bigeminy A type of premature complex that exists when normal complexes and premature complexes occur alternately in a repetitive two-beat pattern, with a pause occurring after each premature complex so that complexes occur in pairs.

bilateral orchiectomy The surgical removal of both testes, typically performed as palliative surgery in patients with prostate cancer. It is not intended to cure the prostate cancer but to arrest its spread by removing testosterone.

bilateral salpingo-oophorectomy (BSO) Surgical removal of both fallopian tubes and both ovaries.

biliary colic Intense pain due to obstruction of the cystic duct of the gallbladder from a stone moving through or lodged within the duct. Tissue spasm occurs in an effort to mobilize the stone through the small duct.

biliary stent A plastic or metal device that is placed percutaneously to keep a duct of the biliary system open in patients experiencing biliary obstruction.

biofilm A complex group of microorganisms that functions within a "slimy" gel coating on medical devices.

biological response modifiers (BRMs) A class of immunomodulating drugs that attempt to modify the course of disease. Also called *biologics*.

biologics See *biological response modifiers*.

biomedical technician Member of the health care team who maintains the safety of adaptive and electronic devices by monitoring their function and making repairs as needed.

biotrauma Inflammatory response–mediated damage to alveoli.

bivalve To cut a cast lengthwise into two equal pieces.

black box warning A governmental designation indicating that a drug has at least one serious side effect and must be used with caution.

bladder ultrasound Less invasive test to determine postvoiding residual urine volumes for the patient with a reflex (upper motor neuron) or uninhibited bladder; often used to measure residual urine in the bladder of patients with spinal cord injury.

blanch To whiten or lighten.

blast effect The damage sustained by the force of an explosion.

blast phase cell Immature cell that divides.

blood pressure (BP) The force of blood exerted against the vessel walls.

blood stem cells Immature, unspecialized (undifferentiated) cells that are capable of becoming any type of blood cell, depending on the body's needs.

bloodborne metastasis The release of tumor cells into the blood; the most common cause of cancer spread.

Blumberg's sign Pain felt on abrupt release of steady pressure (rebound tenderness) over the site of abdominal pain.

blunt trauma A type of trauma resulting from impact forces (e.g., motor vehicle accident, fall, assault).

body mass index (BMI) A measure of nutritional status that does not depend on frame size; indirectly estimates total fat stores within the body by the relationship of weight to height.

bolus feeding A method of tube feeding that involves intermittent feeding of a specified amount of enteral product at specified times during a 24-hour period, typically every 4 hours.

bone biopsy Procedure in which the physician extracts a specimen of bone tissue for microscopic examination to confirm the presence of infection or neoplasm; not commonly done today.

bone mineral density (BMD) The quality of bone that determines bone strength. It peaks between 30 and 35 years of age, when both bone resorption activity and bone-building activity occur at a constant rate. When bone resorption activity exceeds bone-building activity, bone density decreases.

bone reduction Realignment of fractured bone ends for proper healing.

bone remodeling A process in which bone is constantly undergoing changes.

bone resorption Loss of bone density due to demineralization resulting from the release of calcium from storage areas in bones.

bone scan A radionuclide test in which radioactive material is injected for visualization of the entire skeleton; used to detect tumors, arthritis, osteomyelitis, osteoporosis, vertebral compression fractures, and unexplained bone pain.

borborygmus (borborygmi) Bowel sounds, especially loud gurgling sounds, resulting from hypermotility of the bowel.

boring In pain, the type of intense pain that feels as if it is going through the body.

Bouchard's nodes Swelling at the proximal interphalangeal joints in osteoarthritis involving the hands.

bowel retraining A program for patients with neurologic problems that is designed to include a combination of suppository use and a consistent toileting schedule.

bradycardia Slowness of the heart rate; characterized as a pulse rate less than 50 to 60 beats/min.

bradydysrhythmia An abnormal heart rhythm characterized by a heart rate less than 60 beats/min.

bradykinesia Slow or no movement, as seen in a patient with Parkinson disease. Also called *akinesia.*

brain abscess A collection of pus that forms in the extradural, subdural, or intracerebral area of the brain as a result of a purulent infection, usually due to bacteria invading the brain directly or indirectly.

brain attack Stroke; disruption in the normal blood supply to the brain, either as an interruption in blood flow (ischemic stroke) or as bleeding within or around the brain (hemorrhagic stroke). A medical emergency that occurs suddenly, a stroke should be treated immediately to prevent neurologic deficit and permanent disability. Formerly called *cerebrovascular accident,* the National Stroke Association now uses the term *brain attack* to describe stroke.

brain herniation syndrome In the patient with untreated increased intracranial pressure, protrusion (herniation) of the brain downward toward the brainstem or laterally from a unilateral lesion within one cerebral hemisphere, causing irreversible brain damage and possibly death.

breakthrough pain Additional pain that "breaks through" the pain that is being managed by mainstay analgesic drugs.

breast augmentation Cosmetic surgical procedure to enhance the size, shape, or symmetry of the breasts.

breast-conserving surgery Surgical method for breast cancer that removes the bulk of the tumor rather than the entire breast.

Broca's aphasia See *expressive aphasia.*

Broca's area An important speech area of the cerebrum. It is located in the frontal lobe and is composed of neurons responsible for the formation of words, or speech.

bronchoscopy Insertion of a tube in the airway, usually as far as the secondary bronchi, for the purpose of visualizing airway structures and obtaining tissue samples for biopsy or culture.

bruit Swishing sound in the larger arteries (carotid, aortic, femoral, and popliteal) that can be heard with a stethoscope or Doppler probe; may indicate narrowing of the artery and is usually associated with atherosclerotic disease.

B-type natriuretic peptide (BNP) A peptide produced and released by the ventricles when the patient has fluid overload as a result of heart failure (HF).

bulbar Pertaining to the muscles involved in facial expression, chewing, and speech.

bulimia nervosa An eating disorder that is characterized by episodes of binge eating in which the patient ingests a large amount of food in a short time, followed by purging behavior such as self-induced vomiting or excessive use of laxatives and diuretics.

bunion Hallux valgus deformity of the foot in which lateral deviation of the great toe causes the first metatarsal head to become enlarged.

bunionectomy Surgical removal of the hallux valgus deformity (bunion) of the foot.

butterfly rash A dry, scaly raised rash on the face; the major skin manifestation of systemic lupus erythematosus.

C

***C. difficile*–associated disease (CDAD)** Clinical manifestations that are caused by *Clostridium difficile* as a potential result of antibiotic therapy use, especially in older adults.

cachexia Extreme body wasting and malnutrition that develop from an imbalance between food intake and energy use.

calciphylaxis A condition of thrombosis and skin necrosis that can occur in stage 5 chronic kidney disease.

calculi Abnormal formations of a mass of mineral salts that can occur in the body; forms in the kidney when excess calcium precipitates out of solution. Also called *stones.*

calculous cholecystitis Inflammation of the gallbladder usually following and created by obstruction of the cystic duct by a stone (calculus).

callus The loose, fibrous vascular tissue that forms at the site of a fracture as the first phase of healing and is normally replaced by hard bone as healing continues.

calyx The anatomic term for a cuplike structure.

Canadian Triage Acuity Scale (CTAS) A standardized model for triage in which lists of descriptors are used to establish the triage level.

cancellous The softer tissue inside bones that contains large spaces, or trabeculae, that are filled with red and yellow marrow.

candidiasis An infection caused by the fungus *Candida albicans.*

canthus The place where the upper and lower eyelids meet at the corner of either side of the eye.

capillary closing pressure The amount of pressure needed to occlude skin capillary blood flow.

capillary leak syndrome The response of capillaries to the presence of biologic chemicals (mediators) that change blood vessel integrity and allow fluid to shift from the blood in the vascular space into the interstitial tissues.

Caplan's syndrome The presence of pneumoconiosis and rheumatoid nodules in the lungs; noted primarily in coal miners and asbestos workers.

capnography An end-tidal carbon dioxide ($EtCO_2$) monitor.

capsule The layer of fibrous tissue on the outer surface of the kidney, which provides protection and support. The renal capsule itself is surrounded by layers of fat and connective tissue.

carboxyhemoglobin Carbon monoxide on oxygen-binding sites of the hemoglobin molecule.

carcinoembryonic antigen (CEA) An oncofetal antigen that may be elevated in 70% of people with colorectal cancer. CEA is not specifically associated with the colorectal cancer and may be elevated in the presence of other benign or malignant diseases and in smokers. CEA is often used to monitor the effectiveness of treatment and to identify disease recurrence.

carcinogen Any substance that changes the activity of the genes in a cell so that the cell becomes a cancer cell.

carcinogenesis Cancer development.

cardiac axis In electrocardiography (ECG), the direction of electrical current flow in the heart. The relationship between the cardiac axis and the lead axis is responsible for the deflections seen on the ECG pattern.

cardiac catheterization The most definitive but most invasive test in the diagnosis of heart disease; involves passing a small catheter into the heart and injecting contrast medium.

cardiac index A calculation of cardiac output requirements to account for differences in body size; determined by dividing the cardiac output by the body surface area.

cardiac markers Serum studies that include troponin, creatine kinase–MB, and myoglobin.

cardiac output (CO) The volume of blood ejected by the heart each minute; normal range in adults is 4 to 7 L/min.

cardiac rehabilitation The process of actively assisting the patient with cardiac disease to achieve and maintain a productive life while remaining within the limits of the heart's ability to respond to increases in activity and stress. *Phase 1* begins with the acute illness and ends with discharge from the hospital. *Phase 2* begins after discharge and continues through convalescence at home. *Phase 3* refers to long-term conditioning.

cardiac resynchronization therapy (CRT) In patients with some types of heart failure, the use of a permanent pacemaker alone or in combination with an implantable cardioverter-defibrillator to provide biventricular pacing.

cardiac tamponade Compression of the myocardium by fluid that has accumulated around the heart; this compresses the atria and ventricles, prevents them from filling adequately, and reduces cardiac output.

cardiogenic shock Post–myocardial infarction heart failure in which necrosis of more than 40% of the left ventricle has occurred. Also called *class IV heart failure.*

cardiomegaly Enlarged heart.

cardiomyopathy A subacute or chronic disease of cardiac muscle; classified into four categories based on abnormalities in structure and function: dilated, hypertrophic, restrictive, and arrhythmogenic.

cardiopulmonary bypass (CPB) Diversion of the blood from the heart to a bypass machine, where it is heparinized, oxygenated, and returned to the circulation through a cannula placed in the ascending aortic arch or femoral artery to provide oxygenation, circulation, and hypothermia during induced cardiac arrest for coronary artery bypass surgery. This process ensures a motionless operative field and prevents myocardial ischemia.

cardioversion A synchronized countershock that may be performed in emergencies for hemodynamically unstable ventricular or supraventricular tachydysrhythmias or electively for stable tachydysrhythmias that are resistant to medical therapies. The shock depolarizes a critical mass of myocardium simultaneously during intrinsic depolarization and is intended to stop the re-entry circuit and allow the sinus node to regain control of the heart.

care coordination The deliberate organization of and communication about patient care activities among members of the health care team (including the patient) to facilitate continuous health care to meet patient needs.

carina The point at which the trachea branches into the right and left mainstem bronchi.

carpal tunnel syndrome (CTS) A common condition in which the median nerve in the wrist becomes compressed, causing pain and numbness.

carrier (1) A person who harbors an infectious agent without symptoms of active disease; (2) in genetics, a person who has one mutated allele for a recessive genetic disorder. A carrier does not usually have any manifestations of the disorder but can pass the mutated allele to his or her children.

case management The process of assessment, planning, implementation, evaluation, and interaction for patients who have complex health problems and incur a high cost to the health care system. Goals include promoting quality of life, decreasing fragmentation and duplication of care across health care settings, and maintaining cost-effectiveness.

caseation necrosis A type of necrosis in which tissue is turned into a granular mass.

cast A rigid device that immobilizes the affected body part while allowing other body parts to move. It is most commonly used for fractures but may also be applied to correct deformities (e.g., clubfoot) or to prevent deformities (e.g., those seen in some patients with rheumatoid arthritis).

cataract A lens opacity that distorts the image projected onto the retina.

catechol-*O*-methyltransferases (COMTs) Enzymes that inactivate dopamine.

catecholamines Hormones (dopamine, epinephrine, and norepinephrine) released by the adrenal medulla in response to stimulation of the sympathetic nervous system.

catheter-related bloodstream infection (CR-BSI) Health care–acquired bloodstream infection caused by the presence of any type of intravenous catheter.

catheter-related bloodstream infection (CRBSI) prevention bundle An nationally recognized set of evidence-based interventions to prevent CR-BSIs.

cation Ion that has a positive charge.

cell saver system A technique that allows for collection of the person's own red blood cells during surgery, which is then reinfused directly back to the patient via a closed system.

cell-mediated immunity Microbial resistance that is mediated by the action of specifically sensitized T-lymphocytes.

cellular regulation The physiologic processes used to control cellular growth, replication, and differentiation (maturation into a specific cell type) to maintain homeostasis.

cellulitis An acute, spreading, edematous inflammation of the deep subcutaneous tissues; usually caused by infection of a wound or burn.

central IV therapy IV therapy in which a vascular access device (VAD) is placed in a central blood vessel, such as the superior vena cava.

central line–associated bloodstream infection (CLA-BSI) Health care–acquired bloodstream infection caused by the presence of a central intravenous line.

cerebral angiography (arteriography) Visualization of the cerebral circulation (carotid and vertebral arteries) after injecting a contrast medium into an artery (usually the femoral).

cerebral blood flow (CBF) Useful in evaluating cerebral vasospasm; can be measured in many areas of the brain with the use of radioactive substances.

cerebral perfusion pressure (CPP) The pressure gradient over which the brain is perfused. It is influenced by oxygenation, cerebral blood volume, blood pressure, cerebral edema, and intracranial pressure (ICP) and is determined by subtracting the mean ICP from the mean arterial pressure. A cerebral perfusion pressure above 70 mm Hg is generally accepted as an appropriate goal of therapy.

cerebral salt wasting (CSW) The primary cause of hyponatremia in the neurosurgical population; characterized by hyponatremia, decreased serum osmolality, and decreased blood volume. It is thought to result from the extrarenal influence of atrial natriuretic factor.

cerumen The wax produced by glands within the external ear canal; helps protect and lubricate the ear canal.

cervical polyp Tumor that arises from the mucosa and extends to the opening of the cervical os. Polyps result from hyperplasia of the endocervical epithelium, inflammation, or an abnormal local response to hormonal stimulation or localized vascular congestion of the cervical blood vessels. Polyps are the most common benign growth of the cervix.

CHADS₂ scoring system Acronym for <u>C</u>ongestive heart failure, <u>H</u>ypertension, <u>A</u>ge ≥75 years, <u>D</u>iabetes mellitus, <u>S</u>troke. Determines whether a patient with atrial fibrillation needs preventive anticoagulant therapy.

chalazion An inflammation of a sebaceous gland in the eyelid.

chancre The ulcer that is the first sign of syphilis. It develops at the site of entry (inoculation) of the organism, usually 3 weeks after exposure. The lesion may be found on any area of the skin or mucous membranes but occurs most often on the genitalia, lips, nipples, and hands and in the oral cavity, anus, and rectum.

chemotherapy The treatment of cancer with chemical agents that have systemic effects; used to cure and to increase survival time.

chemotherapy-induced peripheral neuropathy (CIPN) The loss of sensory or motor function of peripheral nerves associated with exposure to certain anticancer drugs.

chest tube A drain placed in the pleural space to allow closed–chest drainage, which restores intrapleural pressure and allows re-expansion of the lung after surgery in patients who have undergone thoracotomy (incision of the chest wall).

Cheyne-Stokes respirations Common sign of nearing death in which apnea alternates with periods of rapid breathing.

choked disc See *papilledema.*

cholecystectomy The surgical removal of the gallbladder.

cholecystitis Inflammation of the gallbladder.

cholecystokinin A hormone that stimulates digestive juices and that may work with leptin to increase or decrease appetite.

choledochojejunostomy Surgical anastomosis of the common bile duct with the jejunum.

cholelithiasis The presence of gallstones.

cholesteatoma A benign overgrowth of squamous cell epithelium.

cholesterol Serum lipid that includes high-density lipoproteins and low-density lipoproteins.

cholinergic crisis Overmedication with cholinesterase inhibitors.

cholinesterase inhibitors Drugs that improve cholinergic neurotransmission in the central nervous system by delaying the destruction of acetylcholine by acetylcholinesterase, thus delaying the onset of cognitive decline. These are approved for symptomatic treatment of Alzheimer's disease but do not affect the course of the disease.

chondroitin A supplement that may play a role in strengthening cartilage.

choreiform movement Rapid, jerky movement.

chronic Having a slow onset and symptoms that persist for an extended period.

chronic calcifying pancreatitis (CCP) Alcohol-induced chronic pancreatitis that is characterized by protein precipitates that plug the ducts and lead to ductal obstruction, atrophy, and dilation. The epithelium of the ducts undergoes histologic changes, resulting in metaplasia (cell replacement) and ulceration. This inflammatory process causes fibrosis of the pancreatic tissue.

chronic constrictive pericarditis A fibrous thickening of the pericardium that prevents adequate filling of the ventricles and eventually results in cardiac failure; caused by chronic pericardial inflammation due to tuberculosis, radiation therapy, trauma, kidney failure, or metastatic cancer.

chronic fatigue syndrome (CFS) A chronic illness characterized by severe fatigue for 6 months or longer, usually following flu-like symptoms. At least four of the following criteria are required for diagnosis: sore throat; substantial impairment in short-term memory or concentration; tender lymph nodes; muscle pain; multiple joint pain with redness or swelling; headaches of a new type, pattern, or severity; unrefreshing sleep; and postexertional malaise lasting more than 24 hours.

chronic gastritis A patchy, diffuse inflammation of the mucosal lining of the stomach. Chronic gastritis usually heals without scarring but can progress to hemorrhage and ulcer formation.

chronic health condition A condition that has existed for at least 3 months.

chronic hepatitis Chronic liver inflammation that usually occurs as a result of hepatitis B or C. Superimposed infection with hepatitis D virus (HDV) in patients with chronic hepatitis B may also result in chronic hepatitis. Can lead to cirrhosis and liver cancer.

chronic kidney disease (CKD) A condition characterized by loss of kidney function over time.

chronic obstructive pancreatitis Pancreatitis that develops from inflammation, spasm, and obstruction of the sphincter of Oddi. Inflammatory and sclerotic lesions occur in the head of the pancreas and around the ducts, causing obstruction and backflow of pancreatic secretions.

chronic osteomyelitis Bone infection that persists over a long time due to misdiagnosis or inadequate treatment. Also called *subchronic osteomyelitis*.

chronic pain Pain that persists or recurs for indefinite periods (usually more than 3 months), often involves deep body structures, is poorly localized, and is difficult to describe. Also called *persistent pain*.

chronic pancreatitis A progressive, destructive disease of the pancreas characterized by remissions and exacerbations. Inflammation and fibrosis of the tissue contribute to pancreatic insufficiency and diminished function of the organ.

chronic paronychia Inflammation of the skin around the nail that persists for months. People at risk for chronic paronychia are those with frequent exposure to water, such as homemakers, bartenders, and laundry workers.

chronic pyelonephritis A kidney disorder that results from repeated or continued upper urinary tract infections or the effects of such infections.

chronic stable angina (CSA) Type of angina characterized by chest discomfort that occurs with moderate to prolonged exertion and in a pattern that is familiar to the patient.

chyme The liquid formed when food is transformed during the digestion process in the gastrointestinal tract.

circle of Willis At the base of the brain, the ring formed by the anterior, middle, and posterior cerebral arteries where they are joined together by small communicating arteries.

circumcision The surgical removal of the prepuce or foreskin of the penis.

circumferential Referring to something that completely surrounds an extremity or the thorax.

cirrhosis Liver disease that is characterized by extensive scarring of the liver and that is usually caused by a chronic irreversible reaction to hepatic inflammation and necrosis; disease typically develops insidiously and has a prolonged, destructive course.

classic heat stroke A form of heat stroke in which the body's ability to dissipate heat is significantly impaired; occurs over time as a result of long-term exposure to a hot, humid environment such as a home without air-conditioning in the high heat of the summer.

clinical practice guideline An "official recommendation" based on evidence to diagnose and/or manage a health problem (e.g., pain management).

clinical psychologist Member of the health care team who counsels patients and families on their psychological problems and on strategies to cope with disability.

clinically competent The condition of being legally competent and having decisional capacity.

clonic (rhythmic) Pertaining to a state of alternating muscle stiffness followed by rhythmic jerking motions, as in a tonic-clonic seizure.

clonus The sudden, brief, jerking contraction of a muscle or muscle group often seen in seizures. Also called *myoclonus*.

closed fracture A fracture that does not extend through the skin and therefore has no visible wound. Also called *simple fracture*.

closed reduction A nonsurgical method for managing a simple fracture. While applying a manual pull, or traction, on the bone, the health care provider manipulates the bone ends so that they realign.

closed traumatic brain injury A type of traumatic primary brain injury that occurs as the result of blunt trauma; the integrity of the skull is not violated, and damage to brain tissue depends on the degree and mechanisms of injury.

clotting A complex, multi-step process by which blood forms a protein-based structure (clot) in an appropriate area of tissue injury to prevent excessive bleeding while maintaining whole-body blood flow (perfusion).

clubbing Changes in the tissue beds of the fingers and toes, with the base of the nail becoming spongy; results from chronic oxygen deprivation in the tissue beds.

cluster headache A type of oculotemporal or oculofrontal headache marked by unilateral, excruciating, nonthrobbing pain that is felt deep in and around the eye and may radiate to the forehead, temple, cheek, ear, occiput, or neck. Average duration is 10 to 45 minutes. Headaches occur every 8 to 12 hours and up to 24 hours daily at the same time for about 6 to 8 weeks (hence the term *cluster*), followed by remission for 9 months to a year. Cause and mechanism are unknown but have been attributed to vasoreactivity and oxyhemoglobin desaturation.

clysis See *hypodermoclysis*.

coagulopathy Clotting abnormalities.

cognition The ability of the brain to process, store, retrieve, and manipulate information.

cognitive rehabilitation A way of helping brain-injured patients regain function in areas that are essential for a return to independence and a reasonable quality of life.

cognitive therapist A member of the rehabilitative health care team, usually a neuropsychologist, who works primarily with patients who have experienced head injuries and have cognitive impairments.

cohorting The practice of grouping patients who are colonized or infected with the same pathogen.

cold antibody anemia A form of immunohemolytic anemia (in which the immune system attacks a person's own red blood cells for unknown reasons) that occurs with complement protein fixation on immunoglobulin M (IgM). In this condition, the arteries in the hands and feet constrict profoundly in response to cold temperatures or stress.

cold phase A phase after peripheral nerve trauma resulting in complete denervation in which the skin appears cyanotic, mottled, or reddish blue and feels cool compared with the contralateral unaffected extremity. The cold phase follows the warm phase, which lasts 2 to 3 weeks after injury.

colectomy Surgical removal of part or all of the colon.

collaboration The planning, implementing, and evaluation of patient care using an interdisciplinary (ID) plan of care.

collateral circulation Circulation that provides blood to an area with altered tissue perfusion through smaller vessels that develop and compensate for the occluded vessels.

colon interposition A surgical procedure that may be performed in patients with an esophageal tumor when the tumor involves the stomach or the stomach is otherwise unsuitable for anastomosis. In colon interposition, a section of right or left colon is removed and brought up into the thorax to substitute for the esophagus.

colon resection Surgery performed for colorectal cancer in which the tumor and regional lymph nodes are removed.

colonoscopy The endoscopic examination of the entire large bowel.

colostomy The surgical creation of an opening between the colon and the surface of the abdomen.

colposcopy Examination of the cervix and vagina using a colposcope, which allows three-dimensional magnification and intense illumination of epithelium with suspected disease. This procedure can locate the exact site of precancerous and malignant lesions for biopsy.

comatose Unconscious and cannot be aroused despite vigorous or noxious simulation.

comfort A state of physical well-being, pleasure, and absence of pain or stress.

command center See *emergency operations center.*

commando procedure Mnemonic for combined neck dissection, mandibulectomy, and oropharyngeal resection—a procedure in which the surgeon removes a segment of the mandible with the oral lesion and performs a radical neck dissection.

communicable The ability of an infection, such as influenza, to be transmitted from person to person.

communicating hydrocephalus Form of hydrocephalus that occurs when the flow of cerebrospinal fluid (CSF) is blocked after it exits the ventricles; this form is "communicating" because CSF can still flow between the ventricles, which remain open.

compartment syndrome A condition in which increased tissue pressure in a confined anatomic space causes decreased blood flow to the area, leading to hypoxia and pain.

compensated cirrhosis A form of cirrhosis in which the liver has significant scarring but is still able to perform essential functions without causing significant symptoms.

compensatory mechanism The means of producing compensation. Also called *adaptive mechanism.*

complement activation and fixation Actions triggered by some classes of antibodies that can remove or destroy antigen.

complete spinal cord injury An injury in which the spinal cord has been severed or damaged in a way that eliminates all innervation below the level of the injury.

complex regional pain syndrome (CRPS) A complex disorder that includes debilitating pain, atrophy, autonomic dysfunction (excessive sweating, vascular changes), and motor impairment (most notably muscle paresis), probably caused by an abnormally hyperactive sympathetic nervous system. This syndrome most often results from traumatic injury and commonly occurs in the feet and hands; formerly called *reflex sympathetic dystrophy (RSD).*

compliance In respiratory physiology, a measure of elasticity within the lung. Also, a patient's fulfillment of a caregiver's prescribed course of treatment.

compound fracture See *open fracture.*

compression fracture A fracture that is produced by a loading force applied to the long axis of cancellous bone. These fractures commonly occur in the vertebrae of patients with osteoporosis.

computed tomography coronary angiography (CTCA) 64-slice diagnostic scan used to diagnose coronary artery disease in symptomatic patients.

conductive hearing loss Hearing loss that results from any physical obstruction of sound wave transmission (e.g., a foreign body in the external canal, a retracted or bulging tympanic membrane, or fused bony ossicles).

conductivity The ability of a cell to transmit an electrical stimulus from cell membrane to cell membrane.

congestive heart failure (CHF) Former term for *left-sided heart failure.* Categorized as either systolic heart failure or diastolic heart failure, which may be acute or chronic and mild to severe.

conization The removal of a cone-shaped sample of tissue from the cervix for cytologic study.

conjunctivae The mucous membranes of the eye that line the undersurface of the eyelids (palpebral conjunctiva) and cover the sclera (bulbar conjunctiva).

connective tissue disease (CTD) A group of diseases that are the major focus of rheumatology (the study of rheumatic diseases); most are musculoskeletal disorders.

consensual response In assessing pupillary reaction to light, a slight constriction of the pupil of the eye not being tested when a penlight is brought in from the side of the patient's head and shined into the eye being tested as soon as the patient opens his or her eyes.

consolidation Solidification; lack of air spaces in the lung, such as occurs in pneumonia.

constipation The passage of hard, dry stool fewer than 3 times a week (as defined by the Association of Rehabilitation Nurses).

contact laser prostatectomy (CLP) Procedure for treating benign prostatic hyperplasia that uses laser energy to coagulate excess tissue. Also called *interstitial laser coagulation (ILC).*

Contact Precautions Infection control guidelines from the U.S. Centers for Disease Control and Prevention; used for patients with infections spread by direct contact or contact with items in the patient's environment, such as pediculosis.

contiguous Something in direct contact with, or adjacent to, another area or structure.

continence The ability to voluntarily control emptying the bladder and colon. Continence is a learned behavior whereby a person can suppress the urge to urinate until a socially appropriate location is available.

continuous feeding A method of tube feeding in which small amounts of enteral product are continuously infused (by gravity drip or by a pump or controller device) over a specified time.

continuous femoral nerve blockade A method used to administer anesthesia using an IV moderate sedation agent is used in addition to the neuraxial or PNB drug. PNB may be either a single injection or continuous infusion by a portable pump.

continuous positive airway pressure (CPAP) A respiratory treatment that improves obstructive sleep apnea in patients with heart failure.

contractility The ability of a cell to contract in response to an impulse. In cardiac electrophysiology, the ability of atrial and ventricular muscle cells to shorten their fiber length in response to electrical stimulation, generating sufficient pressure to propel blood forward. Contractility is the mechanical activity of the heart.

contraction The closure of a wound as new collagen replaces damaged tissue, pulling the wound edges inward along the path of least resistance.

contralateral Pertaining to the opposite side.

contrecoup injury Bruising of the brain tissue, with damage occurring on the side opposite the site of impact.

control therapy drugs Drugs used every day, regardless of symptoms, to reduce airway responsiveness to prevent asthma attacks from occurring.

contusion A bruise; when referring to closed head injury, a bruising of brain tissue usually found at the site of impact (coup injury). Compare with *contrecoup injury.*

cor pulmonale Right-sided heart failure caused by pulmonary disease.

cordectomy Excision of a vocal cord in surgery for laryngeal cancer.

cornea The clear layer that forms the external coat on the front of the eye.

corneal abrasion Scrape or scratch of the cornea that disrupts its integrity.

corneal ulceration Deep disruption of the corneal epithelium that extends into the stromal layer and is caused by bacteria, protozoa, or fungi.

coronary artery bypass graft (CABG) A surgical procedure in which occluded coronary arteries are bypassed with the patient's own venous or arterial blood vessels or synthetic grafts.

coronary artery disease (CAD) Disease affecting the arteries that provide blood, oxygen, and nutrients to the myocardium; partial or complete blockage of the blood flow through the coronary arteries, causing ischemia and infarction of the myocardium, angina pectoris, and acute coronary syndromes. Also known as *coronary heart disease* or simply *heart disease.*

coronary artery vasculopathy (CAV) A form of coronary artery disease that presents as diffuse plaque in the arteries of the donor heart in patients who have received a heart transplant.

cortisol The main glucocorticoid produced by the adrenal cortex.

coryza The common cold, or acute viral rhinitis.

cough assist A technique for assisting the tetraplegic patient to cough. Place his or her hands on either side of the rib cage or upper abdomen below the diaphragm; then, as the patient inhales, push upward to help expand the lungs and cough.

craniotomy Surgical incision into the cranium.

creatine kinase (CK) An enzyme specific to cells of the brain, myocardium, and skeletal muscle. Its appearance in the blood indicates tissue necrosis or injury, with levels following a predictable rise and fall during a specified period.

Credé maneuver A technique used to assist in urination in which a patient places his or her hand in a cupped position directly over the bladder area and pushes inward and downward gently as if massaging the bladder to empty.

crepitus A continuous grating sensation caused when irregular cartilage or bone fragments rub together and which may be felt or heard as a joint is put through passive range of motion; also, a crackling sensation that can be felt on a patient's chest, indicating that air is trapped within the tissues.

CREST syndrome In patients with systemic sclerosis, the combination of calcinosis (calcium deposits), Raynaud's phenomenon, esophageal dysmotility, sclerodactyly (scleroderma of the digits), and telangiectasia (spider-like hemangiomas).

cricothyroidotomy Surgical procedure in which an opening is made between the thyroid cartilage and cricoid cartilage ring and results in a tracheostomy. Also called *cricothyrotomy*. The procedure is used in an emergency for access to the lower airways.

crises In the patient with sickle cell disease, periodic episodes of extensive cellular sickling that have a sudden onset and can occur as often as weekly or as seldom as once a year.

critical access hospital A small rural facility of 15 or fewer inpatient beds that provides around-the-clock emergency care services 7 days per week. Considered a necessary provider of health care to community residents who are not close to other hospitals in a given region.

cross-contamination A type of contamination in which organisms from another person or from the environment are transmitted to the patient.

cryotherapy (1) A way of decreasing muscle pain by "cooling down" the area with a local, short-acting gel or cream, such as after physical therapy; (2) in ophthalmologic surgery, use of a freezing probe to repair retinal detachment.

cryptorchidism Failure of the testes to descend into the scrotum.

culture of safety A blame-free approach to improving care in high-risk, error-prone health care organizations using interprofessional collaboration. Patients and families are encouraged to become safety partners in protecting patients from harm.

culture A procedure for identifying a microorganism by cultivating and isolating it in tissue cultures or artificial media.

Curling's ulcer Acute ulcerative gastroduodenal disease, which may develop within 24 hours of a severe burn injury because of reduced gastrointestinal blood flow and mucosal damage.

Cushing's disease (Cushing's syndrome) Hypercortisolism caused by oversecretion of hormones by the adrenal cortex.

Cushing's triad A classic yet late sign of increased intracranial pressure (ICP) manifested by severe hypertension with a widened pulse pressure and bradycardia. As ICP increases, the pulse becomes thready, irregular, and rapid. Cerebral blood flow increases in response to hypertension.

Cushing's ulcer Acute ulcerative gastroduodenal disease that may develop as a result of increased intracranial pressure.

cutaneous (superficial) reflexes Superficial reflexes. Usually the plantar and abdominal reflexes are tested.

cyanosis Bluish or darkened discoloration of the skin and mucous membranes; results from an increased amount of deoxygenated hemoglobin.

cyclic feeding A method of tube feeding similar to continuous feeding (see definition of *continuous feeding*) except the infusion is stopped for a specified time in each 24-hour period ("down time"); the down time typically occurs in the morning to allow bathing, treatments, and other activities.

cystitis Inflammation of the bladder.

cystocele Herniation of the bladder into the vagina.

cytokines Small protein hormones produced by white blood cells.

cytotoxic Having cell-damaging effects.

D

dandruff An accumulation of patchy or diffuse white or gray scales on the surface of the scalp.

death rattle Loud, wet respirations caused by secretions in the respiratory tract and oral cavity of a patient who is near death.

death When illness or trauma overwhelms the compensatory mechanisms of the body and the lungs and heart cease to function.

débridement The removal of infected tissue from a healing wound.

debriefing After a mass casualty incident or disaster, (1) the provision of sessions for small groups of staff in which teams are brought in to discuss effective coping strategies (critical incident stress debriefing), and (2) the administrative review of staff and system performance during the event to determine opportunities for improvement in the emergency management plan.

debris Dead cells and tissues in a wound.

decerebrate posturing Abnormal posturing and rigidity characterized by extension of the arms and legs, pronation of the arms, plantar flexion, and opisthotonos; usually associated with dysfunction in the brainstem area. Also called *decerebration*.

decerebration See *decerebrate posturing*.

decompensated cirrhosis A form of cirrhosis in which liver function is significantly impaired with obvious manifestations of liver failure.

decompressive craniectomy Removal of a section of the skull in the patient with uncontrolled intracranial pressure (ICP); allows for additional space for edema without increasing ICP.

decorticate posturing Abnormal posturing seen in the patient with lesions that interrupt the corticospinal pathways. The arms, wrists, and fingers are flexed with internal rotation and plantar flexion of the legs. Also called *decortication*.

decortication See *decorticate posturing*.

deep tendon reflexes Tested as part of the neurologic assessment. An intact reflex arc is indicated when the muscle contracts in response to the tendon being struck with a reflex hammer.

deep vein thrombophlebitis Presence of a thrombus associated with inflammation in the deep veins, usually in the legs. Compared with superficial thrombophlebitis, it presents a greater risk for pulmonary embolism. Also called *deep vein thrombosis*.

deep vein thrombosis (DVT) Common term for *deep vein thrombophlebitis*.

defibrillation An asynchronous countershock that depolarizes a critical mass of myocardium simultaneously to stop the re-entry circuit, allowing the sinus node to regain control of the heart.

dehiscence A partial or complete separation of the outer layers of a wound, sometimes described as a "splitting open" of the wound.

dehydration Fluid intake less than what is needed to meet the body's fluid needs.

delayed union Term describing a fracture that has not healed within 6 months of injury.

delegation The process of transferring to a competent person the authority to perform a selected nursing task or activity in a selected patient care situation.

delirium An acute state of confusion, usually short-term and reversible within 3 weeks. Often seen among older adults in a hospital or other unfamiliar setting.

dementia A syndrome of slowly progressive cognitive decline with global impairment of intellectual function. The most common type is Alzheimer's disease.

demyelination Destruction of myelin between the nodes of Ranvier; a major pathologic finding in multiple sclerosis or Guillain-Barré syndrome.

depolarization The ability of a cell to respond to a stimulus by initiating an impulse. Also called *excitability*.

depression A response to multiple life stresses, a single situation, a primary disorder, or a problem associated with dementia; this response can range from mild, transient feelings of sadness to a severe sense of helplessness and hopelessness.

dermal papillae Fingerlike projections of dermal tissue that anchor the epidermis to the dermis.

dermatomes Specific areas of the skin that receive sensory input from spinal nerves.

descending tracts Groups of nerves that begin in the brain and end in the spinal cord.

desquamation The shedding or peeling of skin.

diabetic nephropathy A vascular complication of diabetes mellitus that causes permanent damage to kidney tissue and is a leading cause of end-stage kidney disease.

diabetic peripheral neuropathy (DPN) A progressive deterioration of nerves that results in loss of nerve function (sensory perception). A common complication of diabetes, it often involves all parts of the body.

diagnostic peritoneal lavage (DPL) Test that determines the presence of internal bleeding following abdominal trauma.

dialysate The solution used in dialysis. It is composed of water, glucose, sodium chloride, potassium, magnesium, calcium, and bicarbonate; dialysate composition may be altered according to the patient's needs for treatment of electrolyte imbalances.

dialyzer The apparatus used to perform hemodialysis. Also known as the "artificial kidney," it has four parts: a blood compartment, a dialysate compartment, a semipermeable membrane, and an enclosed structure to support the membrane.

diaphragmatic pacing A pacemaker for the phrenic nerve to cause the diaphragm to contract (leading to inhalation). Also known as *phrenic nerve pacing.*

diarrhea A condition in which the stool can be watery and without solid form.

diastole The phase of the cardiac cycle that consists of relaxation and filling of the atria and ventricles; normally about two thirds of the cardiac cycle.

diastolic blood pressure The amount of pressure/force against the arterial walls during the relaxation phase of the heart.

diastolic heart failure Heart failure that occurs when the left ventricle is unable to relax adequately during diastole, which prevents the ventricle from filling with sufficient blood to ensure adequate cardiac output.

Dietary Guidelines for Americans Recommendations made by the USDA and U.S. Department of Health and Human Services to help people maintain nutritional health; updated every 5 years.

Dietary Reference Intakes (DRIs) Nutrition guide developed by the Institute of Medicine of the National Academies that provides a scientific basis for food guidelines in the United States and Canada.

diffuse axonal injury (DAI) A type of closed head injury that is usually related to high-speed acceleration/deceleration, as with motor vehicle crashes. There is significant damage to axons in the white matter, and there are lesions in the corpus callosum, midbrain, cerebellum, and upper brainstem. Patients with severe injury may present with immediate coma, and most survivors require long-term care.

diffuse cutaneous systemic sclerosis Skin thickening on the trunk, face, and proximal and distal extremities in patients with systemic sclerosis.

diffuse light reflex A description of a light reflex that is spotty or multiple because of a changed eardrum shape from either retraction or bulging.

diffusion The spontaneous, free movement of particles (solute) across a permeable membrane down a concentration gradient; that is, from an area of higher concentration to an area of lower concentration.

digestion The mechanical and chemical process in which complex foodstuffs are broken down into simpler forms that can be used by the body.

digital 3D mammography Breast imaging procedure that allows the radiologist to visualize through layers or "slices" of breast tissue, similar to a CT scan.

digoxin toxicity A reaction to therapy with digitalis derivatives (digoxin) that is identified by monitoring serum digoxin and potassium levels (hypokalemia potentiates digitalis toxicity). Signs of toxicity are nonspecific (anorexia, fatigue, changes in mental status). Toxicity may cause dysrhythmia, most commonly premature ventricular contractions.

dilated cardiomyopathy (DCM) A type of cardiomyopathy that involves extensive damage to the myofibrils and interference with myocardial metabolism. There is normal ventricular wall thickness but dilation of both ventricles and impairment of systolic function.

dilation Increase in the diameter of blood vessels.

diplopia Double vision.

direct current stimulation (DCS) The placement of an implantable device to promote bone fusion; used as an adjunct for patients for whom spinal fusion may be difficult.

direct inguinal hernia A sac formed from the peritoneum that contains a portion of the intestine and passes through a weak point in the abdominal wall.

direct response Pupil constriction in response to bringing a penlight in from the side of the patient's head and shining the light in the eye being tested as soon as the patient opens his or her eyes.

directly observed therapy (DOT) A technique in which a health care professional watches the patient swallow prescribed drugs.

disabling health condition Any physical or mental health problem that can cause disability.

disaster triage tag system A system that categorizes triage priority by colored and numbered tags.

disaster A mass casualty incident in which the number of casualties exceeds the resource capabilities of a particular community or hospital facility.

discoid lesion Round lesion in patients who have discoid lupus erythematosus; evident when exposed to sunlight or ultraviolet light.

disease-modifying antirheumatic drugs (DMARDs) Drugs prescribed to slow the progression of mild rheumatoid disease before it worsens, such as hydroxychloroquine, sulfasalazine, or minocycline.

disequilibrium A condition in which the hydrostatic pressure is not the same in the two fluid spaces on either side of a permeable membrane.

disinfection A method of infection control in which the level of disease-causing organisms is reduced but the organisms are not killed; adequate when an item is entering a body area that has resident bacteria or normal flora, such as the respiratory tract.

diskitis Disk inflammation.

dislocation of a joint Occurrence of the articulating surfaces of two or more bones moving away from each other.

dissociate The act of separating and releasing ions.

diverticula Sacs resulting from the herniation of the mucosa and submucosa of a tubular organ into surrounding tissue.

diverticulitis The inflammation of one or more diverticula.

diverticulosis The presence of many abnormal pouchlike herniations (diverticula) in the wall of the intestine.

dizziness A disturbed sense of a person's relationship to space.

DNR Do not resuscitate; order from a physician or other authorized health care provider who instructs that CPR not be attempted in the event of cardiac or respiratory arrest.

dopamine agonist A class of drugs that mimic dopamine. Dopamine agonists stimulate dopamine receptors and are typically the most effective during the first 3 to 5 years of use. Prescribed for the patient with Parkinson disease to reduce dyskinesias (problems with movement).

dose-dense chemotherapy Chemotherapy that uses higher doses more often for aggressive cancer treatment, especially breast cancer.

double-barrel stoma The least common type of colostomy, which is created by dividing the bowel and bringing both the proximal and distal portions to the abdominal surface to create two stomas.

double-contrast barium enema A type of contrast radiography (x-rays) in which the patient's colon and rectum are visualized after a liquid containing barium, and then air, is placed into the colon.

doubling time The amount of time it takes for a tumor to double in size.

Droplet Precautions Infection control guidelines from the U.S. Centers for Disease Control and Prevention; used for patients with infections spread by the droplet transmission route, such as influenza.

drug holiday Period of time lasting up to 10 days in which the patient with Parkinson disease receives no drug therapy.

dual x-ray absorptiometry (DXA or DEXA) A type of radiographic scan that measures bone mineral density in the hip, wrist, or vertebral column; used as a screening and diagnostic tool for diagnosis and for follow-up evaluation of treatment of osteoporosis.

ductal carcinoma in situ (DCIS) An early, noninvasive form of breast cancer in which cancer cells are located within the duct and have not invaded the surrounding fatty breast tissue.

ductal ectasia A benign breast disease caused by dilation and thickening of the collecting ducts in the subareolar area. The ducts become distended and filled with cellular debris, which activates an inflammatory response. It is usually seen in women approaching menopause.

dumping syndrome A constellation of vasomotor symptoms that typically occur within 30 minutes after eating; believed to occur as a result of the rapid emptying of gastric contents into the small intestine, which shifts fluid into the gut and causes abdominal distention. Early manifestations include vertigo, tachycardia, syncope, sweating, pallor, and palpitations.

Dupuytren's contracture A slowly progressive contracture of the palmar fascia that results in flexion of the fourth or fifth digit of the hand and occasionally affects the third digit. Although a fairly common problem, the cause is unknown. It usually occurs in older men, tends to occur in families, and can be bilateral.

durable power of attorney for health care (DPOAHC) A legal document in which a person appoints someone else to make health care decisions in the event he or she becomes incapable of making decisions.

dysarthria Slurred speech.

dysfunctional uterine bleeding (DUB) A nonspecific term to describe bleeding that is excessive or abnormal in amount or frequency without predisposing anatomic or systemic conditions. Such bleeding occurs most often at either end of the span of a woman's reproductive years, when ovulation is becoming established or when it is becoming irregular at menopause.

dyskinesia Difficulty with movement.

dyslexia Problems understanding written language; caused by brain injury or disease.

dysmetria The inability to direct or limit movement.

dyspareunia Painful sexual intercourse.

dyspepsia Indigestion or heartburn following meals.

dysphagia Difficulty in swallowing.

dysphasia Slurred speech.

dyspnea on exertion (DOE) Dyspnea that is associated with activity, such as climbing stairs.

dyspnea Difficulty in breathing or breathlessness.

dysrhythmia A disorder of the heartbeat involving a disturbance in cardiac rhythm; irregular heartbeat.

dystrophic Pertaining to or characterized by dystrophy; abnormal.

dystrophin A muscle protein that maintains muscle integrity by sending signals to coordinate smooth, synchronous muscle fiber contraction. Faulty action of this protein causes muscular dystrophy.

dysuria Painful urination.

E

Eaton-Lambert syndrome A form of myasthenia gravis that affects the muscles of the trunk and the pelvic and shoulder girdles; often observed in combination with small cell carcinoma of the lung. Although weakness increases after exertion, there may be a temporary increase in muscle strength during the first few contractions, followed by a rapid decline.

ecchymoses Large purple, blue, or yellow bruises of the skin resulting from small hemorrhages; these bruises are larger than petechiae.

ecchymotic Pertaining to a bruise.

ECG caliper A measurement tool used in analysis of an electrocardiographic (ECG) rhythm strip.

echocardiography In cardiovascular assessment, the use of ultrasound waves to assess cardiac structure and mobility, particularly of the valves; a noninvasive, risk-free test that is easily performed at the bedside or on an ambulatory care basis.

echolalia Automatic repetition of what another person says.

ectopic Out of place.

ectropion A turning outward and sagging of the eyelid, which is caused by relaxation of the orbicular muscle.

edema Tissue swelling as a result of the accumulation of excessive fluid in the interstitial spaces.

edentulous Without teeth.

efferent arterioles The extremely small blood vessels that carry the remaining blood out of the glomerulus (once the glomerulus has filtered the blood to make urine) and into one of two additional capillary systems (the peritubular capillaries or the vasa recta).

effluent Drainage.

effusion An accumulation of fluid, such as in a joint (where it may limit movement).

ejection fraction The percentage of blood ejected from the heart during systole.

electrical bone stimulation The use of an electronic device (e.g., magnetic coils applied on the skin or over a cast to deliver a pulsed magnetic field) to promote bone union after a fracture. The exact mechanism of action is unknown, but this procedure is based on research showing that bone has inherent electrical properties that are used in healing.

electrocardiogram (ECG) A graphic recording of the electrical current generated by the heart. The ECG provides information about cardiac dysrhythmias, myocardial ischemia, site and extent of myocardial infarction, cardiac hypertrophy, electrolyte imbalances, and effectiveness of cardiac drugs. It is a routine part of cardiovascular evaluation and is a valuable diagnostic test.

electroencephalography (EEG) A recording of the electrical activity of the cerebral hemispheres; it represents the voltage changes in various areas of the brain as determined by recording the difference between two electrodes.

electrolyte A substance in body fluids that carries an electrical charge. Also called an *ion*.

electromyography (EMG) A recording of the electrical activity of peripheral nerves by testing muscle activity.

electrophysiologic study (EPS) In cardiovascular assessment, an invasive procedure performed in a catheterization laboratory during which programmed electrical stimulation of the heart is used to induce and evaluate lethal dysrhythmias and conduction abnormalities to permit accurate diagnosis and effective treatment. The study is used in patients who have survived cardiac arrest, have recurrent tachydysrhythmias, or experience unexplained syncopal episodes.

electrovaporization of the prostate (EVAP) Procedure for treating benign prostatic hyperplasia with high-frequency electrical current to cut and vaporize excess tissue.

elimination The excretion of waste from the body by the GI tract (as feces) and by the kidneys (as urine).

embolectomy Removal of a blood clot.

embolic stroke Damage to the brain when a blood clot forms somewhere in the body (usually the heart) and travels through the bloodstream to block one or more of the arteries supplying the brain.

embolus The occurrence of inflammation and thickening of the vein wall around a clot (thrombus).

emergence Recovery from anesthesia.

emergency medical technician (EMT) Prehospital care provider who supplies basic life-support interventions such as oxygen, basic wound care, splinting, spinal immobilization, and monitoring of vital signs.

emergency medicine physician A member of the emergency health care team with education and training in the specialty of emergency patient management.

emergency operations center (EOC) A designated location in the Hospital Incident Command System (HICS) with accessible communication technology. Also called the *command center*.

emergency preparedness A goal or plan to meet an extraordinary need for hospital beds, staff, drugs, personal protective equipment, supplies, and medical devices such as mechanical ventilators.

Emergency Severity Index (ESI) A standardized model for triage that categorizes both patient acuity and resource utilization into five levels, from most urgent to least urgent.

emergent triage In a three-tiered triage scheme, the category that includes any condition or injury that poses an immediate threat to life or limb, such as crushing chest pain or active hemorrhage.

emetogenic A substance that induces nausea and vomiting.

emmetropia The state of perfect refraction of the eye; with the lens at rest, light rays from a distant source are focused into a sharp image on the retina.

emotional abuse The intentional use of threats, humiliation, intimidation, and isolation to another person.

emotional lability Having uncontrollable emotions; for example, the patient laughs and then cries unexpectedly for no apparent reason.

empyema A collection of pus in the pleural space.

encephalitis An inflammation of the brain parenchyma (brain tissue) and meninges that affects the cerebrum, brainstem, and cerebellum; usually caused by a virus.

endogenous An infection in which organisms are carried by the bloodstream from other areas of infection in the body.

endometrial ablation Procedure for dysfunctional uterine bleeding that removes a built-up uterine lining using a laser, roller ball, or balloon.

endometrial cancer Cancer of the inner uterine lining.

endometriosis The abnormal occurrence of endometrial tissue outside the uterine cavity.

endometritis An infection of the endometrium.

endoscope A tube that allows viewing and manipulation of internal body areas.

endoscopic retrograde cholangiopancreatography (ERCP) The visual and radiographic examination of the liver, gallbladder, bile ducts, and pancreas by means of an endoscope and the injection of radiopaque dye to identify the cause and location of obstruction.

endoscopic variceal ligation (EVL) The application of small "O" bands around the base of esophageal varices to cut off their blood supply. Also called *banding*.

endoscopy The direct visualization of the gastrointestinal tract by means of a flexible fiberoptic endoscope.

endothelin A secretion produced by the endothelial cells when they are stretched.

endovascular stent graft The repair of an abdominal aortic aneurysm using a stent made of flexible material; the stent is inserted through a skin incision into the femoral artery by way of a catheter-based system.

end-stage kidney disease (ESKD) Acute renal failure combined with chronic renal insufficiency, resulting in the inability of the kidney to excrete waste products normally. The patient may need hemodialysis or a kidney transplant.

energy conservation Strategies to reduce the fatigue associated with chronic and disabling conditions, such as allowing rest periods and setting priorities.

engraftment The successful transplantation of cells in the patient's bone marrow.

enophthalmos Backward displacement of the eyeball into the orbit so that the eye appears sunken.

enteroscopy Visualization of the small intestine.

enterostomal feeding tube A tube used for patients who need long-term enteral feeding; the physician directly accesses the gastrointestinal tract using surgical, endoscopic, or laparoscopic techniques.

entropion The turning inward of the eyelid, causing the eyelashes to rub against the eye.

enucleation The surgical removal of the entire eyeball.

envenomation Venom injection from a snakebite.

epididymitis Inflammation of the epididymis.

epidural hematoma An accumulation of clotted blood resulting from arterial bleeding into the space between the dura and the skull; a neurosurgical emergency.

epidural Term for the space between the dura mater and vertebrae; it consists of fat, connective tissue, and blood vessels.

epiglottis A leaf-shaped, elastic structure that is attached along one edge to the top of the larynx; it closes over the glottis during swallowing to prevent food from entering the trachea and opens during breathing and coughing.

epiglottitis Infection or inflammation of the epiglottis and supraglottic structures that results in swelling. If swelling is great enough, the airway can be obstructed.

epilepsy A chronic disorder characterized by recurrent, unprovoked seizure activity; may be caused by an abnormality in electrical neuronal activity, an imbalance of neurotransmitters, or a combination of both.

epistaxis Nosebleed.

erectile dysfunction (ED) The inability to achieve or maintain a penile erection sufficient for sexual intercourse.

ergonomics An applied science in which the workplace is designed to increase worker comfort (thus reducing injury) while increasing efficiency and productivity.

erosion Ulceration.

eructation The act of belching.

erythema migrans A round or oval flat or slightly raised rash.

erythema Redness of the skin.

erythrocyte A red blood cell (RBC). Red blood cells are the major cells in the blood and are responsible for tissue oxygenation.

erythroplakia A velvety red mucosal lesion, most often occurring in the oral cavity.

erythropoiesis The selective maturation of stem cells into mature erythrocytes.

eschar The crust of dead tissue that forms from coagulated particles of destroyed dermis in a patient with a full-thickness burn injury.

escharotomy Incision made through tight eschar to relieve pressure and allow normal blood flow and breathing.

esophageal stricture Narrowing of the esophageal opening.

esophageal varices The distention of fragile, thin-walled esophageal veins due to increased pressure; the increased pressure is a result of portal hypertension, in which the blood backs up from the liver and enters the esophageal and gastric vessels that carry it into the systemic circulation.

esophagectomy The surgical removal of all or part of the esophagus.

esophagitis Inflammation of the esophagus.

esophagogastroduodenoscopy (EGD) The visual examination of the esophagus, stomach, and duodenum by means of a fiberoptic endoscope.

esophagogastrostomy The surgical creation of a communication between the stomach and the esophagus; it involves the removal of part of the esophagus and proximal stomach.

essential hypertension Elevated blood pressure that is not caused by a specific disease. The major risk factor is a family history of hypertension. Also called *primary hypertension*.

euploid Having the correct number of chromosome pairs for the species.

euploidy The normal diploid number for a cell.

eustachian tube Tube that connects the nasopharynx with the middle ear and opens during swallowing to equalize pressure within the middle ear.

euthyroid Having normal thyroid function.

euvolemia A state of balanced fluid intake and output.

evidence-based practice (EBP) A QSEN competency in which the nurse integrates best current evidence with clinical expertise and patient/family preferences and values for delivery of optimal health care.

evisceration The total separation of all layers of a wound and the protrusion of internal organs through the open wound.

evoked potentials Tests to measure the electrical signals to the brain generated by hearing, touch, or sight. Also called *evoked response*.

exacerbation An increase in severity of a disease. Also called *flare-up*.

excitability The ability of a cell to respond to a stimulus by initiating an impulse. Also called *depolarization*. In cardiac electrophysiology, it is the ability of non-pacemaker myocardial cells to respond to an electrical impulse generated from pacemaker cells and to depolarize.

exemplars Selected health problems and issues that are associated with health and professional nursing concepts.

exercise electrocardiography In cardiovascular assessment, a test that assesses cardiovascular response to an increased workload. Also called *exercise tolerance* or a *stress test*. Exercise electrocardiography helps determine the functional capacity of the heart, screens for coronary artery disease, and identifies dysrhythmias that develop during exercise. It also aids in evaluating the effectiveness of antidysrhythmic drugs.

exercise tolerance See *exercise electrocardiography*.

exertional dyspnea Breathlessness or difficulty breathing that develops during activity or exertion.

exertional heat stroke A form of heat stroke with a sudden onset, typically due to strenuous physical activity in hot, humid conditions. Lack of acclimatization to hot weather and wearing clothing too heavy for the environment are common contributing factors.

exogenous hyperthyroidism Hyperthyroidism caused by excessive use of thyroid replacement hormones.

exogenous Originating outside the body.

exophthalmos Abnormal protrusion of the eyeball (proptosis).

expedited partner therapy (EPT) Therapy used to treat chlamydia in which patients are given a drug or prescription with specific instructions for administration to their partners without direct evaluation by a health care provider. Also called *patient-delivered partner therapy*.

exploratory laparotomy A surgical opening of the abdominal cavity to investigate the cause of an obstruction or peritonitis.

exposure (1) The final component of the primary survey that allows for thorough assessment of the trauma patient; (2) in radiation therapy, the amount of radiation that is delivered to a tissue.

expressed gene When a particular gene has been "turned on."

expressed Turned on or activated.

expressive aphasia A type of aphasia resulting from damage in Broca's area of the frontal lobe of the brain. A motor speech problem in which the patient understands what is said but is unable to communicate verbally and has difficulty writing; rote speech and automatic speech, such as responses to a greeting, are often intact. The patient is aware of the deficit and may become frustrated and angry. Also called *Broca's aphasia* or *motor aphasia*.

expressivity In genetics, the degree of expression a person has when a specific autosomal dominant gene is present. The gene is always expressed, but some people have more severe results.

external fixation A system in which pins or wires are passed through skin and bone and connected to a rigid external frame to immobilize a fracture during healing.

external fixator See *external fixation*.

external hemorrhoid A hemorrhoid that lies below the anal sphincter and can be seen on inspection of the anal region.

external otitis A painful irritation or infection of the skin of the external ear, with resulting allergic response or inflammation. When it occurs in patients who participate in water sports, external otitis is called *swimmer's ear*.

external urethral sphincter The sphincter composed of the skeletal muscle that surrounds the urethra.

extracapsular Located outside the joint capsule.

extracellular fluid (ECF) The portion of total body water (about one third) that is in the space outside the cells. This space also includes interstitial fluid, blood, lymph, bone, and connective tissue water, and the transcellular fluids.

extracranial-intracranial bypass A surgical procedure in which the surgeon performs a craniotomy and bypasses the blocked artery by making a graft (bypass) from the first artery to the second artery to establish blood flow around the blocked artery and re-establish blood flow to the involved areas.

extramedullary tumor A tumor found within the spinal dura but outside the cord.

extrapulmonary Involving nonpulmonary tissues.

extravasation Escape of fluids or drugs into the subcutaneous tissue; a complication of intravenous infusion.

extrinsic factor In hematology, an event (e.g., trauma) that occurs outside the blood to cause platelet plugs to form.

extubation The removal of an endotracheal tube.

F

facial paralysis See *Bell's palsy*.

facilitated diffusion Diffusion across a cell membrane that requires the assistance of a transport system or membrane-altering system. Also called *facilitated transport*.

facilitated transport See *facilitated diffusion*.

failed back surgery syndrome (FBSS) A combination of organic, psychological, and socioeconomic factors in patients for whom back surgery is not successful. Discouraged by repeated surgical procedures, these patients must continue long-term nonsurgical management of pain, including nerve blocks.

failure to rescue The inability of nurses or other interprofessional health team members to save a patient's life in a timely manner when a health care issue or medical complication occurs.

fall An unintentional change in body position that results in the patient's body coming to rest on the floor or ground.

fallophobia In some older adults, the fear of falling and sustaining a serious injury.

far point (of vision) The farthest point at which the eye can see an object.

fascia An inelastic tissue that surrounds groups of muscles, blood vessels, and nerves in the body.

fasciculation Abnormal, involuntary twitching of a muscle.

fasciotomy A surgical procedure in which an incision is made through the skin and subcutaneous tissues into the fascia of the affected compartment to relieve the pressure in and restore circulation to the affected area in the patient with acute compartment syndrome.

fat embolism syndrome (FES) A serious complication, usually resulting from a fracture, in which fat globules are released from the yellow bone marrow into the bloodstream. This syndrome usually occurs within 48 hours of the fracture and can result in respiratory failure or death, often from pulmonary edema.

fatigue (stress) fracture A fracture that results from excessive or repeated strain and stress on a bone.

fatty liver Caused by the accumulation of fats in and around the hepatic cells. It may be caused by alcohol abuse or other factors. Also known as *steatosis*.

fecal microbiota transplantation (FMT) A procedure in which healthy normal flora is placed into the lower GI system of the infected patient who does not respond to antibiotic therapy or has recurrent disease .

fecal occult blood test (FOBT) A diagnostic test that measures the presence of blood in the stool from gastrointestinal bleeding; this is a common finding associated with colorectal cancer.

Felty's syndrome The combination of rheumatoid arthritis, hepatosplenomegaly (enlarged liver and spleen), and leukopenia.

femoral hernia A hernia that protrudes through the femoral ring.

fetor hepaticus The distinctive fruity or musty breath odor of chronic liver disease and portal-systemic encephalopathy.

fibrinolysis The breakdown of a clot.

fibrinolytic Drug that targets the fibrin component of the coronary thrombosis; used to dissolve thrombi in the coronary arteries and restore myocardial blood flow; examples include tissue plasminogen activator, anisoylated plasminogen-streptokinase activator complex, and reteplase.

fibroadenoma A solid, slowly enlarging benign mass of connective tissue that is unattached to the surrounding breast tissue and is typically discovered by the patient herself. The mass is usually round, firm, easily movable, nontender, and clearly delineated from the surrounding tissue.

fibrocystic breast condition (FBC) Physiologic nodularity of the breast that is thought to be caused by an imbalance in the normal estrogen-to-progesterone ratio. It is the most common breast problem of women between 20 and 30 years of age.

fibroids See *leiomyomas*.

fibromyalgia syndrome (FMS) A chronic pain syndrome characterized by pain and tenderness at specific sites in the back of the neck, upper chest, trunk, low back, and extremities along with fatigue, sleep disturbances, and headache.

fibrosis Replacement of normal cells with connective tissue and collagen (scar tissue).

fidelity Ethical principle that refers to the agreement that nurses will keep their obligations or promises to patients to follow through with care.

filter The movement of fluid from the space with higher hydrostatic pressure through the membrane into the space with lower hydrostatic pressure.

filtration The movement of fluid through a cell or blood vessel membrane because of hydrostatic pressure differences on both sides of the membrane.

financial abuse Mismanagement or misuse of the patient's property or resources.

first heart sound (S₁) Sound created by the closure of the mitral and tricuspid valves (atrio-ventricular valves).

first intention Healing in which the wound can be easily closed and dead space eliminated without granulation, which thus shortens the phases of tissue repair. Inflammation resolves quickly, and connective tissue repair is minimal, resulting in a thin scar.

fistula An abnormal opening between two adjacent organs or structures.

five cardinal manifestations of inflammation Warmth, redness, swelling, pain, and decreased function.

fixed occlusion Wiring the jaws together in the mouth closed position.

flaccid bladder See *areflexic bladder*.

flaccid paralysis Paralysis of a part of the body that is characterized by loss of muscle tone due to hypotonia; may be seen in the patient who has experienced a brain attack.

flail chest Inward movement of the thorax during inspiration, with outward movement during expiration; results from multiple rib fractures caused by blunt chest trauma that leaves a segment of the chest wall loose.

flat bone Bone that protects vital organs and often contains blood-forming cells, such as the scapula.

flatulence The presence of an excessive amount of gas in the stomach or intestines.

fluid and electrolyte balance The regulation of body fluid, fluid osmolality, and electrolytes by processes such as filtration, diffusion, and osmosis.

fluid overload An excess of body fluid. Also called *overhydration*.

folliculitis A superficial bacterial infection involving only the upper portion of the hair follicle.

forensic nurse examiner (RN-FNE) Emergency department specialist who is trained to recognize evidence of abuse and to intervene on the patient's behalf and who obtains patient histories, collects forensic evidence, and offers counseling and follow-up care for victims of rape, child abuse, and domestic violence.

fracture A break or disruption in the continuity of a bone.

fremitus Vibrations felt on the chest or back when the patient talks.

fremitus Vibration.

frequency (1) The highness or lowness of tones (expressed in hertz). The greater the number of vibrations per second, the higher the frequency (pitch) of the sound; the fewer the number of vibrations per second, the lower the pitch; (2) an urge to urinate frequently in small amounts.

fresh frozen plasma (FFP) Plasma that is frozen immediately after donation so that the clotting factors are preserved.

friable Easily crumbled or damaged.

frostbite A cold injury characterized by the degree of tissue freezing and the resultant damage it produces. Frostbite injuries can be superficial, partial, or full thickness.

frostnip A form of superficial frostbite (typically on the face, fingers, or toes) that produces pain, numbness, and pallor but is easily remedied with the application of warmth and does not induce tissue injury.

Fulmer SPICES A framework that identifies six serious "marker conditions" that can lead to longer hospital stays for patients, higher medical costs, and deaths.

fulminant hepatitis A severe acute and often fatal form of hepatitis caused by failure of the liver cells to regenerate, with progression to necrosis.

furuncle A localized inflammation of the skin caused by bacterial infection, usually *Staphylococcus*, of a hair follicle. Also called a *boil*.

G

gallium scan A test that is similar to a bone scan but that uses the radioisotope *gallium citrate* and is more specific and sensitive in detecting bone problems. This substance also migrates to brain, liver, and breast tissue and therefore is used to examine these structures when disease is suspected.

gamma globulin See *immunoglobulin*.

ganglion A round, cystlike lesion, often overlying a wrist joint or tendon.

gas exchange The process of oxygen transport to the cells and carbon dioxide transport away from the cells through ventilation and diffusion.

gastrectomy The surgical removal of part or all of the stomach.

gastric bypass A type of gastric restriction surgery in which gastric resection is combined with malabsorption surgery. The patient's stomach, duodenum, and part of the jejunum are bypassed so that fewer calories can be absorbed. Also known as a *Roux-en-Y gastric bypass*, or *RNYGB*.

gastric lavage Procedure of irrigating the stomach in which a large-bore nasogastric tube is inserted into the stomach and room-temperature solution is instilled in volumes of 200 to 300 mL. The solution and blood are repeatedly withdrawn manually until returns are clear or light pink and without clots.

gastritis An inflammation of the gastric mucosa (stomach lining).

gastroenteritis An increase in the frequency and water content of stools or vomiting as a result of inflammation of the mucous membranes of the stomach and intestinal tract. It affects primarily the small bowel and can be of either viral or bacterial origin.

gastroesophageal reflux (GER) Condition that occurs as a result of backward flow of stomach contents into the esophagus.

gastroesophageal reflux disease (GERD) An upper gastrointestinal disease caused by the backward flow (reflux) of gastrointestinal contents into the esophagus.

gastrojejunostomy Surgical anastomosis of the stomach to the jejunum.

gastroparesis Delay in gastric emptying.

gastrostomy A stoma created from the abdominal wall into the stomach.

gel phenomenon In patients with rheumatoid arthritis, morning stiffness that lasts between 45 minutes and several hours after awakening.

gender dysphoria Discomfort with one's natal sex.

gender identity A person's inner sense of maleness or femaleness not related to reproductive anatomy.

gender reassignment surgery See *sex reassignment surgery*.

gene The deoxyribonucleic acid (DNA) in the form of chromosomes within the nucleus of each cell that contains the instructions for making all the different proteins any organism makes. Every human cell with a nucleus contains the entire set of human genes.

general anesthesia A reversible loss of consciousness induced by inhibiting neuronal impulses in the central nervous system.

generalized seizure One of the three broad categories of seizure disorders along with partial seizures and unclassified seizures. There are six types: tonic-clonic, tonic, clonic, absence, myoclonic, and atonic (akinetic).

genetics The science concerned with the general mechanisms of heredity and the variation of inherited traits.

genital herpes (GH) An acute, recurring incurable viral disease of the genitalia caused by the herpes simplex virus and transmitted through contact with an infected person. An outbreak typically is preceded by a tingling sensation of the skin followed by the appearance of vesicles (blisters) on the penis, scrotum, vulva, perineum, vagina, cervix, or perianal region. The blisters rupture spontaneously, leaving painful erosions. After the lesions heal, the virus remains dormant, periodically reactivating with a recurrence of symptoms.

genome The complete set of human genes. Each human cell with a nucleus contains the entire set of human genes. The human genome contains about 35,000 individual genes.

genomic health care The application of known genetic variation to enhance health care to individuals and their families.

genomics The science focusing on the function of all of the human DNA, including genes and noncoding DNA regions.

genotype The actual alleles for a genetic trait, not just what can be observed.

genu valgum A deformity in which the knees are abnormally close together and the space between the ankles is increased. Also called *knock-knee*.

genu varum A deformity in which the knees are abnormally separated and the lower extremities are bowed inward. Also called *bowleg*.

Geriatric Depression Scale—Short Form (GDS-SF) A valid and reliable screening tool to help determine if an older patient has clinical depression.

geriatric failure to thrive (GFTT) A complex syndrome including under-nutrition, impaired physical functioning, depression, and cognitive impairment.

geriatric syndromes Major health issues that are associated with late adulthood in community and inpatient settings.

ghrelin The "hunger hormone" that is secreted in the stomach; increases in a fasting state and decreases after a meal.

Glasgow Coma Scale (GCS) An objective and widely accepted tool for neurologic assessment and documentation of level of consciousness. It establishes baseline data for eye opening, motor response, and verbal response. The patient is assessed and assigned a numeric score for each of these areas. A score of 15 represents normal neurologic functioning, and a score of 3 represents a deep coma state.

glaucoma A group of ocular diseases resulting in increased intraocular pressure, causing reduced blood flow to the optic nerve and retina and followed by tissue damage.

glomerulus A series of specialized capillary loops that receive blood from the afferent arteriole and then filter water and small particles from the blood to make urine. The remaining blood leaves the glomerulus via the efferent arteriole.

glossectomy The partial or total surgical removal of the tongue.

glossitis A smooth, beefy red tongue.

glottis The opening between the true vocal cords inside the larynx.

glucagon A hormone secreted by the pancreas that increases blood glucose levels. It is a "counterregulatory" hormone that has actions opposite those of insulin. It causes the release of glucose from cell storage sites whenever blood glucose levels are low.

gluconeogenesis The conversion of proteins and amino acids to glucose in the body.

glucosamine A supplement that may decrease inflammation.

glycemic A term referring to blood glucose.

glycogenesis The production of glycogen in the body.

glycogenolysis The breakdown of glycogen into glucose.

glycoprotein (GP) IIb/IIIa inhibitors Drugs that target the platelet component of the thrombus. They are administered intravenously to prevent fibrinogen from attaching to activated platelets at the site of a thrombus and are given to patients with acute coronary syndromes (especially unstable angina and non–Q-wave myocardial infarction). Examples include abciximab, eptifibatide, and tirofiban.

glycosylated hemoglobin (A1C) A standardized test that measures how much glucose permanently attaches to the hemoglobin molecule. A1C levels greater than 6.5% are diagnostic of diabetes mellitus.

"go bag" See *personal readiness supplies*.

goiter Enlargement of the thyroid gland.

gonadotropins Hormones that stimulate the ovaries and testes to produce sex hormones.

gonads The male and female reproductive endocrine glands. Male gonads are the testes, and female gonads are the ovaries.

goniometer An instrument for measuring angles; also refers to a tool used to measure joint range of motion.

good death A death that is free from avoidable distress and suffering for patients, families, and caregivers; in agreement with patients' and families' wishes; and consistent with clinical practice standards.

gout A systemic disease in which urate crystals deposit in the joints and other body tissues, causing inflammation.

grading System of classifying cellular aspects of a cancer tumor.

granulation The formation of scar tissue for wound healing to occur.

granuloma Growth that develops in the lungs of patients with sarcoidosis and contains lymphocytes, macrophages, epithelioid cells, and giant cells; scar tissue.

Graves' disease Toxic diffuse goiter characterized by hyperthyroidism, enlargement of the thyroid gland, abnormal protrusion of the eyes, and dry, waxy swelling of the front surfaces of the lower legs.

gray (gy) Unit of measurement for an absorbed radiation dose.

gray matter In the spinal cord, neuron cell bodies.

grief The emotional feeling related to the perception of loss.

grommet A polyethylene tube that is surgically placed through the tympanic membrane to allow continuous drainage of middle-ear fluids in the patient with otitis media.

ground substance A lubricant composed of protein and sugar groups that surrounds the dermal cells and fibers and contributes to the skin's normal suppleness and turgor.

guardian A person appointed to make health care decisions for a patient who is determined to not be legally competent.

Guillain-Barré syndrome (GBS) An acute autoimmune disorder characterized by varying degrees of motor weakness and paralysis. It may be referred to by a variety of other names, such as *acute idiopathic polyneuritis* and *polyradiculoneuropathy*.

gynecomastia Abnormal enlargement of the breasts in men.

H

H₂-receptor antagonists A group of drugs that inhibit gastric acid secretion by blocking the effects of histamine on parietal cell receptors in the stomach.

half-life Time it takes for the amount of drug in the body to be reduced by 50%.

halitosis A foul odor of the mouth.

hallux valgus A common deformity of the foot that occurs when the great toe deviates laterally at the metatarsophalangeal joint; sometimes referred to as a *bunion*.

halo fixator A static traction device used for immobilization of the cervical spine. Four pins or screws are inserted into the skull, and a metal halo ring is attached to a plastic vest or cast when the spine is stable, allowing increased patient mobility.

"halo" sign A clear or yellowish ring surrounding a spot of blood.

hammertoe The dorsiflexion of any metatarsophalangeal joint with plantar flexion of the adjacent proximal interphalangeal joint. The second toe is most often affected.

hand hygiene Infection control protocol that refers to both handwashing and alcohol-based hand rubs.

hantavirus pulmonary syndrome A severe and potentially lethal respiratory disease that is a complication of hantavirus infection carried by mice and rats.

health care–associated infection (HAI) Infections associated with the provision of health care; for example, microorganisms can enter the body through the genitourinary tract in patients with indwelling urinary catheters.

heart failure A general term for the inadequacy of the heart to pump blood throughout the body, causing insufficient perfusion of body tissues with vital nutrients and oxygen. Also called *pump failure*.

heart rate (HR) Term referring to the number of times the ventricles contract each minute.

heart transplantation A surgical procedure in which a heart from a donor with a comparable body weight and ABO compatibility is transplanted into a recipient less than 6 hours after procurement. It is the treatment of choice for patients with severe dilated cardiomyopathy and may be considered for patients with restrictive cardiomyopathy.

heat exhaustion A syndrome primarily caused by dehydration from heavy perspiration and inadequate fluid and electrolyte consumption during heat exposure over hours to days; if left untreated, can be a precursor to heat stroke.

heat stroke A true medical emergency in which the victim's heat regulatory mechanisms fail and are unable to compensate for a critical elevation in body temperature; if uncorrected, organ dysfunction and death will ensue.

Heberden's nodes Swelling at the distal interphalangeal joints in osteoarthritis that involves the hands.

hematemesis The vomiting of blood.

hematochezia The passage of red blood via the rectum.

hematocrit The percentage of packed red blood cells per deciliter of blood.

hematogenous See *endogenous*.

hematogenous tuberculosis A form of tuberculosis that spreads throughout the body when a large number of organisms enter the blood. Also called *miliary tuberculosis*.

hematopoiesis The production of blood cells, which occurs in the red marrow of bones.

hematuria Blood in the urine.

hemianopsia Blindness in half of the visual field of one or both eyes. Also called *hemianopia*.

hemiarthroplasty Surgical replacement of part of the shoulder joint, typically the humeral component, as an alternative to total shoulder arthroplasty.

hemiparesis Weakness on one side of the body.

hemiplegia Paralysis on one side of the body.

hemoconcentration Elevated plasma levels of hemoglobin, hematocrit, serum osmolarity, glucose, protein, blood urea nitrogen, and electrolytes that occur when only the water is lost and other substances remain.

hemodilution Excessive water in the vascular space.

hemoglobin A (HbA) Normal adult hemoglobin. The molecule has two alpha chains and two beta chains of amino acids.

hemoglobin S (HbS) An abnormal beta chain of hemoglobin associated with sickle cell disease that is sensitive to low oxygen content of red blood cells.

hemolytic anemia Anemia caused by the destruction of red blood cells.

hemolytic The characteristic of destroying red blood cells.

hemoptysis Coughing up blood or blood-stained sputum.

hemorrhoid Unnaturally swollen or distended vein in the anorectal region.

hemorrhoidectomy The excision of a hemorrhoid.

hemostasis The multistep process of controlled blood clotting.

hemothorax Bleeding into the chest cavity.

heparin-induced thrombocytopenia (HIT) The aggregation of platelets into "white clots" that can cause thrombosis, usually in the form of an acute arterial occlusion; occurs with heparin administration. Also called *white clot syndrome*.

hepatic encephalopathy See *portal-systemic encephalopathy*.

hepatitis A Hepatitis that is caused by the hepatitis A virus (HAV) and is characterized by a mild course similar to that of a typical viral syndrome and often goes unrecognized. It is spread via the fecal-oral route by oral ingestion of fecal contaminants. Sources of infection include contaminated water, shellfish caught in contaminated water, and food contaminated by infected food handlers. The virus may also be spread by oral-anal sexual activity. The incubation period is usually 15 to 50 days. The disease is usually not life threatening but may be more severe in people older than 40 years. It can also complicate pre-existing liver disease.

hepatitis B A form of hepatitis that is caused by the hepatitis B virus (HBV), which is shed in the body fluids of infected people and asymptomatic carriers. It is spread through unprotected sexual intercourse with an infected partner, needle sharing, blood transfusions, and other modes. Symptoms usually occur within 25 to 180 days of exposure and include nausea, fever, fatigue, joint pain, and jaundice. Most adults who get hepatitis B recover, clear the virus from their bodies, and develop immunity; however, up to 10% of patients with the disease do not develop immunity and become carriers.

hepatitis C Hepatitis that is caused by the hepatitis C virus (HCV). Transmission is blood to blood, most commonly by needle sharing or needlestick injury with contaminated blood. The rate of sexual transmission is very low; it is not spread by casual contact and is rarely transmitted from mother to fetus. The average incubation period is 7 weeks. Most people are asymptomatic and are not diagnosed until long after the initial exposure when an abnormality is detected during a routine laboratory evaluation or when symptoms of liver impairment appear. Hepatitis C causes chronic inflammation in the liver that eventually causes the hepatocytes to scar and may progress to cirrhosis.

hepatitis carrier Person who has had hepatitis B but has not developed immunity. Hepatitis carriers can infect others even though they are not sick and demonstrate no obvious signs of disease. Chronic carriers are at high risk for cirrhosis and liver cancer.

hepatitis D The hepatitis D virus (HDV) co-infects with hepatitis B virus (HBV) and needs the presence of HBV for viral replication. HDV can co-infect a patient with HBV or can occur as a superinfection in a patient with chronic HBV. Superinfection usually develops into chronic HDV infection. The incubation period is 14 to 56 days. As with HBV, the disease is transmitted primarily by parenteral routes.

hepatitis E Hepatitis E virus (HEV) was originally identified by its association with waterborne epidemics of hepatitis in the Indian subcontinent. Since then, it has occurred in epidemics in Asia, Africa, the Middle East, Mexico, and Central and South America, typically after heavy rains and flooding. In the United States, hepatitis E has been found only in travelers returning from endemic areas. The virus is transmitted via the fecal-oral route, and the clinical course resembles that of hepatitis A. HEV has an incubation period of 15 to 64 days. There is no evidence at this time of a chronic form of hepatitis E.

hepatitis The widespread inflammation of liver cells.

hepatocyte Liver cell.

hepatomegaly Enlargement of the liver.

hepatorenal syndrome (HRS) A state of progressive oliguric renal failure associated with hepatic failure, resulting in functional impairment of kidneys with normal anatomic and morphologic features. It indicates a poor prognosis for the patient with hepatic failure and is often the cause of death in patients with cirrhosis.

hereditary chronic pancreatitis Pancreatitis that may be associated with *SPINK1* and *CFTR* gene mutations.

heritability The risk that a disorder can be transmitted to one's children in a recognizable pattern.

hernia A weakness in the abdominal muscle wall through which a segment of the bowel or other abdominal structure protrudes.

herniated nucleus pulposus (HNP) The protrusion (herniation) of the pulpy material from the center of a vertebral disk; herniated disks occur most often between the fourth and fifth lumbar vertebrae (L4-5) but may occur at other levels. A herniation in the lumbosacral area can press on the adjacent spinal nerve (usually the sciatic nerve), causing severe burning or stabbing pain into the leg or foot, or it may press on the spinal cord itself, causing leg weakness and bowel and bladder dysfunction. The specific area of pain depends on the level of herniation.

hernioplasty Surgical repair of a hernia in which the surgeon reinforces the weakened outside muscle wall with a mesh patch.

herniorrhaphy The surgical repair of a hernia.

heterotopic ossification Abnormal bony overgrowth, often into muscle; seen as a complication of prolonged immobility in patients with spinal cord injury.

hiatal hernia Protrusion of the stomach through the esophageal hiatus of the diaphragm and into the thorax. Also called *diaphragmatic hernia*.

high altitude disease (HAD) See *high altitude illnesses*.

high altitude illnesses Pathophysiologic responses in the body caused by exposure to low partial pressure of oxygen at high elevations.

high altitude pulmonary edema (HAPE) A form of acute mountain sickness often seen with high altitude cerebral edema. Clinical indicators include persistent dry cough, cyanosis of the lips and nail beds, tachycardia and tachypnea at rest, and rales auscultated in one or both lungs. Pink, frothy sputum is a late sign.

high-alert drug A drug that has an increased risk for causing patient harm if given in error.

high-density lipoproteins (HDLs) Part of the total cholesterol value that should be more than 45 mg/dL for men and more than 55 mg/dL for women; "good" cholesterol.

highly sensitive C-reactive protein (hsCRP) A serum marker of inflammation and a common and critical component to the development of atherothrombosis.

high-output heart failure Heart failure that occurs when cardiac output remains normal or above normal. It is usually caused by increased metabolic needs or hyperkinetic conditions such as septicemia (fever), anemia, and hyperthyroidism. This type of heart failure is different from left- and right-sided heart failure, which are typically low-output states, and is not as common as other types.

hilum The area of the kidney in which the renal artery and nerve plexus enter and the renal vein and ureter exit. This area is not covered by the renal capsule.

hirsutism Abnormal growth of body hair, especially on the face, chest, and the linea alba of the abdomen of women.

homeostasis The narrow range of normal conditions (e.g., body temperature, blood electrolyte values, blood pH, blood volume) in the human body; the tendency to maintain a constant balance in normal body states.

homeostatic mechanism A safeguard or control mechanism within the human body that prevents dangerous changes.

homocysteine An essential sulfur-containing amino acid that is produced when dietary protein breaks down; elevated values (greater than 15 mmol/L) may be a risk factor for the development of cardiovascular disease.

homonymous hemianopsia Condition in which there is blindness in the same side of both eyes.

hordeolum An infection of the sweat glands in the eyelid.

hormone Chemical produced in the body that exerts its effects on specific tissues known as *target tissues*.

hospice An interdisciplinary approach to facilitate quality of life and a "good" death for patients near the end of their lives, with care provided in a variety of settings.

Hospital Incident Command System (HICS) An organizational model for disaster management in which roles are formally structured under the hospital or long-term care facility incident commander, with clear lines of authority and accountability for specific resources.

hospital incident commander As defined in a hospital's emergency response plan, the person (either an emergency physician or administrator) who assumes overall leadership for implementing the institutional plan at the onset of a mass casualty incident. The hospital incident commander has a global view of the entire situation, facilitates patient movement through the system, and brings in resources to meet patient needs.

hospitalist Family practitioner or internist employed by a hospital.

human leukocyte antigen (HLA) Antigen that is present on the surfaces of nearly all body cells as a normal part of the person and acts as an antigen only if it enters another person's body.

human papilloma virus (HPV) test A test that can identify many high-risk types of HPV associated with the development of cervical cancer.

humoral immunity A type of immunity provided by antibodies circulating in body fluids.

Huntington disease (HD) A hereditary disorder transmitted as an autosomal dominant trait at the time of conception (formerly called *Huntington chorea*). Men and women between 35 and 50 years of age are affected; clinical onset is gradual. The two main symptoms are progressive mental status changes (leading to dementia) and choreiform movements (rapid, jerky movements) in the limbs, trunk, and facial muscles.

hydrocephalus The abnormal accumulation of cerebrospinal fluid within the skull.

hydronephrosis Abnormal enlargement of the kidney caused by a blockage of urine lower in the tract and filling of the kidney with urine.

hydrophilic Tending to absorb water readily.

hydrophobic Not readily absorbing water; waterproof.

hydrostatic pressure The force of the weight of water molecules pressing against the confining walls of a space.

hydrotherapy The application of water for treatment of injury or disease.

hydroureter Abnormal distention of the ureter.

hyperacusis An intolerance for sound levels that do not bother other people.

hyperaldosteronism Excessive mineralocorticoid production.

hypercalcemia A total serum calcium level above 10.5 mg/dL or 2.75 mmol/L, which can cause fatigue, anorexia, nausea and vomiting, constipation, polyuria, and serious damage to the urinary system.

hypercapnia Increased arterial carbon dioxide levels.

hypercarbia Increased partial pressure of arterial carbon dioxide ($PaCO_2$) levels.

hypercellularity An abnormal number of cells.

hypercoagulability Increased clotting ability.

hyperemia Increased blood flow to an area.

hyperesthesia Abnormally increased sensation.

hyperextension A mechanism of injury that occurs when a part of the body is suddenly accelerated and then decelerated, causing extreme extension.

hyperflexion A mechanism of injury that occurs when a part of the body is suddenly and forcefully accelerated forward, causing extreme flexion.

hyperglycemia Abnormally high levels of blood glucose.

hyperinsulinemia Chronic high blood insulin levels.

hyperkalemia An elevated level of potassium in the blood.

hyperlipidemia An elevation of serum lipid (fat) levels in the blood.

hypermagnesemia A serum magnesium level above 2.1 mEq/L.

hypernatremia An excessive amount of sodium in the blood.

hyperopia An error of refraction that occurs when the eye does not refract light enough, causing images to fall (converge) behind the retina and resulting in poor near vision. Also called *farsightedness*.

hyperosmotic Describes fluids with osmolarities (solute concentrations) greater than 300 mOsm/L; hyperosmotic fluids have a greater osmotic pressure than do isosmotic fluids and tend to pull water from the isosmotic fluid space into the hyperosmotic fluid space until an osmotic balance occurs. Also called *hypertonic*.

hyperpharmacy See *polypharmacy*.

hyperphosphatemia A serum phosphorus level above 4.5 mg/dL.

hyperpituitarism Hormone oversecretion that occurs with pituitary tumors or hyperplasia.

hyperplasia Growth that causes tissue to increase in size by increasing the number of cells; abnormal overgrowth of tissue.

hyperpnea An abnormal increase in the depth of respiratory movements.

hypersensitivity An overreaction to a foreign substance.

hypertension A cardiovascular condition pertaining to people who have a systolic blood pressure of 140 mm Hg or higher or a diastolic blood pressure of 90 mm Hg or higher or who take medication to control blood pressure; approximately 1 of every 5 Americans has hypertension.

hypertensive crisis A severe elevation in blood pressure (greater than 180/120 mm Hg) that can cause damage to organs such as the kidneys or heart.

hyperthermia Elevated body temperature; fever.

hyperthyroidism A condition caused by excessive production of thyroid hormone.

hypertonia A condition of excessive muscle tone, which tends to cause fixed positions or contractures of the involved extremities and restricted range of motion of the joints.

hypertonic See *hyperosmotic*.

hypertriglyceridemia Elevated levels (150 mg/dL or above) of triglyceride in the blood.

hypertrophic cardiomyopathy (HCM) A type of cardiomyopathy that involves disarray of the myocardial fibers and asymmetric ventricular hypertrophy; leads to a stiff left ventricle that results in diastolic filling abnormalities.

hypertrophy The enlargement or overgrowth of an organ; tissue increases in size by the enlargement of each cell.

hyperuricemia An excess of uric acid in the blood.

hyperventilation A state of increased rate and depth of breathing.

hyperviscous The quality of being thicker than normal.

hypervolemia Increased plasma volume; or fluid excess.

hypocalcemia A total serum calcium level below 9.0 mg/dL or 2.25 mmol/L.

hypocapnia Decreased arterial carbon dioxide levels.

hypocarbia $Paco_2$ less than 40 to 45 mm Hg or decreased partial pressure of carbon dioxide in arterial blood.

hypodermoclysis The slow infusion of isotonic fluids into subcutaneous tissue.

hypoesthesia Abnormally decreased sensation.

hypoglycemia Abnormally low levels of glucose in the blood.

hypokalemia A decreased serum potassium level; a common electrolyte imbalance.

hypomagnesemia A low serum magnesium level, usually lower than 1.8 mEq/L or 0.74 mmol/L.

hyponatremia A serum sodium level below 136 mEq/L (mmol/L).

hypo-osmotic Describes fluids with osmolarities of less than 270 mOsm/L. Hypo-osmolar fluids have a lower osmotic pressure than isosmotic fluids, and water tends to be pulled from the hypo-osmotic fluid space into the isosmotic fluid space until an osmotic balance occurs. Also called *hypotonic*.

hypophonia Soft voice.

hypophosphatemia Inadequate levels of phosphate in the blood (below 3.0 mg/dL).

hypophysectomy Surgical removal of the pituitary gland.

hypoproteinemia A decrease in serum proteins.

hypothalamic-hypophysial portal system The small, closed circulatory system that the hypothalamus shares with the anterior pituitary gland; it allows hormones produced in the hypothalamus to travel directly to the anterior pituitary gland.

hypothalamus A structure within the brain; an integral part of autonomic nervous system control (controlling temperature and other functions) that is essential in intellectual function.

hypothermia A core body temperature less than 95° F (35° C).

hypotonia An abnormal condition of inadequate muscle tone, with an inability to maintain balance.

hypotonic See *hypo-osmotic*.

hypoventilation A state in which gas exchange at the alveolar-capillary membrane is inadequate so that too little oxygen reaches the blood and carbon dioxide is retained.

hypovolemia Abnormally decreased volume of circulating fluid in the body; fluid deficit.

hypoxemia (hypoxemic) Decreased blood oxygen levels; hypoxia.

hypoxia A reduction of oxygen supply to the tissues.

hysterosalpingogram An x-ray of the cervix, uterus, and fallopian tubes that is performed after injection of a contrast medium. This test is used in infertility workups to evaluate tubal anatomy and patency and uterine problems such as fibroids, tumors, and fistulas.

hysteroscopy Examination of the interior of the uterus and cervical canal using an endoscope.

I

icterus Yellow discoloration of the sclerae.

idiopathic chronic pancreatitis Pancreatitis that may be associated with *SPINK1* and *CFTR* gene mutations.

idiopathic seizure See *unclassified seizure*.

ileostomy The surgical creation of an opening into the ileum, usually by bringing the end of the terminal ileum through the abdominal wall and forming a stoma, or ostomy.

immediate memory Short-term or new memory. Test by asking the patient to repeat two or three unrelated words to make sure they were heard; after about 5 minutes, while continuing the examination, ask the patient to repeat the words.

immunity Resistance to infection; usually associated with the presence of antibodies or cells that act on specific microorganisms.

immunocompetent Having proper functioning of the body's ability to maintain itself and defend against disease.

immunoglobulin Antibody. Also called *gamma globulin*.

impermeable Not porous.

implanted port A device used for long-term or frequent infusion therapy; consists of a portal body, a dense septum over a reservoir, and a catheter that is surgically implanted on the upper chest or upper extremity.

inactivation The process of binding an antibody to an antigen to cover the antigen's active site and to make the antigen harmless without destroying it. Also called *neutralization*.

incisional hernia Protrusion of the intestine at the site of a previous surgical incision resulting from inadequate healing. Most often caused by postoperative wound infections, inadequate nutrition, and obesity. Also called *ventral hernia*.

incomplete spinal cord injury An injury in which the spinal cord has been damaged in a way that allows some function or movement below the level of the injury.

incontinence Involuntary loss of urine or stool severe enough to cause social or hygienic problems.

independent living skills See *instrumental activities of daily living (IADLs)*.

indirect inguinal hernia A sac formed from the peritoneum that contains a portion of the intestine or omentum. The hernia pushes downward at an angle into the inguinal canal. In males, indirect inguinal hernias can become large and often descend into the scrotum.

indolent Slow-growing.

induration Hardening.

infarction Necrosis, or cell death.

infective endocarditis A microbial infection (e.g., viruses, bacteria, fungi) involving the endocardium; previously called *bacterial endocarditis*.

inferior vena cava filtration Surgical procedure in which the surgeon inserts a filter device percutaneously into the inferior vena cava of a patient with recurrent deep vein thrombosis (to prevent pulmonary emboli) or pulmonary emboli that do not respond to medical treatment. The device is meant to trap emboli in the inferior vena cava before they progress to the lungs. Holes in the device allow blood to pass through, thus not significantly interfering with the return of blood to the heart.

inferior wall myocardial infarction A type of myocardial infarction that occurs in patients with obstruction of the right coronary artery, causing significant damage to the right ventricle.

infiltrating ductal carcinoma The most common type of breast cancer; it originates in the mammary ducts and grows in the epithelial cells lining these ducts.

infiltration The leakage of IV solution into the tissues around the vein.

inflammatory breast cancer A rare but highly aggressive form of invasive breast cancer. Symptoms include swelling, skin redness, and pain in the breasts.

inflammatory cytokines Proteins produced primarily by white blood cells that assist in the inflammatory and immune responses of the body (e.g., tumor necrosis factor, interleukins).

inflow disease Chronic peripheral arterial disease with obstruction at or above the common iliac artery, abdominal aorta, or profunda femoris artery. The patient experiences discomfort in the lower back, buttocks, or thighs after walking a certain distance. The pain usually subsides with rest.

informatics A QSEN competency in which the nurse uses information and technology to communicate, manage knowledge, mitigate error, and support decision making.

infratentorial Located below the tentorium of the cerebellum.

infusate A solution that is infused into the body.

infusion therapy The delivery of parenteral medications and fluids through a variety of catheter types and locations using multiple techniques and procedures, such as intravenous and intra-arterial therapy to deliver solutions into the vascular system.

inpatient rehabilitation facilities (IRFs) Free-standing rehabilitation hospitals, rehabilitation or skilled units within hospitals (e.g., transitional care units), and skilled nursing facilities to which the patient is typically admitted for 1 to 3 weeks or longer.

inpatient A patient who is admitted to a hospital.

insensible water loss Water loss from the skin, lungs, and stool that cannot be controlled.

instrumental activities of daily living (IADLs) Special activities performed in the course of a day such as using the telephone, shopping, preparing food, and housekeeping. Also called *independent living skills.*

insufflation The practice of injecting gas or air into a cavity before surgery to separate organs and improve visualization.

intensity A quality of sound that is expressed in decibels; generally, having a high degree of energy or activity.

intensivist A physician who specializes in critical care.

intention tremor A tremor that occurs when performing an activity.

interbody cage fusion Cagelike spinal device that is implanted into the space where a disk was removed. Bone graft tissue grows into and around the cage and creates a stable spine at that level.

intercostally Located between the ribs.

intermittent claudication A characteristic leg pain experienced by patients with chronic peripheral arterial disease. Typically, patients can walk only a certain distance before a cramping muscle pain forces them to stop. As the disease progresses, the patient can walk only shorter and shorter distances before pain recurs. Ultimately, pain may occur even at rest.

internal derangement A broad term for disturbances of an injured knee joint.

internal fixation The use of metal pins, screws, rods, plates, or prostheses to immobilize a fracture during healing. The surgeon makes an incision (open reduction) to gain access to the broken bone and implants one or more devices.

internal hemorrhoid A hemorrhoid that is located above the anal sphincter and cannot be seen on inspection of the perineal area.

internal urethral sphincter The smooth detrusor muscle that lines the interior of the bladder neck.

interstitial cystitis A bladder inflammation of unknown etiology that occurs predominantly in women and is characterized by urinary frequency and pain on bladder filling.

interstitial fluid A portion of the extracellular fluid that is between cells, sometimes called the *third space.*

interstitial laser coagulation (ILC) Procedure for treating benign prostatic hyperplasia that uses laser energy to coagulate excess tissue. Also called *contact laser prostatectomy (CLP).*

intra-abdominal hypertension (IAH) Condition of sustained or repeated intra-abdominal pressure of 12 mm Hg or higher.

intra-abdominal pressure Pressure contained within the abdominal cavity.

intra-aortic balloon pump (IABP) An intra-aortic counterpulsation device. It may be used as an invasive intervention to improve myocardial perfusion during an acute myocardial infarction, to reduce preload and afterload, and to facilitate left ventricular ejection. It is also used when patients do not respond to drug therapy with improved tissue perfusion, decreased workload of the heart, and increased cardiac contractility.

intra-arterial infusion therapy The use of catheters placed into arteries to obtain repeated arterial blood samples, to monitor various hemodynamic pressures continuously, and to infuse chemotherapy agents or fibrinolytics.

intracapsular Located within the joint capsule.

intracellular fluid (ICF) The portion of total body water (about two thirds) that is found inside the cells.

intracerebral hemorrhage Bleeding within the brain tissue caused by the tearing of small arteries and veins in the subcortical white matter.

intracorporeal Situated or occurring inside the body.

intramedullary tumor Tumor originating within the spinal cord in the central gray matter and anterior commissure. It is often malignant.

intraocular pressure (IOP) Pressure of the fluid within the eye; may be measured by methods that involve direct contact with the eye or by noncontact techniques.

intraoperative During surgery.

intraosseous (IO) therapy Infusion therapy that is delivered to the vascular network in the long bones.

intraperitoneal (IP) infusion therapy The administration of antineoplastic agents into the peritoneal cavity.

intrapulmonary Within the respiratory tract.

intrarenal/intrinsic renal failure Decreased renal function resulting from damage to the glomeruli, interstitial tissue, or tubules. It can contribute to acute renal failure.

intrathecal Referring to the spine.

intravascular ultrasonography (IVUS) In cardiac catheterization, the use of a flexible catheter with a miniature transducer that emits sound waves. Sound waves are reflected off the plaque and the arterial wall, creating an image of the blood vessel; used as an alternative to injecting a contrast medium into the coronary arteries.

intravenous (systemic) fibrinolytic therapy The intravenous administration of thrombolytic agents to dissolve a thrombus.

intravesical Situated inside the bladder.

intrinsic factor A substance normally secreted by the gastric mucosa and needed for intestinal absorption of vitamin B_{12}. A deficiency of intrinsic factor and the resulting failure to absorb vitamin B_{12} lead to pernicious anemia.

intussusception The telescoping of a segment of the intestine within itself.

invasive hemodynamic monitoring System used in critical care areas to provide quantitative information about vascular capacity, blood volume, pump effectiveness, and tissue perfusion. It directly measures pressures in the heart and great vessels.

ion A substance found in body fluids that carries an electrical charge. Also called *electrolyte.*

iontophoresis A treatment for lower back pain in which a small electrical current and dexamethasone are typically used.

ipsilateral Occurring on the same side.

iris The colored portion of the external eye; its center opening is the pupil. Muscles of the iris contract and relax to control pupil size and the amount of light entering the eye.

irreducible hernia A hernia that cannot be reduced or placed back into the abdominal cavity; requires immediate surgical evaluation.

irregular bone Bone that has a unique shape, such as the carpal bones of the wrist.

irritability An overresponse to stimuli.

irritable bowel syndrome (IBS) A chronic gastrointestinal disorder characterized by chronic or recurrent diarrhea, constipation, and/or abdominal pain and bloating. Also called *spastic colon, mucous colon,* or *nervous colon.*

ischemia Blockage of blood flow through a blood vessel resulting in a lack of oxygen. Prolonged severe ischemia can cause irreversible damage to tissue.

ischemic stroke A type of brain attack caused by occlusion of a cerebral artery by either a thrombus or an embolus. About 80% of all brain attacks are ischemic.

ischemic Cell dysfunction or death from a lack of oxygen resulting from decreased blood flow in a body part.

isoelectric Having equal electric potentials, such as in the heart.

isosmotic Having the same osmotic pressures. Also called *isotonic* or *normotonic*.

isotonic See *isosmotic*.

J

jaundice A syndrome characterized by excessive circulating bilirubin levels. Liver cells cannot effectively excrete bilirubin, and skin and mucous membranes become characterized by a yellow coloration.

jejunostomy The surgical creation of an opening between the jejunum and the surface of the abdominal wall.

joint The place at which two or more bones come together. Also referred to as "articulation" of the joint. The primary function is to provide movement and flexibility in the body.

jugular venous distention (JVD) Enlargement of the jugular vein of the neck; caused by an increase in jugular venous pressure.

juxtaglomerular complex Specialized cells that produce and store renin in the afferent arteriole, efferent arteriole, and distal collecting tubule; taken together, the juxtaglomerular cells and the macula densa.

K

karyotype Technique used to make an organized arrangement of all the chromosomes within one cell during the metaphase section of mitosis.

keratin The protein produced by keratinocytes; makes the outermost skin layer waterproof.

keratinocytes Basal skin cells attached to the basement membrane of the epidermis that undergo cell division and differentiation to continuously renew skin tissue integrity and maintain optimal barrier function. As basal cells divide, keratinocytes are pushed upward and flattened to form the stratified layers of the epithelium (Malpighian layers).

keratoconjunctivitis sicca A condition of the eyes that results from changes in tear composition, lacrimal gland malfunction, or altered tear distribution. Also called *dry eye syndrome*.

keratoconus The degeneration of the corneal tissue resulting in abnormal corneal shape.

keratoplasty Corneal transplant. The surgical removal of diseased corneal tissue and replacement with tissue from a human donor cornea.

ketogenesis The conversion of fats to acids in the body.

ketone bodies Substances, including acetone, that are produced as by-products of the incomplete metabolism of fatty acids. When insulin is not available (as in uncontrolled diabetes mellitus), they accumulate in the blood and cause metabolic acidosis. Also called *ketones*.

knee height caliper Device that uses the distance between the patella and heel to estimate height.

Kupffer cells Phagocytic cells that are part of the body's reticuloendothelial system and that are involved in the protective function of the liver. Kupffer cells engulf harmful bacteria and anemic red blood cells.

Kussmaul respiration A type of breathing that occurs when excess acids caused by the absence of insulin increase hydrogen ion and carbon dioxide levels in the blood. This state triggers an increase in the rate and depth of respiration in an attempt to excrete more carbon dioxide and acid.

kwashiorkor Lack of protein quantity and quality in the presence of adequate calories. Body weight is somewhat normal, and serum proteins are low.

kyphoplasty A minimally invasive surgery for managing vertebral fractures in patients with osteoporosis. Bone cement is injected into the fracture site to provide pain relief, and an inflated balloon is used to restore height to the vertebra.

L

labyrinthectomy Surgical removal of the labyrinth; used as a radical treatment of Ménière's disease when medical therapy is ineffective and the patient already has significant hearing loss.

labyrinthitis An infection of the labyrinth of the ear; may occur as a complication of acute or chronic otitis media.

laceration A type of wound characterized by tearing or mangling and usually caused by sharp objects and projectiles.

lacrimal gland A small gland that produces tears; located in the upper outer part of each ocular orbit.

lacto-ovo-vegetarian A vegetarian diet pattern in which milk, cheese, eggs, and dairy foods are eaten but meat, fish, and poultry are avoided.

lactose intolerance The inability to convert lactose (found in milk and dairy products) to glucose and galactose in the body.

lacto-vegetarian A vegetarian diet pattern in which milk, cheese, and dairy foods are eaten but meat, fish, poultry, and eggs are avoided.

laparoscopy A minimally invasive procedure in which the surgeon makes several small incisions near the umbilicus through which a small endoscope is placed to examine the abdomen; direct examination of the pelvic cavity through an endoscope.

laparotomy An open surgical approach in which a large abdominal incision is made.

laryngectomee A person who has had a laryngectomy.

laryngopharynx The area behind the larynx that extends from the base of the tongue to the esophagus. It is the critical dividing point at which solid foods and fluids are separated from air.

larynx The "voice box"; it is composed of several cartilages and is located above the trachea and just below the throat at the base of the tongue; part of the upper respiratory tract.

laser An acronym for light amplification by stimulated emission of radiation. As a surgical tool, a laser emits a high-powered beam of light that cuts tissue more cleanly than do scalpel blades. A laser creates intense heat, rapidly clots blood vessels or tissue, and turns target tissue (e.g., a tumor) into vapor.

latency period The time between the initiation of a cell and the development of an overt tumor.

latex allergy Reactions to exposure to latex in gloves and other medical products; reactions include rashes, nasal or eye symptoms, and asthma.

latrodectism A syndrome caused by the venom of a black widow spider bite in which neurotransmitter releases from nerve terminals to cause severe abdominal pain, muscle rigidity and spasm, hypertension, and nausea and vomiting.

lead axis In electrocardiography, the imaginary line that joins the positive and negative poles of the lead systems.

lead In an ECG, the provider of one view of the heart's electrical activity.

left shift An increase in the band cells (immature neutrophils) in the white blood cell differential count; an early indication of infection.

left-sided heart (ventricular) failure Inadequacy of the left ventricle of the heart to pump adequately; results in decreased tissue perfusion from poor cardiac output and pulmonary congestion from increased pressure in the pulmonary vessels; typical causes include hypertensive, coronary artery, or valvular disease involving the mitral or aortic valve. Most heart failure begins with failure of the left ventricle and progresses to failure of both ventricles.

legally competent A legal term used to describe a person 18 years of age or older, a pregnant or a married minor, a legally emancipated (free) minor who is self-supporting, or a person not declared incompetent by a court of law.

leiomyomas Benign, slow-growing solid tumors of the uterine myometrium (muscle layer). These are the most commonly occurring pelvic tumors. Also called *myomas* and *fibroids*.

lens The circular, convex structure of the eye that lies behind the iris and in front of the vitreous body. Normally transparent, the lens bends the rays of light entering through the pupil so that they focus on the retina. The curve of the lens changes to focus on near or distant objects.

leptin A hormone that is released by fat cells and possibly by gastric cells; it also acts on the hypothalamus to control appetite.

lethargic Drowsy but easily awakened.

leukemia A type of cancer with uncontrolled production of immature white blood cells in the bone marrow; the bone marrow becomes overcrowded with immature, nonfunctional cells, and the production of normal blood cells is greatly decreased.

leukocyte White blood cell (WBC); this immune system cell protects the body from the effects of invasion by organisms.

leukopenia A reduction in the number of white blood cells.

leukoplakia White, patchy lesions on a mucous membrane.

level of consciousness (LOC) The degree of alertness or the amount of stimulation needed to engage a patient's attention and can range from *alert* to *coma*.

levels of evidence Term used to refer to the status, rank, or strength of evidence.

LGBTQ Acronym for "lesbian, gay, bisexual, transgender, and queer/questioning" culture.

libido Sexual desire.

lichenified An abnormal thickening of the skin to a leathery appearance; can occur in patients with chronic dermatitis because of their continual rubbing of the area to relieve itching.

Lichtenberg figures Branching or ferning marks that appear on the skin as a result of a lightning strike. Also called *keraunographic markings* or *erythematous arborization*.

life review A structured process of reflecting on one's life that is often facilitated by an interviewer.

ligament Connective tissue that attaches bones to other bones at joints.

light reflex The reflection of the otoscope's light off the eardrum in the form of a clearly demarcated triangle of light in the normal ear.

limited cutaneous systemic sclerosis Thick skin that is usually limited to sites distal to the elbow and knee but also involves the face and neck.

lipid Fat, including cholesterol and triglycerides, that can be measured in the blood.

lipolysis The decomposition or splitting up of fat to provide fuel for energy when liver glucose is unavailable.

liposuction A cosmetic procedure to reduce the amount of adipose tissue in selected areas of the body.

literacy challenged An individual who has a low reading level ability.

lithotripsy The use of sound, laser, or dry shock wave energy to break a kidney stone into small fragments. Also called *extracorporeal shock wave lithotripsy*.

living will A legal document that instructs physicians and family members about what life-sustaining treatment is wanted (or not wanted) if the patient becomes unable to make decisions.

lobectomy Surgical removal of an entire lung lobe.

lobular carcinoma in situ (LCIS) A noninvasive form of breast cancer that does not show up as a calcified cluster on a mammogram and is therefore most often diagnosed incidentally during a biopsy for another problem.

local anesthesia Anesthesia that is delivered by applying it to the skin or mucous membranes of the area to be anesthetized or by injecting it directly into the tissue around an incision, wound, or lesion.

locus The specific chromosome location for a gene.

log rolling Turning technique in which the patient turns all at once while his or her back is kept as straight as possible.

long bone Bone that is cylindric with rounded ends and often bears weight, such as the femur.

loop electrosurgical excision procedure (LEEP) Diagnostic procedure/treatment in which a thin loop-wire electrode that transmits a painless electrical current is used to cut away affected cervical cancer tissue.

lordosis The anterior concavity in the curvature of the lumbar and cervical spine when viewed from the side; a common finding in pregnancy and abdominal obesity.

Lou Gehrig's disease See *amyotrophic lateral sclerosis (ALS)*.

low back pain (LBP) Pain in the lumbosacral region of the back caused by muscle strain or spasm, ligament sprain, disk degeneration, or herniation of the nucleus pulposus from the center of the disk. Herniated disks occur most

often between the fourth and fifth lumbar vertebrae (L4-5) but may occur at other levels.

low-density lipoproteins (LDLs) Part of the total cholesterol value that should be less than 130 mg/dL; "bad" cholesterol.

lower esophageal sphincter (LES) The portion of the esophagus proximal to the gastroesophageal junction; when at rest, the sphincter is closed to prevent reflux of gastric contents into the esophagus.

lower urinary tract symptoms (LUTS) Symptoms that occur as a result from prostatic hyperplasia, such as urinary retention and overflow incontinence, or urinary leaking.

low-intensity pulsed ultrasound A method using ultrasonic waves to promote bone union in slow-healing fractures or for new fractures as an alternative to surgery.

low-profile gastrostomy device (LPGD) A gastrostomy device that uses a firm or balloon-style internal bumper or retention disk; an antireflux valve keeps gastric contents from leaking onto the skin.

loxoscelism Systemic effects from the injected toxin of a spider bite.

lumbar puncture (spinal tap) The insertion of a spinal needle into the subarachnoid space between the third and fourth (sometimes the fourth and fifth) lumbar vertebrae to withdraw spinal fluid for analysis.

lumen The inside cavity of a tube or tubular organ, such as a blood vessel or airway.

lung compliance The quality of elasticity of the lungs.

lunula The white crescent-shaped portion of the nail at the lower end of the nail plate.

lurch An abnormality in the swing phase of gait; occurs when the muscles in the buttocks or legs are too weak to allow the person to change weight from one foot to the other.

Lyme disease A systemic infectious disease that is caused by the spirochete *Borrelia burgdorferi* and results from the bite of an infected deer tick. Signs and symptoms include a large "bull's-eye" circular rash, malaise, fever, headache, and muscle or joint aches.

lymphadenopathy Persistently enlarged lymph nodes.

lymphedema Abnormal accumulation of protein fluid in the subcutaneous tissue of the affected limb after a mastectomy.

lymphoblastic Pertaining to abnormal leukemic cells that come from the lymphoid pathways and develop into lymphocytes.

lymphocytic Pertaining to abnormal leukemic cells that come from the lymphoid pathways.

lymphokine Cytokine produced by T-cells.

lysis Breakage, for example, of a cell membrane.

M

macrocytic anemia A form of vitamin B_{12} deficiency anemia characterized by abnormally large precursor cells.

macrovascular Referring to large blood vessels.

macular degeneration The deterioration of the macula, the area of central vision.

macular Referring to a macula, a discolored spot on the skin that is not raised above the surface.

magnesium (Mg^{2+}) A mineral that forms a cation when dissolved in water.

magnetoencephalography (MEG) A noninvasive imaging technique that measures the magnetic fields produced by electrical activity in the brain via extremely sensitive devices such as superconducting quantum interference devices (SQUIDs).

malabsorption A syndrome associated with a variety of disorders and intestinal surgical procedures and characterized by impaired intestinal absorption of nutrients.

malignant cell growth Altered cell growth that is serious and, without intervention, leads to death; cancer.

malignant hypertension A severe type of elevated blood pressure that rapidly progresses, with systolic blood pressure greater than 200 mm Hg and diastolic blood pressure greater than 150 mm Hg (greater than 130 mm Hg when there are pre-existing complications).

malignant transformation The process of changing a normal cell into a cancer cell.

malignant Referring to cancer.

mammography An x-ray of the soft tissue of the breast.

mandibulectomy Surgical removal of the jaw.

marasmic-kwashiorkor A combined protein and energy malnutrition that often presents clinically when metabolic stress is imposed on a chronically starved patient.

marasmus A calorie malnutrition in which body fat and protein are wasted but serum proteins are often preserved.

marsupialization Surgical formation of a pouch that is a new duct opening.

mass casualty event A situation affecting the public health that is defined based on the resource availability of a particular community or hospital facility. When the number of casualties exceeds the resource capabilities, a disaster situation is recognized to exist.

mastication The process of chewing.

mastoiditis An acute or chronic infection of the mastoid air cells caused by untreated or inadequately treated otitis media.

maze procedure An open chest surgical technique often performed with coronary artery bypass grafting for patients in atrial fibrillation with decompensation.

mean arterial pressure (MAP) The arterial blood pressure (between 60 and 70 mm Hg) necessary to maintain perfusion of major body organs, such as the kidneys and brain.

mechanical débridement Method of débriding a wound by mechanical entrapment and detachment of dead tissue.

mechanical obstruction The physical obstruction of the bowel by disorders outside the intestine (e.g., adhesions or hernias) or by blockages in the lumen of the intestine (e.g., tumors, inflammation, strictures, or fecal impactions).

mechanism of injury (MOI) The method by which a traumatic event occurred.

mediastinal shift A shift of central thoracic structures toward one side; seen on chest x-ray.

mediastinitis Infection of the mediastinum.

medical command physician As defined in a hospital's emergency response plan, the person responsible for determining the number, acuity, and medical resource needs of victims arriving from the incident scene and for organizing the emergency health care team response to injured or ill patients.

medical harm Physician incidents and all errors caused by members of the health care team or system that lead to patient injury or death.

medical nutrition supplements (MNSs) Enteral products taken by patients who cannot consume enough nutrients in their usual diet (e.g., Ensure, Boost).

medication overuse headache See *rebound headache.*

medication reconciliation A formal evaluative process in which the patient's actual current medications are compared with his or her prescribed medications at time of admission, transfer, or discharge to identify and resolve discrepancies.

medulla A general term for the most interior portion of an organ or structure.

melena Blood in the stool, with the appearance of black tarry stools.

memory cell A type of B-lymphocyte that remains sensitized but does not start to produce antibodies until the next exposure to the same antigen.

Ménière's disease Tinnitus, one-sided sensorineural hearing loss, and vertigo that is related to overproduction or decreased reabsorption of endolymphatic fluid and causes a distortion of the entire inner canal system.

meninges The immediate protective covering of the brain and the spinal cord.

meningioma A type of benign brain tumor that arises from the coverings of the brain (the meninges) and causes compression and displacement of adjacent brain tissue.

meningitis Inflammation, usually bacterial or viral, of the arachnoid and pia mater of the brain and spinal cord and the cerebrospinal fluid. May be caused by bacteria or viruses; symptoms are the same regardless of the causative organism.

meniscectomy Surgical excision of a meniscus, as in a knee joint.

menses The monthly flow of blood from the genital tract of women.

metabolic syndrome A collection of related health problems with insulin resistance as a main feature. Other features include obesity, low levels of physical activity, hypertension, high blood levels of cholesterol, and elevated triglyceride levels. Metabolic syndrome increases the risk for coronary heart disease. Also called *syndrome X.*

metastasis The growth and spread of cancer.

metastasize To spread cancer from the main tumor site to many other body sites.

metastatic Referring to disease, such as cancer, that transfers from one organ to another organ or part not directly connected; pertains to additional tumors that form after cancer cells move from the primary location by breaking off from the original group and establishing remote colonies.

methemoglobinemia The conversion of normal hemoglobin to methemoglobin.

microalbuminuria The presence of very small amounts of albumin in the urine that are not measurable by a urine dipstick or usual urinalysis procedures. Specialized assays are used to analyze a freshly voided urine specimen for microscopic levels of albumin.

microbiome The genomes of all the microorganisms that coexist in and on an adult and can affect cellular regulation.

microcytic Abnormally small in size, such as an abnormally small red blood cell.

microvascular decompression A surgical procedure to relieve the pain of trigeminal neuralgia by relocating a small artery that compresses the trigeminal nerve as it enters the pons. The surgeon carefully lifts the loop of the artery off the nerve and places a small silicone sponge between the vessel and the nerve.

microvascular Referring to small blood vessels.

midline catheter A type of catheter that is 6 to 8 inches long and inserted through the veins of the antecubital fossa; used in therapies lasting from 1 to 4 weeks.

migraine headache An episodic familial disorder manifested by a unilateral, frontotemporal, throbbing pain that is often worse behind one eye or ear. It is often accompanied by a sensitive scalp, anorexia, photophobia, and nausea with or without vomiting. Three categories of migraine headache are migraines with aura, migraines without aura, and atypical migraines.

migratory arthritis In the early stage of rheumatoid arthritis, symptoms that are migrating or involve more joints.

miliary tuberculosis See *hematogenous tuberculosis.*

minimally invasive direct coronary artery bypass (MIDCAB) Surgical procedure that does not require cardiopulmonary bypass and may be used for patients with a lesion of the left anterior descending artery. Also known as "keyhole" surgery.

minimally invasive esophagectomy (MIE) A laparoscopic surgical procedure to remove part of the esophagus; may be performed in patients with early-stage cancer.

minimally invasive inguinal hernia repair (MIIHR) Surgical repair of an inguinal hernia through a laparoscope, which is the treatment of choice.

minimally invasive surgery (MIS) A general term for any surgery performed using laparoscopic technique.

Minimum Data Set (MDS) 3.0 Interdisciplinary tool required by the U.S. Centers for Medicare and Medicaid Services (CMS) to assess patients (residents) in nursing homes.

miosis Constriction of the pupil of the eye.

mitosis Cell division.

mitotic index The percentage of actively dividing cells within a tumor.

mitral regurgitation Inability of the mitral valve to close completely during systole, which allows the backflow of blood into the left atrium when the left ventricle contracts; usually due to fibrosis and calcification caused by rheumatic disease. Also called *mitral insufficiency.*

mitral stenosis Thickening of the mitral valve due to fibrosis and calcification and usually caused by rheumatic fever. The valve leaflets fuse and become stiff, the chordae tendineae contract, and the valve opening narrows, preventing normal blood flow from the left atrium to the left ventricle. As a result, left atrial pressure rises, the left atrium dilates, pulmonary artery pressures increase, and the right ventricle hypertrophies.

mitral valve prolapse (MVP) Dysfunction of the mitral valve that occurs because the valvular leaflets enlarge and prolapse into the left atrium during systole; usually benign but may progress to pronounced mitral regurgitation.

mixed conductive-sensorineural hearing loss A profound hearing loss that results from a combination of both conductive and sensorineural types of hearing loss.

mobility The ability of an individual to perform purposeful physical movement of the body.

modifiable risk factor A factor in disease development that can be altered or controlled by the patient. Examples include elevated serum cholesterol levels, cigarette smoking, hypertension, impaired glucose tolerance, obesity, physical inactivity, and stress.

monokine Cytokine made by macrophages, neutrophils, eosinophils, and monocytes.

morbid obesity A weight that has a severely negative effect on health; usually more than 100% above ideal body weight or a body mass index greater than 40.

morbidity An illness or an abnormal condition or quality.

mortality Death.

Morton's neuroma Plantar digital neuritis, a condition in which a small tumor grows in a digital nerve of the foot. The patient usually describes the pain as an acute, burning sensation in the web space that involves the entire surface of the third and fourth toes.

motor aphasia See *expressive aphasia.*

motor cortex Area in the frontal lobe of the brain that controls voluntary movement.

motor end plate The junction of a peripheral motor nerve and the muscle cells that it supplies.

motor Facilitating movement.

mourning The outward social expression of loss.

MR elastography A noninvasive diagnostic procedure that provides information about tissue stiffness by assessing qualities of shear waves generated into the tissue.

mucositis Open sores on mucous membranes.

multi-casualty event A disaster event in which a limited number of victims or casualties are involved and can be managed by a hospital using local resources.

multigated blood pool scanning In nuclear cardiology, cardiac blood pool imaging is a noninvasive test to evaluate cardiac motion and calculate ejection fraction by using a computer to synchronize the patient's electrocardiogram with pictures obtained by a gamma-scintillation camera. In multigated blood pool scanning, the computer breaks the time between R waves into fractions of a second, called "gates." The camera records blood flow through the heart during each gate. By analyzing information from multiple gates, the computer can evaluate ventricular wall motion and calculate ejection fraction (percentage of the left ventricular volume that is ejected with each contraction) and ejection velocity.

multiple organ dysfunction syndrome (MODS) The sequence of inadequate blood flow to body tissues, which deprives cells of oxygen and leads to anaerobic metabolism with acidosis, hyperkalemia, and tissue ischemia; this is followed by dramatic changes in vital organs and leads to the release of toxic metabolites and destructive enzymes.

multiple sclerosis (MS) A chronic autoimmune disease that affects the myelin sheath and conduction pathway of the central nervous system. It is one of the leading causes of neurologic disability in persons 20 to 40 years of age.

murmur Abnormal heart sound that reflects turbulent blood flow through normal or abnormal valves; murmurs are classified according to their timing in the cardiac cycle (systolic or diastolic) and their intensity depending on their level of loudness.

muscle biopsy The extraction of a muscle specimen for the diagnosis of atrophy (as in muscular dystrophy) and inflammation (as in polymyositis).

muscular dystrophy (MD) A group of degenerative myopathies characterized by weakness and atrophy of muscle without nervous system involvement. At least nine types have been clinically identified and can be broadly categorized as slowly progressive or rapidly progressive.

mutation A change in deoxyribonucleic acid (DNA) that is passed from one generation to another.

myalgia Muscle aches/muscle pain.

myasthenia gravis (MG) A chronic autoimmune disease of the neuromuscular junction. It is characterized by remissions and exacerbations, with fatigue and weakness primarily in the muscles innervated by the cranial nerves and in the skeletal and respiratory muscles. It ranges from mild disturbances of the ocular muscles to a rapidly developing, generalized weakness that may lead to death from respiratory failure.

myasthenic crisis Undermedication with cholinesterase inhibitors.

mydriasis Dilation of the pupil of the eye.

myelin sheath A white, lipid covering of the axon.

myelocytic Pertaining to leukemias in which the abnormal cells come from the myeloid pathways.

myelogenous Pertaining to leukemias in which the abnormal cells come from the myeloid pathways.

myelography Radiography of the spine after injection of contrast medium into the subarachnoid space of the spine; used to visualize the vertebral column, intervertebral disks, spinal nerve roots, and blood vessels.

myocardial hypertrophy Enlargement of the myocardium.

myocardial infarction (MI) Injury and necrosis of myocardial tissue that occurs when the tissue is abruptly and severely deprived of oxygen; usually caused by atherosclerosis of a coronary artery, rupture of the plaque, subsequent thrombosis, and occlusion of blood flow.

myocardial nuclear perfusion imaging (MNPI) The use of radionuclide techniques in which radioactive tracer substances are used to view, record, and evaluate cardiovascular abnormalities; useful for detecting myocardial infarction

and decreased myocardial blood flow and for evaluating left ventricular ejection.

myocardium The heart muscle.

myoglobin A low–molecular-weight heme protein found in cardiac and skeletal muscle; an early marker of myocardial infarction.

myoglobinuria The release of muscle myoglobulin into the urine.

myomas See *leiomyomas*.

myomectomy The surgical removal of leiomyomas with preservation of the uterus.

myopathy A problem in muscle tissue.

myopia An error of refraction that occurs when the eye over-refracts or over-bends the light and focuses images in front of the retina; this results in normal near vision but poor distance vision. Also called *nearsightedness*.

myositis Inflammation of a muscle.

myosplint Electrical stimulation of tension splints in the heart to help the ventricle change to a more normal shape in the patient with heart failure; under investigation in Europe and the United States.

myringoplasty Surgical reconstruction of the eardrum.

myringotomy The surgical creation of a hole in the eardrum; performed to drain middle-ear fluids and relieve pain in the patient with otitis media (middle-ear infection).

myxedema coma A rare, serious complication of untreated or poorly treated hypothyroidism in which decreased metabolism causes the heart muscle to become flabby and the chamber size to increase, resulting in decreased cardiac output and decreased perfusion to the brain and other vital organs.

myxedema Dry, waxy swelling of the skin that is accompanied by nonpitting edema (especially around the eyes, in the hands and feet, and between the shoulder blades) and is associated with primary hypothyroidism.

N

nadir In cancer treatment therapy, the period of greatest bone marrow suppression, when the patient's platelet count may be very low.

nasoduodenal tube (NDT) A tube that is inserted through a nostril and into the small intestine.

nasoenteric tube (NET) Any feeding tube that is inserted nasally and then advanced into the gastrointestinal tract.

nasogastric (NG) tube A tube that is inserted through a nostril and into the stomach for liquid feeding or for withdrawing gastric contents.

nasotracheal The route for inserting a tube into the trachea via the nose.

natal sex A person's genital anatomy present at birth. Also known as *biological sex*.

National Patient Safety Goals (NPSGs) Goals published by The Joint Commission that require health care organizations to focus on specific priority safety practices.

natural chemical débridement Method of débriding a wound by creating an environment that promotes self-digestion of dead tissues by bacterial enzymes.

near point of vision The closest distance at which the eye can see an object clearly.

near-drowning Recovery after submersion in a liquid medium (usually water); this term is no longer used because language that describes drowning incidents has been standardized.

near-syncope Dizziness with an inability to remain in an upright position.

necrotizing hemorrhagic pancreatitis (NHP) Inflammation of the pancreas that is characterized by diffusely bleeding pancreatic tissue with fibrosis and tissue death. This form affects about 20% of patients with pancreatitis.

needle thoracostomy A quick, temporary method of chest decompression in which a large-bore needle is used to vent trapped air pending chest tube insertion.

negative deflection In electrocardiography, the flow of electrical current in the heart (cardiac axis) away from the positive pole and toward the negative pole.

negative feedback control mechanism The condition of maintaining a constant output of a system by exerting an inhibitory control on a key step by a product of that system. Used in a series of reactions that control hormone secretion and cellular activity based on responses to correct any movement away from normal function. An example of a simple negative feedback hormone response is the control of insulin secretion in which the action of insulin (decreasing blood glucose levels) is the opposite of the condition that stimulated insulin secretion (elevated blood glucose levels).

negative nitrogen balance A net loss of protein that occurs when the breakdown (degradation) of protein exceeds buildup (synthesis).

neglect In nursing, failure to provide for a patient's basic needs.

neoadjuvant therapy Treatment of a cancerous tumor with chemotherapy to shrink the tumor before it is surgically removed.

neoplasia Any new or continued cell growth not needed for normal development or replacement of dead and damaged tissues.

nephrectomy The surgical removal of the kidney.

nephrolithiasis The formation of stones in the kidney.

nephron The "working" unit of the kidney where urine is formed from blood. Each kidney consists of about 1 million nephrons, and each nephron separately makes urine. There are two types of nephrons: cortical and juxtamedullary.

nephropathy Pathologic change in the kidney that reduces kidney function and leads to renal failure.

nephrosclerosis Thickening in the nephron blood vessels that results in narrowing of the vessel lumen, with decreased renal blood flow and chronically hypoxic kidney tissue.

nephrostomy The surgical creation of an opening directly into the kidney; performed to divert urine externally and prevent further damage to the kidney when a stricture is causing hydronephrosis and cannot be corrected with urologic procedures.

nephrotic syndrome (NS) A condition of increased glomerular permeability that allows larger molecules to pass through the membrane into the urine and be removed from the blood.

This process causes massive loss of protein into the urine, edema formation, and decreased plasma albumin levels.

neuraxial Referring to the epidural or spinal area.

neuritic plaques Degenerating nerve terminals found particularly in the hippocampus, an important part of the limbic system, and marked by increased amounts of an abnormal protein called *beta amyloid;* a characteristic change of the brain found in patients with Alzheimer's disease.

neurofibrillary tangles Tangled masses of fibrous elements throughout the neurons; a classic finding at autopsy in the brains of patients with Alzheimer's disease.

neurogenic shock Hypotension and bradycardia associated with cervical spinal injuries and caused by a loss of autonomic function. The patient is at greatest risk in the first 24 hours after injury.

neuroglia cells Cells of varying size and shape that provide protection, structure, and nutrition for the neurons.

neurohypophysis The posterior lobe of the pituitary gland that stores hormones produced in the hypothalamus.

neuroma A sensitive tumor consisting of nerve cells and nerve fibers.

neuron Excitable nerve cell that processes and transmits information through electrical and chemical signals.

neuropathic pain A type of chronic noncancer pain that results from a nerve injury. Examples of causes include diabetic neuropathy, postherpetic neuralgia, radiculopathy (spinal nerve damage), and trigeminal neuralgia. Neuropathic pain is described as burning, shooting, stabbing, and the sensation of "pins and needles."

neuropathy A problem in nerve tissue that can cause muscle weakness.

neurotransmitter Regulatory chemical that exerts inhibitory (slowing down) or excitatory (speeding up) activity at postsynaptic nerve cell membranes. Acetylcholine, norepinephrine, epinephrine, dopamine, and serotonin are neurotransmitters.

neurovascular assessment Assessment of the neuromuscular system that includes inspection of skin color, temperature, and capillary refill distal to an injury, surgical procedure, or cast. Palpation of pulses in the extremities below level of injury and assessment of sensation, movement, and pain in the injured part give a complete assessment.

neutralization See *inactivation.*

neutropenia Decreased numbers of leukocytes, especially neutrophils, which causes immunosuppression.

neutrophilia Increased number of circulating neutrophils.

nevus A mole; a benign skin growth of the pigment-forming cells.

new-onset angina Cardiac chest pain that occurs for the first time.

nitroglycerin (NTG) A drug prescribed for patients with angina. It increases collateral blood flow, redistributes blood flow toward the subendocardium, and causes dilation of the coronary arteries.

nits Lice eggs.

N-methyl-D-aspartate (NMDA) receptor antagonist A group of drugs that block excess amounts of glutamate, which damages nerve cells in the brain; used to treat Alzheimer's disease.

nociception Term used to describe how pain becomes a conscious experience.

nociceptive pain Pain related to the skin, musculoskeletal structures, or body organs.

nociceptors Sensory neurons that respond to pain or other noxious stimuli.

nocturia The need to urinate excessively at night. Also called *nocturnal polyuria.*

nocturnal polyuria See *nocturia.*

nonadherence In health care, accidental failure by a patient to take medication.

noncompliance In health care, deliberate failure by a patient to take medication.

nonmaleficence Ethical principle that emphasizes the importance of preventing harm and ensuring the patient's well-being.

nonmechanical obstruction Intestinal obstruction that does not involve a physical obstruction in or outside the intestine. Instead, decreased or absent peristalsis results in a slowing of the movement or a backup of intestinal contents. This is also known as *paralytic ileus* or *adynamic ileus* because it is a result of neuromuscular disturbance.

nonmodifiable risk factor Factor in disease development that cannot be altered or controlled by the patient. Examples include age, gender, family history, and ethnic background.

non–ST-segment elevation myocardial infarction (NSTEMI) Myocardial infarction in which the patient typically has ST and T-wave changes on a 12-lead ECG; this indicates myocardial ischemia.

nonsustained ventricular tachycardia (NSVT) Occurrence of three or more successive premature ventricular complexes.

nontunneled percutaneous central venous catheter (CVC) A type of catheter, usually 15 to 20 cm long and with dual or triple lumens, that is inserted through the subclavian vein in the upper chest or through the jugular veins in the neck using sterile technique.

nonurgent In a three-tiered triage scheme, the category that includes patients who can generally tolerate waiting several hours for health care services without a significant risk of clinical deterioration, such as those with sprains, strains, or simple fractures.

normal flora The microorganisms living in or on the human host without causing disease; the bacteria that are characteristic of each body location. Normal flora often compete with and prevent infection from unfamiliar microorganisms attempting to invade a body site.

normal sinus rhythm (NSR) The rhythm originating from the sinoatrial node (dominant pacemaker), with atrial and ventricular rates of 60 to 100 beats/min and regular atrial and ventricular rhythms.

normotonic See *isosmotic.*

North American pit vipers The Crotalidae, one of two families of indigenous poisonous snakes in North America; named for the characteristic depression between each eye and nostril. They include rattlesnakes, copperheads, and water moccasins and account for most poisonous snakebites in the United States.

nosocomial (infection) Acquired in an inpatient health care setting; for example, infections that were not present at hospital admission. Also called *hospital-acquired infections* and *health care–associated infections.*

nothing by mouth (NPO) No eating, drinking (including water), or smoking.

nuchal rigidity Stiff neck, which can be a sign of cerebrospinal fluid leak; nuchal rigidity is not checked until a spinal cord injury has been ruled out.

nucleotide The final form of a base that actually gets put into the strand of deoxyribonucleic acid. A nucleoside becomes a complete nucleotide by the attachment of phosphate groups.

nursing assistant A member of the rehabilitative health care team who assists the registered nurse in the care of patients.

nursing technician See *nursing assistant.*

nutrition The process of ingesting and using food and fluids to grow, repair, and maintain optimal body functions.

nutritional screening A screening by the health care provider that includes visual inspection, measured height and weight, weight history, usual eating habits, ability to chew and swallow, and any recent changes in appetite or food intake. The screening is a way to determine which patients need more extensive nutritional assessment.

nutritional status Reflects the balance between nutrient requirements and intake.

nystagmus Involuntary rapid eye movements.

O

obesity An increase in body weight at least 20% above the upper limit of the normal range for ideal body weight, with an excess amount of body fat; in an adult, a body mass index greater than 30.

obligatory urine output The minimum amount of urine per day needed to dissolve and excrete toxic waste products.

obstipation The inability to pass stool; intractable constipation.

obstruction Blockage.

obstructive jaundice Jaundice caused by an impediment to the flow of bile from the liver to the duodenum; may be caused by edema of the ducts or gallstones.

obstructive sleep apnea A breathing disruption during sleep that lasts at least 10 seconds and occurs a minimum of 5 times in an hour.

Occupational Safety and Health Administration (OSHA) A federal agency that protects workers from injury or illness at their place of employment.

occupational therapist (OT, OTR) A member of the rehabilitation health care team who works to develop the patient's fine motor skills used for activities of daily living and the skills related to coordination and cognitive retraining.

odynophagia Pain on swallowing.

oligomenorrhea Scant or infrequent menses.

oligospermia Low sperm count.

oliguria Scant urine output. Usually less than 400 mL per day.

oliguria Decreased excretion of urine in relation to amount of fluid intake; usually defined as urine output less than 400 mL/day.

oncogene Proto-oncogene that has been "turned on" and can cause cells to change from normal cells to cancer cells.

oncogenesis Cancer development.

oncovirus Virus that causes cancer.

oophorectomy Surgical removal of the ovary.

open fracture A fracture in which the skin surface over the broken bone is disrupted, causing an external wound. Also called *compound fracture*.

open reduction The reduction of a fracture after surgical incision into the site to allow direct visualization of the fracture. See *internal fixation*.

open traumatic brain injury A type of traumatic primary brain injury that occurs with a skull fracture or when the skull is pierced by a penetrating object. The integrity of the brain and the dura is violated, and there is exposure to outside contaminants, with damage to the underlying vessels, dural sinus, brain, and cranial nerves.

opportunistic infection Infection caused by organisms that are present as part of the normal environment and would be kept in check by normal immune function.

optic disc The point at the inside back of the eye where the optic nerve enters the eyeball. It appears as a creamy pink to white depressed area in the retina and contains only nerve fibers and no photoreceptor cells.

optic fundus The area at the inside back of the eye that can be seen with an ophthalmoscope.

optic nerve The nerve of sight; connects the optic disc to the brain.

orbit The bony socket of the skull that surrounds and protects the eye along with the attached muscles, nerves, vessels, and tear-producing glands.

orchiectomy The surgical removal of one or both testes.

orchitis An acute testicular inflammation resulting from trauma or infection.

orexin Neuropeptide that is an appetite stimulant.

organ donor An individual who has consented to donating one or more organs when he or she dies.

orotracheal The route for inserting a tube into the trachea via the mouth.

orthopnea Shortness of breath that occurs when lying down but is relieved by sitting up.

orthostatic hypotension A decrease in blood pressure (20 mm Hg systolic and/or 10 mm Hg diastolic) that occurs during the first few seconds to minutes after changing from a sitting or lying position to a standing position. Also called *postural hypotension*.

orthostatic Pertaining to or caused by standing erect.

orthotopic The most common type of transplantation procedure in which a diseased organ is removed and a donor organ is grafted in its place. For example, during heart transplantation, the surgeon removes the diseased heart and leaves the posterior walls of the patient's atria, which serve as the anchor for the donor heart; anastomoses

are made between the recipient and donor atria, aorta, and pulmonary arteries.

osmolality The number of milliosmoles in a kilogram of solution.

osmolarity The number of milliosmoles in a liter of solution.

osmosis The movement of a solvent across a semipermeable membrane (a membrane that allows the solvent but not the solute to pass through) from a lesser to a greater concentration.

ossiculoplasty Replacement of the ossicles within the middle ear.

osteitis deformans See *Paget's disease*.

osteoarthritis Noninflammatory form of arthritis characterized by the progressive deterioration and loss of cartilage in one or more joints; most common form of arthritis.

osteoblast Cell associated with formation of bone.

osteoclast Cell associated with destruction or resorption of bone.

osteocyte Bone cell.

osteomalacia Abnormal softening of the bone tissue characterized by inadequate mineralization of osteoid. It is the adult equivalent of rickets (vitamin D deficiency) in children.

osteomyelitis An inflammation of bone tissue caused by pathogenic microorganisms; produces an increased vascularity and edema often involving the surrounding soft tissues.

osteonecrosis The death of bone tissue, usually because the blood supply to the bone is disrupted. Usually a complication of a hip fracture or any fracture in which there is displacement of bone.

osteopenia A condition of low bone mass that occurs when there is a disruption in the bone remodeling process.

osteophyte Bone spur.

osteoporosis A metabolic disease in which bone demineralization results in decreased density and subsequent fractures.

osteotomy Surgical resection of bone.

ostomate A patient with an ostomy.

ostomy The surgical creation of an opening, usually referring to an opening in the abdominal wall; stoma.

otorrhea Ear discharge.

otosclerosis Irregular bone growth around the ossicles.

otoscope An instrument used to examine the ear; consists of a light, a handle, a magnifying lens, and a pneumatic bulb for injecting air into the external canal to test mobility of the eardrum.

ototoxic Having a toxic effect on the inner ear structures.

outflow disease Chronic peripheral arterial disease with obstruction at or below the superficial femoral or popliteal artery. The patient experiences burning or cramping in the calves, ankles, feet, and toes after walking a certain distance; the pain usually subsides with rest.

outpatient A patient who goes to the hospital for treatment and returns home on the same day.

overflow urinary incontinence The involuntary loss of urine when the bladder is overdistended.

overweight An increase in body weight for height compared with a reference standard (e.g., the Metropolitan Life height and weight tables) or 10% greater than ideal body weight. However,

this weight may not reflect excess body fat, which in an adult is a body mass index of 25 to 30.

ovoid pupil In evaluating pupils for size and reaction to light, the midstage between a normal-size pupil and a dilated pupil; indicates the development of increased intracranial pressure.

oxygen concentrator A machine that removes nitrogen, water vapor, and hydrocarbons from room air. Also known as *oxygen extractor*.

oxygen dissociation The transfer of oxygen from hemoglobin to tissues.

P

P wave In the electrocardiogram, the deflection representing atrial depolarization.

pack-years The number of packs of cigarettes per day multiplied by the number of years the patient has smoked; used in recording a patient's smoking history.

Paget's disease A metabolic disorder of bone remodeling, or turnover, in which increased resorption or loss results in bone deposits that are weak, enlarged, and disorganized. Also known as *osteitis deformans*.

pain An unpleasant sensory and emotional experience associated with actual or potential tissue damage; the most reliable indication of pain is the patient's self-report.

palliation Relieving symptoms.

palliative care A compassionate and supportive approach to patients and families who are living with life-threatening illnesses; involves a holistic approach that provides relief of symptoms experienced by the dying patient.

palpitations A feeling of fluttering in the chest, an unpleasant awareness of the heartbeat, or an irregular heartbeat; may result from a change in heart rate or rhythm or from an increase in the force of heart contractions.

pancreatic abscess A collection of purulent material that results from extensive inflammatory necrosis of the pancreas after infection by organisms such as *Escherichia coli*; the most serious complication of pancreatitis. It is fatal if left untreated.

pancreatic pseudocyst A false cyst, so named because, unlike a true cyst, it does not have an epithelial lining. It is an encapsulated saclike structure that forms on or surrounds the pancreas and develops as a complication of acute or chronic pancreatitis. It may contain up to several liters of straw-colored or dark-brown viscous fluid, the enzymatic exudate of the pancreas.

pancreaticojejunostomy Surgical anastomosis of the pancreatic duct with the jejunum.

pancytopenia A deficiency of all three cell types (red blood cells, white blood cells, and platelets) of the blood.

pandemic A general epidemic spread over a wide geographic area and affecting a large proportion of the population.

panniculectomy The surgical removal of any panniculus, most often the abdominal apron; usually done as a follow-up to bariatric surgery in an obese patient.

panniculitis Infection of the panniculus.

panniculus A layer of membrane; also used to refer to skinfold areas in the obese patient.

pannus Vascular granulation tissue composed of inflammatory cells that forms in a joint space; erodes articular cartilage and eventually destroys bone.

Papanicolaou test (Pap smear) A cytologic study that is effective in detecting precancerous and cancerous cells obtained from the cervix.

papilla The anatomic term for a small, nipple-shaped projection or structure.

papilledema Edema and hyperemia of the optic disc; a sign of increased intracranial pressure found on ophthalmoscopic examination. Also called a *choked disc.*

papilloma A pedunculated outgrowth of tissue.

papillotomy An incision of a papilla, a small nipple-shaped projection or structure.

papular Referring to a papule, a small, solid elevation of the skin.

paracentesis A procedure in which the physician inserts a trocar catheter into the abdomen to remove and drain ascitic fluid from the peritoneal cavity.

paradoxical blood pressure An exaggerated decrease in systolic pressure by more than 10 mm Hg during the inspiratory phase of the respiratory cycle (normal is 3 to 10 mm Hg); clinical conditions that may produce a paradoxical blood pressure include pericardial tamponade, constrictive pericarditis, and pulmonary hypertension. Also known as *paradoxical pulse* and *pulsus paradoxus.*

paradoxical chest wall movement The "sucking inward" of the loose chest area during inspiration and a "puffing out" of the same area during expiration in a patient with a flail chest.

paradoxical pulse See *paradoxical blood pressure.*

paradoxical splitting Abnormal splitting of the S_2 heart sound heard in patients with severe myocardial depression; causes early closure of the pulmonic valve or a delay in aortic valve closure.

paralysis Absence of movement.

paralytic ileus Absence of peristalsis.

paramedic Prehospital care provider for patients who require care that exceeds basic life support resources. Advanced life support (ALS) may include cardiac monitoring, advanced airway management and intubation, establishing IV access, and administering drugs en route to the emergency department.

paranasal sinuses The air-filled cavities within the bones that surround the nasal passages. Lined with ciliated membrane, the sinuses provide resonance during speech and decrease the weight of the skull.

paraparesis Weakness that involves only the lower extremities, as seen in lower thoracic and lumbosacral injuries or lesions.

paraplegia Paralysis that involves only the lower extremities, as seen in lower thoracic and lumbosacral injuries or lesions.

paresis Weakness.

paresthesia Abnormal or unusual nerve sensations of touch, such as tingling and burning.

parietal cells Cells lining the wall of the stomach that secrete hydrochloric acid and produce intrinsic factor.

Parkinson disease (PD) A debilitating neurologic disease that affects motor ability and is characterized by four cardinal symptoms: tremor, rigidity, akinesia (slow movement), and postural instability. It is the third most common neurologic disorder of older adults. Also called *paralysis agitans.*

parotidectomy The surgical removal of the parotid glands.

paroxysmal nocturnal dyspnea (PND) In the patient with heart disease, difficulty breathing that develops after lying down for several hours and causes the patient to awaken abruptly with a feeling of suffocation and panic. Occurs because the heart is unable to compensate for the increased volume when blood from the lower extremities is redistributed to the venous system, which increases venous return to the heart. A diseased heart is ineffective in pumping the additional fluid into the circulatory system, and pulmonary congestion results.

paroxysmal supraventricular tachycardia (PSVT) A form of supraventricular tachycardia that occurs when the rhythm is intermittent; it is initiated suddenly by a premature complex, such as a premature atrial complex, and terminated suddenly with or without intervention.

partial left ventriculectomy (PLV) A ventricular reconstructive procedure that involves removing a triangle-shaped section of the weakened heart in the left lateral ventricle to reduce the ventricle's diameter and decrease wall tension. Also known as *heart reduction surgery* and *Batista procedure.*

partial seizure One of the three broad categories of seizure disorders along with generalized seizure and unclassified seizure. Partial seizures are of two types: complex and simple. Partial seizures begin in a part of one cerebral hemisphere; some can evolve into generalized tonic-clonic, tonic, or clonic seizures. They are most often seen in adults and in general are less responsive to medical treatment. Also called *focal seizures* or *local seizures.*

passive euthanasia See *withdrawing or withholding life-sustaining therapy.*

passive immunity Resistance to infection that is of short duration (days or months) and either natural by transplacental transfer from the mother or artificial by injection of antibodies (e.g., immunoglobulin).

patellofemoral pain syndrome (PFPS) A health problem that occurs most often in people who are runners or who overuse their knee joints. For that reason, it is sometimes referred to as "runner's knee." These patients describe pain as being behind or around their patella (knee cap) in one or both knees.

pathogen Any microorganism capable of producing disease.

pathogenicity The ability to cause disease.

pathologic (spontaneous) fracture A fracture that occurs after minimal trauma to a bone that has been weakened by a disease such as bone cancer or osteoporosis.

patient-centered care A QSEN competency in which the nurse recognizes the patient or designee as the source of control and full partner in providing compassionate and coordinated care based on respect for the patient's preferences, values, and needs.

patient-controlled analgesia A method that allows the patient to control the dosage of opioid analgesic received by using an infusion pump to deliver the desired amount of medication through a conventional IV route.

PDSA Acronym for plan, do, study, act, which is one of the steps of the evidence-based practice improvement (EBPI) model.

peaceful death A death that is free from avoidable distress and suffering for patients and families, is in agreement with patients' and families' wishes, and is consistent with clinical practice standards.

pedal Pertaining to the feet.

pediculosis An infestation by human lice.

pedigree A graph of a family history for a specific trait or health problem over several generations.

pelvic inflammatory disease (PID) Any infection of the pelvis involving the upper genital tract beyond the cervix in women. It occurs when organisms from the lower genital tract migrate from the endocervix upward through the uterine cavity into the fallopian tubes.

pelvic organ prolapse (POP) Condition in which the sling of muscles and tendons that support the pelvic organs becomes weak and is no longer able to hold them in place.

penetrance In genetics, how often or how well a gene is expressed when it is present within a population.

penetrating trauma Injuries caused by piercing; classified by the velocity of the vehicle (e.g., knife or bullet) causing the injury. Low-velocity injuries from knife wounds cause damage directly at the site; high-velocity injuries from gunshot wounds cause both direct and indirect damage. Also called *penetrating injury.*

peptic ulcer disease (PUD) The impairment of gastric mucosal defenses so that they no longer protect the epithelium from the effects of acid and pepsin.

peptic ulcer A mucosal lesion of the stomach or duodenum.

percutaneous alcohol septal ablation Surgical procedure for hypertrophic cardiomyopathy (HCM) in which alcohol is injected into a target septal branch of the left anterior descending coronary artery to produce a small septal infarction. This procedure also widens the left ventricular outflow tract.

percutaneous coronary intervention (PCI) See *percutaneous transluminal coronary angioplasty (PTCA).*

percutaneous endoscopic gastrostomy (PEG) A stoma created from the abdominal wall into the stomach for insertion of a short feeding tube.

percutaneous stereotactic rhizotomy (PSR) Procedure performed under general anesthesia to treat trigeminal neuralgia; a hollow needle is passed through the inside of the patient's cheek into the trigeminal nerve fibers, and a heating current (radiofrequency thermocoagulation) goes through the needle to destroy some of the fibers.

percutaneous transhepatic cholangiography (PTC) The radiographic study of the biliary duct system using an iodinated dye instilled via a percutaneous needle inserted through the liver into the intrahepatic ducts. It may be performed when a patient has jaundice or persistent upper abdominal pain, even after cholecystectomy, but it is rarely performed as a diagnostic procedure.

percutaneous transluminal coronary angioplasty (PTCA) A nonsurgical method of improving arterial flow by opening the vessel lumen and creating a smooth inner vessel surface. One or more arteries are dilated with a balloon catheter advanced through a cannula, which is inserted into or above an occluded or stenosed artery. Also called *percutaneous vascular intervention* and *percutaneous coronary intervention (PCI)*.

percutaneous vascular intervention See *percutaneous transluminal coronary angioplasty.*

percutaneous Performed through the skin and other tissues.

perfusion Adequate arterial blood flow to the peripheral tissues (peripheral perfusion) and blood that is pumped by the heart to oxygenate major body organs (central perfusion).

pericardial effusion Complication of pericarditis that occurs when the space between the parietal and visceral layers of the pericardium fills with fluid.

pericardial friction rub An abnormal sound that originates from the pericardial sac and occurs with the movements of the heart during the cardiac cycle; usually transient and a sign of inflammation, infection, or infiltration; may be heard in patients with pericarditis resulting from myocardial infarction, cardiac tamponade, or post-thoracotomy.

pericardiectomy Surgical excision of the pericardium (the sac around the heart).

pericardiocentesis Withdrawal of pericardial fluid through a catheter inserted into the pericardial space to relieve the pressure on the heart.

pericarditis An inflammation of the tissue (pericardium) surrounding the heart.

perichondrium A tough, fibrous tissue layer that surrounds the ear cartilage and gives shape to the pinna.

periodontal disease Gum disease in which mandibular bone loss has occurred.

perioperative The operative experience consisting of the preoperative, intraoperative, and postoperative time periods.

peripheral blood stem cells (PBSCs) Stem cells that are collected from peripheral blood for transplantation into the patient.

peripheral chemoreceptors Several 1- to 2-mm collections of tissue identified in the carotid arteries and along the aortic arch.

peripheral IV therapy IV therapy in which a vascular access device (VAD) is placed in a peripheral vein, usually in the arm.

peripheral vascular disease (PVD) Any disorder that alters the natural flow of blood through the arteries and veins of the peripheral circulation.

peripherally inserted central catheter (PICC) A long catheter inserted through a vein of the antecubital fossa (inner aspect of the bend of the arm) or the middle of the upper arm.

peritonitis Acute inflammation of the visceral/parietal peritoneum and endothelial lining of the abdominal cavity, or peritoneum.

peritonsillar abscess (PTA) A complication of acute tonsillitis. The infection spreads from the tonsil to the surrounding tissue, which forms an abscess.

periungual lesion Skin lesion around the nail bed.

permeable The quality of being porous.

pernicious anemia A form of megaloblastic anemia caused by failure to absorb vitamin B_{12} because of a deficiency of intrinsic factor (normally secreted by the gastric mucosa) needed for intestinal absorption of vitamin B_{12}.

PERRLA An acronym that stands for the phrase "*P*upils should be *e*qual in size, *r*ound and *r*egular in shape, and react to *l*ight and *a*ccommodation."

personal emergency preparedness plan An individual plan that outlines specific arrangements in the event of disaster, such as childcare, pet care, and older adult care.

personal protective equipment (PPE) Infection control protocol that refers to the use of gloves, isolation gowns, face protection, and respirators with N95 or higher filtration.

personal readiness supplies A preassembled disaster supply kit for the home and/or automobile that contains clothing and basic survival supplies. Also called a "*go bag.*"

petechiae Pinpoint red spots on the mucous membranes, palate, conjunctivae, or skin.

pH monitoring examination The most accurate testing method of diagnosing GERD, accomplished by placing a small catheter into the distal esophagus or esophageal wall (depending on the specific technique). The patient then records a diary of activities and symptoms over a 24- to 48-hour period while pH is continuously monitored.

pH A measure of the free hydrogen ion level in body fluid.

phagocytosis The process of engulfing, ingesting, killing, and disposing of an invading organism by neutrophils and macrophages; a key process of inflammation.

Phalen's maneuver Test to determine the presence of carpal tunnel syndrome (CTS); a positive test for CTS causes paresthesia in the medial nerve distribution of the palm of the hand in 60 seconds.

phantom limb pain (PLP) A frequent complication of amputation in which the patient perceives sensation in the absent (amputated) foot or hand. This sensation usually diminishes over time.

pharmacist Member of the health care team who oversees the prescription and preparation of medications and provides the team with essential information regarding drug safety.

pharmacologic stress echocardiogram A form of echocardiography in which either dobutamine (increases heart's contractility) or adenosine (dilates coronary arteries) is given to the patient; usually used when patients cannot tolerate exercise.

phenotype Any genetic characteristic that can actually be observed or, in some cases, determined by laboratory test.

pheochromocytoma A tumor of the adrenal medulla, which can cause excessive secretion of catecholamines.

phlebitis Inflammation of a vein, which can predispose patients to thrombosis.

phlebothrombosis Presence of a thrombus in a vein without inflammation.

phonophobia Abnormal sensitivity to sound.

phonophoresis Treatment for back pain in which a topical drug (e.g., lidocaine, hydrocortisone) is applied followed by continuous ultrasound for 10 minutes.

photophobia Abnormal sensitivity to light.

photopsia The appearance of bright flashes of light due to the onset of retinal detachment.

physiatrist A physician who specializes in rehabilitative medicine.

physical abuse The use of a physical force, such as hitting, burning, pushing, and molesting the patient, that results in bodily injury.

physical therapist (PT, RPT) A member of the rehabilitation health care team who helps the patient achieve mobility and who teaches techniques for performing certain activities of daily living.

piggyback set See *secondary administration set.*

pitting Indentation of the skin; often occurs with edema.

pituitary Cushing's disease Oversecretion of ACTH by the anterior pituitary gland, which causes hyperplasia of the adrenal cortex in both adrenal glands and an excess of most hormones secreted by the adrenal cortex.

placebo Any medication or procedure, including surgery, that produces an effect in a patient because of its implicit or explicit intent and not because of its specific physical or chemical properties.

Plan-Do-Study-Act (PDSA) A specific systematic model of quality improvement.

plantar fasciitis An inflammation of the plantar fascia, which is located in the area of the arch of the foot. It is often seen in athletes, especially runners.

plasma cell A short-lived B-lymphocyte that begins to function immediately to produce antibodies against sensitizing antigens.

plasmapheresis The separation of plasma from whole blood, after which the blood cells are returned to the patient without the plasma to eliminate antibodies.

plethoric A flushed appearance of the skin.

pleura The continuous smooth membrane composed of two surfaces that totally enclose the lungs.

pleural effusion Fluid in the pleural space.

pleuritic chest pain A stabbing pain on taking a deep breath.

plexus Cluster of nerves.

ploidy The number and appearance of chromosomes; used to describe cancer cells.

pluripotent stem cell The precursor cell involved in the production of red blood cells.

pneumonectomy Removal of an entire lung, including all blood vessels.

pneumonia Excess fluid in the lungs resulting from an inflammatory process that can include infection.

pneumothorax Air in the pleural (chest) cavity.

podagra Inflammation of the metatarsophalangeal joint of the great toe.

point of maximal impulse (PMI) See *apical impulse.*

polycystic kidney disease (PKD) An inherited disorder in which fluid-filled cysts develop in the kidneys.

polycythemia vera (PV) A disease that involves massive production of red blood cells, leukocytes, and platelets.

polydipsia Excessive intake of water.

polymedicine The use of many drugs to treat multiple health problems for older adults.

polymorphism A variation in form.

polyp An abnormal outgrowth from a mucous membrane.

polyphagia Excessive eating.

polypharmacy The use of many drugs to treat multiple health problems for older adults. Also known as *hyperpharmacy.*

polyuria Frequent and excessive urination.

pores Openings or spaces.

portal hypertension An abnormal persistent increase in pressure within the portal vein; a major complication of cirrhosis.

portal hypertensive gastropathy A complication that can occur in patients with portal hypertension, with or without esophageal varices. Slow gastric mucosal bleeding may result in chronic slow blood loss, occult positive stools, and anemia.

portal-systemic encephalopathy (PSE) A clinical disorder seen in hepatic failure and cirrhosis; it is manifested by neurologic symptoms and is characterized by an altered level of consciousness, impaired thinking processes, and neuromuscular disturbances. Also called *hepatic encephalopathy* and *hepatic coma.*

positive deflection In electrocardiography, the flow of electrical current in the heart (cardiac axis) toward the positive pole.

positive inotropic agents Drugs that increase myocardial contractility; such drugs are prescribed to improve cardiac output.

postanesthesia care unit (PACU) Recovery room.

postcholecystectomy syndrome (PCS) The occurrence of the clinical manifestations of biliary tract disease following cholecystectomy; caused by residual or recurring calculi, inflammation, or stricture of the common bile duct.

post-concussion syndrome A group of clinical manifestations following a concussion that consist of personality changes, irritability, headaches, dizziness, restlessness, nervousness, insomnia, memory loss, and depression. The prolonged pattern is classified as post-trauma syndrome.

posterior colporrhaphy The surgical procedure to repair a rectocele by strengthening pelvic supports and reducing the bulging.

posteroanterior Back to front; position for standard chest x-rays.

postherpetic neuralgia Pain that persists after herpes zoster lesions have resolved.

postictal stage Referring to the time immediately after a seizure.

postoperative period After surgery.

postpericardiotomy syndrome Symptoms, including pericardial and pleural pain, pericarditis, friction rub, elevated temperature and white blood cell count, and dysrhythmias, that occur in patients after cardiac surgery; may occur days to weeks after surgery and seems to be associated with blood that remains in the pericardial sac.

postrenal failure Decrease in renal function related to an obstruction in the flow of urine. It can progress to acute renal failure.

postural hypotension See *orthostatic hypotension.*

posture A person's body build and alignment when standing and walking.

post-void residual (PVR) The amount of urine remaining in the bladder within 20 minutes after voiding.

power air purifying respirator (PAPR) Device with a high efficiency particulate air (HEPA) filter and battery to promote positive pressure air flow; more effective than an N95 respirator.

PQRST A mnemonic (memory device) that may help in the current problem assessment of patients with gastrointestinal tract disorders. The letters represent these areas: P, precipitating or palliative (What brings it on? What makes it better or worse?); Q, quality or quantity (How does it look, feel, or sound?); R, region or radiation (Where is it? Does it spread anywhere?); S, severity scale (How bad is it [on a scale of 0 to 10]? Is it getting better, worse, or staying the same?); T, timing (Onset, duration, and frequency?).

PR interval In the electrocardiogram, the interval measured from the beginning of the P wave to the end of the PR segment; represents the time required for atrial depolarization as well as impulse delay in the atrioventricular node and travel time to the Purkinje fibers.

PR segment In the electrocardiogram, the isoelectric line from the end of the P wave to the beginning of the QRS complex, when the electrical impulse is traveling through the atrioventricular node, where it is delayed.

Prader-Willi syndrome (PWS) A complex neurodevelopmental genetic disorder that results from a hypothalamic-pituitary dysfunction that prevents appetite control. Patients with this syndrome are typically morbidly obese.

prandial (insulin secretion) The increased levels of insulin that are secreted after eating. Within 10 minutes of eating, an early burst of insulin secretion occurs, which is followed by an increasing insulin release that lasts as long as hyperglycemia is present.

prealbumin (PAB) A protein secreted by the liver that binds thyroxine.

precipitation The formation of large, insoluble antigen-antibody complexes during the antibody-binding process.

prediabetes An impaired fasting glucose (IFG) or impaired glucose tolerance (IGT).

prehospital care provider Typically, any of the first caregivers encountered by the patient if he or she is transported to the emergency department by an ambulance or helicopter.

preictal phase Referring to events that a patient experiences before a seizure, such as the presence of an aura.

pre-infarction angina Chest pain that occurs in the days or weeks before a myocardial infarction.

preload The degree of myocardial fiber stretch at the end of diastole and just before contraction; determined by the amount of blood returning to the heart from both the venous system (right heart) and the pulmonary system (left heart).

premature atrial complex (contraction) (PAC) In the electrocardiogram, an early complex that occurs when atrial tissue becomes irritable. This ectopic focus fires an impulse before the next sinus impulse is due, thus usurping the sinus pacemaker. The premature P wave from the atrial focus is early and has a shape different from that of the P wave generated from the sinus node.

premature complex In the electrocardiogram, an early complex that occurs when a cardiac cell or cell group other than the sinoatrial node becomes irritable and fires an impulse before the next sinus impulse is generated. After the premature complex, there is a pause before the next normal complex, which creates an irregularity in the rhythm.

premature ventricular complex (PVC) In the electrocardiogram, an early ventricular complex is followed by a pause that results from increased irritability of ventricular cells. The QRS complexes may be unifocal or uniform (of the same shape), or multifocal or multiform (of different shapes).

preoperative Before surgery.

prerenal failure Condition that causes inadequate kidney perfusion; can progress to acute renal failure.

presbycusis The loss of hearing, especially for high-pitched sounds; occurs as a result of aging.

presbyopia An age-related impairment of vision characterized by a loss of lens elasticity and the ability of the eye to accommodate. The near point of vision increases, and near objects must be placed farther from the eye to be seen clearly.

presence A type of communication that consists of listening and acknowledging the legitimacy of the patient's and/or family's pain.

pressure ulcer Tissue damage caused when the skin and underlying soft tissue are compressed between a bony prominence and an external surface for an extended period; commonly occurs over the sacrum, hips, and ankles.

pretibial myxedema Dry, waxy swelling of the front surfaces of the lower legs.

pretibial Pertaining to the front of the leg below the knee.

primary angle-closure glaucoma A form of glaucoma characterized by a narrowed angle and forward displacement of the iris so that movement of the iris against the cornea narrows or closes the chamber angle, obstructing the outflow of aqueous humor. It can have a sudden onset and is an emergency. Also called *closed-angle glaucoma, narrow-angle glaucoma,* or *acute glaucoma.*

primary arthroplasty A total joint arthroplasty procedure that has been performed for the first time.

primary gout The most common type of gout; results from one of several inborn errors of purine metabolism.

primary lesions In describing skin disease, the initial reaction to a problem that alters one of the structural components of the skin.

primary open-angle glaucoma (POAG) The most common form of primary glaucoma; characterized by reduced outflow of aqueous humor through the chamber angle. Because the fluid cannot leave the eye at the same rate it is produced, intraocular pressure gradually increases.

primary prevention Strategies used to avoid or delay the actual occurrence of a specific disease.

primary progressive multiple sclerosis (PPMS) A type of multiple sclerosis (MS) that involves a steady and gradual neurologic deterioration without remission of symptoms. Patients with this type of MS are usually between 40 and 60 years of age at onset of the disease and experience progressive disability with no acute attacks.

primary survey Priorities of care addressed in order of immediate threats to life as part of the initial assessment in the emergency department. Survey is based on an "ABC" mnemonic with "D" and "E" added for trauma patients: airway/cervical spine (A), breathing (B), circulation (C), disability (D), and exposure (E).

primary tumor The original tumor, usually identified by the tissue from which it arose (parent tissue), such as in breast cancer or lung cancer.

progressive multifocal leukoencephalopathy (PML) Rare disease affecting the white matter of the brain caused by a virus that attacks the cells that make myelin; occurs most often in patients who are immunosuppressed.

progressive-relapsing multiple sclerosis (PRMS) A type of multiple sclerosis (MS) that occurs in only 5% of patients with MS. It is characterized by the absence of periods of remission, and the patient's condition does not return to baseline. Progressive cumulative symptoms and deterioration occur over several years.

proliferative diabetic retinopathy A form of retinopathy associated with diabetes mellitus in which a network of fragile new blood vessels develops, leaking blood and protein into surrounding tissue. The new blood vessels are stimulated by retinal hypoxia that results from poor capillary perfusion of the retinal tissues. New blood vessels grow in the retina, onto the iris, and into the back of the vitreous. The vitreous contracts and pulls away from the retina, causing blood vessels to break and bleed into the vitreous.

promoter In oncology, a substance that promotes or enhances growth of the initiated cancer cell; may be a hormone, drug, or chemical.

pronator drift Occurs in a patient with muscle weakness due to cerebral or brainstem reasons. The arm on the weak side tends to fall, or "drift," with the palm pronating (turning inward) after the patient has closed his or her eyes and held the arms perpendicular to the body with the palms up for 15 to 30 seconds; part of the neurologic assessment.

prophylactic mastectomy Highly controversial practice of surgically removing the breast in order to reduce the risk of breast cancer.

proportionate palliative sedation A care management approach involving the administration of drugs such as benzodiazepines for the purpose of lowering patient consciousness.

proprioception (proprioceptive) Awareness of body position and movement.

prosopagnosia The inability to recognize oneself and other familiar faces; occurs in patients in the later stages of Alzheimer's disease.

prostaglandins Chemicals that are produced in the cells and cause inflammation and swelling.

prostate artery embolization A procedure in which the interventional radiologist threads a small vascular catheter into the prostate's arteries and injects particles blocking some of the blood flow to shrink the prostate gland.

prostate-specific antigen (PSA) A glycoprotein produced solely by the prostate. The normal blood level of PSA is less than 4 ng/mL; levels are higher in patients with increased prostatic tissue as a result of benign prostatic hyperplasia, prostatic infarction, prostatitis, and prostate cancer. Levels associated with prostate cancer are usually much higher than those occurring with other prostate tissue enlargement.

prostatitis Inflammation of the prostate.

protein synthesis The process by which genes are used to make the proteins needed for physiologic function.

protein-calorie malnutrition (PCM) A disorder of nutrition that may present in three forms: marasmus, kwashiorkor, and marasmic-kwashiorkor. Also called *protein-energy malnutrition*.

protein-energy malnutrition (PEM) See *protein-calorie malnutrition*.

proteinuria The presence of protein in the urine.

proteolysis The breakdown of proteins to provide fuel for energy when liver glucose is unavailable.

proton pump inhibitor (PPI) A group of drugs that inhibit the proton pump in the stomach to decrease gastric acid production.

pruritus An unpleasant itching sensation.

psoriasis A chronic autoimmune disorder of the skin with exacerbations and remissions. It results from overstimulation of the immune system (Langerhans' cells) in the skin that activates T-lymphocytes. The features include increased skin cell division in patchy areas forming scaly plaques.

psoriatic arthritis (PsA) A syndrome of inflammatory arthritis associated with psoriasis, the skin condition characterized by a scaly, itchy rash.

psychiatric crisis nurse team An emergency department specialty team whose nurses interact with patients and families in crisis.

psychotropic drugs Antipsychotic and neuroleptic drugs. These are appropriately given to patients with emotional and behavioral health problems (e.g., hallucinations and delusions) that accompany dementia but are sometimes inappropriately used for agitation, combativeness, or restlessness. They are considered chemical restraints because they decrease mobility and patients' ability to care for themselves.

ptosis Drooping of the eyelid.

pulmonary artery occlusive pressure (PAOP) See *pulmonary artery wedge pressure*.

pulmonary artery wedge pressure (PAWP) Measurement of pressure in the left atrium using a balloon-tipped catheter introduced into the pulmonary artery. When the balloon at the catheter tip is inflated, the catheter advances and wedges in a branch of the pulmonary artery. The tip of the catheter is able to sense pressures transmitted from the left atrium, which reflect left ventricular end-diastolic pressure. Also called *pulmonary artery occlusive pressure*.

pulmonary autograph The relocation of the patient's own pulmonary valve to the aortic position for aortic valve replacement (Ross procedure).

pulmonary embolism (PE) A collection of particulate matter, most commonly a blood clot, that enters venous circulation and lodges in the pulmonary vessels, obstructing pulmonary blood flow and leading to decreased systemic oxygenation, pulmonary tissue hypoxia, and potential death.

pulmonary empyema A collection of pus in the pleural space most commonly caused by a pulmonary infection.

pulse deficit The difference between the apical and peripheral pulses.

pulse pressure The difference between the systolic and diastolic pressures.

pulse therapy Any therapy given at a high dose for a short duration.

pulsus alternans A type of pulse in which a weak pulse alternates with a strong pulse despite a regular heart rhythm; seen in patients with severely depressed cardiac function.

punctum The opening through which tears drain; located at the nasal side of the eyelid edges.

pupil The opening through which light enters the eye; located in the center of the iris of the eye.

Purkinje cells In the cardiac conduction system, the cells that make up the bundle of His, bundle branches, and terminal Purkinje fibers. These cells are responsible for the rapid conduction of electrical impulses throughout the ventricles, leading to ventricular depolarization and subsequent ventricular muscle contraction.

purpura Purple patches on the skin that may be caused by blood disorders, vascular abnormalities, or trauma.

pyelolithotomy The surgical removal of a stone from the kidney.

pyelonephritis A bacterial infection in the kidney and renal pelvis (the upper urinary tract).

pyloromyotomy An incision through the serosa and muscularis of the pylorus, down to the mucosa; created to prevent gastric motility disturbances in patients who have undergone esophagectomy.

pyuria The presence of white blood cells (pus) in the urine.

Q

QRS complex In the electrocardiogram, the portion consisting of the Q, R, and S waves, representing ventricular depolarization.

QRS duration In the electrocardiogram, the time required for depolarization of both ventricles; measured from the beginning of the QRS complex to the J point (the junction at which the QRS complex ends and the ST segment begins).

QT interval In the electrocardiogram, the time from the beginning of the QRS complex to the end of the T wave. It represents the total time required for ventricular depolarization and repolarization.

quadriceps-setting exercise Postoperative leg exercise performed by straightening the legs and pushing the back of the knees into the bed.

quadrigeminy A type of premature complex consisting of a repetitive four-beat pattern; usually occurs as three sequential normal complexes followed by a premature complex and a pause, with the same pattern repeating itself in a four-beat pattern.

quadriparesis Weakness that involves all four extremities; seen with cervical spinal cord injury.

qualitative question A clinical question that focuses on the meanings and interpretations of human phenomena or experience of people and usually analyzes the content of what a person says during an interview or what a researcher observes.

quality improvement A QSEN competency in which the nurse uses data to monitor the outcomes of care processes and uses improvement methods to design and test changes to continuously improve the quality and safety of health care systems.

quantitative question A clinical question that asks about the relationship between or among defined, measurable phenomena and includes statistical analysis of information that is collected to answer a question.

R

radiation dose The amount of radiation absorbed by the tissue.

radiation proctitis Rectal mucosa inflammation that results from external beam radiation therapy.

radical cystectomy Removal of the bladder and surrounding tissue with urinary diversion.

radicular Referring to a nerve root.

radiculopathy Referring to radicular pain; spinal nerve root involvement.

radiofrequency catheter ablation An invasive procedure that uses radiofrequency waves to abolish an irritable focus that is causing a supraventricular or ventricular tachydysrhythmia.

Rapid Response Team Team of critical care experts who save lives and decrease the risk for harm by providing care to patients before a respiratory or cardiac arrest occurs. Also called *Medical Emergency Team.*

rapidly progressive glomerulonephritis A primary inflammation of the glomeruli, nephrons, and kidney tissue that develops over several weeks to months.

RBC Red blood cell.

rebound headache Headache that occurs as a side effect of a drug that has relieved an initial migraine headache. Also called *medication overuse headache.*

recall memory Recent memory, which can be tested during the history taking by asking about items such as the dates of clinic or physician appointments.

receptive aphasia A type of aphasia caused by injury to Wernicke's area in the temporoparietal area of the brain and characterized by an inability to understand the spoken and written word; reading and writing ability are equally affected. Although the patient can talk, the language is often meaningless and neologisms (made-up words) are common parts of speech. Also called *Wernicke's aphasia* or *sensory aphasia.*

reconstructive plastic surgery Type of plastic surgery that corrects or improves functional defects that have occurred as a result of congenital problems, trauma and scarring, or other types of therapy.

recreational therapist A member of the health care team who works to help patients continue or develop hobbies or interests. Also called *activity therapist.*

rectocele A protrusion of the rectum through a weakened vaginal wall.

red reflex A reflection of light on the retina seen as a red glare during ophthalmoscopic examination. An absent red reflex may indicate a lens opacity or cloudiness of the vitreous.

redirection An intervention to help with communication problems in patients with dementia; consists of attracting the patient's attention before conversing, keeping the environment as free of distractions as possible, and speaking directly to the patient in a distinct manner using clear and short sentences.

reducible hernia A hernia that can be placed back into the abdominal cavity by gentle pressure.

reduction mammoplasty Breast reduction surgery in which the surgeon removes excess breast tissue and then repositions the nipple and remaining skin flaps to produce an optimal cosmetic effect.

Reed-Sternberg cell A specific cancer cell type, found in lymph nodes, that is a marker for Hodgkin's lymphoma.

re-epithelialization In partial-thickness (superficial) wounds involving damage to the epidermis and upper layers of the dermis, a form of healing by means of the production of new skin cells by undamaged epidermal cells in the basal layer of the dermis.

refeeding syndrome Life-threatening metabolic complication that can occur when nutrition is restarted for a patient who is in a starvation state.

reflex arc A closed circuit of spinal and peripheral nerves that requires no control by the brain.

reflex sympathetic dystrophy (RSD) See *complex regional pain syndrome.*

reflux esophagitis Damage to the esophageal mucosa, often with erosion and ulceration, in patients with gastroesophageal reflux disease.

reflux Reverse or backward flow.

refraction The bending of light rays.

refractory hypoxemia Low blood oxygen levels that persist even when 100% oxygen is given.

regional anesthesia A type of local anesthesia that blocks multiple peripheral nerves in a specific body region.

registered dietitian (RD) Member of the health care team who ensures that patients meet their nutritional needs. Also called *nutritionist.*

regurgitation Flowing in the opposite direction from normal, as the occurrence of warm fluid traveling up the throat, unaccompanied by nausea, in the patient with gastroesophageal reflux disease.

rehabilitation assistants Assistants to rehabilitation therapists.

rehabilitation case manager Nurse or other health care professional who coordinates health care for patients undergoing rehabilitation in home or acute care settings.

rehabilitation nurse Nurse who coordinates the efforts of health care team members for patients undergoing rehabilitation in the inpatient setting; may be designated as the patient's case manager.

rehabilitation therapists The collective group of physical therapists (PTs), occupational therapists (OTs), and speech-language pathologists (SLPs).

rehabilitation The process of learning to live with chronic and disabling conditions by returning the patient to the fullest possible physical, mental, social, vocational, and economic capacity.

reinfusion system A technique that allows for collection of red blood cells from a joint drain over a specific time frame, which then can be reinfused directly back into the patient's systemic circulation.

relapsing-remitting multiple sclerosis (RRMS) A type of multiple sclerosis that occurs in 85% of cases and is characterized by a mild or moderate course, depending on the degree of disability. Relapses develop over 1 to 2 weeks and resolve over 4 to 8 months, after which the patient returns to baseline.

reliever drugs Drugs used in asthma therapy to stop an asthma attack once it has started.

religions Formal belief systems that provide a framework for making sense of life, death, and suffering and responding to universal spiritual questions; a formal expression of spirituality.

relocation stress syndrome Physiologic or psychosocial distress following transfer from one environment to another, such as after admission to a hospital or nursing home. Also called *relocation trauma.*

reminiscence The process of randomly reflecting on memories of events in one's life.

remote memory Long-term memory of events; can be tested by asking patients about their birth date, schools attended, city of birth, or anything from the past that can be verified.

renal colic Severe pain associated with distention or spasm of the ureter, such as with an obstruction or the passing of a stone; the pain radiates into the perineal area, groin, scrotum, or labia. Pain may be intermittent or continuous and may be accompanied by pallor, diaphoresis, and hypotension.

renal columns Cortical tissue that dips into the interior of the kidney and separates the pyramids in the medulla. Also called *columns of Bertin.*

renal cortex The outermost layer of functional kidney tissue lying beneath the renal capsule.

renal osteodystrophy The problems in bone metabolism and structure caused by renal failure–induced hypocalcemia and hyperphosphatemia.

renal pelvis The expansion from the upper end of the ureter into which the calices of the kidney open.

renal threshold The limit to the amount of glucose that the kidney can reabsorb as glucose is filtered from the blood. Also called the *transport maximum*.

renin A hormone that is produced in the juxtaglomerular complex of the kidney and that helps regulate blood flow, glomerular filtration rate, and blood pressure. Renin is secreted when sensing cells (macula densa) in the distal convoluted tubule sense changes in blood volume and pressure.

repetitive stress injury (RSI) Injury caused by repeated movements of the same part of the body (e.g., carpal tunnel syndrome).

replication The reproduction of DNA that occurs each time a cell divides.

resident An individual who lives in an inpatient facility and has all the rights of anyone living in his or her home.

residuals Amount of feeding that remains in the stomach after enteral nutrition.

resistin A hormone produced by fat cells that creates resistance to insulin activity.

resorption In referring to bone, the loss of bone minerals and density; the release of free calcium from bone storage sites directly into the extracellular fluid.

restorative aide A member of the health care team, often with the nursing department, who assists the therapists, especially in the long-term care setting.

restraint Any device (physical restraint) or drug (chemical restraint) that prevents the patient from moving freely.

restrictive (lung disorder) Any lung disorder that prevents good expansion and recoil of the gas exchange unit.

restrictive cardiomyopathy A form of cardiomyopathy that restricts the filling of the ventricles; a type of lung disease that prevents good expansion and recoil of the gas exchange unit.

resurfacing Regrowth of new skin cells across the open area of a wound as it heals.

resuscitation phase The first phase of a burn injury, beginning at the onset of injury and continuing to about 48 hours.

rete pegs The fingers of epidermal tissue that project into the dermis.

reticular activating system (RAS) Special cells throughout the brainstem that constitute the system that controls awareness and alertness.

retina The innermost layer of the eye, made up of sensory receptors that transmit impulses to the optic nerve. It contains blood vessels and two types of photoreceptors called *rods* and *cones*. Rods work at low light levels and provide peripheral vision; cones are active at bright light levels and provide color and central vision.

retinal detachment Separation of the retina from the epithelium.

retinal hole A break in the retina; can be caused by trauma or can occur with aging.

retinal tear Jagged and irregularly shaped break in the retina resulting from traction on the retina.

retinopathy Inflammation of the retina. Also used as a general term for vision problems.

retrograde Going against the normal direction of flow.

retroviruses The family of viruses that includes the human immune deficiency virus.

revision arthroplasty Surgical replacement of a prosthesis that has loosened and is causing pain.

rhabdomyolysis The breakdown or disintegration of muscle tissue; associated with excretion of myoglobin in the urine.

rheumatic carditis Inflammatory lesions in the heart due to a sensitivity response that develops after an upper respiratory tract infection with group A beta-hemolytic streptococci, which occurs in about 40% of patients with rheumatic fever. Inflammation results in impaired contractile function of the myocardium, thickening of the pericardium, and valvular damage. Also called *rheumatic endocarditis*.

rheumatic disease Any disease or condition involving the musculoskeletal system.

rheumatoid arthritis (RA) A chronic, progressive, systemic, inflammatory autoimmune disease process that primarily affects the synovial joints; one of the most common connective tissue diseases and the most destructive to the joints.

rhinitis An inflammation of the nasal mucosa.

rhinoplasty A surgical reconstruction of the nose done for cosmetic purposes and improvement of airflow.

rhinorrhea Watery drainage from the nose; a "runny" nose.

rhinosinusitis An inflammation of the mucous membranes of one or more of the sinuses; usually seen with rhinitis, especially the common cold (coryza).

rickets Vitamin D deficiency in children.

right-sided heart (ventricular) failure The inability of the right ventricle to empty completely, resulting in increased volume and pressure in the systemic veins and systemic venous congestion with peripheral edema.

robotic technology Technology that provides mechanical parts for extremities when they are not functional or have been amputated.

Romberg sign Swaying or falling when the patient is standing with arms at the sides, feet and knees close together, and eyes closed; a test of equilibrium in neurologic assessment.

rotation A mechanism of injury in which the head is turned excessively beyond the normal range.

rubor Dusky red discoloration of the skin.

rugae Folds, as of a mucous membrane.

S

S₃ gallop The third heart sound; an early diastolic filling sound that indicates an increase in left ventricular pressure and may be heard on auscultation in patients with heart failure.

safer sex practices Interventions that reduce the risk of nonintact skin or mucous membranes coming in contact with infected body fluids and blood, such as using a condom.

safety A QSEN competency in which the nurse minimizes risk of harm to patients and providers through both system effectiveness and individual performance.

Salem sump tube Tube inserted through the nose and placed into the stomach that is attached to low continuous suction. It has a vent ("pigtail") that prevents the stomach mucosa from being pulled away during suctioning.

salpingitis Infection of the fallopian tube.

sanguineous Having a bloody appearance.

sarcoidosis A granulomatous disorder of unknown cause that can affect any organ but most often involves the lung.

SBAR Acronym for a formal method of communication between two or more members of the health care team. It is used most often when there is an unmet patient need or problem but can also be used to communicate continuing care issues when a patient is discharged from one agency to another. It consists of four steps: Situation, Background, Assessment, Recommendation.

scabies A contagious skin disease caused by mite infestations.

sclera The external white layer of the eye.

scleroderma See *systemic sclerosis*.

sclerotherapy The injection of a sclerosing agent via a catheter, usually in an endoscopic procedure, to stop variceal bleeding.

sclerotic Hard, or hardening.

scoliosis An abnormal lateral curve in the spine, which normally should be a straight vertical line.

scotomas Changes in peripheral vision.

sebum A mildly bacteriostatic, fat-containing substance produced by the sebaceous glands. Sebum lubricates the skin and reduces water loss from the skin surface.

second intention Healing of deep tissue injuries or wounds with tissue loss in which a cavity-like defect requires gradual filling of the dead space with connective tissue, which prolongs the repair process.

secondary administration set A short conduit that is attached to the primary administration set at a Y-injection site and is used to deliver intermittent medications. Also called a *piggyback set*.

secondary gout Gout involving hyperuricemia.

secondary hypertension Elevated blood pressure that is related to a specific disease (e.g., kidney disease) or medication (e.g., estrogen).

secondary lesion Describing skin disease in terms of changes in the appearance of the primary lesion. These changes occur with progression of an underlying disease or in response to a topical or systemic therapeutic intervention.

secondary prevention Early detection of a disease or condition, sometimes before signs and symptoms are evident, to prevent or limit permanent disability or death.

secondary progressive multiple sclerosis (SPMS) A type of multiple sclerosis that begins with a relapsing-remitting course and later becomes steadily progressive. Attacks and partial recoveries may continue to occur.

secondary survey In the emergency department, a more comprehensive head-to-toe assessment performed to identify other injuries or medical issues that need to be managed or that might impact the course of treatment.

secondary tumor Additional tumor that is established when cancer cells move from the primary location to another area in the body. Also called *metastatic tumor*.

seizure An abnormal, sudden, excessive, uncontrolled electrical discharge of neurons within the brain that may result in an alteration in consciousness, motor or sensory ability, and/or behavior. A single seizure may occur for no known reason; however, seizures may be due to a pathologic condition of the brain, such as a tumor.

self-tolerance In immunology, the ability to recognize self cells versus non-self cells, which is necessary to prevent healthy body cells from being destroyed along with invading cells.

Sengstaken-Blakemore tube Tube similar to a nasogastric tube that is placed through the nose and into the stomach in which an attached balloon is inflated to apply pressure to bleeding variceal areas of the esophagus.

sensitivity The likelihood that infecting bacterial organisms will be killed or stopped by a particular antibiotic drug. Sensitivity is determined by testing different antibiotics against the organisms. Organisms are sensitive if the antibiotic is effective in stopping their growth; organisms are resistant if the antibiotic is not effective.

sensorineural hearing loss Hearing loss that results from a defect in the cochlea, the eighth cranial nerve, or the brain itself. Exposure to loud noises and music may cause this type of hearing loss as a result of damage to the cochlear hair cells.

sensory aphasia See *receptive aphasia*.

sensory perception The ability to perceive and interpret sensory input into one or more meaningful responses. Sensory input is usually received through the five major senses of vision, hearing, smell, taste, and touch.

sensory Facilitating sensation.

sentinel event As defined by The Joint Commission, an unexpected occurrence involving serious physical or psychological injury or the risk thereof and requiring an intense analysis of the contributing factors and corrective action.

sepsis Systemic infection.

septic shock The type of shock that occurs when large amounts of toxins and endotoxins produced by bacteria are released into the blood, causing a whole-body inflammatory reaction.

septicemia Systemic disease associated with sepsis; the presence of pathogens in the blood.

sequestrum A piece of necrotic bone that has separated from surrounding bone tissue; a common complication of osteomyelitis.

serologic testing Laboratory testing that is performed to identify pathogens by detecting antibodies to the organism.

serositis Inflammation of a serous membrane, such as the pleura or peritoneum.

serous Having a serum-like appearance, or yellow color.

serum sickness A type III hypersensitivity reaction that develops first as a skin rash and occurs within 3 to 21 days of the administration of antivenin (Crotalidae) polyvalent. This allergic response is often accompanied by other manifestations such as fever, arthralgias (joint pains), and pruritus (itching).

severe acute respiratory syndrome (SARS) An easily spread respiratory infection first identified in China in November 2002. At first appearing as an atypical pneumonia, it is caused by a new, more virulent form of coronavirus, and there is no known effective treatment.

severe sepsis The progression of sepsis with an amplified inflammatory response.

sex chromosomes The pair of chromosomes containing the genes for sexual differentiation in humans. In males, the sex chromosomes are an X and a Y; in females, the sex chromosomes are two Xs.

sex reassignment surgery (SRS) Surgery, particularly procedures that affect the external or internal genitalia, that transitions an individual from one's natal sex to one's inner gender identity. Also known as *gender reassignment surgery*.

sexuality An integration of the physiologic, emotional, and social aspects of well-being related to intimacy, self-concept, and role relationships.

sexually transmitted infections (STIs) Any of a group of diseases caused by infectious organisms that have been passed from one person to another through intimate contact. Some organisms that cause these diseases are transmitted only through sexual contact. Other organisms are transmitted by parenteral exposure to infected blood, fecal-oral transmission, intrauterine transmission to the fetus, and perinatal transmission from mother to neonate. Also known as *sexually transmitted diseases (STDs)*.

SHARE Acronym standing for **S**tandardize critical content, **H**ardwire within your system, **A**llow opportunity to ask questions, **R**einforce quality and measurement, **E**ducate and coach.

shift to the left An increased number of immature neutrophils found on a differential count in patients with infections; can be characterized by changes in percentages of different types of leukocytes. Also known as *left shift*.

shock The whole-body response to poor tissue oxygenation. Any problem that impairs oxygen delivery to tissues and organs can start the syndrome of shock and lead to a life-threatening emergency.

short bone Bone that is small and bears little or no weight, such as the phalanges (fingers and toes).

short peripheral catheter A catheter that consists of a plastic cannula built around a sharp stylet for venipuncture, which extends slightly beyond the cannula and is advanced into the vein.

sialagogue An agent that stimulates the flow of saliva.

simple fracture See *closed fracture*.

single-photon emission computed tomography (SPECT) A diagnostic tool using a radiopharmaceutical (agent that enables radioisotopes to cross the blood-brain barrier) that is administered by IV injection, after which the patient is scanned.

sinoatrial (SA) node In the cardiac conduction system, the primary pacemaker of the heart; located close to the epicardial surface of the right atrium near its junction with the superior vena cava. It can spontaneously and rhythmically generate electrical impulses at a rate of 60 to 100 beats/min. Also called the *sinus node*.

sinus arrhythmia A variant of normal sinus rhythm that results from changes in intrathoracic pressure during breathing; heart rate increases slightly during inspiration and decreases slightly during exhalation. Atrial and ventricular rates are between 60 and 100 beats/min, and atrial and ventricular rhythms are irregular.

sinus bradycardia A cardiac dysrhythmia caused by a decreased rate of sinus node discharge, with a heart rate that is less than 60 beats/min.

sinus tachycardia A cardiac dysrhythmia caused by an increased rate of sinus node discharge, with a heart rate that is more than 100 beats/min.

sinusitis An inflammation of the mucous membranes of the sinuses.

SIRS Acronym for systemic inflammatory response syndrome, an inflammatory state affecting the whole body.

Sjögren's syndrome In patients with advanced rheumatoid arthritis, the triad of dry eyes, dry mouth, and dry vagina caused by the obstruction of secretory ducts and glands by inflammatory cells and immune complexes.

skilled nursing facility (SNF) Part of either a hospital or long-term care (nursing home) setting in which care is reimbursed through Medicare Part A for the first 21 days after admission.

skinfold measurement Measurement that estimates body fat.

smart pump An infusion pump with dosage calculation software.

social justice Ethical principle that refers to equality and fairness—that all patients should be treated equally and fairly, regardless of age, gender, religion, race, ethnicity, or education.

social worker Member of the health care team who helps patients identify support services and resources and who coordinates transfers to or discharges from the rehabilitation setting.

sodium (Na⁺) A mineral that is the major cation in the extracellular fluid and maintains extracellular fluid (ECF) osmolarity.

solute A particle dissolved or suspended in the water portion (solvent) of body fluids; a solution consists of a solute and a solvent.

solvent The water portion of fluids.

spastic bladder Incontinence characterized by sudden, gushing voids, usually without completely emptying the bladder; caused by neurologic problems affecting the upper motor neuron, such as with spinal cord injuries above the twelfth thoracic vertebra.

spastic paralysis Paralysis of a part of the body that is characterized by spasticity of muscles due to hypertonia; may be seen in the patient who has experienced a brain attack.

specialized nutrition support (SNS) Total nutritional intake orally or intravenously with commercially prepared products (either total enteral nutrition or total parenteral nutrition).

speech-language pathologist (SLP) A member of the rehabilitation health care team who evaluates and retrains patients with speech, language, or swallowing problems.

sphincter of Oddi The sheath of muscle fibers surrounding the papillary opening of the duodenum.

sphincterotomy A procedure for opening a sphincter.

spider angiomas See *telangiectasias.*

spinal cord stimulation An invasive stimulation technique that provides pain control by applying an electrical field over the spinal cord.

spinal fusion (arthrodesis) A surgical procedure to stabilize the spine after repeated laminectomies have been unsuccessful. Chips of bone are removed (typically from the iliac crest) or are obtained from donor bone; the chips are grafted between the vertebrae for support and to strengthen the back.

spinal shock syndrome Loss of reflex activity below the level of a spinal lesion; occurs immediately after injury as a result of disruption in the communication pathways between the upper motor neurons and the lower motor neurons. Also called *spinal shock.*

spinal shock See *spinal shock syndrome.*

spinal stenosis Narrowing of the spinal canal; typically seen in people older than 60 years.

spiritual counselor Counselor who specializes in spiritual assessments and care, usually a member of the clergy.

spirituality The connection to self, others, the environment, and a "higher power."

splenectomy Surgical removal of the spleen.

splenomegaly Enlargement of the spleen.

splint Any object or device that extends to the joints above and below a fracture to immobilize it.

splinter hemorrhage Black longitudinal line or small red streak on the distal third of the nail bed; seen in patients with infective endocarditis.

spondee Two-syllable words in which there is generally equal stress on each syllable, such as *airplane, railroad,* and *cowboy;* used in testing speech reception threshold.

spondylolisthesis Condition in which one vertebra slips forward on the one below it, often as a result of spondylolysis. This problem causes pressure on the nerve roots, leading to pain in the lower back and into the buttocks.

spondylolysis A defect in one of the vertebrae; usually found in the lumbar spine.

spontaneous bacterial peritonitis (SBP) Bacterial infection of the abdominal peritoneum caused by ascites; often seen in patients with cirrhosis of the liver.

spore An encapsulated inactive organism.

sprain Excessive stretching of a ligament.

ST segment In the electrocardiogram, the line (normally isoelectric) representing early ventricular repolarization. It occurs from the J point to the beginning of the T wave.

staging System of classifying clinical aspects of a cancer tumor.

Standard Precautions Infection control guidelines from the U.S. Centers for Disease Control and Prevention stating that all body excretions, secretions, and moist membranes and tissues are potentially infectious; combines protective measures from Universal Precautions and Body Substance Isolation.

stasis dermatitis In patients with venous insufficiency, discoloration of the skin along the ankles, which may extend up to the calf.

stasis ulcer In patients with long-term venous insufficiency, ulcer formed as a result of edema or minor injury to the limb; typically occurs over the malleolus.

status epilepticus Prolonged seizures lasting more than 5 minutes or repeated seizures over the course of 30 minutes; a potential complication of all types of seizures.

steatorrhea An excessive amount of fat in the stool.

ST-elevation myocardial infarction (STEMI) Myocardial infarction in which the patient typically has ST elevation in two contiguous leads on a 12-lead ECG; this indicates myocardial infarction/necrosis.

stem cell An immature, undifferentiated cell produced by the bone marrow.

stent A small tube that is placed in a tubular structure to dilate it; a wirelike device that may be used along with percutaneous transluminal angioplasty to help keep the vessel open.

stereotactic pallidotomy A surgical treatment for the patient with Parkinson disease when drugs are ineffective in symptom management. An electrode is used to create a lesion in a targeted area within the pallidum, with the goal of reducing tremor and rigidity.

sterilization A method of infection control in which all living organisms and bacterial spores are destroyed; used on items that invade human tissue where bacteria are not commonly found.

stoma The surgical creation of an opening; usually refers to an opening in the abdominal wall.

stomatitis Inflammation of the oral mucosa; characterized by painful single or multiple ulcerations that impair the protective lining of the mouth. The ulcerations are commonly referred to as "canker sores."

strain Excessive stretching of a muscle or tendon when it is weak or unstable; sometimes referred to as "muscle pulls."

strangulated hernia A tightly constricted hernia that compromises the blood supply to the herniated segment of the bowel as a result of pressure from the hernial ring (the band of muscle around the hernia); leads to ischemia and obstruction of the bowel loop, with necrosis of the bowel and possibly bowel perforation.

strangulated obstruction Intestinal obstruction with compromised blood flow.

stratum corneum The outermost layer of the skin.

stress test See *exercise electrocardiography.*

stress ulcers Multiple shallow erosions of the proximal stomach and occasionally the duodenum.

stress urinary incontinence (SUI) Loss of urine during activities that increase intra-abdominal pressure, such as laughing, coughing, sneezing, or lifting heavy objects.

striae Reddish purple streaks on the skin. Also called *stretch marks.*

stricture Narrowing.

stridor A high-pitched crowing sound caused by laryngospasm or edema above or below the glottis; heard during respiration.

stroke volume (SV) The amount of blood ejected by the left ventricle during each heartbeat.

stroke See *brain attack.*

stuporous Arousable only with vigorous or painful stimulation.

subarachnoid space Term for the space between the arachnoid mater and pia mater of the spinal cord. Also called *subarachnoid.*

subcutaneous emphysema The presence of bubbles under the skin because of air trapping; an uncommon late complication of fracture.

subcutaneous infusion therapy Infusion therapy that is delivered under the skin when patients cannot tolerate oral medications, when intramuscular injections are too painful, or when vascular access is not available.

subcutaneous nodule Characteristic round, movable, nontender swelling under the skin of the arm or fingers in patients with severe rheumatoid arthritis.

subdural hematoma (SDH) The collection of clotted blood that typically results from venous bleeding into the space beneath the dura and above the arachnoid.

subdural space Term for the space between the dura mater and the middle layer (arachnoid).

subluxation Partial joint dislocation.

submucous resection (SMR) Surgical procedure to straighten a deviated septum when chronic symptoms or discomfort occur. Also called *nasoseptoplasty.*

submucous resection Surgical procedure to straighten a deviated septum.

substernally Located below the ribs.

subtotal thyroidectomy The surgical removal of part of the thyroid tissue.

sundowning In patients with Alzheimer's disease, increased confusion at night or when excessively fatigued.

superinfection Reinfection or a second infection of the same type.

supervision Guidance or direction, evaluation, and follow-up by the nurse to ensure that the task or activity is performed appropriately.

supratentorial Located within the cerebral hemispheres, in the area above the tentorium of the cerebellum; the tentlike fold of dura that surrounds the cerebellar hemisphere and supports the occipital lobe.

supraventricular tachycardia (SVT) A form of tachycardia that involves the rapid stimulation of atrial tissue at a rate of 100 to 280 beats/min. It is most often due to a re-entry mechanism in which one impulse circulates repeatedly throughout the atrial pathway, re-stimulating the atrial tissue at a rapid rate.

surfactant A fatty protein secreted by type II pneumocytes to reduce surface tension in the alveoli.

surveillance Term used to describe the tracking of infections by health care agencies.

susceptibility The risk of the host to infection; may be increased by the breakdown of host defenses against pathogens.

swimmer's ear See *external otitis.*

sympathectomy Surgical cutting of the sympathetic nerve branches via endoscopy through a small axillary incision.

sympathetic tone A state of partial blood vessel constriction caused when nerves from the sympathetic division of the autonomic nervous system continuously stimulate vascular smooth muscle.

synapse The area through which impulses are transmitted to their eventual destination.

syncope Transient loss of consciousness (blackouts), most commonly caused by decreased perfusion to the brain.

syndrome of inappropriate antidiuretic hormone (SIADH) Persistent hyponatremia, hypovolemia, and inappropriately elevated urine osmolality that occurs when vasopressin (antidiuretic hormone) is secreted even when plasma osmolarity is low or normal.

synovectomy The surgical removal of synovium.

synovial joint Type of joint lined with synovium, a membrane that secretes synovial fluid for lubrication and shock absorption.

synovitis Inflammation of synovial membrane.

syphilis A complex sexually transmitted disease that can become systemic and cause serious complications and even death. It is caused by the spirochete *Treponema pallidum,* which is found in the mouth, intestinal tract, and genital areas of people and animals. The infection is usually transmitted by sexual contact, but transmission can occur through close body contact and kissing.

syringe pump Pump for infusion therapy that uses a battery-powered piston to push the plunger continuously at a selected mL/hr rate; limited to small-volume continuous or intermittent infusions.

systemic lupus erythematosus (SLE) A chronic, progressive inflammatory connective tissue disorder that can cause major body organs and systems to fail; characterized by spontaneous remissions and exacerbations.

systemic sclerosis (SSc) A chronic connective tissue disease characterized by inflammation, fibrosis, and sclerosis of the skin and vital organs. Also called *scleroderma* and formerly called *progressive systemic sclerosis.*

systemic Affecting the body system as a whole.

systole The phase of the cardiac cycle that consists of the contraction and emptying of the atria and ventricles.

systolic blood pressure The amount of pressure/force generated by the left ventricle to distribute blood into the aorta with each contraction of the heart.

systolic heart failure (systolic ventricular dysfunction) Heart failure that results when the heart is unable to contract forcefully enough during systole to eject adequate amounts of blood into the circulation.

T

T wave In the electrocardiogram, the deflection that follows the ST segment and represents ventricular repolarization.

tachycardia An excessively fast heart rate; characterized as a pulse rate greater than 100 beats/min.

tachydysrhythmia An abnormal heart rhythm with a rate greater than 100 beats/min.

tactile (vocal) fremitus A vibration of the chest wall produced when the patient speaks; can be palpated on the chest wall.

target tissues The tissues that respond specifically to a given hormone.

taut Tightly stretched.

teamwork and collaboration A QSEN competency in which the nurse functions effectively within nursing and interprofessional teams, fostering open communication, mutual respect, and shared decision making to achieve quality patient care.

telangiectasias Vascular lesions with a red center and radiating branches. Also called *spider angiomas, spider nevi,* or *vascular spiders.*

telemetry In electrocardiography (ECG), the use of a battery-powered transmitter system for monitoring an ambulatory patient; allows freedom of movement within a certain radius without losing transmission of the ECG.

temporal field blindness A decrease in lateral peripheral vision.

temporary pacing A nonsurgical intervention for cardiac dysrhythmia that provides a timed electrical stimulus to the heart when either the impulse initiation or the intrinsic conduction system of the heart is defective.

tendon transplant Removal of a tendon from one part of the body and transplantation into the affected area to replace a ruptured tendon that cannot be repaired surgically.

tendon Any one of many bands of tough, fibrous tissue that attach muscles to bones.

tenesmus Straining, especially painful straining to defecate.

tension pneumothorax A life-threatening complication of pneumothorax in which air continues to enter the pleural space during inspiration and does not exit during expiration.

teratogenic Tending to produce birth defects.

tetany Continuous contractions of muscle groups; hyperexcitability of nerves and muscles.

tetraplegia Another term for *quadriplegia* (paralysis that involves all four extremities).

thalamotomy An alternative to stereotactic pallidotomy as a surgical treatment for the patient with Parkinson disease; uses thermocoagulation of brain cells to reduce tremor. Usually only unilateral surgery is performed to benefit the side of the body most affected by the disease.

thalamus A structure within the brain; functions as the "central switchboard" for the central nervous system.

thallium scan A test that is similar to a bone scan but uses the radioisotope *thallium* and is more sensitive in diagnosing the extent of disease in patients with osteosarcoma.

The Joint Commission An organization that offers peer evaluation for accreditation every 3 years for all types of health care agencies that meet their standards. Formerly known as the *Joint Commission for Accreditation of Healthcare Organizations (JCAHO).*

therapeutic hypothermia Treatment that lowers the body core temperature to reduce the risk of cell, tissue, and organ damage from a low or absent blood flow. Usually follows cardiac arrest.

thermotherapy Technique for treating benign prostatic hyperplasia that uses a variety of heat methods to destroy excess prostate tissue.

third intention Delayed primary closure of a wound with a high risk for infection. The wound is intentionally left open for several days until inflammation has subsided and is then closed by first intention.

thoracentesis The aspiration of pleural fluid or air from the pleural space.

threshold In evaluating hearing, the lowest level of intensity at which pure tones and speech are heard by a patient; in general, the lowest level at which a stimulus is perceived.

thrombectomy Removal of a clot (thrombus) from a blood vessel.

thrombocytopenia A reduction in the number of blood platelets below the level needed for normal coagulation, resulting in an increased tendency to bleed.

thrombophlebitis The presence of a thrombus associated with inflammation; usually occurs in the deep veins of the lower extremities.

thrombosis The formation of a blood clot (thrombus) within a blood vessel.

thrombotic stroke Damage to the brain when blood flow is impaired from a clot, resulting in blockage to one or more of the arteries supplying blood to the brain.

thrombus A blood clot believed to result from an endothelial injury, venous stasis, or hypercoagulability.

thymectomy Removal of the thymus gland.

thymoma An encapsulated tumor of the thymus gland.

thyrocalcitonin (TCT) A hormone produced and secreted by the parafollicular cells of the thyroid gland to help regulate serum calcium levels; secreted in response to excess plasma calcium.

thyroid storm (thyroid crisis) A life-threatening event that occurs in patients with uncontrolled hyperthyroidism and is usually caused by Graves' disease. Key manifestations include fever, tachycardia, and systolic hypertension.

thyroiditis Inflammation of the thyroid gland.

thyrotoxicosis The condition caused by excessive amounts of thyroid hormones.

thyroxine (T_4) A hormone that is produced by the follicular cells of the thyroid gland and that increases metabolism.

Tinel's sign Test that confirms a diagnosis of carpal tunnel syndrome; a positive test causes palmar paresthesias when the area of the median nerve is tapped lightly.

tinnitus A continuous ringing or noise perception in the ears.

tissue integrity The intactness of the structure and function of the integument (skin and subcutaneous tissue) and mucous membranes.

titration Adjustment of IV fluid rate on the basis of the patient's urine output plus serum electrolyte values.

TNM (tumor, node, metastasis) System developed by the American Joint Committee on Cancer to describe the anatomic extent of cancers.

toe brachial pressure index (TBPI) Toe systolic pressure divided by brachial (arm) systolic pressure; may be performed instead of or in addition to ankle-brachial index to determine arterial perfusion in the feet and toes.

toll-like receptors (TLRs) Receptors on immune system cells of humans and other animals that interact with the surface of any invading organism and allow recognition of non-self so actions are taken to rid the body of this invader.

tonic phase Pertaining to a state of stiffening or rigidity of the muscles, particularly of the arms and legs, and immediate loss of consciousness of a tonic-clonic seizure.

tonsillitis An inflammation and infection of the tonsils and lymphatic tissues located on each side of the throat.

tophi A collection of uric acid crystals that form hard irregular, painless nodules on the ears, arms, and fingers of patients with gout.

topical chemical débridement Method of débriding a wound by applying topical enzyme preparations to loosen necrotic tissue.

torn meniscus Tear of the knee meniscus (medial or lateral) in which the patient typically has pain, swelling, and tenderness in the knee.

torsades de pointes A type of ventricular tachycardia that is related to a prolonged QT interval.

total hysterectomy Removal of the uterus and cervix; the procedure may be vaginal or abdominal.

total joint arthroplasty (TJA) Surgical creation of a joint, or total joint replacement; commonly performed in patients with osteoarthritis. Also called *total joint replacement (TJR)*.

total joint replacement (TJR) See *total joint arthroplasty*.

total parenteral nutrition (TPN) Provision of intensive nutritional support for an extended time; delivered to the patient through access to central veins, usually the subclavian or internal jugular veins.

total thyroidectomy The surgical removal of all of the thyroid tissue.

touch discrimination Part of the neurologic examination. The patient closes his or her eyes while the practitioner touches the patient with a finger and asks that the patient point to the area touched.

toxic and drug-induced hepatitis Liver inflammation resulting from exposure to hepatotoxins (e.g., industrial toxins, alcohol, and medications).

toxic epidermal necrolysis (TEN) A rare acute drug reaction of the skin that results in diffuse erythema and blister formation, with mucous membrane involvement and systemic toxicity.

toxic megacolon Acute enlargement of the colon along with fever, leukocytosis, and tachycardia; usually associated with ulcerative colitis.

toxic multinodular goiter Hyperthyroidism caused by multiple thyroid nodules, which may be enlarged thyroid tissues or adenomas, and a goiter that has been present for several years.

toxic shock syndrome (TSS) A severe illness caused by a toxin produced by certain strains of *Staphylococcus aureus*. It was first recognized in 1980 as related to menstruation and tampon use. It is characterized by abrupt onset of a high fever and headache, sore throat, vomiting, diarrhea, generalized rash, and hypotension. The most common manifestations are skin changes (initially a rash that resembles a severe sunburn and changes to a macular erythema similar to a drug-related rash).

toxidrome A syndrome related to drug toxicity.

toxin Protein molecule released by bacteria that affects host cell at a distant site. Continued multiplication of a pathogen is sometimes accompanied by toxin production.

trabeculation An abnormal thickening of the bladder wall caused by urinary retention and obstruction.

tracheostomy The (tracheal) stoma, or opening, that results from a tracheotomy.

tracheotomy The surgical incision into the trachea for the purpose of establishing an airway.

trachoma A chronic conjunctivitis caused by *Chlamydia trachomatis*.

traction The application of a pulling force to a part of the body to provide reduction, alignment, and rest.

transcellular fluid Any of the fluids in special body spaces, including cerebrospinal fluid, synovial fluid, peritoneal fluid, and pleural fluid.

transcutaneous electrical nerve stimulation (TENS) A battery-operated device capable of delivering small electrical currents through electrodes applied to an area of the body to relieve pain.

transcutaneous pacing Temporary pacing that is accomplished through the application of two large external electrodes.

transesophageal echocardiography (TEE) A form of echocardiography performed transesophageally (through the esophagus); an ultrasound transducer is placed immediately behind the heart in the esophagus or stomach to examine cardiac structure and function.

transferrin An iron-transport protein that can be measured directly or calculated as an indirect measurement of total iron-binding capacity.

transgender Patients who self-identify as the opposite gender or a gender that does not match their natal sex.

transient ischemic attack (TIA) A brief attack (lasting a few minutes to less than 24 hours) of focal neurologic dysfunction caused by a brief interruption in cerebral blood flow, possibly resulting from cerebral vasospasm or transient systemic arterial hypertension. Repeated attacks may damage brain tissue; multiple attacks indicate significant increased risk for brain attack.

transition manager A role of the professional nurse to facilitate continuity of care for patients as they transfer among health care settings and the community.

transmyocardial laser revascularization A new surgical procedure for patients with unstable angina and inoperable coronary artery disease with areas of reversible myocardial ischemia. After a single-lung intubation, a left anterior thoracotomy is performed and the heart is visualized. A laser is used to create 20 to 24 long, narrow channels through the left ventricular muscle to the left ventricle. The channels eventually allow oxygenated blood to flow from the left ventricle during diastole to nourish the muscle.

transport maximum See *renal threshold*.

transsexual A person who has modified his or her natal body to match the appropriate gender identity, either through cosmetic, hormonal, or surgical means.

transurethral microwave therapy (TUMT) Procedure for treating benign prostatic hyperplasia using high temperatures to heat and destroy excess tissue.

transurethral needle ablation (TUNA) Procedure for treating benign prostatic hyperplasia using low radiofrequency energy to shrink the prostate.

transurethral resection of the prostate (TURP) The traditional "closed" surgical procedure for removal of the prostate. In this procedure, the surgeon inserts a resectoscope (an instrument similar to a cystoscope, but with a cutting and cauterizing loop) through the urethra. The enlarged portion of the prostate gland is then resected in small pieces.

trauma center Specialty care facility that provides competent and timely trauma services to patients depending on its designated level of capability.

trauma system An organized and integrated approach to trauma care designed to ensure that all critical elements of trauma care delivery are aligned to meet the injured patient's needs.

trauma Bodily injury.

triage officer In a hospital's emergency response plan, the person who rapidly evaluates each patient who arrives at the hospital. In a large hospital, this person is generally a physician who is assisted by triage nurses; however, a nurse may assume this role when physician resources are limited.

triage In the emergency department, sorting or classifying patients into priority levels depending on illness or injury severity, with the highest acuity needs receiving the quickest evaluation and treatment.

trigeminy A type of premature complex consisting of a repetitive three-beat pattern; usually occurs as two sequential normal complexes followed by a premature complex and a pause, with the same pattern repeating itself in triplets.

trigger points In patients with fibromyalgia syndrome, tender areas that can typically be palpated to elicit pain in a predictable, reproducible pattern.

triglycerides Serum lipid profile that includes the measurement of cholesterol and lipoproteins.

triiodothyronine (T₃) A hormone produced by the follicular cells of the thyroid gland.

troponin A myocardial muscle protein released into the bloodstream after injury to myocardial muscle. Because it is not found in healthy patients, any rise in values indicates cardiac necrosis or acute myocardial infarction.

truss A device, usually a pad made with firm material, that is held in place over the hernia with a belt to keep the abdominal contents from protruding into the hernial sac.

tuberculosis (TB) A highly communicable disease caused by *Mycobacterium tuberculosis*. It is the most common bacterial infection worldwide.

tumescence The condition of being swollen.

tunneled central venous catheter A type of catheter used for long-term infusion therapy in which a portion of the catheter lies in a subcutaneous tunnel, separating the points where the catheter enters the vein from where it exits the skin.

turbidity Cloudiness of a solution.

turbinates Three bony projections that protrude into the nasal cavities from the walls of the internal portion of the nose.

turgor The condition of being swollen and congested; indicates the amount of skin elasticity; the normal resiliency of a pinched fold of skin.

type A gastritis A type of gastritis that refers to an inflammation of the glands, fundus, and body of the stomach.

type B gastritis A type of gastritis that affects the glands of the antrum and may involve the entire stomach.

tyrosine kinase inhibitors (TKIs) Drugs with the main action of inhibiting activation of tyrosine kinases. There are many different TKIs. Some are unique to the cell type; others may be present only in cancer cells that express a specific gene mutation. As a result, the different TKI drugs are effective in disrupting the growth of some cancer cell types and not others.

U

U wave In the electrocardiogram, the deflection that follows the T wave and may result from slow repolarization of ventricular Purkinje fibers. When present, it is of the same polarity as the T wave, although generally smaller. Abnormal prominence of the U wave suggests an electrolyte abnormality or other disturbance.

ulcerative colitis (UC) A chronic inflammatory process that affects the mucosal lining of the colon or rectum; one of a group of bowel diseases of unknown etiology characterized by remissions and exacerbations. It can result in loose stools containing blood and mucus, poor absorption of vital nutrients, and thickening of the colon wall.

umbilical hernia Protrusion of the intestine at the umbilicus; can be congenital or acquired. Congenital umbilical hernias appear in infancy. Acquired umbilical hernias directly result from increased intra-abdominal pressure and are most commonly seen in obese people.

unclassified seizure One of the three broad categories of seizure disorders along with *partial seizure* and *generalized seizure*. They occur for no known reason, do not fit into the generalized or partial classifications, and account for about half of all seizure activity. Also called *idiopathic seizure*.

uncus The inner part of the temporal lobe of the brain that can move downward and cause pressure on the brainstem; the vital sign center.

undermining Separation of the skin layers at the wound margins from the underlying granulation tissue.

unilateral body neglect syndrome In the patient who has had a brain attack, an unawareness of the existence of the paralyzed side. For example, the patient may believe he or she is sitting up straight when actually he or she is leaning to one side. Another typical example is the patient who washes or dresses only one side of the body.

Unna boot A wound dressing constructed of gauze moistened with zinc oxide; used to promote venous return in the ambulatory patient with a stasis ulcer and to form a sterile environment for the ulcer. The boot is applied to the affected limb, from the toes to the knee, after the ulcer has been cleaned with normal saline solution and covered with an elastic wrap. The dressing hardens like a cast.

upper endoscopy See *esophagogastroduodenoscopy*.

upper esophageal sphincter (UES) The ringlike band of muscle fibers at the upper end of the esophagus. When at rest, the sphincter is closed to prevent air from entering into the esophagus during respiration.

upper GI (gastrointestinal) radiographic series The radiographic visualization of the gastrointestinal tract from the oral part of the pharynx to the duodenojejunal junction; used to detect disorders of structure or function of the esophagus (barium swallow), stomach, or duodenum.

uremia The accumulation of nitrogenous wastes in the blood (azotemia); a result of renal failure, with clinical symptoms including nausea and vomiting.

uremic frost A layer of urea crystals from evaporated sweat; may appear on the face, eyebrows, axilla, and groin in patients with advanced uremic syndrome.

uremic syndrome The systemic clinical and laboratory manifestations of end-stage kidney disease.

ureterolithiasis Formation of stones in the ureter.

ureteropelvic junction (UPJ) The narrow area in the upper third of the ureter at the point at which the renal pelvis becomes the ureter.

ureteroplasty Surgical repair of the ureter.

ureterovesical junction (UVJ) The point at which each ureter becomes narrow as it enters the bladder.

urethral meatus The opening at the endpoint of the urethra.

urethral stricture An obstruction that occurs low in the urinary tract due to decreased diameter of the urethra, causing bladder distention before hydroureter and hydronephrosis.

urethritis An inflammation of the urethra that causes symptoms similar to urinary tract infection.

urethroplasty Surgical treatment of the urethral stricture to remove the affected area with or without grafting to create a larger opening.

urgency The feeling that urination will occur immediately.

urgent triage In a three-tiered triage scheme, the category that includes patients who should be treated quickly but in whom an immediate threat to life does not currently exist, such as those with abdominal pain or displaced fractures or dislocations.

urinary tract infection (UTI) An infection in the normally sterile urinary system. The unobstructed and complete passage of urine from the renal and urinary systems is critical in maintaining a sterile urinary tract. When any structural abnormality is present, the risk for damage as a result of infection is greatly increased.

urolithiasis The presence of calculi (stones) in the urinary tract.

urosepsis The spread of an infection from the urinary tract to the bloodstream, resulting in systemic infection accompanied by fever, chills, hypotension, and altered mental status.

urticaria A transient vascular reaction of the skin marked by the development of wheals (hives).

uterine artery embolization Treatment for leiomyomas in which a radiologist uses a percutaneous catheter inserted through the femoral artery to inject polyvinyl alcohol pellets into the uterine artery. The resulting blockage starves the tumor of circulation, allowing it (or them) to shrink.

uterine prolapse Downward displacement of the uterus into the vagina.

uvea The middle layer of the eye, which consists of the choroid, ciliary body, and iris. The choroid has many blood vessels that supply nutrients to the retina.

V

vagal maneuver Nonsurgical management of cardiac dysrhythmias that is intended to induce vagal stimulation of the cardiac conduction system, specifically the sinoatrial and atrioventricular nodes. Vagal maneuvers may be attempted to terminate supraventricular tachydysrhythmia.

vaginoplasty The construction of a new vagina in a male-to-female patient, usually with inverted penile tissue or a colon graft, and the creation of a clitoris and labia using scrotal or penile tissue and skin grafts.

validation therapy For the patient with moderate or severe Alzheimer's disease, the process of recognizing and acknowledging the patient's feelings and concerns without reinforcing an erroneous belief (e.g., if the patient is looking for his or her deceased mother).

Valsalva maneuver A form of vagal stimulation of the cardiac conduction system in which the health care provider instructs the patient to bear down as if straining to have a bowel movement.

valvular regurgitation Regurgitation of any heart valve. See also *mitral regurgitation*.

variant (Prinzmetal's) angina A type of angina caused by coronary vasospasm (vessel spasm); usually associated with elevation of the ST segment on an electrocardiogram obtained during anginal attacks.

varicose veins Distended, protruding veins that appear darkened and tortuous; common in patients older than 30 years whose occupations require prolonged standing. As the vein wall weakens and dilates, venous pressure increases and the valves become incompetent (defective). The incompetent valves enhance the vessel dilation, and the veins become tortuous and distended.

vascular access device (VAD) A catheter; a plastic tube placed in a blood vessel to deliver fluids and medications.

vasculitis Blood vessel inflammation.

vasoconstriction Decrease in diameter of blood vessels.

vasopressin Secretion of the posterior pituitary gland. Also known as *antidiuretic hormone* or *ADH*.

vasospasm A sudden and transient constriction of a blood vessel.

Vaughn-Williams classification System used to categorize antidysrhythmic agents according to their effects on the action potential of cardiac cells.

vegan A vegetarian diet pattern in which only foods of plant origin are eaten.

venous beading A complication of diabetes; the abnormal appearance of retinal veins in which areas of swelling and constriction along a segment of vein resemble links of sausage. Such bleeding occurs in areas of retinal ischemia and is a predictor of proliferative diabetic retinopathy.

venous insufficiency Alteration of venous efficiency by thrombosis or defective valves; caused by prolonged venous hypertension, which stretches the veins and damages the valves, resulting in further venous hypertension, edema, and, eventually, venous stasis ulcers, swelling, and cellulitis.

venous thromboembolism (VTE) A term that refers to both deep vein thrombosis and pulmonary embolism; obstruction by a thrombus.

ventilator-associated events (VAEs) Complications of ventilator therapy that result in a significant and sustained deterioration in oxygenation (greater than 20% increase in the daily minimum fraction of inspired oxygen or an increase of at least 3 cm H_2O in the daily minimum positive end-expiratory pressure [PEEP] to maintain oxygenation).

ventilator-associated lung injury (VALI) Damage from prolonged ventilation causing loss of surfactant, increased inflammation, fluid leakage, and noncardiac pulmonary edema. Also known as *ventilator-induced lung injury*.

ventilator-induced lung injury (VILI) See *ventilator-associated lung injury*.

ventral hernia See *incisional hernia*.

ventricular asystole The complete absence of any ventricular rhythm. There are no electrical impulses in the ventricles and therefore no ventricular depolarization, no QRS complex, no contraction, no cardiac output, and no pulse, respirations, or blood pressure. The patient is in full cardiac arrest.

ventricular fibrillation (VF) A cardiac dysrhythmia that results from electrical chaos in the ventricles; impulses from many irritable foci fire in a totally disorganized manner so that ventricular contraction cannot occur; there is no cardiac output or pulse and therefore no cerebral, myocardial, or systemic perfusion. This rhythm is rapidly fatal if not successfully terminated within 3 to 5 minutes.

ventricular gallop An abnormal third heart sound that arises from vibrations of the valves and supporting structures and is produced during the rapid passive filling phase of ventricular diastole when blood flows from the atrium to a noncompliant ventricle. In patients older than 35 years, it is an early sign of heart failure or ventricular septal defect.

ventricular remodeling (1) Progressive myocyte (myocardial cell) contractile dysfunction over time; results from activation of the renin-angiotensin system caused by reduced blood flow to the kidneys, a common occurrence in low-output states; (2) after a myocardial infarction, permanent changes in the size and shape of the left ventricle due to scar tissue; such remodeling may decrease left ventricular function, cause heart failure, and increase morbidity and mortality.

ventricular tachycardia (VT) An abnormal heart rhythm that occurs with repetitive firing of an irritable ventricular ectopic focus, usually at a rate of 140 to 180 beats/min or more.

ventriculomyomectomy The surgical excision of a portion of the hypertrophied ventricular septum to create a widened outflow tract in patients with obstructive hypertrophic cardiomyopathy. Also called *ventricular septal myectomy*.

veracity Ethical principle that requires that the nurse is obligated to tell the truth to the best of his or her knowledge.

vertebroplasty A minimally invasive surgery for managing vertebral fractures in patients with osteoporosis. Bone cement is injected directly into the fracture site to provide immediate pain relief.

vertigo A sense of spinning movement that may result from diseases of the inner ear.

vesicant medications Drugs that cause severe tissue damage if they escape into the subcutaneous tissue; also referred to as vesicants.

vesicants Chemicals or drugs that cause tissue damage on direct contact or extravasation.

vesicle In health care, a small bladder or blister.

vestibule A longitudinal area between the labia minora, the clitoris, and the vagina that contains Bartholin glands and the openings of the urethra, Skene's glands (paraurethral glands), and vagina.

viral hepatitis Inflammation of the liver that results from an infection caused by one of five major categories of viruses (hepatitis A, B, C, D, or E). Viral hepatitis is the most common type and can be either acute or chronic.

viral load testing Test that measures the presence of human immune deficiency virus genetic material (ribonucleic acid) or other viral proteins in the patient's blood.

Virchow's triad The occurrence of stasis of blood flow, endothelial injury, or hypercoagulability; often associated with thrombus formation.

viremia The presence of viruses in the blood.

virilization The presence of male secondary sex characteristics.

virtual colonoscopy A noninvasive alternative to the colonoscopy procedure. A scanner is used to view the colon.

virulence A term used to describe the frequency with which a pathogen causes disease (degree of communicability) and its ability to invade and damage a host. Virulence can also indicate the severity of the disease; often used as a synonym for *pathogenicity*.

visceral proteins Proteins such as albumin that circulate in the bloodstream and may be produced by the liver.

vitiligo An abnormality of the skin characterized by patchy areas of pigment loss with increased pigmentation at the edges. It is seen with primary hypofunction of the adrenal glands and is due to autoimmune destruction of melanocytes in the skin.

vitreous body The clear, thick gel that fills the vitreous chamber of the eye (the space between the lens and the retina). This gel transmits light and shapes the eye.

vocational counselor A member of the rehabilitative health care team who assists the patient with job placement, training, or further education.

volutrauma Damage to the lung by excess volume delivered to one lung over the other.

volvulus Obstruction of the bowel caused by twisting of the bowel.

vulva The external female genitalia.

vulvovaginitis Inflammation of the lower genital tract resulting from a disturbance of the balance of hormones and flora in the vagina and vulva.

W

warm antibody anemia A form of immunohemolytic anemia (in which the immune system attacks a person's own red blood cells for unknown reasons) that occurs with immunoglobulin G antibody excess and may be triggered by drugs, chemicals, or other autoimmune problems.

warm phase A phase lasting 2 to 3 weeks after peripheral nerve trauma resulting in complete denervation; the extremity is warm, and the skin appears flushed or rosy. The warm phase is gradually superseded by a cold phase.

water brash Reflex salivary hypersecretion that occurs in response to reflux in the patient with gastroesophageal reflux disease.

WBC White blood cell.

weaning The process of going from ventilatory dependence to spontaneous breathing.

wedge resection Removal of small, localized areas of disease.

Wernicke's aphasia See *receptive aphasia*.

Wernicke's area An important speech area of the cerebrum. It is located in the temporal lobe and plays a significant role in higher-level brain function. It enables the processing of words into coherent thought and recognition of the idea behind written or printed words (language).

Whipple procedure (radical pancreaticoduodenectomy) A surgical treatment for cancer of the head of the pancreas. The procedure entails removal of the proximal head of the pancreas, the duodenum, a portion of the jejunum, the stomach (partial or total gastrectomy), and the gallbladder, with anastomosis of the pancreatic duct (pancreaticojejunostomy), the common bile duct (choledochojejunostomy), and the stomach (gastrojejunostomy) to the jejunum.

white matter In the spinal cord, myelinated axons that surround the gray matter (neuron cell bodies).

Williams position A position in which the patient lies in the semi-Fowler's position and flexes the knees to relax the muscles of the lower back and relieve pressure on the spinal nerve root. This is typically more comfortable and therapeutic for the patient with low back pain.

withdrawing or withholding life-sustaining therapy The withdrawal or withholding of one or more therapies that might prolong the life of a person who cannot be cured by the therapy; the withdrawal of therapy does not directly cause death. Formerly called *passive euthanasia*.

work-related musculoskeletal disorders (MSDs) Disorders caused by heavy lifting and dependent transfers by staff members.

X

xenograft Tissue transplanted (grafted) from another species; for example, a heart valve transplanted from a pig to a human.

xerosis Abnormally dry skin.

xerostomia Abnormal dryness of the mouth caused by a severe reduction in the flow of saliva.

x-ray Radiation that is generated by machine.

Z

Zika virus A virus carried by mosquitoes that has affected people in over a dozen countries, including the United States, and can cause microcephaly (abnormally small heads) in newborns and Gullain-Barré syndrome in adults.

NCLEX® EXAMINATION CHALLENGES ANSWER KEY

Chapter 3
3-1   B
3-2   A, B, D, E, F
3-3   B
3-4   B

Chapter 4
4-1   A, B, D
4-2   A, C, D, E
4-3   0.2
4-4   A

Chapter 5
5-1   C
5-2   B
5-3   C, D, E

Chapter 6
6-1   B
6-2   B, C, D
6-3   D

Chapter 7
7-1   D
7-2   B

Chapter 8
8-1   D
8-2   A, C, D
8-3   B

Chapter 9
9-1   D
9-2   A, B, C, D, E, G
9-3   B, C, D, E

Chapter 10
10-1   D
10-2   A, C
10-3   A, B, C, D, F, G

Chapter 11
11-1   C
11-2   A
11-3   B, D, E, F
11-4   D
11-5   B

Chapter 12
12-1   D
12-2   B, D, E
12-3   B

Chapter 13
13-1   D
13-2   125

Chapter 14
14-1   C
14-2   B, C, F
14-3   C

Chapter 15
15-1   D
15-2   B, C, D, F
15-3   B
15-4   A

Chapter 16
16-1   A
16-2   D
16-3   C, D
16-4   C

Chapter 17
17-1   B, D, E
17-2   C

Chapter 18
18-1   A, C, E
18-2   A, D, E
18-3   A
18-4   A, B, C, D, E
18-5   A, C, D, E
18-6   C

Chapter 19
19-1   B
19-2   B, C, F
19-3   D

Chapter 20
20-1   A, D

Chapter 21
21-1   A, D, E
21-2   A
21-3   A, E, F

Chapter 22
22-1   A, D, E
22-2   B
22-3   A, C, D
22-4   C

Chapter 23
23-1   A, E
23-2   B, E

Chapter 24
24-1   B
24-2   B
24-3   A, B, D, E, F, G

Chapter 25
25-1   C
25-2   D
25-3   A, B, F
25-4   C

Chapter 26
26-1   D
26-2   D
26-3   A, C, D
26-4   B, D, E

Chapter 27
27-1   C
27-2   A, D
27-3   A, C, D, F
27-4   B

Chapter 28
28-1   C
28-2   A, C, D, F
28-3   C

Chapter 29
29-1   B, D, F
29-2   A, F
29-3   A

Chapter 30
30-1   C
30-2   A, B, D, G
30-3   A
30-4   B
30-5   D

Chapter 31
31-1   B, C, E
31-2   A, D, E
31-3   B
31-4   B

Chapter 32
32-1   A, E, F
32-2   C, D, E, G, H
32-3   C, E, G

Chapter 33
33-1   B, C, E, F
33-2   C
33-3   B

Chapter 34
34-1   B
34-2   C
34-3   D

Chapter 35
35-1   A, C, D, E
35-2   A
35-3   D
35-4   C

Chapter 36
36-1   A, B, C, E
36-2   A
36-3   D
36-4   A
36-5   A, D, E

Chapter 37
37-1   A
37-2   A, B, D, E, H
37-3   D
37-4   C

Chapter 38
38-1   B, D, F
38-2   C, E, F
38-3   B

Chapter 39
39-1   D
39-2   B, E
39-3   C

Chapter 40
40-1   A
40-2   A, B, H
40-3   C
40-4   B

Chapter 41
41-1   B, E
41-2   B
41-3   B
41-4   A

Chapter 42
42-1   B, D, E
42-2   B
42-3   C
42-4   B
42-5   C, D, E, F

Chapter 43
43-1   A
43-2   D
43-3   B
43-4   A, B, C, D, E

Chapter 44
44-1   A, C, D, E
44-2   A, B, D
44-3   D

Chapter 45
45-1   B, C, D, E
45-2   B
45-3   C
45-4   C
45-5   B

Chapter 46
46-1   A
46-2   A, B, C, F

Chapter 47
47-1   C
47-2   B
47-3   D
47-4   A, B, E
47-5   C

Chapter 48
48-1   D
48-2   C
48-3   C, E
48-4   C

Chapter 49
49-1   A, B, D, E
49-2   D

Chapter 50
50-1   A, B, C, D, E, F
50-2   D
50-3   C
50-4   B

Chapter 51
51-1   B
51-2   B, C, D, E
51-3   D
51-4   A

Chapter 52
52-1   B, D, E
52-2   B
52-3   A, C, D, E, F

Chapter 53
53-1   D
53-2   B
53-3   C
53-4   A, D, F
53-5   A

Chapter 54
54-1   B
54-2   C
54-3   A
54-4   B, E

Chapter 55
55-1   A, B, E
55-2   A
55-3   B
55-4   C

Chapter 56
56-1   D
56-2   B
56-3   B, C, E
56-4   A, B, C, E

Chapter 57
57-1   B, C, D
57-2   A, B, C
57-3   B
57-4   A
57-5   B, C

Chapter 58
58-1   B
58-2   B, D, E
58-3   C

Chapter 59
59-1   B, E
59-2   A, D, E
59-3   D
59-4   C
59-5   C

Chapter 60
60-1   41
60-2   A, B, C, D
60-3   B, C, D

Chapter 61
61-1   A
61-2   B, C, E, F

Chapter 62
62-1   A, C, D, E
62-2   C
62-3   D

Chapter 63
63-1   B
63-2   A
63-3   B, C, D, H
63-4   C

Chapter 64
64-1   A, C, G, H
64-2   C
64-3   D
64-4   B

Chapter 65
65-1   B, C, E, F
65-2   A
65-3   B, D, F
65-4   D

Chapter 66
66-1   B, C, D, G
66-2   D
66-3   C, E, F, G
66-4   A
66-5   C

Chapter 67
67-1   B
67-2   C
67-3   A
67-4   A, D, E, F, H
67-5   B, C, D, E, F, G

Chapter 68
68-1   B
68-2   A, E, F, G
68-3   D
68-4   A
68-5   D
68-6   C

Chapter 69
69-1   D
69-2   C

Chapter 70
70-1   D
70-2   A, C, E

Chapter 71
71-1   B
71-2   B

Chapter 72
72-1   775
72-2   C
72-3   A
72-4   D

Chapter 73
73-1   A, B, D, E
73-2   A, B

Chapter 74
74-1   C
74-2   A, B, C, E

A

Abatacept, 323*b*, 369, 370*b*
Abdomen
 assessment of, 803
 auscultation of, 1067, 1123, 1128–1129
 chronic pancreatitis findings in, 1203
 distention of, 1124, 1162–1163, 1222
 inspection of, 1067
 palpation of, 1067–1068
 percussion of, 1067
 quadrants of, 1066–1068, 1066*f*, 1067*t*
 sickle cell disease effects on, 810
 ultrasound of, 1123
Abdominal aortic aneurysms, 739–740
Abdominal breathing, 578, 578*b*
Abdominal hernias, 1137–1138, 1137*f*
Abdominal obesity, 1287
Abdominal pain
 acute pancreatitis as cause of, 1199–1201
 appendicitis as cause of, 1147–1148
 cholecystitis as cause of, 1193
 Crohn's disease as cause of, 1159
 in pancreatic cancer, 1206
Abdominal thrust maneuver, 561*f*
Abdominal ultrasonography, 1163, 1515
Abdominal x-rays, for peritonitis evaluation, 1146
Abdominoperineal transition, 1130
Abducens nerve, 844*t*
Abduction, 1010*f*
ABI. *See* Ankle-brachial index
AbioCor Implantable Replacement Heart, 701*f*
Above-the-knee amputation, 1051, 1054, 1055*f*
Abscess
 anorectal, 1164–1165
 definition of, 880–881
 pancreatic, 1205
 peritonsillar, 611
 renal, 1373
 in ulcerative colitis, 1151*t*
Absolute neutrophil count, 293
Absorbable sutures, 267
Absorption, 1062
Absorptive atelectasis, 530, 531*b*
A1C. *See* Glycosylated hemoglobin

Acalculia, 933
Acalculous cholecystitis, 1192
Acarbose, 1118, 1292*b*–1293*b*
Accelerated graft atherosclerosis, 301
Acceleration-deceleration injury, 941, 941*f*, 1035–1036
Accessory muscles of respiration, 511
Accessory nerve, 844*t*
Accidents. *See also* Motor vehicle accidents
 chronic and disabling health conditions caused by, 87
 in older adults, 33–34
Acclimatization, 145
Accommodation, 960
AccuVein AV300, 203*f*
Acetaminophen
 dosing of, 307*b*
 hepatotoxicity caused by, 55
 osteoarthritis uses of, 307, 307*b*
 pain management uses of, 55, 307
Acetazolamide, for acute mountain sickness, 146
Acetic acid, 186
Acetylcholine, 868
Acetylcholine receptors, 917
Achlorhydria, 1115
Acid(s)
 definition of, 186
 formation of, 190
 sources of, 188
Acid deficit, 195–196
Acid-base assessment, 188*b*
Acid-base balance
 acids, 186
 assessment of, 14
 bases, 186
 buffers, 186–189, 186*f*–187*f*
 chemistry of, 186–187
 definition of, 13, 185
 importance of, 185
 maintenance of, 185–190
 postoperative, 276
 promotion of, 14
 regulatory actions and mechanisms, 188–190
  chemical, 188–189, 189*t*
  kidneys, 189*t*, 190
  respiratory, 189–190, 189*f*, 189*t*
 scope of, 14*f*
Acid-base imbalances
 acidosis. *See* Acidosis
 alkalosis. *See* Alkalosis
 arterial blood gas monitoring of, 14
 compensatory mechanisms for, 14, 190
 definition of, 13, 190

Acid-base imbalances (*Continued*)
 interventions for, 14
 kidney compensation for, 190
 physiologic consequences of, 14
 prevention of, 14
 respiratory compensation for, 190
 risk factors for, 13–14
Acidic pH, 186*f*
Acidosis
 assessment of, 192–194
 in chronic kidney disease, 1400
 complications of, 195
 definition of, 13
 laboratory assessment of, 193–194
 lactic, 191–192
 metabolic, 13, 191, 191*t*, 193–195, 193*b*, 1122
 metabolic/respiratory, 192
 pathophysiology of, 190–192, 191*t*
 potassium levels in, 194
 psychosocial assessment of, 193
 respiratory, 13, 191*t*, 192, 194–195
 signs and symptoms of, 192–193, 193*b*
Acinus, 510, 511*f*
Acitretin, 333, 465*b*
ACLS. *See* Advanced cardiac life support
Acorn cardiac support device, 702
Acoustic neuroma, 951, 996
Acquired immunity, 295, 298
Acquired immunodeficiency syndrome. *See also* Human immunodeficiency virus infection
 assessments in, 356*b*
 defining conditions for, 340*t*
 diagnostic criteria for, 339
 diarrhea management in, 354
 features of, 346*b*
 health care resources for, 357
 high-risk populations for, 340
 human immunodeficiency virus infection versus, 338
 incidence of, 340
 infection control in, 357*b*
 Kaposi's sarcoma associated with, 347, 348*f*, 354–355
 malignant lymphomas associated with, 347–348
 pathophysiology of, 337–340
 prevalence of, 340
 psychosocial preparation in, 356–357
 seizures in, 355
Acromegaly, 1247, 1247*f*, 1248*b*
Actemra. *See* Tocilizumab
Acticoat, 501*b*
Actinic keratosis, 475, 475*t*

Actinic lentigo, 435*f*
Actiq. *See* Fentanyl
Activated partial thromboplastin time, 619–620
Active immunity, 21–22, 298, 414
Active listening, 158
Active range of motion, 1010
Activities of daily living
 in Alzheimer's disease patients, 863
 assessment of, 1009–1010
 definition of, 23, 92, 96
 dyspnea and, 517*t*
 rehabilitation for, 96
 self-management education for performing, 100
Activity therapists, 89
Acupressure, 876
Acupuncture, 876
Acute abdomen series, 1070
Acute adrenal insufficiency, 1253, 1253*b*
Acute arterial occlusion, 737
Acute chest syndrome, 810, 812
Acute compartment syndrome, 1033–1034, 1034*b*, 1044–1045, 1044*b*
Acute coronary syndromes
 angina pectoris. *See* Angina pectoris
 antiplatelet agents for, 777, 777*b*
 assessment of, 772–774
 cardiac rehabilitation for, 779, 792
 coping with, 779
 coronary artery disease. *See* Coronary artery disease
 definition of, 769–770
 description of, 655
 drug therapy for, 774–775, 776*b*
 dysrhythmias caused by, 779–780
 etiology of, 771
 functional ability promotion in, 778–779
 genetic risks of, 771, 771*b*
 health care resources for, 792
 incidence of, 772
 medical assistance indications in, 791–792
 myocardial infarction. *See* Myocardial infarction
 nitrates for, 776*b*
 pathophysiology of, 769–771
 percutaneous coronary intervention for, 778
 physical assessment of, 772–773
 prevalence of, 772
 signs and symptoms of, 772–773
Acute gastritis, 1104–1105, 1105*b*
Acute glomerulonephritis, 1376–1378, 1376*t*

Acute hematogenous infection, 1022–1023

Acute kidney injury
assessment of, 1393–1394
chronic kidney disease versus, 1391t
classification of, 1391t, 1392
complications from, 1392t
contributing factors, 1392t
definition of, 1391
diseases and conditions contributing to, 1392t
drug therapy for, 1396
end-stage renal disease secondary to, 1398
etiology of, 1391–1392
features of, 1391t
health promotion and maintenance, 1393
history-taking for, 1393–1394
imaging assessment of, 1394
incidence of, 1392–1393
interventions for, 1395–1398
KDIGO classification system for, 1391t
kidney biopsy of, 1394
kidney replacement therapy for, 1397–1398, 1397f
laboratory assessment of, 1394, 1395b
nephrotoxic substances that cause, 1393t
nutrition therapy for, 1396–1397
in older adults, 1394b
oliguria associated with, 1396, 1423
pathophysiology of, 1391–1393
physical assessment of, 1394
prevalence of, 1392–1393
renal replacement therapy for, 1397, 1397f
signs and symptoms of, 1394

Acute leukemia
consolidation therapy for, 820–821
description of, 817, 819b
drug therapy for, 820–821
induction therapy for, 820

Acute lung injury, 626
Acute lymphocytic leukemia, 814t
Acute mountain sickness, 145–146, 145b–146b
Acute myelogenous leukemia, 814t, 820
Acute osteomyelitis, 1023, 1023b
Acute otitis media, 991
Acute pain, 46–47, 46t, 52
Acute pain transfusion reaction, 836

Acute pancreatitis
abdominal pain associated with, 1199–1201
alcohol consumption as cause of, 1200
assessment of, 1199–1200
autodigestion in, 1198f

Acute pancreatitis (Continued)
care coordination for, 1202
complications of, 1197–1198, 1198t, 1201
death caused by, 1199
definition of, 1197
drug therapy for, 1200–1201
endoscopic retrograde cholangiopancreatography-related trauma as cause of, 1199
etiology of, 1199
gallstones as cause of, 1201
genetic risk of, 1199
history-taking for, 1199
home care management of, 1202
imaging assessment of, 1200
incidence of, 1199
interventions for, 1200–1201
laboratory assessment of, 1200, 1200t
multi-system organ failure caused by, 1198
nonsurgical management of, 1200–1201
nutrition promotion in, 1201
in older adults, 1199
paralytic ileus secondary to, 1201b
pathophysiology of, 1197–1199
physical assessment of, 1199
prevalence of, 1199
psychosocial assessment of, 1200
respiratory status monitoring in, 1201b
shock caused by, 1198, 1199b
signs and symptoms of, 1199
surgical management of, 1201
transition management for, 1202
ultrasonography of, 1200

Acute paronychia, 442
Acute peripheral arterial occlusion, 737–738
Acute promyelocytic leukemia, 814t
Acute radiation cystitis, 1485

Acute respiratory distress syndrome
acute lung injury in, 626
acute pancreatitis as risk factor for, 1198
assessment of, 627
in burn injury, 497
causes of, 626t
definition of, 626
diagnostic assessment of, 627
drug therapy for, 628
etiology of, 626, 626t
extracorporeal membrane oxygenation for, 628
fluid therapy for, 628
genetic risks for, 626, 627b
health promotion and maintenance for, 627
incidence of, 626
interventions for, 627–628

Acute respiratory distress syndrome (Continued)
nutrition therapy for, 628
pathophysiology of, 626
positive end-expiratory pressure for, 627
prevalence of, 626
in sepsis, 764
signs and symptoms of, 627

Acute respiratory failure, 624–626, 625t
Acute sialadenitis, 1084–1085
Acute stress disorder, 156, 156b, 158
Acute transfusion reaction, 835–836
Acute transplant rejection, 301
Acute tubular necrosis, 1392

Acyclovir
for encephalitis, 884
for genital herpes, 1507

Adalimumab, 323b, 466b, 1153
Adam's apple, 510
Addiction, opioid, 58
Addisonian crisis, 1253
Addison's disease, 1253–1254
Adduction, 1010f
Adefovir, 1185t
A-delta fibers, 47–48, 49f

Adenocarcinomas. See also Cancer
colorectal, 1127
endometrial, 1465

Adenohypophysis, 1236, 1237f
Adenomas, 1126
Adenomatous polyposis coli gene, 1127b
Adenosine, 677b–678b, 678
Adenosine triphosphate, 802
Adipokines, 1225
Adiponectin, 1225
Adjustable gastric band, laparoscopic, 1229, 1230f
Adjuvant analgesics, 55, 63–65
ADLs. See Activities of daily living
Administration sets, for infusion therapy
add-on devices, 209–210
definition of, 209
filters used with, 210
intermittent, 209
needleless connection devices, 210–211, 210f, 214
secondary, 209, 209f
slip lock, 210

Administrative review, 157
Adrenal cortex, 1235t, 1237–1238
Adrenal crisis, 1253

Adrenal gland(s)
anatomy of, 1237–1238
hypofunction of, 1253–1255, 1254b–1255b, 1254f
laboratory assessment of, 1255b

Adrenal gland disorders
Cushing's disease. See Cushing's disease
hyperaldosteronism, 1260–1261
pheochromocytoma, 1261–1262

Adrenal glucocorticoids, 1006

Adrenal insufficiency, 1386
acute, 1253, 1253b
features of, 1254b
primary, 1253t
secondary, 1253t
sepsis as cause of, 765

Adrenal medulla, 1238
Adrenalectomy, 1259

Adrenergic agonists, for glaucoma, 966b

Adrenocorticotropic hormone
deficiency of, 1246, 1246b
description of, 1235t, 1236, 1238, 1254
overproduction of, 1248b

Advance directives, 104–115, 241, 263, 705

Advanced cardiac life support
certifications in, 120t, 123
dysrhythmias treated with, 687

Advanced life support providers, 119

Advanced practice nurses
in rehabilitation settings, 88
trauma, 131

Adventitious breath sounds, 519, 521t

Adverse drug events, 42b, 111b

Adverse events
definition of, 4–5
as sentinel events, 4–5

Adynamic ileus, 1122
Aerobic exercise, 32
Aerophagia, 1095
Afatinib, 589t
Afferent arterioles, 1322–1323
Afferent neurons, 840
Affordable Care Act, 118

African Americans
Alzheimer's disease in, 859b, 864b
angioedema in, 362b
hypertension in, 722b
sickle cell disease in, 809

"Africanized" bees, 137

Afterload
definition of, 645
drugs that affect, 698

Age-related macular degeneration, 979

Agglutination, 297

Aging. See also Older adults
cancer risks associated with, 380
cardiovascular system affected by, 646, 647b
endocrine system changes associated with, 1240, 1241b
eye changes associated with, 961, 961b
fluid balance affected by, 165b
gastrointestinal system changes associated with, 1064, 1064b
hearing affected by, 986
hematologic system changes associated with, 800, 800b

Aging *(Continued)*
  immune system affected by, 291*b*
  immunity changes caused by, 290, 300
  musculoskeletal system affected by, 1007–1008, 1007*b*
  neurologic changes associated with, 234*b*, 844–845, 845*b*
  renal system changes associated with, 234*b*, 1328–1329, 1328*b*
  reproductive system changes associated with, 1431, 1431*b*
  respiratory changes associated with, 512, 513*b*
  skin changes associated with, 234*b*, 433, 652
  spinal cord injury and, 902*b*
  urinary system changes associated with, 234*b*, 1328–1329
Agitated delirium, 111
Agnosia, 860, 933
Agraphia, 933
AIDS. *See* Acquired immunodeficiency syndrome
AIDS dementia complex, 348
AIDS wasting syndrome, 348
Air embolism, 214–215
Air trapping, 572
Airborne infection isolation room, 416
Airborne precautions, 419, 420*t*, 609
Airborne transmission
  description of, 416
  precautions for, 419, 420*t*, 609
Air-fluidized beds, 97
Airway. *See also* Upper airway
  anatomy of, 510, 511*f*
  in angioedema patients, 363
  artificial
    description of, 273
    suctioning of, 541–542, 541*b*
  burn injury of, 489–490
  clearance of, in tuberculosis, 607–608
  narrowing of, 565*f*
  postoperative maintenance of, 280
  primary survey of, 129, 131*t*
  in spinal cord injury patients, 897–898
  in traumatic brain injury patients, 948–949
Airway obstruction
  burn injury as cause of, 490*t*, 494
  head and neck cancer as cause of, 549–553
  monitoring for, 629*b*
  pathophysiology of, 563
  in pneumonia, 604
  respiratory acidosis caused by, 192
  upper, 560–561, 561*f*
Airway pressure-release ventilation, 627
Airway secretions, 129
AKI. *See* Acute kidney injury
Akinesia, 868

Alanine aminotransferase, 1068, 1069*b*, 1174, 1200
Albiglutide, 1292*b*–1293*b*
Albumin
  functions of, 796
  laboratory testing for, 1069*b*
  in malnutrition assessments, 25
  serum, 1217
Albuminuria, 1283, 1399
Albuterol
  asthma treated with, 569*b*–570*b*
  bronchospasm treated with, 365
Alcohol consumption, 610
  blood glucose levels affected by, 1299
  cirrhosis caused by, 1172
  surgical risks associated with, 232–233
Aldosterone
  deficiency of, 1255
  description of, 485, 1237, 1323
  fluid balance regulation by, 165
  sodium reabsorption affected by, 1326
Aldosterone antagonists, for heart failure, 700
Alectinib, 589*t*
Alefacept, 333
Alendronate, 1021
Alexia, 933
Alirocumab, 730–731
Alkaline pH, 187*f*
Alkaline phosphatase, 1011, 1069*b*
Alkaline reflux gastropathy, 1118
Alkalis, 487
Alkalosis
  definition of, 13
  metabolic, 13, 193*b*, 196, 196*t*, 1122
  pathophysiology of, 195–196, 196*t*
  relative, 195
  respiratory, 13, 196, 196*t*
Alkylating agents, 391
Alleles, 74–75, 75*f*, 79
Allergens, 360–361, 364*b*
Allergic rhinosinusitis, 365–366
Allergy/allergies
  to anesthesia, 263
  atopic, 360–361
  breathing affected by, 516
  definition of, 360
  food, 234–235, 1212*b*
  history-taking, 1008
  latex, 234–235, 419
  preoperative evaluation for, 234–235
Allogeneic bone marrow transplantation, 822
Allogeneic stem cells, 822
Allografts, 499
Allopurinol, 331–332, 1364
Alopecia
  chemotherapy as cause of, 395, 400, 588, 1467
  drugs as cause of, 820

Alosetron, 1136–1137, 1137*b*
5-Alpha reductase inhibitors, 1477, 1498
Alpha$_1$-antitrypsin deficiency, 573, 573*b*, 573*t*
Alpha-fetoprotein, 1186–1187
Alpha-glucosidase inhibitors, 1292*b*–1293*b*, 1293
Alteplase, 935, 936*b*
Altitude-related illnesses, 145–146, 145*b*–146*b*
Aluminum hydroxide, 1091, 1106*b*–1107*b*
Alveolar ducts, 510
Alveolar edema, 486
Alveolar-capillary diffusion, 192
Alveoli
  age-related changes in, 513*b*
  anatomy of, 510
Alzheimer's disease
  abuse concerns in, 865–866
  accident prevention in, 864–865
  activities of daily living in, 863
  in African Americans, 859*b*, 864*b*
  antidepressants for, 864
  assessment of, 860–861
  behavior changes associated with
    description of, 861
    management of, 862–864, 865*t*
  care coordination for, 866–867
  caregivers for, 866, 866*b*–867*b*
  cholinesterase inhibitors for, 864
  cognitive changes associated with, 860–861
  cognitive stimulation training for, 862
  communication methods for, 863*b*, 865
  complementary and integrative health for, 863
  depression in, 864
  drug therapy for, 863–864
  elder abuse concerns, 865–866
  etiology of, 858
  family caregivers for, 866, 866*b*
  genetic risk of, 858, 859*b*
  genetic testing for, 861
  health care resources for, 867
  health promotion and maintenance for, 859
  in Hispanics, 866*b*
  history-taking for, 860
  imaging assessments for, 861
  incidence of, 859
  injury prevention in, 864–865
  laboratory assessments for, 861
  memory impairments associated with, 860, 862
  neuritic plaques associated with, 858, 859*f*
  neurofibrillary tangles associated with, 858, 859*f*
  neuropsychiatric symptoms associated with, 861

Alzheimer's disease *(Continued)*
  nonpharmacologic management of, 862–863
  pathophysiology of, 857–859
  personality changes associated with, 861
  physical assessment of, 860–861
  prevalence of, 859
  psychosocial assessment of, 861
  psychotropic drugs in, 864
  reminiscence therapy for, 862
  risk factors for, 858, 859*b*
  Safe Return Program for, 867
  screening for, 860–861
  self-management education for, 866–867
  self-management skills associated with, 861
  sexual disinhibition associated with, 861
  signs and symptoms of, 860–861
  stages of, 860, 860*b*
  transition management for, 866–867
  validation therapy for, 863
  vascular dementia versus, 858*t*
  in veterans, 859*b*, 867*b*
  wandering associated with, 864, 864*b*
Amantadine, 871
Ambulation
  assistive devices for, 95, 95*f*
  after burn injury, 503
  nurse-initiated protocol for, 24*b*
Ambulatory aids, 23
Ambulatory care rehabilitation, 88
Ambulatory pumps, 211
Ambulatory surgical centers, 228, 271
Amebiasis, 1165–1166
Amebic meningoencephalitis, 883
Amenorrhea, 1173, 1246
American Chronic Pain Association, 52–53
American Nurses Association
  Code of Ethics, 9*t*, 1492
  ethics as defined by, 8–9
American Nurses Credentialing Center's Magnet Recognition, 7
American Occupational Therapy Association, 93
American Physical Therapy Association, 93
American Sign Language, 1001
American Society of Anesthesiologists Physical Status Classification system, 230–232, 233*t*, 257
Americans with Disabilities Act, 92
Amevive. *See* Alefacept
AMI. *See* Antibody-mediated immunity
Amino acids, 76, 76*f*
Aminocaproic acid, 620
Aminosalicylates, 1152, 1153*t*

5-Aminosalicylates, 1152, 1153t
Amiodarone, 200b, 677b–678b, 708
Amitriptyline, 1137
Ammonia, 190, 1068, 1073b
Ammonium, 190
Amnesia, 257
Amoxicillin, 612b, 1359b
Amoxicillin/clavulanate, 1359b
Amphiarthrodial joints, 1006
Amputation
    above-the-knee, 1051, 1054,
        1055f
    assessment of, 1052–1053
    bandaging of stump, 1054, 1055f
    below-the-knee, 1051, 1051f, 1054,
        1055f
    care coordination for, 1055–1056,
        1056b
    complications of, 1051–1052
    contracture prevention in, 1054
    definition of, 1050
    diagnostic assessment of, 1052
    emergency care for, 1053
    health care resources for, 1056,
        1056t
    health promotion and
        maintenance for, 1052
    home care management of, 1055,
        1056b
    infection prevention after, 1054
    levels of, 1051, 1051f
    lower-extremity, 1051, 1051b,
        1051f
    mobility promotion after,
        1053–1054
    pain caused by, 1051, 1053
    physical assessment of, 1052
    psychosocial assessment of, 1052,
        1052b
    self-esteem promotion in,
        1054–1055
    self-management education for,
        1055–1056
    signs and symptoms of,
        1052–1056
    Syme, 1051, 1051f
    tissue perfusion monitoring after,
        1053
    transition management for,
        1055–1056, 1056b
    traumatic, 1050, 1053
    types of, 1050
AMS. See Acute mountain sickness
Amylase
    serum, 1062, 1068, 1069b
    urine, 1068
Amylin analogs, 1292b–1293b,
    1293–1294
Amyloid beta protein precursor, 861
Amyotrophic lateral sclerosis, 889t
Anaergy, 607
Anaerobic conditions, 188
Anaerobic metabolism, 191–192
Anakinra, 323b
Anal canal, 1064

Anal disorders
    anal fissure, 1165
    anal fistula, 1165
    anorectal abscess, 1164–1165
    parasitic infections, 1165–1166
Anal intercourse, 342
Analgesia. See also Opioid analgesics;
        specific analgesics
    definition of, 257
    intraspinal, 61–62
    intrathecal, 61–62, 62b
    multimodal, 54–55
    patient-controlled, 55, 283–284
    preemptive, 54
Analgesic trial, 59b
Anamnestic response, 298
Anaphylaxis
    antihistamines for, 365
    assessment of, 364
    definition of, 361, 753
    emergency care of, 365b
    epinephrine injectors for, 363f,
        364b, 365
    features of, 364b
    health promotion and
        maintenance for, 363–364
    interventions for, 364–365, 365b
    pathophysiology of, 363
Anaplasia, 374
Anaplastic carcinoma, 1275
Anasarca, 651, 1394
Anastomosis, 1131
Anatomic dead space, 531–532
Androblastomas, 1487
Androderm, 1498
AndroGel, 1498
Androgen deprivation therapy,
    1485
Androgens
    description of, 1006
    hypopituitarism treated with,
        1247
Anemia
    aplastic, 814t, 815–816
    autoimmune hemolytic, 815
    causes of, 814t
    chemotherapy as cause of, 397
    in chronic kidney disease, 1401
    cold antibody, 815
    in Crohn's disease, 1159
    definition of, 813
    fatigue associated with, 802
    folic acid deficiency, 814–816,
        814t
    glucose-6-phosphate
        dehydrogenase deficiency,
        814t, 815–816
    immunohemolytic, 815–816
    iron deficiency, 814–816, 814t,
        815b
    management of, 815–816
    megaloblastic, 814
    in older adults, 803
    pernicious, 814, 1104–1105
    sickle cell. See Sickle cell disease

Anemia (Continued)
    types of, 814
    vitamin B_{12} deficiency, 814, 814t,
        815f, 816
    warm antibody, 815
Aneroid pressure manometer, 541f
Anesthesia
    allergies to, 263
    definition of, 256
    epidural, 261t, 262f, 275, 275b
    general, 257–260, 258t–259t, 260b,
        275
    local, 260–261
    moderate sedation, 261–262, 262t
    previous experiences with, 234
    providers of, 256–257
    regional, 260–261, 261f–262f, 261t
    selection criteria for, 256–257
    spinal, 261t, 262f, 275, 275b
    total hip arthroplasty, 310
Anesthesiologist, 253t, 256
Anesthesiologist assistant, 256
Aneuploid, 74
Aneuploidy, 374, 376–377
Aneurysm(s)
    abdominal aortic, 739–740
    arterial, 738–740, 739f
    arteriovenous fistula, 1415
    assessment of, 739
    atherosclerosis as cause of,
        738–739
    definition of, 738, 929
    dissecting, 738–739
    femoral, 740
    interventions for, 739–740
    nonsurgical management of, 739
    pathophysiology of, 738–739
    peripheral arteries, 740
    surgical management of, 739–740
    thoracic aortic, 738–739
Aneurysmectomy, 739
Angina pectoris, 650t
    atypical, 773b
    chronic stable, 768–769
    definition of, 768–769
    features of, 773b
    new-onset, 770
    nitroglycerin for, 774–775
    pre-infarction, 770
    Prinzmetal's, 770
    self-management education for,
        792b
    unstable, 769–770
    variant, 770, 774
Angioedema, 361–366, 362b, 362f
Angiogenesis inhibitors, 404t, 405
Angiography, 657
Angiotensin I, 1237
Angiotensin II, 167, 1237, 1326
Angiotensin receptor blockers
    afterload affected by, 698
    hypertension treated with, 167,
        725b, 726–727
Angiotensin receptor neprilysin
    inhibitor, 698

Angiotensin-converting enzyme
    inhibitors
    afterload affected by, 698
    albuminuria treated with, 1308
    hypertension managed with, 167,
        725b, 726
Angiotensinogen, 167, 1237, 1324f
Anions, 172
Anisocoria, 963
Ankle fracture, 1043, 1049
Ankle-brachial index, 653, 733, 1052
Ankylosing spondylitis, 334t
Anomia, 860
Anorectal abscess, 1164–1165
Anorexia, 1065
Anorexia nervosa, 1216
Anorexins, 1225
ANP. See Atrial natriuretic peptide
Antacids
    for gastroesophageal reflux
        disease, 1090–1091
    for peptic ulcer disease,
        1106b–1107b, 1112
Antalgic gait, 1009
Anterior cerebral artery
    anatomy of, 841
    stroke involving, 933b
Anterior cervical diskectomy and
    fusion, 909–910, 910b
Anterior colporrhaphy, 1349t, 1465
Anterior pituitary gland
    hormones produced by, 1235t,
        1237t, 1245–1246
    hyperfunction of, 1248b
Anterior wall myocardial infarction,
    771
Anthralin, 464
Anthrax
    bioterrorism uses of, 428, 466b
    cutaneous, 466–468, 467f
    inhalation, 611–612, 612b
Anthropometric measurements,
    1213–1215
Anti-androgen drugs, 1485
Antibiotics
    dyspnea treated with, 110
    gastroenteritis treated with, 1149
    nonabsorbable, 1178–1179
    pelvic inflammatory disease
        treated with, 1516, 1516b
    preoperative prophylaxis, 247
Antibody
    antigen and, interactions between,
        296–298
    classification of, 298, 298t
    monoclonal. See Monoclonal
        antibodies
    production of, 297
Antibody-antigen binding, 297, 297f
Antibody-mediated immune system,
    417
Antibody-mediated immunity
    acquiring of, 298–299
    antigen-antibody interactions in,
        296–298

Antibody-mediated immunity
(*Continued*)
  B-lymphocytes in, 295–296
  cells involved in, 292*t*, 797*t*
  definition of, 295
  description of, 22, 290–291
  sequence of, 296*f*
Anticholinergics
  Parkinson disease treated with,
    871
  respiratory secretions during
    dying treated with, 110
  urinary incontinence treated with,
    1349
Anticoagulants. *See also specific drug*
  best practices for, 744*b*
  clotting inadequacies treated with,
    16
  direct thrombin inhibitors, 801
  heparin-induced
    thrombocytopenia treated
    with, 832
  indirect thrombin inhibitors, 801
  injury prevention in patients
    using, 623*b*
  mechanism of action, 801
Anticoagulation
  blood tests for monitoring, 634*t*
  during hemodialysis, 1413
Anticonvulsants
  fibromyalgia treated with, 333
  pain management uses of, 63–64
Anti-cyclic citrullinated peptide, 320
Antidepressants. *See also specific
    antidepressants*
  in Alzheimer's disease patients,
    864
  pain management uses of, 63–64
Antidiuretic hormone
  age-related changes in, 1241*b*
  deficiency of, 1246*b*, 1250
  fluid balance regulation by,
    165–166
  secretion of, 407
  syndrome of inappropriate. *See*
    Syndrome of inappropriate
    antidiuretic hormone
Antidysrhythmics, 677*b*–678*b*,
    685–686
Antiembolism stockings, 244
Antiemetics, 399
Antiepileptic drugs
  dry mouth caused by, 26
  migraine headaches treated with,
    875
  pain management uses of,
    63–64
  seizures treated with, 111,
    877–878, 878*b*
Anti-factor Xa test, 805
Antigen
  antibody and, interactions
    between, 296–298
  inactivation of, 297
  sensitization to, 297

Antigen recognition, 296
Antihemophilic factor, 798*t*
Antihistamines
  anaphylaxis treated with, 365
  pruritus treated with, 463
  rhinosinusitis treated with, 611,
    611*b*
Antimetabolites, 391, 391*t*
Antimicrobial-resistant infection,
    421, 421*b*
Antimicrobials
  fever treated with, 425
  infective endocarditis treated with,
    712
  sensitivity testing for, 424
Antimitotic agents, 391, 391*t*
Antinuclear antibodies, 326
Antinuclear antibody test, 320
Antiplatelet agents
  acute coronary syndromes treated
    with, 777, 777*b*
  clotting inadequacies treated
    with, 16
  injury prevention in patients
    using, 623*b*
  mechanism of action, 801–802
  peripheral arterial disease treated
    with, 734–737
Antipsychotic drugs
  adverse drug events caused by,
    42*b*, 111*b*
  in Alzheimer's disease patients,
    864
  indications for, 41
  in older adults, 41, 42*b*
Antipyretic drugs, 426
Antithymocyte globulin, 302*b*
α₁-Antitrypsin, 83
Anuria, 18, 1362
Anxiety
  in angioedema patients, 363
  in chronic kidney disease,
    1410–1411
  in chronic obstructive pulmonary
    disease, 580
  in head and neck cancer, 553
  in hearing loss patients, 1001
  management of, 622–623,
    1410–1411
  postoperative, 280
  preoperative, 237, 246
  in pulmonary embolism,
    622–623
  signs and symptoms of, 280
  surgery-related, 17
  in tuberculosis patients, 609
Anzemet, 399
AORN. *See* Association of
    periOperative Registered Nurses
Aorta
  blood flow in, 642
  dissection of, 740–741
Aortic regurgitation, 706*b*, 707
Aortic stenosis, 706–707, 706*b*
Aortic valvuloplasty, 708

Aortofemoral bypass surgery, 735,
    736*f*
APC gene, 382
Aphasia, 91, 860, 933, 938, 938*t*
Apheresis, for polycythemia vera,
    816
Aphthous stomatitis, 1076
Aphthous ulcers, 1076
Apical impulse, 654
Aplastic anemia, 814*t*, 815–816
Apo-Acetazolamide. *See*
    Acetazolamide
Apocrine sweat glands, 433
Apolipoprotein E, 1225
Apolipoprotein E4, 861
Apoptosis, 373
Appendectomy, 1148
Appendicitis, 1147–1148, 1147*b*,
    1148*f*
Appendix, 1064
Appetite, 1225
Apraxia, 860, 934
Apremilast, 369
aPTT. *See* Activated partial
    thromboplastin time
Aquacel Ag, 501*b*
Aqueous humor
  creation of, 972
  definition of, 958
  flow of, 959*f*
Arachidonic acid, 295
Arachnoid, 840
Arava. *See* Leflunomide
Arboviruses, 883
Archiving, 350
Arcus senilis, 435*f*, 961
ARDS. *See* Acute respiratory distress
    syndrome
Areflexic bladder, 97–98, 98*t*
Aromatase inhibitors, 1452
Aromatherapy, 109, 111
Around-the-clock dosing, of
    analgesics, 54–55, 59*b*
Arrhythmogenic right ventricular
    cardiomyopathy, 715
Arterial aneurysms, 738–740, 739*f*
Arterial baroreceptors, 721
Arterial blood gas
  analysis of, 521, 522*b*
  monitoring of
    acid-base imbalance, 14
    gas exchange assessments, 21
    postoperative, 280
Arterial embolization, 711
Arterial pulses, 653, 653*f*
Arterial system, 645–646
Arterial thrombosis, 16*b*
Arterial ulcers, 732–733, 734*b*
Arterial vasoconstriction, 694
Arteriography, 657
Arteriosclerosis
  assessment of, 729–730
  definition of, 728
  pathophysiology of, 728–729
Arteriotomy, 738

Arteriovenous fistulas, 1413,
    1414*f*–1415*f*, 1414*t*–1415*t*,
    1415*b*
Arteriovenous grafts, 1413, 1414*f*,
    1414*t*–1415*t*, 1415*b*
Arteriovenous malformation, 929,
    935, 952
Arteriovenous shunt, 1414*f*
Arthritis
  definition of, 305
  disease-associated, 332–333, 333*t*
  energy conservation in, 324*b*
  osteoarthritis. *See* Osteoarthritis
  psoriatic, 332–333
  rheumatoid. *See* Rheumatoid
    arthritis
Arthritis Foundation, 317, 324, 328,
    334
Arthrocentesis, for rheumatoid
    arthritis, 321
Arthrodesis, 906
Arthrogram, 1011
Arthropod bites, 136–137, 137*b*,
    137*f*, 138*t*–140*t*
Arthroscope, 1013
Arthroscopy
  complications of, 1014
  follow-up care after, 1014, 1014*b*
  musculoskeletal system
    applications of, 1013–1014,
    1013*f*
  patient preparation for, 1013
  procedure for, 1014
Articular cartilage, 1006–1007
Artifacts, electrocardiogram, 670
Artificial airway
  description of, 273
  suctioning of, 541–542, 541*b*
Artificial skin, 499
Ascending colostomy, 1131*f*
Aschoff bodies, 714
Ascites, 1170, 1173, 1173*f*, 1202,
    1206
Aseptic meningitis, 881
Aspartate aminotransferase, 1068,
    1069*b*, 1174
Aspiration
  during drowning, 147
  in head and neck cancer, 553
  nasogastric feeding tube as cause
    of, 553
  precautions for, 1081*b*
  during swallowing, 543*b*
Aspirin
  mechanism of action, 801–802
  myocardial infarction treated with,
    776–777
  stroke prophylaxis using, 937
Assist-control ventilation, 631
Assistive/adaptive devices
  for ambulation, 95–96, 95*f*, 96*t*
  for self-care, 96
  types of, 96*t*
Association of periOperative
    Registered Nurses, 229, 251

Association of Rehabilitation Nurses, 93
Asterixis, 1173, 1378
Asthma
    action plan for, 567–568
    assessment of, 565–567
    barrel chest associated with, 566, 567f
    deaths caused by, 563
    definition of, 563
    drug therapy for
        anti-inflammatory agents, 569b–571b, 571
        bronchodilators, 568–571, 569b–570b
        cholinergic antagonists, 569b–570b, 571
        corticosteroids, 569b–570b, 571
        cromones, 569b–570b, 571
        leukotriene modifiers, 569b–570b, 571
        metered dose inhaler for, 568–570, 570b, 570f
        step system for, 566b
        xanthines, 571
    etiology of, 563–565
    exercise for, 571
    features of, 566b
    gas exchange affected by, 21
    gastroesophageal reflux disease as trigger of, 565
    genetic risk of, 563–565
    history-taking for, 565
    incidence of, 565, 565b
    inflammation as trigger of, 565
    laboratory assessment of, 567
    oxygen therapy for, 571
    pathophysiology of, 563–565, 564f
    physical assessment of, 566–567, 567f
    prevalence of, 565, 565b
    pulmonary function tests for, 567
    self-management education for, 567–568, 568b, 568f
    signs and symptoms of, 566–567, 567f
    status asthmaticus, 572
Astigmatism, 960, 980–981
Asymptomatic bacterial urinary tract infection, 1354
Ataxia, 145–146, 933–934, 946
Atelectasis, 233–234
    absorptive, 530, 531b
Atelectrauma, 635
Atherectomy
    for coronary artery disease, 784
    for peripheral arterial disease, 735
Atherosclerosis
    aneurysms caused by, 738–739
    assessment of, 729–730
    complementary and integrative health for, 731
    coronary artery disease caused by, 771
    cross-section of, 769f

Atherosclerosis (Continued)
    definition of, 728, 928
    drug therapy for, 730–731, 730t
    incidence of, 729
    interventions for, 730–731
    nutrition therapy for, 730
    pathophysiology of, 728–729, 729f
    physical activity for, 730
    plaque, 928
    risk factors for, 729t
    statins for, 731b
    triglycerides in, 729–730
Atopic allergy, 360–361
Atopic dermatitis, 462, 463b
Atrial dysrhythmias
    atrial fibrillation. See Atrial fibrillation
    description of, 675–676
    drug therapy for, 677b–678b
    premature atrial complexes, 676
    supraventricular tachycardia, 676–678
Atrial fibrillation
    assessment of, 679
    biventricular pacing for, 681
    clotting inadequacies associated with, 15
    definition of, 678
    drug therapy for, 679–680
    electrocardiographic findings, 679f
    etiology of, 679
    genetic risk of, 679
    heart failure in, 680–681
    incidence of, 679
    interventions for, 679–680
    pathophysiology of, 678–679
    permanent, 679
    persistent, 679
    prevalence of, 679
    pulmonary embolism risks in, 680b
    stroke risks in, 16
    valvular heart disease and, 708
Atrial gallop, 654–655
Atrial kick, 665
Atrial natriuretic peptide, 166
Atrioventricular junctional area, 665
Atrioventricular valves, 642–643
Atrophic gastritis, 1104, 1115
Atrophic glossitis, 1118
Atrophy, 438f
Atropine sulfate, 677b–678b, 898
Atypical angina, 773b
Atypical chest pain, 1089
Atypical migraines, 873–874
Audiometry, 990–991
Audioscopy, 989
Auditory brainstem-evoked response, 991
Auditory evoked potentials, 855
Auscultation
    of abdomen, 1067, 1123
    of cardiovascular system, 654–655
    of heart sounds, 654–655
    of lungs, 519, 520f

Autoamputation of the distal digits, 329–330
Autoantibodies, 367
Auto-contamination, 820
Autodigestion, 1104, 1198f
Autoimmune diseases
    antiproliferative drugs for, 368–369, 370b
    calcineurin inhibitors for, 369, 370b
    corticosteroids for, 368
    cytotoxic drugs for, 368
    description of, 368
    disease-modifying antirheumatic drugs for, 368–369, 370b
    immunosuppressive therapy for, 368–369, 370b
Autoimmune hemolytic anemia, 815
Autoimmune pancreatitis, 1202
Autoimmune thrombocytopenic purpura, 830–831
Autoimmunity
    disorders with, 367t
    incidence of, 367
    pathophysiology of, 367–368
    self-reactions, 368
Autologous blood donation
    intraoperative, 263, 264b
    preoperative, 235
Autologous blood transfusions, 836
Automated external defibrillator
    dysrhythmias treated with, 686–687, 687f
    illustration of, 687f
    ventricular fibrillation treated with, 685
Automated peritoneal dialysis, 1419–1420, 1419f–1420f
Automaticity, 665
Autonomic dysreflexia, 896, 896b, 898, 898b
Autonomic hyperreflexia, 896
Autonomic nervous system, 646, 842–844
Autonomic neuropathy, 1285, 1285t, 1305
Autonomy, 9
Autoregulation, 945
Autosomal dominant pattern of inheritance, 78–79, 78t
Autosomal recessive pattern of inheritance, 78t, 79, 79f
Autosomal-dominant polycystic kidney disease, 1380, 1380b, 1380f
Autosomes, 74
Avascular necrosis, 1021, 1035, 1047
Axial loading, 894, 895f
Axillary lymph node dissection, 1447
Axillofemoral bypass surgery, 735–736, 736f
Axon, 840, 840f
Azathioprine
    autoimmune diseases treated with, 368
    immunosuppression uses of, 302b

Azithromycin
    for chlamydia infection, 1512
    for gonorrhea, 1513
Azoospermia, 1487–1488
Azotemia, 1392, 1398

B
B cells
    in antibody-mediated immunity, 295–296, 797t
    differentiation of, 295f
    types of, 297
Babinski's sign, 848
Bacille Calmette- Guérin vaccine, 606–607
Bacillus anthracis, 611–612
Back pain
    acute, 903–904
    areas commonly affected by, 903
    assessment of, 904–905
    care coordination for, 908–909
    chronic, 903
    contributing factors for, 904b
    diskectomy for, 906
    exercises for, 906b
    health care resources for, 909
    health promotion and maintenance for, 904
    home care management of, 908
    imaging assessment of, 905
    laminectomy for, 906
    laser-assisted laparoscopic lumbar diskectomy for, 906
    microdiskectomy for, 906
    minimally invasive surgery for, 906
    nonsurgical management of, 905–906, 906b
    pathophysiology of, 903–904
    physical assessment of, 904–905
    prevalence of, 903
    prevention of, 904b, 908b
    self-management education for, 908–909
    subacute, 903–904
    surgical management of, 906–908, 907b
    transition management for, 908–909
Bacteremia
    catheter-acquired, 415–416
    description of, 1356–1357
Bacterial gastroenteritis, 1148t, 1149
Bacterial infections
    of skin, 466–468, 466f, 467b
    skin cultures for, 444
Bacterial overgrowth, of intestine, 1142
Bacterial peritonitis, 1122
Bacteriuria, 1354
Bad death, 103
Bag-valve-mask ventilation, 129
Baker's cysts, 319
Balance
    assessment of, 991
    testing of, 849–850

Ball-and-socket joints, 1007
Balloon brachytherapy, 1451
Balloon valvuloplasty, 708
Band neutrophils, 292–293
Bandemia, 280, 293
Bar code-point of care system, 833
Bar-code medication administration
    as best safety practice, 4
    description of, 8
    example of, 4f
Bariatric surgery, 1229–1231
Barium enema, 1152
Barium swallow study, 1089, 1093, 1096
Baroreceptors, 646, 754
Barotrauma, 635, 995
Barrel chest
    in asthma, 566, 567f
    in chronic obstructive pulmonary disease, 576
Barrett's epithelium, 1088
Barrett's esophagus, 1095, 1115
Bartholin glands, 1429
Basal cell carcinoma, 475t, 476, 476f, 1079
Basal ganglia, 868
Base, 73, 186
Base deficit, 191
Base excess, 191
Base pairs, 73
Basic cardiac life support, 686
Basic life support, 120t, 123
Basilar artery, 841
Basilar skull fracture, 880–881, 946
Basiliximab, 302b
Basophils, 293–294, 361, 565, 797t
Batista procedure, 702
Beau's grooves, 443t
Bedaquiline fumarate, 609
Bedbugs, 471
Bedside sonography, 1336–1337, 1337f
Bee stings, 137, 137b, 138t–140t
Beers criteria, 35, 36t
Behavior, Alzheimer's disease-related changes in
    description of, 861
    management of, 862–864, 865t
Belimumab, 328
Bell's palsy. See Facial paralysis
Below-the-knee amputations, 1051, 1051f, 1054, 1055f
Beneficence, 9
Benign cellular growth, 14
Benign prostatic hyperplasia
    assessment of, 1474–1477, 1475f–1476f
    care coordination for, 1481
    complementary and integrative health for, 1477
    concept map for, 1477f–1478f
    drug therapy for, 1477
    etiology of, 1474
    genetic risk of, 1474

Benign prostatic hyperplasia (Continued)
    health care resources for, 1481
    history-taking for, 1474
    home care management of, 1481
    incidence of, 1474
    International Prostate Symptom Score, 1474, 1475f–1476f
    interventions for, 1477–1480
    laboratory assessment of, 1476–1477
    lower urinary tract symptoms associated with, 1474, 1477
    nonsurgical management of, 1477–1479
    pathophysiology of, 1474, 1474f
    physical assessment of, 1474–1476
    prevalence of, 1474
    prostate artery embolization, 1479
    prostate cancer and, 1482f
    psychosocial assessment of, 1476
    quality of life after, 1481b
    self-management education for, 1481
    signs and symptoms of, 1474–1476
    surgical management of, 1479–1480, 1480b, 1480f
    transition management for, 1481
    transurethral resection of the prostate for, 1479–1480, 1480b, 1480f
    urinary retention caused by, 18
Benign tumor cells, 373–374
Benlysta. See Belimumab
Benzathine penicillin G, for syphilis, 1509, 1509b
Benzocaine spray, 525
Benzodiazepines
    chemotherapy-induced nausea and vomiting treated with, 399b
    overdose of, 281b
    shivering managed with, 135
Bereavement, 108
Beta amyloid, 858
Beta blockers
    acute coronary syndromes treated with, 776b
    atrial fibrillation treated with, 680
    glaucoma treated with, 966b
    heart failure treated with, 700
    hemorrhage treated with, 1177
    hypertension treated with, 725b, 727
    migraine headaches prophylaxis using, 875
    myocardial infarction treated with, 777
    types of, 677b–678b
Beta cells, 72
Beta particles, 387, 387f
Bevacizumab, 405, 589t, 1130

Bicarbonate
    absorption of, 1325
    description of, 187
    overelimination of, 192
    renal movement of, 190
    sources of, 188
    underproduction of, 192
Bichloroacetic acid, 1511
Bigeminy, 671
Biguanides, 1291, 1292b–1293b
Bilateral salpingo-oophorectomy, 1461t, 1466–1467
Bile, 1064
Bile acid breath test, 1141
Bile reflux gastropathy, 1118
Bile salt deficiencies, 1141
Bi-level positive airway pressure, 535, 631
Biliary cirrhosis, 1170
Biliary colic, 1193, 1193b
Biliary obstruction, 1170
Biliary stents, 1207
Biliary system
    components of, 1191
    gallbladder. See Gallbladder
    liver. See Liver
    obstruction of, 1191
    pancreas. See Pancreas
Bilirubin, 1068, 1069b
BIMS. See Brief Interview for Mental Status
Binge eating, 1216
Biofilm, 421, 991
Biologic dressings, 499
Biologic heart valve replacement, 709–710
Biological response modifiers
    bone marrow suppression treated with, 396
    cancer treated with, 401–402
    connective tissue diseases treated with, 323b
    Crohn's disease treated with, 1153, 1159
    interferons, 402, 402t
    interleukins, 402, 402t
    psoriatic arthritis treated with, 332–333
    renal cell carcinoma treated with, 1386
    rheumatoid arthritis treated with, 321–322, 323b
    self-management education for, 1156
    side effects of, 402
    ulcerative colitis treated with, 1153
Biopsy
    bone, 1013, 1013b
    bone marrow. See Bone marrow aspiration and biopsy
    breast, 1438, 1446
    cervical, 1437, 1437b
    endometrial, 1437–1438, 1466
    excisional, 445

Biopsy (Continued)
    hepatitis diagnosis using, 1184
    intraoral, 1080
    kidney, 1340–1341
    lung. See Lung biopsy
    muscle, 1013
    needle, 1243
    prostate, 1438
    punch, 445
    reproductive system assessments, 1437–1438, 1437b
    shave, 445
    skin, 445
Bioterrorism, 427–428, 466b
Biotherapy
    head and neck cancer treated with, 549–550
    non-Hodgkin's lymphoma treated with, 829
    skin cancer treated with, 477
Biotrauma, 635
BiPAP. See Bi-level positive airway pressure
Biphenotypic leukemia, 818
Bisacodyl, 99
Bismuth subsalicylate, 1112
Bisphosphonates
    bone tumors treated with, 1026
    osteoporosis treated with, 1021, 1021b
Bitemporal hemianopia, 934f
Bites
    arthropod, 136–137, 137b, 137f, 138t–140t
    snakebites, 135–137, 136b, 136f–137f, 136t, 138t–140t
    spider, 136–137, 137b, 137f, 138t–140t
Bivalirudin, 744, 784
Biventricular pacemaker, 675
Biventricular pacing, 681
Black box warnings, 1291
Black widow spider bite, 136–137, 137b, 137f, 138t–140t
Bladder
    anatomy of, 1327, 1327f
    capacity of, 98
    distention of, 1331
    function of, 1327
    neurogenic, 98t
    transitional cell carcinoma of, 1366
    trauma to, 1369
Bladder cancer, 380b
Bladder scanners, 1336–1337, 1337f
Bladder suspension procedure, 1348
Bladder training, for urinary incontinence, 1350–1351, 1351b
BladderScan, 98
Blanch, 483
Blast phase cells, 820
Bleeding. See also Hemorrhage
    in high-risk patients, 827b
    laboratory tests for, 805

Bleeding *(Continued)*
  in leukemia, 825, 825*b*
  management of, in pulmonary embolism, 622
  upper gastrointestinal. *See* Upper gastrointestinal bleeding
Blink reflex, 963
Blood
  accessory organs in formation of, 797–798
  components of, 796–797
  infusion therapy of, 200
  spleen in formation of, 797
Blood administration set, 834*f*
Blood cells
  growth of, 797*f*
  laboratory assessment of, 803–805, 804*b*
  types of, 796
Blood clot embolism, 1034*b*
Blood donation, autologous
  intraoperative, 263, 264*b*
  preoperative, 235
Blood glucose
  alcohol consumption effects on, 1299
  continuous monitoring of, 1298–1299
  exercise effects on, 1311
  fasting levels of, 1281*f*, 1282
  glycosylated hemoglobin and, 1289*t*
  in hospitalized patients, 1301–1302
  monitoring of, 1296*f*, 1298–1300, 1311
  self-monitoring of, 1298, 1317
Blood osmolarity, 1332
Blood pH, 13–14, 188
Blood pressure
  ambulatory monitoring of, 728
  calculation of, 720–721
  definition of, 645
  determinants of, 645
  diastolic, 646
  elevated. *See* Hypertension
  as hydrostatic filtering force, 161
  lifestyle modifications for, 1284
  management of, 1284, 1381–1382
  measurement of, 652–653, 781, 1284
  mechanisms that influence, 720–721
  normal range for, 720
  paradoxical, 652–653
  in polycystic kidney disease, 1381–1382
  regulation of, 646
  renal regulation of, 646
  screening of, 722*f*
  systolic, 646
Blood stem cells, 796, 796*f*
Blood thinners, 801

Blood transfusion. *See also* Transfusion
  allergies to, 263
  autologous, 836
  cell savers, 235, 310
  indications for, 832*t*
  infusion therapy for, 200
  in older adults, 834*b*
  reactions to, 835–836
  red blood cells, 834–835
    compatibility determinations for, 834, 834*t*
    indications for, 832*t*, 834–835
    sickle cell disease treated with, 812
  reinfusion system, 310
  responsibilities in, 832–834
  safety in, 833*b*
  setup for, 832, 834*f*
  types of, 834–835
Blood urea nitrogen, 1331–1332, 1332*b*
Blood urea nitrogen to serum creatinine ratio, 1332, 1332*b*
Bloodborne metastasis, 375
Bloodborne Pathogen Standards, 202
Blood-brain barrier, 390–391, 841
Bloodstream infections, 416, 423
BLS. *See* Basic life support
Blumberg's sign, 1194
Blunt trauma, 129
BMI. *See* Body mass index
BNP. *See* Brain natriuretic peptide
Boceprevir, 1185*t*
Body fat, 1225
Body fluids. *See also* Fluid(s)
  chemistry of, 187–188, 188*b*
  electrolytes in, 173*f*
  pH of, 185–186
Body image, 92, 1019
Body mass index, 1215, 1215*b*, 1225
Body temperature
  in heat stroke victims, 134
  normal, 482
Body water
  insensible loss of, 165
  total, 160, 161*f*
Bolus feeding, 1221
Bone
  cancellous tissue of, 1005
  classification of, 1005
  flat, 1005
  function of, 1005–1006
  haversian system of, 1005, 1005*f*
  healing of, 1032, 1033*b*, 1033*f*
  irregular, 1005
  long, 1005, 1005*f*
  matrix of, 1005
  minerals and hormones associated with, 1006
  resorption of, 1006, 1239, 1276
  short, 1005
  structure of, 1005, 1005*f*
  vascularity of, 1005

Bone banking, 1043
Bone biopsy, 1013, 1013*b*
Bone marrow
  age-related changes in, 800
  blood stem cells produced by, 796, 796*f*
  chemotherapy-induced suppression of, 396–398
  functions of, 795–796
  harvesting of, 823
  stem cell production in, 290, 291*f*
  transplantation of, 822
Bone marrow adipose tissue, 1019
Bone marrow aspiration and biopsy
  description of, 806
  leukemia diagnosis using, 820, 820*f*
Bone mineral density, 1016, 1019
Bone morphogenetic protein-2, 1017*b*
Bone reduction, 1038
Bone scan, 1011
Bone tumors
  assessment of, 1025–1026
  benign, 1024–1025
  care coordination for, 1027–1028
  chondroma, 1024–1025
  chondrosarcoma, 1025
  drug therapy for, 1026
  Ewing's sarcoma, 1025
  fibrosarcoma, 1025
  giant cell tumor, 1025
  health care resources for, 1028
  home care management of, 1027
  interventional radiology for, 1026
  interventions for, 1026–1027
  malignant, 1025
  metastatic, 1028
  nonsurgical management of, 1026
  osteochondroma, 1024
  osteosarcoma, 1012, 1025
  pain management in, 1027–1028
  pathophysiology of, 1024–1025
  radiation therapy for, 1026
  radical resection of, 1026
  self-management education for, 1027–1028
  surgical management of, 1026–1027
  transition management for, 1027–1028
Bone turnover markers, 1019, 1019*t*
Bony ossicles, 984, 985*f*–986*f*
Borborygmus, 1067, 1123
Bordetella pertussis, 613
Borrelia burgdorferi, 332
Bortezomib, 405
Bosentan, 330, 585
Bowel continence, 99
Bowel elimination
  assessment of, 90*t*, 91
  description of, 18, 18*f*
  rehabilitation for, 99

Bowel preparation, preoperative, 242
Bowel retraining programs, 99
Bowel sounds, 276, 1067, 1199
Bowel strictures, 1161
Bowman's capsule, 1323, 1324*f*
Brachial plexus injury, 267*b*
Brachytherapy
  balloon, 1451
  description of, 388
  endometrial cancer treated with, 1466–1467, 1466*b*
  interstitial, 1451
  oral cancer treated with, 1081
  prostate cancer treated with, 1485
Braden Scale for Predicting Pressure Sore Risk, 42, 457*t*
Bradycardia
  heart rate in, 670
  sinus, 673*f*–674*f*, 674–675
Bradydysrhythmias, 671–672
BRAF gene, 477
Brain
  age-related changes in, 858
  anatomy of, 840–841, 840*f*
  cerebellum, 841
  cerebrum, 840–841
  circulation in, 841, 842*f*
  diencephalon, 840, 840*f*
  frontal lobe of, 841*t*
  occipital lobe of, 841*t*
  in older adults, 858
  parietal lobe of, 841*t*
  temporal lobe of, 841*t*
Brain cancer, 376*t*
Brain death, 947
Brain disorders
  Alzheimer's disease. *See* Alzheimer's disease
  encephalitis, 883–884, 884*b*
  meningitis. *See* Meningitis
  migraine headaches. *See* Migraine headaches
  Parkinson disease. *See* Parkinson disease
  seizures. *See* Seizures
Brain herniation syndromes, 942–943, 943*f*
Brain injuries
  hypotension as cause of, 941
  secondary causes of, 941–943
  traumatic. *See* Traumatic brain injury
Brain natriuretic peptide, 166
Brain tumors
  assessment of, 951
  care coordination for, 955
  cerebral tumors, 950
  classification of, 950–951, 951*t*
  clinical features of, 951*b*
  craniotomy for, 952–953, 954*t*
  drug therapy for, 952
  etiology of, 951
  genetic risk of, 951
  increased intracranial pressure caused by, 954

Brain tumors (Continued)
infratentorial, 950, 953
interventions for, 951–954
meningiomas, 951
nonsurgical management of, 952
pathophysiology of, 950–951
pituitary, 951
stereotactic radiosurgery for, 952, 952f
supratentorial, 950
surgical management of, 952–954
transition management for, 955
Brainstem
anatomy of, 841, 841t
assessment of, 848
traumatic injuries to, 945
BRCA1 gene, 81, 83, 382, 1432
BRCA2 gene, 79, 382, 1432
Breakthrough pain, 54–55
Breast(s)
anatomy of, 1429–1430
biopsy of, 1438, 1446
clinical examination of, 1443, 1456
large-breasted women, 1456
lymphatic drainage of, 1430f
mammography of, 1435–1436
reduction mammoplasty of, 1456
small-breasted women, 1456
ultrasonography of, 1446
Breast augmentation
description of, 1456
in male-to-female transgender patients, 1499
Breast cancer, 376t
adjuvant therapy for, 1450–1451
aromatase inhibitors for, 1452
assessment of, 1445–1455
axillary lymph node dissection for, 1447
BRCA1 gene, 81, 83, 1442b
BRCA2 gene, 79, 1442b
breast-conserving surgery for, 1447, 1448f
care coordination for, 1452–1454
chemotherapy for, 1451–1452
complementary and integrative health for, 1446–1447, 1447t
coping strategies for, 1452
diagnostic assessment of, 1446
drug therapy for, 1451–1452
ductal carcinoma in situ, 1441
early detection of, 83
etiology of, 1442
genetic risk of, 1442, 1442b
health care resources for, 1454
health promotion and maintenance for, 1443–1445
in high-risk women, 1443–1445
history-taking for, 1445
home care management of, 1452–1453
imaging assessment of, 1446
incidence of, 1442–1443

Breast cancer (Continued)
infiltrating ductal carcinoma, 1441
inflammatory, 1441
interventions for, 1446–1454
invasive, 1440–1441, 1441f
laboratory assessment of, 1445–1446
in lesbian and bisexual women, 1446b
lobular carcinoma in situ, 1441
magnetic resonance imaging of, 1446
mammographic screening for, 1443, 1446
mastectomy for
adjuvant therapy after, 1450–1451
breast reconstruction after, 1449–1450, 1450t, 1451b
exercises after, 1451b
modified radical, 1448, 1448f
postoperative teaching for, 1453–1454
prophylactic, 1444
total, 1448f
in men, 1441
metastasis of, 1440–1441, 1446–1452
noninvasive, 1440–1441
nonsurgical management of, 1446–1447
pathophysiology of, 1440–1443
physical assessment of, 1445
prevalence of, 1442–1443
prophylactic mastectomy for, 1444
psychosocial assessment of, 1445
psychosocial preparation for, 1454
radiation therapy for, 1451
risk factors for, 1442, 1442t
screening for, 382, 1441, 1443
selective estrogen receptor modulators for, 1452
self-management education for, 1453–1454
sexuality issues, 1445
signs and symptoms of, 1445
stem cell transplantation for, 1452
surgical management of, 1447–1452, 1448b, 1448f, 1453b
survival rates for, 1442–1443
targeted therapy for, 1452
transition management for, 1452–1454
in young women, 1441
Breast disorders
benign, 1455–1456, 1455t
cancer. See Breast cancer
fibroadenoma, 1455, 1455t
fibrocystic breast condition, 1455–1456, 1455t
in large-breasted women, 1456
in small-breasted women, 1456

Breast implants, 1450t, 1456
Breast mass, 1445, 1445b
Breast reconstruction, 1449–1450, 1450t, 1451b
Breast self-examination, 1443, 1444b, 1456
Breast-conserving surgery, 1447, 1448f
Breath sounds, 519, 520t, 897b
Breathing
allergy effects on, 516
in lung cancer, 587
postoperative exercises, 281
primary survey of, 129, 131t
purpose of, 509
techniques in, for chronic obstructive pulmonary disease, 578, 578b
Brief Interview for Mental Status, 91, 861
BRMs. See Biological response modifiers
Broca's aphasia, 938
Bromocriptine, 870–871, 1248, 1248b
Bronchi, 510, 511f
Bronchial sounds, 520t
Bronchioles, 510, 511f
Bronchodilators
asthma treated with, 568–571, 569b–570b
bronchospasm treated with, 110, 604
Bronchogenic carcinomas, 586
Bronchopneumonia, 599
Bronchoscopy, 494, 525
Bronchospasm, 565
in artificial airway suctioning, 542
interventions for, 365
Bronchovesicular sounds, 520t
Brown recluse spider bite, 136–137, 137b, 137f, 138t–140t
Bruits, 653, 723, 729, 1067, 1330
Buerger's disease, 741t
Buffers, 186–189, 186f–187f
Bulimia nervosa, 1216
Bullae, 572
Bullae, 572
Bumetanide, 699
Bundle of His, 665
Bunion, 1028, 1028f
Bunionectomy, 1028–1029
Bupropion, for smoking cessation, 515, 515b
Burkholderia cepacia, 583
Burn injury
acute phase of, 497–504
acute respiratory distress syndrome in, 497
age-related complications that affect, 490b
airway maintenance in, 493–494

Burn injury (Continued)
airway obstruction caused by, 490t
ambulation after, 503
assessment of
cardiopulmonary, 497
cardiovascular, 491
gastrointestinal, 492
imaging, 493
immune, 497–498
kidney, 491–492
laboratory, 492, 493b
musculoskeletal, 498
neuroendocrine, 497
physical, 489–493
respiratory, 489–491
in resuscitation phase, 489–493
skin, 492
urinary, 491–492
capillary response to, 485, 485f
carbon monoxide poisoning secondary to, 490, 491t
cardiac changes caused by, 485–486
cardiovascular assessment of, 491
care coordination for, 505
chemical, 487
circumferential, 484
classification of, 482
compensatory responses for, 486
compression dressings in, 503–504, 504f
contact, 486
contracture prevention after, 503–504, 503b, 504f
deaths caused by, 488
deep full-thickness, 482t, 485, 485f
deep partial-thickness, 483–484
depth of, 482–485, 482t
direct airway injury caused by, 489–490
dry heat as cause of, 486
electrical, 487–488, 487f–488f
emergency management of, 489b
escharotomies for, 484, 494–496, 496f
etiology of, 486–488
fluid resuscitation for, 494–495, 495b
fluid shift after, 485, 485f
full-thickness, 482t, 484–485, 484f
gastrointestinal assessment of, 492
gastrointestinal changes caused by, 486
health care resources for, 505
health promotion and maintenance for, 488–489
history-taking for, 489
home care management of, 505
hypovolemic shock prevention in, 494–496
immunologic changes caused by, 486
incidence of, 488

Burn injury (Continued)
  inhalation injury caused by, 490t
  laboratory assessment of, 492, 493b
  metabolic changes caused by, 486
  minor, 483t
  mobility after, 502–504
  moderate, 483t
  moist heat as cause of, 486
  oxygen therapy for, 494
  oxygenation support in, 493–497
  pain management in, 491
  partial-thickness, 482t, 483–484, 484f
  pathophysiology of, 481–488
  patient positioning, 503
  prevalence of, 488
  psychosocial preparation in rehabilitative phase of, 505
  pulmonary changes caused by, 486
  pulmonary fluid overload associated with, 491
  radiation, 488
  rehabilitative phase of, 504–506
  respiratory assessment of, 489–491
  resuscitation phase of
    assessment in, 489–493
    overview of, 486, 489
  rule of nines for, 492, 492f
  scald, 486
  self-esteem promotion in, 504
  self-management education for, 505
  skin changes caused by, 481–485, 484f, 492
  smoke poisoning caused by, 491
  superficial-thickness, 482–483, 482t, 484f
  thermal, 488, 490
  tissues involved in, 483f
  total body surface area of, 489, 492
  transition management for, 505
  vascular changes caused by, 485
  weight loss minimization after, 502
  wound care management in
    biosynthetic dressings for, 499
    dressings for, 499
    enzymatic débridement, 499
    excision, 500
    hydrotherapy, 498–499
    mechanical debridement, 498–499
    nonsurgical, 498–499
    skin grafts, 500–501
    surgical, 499–501
  wound infections secondary to
    drug therapy for, 501–502, 501b
    indicators of, 498t
    nonsurgical management of, 501–502
    potential for, 501–502
    surgical management of, 502
  wound sepsis, 497–498, 498t

Burnout, 124
Butorphanol tartrate, 284b
Butterfly needles, 203–204
"Butterfly" rash, 326–327, 327f

C
C fibers, 47–48, 49f
CA-125, 1468
CA19-9, 1068, 1069b
CABG. See Coronary artery bypass graft
Cachexia, 1216
Café au lait spots, 79
CAHs. See Critical care access hospitals
Calcineurin inhibitors
  autoimmune diseases treated with, 369, 370b
  immunosuppression uses of, 302b
Calcipotriene, 464–465
Calcitonin, 1006
Calcitriol, 1277
Calcium
  absorption of, 179
  in bone, 1006
  bound, 179
  chronic kidney disease effects on, 1400, 1400f
  description of, 179–181
  free, 179
  imbalances of
    hypercalcemia, 181, 181t
    hypocalcemia, 179–181, 180f, 180t, 196
    in postmenopausal women, 180b
  laboratory testing for, 1069b
  in older adults, 165b
  osteoporosis prevention with, 1020–1021, 1021b
  parathyroid hormone effects on, 179, 1239, 1275
  serum levels of, 164t
Calcium carbonate, 1020, 1112
Calcium channel blockers
  chronic stable angina treated with, 777
  coronary spasm prevention using, 717
  high-altitude pulmonary edema treated with, 146
  hypertension treated with, 725b, 726
  migraine headaches prophylaxis using, 875
  types of, 677b–678b
Calculous cholecystitis, 1192
Calf circumference, 1215
Callus, 1029t
Caloric testing, 991
CAM. See Confusion Assessment Method
Campylobacter enteritis, 1148t
Canada Food Guide, 1212

Canadian Hospice Care Association, 113–114
Canadian Triage Acuity Scale, 124
Canagliflozin, 1292b–1293b
Canal of Schlemm, 958
Cancellous tissue, 1005
Cancer. See also Adenocarcinomas; Oncologic emergencies; Tumor(s)
  cardiac function affected by, 386
  cervical, 1469–1470, 1470b
  chemoprevention of, 382
  classification of, 375–376, 377t
  clotting affected by, 385
  colorectal. See Colorectal cancer
  development of, 375–382
  dietary factors associated with, 379, 379b
  emergencies caused by. See Oncologic emergencies
  endometrial, 1465–1467, 1465t, 1466b
  etiology of, 377–381
  external factors that cause, 378t, 379
  gastric. See Gastric cancer
  gastrointestinal function affected by, 385
  gene mutations associated with, 382
  genetic risk of, 377–381, 380b
  genetic testing for, 380–382
  grading of, 376–377, 377t
  head and neck. See Head and neck cancer
  immunity affected by, 385
  incidence of, 378f, 380, 381b
  liver, 1186–1187
  lung. See Lung cancer
  management of. See Cancer management
  metastasis of. See Metastasis
  motor deficits caused by, 385
  nasal, 556
  nutrition support for, 385
  in older adults, 380b
  oral. See Oral cancer
  ovarian, 1467–1469, 1467t
  pain caused by, 385–386
  pancreatic. See Pancreatic cancer
  pathophysiology of, 372–374
  peripheral nerve function affected by, 385
  personal factors associated with, 380–381
  physical function affected by, 384–386
  prevalence of, 372
  prevention of, 381–382
  primary prevention of, 381–382
  prostate. See Prostate cancer
  race-based incidence of, 381b
  radiation exposure as cause of, 379
  respiratory function affected by, 386

Cancer (Continued)
  risk factors for, 380–381
  screening for, 382
  secondary prevention of, 382
  sensory deficits caused by, 385
  skin. See Skin cancer
  staging of, 376–377, 378t
  testicular. See Testicular cancer
  thyroid, 1275
  TNM staging of, 377, 378t
  tobacco use as cause of, 379
  urothelial. See Urothelial cancer
  vaccinations for prevention of, 382
  warning signs of, 380t
Cancer cells, 387
Cancer management
  angiogenesis inhibitors, 404t, 405
  biological response modifiers, 401–402
  brachytherapy. See Brachytherapy
  chemotherapy. See Chemotherapy
  cytotoxic systemic therapy. See Chemotherapy
  epidermal growth factor/receptor inhibitors, 404t, 405
  hormonal manipulation, 406–407, 406t
  immunotherapy, 401–403, 402t
  monoclonal antibodies, 402–403
  multikinase inhibitors, 404t, 405
  photodynamic therapy, 405–406
  proteasome inhibitors, 404t, 405
  radiation therapy. See Radiation therapy
  small molecule inhibitor targeted therapy, 403–405, 403f–404f, 404t
  surgery, 386–387
  tyrosine kinase inhibitors, 404t, 405
  vascular endothelial growth factor/receptor inhibitors, 404t, 405
Cancer pain
  chronic, 47
  intrathecal pump for, 62b
  self-management education for, 68
Cancer therapy symptom distress, 395
Candida albicans, 346–347, 468, 1076
Candidiasis, 346–347, 347f, 467b, 468, 1076–1077, 1076b, 1077f
Cane, 1044
Cangrelor, 783–784
Canker sores, 1076
Canthus, 958
Capillaries
  hydrostatic pressure in, 162
  structure of, 162f
Capillary closing pressure, 451
Capillary leak syndrome, 485, 753
Capnography, 523, 523f, 524b
Capnometry, 523, 1222

Capsaicin, 308, 1307
Capsule endoscopy, 1071–1072
Carbapenem-resistant
    Enterobacteriaceae, 422–423
Carbohydrate counting, 1300
Carbohydrate metabolism, 188
Carbon dioxide
    blood pH determined by, 188
    definition of, 187
    description of, 508–509
    hydrogen ions and, 187–188
    metabolism effects on, 189
Carbon monoxide poisoning, 490,
    491*t*
Carbonic acid, 187, 187*f*
Carbonic anhydrase equation, 187*f*
Carbonic anhydrase inhibitors,
    974–975
Carboxyhemoglobin, 233–234
Carcinoembryonic antigen, 1068,
    1069*b*, 1129
Carcinogenesis. *See also* Cancer
    chemical, 379
    definition of, 375, 377–378
    physical, 379
    viral, 378*t*, 379
Carcinogens, 375, 378, 381
Cardiac arrest
    hypothermic, 143–144
    lightning injury as cause of, 141
    spinal anesthesia as cause of, 261
Cardiac axis, 666, 666*f*
Cardiac blood pool imaging, 661
Cardiac catheterization, 657–659,
    657*t*–658*t*, 658*f*
Cardiac conduction system, 664–665,
    665*f*
Cardiac cycle, 644–645, 644*f*
Cardiac muscle, 1007
Cardiac output
    burn injury effects on, 485–486
    calculation of, 645
    decreased, 25
    definition of, 645
    determinants of, 720–721
    diuretics effect on, 495
    in valvular heart disease, 708
Cardiac rehabilitation, 779, 790, 792
Cardiac resynchronization therapy,
    701
Cardiac tamponade, 713–714, 788
Cardiac valves, 642, 643*f*
Cardinal positions of gaze, 964, 964*f*
Cardiogenic shock
    acute coronary syndrome as cause
        of, 782
    etiology of, 753
    risk factors for, 752*t*, 756*b*
CardioMEMS implantable
    monitoring system, 701
Cardiomyopathy
    arrhythmogenic right ventricular,
        715
    assessment of, 715
    dilated, 714, 715*t*

Cardiomyopathy (Continued)
    heart transplantation for, 716–717,
        717*f*
    hypertrophic, 714–716, 715*t*
    interventions for, 715–717
    myomectomy and ablation for,
        716
    nonsurgical management of,
        715–716
    pathophysiology of, 714–715, 715*t*
    percutaneous alcohol septal
        ablation for, 716
    restrictive, 714–715, 715*t*
    signs and symptoms of, 715*t*
    surgical management of, 716–717
    treatment of, 715*t*
    uremic, 1401
Cardiopulmonary bypass, 143, 785,
    786*f*
Cardiopulmonary resuscitation, 129,
    686–687
Cardiovascular autonomic
    neuropathy, 1285
Cardiovascular disease
    contributory factors for, 649*b*
    description of, 642
    diabetes mellitus as risk factor for,
        1283–1284
    orthopnea associated with,
        649–650
    risk factors for, 646–648,
        1283–1284
    sedentary lifestyle as risk factor
        for, 647–648
    smoking as cause of, 647
Cardiovascular system. *See also*
    Heart
    acidosis effects on, 192, 193*b*
    age-related changes in, 646, 647*b*
    alkalosis effects on, 196, 196*b*
    arterial system, 645–646
    assessment of, 90, 90*t*, 802–803
        angiography, 657
        cardiac catheterization,
            657–659, 657*t*–658*t*, 658*f*
        computed tomography, 661
        current health problems,
            649–651
        diagnostic, 655–661
        echocardiography, 660
        electrocardiography, 659
        exercise electrocardiography,
            659–660, 660*f*
        extremities, 652
        family history, 649
        functional history, 651
        general appearance, 651
        genetic risk, 649
        history-taking, 646–651
        laboratory, 655–661, 656*b*
        magnetic resonance imaging,
            661
        myocardial nuclear perfusion
            imaging, 661
        nutrition history, 648–649

Cardiovascular system (Continued)
    physical, 651–655
    positron emission tomography,
        661
    psychosocial, 655
    serum lipids, 656
    skin, 651–652
    in spinal cord injury, 896
    in stroke patients, 934
    transesophageal
        echocardiography, 660
    auscultation of, 654–655
    burn injury effects on, 485–486,
        491
    dehydration effects on, 168
    emotional behaviors' effect on,
        646
    fluid overload effects on, 171*f*
    functions of, 641
    hypercalcemia effects on, 181
    hyperkalemia effects on, 178
    hypernatremia effects on, 175
    hypocalcemia effects on, 180
    hypokalemia effects on, 176
    hypomagnesemia effects on, 182
    hyponatremia effects on, 174
    inspection of, 653, 654*f*
    leukemia effects on, 819
    lightning injury effects on, 141
    nutrition assessments, 1213*b*
    in older adults, 222–223, 234*b*,
        647*b*
    postoperative assessments of, 274
    postoperative procedures and
        exercises for, 244–246
    preoperative assessment of, 236
    sickle cell disease effects on, 810
    venous system, 646
Cardioversion, 680–681
Care coordination, 3. *See also specific
    disorder, care coordination for*
Carotenoids, 979
Carotid artery angioplasty with
    stenting, 936
Carotid sinus massage, 678
Carpal tunnel syndrome, 1057–1059,
    1058*b*
Carrier, 79, 414
Case management
    of emergency department
        patients, 125
    purpose of, 3
Case manager
    care coordination by, 3
    in emergency departments,
        119–120, 125
    functions of, 3
    rehabilitation, 88
Caseation necrosis, 605
Cast (orthopedic)
    bivalving of, 1039
    circulation impairment caused by,
        1040
    definition of, 1039
    fiberglass, 1039, 1039*f*

Cast (orthopedic) (Continued)
    fractures treated with, 1039–1040,
        1039*f*
    infection concerns with,
        1039–1040
    removal of, 1045*b*
Cast (urine), 1335
Catabolism, 486, 1396
Cataracts
    assessment of, 969
    care coordination for, 971
    definition of, 958, 968
    etiology of, 960*t*, 968
    eye injury as risk factor for, 961
    genetic risks of, 968
    health care resources for, 971
    health promotion and
        maintenance for, 960*t*
    history-taking for, 969
    home care management of, 962*b*,
        971, 971*f*
    incidence of, 968
    interventions for, 969–971, 970*f*
    pathophysiology of, 968
    phacoemulsification for, 970, 970*f*
    physical assessment of, 969
    prevalence of, 968
    psychosocial assessment of, 969
    self-management education for,
        971
    signs and symptoms of, 969*f*
    surgery for, 969–971, 970*f*
    transition management for, 971
    ultraviolet light exposure and, 961
    visual impairment caused by,
        969*f*
Catechol O-methyltransferase
    inhibitors, 870
Catecholamines, 770
    adrenal medulla secretion of, 1238
    stress response activated by, 486
Catheter(s)
    central venous. *See* Central venous
        catheters
    complications of, 226
    dialysis, 1397, 1397*f*, 1414*t*
    dressings with, 212–214
    embolism caused by, 219*t*–220*t*
    epidural, 226
    flushing of, 214–215
    hemodialysis, 208
    intraperitoneal infusion therapy,
        225
    intraspinal, 226
    midline, 204–205, 204*f*, 213
    peripherally inserted central,
        205–206, 205*f*, 206*b*, 212–213
    peritoneal dialysis, 1418*f*, 1420*b*
    securing of, 212–214, 213*f*, 222*b*
    short peripheral, 202–204,
        202*f*–203*f*, 202*t*, 203*b*,
        214–215
    subclavian dialysis, 1397*f*
    urinary tract infections caused by,
        415, 415*b*, 421, 1355–1356

Catheter-acquired bacteremia, 415–416
Catheter-associated urinary tract infection, 415, 415b, 421, 1356b, 1423, 1500
Catheter-related bloodstream infection, 204–206, 211–212, 216, 216t, 220t–221t
Cations, 172
CAUTIs. See Catheter-associated urinary tract infection
Caval-atrial junction, 205
CBT. See Cognitive-behavioral therapy
CCR5 antagonists, 351b–352b
CD16+ cells, 299
CD4+ T-cells, 337–339
Cecum, 1064
Cefaclor, 1359b
Cefdinir, 1359b
Cefpodoxime, 1359b
Ceftriaxone, 1513–1514
Celecoxib, 321
Celiac disease, 1164, 1164b
Cell(s)
    abnormal, 373–374, 374t
    biology of, 372–373, 373f
    cancer, 373–374, 374t
    features of, 374t
    malignant transformation of, 375
    mitosis of, 373
    plasma membrane of, 290f
    specific morphology of, 373, 373f
Cell cycle, 373, 373f
Cell differentiation, 14
Cell replication, 14
Cell salvage, 235
Cell savers, 235, 310
Cell-mediated immunity
    cells involved in, 292t, 299–300, 797t
    cytokines in, 299–300, 300t
    description of, 22, 290–291, 299
    protection provided by, 300
    tuberculosis and, 605
Cellular growth
    benign, 14
    definition of, 14
Cellular regulation
    definition of, 14, 71, 372
    impaired, 14–15
    orderly and well-regulated growth of, 373
    promotion of, 15
    proteins involved in, 373
Cellulitis, 28, 453, 466, 467b
Center for Epidemiological Studies Depression-Revised, 850–851
Centers for Disease Control and Prevention, 414
Central cyanosis, 651

Central intravenous therapy
    hemodialysis catheters, 208
    implanted ports, 207–208, 207f–208f
    peripherally inserted central catheters, 205–206, 205f, 206b, 212–213
    tunneled central venous catheters, 207, 207f, 213, 226
    vascular access devices for, 205
Central line-associated bloodstream infections, 205, 762
Central nervous system
    acidosis effects on, 193, 193b
    alkalosis effects on, 196, 196b
    assessment of, 803
    brain. See Brain
    components of, 840–842
    function of, 840–842
    hypernatremia effects on, 175
    hypokalemia effects on, 176
    hypomagnesemia effects on, 182
    leukemia effects on, 819
    lightning injury effects on, 142
    sickle cell disease effects on, 810
    spinal cord, 842
    structure of, 840–842
Central nervous system disorders
    Alzheimer's disease. See Alzheimer's disease
    encephalitis, 883–884, 884b
    meningitis. See Meningitis
    migraine headaches. See Migraine headaches
    multiple sclerosis. See Multiple sclerosis
    Parkinson disease. See Parkinson disease
    seizures. See Seizures
Central perfusion, 25
Central venous catheters
    blood samples obtained from, 215
    central line-associated bloodstream infection with, 205
    complications of, 220t–221t
    dislodgement of, 220t–221t
    home care of, 826b
    migration of, 220t–221t
    nontunneled percutaneous, 206–207, 206f, 215
    rupture of, 220t–221t
    tunneled, 207, 207f, 213, 226
Central venous pressure, 653, 1396
Cerebellar pontine angle tumors, 951
Cerebellum
    anatomy of, 841
    function assessments, 849–850
Cerebral aneurysms, 1380
Cerebral angiography, 852–853, 852b
Cerebral cortex, 841, 841t

Cerebral edema
    high-altitude, 145–146, 145b–146b
    pathophysiology of, 950
Cerebral functioning, 274–275
Cerebral hemispheres, 840–841
Cerebral hypoxia, 758
Cerebral perfusion, 935–938
Cerebral vasospasm, 937
Cerebrospinal fluid
    functions of, 841
    leakage of, 907b, 946
    lumbar puncture examination of, 855
Cerebrovascular disease, 1284
Cerebrum
    anatomy of, 840–841
    assessment of, 848
    hyponatremia-related changes, 174
    tumors of, 950
Certifications, for emergency nursing, 120t, 123
Certified registered nurse anesthetist, 253t, 256
Certified wound, ostomy, continence nurse, 1130, 1131t, 1153, 1156–1157
Certolizumab, 1160b
Cerumen
    definition of, 984
    impaction of, 995b
    pathophysiology of, 994
    removal of, 987b, 994–995, 994b, 994f
Cervarix, 1469, 1511
Cervical ablation, 1470, 1470b
Cervical biopsy, 1437, 1437b
Cervical cancer, 1469–1470, 1470b
Cervical collar, 899, 899f, 945
Cervical intraepithelial neoplasia, 1469
Cervical lymph nodes
    anatomy of, 1080, 1080f
    metastasis to, 1082
Cervical neck pain, 909–910, 910b
Cervical spinal cord injury, 896–897
Cervical spine, 319b
Cervix, 1429. See also specific cervical entries
Cetuximab, 1130
Chagas disease, 1166
Charcot foot, 1304, 1305f
Checklist of Nonverbal Pain Indicators, 54
CHEK2 gene, 382
Chemical burns, 487
Chemical carcinogenesis, 379
Chemical débridement, 457, 457t
Chemoprevention, 382
Chemoradiation, for head and neck cancer, 549
Chemotherapy
    breast cancer treated with, 1451–1452
    cardiac function affected by, 386

Chemotherapy (Continued)
    cervical cancer treated with, 1470
    colorectal cancer treated with, 1130
    combination, 392
    drugs used in
        administration of, 392
        categories of, 391–392, 391t
        disposal of, 394
        dose-dense, 392
        intra-arterial infusion of, 225
        oral, 393–394, 393t, 394b
    endometrial cancer treated with, 1467
    esophageal tumors treated with, 1097
    gastric cancer treated with, 1116
    head and neck cancer treated with, 549
    intra-arterial infusion of, 392
    intrathecal administration of, 392
    intravenous administration of, 392
    intraventricular administration of, 392
    intravesicular administration of, 392
    liver cancer treated with, 1187
    lung cancer treated with, 588
    oral cancer treated with, 1080–1081
    pancreatic cancer treated with, 1206–1207
    polycythemia vera treated with, 816–817
    prostate cancer treated with, 1485
    protections during administration of, 392
    psychosocial issues during, 395–396
    side effects of, 395–396, 1119
        alopecia, 395, 400
        anemia, 397
        bone marrow suppression, 396–398
        cognitive function changes, 400–401
        extravasation, 392–393
        mucositis, 395, 399–400, 400b
        myelosuppression, 396–398, 397b
        nausea and vomiting, 398–399, 399b
        neutropenia, 395, 396b
        peripheral neuropathy, 385, 401, 401b
        short-term, 395
        thrombocytopenia, 397–398
    testicular cancer treated with, 1488–1489
    urothelial cancer treated with, 1366
Cherry angiomas, 439, 439f

Chest
  auscultation of, 1242
  landmarks of, 518f
  palpation of, 518–519
Chest expansion
  assessment of, 518
  inadequate, 192
  postoperative exercises for, 243, 244b
  semi-Fowlers position for, 21
Chest pain, 517. See also Angina pectoris
  atypical, 1089
Chest physiotherapy, 583
Chest trauma
  flail chest, 637, 637f
  fractures caused by, 1049–1050
  pulmonary contusion, 636
  rib fracture, 636–637
Chest tubes
  drainage systems for, 590–592, 591f, 592b
  placement of, 590–592, 590f
Chest x-rays
  acute respiratory distress syndrome evaluations, 627
  chronic obstructive pulmonary disease evaluations using, 577
  pneumonia evaluations using, 603
  preoperative, 237
  respiratory system assessment using, 521
Cheyne-Stokes respirations, 107
Chimerism, 824
Chlamydia infection, 1511–1512
Chlamydia trachomatis, 1511–1512
Chlorhexidine, 216–222
Chloride
  in older adults, 165b
  serum levels of, 164t
Cholecystectomy
  cholecystitis treated with, 1195–1197
  laparoscopic, 1195–1196
  postcholecystectomy syndrome, 1196, 1196t
  traditional, 1196–1197
Cholecystitis
  acalculous, 1192
  acute, 1192
  acute pancreatitis caused by, 1201
  assessment of, 1193–1194
  calculous, 1192
  care coordination for, 1197
  cholecystectomy for, 1195–1197
  chronic, 1192, 1194
  definition of, 1191
  diagnostic assessment of, 1194
  drug therapy for, 1195
  etiology of, 1192
  extracorporeal shock wave lithotripsy for, 1195
  features of, 1193b

Cholecystitis (Continued)
  genetic risk of, 1192
  hepatobiliary scan for, 1194
  icterus as cause of, 1192
  illustration of, 1192f
  incidence of, 1193
  jaundice associated with, 1192
  nonsurgical management of, 1195
  nutrition promotion in, 1194
  pain management in, 1194–1197
  pathophysiology of, 1191–1193
  percutaneous transhepatic biliary catheter for, 1195
  physical assessment of, 1193–1194
  prevalence of, 1193
  risk factors for, 1193t
  signs and symptoms of, 1193–1194
  surgical management of, 1195–1197
  transition management for, 1197
  ultrasonography of, 1194
Cholecystokinin, 1225
Cholecystotomy, 1195
Choledochojejunostomy, 1207
Cholelithiasis, 1192, 1195
Cholesterol, 656, 1069b
Cholesterol stones, 1192
Cholinergic agonists, 966b
Cholinergic antagonists, 569b–570b, 571
Cholinergic crisis, 918–920, 920t
Cholinesterase inhibitors
  Alzheimer's disease treated with, 864
  myasthenia gravis treated with, 919–920
  Parkinson disease treated with, 871
Chondroitin, 309
Chondroma, 1024–1025
Chondrosarcoma, 1025
Choreiform movements, 868
Choroid, 957
Christianity, 112t
Christmas disease, 831
Christmas factor, 798t
Chromatographic assays, 1243
Chromosomes
  formation of, 73, 73f
  genes in, 72
  locus of, 72
  number of, 72, 74
  sex, 74, 75f
  structure of, 74
Chronic airflow limitation, 564f, 572f, 635
Chronic back pain, 903
Chronic bacteriuria, 98
Chronic bronchitis, 573, 576
Chronic calcifying pancreatitis, 1202
Chronic cholecystitis, 1192, 1194
Chronic constrictive pericarditis, 712–713

Chronic gastritis, 1104–1105, 1105b
Chronic glomerulonephritis, 1378
Chronic health conditions, 86–87
Chronic hepatitis, 1182
Chronic kidney disease
  acidosis in, 1400
  acute kidney injury versus, 1391t
  albuminuria secondary to, 1399
  anxiety management in, 1410–1411
  assessment of, 1403–1404
  cardiac changes caused by, 1401, 1403–1404
  cardiac function in, 1407
  care coordination for, 1424–1425, 1425b
  causes of, 1401, 1402t
  cognitive changes associated with, 1401
  concept map for, 1405f–1406f
  definition of, 1398
  depression secondary to, 1411
  dietary restriction for, 1407t
  end-stage kidney disease progression of, 1398–1399
  etiology of, 1401, 1402t
  fatigue associated with, 1409–1410
  features of, 1391t
  fluid restriction for, 1405
  fluid volume management in, 1405, 1405b
  gastrointestinal changes associated with, 1401, 1404
  genetic risk of, 1401
  health care resources for, 1425
  health promotion and maintenance of, 1402, 1402b
  heart failure in, 1401
  hematologic changes associated with, 1401, 1404
  hemodialysis for
    anticoagulation during, 1413
    arteriovenous fistulas, 1413, 1414f–1415f, 1414t–1415t, 1415b
    arteriovenous grafts, 1413, 1414f, 1414t–1415t, 1415b
    cardiac events during, 1417
    care after, 1416, 1416b
    complications of, 1416–1417
    description of, 1411
    dialyzers, 1412–1413, 1412f, 1417
    hemofiltration versus, 1413f
    home care management of, 1424
    infectious disease transmission during, 1417
    nursing care during, 1416
    patient selection, 1411–1412
    peritoneal dialysis versus, 1411t
    procedure, 1412–1413, 1412f–1413f

Chronic kidney disease (Continued)
  self-management education for, 1424–1425
  settings, 1412
  temporary vascular access, 1416
  vascular access, 1413–1416, 1414f, 1414t–1415t
  history-taking for, 1403
  home care management of, 1424
  hospitalization for, 1402–1403
  hyperkalemia risks, 1400
  hyperlipidemia in, 1401
  hypertension in, 1401, 1407
  hyponatremia risks, 1400
  imaging assessment of, 1404
  immunity changes associated with, 1401
  incidence of, 1401
  infection prevention in, 1408
  injury prevention in, 1408–1409
  kidney changes caused by, 1399–1400
  kidney replacement therapies for, 1411–1424, 1411t, 1412f–1415f
  indications for, 1411
  kidney transplantation for
    acute rejection, 1423–1424, 1423t
    assessments after, 1425b
    candidate selection criteria, 1421
    chronic rejection, 1423–1424, 1423t
    complications of, 1423–1424, 1423t
    donors, 1421–1422, 1422f
    hyperacute rejection, 1423–1424, 1423t
    immunosuppressive drug therapy in, 1424
    incidence of, 1421
    living related donors, 1421, 1423
    operative procedures, 1422–1423, 1422f
    postoperative care, 1423
    preoperative care, 1422
    rejection, 1423–1424, 1423t
    self-management education after, 1425
  laboratory assessment of, 1404
  metabolic changes caused by, 1400–1401, 1400f
  nutrition in, 1407–1408, 1407t
  opioid analgesic dosing in, 1409
  pathophysiology of, 1398–1401
  patient and family education about, 1402b
  pericarditis in, 1401
  peritoneal dialysis for
    automated, 1419–1420, 1419f–1420f
    catheters, 1418f, 1420b

Chronic kidney disease *(Continued)*
  complications of, 1420–1421
  continuous ambulatory, 1418, 1419f
  continuous-cycle, 1419
  description of, 1408, 1417
  dialysate additives, 1418
  dialysate leakage during, 1420
  hemodialysis versus, 1411t
  home care management of, 1424
  intermittent, 1420
  nursing care during, 1421
  patient selection, 1417
  peritonitis caused by, 1420, 1420b
  procedure, 1417–1418, 1418f
  self-management education for, 1425
  types of, 1418–1420, 1418f–1419f
  phosphorus restriction in, 1408
  physical assessment of, 1403–1404
  polycystic kidney disease progression to, 1382
  potassium restriction in, 1408
  prevalence of, 1401
  prevention of, 1375
  priority problems for, 1404–1405
  protein restriction in, 1407–1408
  psychosocial preparation in, 1425
  pulmonary edema prevention in, 1405–1407
  respiratory symptoms of, 1404
  self-management education for, 1424–1425
  signs and symptoms of, 1403–1404, 1403b
  skeletal symptoms of, 1404
  sodium restriction in, 1408
  stages of, 1398–1399, 1399t
  transition management for, 1424–1425, 1425b
  uremic encephalopathy associated with, 1403
  urinary output affected by, 18
  vitamin supplementation for, 1408, 1410b
Chronic lymphocytic leukemia, 814t, 821
Chronic myelogenous leukemia, 814t
Chronic obstructive pancreatitis, 1202
Chronic obstructive pulmonary disease
  acid-base imbalances caused by, 13–14
  activity improvements in, 580
  alpha$_1$-antitrypsin deficiency as risk factor for, 573, 573b, 573t
  anxiety management in, 580
  assessment of, 574–577
  barrel chest associated with, 576

Chronic obstructive pulmonary disease *(Continued)*
  breathing techniques for, 578, 578b
  cardiac changes associated with, 576
  care coordination for, 581, 581b
  chronic bronchitis, 573, 576
  complications of, 573–574
  diagnostic assessments, 577, 577t
  digital clubbing associated with, 576, 576f
  drug therapy for, 578–579
  dry powder inhalers for, 579
  dyspnea in, 576, 580
  effective coughing for, 578
  emphysema, 572–573, 572f
  etiology of, 573
  exercise for, 579
  gas exchange affected by, 21, 21f
  genetic risks, 573
  health care resources for, 581, 581b
  health promotion and maintenance for, 574
  history-taking for, 574
  home care management of, 581, 581b
  hydration for, 579
  imaging assessment of, 577
  incidence of, 573
  laboratory assessment of, 576–577
  monitoring of, 578
  nonsurgical management of, 577–579
  oxygen therapy for, 578
  pathophysiology of, 572–574
  patient positioning with, 574, 576f, 578
  physical assessment of, 574–576
  prevalence of, 573
  psychosocial assessment of, 576
  pulmonary rehabilitation for, 579
  respiratory acidosis associated with, 195
  respiratory infections in, 573, 581
  self-care management of, 581
  severity assessments, 577t
  signs and symptoms of, 574–576
  smoking as cause of, 14, 21, 573
  stepped therapy for, 579
  suctioning in, 579
  surgical management of, 579–580
  transition management for, 581, 581b
  vibratory positive expiratory pressure device for, 579, 579f
  weight loss prevention in, 580
Chronic osteomyelitis, 1023–1024, 1023b
Chronic otitis media, 991

Chronic pain
  description of, 46–47
  epidural infusion for, 225
  in older adults, 56b
  psychosocial factors that affect, 52
  self-management education for, 68
Chronic pancreatitis, 1202–1204, 1203b–1204b
Chronic paronychia, 442
Chronic renal failure. *See* Chronic kidney disease
Chronic stable angina pectoris, 768–769
Chronic tophaceous gout, 331
Chronic transplant rejection, 301
Chronic venous insufficiency, 746–747
Chvostek's sign, 180, 180f, 182, 1201, 1277
Chyme, 1062–1063
Cigarette smoking. *See* Smoking
Ciliary body, 957
Cimex lectularius, 471
Cinacalcet, 1276–1277, 1408, 1410b
Ciprofloxacin, 612b, 1359b
Circle of Willis, 841, 842f
Circulation, 129–130, 131t
Circulator, 253t
Circumcision, 1430
Circumduction, 1010f
Cirrhosis
  abdominal assessment of, 1173
  advanced, 1173
  alcohol use as cause of, 1172
  ascites caused by, 1170, 1173, 1173f
  assessment of, 1172–1175
  biliary, 1170
  biliary obstruction caused by, 1170
  care coordination for, 1179–1180
  causes of, 1170t
  clotting factors affected by, 15
  compensated, 1170, 1173
  complications of, 1170–1172
  concept map for, 1175f–1176f
  decompensated, 1170
  definition of, 1169
  diagnostic assessment of, 1174–1175
  drug therapy for, 1175
  esophageal varices caused by, 1170
  esophagogastroduodenoscopy evaluations, 1175
  etiology of, 1172
  fluid volume management in, 1175–1177
  gastroesophageal varices caused by, 1170
  genetic risk of, 1172
  health care resources for, 1180
  hemorrhage management in, 1177–1178

Cirrhosis *(Continued)*
  hepatic encephalopathy caused by, 1170–1171, 1171t, 1178–1179
  hepatitis B as cause of, 1172
  hepatitis C as cause of, 1172
  hepatitis D as cause of, 1172
  hepatorenal syndrome caused by, 1171
  history-taking for, 1172
  home care management of, 1179, 1179b
  imaging assessment of, 1174
  jaundice secondary to, 1170
  laboratory assessment of, 1174, 1174t
  Laennec's, 1170
  magnetic resonance elastography of, 1174
  magnetic resonance imaging of, 1174
  nutrition therapy for, 1175
  paracentesis for, 1175–1177, 1177b
  physical assessment of, 1173
  portal hypertension caused by, 1170
  postnecrotic, 1170
  primary biliary, 1170
  psychosocial assessment of, 1173–1174
  respiratory support in, 1177
  self-management education for, 1179–1180, 1179b
  signs and symptoms of, 1173
  transition management for, 1179–1180
  transjugular intrahepatic portal-systemic shunt for, 1177–1178
  types of, 1170
CKD. *See* Chronic kidney disease
CLASBI. *See* Central line-associated bloodstream infection
Clean-catch urine specimen, 1334t
Clinical breast examination, 382, 1443, 1456
Clinical competence, 36
Clinical judgment, 8
Clinical psychologists, 89
Clitoris, 1429
Clock Drawing Test, 861
Clonus, 849
Closed fracture, 1032, 1032f
Closed reduction and immobilization, of fractures, 1038–1040
Closed-loop obstruction, 1122
Clostridium difficile
  microbiome changes and, 77
  stool tests for, 1068–1070
Clostridium difficile-associated disease, 428
Clostridium tetani, 501
Clot lysis, 15
Clothing, 142

Clotting
    anti-clotting forces, 799–800
    assessment of, 16
    cancer effects on, 385
    definition of, 15, 795, 798
    drugs that affect, 801t
    inadequate, 15–16
    laboratory testing for, 16
    nutrition effects on, 802
    promotion of, 16
    scope of, 15, 15f
Clotting cascade, 15, 798, 799f, 800
Clotting factors, 798–799, 798t
Clubbing, of nails, 443t, 652
CNPI. See Checklist of Nonverbal
    Pain Indicators
Coagulation, 805. See also Clotting
Co-analgesics, 55, 63
Co-carcinogens, 379
Coccidioidomycosis, 613
Cochlea, 986
Cochlear implantation, 999
Code of Ethics, American Nurses
    Association, 9, 9t, 1492
Codeine, 61, 77, 284b
Co-dominant, 75
Coercion, 81–82
Cognition
    acidosis effects on, 193
    age-related changes in, 844
    Alzheimer's disease-related
        changes in, 860–861
    assessment of, 847, 847b
        before rehabilitation, 91
        description of, 17
    chemotherapy effects on,
        400–401
    chronic kidney disease effects on,
        1401
    definition of, 16, 860
    diabetes mellitus effects on,
        1286
    in human immunodeficiency
        virus infection, 355
    in hypothyroidism, 1273
    inadequate
        description of, 17
        in older adults, 35–38
        pain assessment challenges
            caused by, 53–54, 53t
    promotion of, 17
    scope of, 16
    sleep deprivation effects on, 846
    stroke effects on, 932–933
Cognitive impairment
    in multiple sclerosis, 892b
    pain management for, 59b
    safe environment for, 17b
Cognitive rehabilitation, 948
Cognitive retraining, 1043
Cognitive therapists, 89
Cognitive-behavioral therapy,
    66–67
Cogwheel rigidity, 869
Cohorting, 421

Cold antibody anemia, 815
Cold-related injuries
    frostbite, 144–145, 144b, 144f
    health promotion and
        maintenance for, 142
    hypothermia, 142–144, 143b
Colectomy, 1130
Collagen
    in dermis, 431–432
    in wound dressings, 499
Collagenase, 501b
Collateral circulation, 733
Colles' fracture, 1046, 1046f, 1057
Colloids, 170
Colon interposition, 1098–1099
Colon resection, 1130
Colon tumors, 1130t
Colonization, 455
Colonoscopy
    American Cancer Society
        recommendations for, 1072
    colorectal cancer diagnosis using,
        1128b, 1129
    description of, 382
    follow-up care for, 1072, 1073b
    gastrointestinal system
        assessments using, 1072–1073
    patient preparation for, 1072
    procedure for, 1072
    ulcerative colitis evaluations using,
        1152
    virtual, 1073
Colony-stimulating factor, 294–295,
    826
Color vision
    age-related changes in, 961b
    testing of, 964
Colorectal cancer
    adenocarcinomas, 1127
    assessment of, 380b, 1128–1129
    care coordination for, 1133–1135
    chemotherapy for, 1130
    colonoscopy of, 1128b, 1129
    colostomy for, 1130, 1131f–1132f,
        1131t, 1132, 1134–1135,
        1134b
    etiology of, 1127–1128
    fecal occult blood test for,
        1128–1129, 1128b
    genetic risk of, 1127–1128, 1133b
    grief management in, 1132–1133
    health care resources for, 1135
    health promotion and
        maintenance for, 1128
    hereditary nonpolyposis, 1126,
        1127b, 1466
    history-taking for, 1128
    home care management of,
        1133
    imaging assessment of, 1129
    incidence of, 1128
    interventions for, 1129–1132
    laboratory assessment of, 1129
    metastasis of, 376t, 1127,
        1129–1132

Colorectal cancer (Continued)
    minimally invasive surgery for,
        1130, 1132
    nonsurgical management of,
        1129–1130
    pathophysiology of, 1126–1128
    physical assessment of, 1128–1129,
        1129f
    prevalence of, 1128
    psychosocial assessment of, 1129
    psychosocial concerns in patients
        with, 1134–1135
    radiation therapy for, 1129–1130
    risk factors for, 1127–1128
    screening for, 1070, 1128, 1128b
    self-management education for,
        1133–1135
    sigmoidoscopy of, 1128b, 1129
    signs and symptoms of,
        1128–1129, 1129f
    sites of, 1127f
    staging of, 1129
    surgical management of,
        1130–1132
    transition management for,
        1133–1135
    ulcerative colitis and, 1151t
    vascular endothelial growth factor
        inhibitors for, 1130
Colostomy, for colorectal cancer,
    1130, 1131f–1132f, 1131t, 1132,
    1134–1135, 1134b
Colporrhaphy, 1465
Colposcopy, 1436, 1469–1470
Comatose, 846
Combination antiretroviral therapy,
    342–343, 350–353
Combination chemotherapy, 392
Comfort
    decreased, 17–18
    definition of, 17
    in pericarditis patients, 713
    scope of, 17
    for urinary tract infections, 1359
Coming out, 1493t
Commando procedure, 1082
Common bile duct, 1064
Communicable infections, 414
Communicating hydrocephalus,
    943
Communication
    with Alzheimer's disease patients,
        863b, 865
    by emergency nurse, 123
    hand-off, 119–120
    with hearing-impaired patients,
        998b, 1001–1002
    in patient unable to speak, 550b
    with stroke patients, 938
    in tracheostomy patients, 543–544
Community-acquired pneumonia,
    599t–600t
Community-associated
    methicillin-resistant
    Staphylococcus aureus, 422

Compartment syndrome
    acute, 1033–1034, 1034b,
        1044–1045, 1044b
    definition of, 224
    description of, 738
    fasciotomy for, 1044–1045
    fractures as cause of, 1033–1034,
        1034b, 1044–1045, 1044b
    frostbite as cause of, 144–145
    in intraosseous therapy, 224
Compassion fatigue, 124
Compensated cirrhosis, 1170, 1173
Competence, 36
Competencies
    core. See Core competencies
    genetic, 72, 72t
Complement activation and fixation,
    297
Complement system, 294
Complementary and integrative
    health
    agitation treated with, 111
    Alzheimer's disease managed with,
        863
    atherosclerosis treated with, 731
    benign prostatic hyperplasia
        managed with, 1477
    breast cancer managed with,
        1446–1447, 1447t
    endometrial cancer treated with,
        1467
    gastritis managed with, 1107t
    human immunodeficiency virus
        infection treated with,
        353–354
    hypertension managed with, 723
    irritable bowel syndrome
        managed with, 1137
    migraine headaches managed
        with, 875–876
    multiple sclerosis managed with,
        892
    after myocardial infarction, 791
    nausea and vomiting treated with,
        111
    obesity managed with, 1229
    osteoarthritis managed with,
        308–309
    pain management use of, 109, 285,
        308–309, 496
    peptic ulcer disease managed with,
        1107t, 1112–1113
    rheumatoid arthritis managed
        with, 324
    sickle cell disease treated with,
        811–812
    ulcerative colitis managed with,
        1153
Complete blood count, 803, 1068
Complete fracture, 1032
Complex patterns of inheritance,
    78t, 80
Complex regional pain syndrome,
    1035, 1041–1042
Compound fracture, 1032

Compression dressings, 503–504, 504f
Compression fracture, 1032, 1033f
Computed tomography
  cardiovascular system evaluations using, 661
  contrast-enhanced, 1338
  ear assessments using, 990
  gastrointestinal system assessments using, 1070
  musculoskeletal system assessments using, 1011
  neurologic system evaluations using, 853
  renal system assessments, 1337–1338, 1337t, 1338b
  reproductive system assessments, 1435
  respiratory system assessment using, 521–522
  urinary stones on, 1363f
  vision assessments, 965
Computed tomography angiography, 661, 853
Computed tomography colonography, 1073
Computed tomography coronary angiography, 774
Computed tomography perfusion study, 853
Computed tomography-based absorptiometry, 1019
Computed tomography–magnetic resonance imaging, 853–854
Concussion, 949b. See also Traumatic brain injury
Condoms, 1508b
Conductive hearing loss, 989, 996–997, 997t
Conductivity, 665
Condylomata acuminata, 1510–1511, 1510f
Cones, 957–958
Confidentiality, 81, 83
Confrontation test, 964
Confusion, 40–42
Confusion Assessment Method, 17, 38, 38t, 91
Congestive heart failure, 692
Conivaptan, 954, 1252b
Conization, 1437
Conjunctivae, 958
Connective tissue diseases
  ankylosing spondylitis, 334t
  biological response modifiers for, 323b
  characteristics of, 304–305
  dermatomyositis, 334t
  fibromyalgia syndrome, 333–334
  gout, 330–332, 331f
  laboratory assessments, 320–321, 320b
  lupus erythematosus. See Lupus erythematosus; Systemic lupus erythematosus

Connective tissue diseases (Continued)
  Lyme disease, 332, 333b
  Marfan syndrome, 334t
  osteoarthritis. See Osteoarthritis
  polymyalgia rheumatica, 334t
  polymyositis, 334t
  psoriatic arthritis, 332–333
  Reiter's syndrome, 334t
  rheumatoid arthritis. See Rheumatoid arthritis
  systemic necrotizing vasculitis, 334t
  systemic sclerosis, 326b, 329–330, 330b
  temporal arteritis, 334t
Conn's syndrome, 1260–1261
Consciousness
  definition of, 846
  level of. See Level of consciousness
Consensual response, 848, 963
Consent, informed, 239–241, 240f
Consolidation, 599
Constipation
  definition of, 18
  diabetes mellitus as cause of, 1285
  interventions for, 19
  nausea and vomiting caused by, 111
  in older adults, 31
  opioid analgesics as cause of, 63t
  in polycystic kidney disease, 1382
  postoperative, 277
  prevention of, 19, 1382
  risk factors for, 18, 31
Contact burns, 486
Contact dermatitis, 462, 463b
Contact transmission
  description of, 416
  precautions for, 419, 420t
Contiguous osteomyelitis, 1023
Continence, 18, 1327, 1343
Continuous ambulatory peritoneal dialysis, 1418, 1419f
Continuous bladder irrigation system, 1479, 1480f
Continuous blood glucose monitoring, 1298–1299
Continuous femoral nerve blockade, 315
Continuous kidney replacement therapies, 1397–1398
Continuous passive motion machine, 315, 315f, 316b, 1027
Continuous peripheral nerve block, 65
Continuous positive airway pressure
  heart failure treated with, 701
  indications for, 535, 536f, 559, 632
Continuous quality improvement, 7
Continuous sutures, 268f
Continuous tube feeding, 1221
Continuous venovenous hemofiltration, 1398

Continuous venovenous hemofiltration and dialysis, 1398
Continuous-cycle peritoneal dialysis, 1419
Contractility
  definition of, 665
  drugs that enhance, 699–700
Contractures
  after amputation, 1054
  prevention of, in burn injury patients, 503–504, 503b, 504f
  in spinal cord injury patients, 900–901
  Volkmann's, 1034
Contrast agents, 1338, 1338b
Contrast-induced nephropathy, 1338
Convergence, 960
Coombs' tests, 805
COPD. See Chronic obstructive pulmonary disease
Coping, 32–33, 655, 779, 1452
Copperhead snake bite, 136, 136f, 138t–140t
Cor pulmonale, 573–574, 574b, 584
Coral snakes, 136, 137f, 138t–140t
Cordectomy, 550, 551t
Core competencies
  clinical judgment, 8
  emergency nursing, 122–123
  ethics. See Ethics
  evidence-based practice, 7
  health care disparities, 10–11, 11t
  health care organizations. See Health care organizations
  informatics, 7–8
  patient-centered care, 2–3
  quality and safety education for, 2
  quality improvement, 7
  safety, 3–5
  teamwork, 5–6, 5t
  technology, 7–8
Core Measures, 7
Corn, 1029t
Cornea
  abrasion of, 977
  age-related changes in, 961b
  anatomy of, 958, 958f
  assessment of, 963
  infection of, 977
  lacerations of, 982
  opacities of, 977–979, 978f
  staining of, 965
  transplantation of, 978f
  ulceration of, 977
Corneal light reflex, 964
Corneal ring placement, 981
Coronary arteries
  anatomy of, 643, 643f
  atherosclerotic, 769f
Coronary arteriography, 658

Coronary artery bypass grafting
  bleeding after, 788b
  candidates for, 785
  cardiopulmonary bypass, 785, 786f
  complications of, 787–788
  description of, 784
  electrolyte imbalance after, 787
  endovascular vessel harvesting for, 789
  fluid imbalance after, 787
  health care resources for, 792
  home care management after, 789–790
  hypertension after, 787–788
  hypothermia after, 787
  indications for, 785
  internal mammary artery used in, 784–786
  mechanical ventilation after, 788
  mediastinitis after, 788–789
  methods of, 787f
  minimally invasive, 789
  off-pump, 789
  in older adults, 790b
  operative procedures, 785–786
  pain management after, 788
  postoperative care for, 786–789
  postpericardiotomy syndrome after, 789
  preoperative care for, 785
  self-management education for, 790–791
  special care unit transfer after, 788–789
  sternal wound infection as cause of, 785, 788–789
  sternotomy pain after, 788
  surgical site infections after, 786b
Coronary artery calcification, 661
Coronary artery disease
  atherosclerosis as risk factor for, 771. See also Atherosclerosis
  coronary artery bypass graft for. See Coronary artery bypass graft
  definition of, 768
  health promotion and maintenance for, 772
  home care management of, 789–790
  incidence of, 647
  percutaneous coronary intervention for, 783–784, 784f
  physical activity recommendations for, 791b
  prevention of, 771b
  risk factors for, 771–772, 772b, 790–791
  stents for, 783
  waist circumference and, 1225
  in women, 772b
Coronary artery vasculopathy, 717

Coronary heart disease. *See* Coronary artery disease

Coronary sinus, 642

Corpus callosum, 840–841

Cortical nephrons, 1323

Corticosteroids
asthma treated with, 569b–570b, 571
autoimmune diseases treated with, 368
chemotherapy-induced nausea and vomiting treated with, 399b
idiopathic pulmonary fibrosis treated with, 586
immunosuppression uses of, 302b
inflammation treated with, 462
psoriasis treated with, 464
side effects of, 324

Corticotropin-releasing hormone, 1236, 1238, 1260

Cortisol, 1237–1238, 1255, 1260b

Cosentyx. *See* Secukinumab

Costovertebral angle, 1330

Cough/coughing
for chronic obstructive pulmonary disease, 578
description of, 516
in spinal cord injury patients, 897–898, 898f

Counterimmunoelectrophoresis, 882

CPAP. *See* Continuous positive airway pressure

CPB. *See* Cardiopulmonary bypass

C-peptide, 1289

Crackles, 521t, 601, 696, 1089

Cranberry juice, 1359

Cranial nerves
assessment of, 847–848, 934
description of, 842, 844t
Guillain-Barré syndrome involvement of, 914
stroke-related effects to, 934

Cranial polyneuritis, 924

Craniotomy, for brain tumors, 952–953, 954t

CRBSI. *See* Catheter-related bloodstream infection

C-reactive protein, 1283

Creatinine, serum, 1331

Creatinine clearance, 1335–1336
chronic kidney disease effects on, 1400
gender differences in, 57b
test for, 34

Credé maneuver/method, 98, 1352

Crepitus, 305–306, 518

CREST syndrome, 329

Cricoid cartilage, 510

Cricothyroid membrane, 510

Cricothyroidotomy, 510, 558, 560–561

Critical access hospitals, 117

Critical care access hospitals, 9

Critical incident stress debriefing, 156–157

Crizotinib, 589t

Crohn's disease
abdominal assessments in, 1159
abdominal pain associated with, 1159
anemia associated with, 1159
assessment of, 1159
biologic response modifiers for, 1153, 1159
care coordination for, 1161–1162
clinical presentation of, 1158
complications of, 1151t, 1158
definition of, 1157–1158
drug therapy for, 1159, 1160b
family history of, 1158b
fistulas associated with, 1158, 1158f, 1160, 1160b, 1162
glucocorticoids for, 1160
health teaching plan for, 1161–1162
home care assessment for, 1158b
incidence of, 1158
interventions for, 1159–1161
magnetic resonance enterography of, 1159
nonsurgical management of, 1159–1160
nutrition therapy for, 1159–1160
pathophysiology of, 1157–1158
psychosocial assessment of, 1159
risk factors for, 1158b
signs and symptoms of, 1159
skip lesions associated with, 1157–1158
surgical management of, 1161
transition management for, 1161–1162
ulcerative colitis versus, 1150t

Cromones, 569b–570b, 571

Cross-bridges, 644

Cross-contamination, 820–822

CRPS. *See* Complex regional pain syndrome

Crusts, 438f

Crutches, 1043–1044, 1044f

Cryopexy, 979

Cryosurgery, 477

Cryotherapy, 66, 315
cervical cancer treated with, 1470
condylomata acuminata treated with, 1511
mucositis treated with, 400
oral cancer treated with, 1081

Cryptococcosis, 347

Cryptococcus neoformans
description of, 347
meningitis caused by, 881

Cryptorchidism, 1487

Cryptosporidium, 1166

Cryptosporidiosis, 346

Crystalloids
dehydration treated with, 170
hypovolemic shock treated with, 758–759

CSF. *See* Colony-stimulating factor

CTAS. *See* Canadian Triage Acuity Scale

CTD. *See* Connective tissue diseases

CTS. *See* Carpal tunnel syndrome

Cultural safety, 2

Culturally competent care, 152b

Culture (microorganism), 424, 444

Culture of safety, 4–5

Curative surgery, 386

Curettage and electrodesiccation, 477

Curling's ulcer, 486, 1108

Cushing's disease
adrenal, 1256
assessment of, 1256–1257
care coordination for, 1260
conditions that cause, 1256t
cortisol replacement therapy for, 1260b
description of, 1247, 1248b
dexamethasone suppression testing for, 1257
etiology of, 1256
features of, 1256, 1257b
fluid retention in, 1258
gastrointestinal bleeding in, 1259
health care resources for, 1260
home care management of, 1260
imaging assessment of, 1257
incidence of, 1256
infection prevention in, 1259–1260
injury prevention in, 1259
interventions for, 1258–1260
laboratory assessment of, 1257
nonsurgical management of, 1258
nutrition therapy for, 1258
pathologic fractures in, 1259
pathophysiology of, 1255–1256
physical assessment of, 1256–1257
pituitary, 1256
prevalence of, 1256
psychosocial assessment of, 1257
self-management education for, 1260
signs and symptoms of, 1256–1257
surgical management of, 1258–1259
transition management for, 1260

Cushing's syndrome, 721

Cushing's triad, 945

Cushing's ulcer, 1108

Cutaneous anthrax, 466–468, 467f

Cutaneous reflexes, 848

Cuticle, 432f, 433

Cyanosis, 443, 802b
central, 651
definition of, 651

CyberKnife, 952

Cyclic tube feeding, 1221

Cyclin D1, 1095b

Cyclooxygenase, 295

Cyclosporine, 302b, 1303

CYP450 enzymes, 57b

CYP2C9, 77

CYP2C19, 77

CYP2D6, 77, 77b

Cyst(s)
in fibrocystic breast condition, 1455
illustration of, 438f

Cystic fibrosis
assessment of, 582
chest physiotherapy for, 583
exacerbation therapy for, 583
gene therapy for, 583
genetics of, 582b
high-frequency chest wall oscillation for, 583, 583f
lung transplantation for, 583
nonsurgical management of, 582–583
pathophysiology of, 581–582
surgical management of, 583–584
sweat chloride test for, 582

Cystinuria, 1362t, 1365

Cystitis. *See also* Urinary tract infections
acute radiation, 1485
assessment of, 1357–1359
definition of, 1354
description of, 1329
diagnostic assessment of, 1358–1359
etiology of, 1354–1357
fungal infections as cause of, 1356
genetic risk of, 1354–1357
infectious, 1355
interstitial, 1354, 1356
noninfectious, 1356
pathophysiology of, 1354–1357
signs and symptoms of, 1358
surgical management of, 1359

Cystocele, 1352, 1464, 1464f

Cystogram, 1339

Cystography, 1337t, 1339

Cystometrography, 1340

Cystoscopy, 1339, 1358–1359, 1367

Cystourethrography, 1337t, 1339

Cystourethroscopy, 1339

Cytokines
in cell-mediated immunity, 299–300, 300t
definition of, 299
types of, 300t

Cytomegalovirus, 347

Cytoreductive surgery, 386

Cytotoxic drugs, 368

Cytotoxic edema, 942

Cytotoxic systemic therapy, 390–391. *See also* Chemotherapy

Cytotoxic T lymphocyte-associated protein 4, 367, 369, 477

Cytotoxic T-cells, 299, 797t

D

Dabigatran, 680, 801
Dacarbazine, 399
Daclizumab, 302b
Dalfampridine, 891
Dandruff, 441
Dantrolene sodium, 258–259
Dapagliflozin, 1292b–1293b
Darbepoetin alfa, 397, 402t
Dark-skin patients
  cyanosis in, 651, 802b
  jaundice in, 444
  oxygen saturation in, 516b
  pallor in, 802b
Dawn phenomenon, 1296
D-dimer test, 743
Death
  approaching, 107–108, 107b–108b
  definition of, 104
  direct causes of, 104
  in emergency department, 126–127
  leading causes of, 104t
  overview of, 103–104
  peaceful, 103
  physical manifestations of, 113b
  postmortem care after, 114, 114b
  pronouncement of, 114b
  without dignity, 103
Death rattle, 110
Débridement, of wound, 457, 457t
Debriefing, 156–157
Decadron. See Dexamethasone
Decerebrate posturing, 848, 848f, 946
Decerebration, 848, 848f
Decibel scale, 990
Decisional capacity, 36
Decompensated cirrhosis, 1170
Decorticate posturing, 848, 848f, 946
Decortication, 848, 848f
Deep brain stimulation, for Parkinson disease, 872
Deep breathing, 244b
Deep tendon reflexes, 848
Deep vein thrombophlebitis, 742
Deep vein thrombosis
  anticoagulants for, 743–745
  care coordination for, 746
  D-dimer test for, 743
  definition of, 742
  diagnostic assessment of, 743
  drug therapy for, 743–745
  fractures as risk factor for, 1034–1035
  health care resources for, 746
  home care management of, 746
  impedance plethysmography for, 743
  incidence of, 742
  low-molecular-weight heparin for, 744–745
  nonsurgical management of, 743–745
  novel oral anticoagulants for, 745

Deep vein thrombosis (Continued)
  pneumatic compression devices for prevention of, 245, 245f
  postoperative, 281
  prevalence of, 742
  prevention of, 23, 281, 744
  pulmonary embolism caused by, 617
  self-management education for, 746, 746b
  signs and symptoms of, 742–743
  surgical management of, 745–746
  thrombolytic therapy for, 745
  transition management for, 746
  unfractionated heparin for, 744
  venous duplex ultrasonography for, 743
  warfarin for, 745
Defecation, 1064, 1204
Defense mechanisms, 92
Defibrillation
  automated external defibrillator
    dysrhythmias treated with, 686–687, 687f
    illustration of, 687f
    ventricular fibrillation treated with, 685
  definition of, 686
  implantable cardioverter/defibrillator, 686, 688b
Dehiscence, wound, 277, 278f, 282–283
Dehydration
  assessment of, 168–169, 1084
  care coordination for, 170
  in diabetes mellitus, 1283
  drug therapy for, 170
  fluid compartments affected by, 168f
  fluid replacement for, 169–170, 170t
  gender differences, 164b
  health promotion and maintenance of, 168
  injury prevention in patients with, 170
  interventions for, 169–170, 169b
  intravenous solutions for, 170, 170t
  isotonic, 167–168
  laboratory assessment of, 169
  in older adults, 167b, 1194b
  oral rehydration solutions for, 170
  pathophysiology of, 167–168, 167t
  prevention of, 1314
  relative, 167
  safety considerations in, 170
  signs and symptoms of, 168–169
  systemic changes associated with, 168–169
  transition management for, 170
  weight loss as sign of, 168
Delayed gastric emptying, 1118

Delayed union, of fracture, 1035
Delegation, 6
Delirium
  definition of, 16
  dementia versus, 20t
  in older adults, 38
  pain assessment challenges associated with, 53–54, 53t
  types of, 38
Delirium tremens, 232–233
Delta hepatitis, 1181
Dementia
  Alzheimer's disease, 857–858. See also Alzheimer's disease
  clinical features of, 858t
  definition of, 16, 857–858
  delirium versus, 20t
  emergency department visits for, 126b
  multi-infarct, 37
  in older adults, 37
  pain assessment challenges associated with, 53–54, 53t
  vascular, 857–858, 858t
  in veterans, 126b
Demerol. See Meperidine
Demyelination, 912–913
Dendrites, 839–840, 840f
Denial, 655
Denosumab, 1021, 1026
Deoxyribonucleic acid. See DNA
Depression, 1010f
  in Alzheimer's disease, 864
  in chronic kidney disease patients, 1411
  cognitive changes caused by, 850–851
  in older adults, 36–37, 37f
  post-stroke, 939
  screening tool for, 850–851
  selective serotonin reuptake inhibitors for, 37
  situational, 36
  after stroke, 939
Dermal appendages, 481–482
Dermal papillae, 432
Dermatitis
  atopic, 462, 463b
  contact, 462, 463b
  incontinence-associated, 1352
  radiation, 389
Dermatomes, 842, 843f, 896
Dermatomyositis, 334t
Dermatophytosis, 467b, 468
Dermis
  age-related changes, 434b
  anatomy of, 432
  definition of, 431
  functions of, 433t
Descending colostomy, 1131f
Desmopressin acetate, 1251, 1477
Detrusor hyperreflexia, 1345t
Dexamethasone, 146
Dexamethasone suppression testing, 1257

Dextran, 898
Diabetes insipidus, 1246b, 1250–1251, 1250b
Diabetes mellitus
  assessment of, 1288–1289
  blood glucose in
    continuous monitoring of, 1298–1299
    decreases of, 1309
    exercise effects on, 1311
    in hospitalized patients, 1301–1302
    levels of, 1281f
    monitoring of, 1296f, 1298–1300, 1311
    self-monitoring of, 1298, 1317
    therapy target goals for, 1298
  care coordination for, 1316–1318, 1316t, 1318b, 1318t
  Charcot foot deformity in, 1304, 1305f
  classification of, 1281–1282, 1281t
  complications of
    acute, 1283
    cardiovascular disease, 1283–1284
    cerebrovascular disease, 1284
    chronic, 1283–1286
    cognitive dysfunction, 1286
    constipation, 1285
    description of, 1280
    diabetic autonomic neuropathy, 1285, 1285t, 1305
    diabetic nephropathy, 1286, 1384–1385
    diabetic retinopathy, 1284, 1284b
    exercise adjustments for, 1301
    hyperglycemia, 1281
    hyperglycemic-hyperosmolar state, 1300b, 1313t, 1314–1316, 1314b, 1315f
    hyperlipidemia, 1280
    hypoglycemia. See Diabetes mellitus, hypoglycemia in
    immunity reductions, 1284
    ketoacidosis. See Diabetic ketoacidosis
    kidney disease, 1308
    macrovascular, 1283–1284
    microvascular, 1283–1286
    peripheral neuropathy, 1284–1285, 1285t, 1304–1307, 1305f
    sexual dysfunction, 1286
    stroke, 1284
    surgical complications secondary to, 1303
  concept map for, 1289f–1290f
  definition of, 1280
  dehydration associated with, 1283
  diagnosis of, 1288–1289, 1288t
  drug therapy for
    alpha-glucosidase inhibitors, 1292b–1293b, 1293

Diabetes mellitus (Continued)
amylin analogs, 1292b–1293b, 1293–1294
biguanides, 1291, 1292b–1293b
DPP-4 inhibitors, 1292b–1293b, 1293
examples of, 1292b–1293b
incretin mimetics, 1292b–1293b, 1293
insulin. See Diabetes mellitus, insulin for
metformin, 1291, 1291b
overview of, 1291–1299
patient education regarding, 1297–1298
selection of, 1291
sodium-glucose cotransport inhibitors, 1292b–1293b, 1294
thiazolidinediones, 1291, 1292b–1293b
in ethnic minorities, 1292b–1293b
etiology of, 1286–1287
exercise therapy for, 1300–1301, 1301b
foot care in, 1304–1307, 1305f–1306f, 1306b–1307b
foot deformities in, 1304–1307, 1305f–1306f, 1306b
foot ulcers associated with, 1305–1306
genetic risk of, 1286–1287, 1286b
gestational, 1281t, 1288
glycosylated hemoglobin in, 1289, 1289t
health promotion and maintenance for, 1287–1288
history-taking for, 1288
home care management of, 1317–1318, 1318b
hypoglycemia in
definition of, 1308–1309
drug therapy for, 1311
home care management of, 1310b
interventions for, 1309–1311
nutrition therapy for, 1310–1311
in older adults, 1312b
patient and family education about, 1311
patient education about, 1317
prevention of, 1308–1311
signs and symptoms of, 1308–1309, 1309t
incidence of, 1287
insulin for. See also Insulin
absorption of, 1295–1296
alternative administration methods for, 1296–1297
complications of, 1296, 1296f
continuous subcutaneous infusion of, 1294, 1296, 1296f
injection areas and sites, 1295f

Diabetes mellitus (Continued)
injection devices for, 1297
Lispro, 1294
long-acting, 1295t
mixing of, 1296
pen-type injectors for, 1297–1298
rapid-acting, 1295t, 1296
regimens, 1294–1295
short-acting, 1295t
stimulators of, 1291–1294, 1292b–1293b
storage of, 1297
subcutaneous administration of, 1297b
syringes for, 1297
types of, 1294
islet cell transplantation for, 1303
laboratory assessment of, 1288–1289, 1288b
learning needs assessments in, 1316, 1316t
lifestyle considerations for, 1288
meal planning for, 1300
medical nutrition therapy for, 1299–1300
nonsurgical management of, 1291–1302
nutrition therapy for, 1299–1301, 1299t
in older adults, 1300b
oral glucose tolerance testing for, 1289
pain management in, 1307
pancreatic transplantation for, 1302–1303
patient education about, 1317
polydipsia associated with, 1283
polyphagia associated with, 1283
polyuria associated with, 1283
prevalence of, 1287, 1292b–1293b
psychosocial preparation of, 1317
screening for, 1289
self-management education about, 1318t
signs and symptoms of, 1283
surgical management of, 1302–1304
survival skills information for patients with, 1316
testing for, 1287t
transition management for, 1316–1318, 1316t, 1318b, 1318t
type 1
etiology of, 1286
exercise therapy for, 1300–1301, 1301b
features of, 1281t, 1286t
genetic risk of, 1286b
hypoglycemic unawareness associated with, 1309
type 2 versus, 1286t

Diabetes mellitus (Continued)
type 2
etiology of, 1286–1287
features of, 1281t, 1286t
meal planning for, 1300
metabolic syndrome as risk factor for, 1287
prevalence of, 1287
testing for, 1287t
type 1 versus, 1286t
in veterans, 1291b
ulcers associated with, 732–733, 734b, 1305–1306
vision loss secondary to, 1307–1308
Diabetic autonomic neuropathy, 1285, 1285t
Diabetic ketoacidosis
acidosis management in, 1313–1314
characteristics of, 1311–1312
drug therapy for, 1313
hyperglycemic-hyperosmolar state versus, 1313t, 1314
interventions in, 1313–1314
pathophysiology of, 1312f
patient and family education about, 1314
signs and symptoms of, 1312–1313
Diabetic nephropathy, 1286, 1384–1385
Diabetic peripheral neuropathy, 1284–1285, 1285t, 1304–1307, 1305f
Diabetic retinopathy, 1284, 1284b
Diagnostic surgery, 386
Dialysate, 1412
Dialysis. See Hemodialysis; Peritoneal dialysis
Dialysis catheters, 1397, 1397f, 1414t
Dialysis disequilibrium syndrome, 1417
Dialyzer, 1412–1413, 1412f, 1417
Diamox. See Acetazolamide
Diaphragmatic breathing, 244b, 578, 578b
Diaphragmatic hernias. See Hiatal hernias
Diarrhea
antidiarrheal drugs for, 1153
best practices for, 19b
definition of, 18
Escherichia coli, 1148t
fluid and electrolyte imbalances caused by, 18
in human immunodeficiency virus infection, 354
interventions for, 19, 19b
skin care in, 1142b
in total enteral nutrition patients, 1223
in ulcerative colitis, 1152–1155
Diarthrodial joints, 1006–1007
Diascopy, 445

Diastole, 644, 706
Diastolic blood pressure, 646
Diastolic heart failure, 692
Diastolic murmurs, 655
Diazoxide, 1311
DIC. See Disseminated intravascular coagulation
Diencephalon, 840, 840f
Diet. See also Nutrition
chronic kidney disease managed with, 1407t
dumping syndrome managed with, 1118t
gastritis managed with, 1104–1105
gluten-free, 1164
hemorrhoids managed with, 1140
irritable bowel syndrome managed with, 1136
liquid formula, 1227
low-energy, 1228
novelty, 1228
nutritionally balanced, 1228
obesity managed with, 1227–1228
peptic ulcer disease managed with, 1112, 1112b
preoperative restrictions for, 241
urolithiasis treated with, 1365, 1366t
very-low-calorie, 1227
Dietary Guidelines for Americans, 1211, 1212t
Dietary Reference Intakes, 1211
Di-2-ethylhexylphthalate, 209
Diffusion, 162–163, 162f, 1412
Diffusion imaging, 853
Digestion, 1062
Digital breast tomosynthesis, 1446
Digital clubbing, 576, 576f
Digital 3D mammography, 1436, 1446
Digital rectal examination, 382, 1346–1347, 1474, 1483
Digoxin, 677b–678b
in chronic kidney disease patients, 1409b
heart failure treated with, 700, 700b
hypokalemia caused by, 176
toxicity caused by, 700b
Dihydroergotamine, 875
Dihydrotestosterone, 1481–1482
Dilated cardiomyopathy, 714, 715t
Dilation, 752
Dilaudid. See Hydromorphone
Dilutional hyponatremia, 1251
"Dinner fork" deformity, 1046, 1046f
Diphosphoglycerate, 512
Diplopia, 892, 917, 1246–1247
Direct commissurotomy, 709
Direct inguinal hernia, 1137, 1137f
Direct ophthalmoscopy, 966t
Direct response, 848
Direct thrombin inhibitors, 16, 617–618, 620, 801

Directed blood donation, 235
Directly observed therapy, 423, 610
Disability examination, 130, 131*t*
Disabling health conditions, 86–87
Disaster
  definition of, 149
  external, 149–151
  internal, 149
  nursing roles in, 155
  types of, 149–150
Disaster Medical Assistance Team, 153
Disaster triage tag system, 152, 152*b*
Discharge planning, 235
Discoid lesions, 327
Discoid lupus erythematosus, 326–328, 328*b*
Discomfort, 17
Disease-modifying antirheumatic drugs, 322, 368–369, 370*b*
Disequilibrium, 161
Disinfection, 418
Diskectomy
  back pain treated with, 906
  cervical neck pain treated with, 909–910, 910*b*
Dissecting aneurysms, 738–739
Disseminated intravascular coagulation
  assessment of, 763–764
  definition of, 761
  as oncologic emergency, 407
Distal convoluted tubule, 1323, 1325
Distal interphalangeal joint, 1009, 1009*f*
Distal radius fracture, 1046–1047, 1046*f*
Distal symmetric polyneuropathy, 1285*t*
Distraction, 66–67
Distress
  at end of life, 107–108
  refractory symptoms of, 111
  symptoms of, 108–111
Distributive shock
  chemical-induced, 753
  etiology of, 753
  risk factors for, 752*t*, 756*b*
Diuretics
  cardiac output affected by, 495
  fluid overload treated with, 20
  heart failure treated with, 699
  hypertension treated with, 725*b*, 726
  loop, 699*b*, 701
  potassium excretion caused by, 177
  potassium-sparing, 177, 699, 701
  syndrome of inappropriate antidiuretic hormone treated with, 1252
  thiazide, 699, 725*b*

Diverticula
  esophageal, 1101
  intestinal, 1162–1164, 1162*f*, 1163*b*
Diverticular disease, 1162–1164, 1162*f*, 1163*b*
Diverticulitis, 1162, 1164
Diverticulosis, 1162–1163
Diving reflex, 147
DLE. *See* Discoid lupus erythematosus
DMAIC model, 7
DMARDs. *See* Disease-modifying antirheumatic drugs
DMAT. *See* Disaster Medical Assistance Team
DNA
  base pairs of, 73
  bases of, 73
  complementary strands of, 73, 73*f*
  double-stranded, 73, 73*f*
  forms of, 73*f*
  replication of, 73–74, 74*f*
  structure of, 72–73, 73*f*
DNR order. *See* Do-not-resuscitate order
Dobutamine, 700, 783*b*
Docusate sodium, 1140
Dofetilide, 677*b*–678*b*
Dolophine. *See* Methadone
Do-not-attempt-to-resuscitate order, 104–106
Do-not-resuscitate order, 104–106, 263
Dopamine
  for myocardial infarction, 783*b*
  in Parkinson disease, 868
Dopamine agonists
  adverse effects of, 870*b*
  Parkinson disease treated with, 870–871, 870*b*
  restless legs syndrome treated with, 923
Dose-dense chemotherapy, 392
Double-barrel colostomy, 1131*f*
Double-barrel stoma, 1132
Double-contrast barium enema, 1070
Doubling time, 377
Douching, 1500
Dowager's hump, 1018, 1018*f*
Down syndrome, 988
Doxycycline, 612*b*
DPOAHC. *See* Durable power of attorney for health care
DPP-4 inhibitors, 1292*b*–1293*b*, 1293
Drain(s)
  postoperative, 277–278, 279*f*
  preoperative preparation for, 242
  types of, 279*f*
Drainage systems, for chest tubes, 590–592, 591*f*, 592*b*

Dressings
  biologic, 499
  biosynthetic, 499
  burn wound, 499
  with catheters, 212–214
  postoperative, 277–278, 278*f*, 281–282
  pressure, 267, 457–458
  synthetic, 499, 500*f*
  tracheostomy, 543, 543*f*
  transparent film, 499, 500*f*
  for venous stasis ulcers, 747
DRIs. *See* Dietary Reference Intakes
Driving safety, for older adults, 34, 34*b*
Dronedarone, 677*b*–678*b*
Droplet transmission
  description of, 416
  precautions for, 419, 420*t*
Drowning, 147, 147*b*
Drug(s). *See also specific drug*
  absorption of, 34
  acute pancreatitis treated with, 1200–1201
  age-related changes in metabolism of, 34
  allergic rhinosinusitis treated with, 365
  Alzheimer's disease treated with, 863–864
  angioedema treated with, 363
  assessment of, 35
  Beers criteria for, 35, 36*t*
  benign prostatic hyperplasia treated with, 1477
  bone tumors treated with, 1026
  brain tumors treated with, 952
  breast cancer treated with, 1451–1452
  cholecystitis treated with, 1195
  cirrhosis treated with, 1175, 1178–1179
  copayments for, 10
  Crohn's disease treated with, 1159, 1160*b*
  dehydration treated with, 170
  diabetes insipidus caused by, 1250
  diabetes mellitus treated with. *See* Diabetes mellitus, drug therapy for
  dialyzable, 1416*t*
  discoid lupus erythematosus managed with, 327–328
  distribution of, 34
  excretion of, 34
  fluid overload treated with, 172
  genital herpes treated with, 1507
  gout treated with, 331–332
  half-life of, 58–59
  hemorrhage treated with, 1177
  hepatitis B treated with, 1185*t*
  hepatitis C treated with, 1185*t*
  hepatitis treated with, 1184
  hypercalcemia treated with, 181

Drug(s) *(Continued)*
  hyperkalemia treated with, 178
  hypernatremia treated with, 175
  hyperpituitarism treated with, 1248
  hyperthyroidism treated with, 1267–1268, 1268*b*
  hypocalcemia treated with, 180
  hypokalemia treated with, 176
  hyponatremia treated with, 174
  infusion therapy, 201
  malabsorption treated with, 1142
  malnutrition treated with, 1219
  metabolism of, 34
  migraine headaches treated with, 874–875
  obesity caused by, 1226
  obesity treated with, 1228–1229
  osteoporosis treated with, 1020–1022
  ototoxicity caused by, 26
  peptic ulcer disease treated with, 1106*b*–1107*b*, 1111–1112
  peristalsis promotion using, 286
  preoperative, 241–242, 247, 257
  respiratory acidosis treated with, 195
  self-administration of, by older adults, 35, 35*f*
  stomatitis treated with, 1077–1078
  syndrome of inappropriate antidiuretic hormone treated with, 1252
  systemic lupus erythematosus managed with, 327–328
  transplant rejection treated with, 302*b*
  trigeminal neuralgia treated with, 924
  ulcerative colitis treated with, 1152–1153
  wound infection treated with, 282
Drug eruption, 463*b*
Drug holiday, 871
Drug reconciliation, 287
Drug-eluting stents, 783
Drug-induced hepatitis, 1180
Dry age-related macular degeneration, 979
Dry heat, 486
Dry powder inhalers
  asthma managed with, 570, 571*b*
  chronic obstructive pulmonary disease treated with, 579
Dual x-ray absorptiometry, 1019
Ductal carcinoma in situ, 1441
Ductal ectasia, 1455*t*
Dulaglutide, 1292*b*–1293*b*
Dulcolax. *See* Bisacodyl
Dumping syndrome, 1117–1119, 1118*t*
Duodenum
  anatomy of, 1064
  ulcers of, 1107–1108, 1108*f*, 1110

Dupuytren's contracture, 1028, 1028f
Dura mater, 840
Durable power of attorney for health care, 104, 105f
Duragesic. See Fentanyl
Dwarfism, 1006
Dying. See also End of life
    comfort during, 107, 107b
    dyspnea during, 109–111, 110b
    ethics and, 114–115
    grieving during, 112–114
    life review during, 112
    overview of, 103–104
    pain management during, 108–109
    pathophysiology of, 104
    as process, 112
    psychosocial assessment of, 108b
    reminiscence during, 112
    signs and symptoms of, 107–108, 107b
    storytelling during, 112
    weakness during, 109
Dysarthria, 938
Dyskinesias, 870, 872
Dyslexia, 933
Dyspareunia, 1165, 1246, 1515
Dyspepsia, 1065, 1088–1089, 1105, 1110, 1193
Dysphagia, 109, 917, 934, 1077, 1089, 1096, 1217b, 1275
Dysphasia, 91
Dyspnea, 517, 517t
    in asthma, 566
    in chronic obstructive pulmonary disease, 576, 580
    during dying, 109–111, 110b
    exertional, 695
    in follicular carcinoma, 1275
    in heart failure, 695
    in lung cancer, 593
    paroxysmal nocturnal, 517, 650, 695
    pathophysiology of, 110
    visual analog scale for, 576, 576f
Dyspnea on exertion, 649
Dysrhythmias
    acute coronary syndromes as cause of, 779–780
    atrial. See Atrial dysrhythmias
    bradydysrhythmias, 671–672
    care coordination for, 681–684
    in chronic obstructive pulmonary disease, 574
    definition of, 671
    etiology of, 672
    home care management of, 681–682
    in older adults, 682b
    pathophysiology of, 671–672
    patient care for, 672b
    premature complexes, 671
    prevention of, 682b
    self-management education for, 682

Dysrhythmias (Continued)
    sinus, 672–675
    sinus tachycardia, 673, 673f
    tachydysrhythmias, 668b, 672
    transition management for, 681–684
    ventricular. See Ventricular dysrhythmias
Dystrophic nails, 441
Dysuria, 236, 1381

E
Ear(s). See also Hearing
    age-related changes, 986, 987b
    anatomy of, 984–986, 985f
    assessment of, 988–989, 989f
    diagnostic assessment of, 990–991
    external, 984, 985f, 988
    foreign bodies in, 994–995, 994b, 994f
    imaging assessment of, 990
    inner, 985–986
    irrigation of, 994b, 994f
    middle, 984–985, 985f
    otoscopic assessment of, 988–989, 989f
    physical assessment of, 988–989, 989f
Ear disorders
    acoustic neuroma, 951, 996
    external otitis, 993–994, 993b, 994f
    mastoiditis, 995
    Ménière's disease, 986–987, 995–996
    otitis media, 991–993, 992f, 1023b
    tinnitus, 987, 995
    trauma, 995, 1000b
Ear infection, 1000b
Ear surgery, 993b
Eardrops, 993b
Eardrum
    anatomy of, 984–985, 986f
    otoscopic examination of, 988–989, 989f
Earwax. See Cerumen
Eating disorders, 1216
Eaton-Lambert syndrome, 918
Ebola virus, 151, 427, 427t
EBP. See Evidence-based practice
EBPI. See Evidence-based practice improvement
Ecchymoses, 439, 802, 830, 1036, 1173
Eccrine sweat glands, 433
Echocardiography
    description of, 660
    valvular heart disease evaluations, 707
Edema
    assessment of, 652
    cerebral. See Cerebral edema
    formation of, 162
    in heart failure, 696b
    increased intracranial pressure caused by, 942

Edema (Continued)
    pitting, 171f, 652f
    pulmonary. See Pulmonary edema
    skin effects of, 437
Edentulous, 1218
Edrophonium chloride, 918–919, 919b
Efferent arterioles, 1323
Efferent neurons, 840
EGD. See Esophagogastroduodenoscopy
EHR. See Electronic health record
Ejection fraction, 692
Elastase, 1197
Elder abuse and neglect. See also Older adults
    in Alzheimer's disease patients, 865–866
    description of, 39, 39t
Elective surgery, 232t
Electrical bone stimulation, 1043
Electrical burn injuries, 487–488, 487f–488f
Electrical cardioversion, 680–681
Electrical safety, 252
Electrical stimulation, 458–459
Electrocardiogram
    artifacts on, 670
    burn injury evaluations, 491
    graph paper for, 667, 668f
    normal sinus rhythm, 671, 671f
    P wave of, 665
    preoperative, 238
    rhythm analysis, 670–671
Electrocardiogram caliper, 670–671
Electrocardiography
    complexes, 667–670, 669f
    continuous monitoring using, 667
    description of, 659, 665–666
    electrode positioning for, 666, 666f, 668b
    lead systems for, 666–667, 666f
    premature ventricular contractions on, 683f
Electroencephalography, 854
Electrolarynx, 552, 552f
Electrolyte(s). See also specific electrolyte
    abnormal levels of, 164t
    in body fluids, 173f
    deficit of, 20
    definition of, 19, 172
    excess of, 20
    in gastrointestinal tract dysfunction, 1068
    levels of, 164t, 165b, 173f
    in older adults, 165b
    plasma levels of, 165b
    serum levels of, 164t
    in urine, 1336
Electrolyte balance
    anatomy of, 160–164
    assessment of, 20
    definition of, 19

Electrolyte balance (Continued)
    homeostatic mechanisms in, 160
    laboratory testing for, 20
    physiology of, 160–164
    postoperative, 276
    promotion of, 20
    renin-angiotensin II pathway in, 166–167, 166f
    scope of, 19
Electrolyte imbalances
    after coronary artery bypass grafting, 787
    diarrhea caused by, 18
    hypercalcemia, 181, 181t
    hyperkalemia, 178–179, 178t, 179b, 192, 237
    hypermagnesemia, 182, 182t
    hypernatremia, 174–175, 175t
    hypocalcemia, 179–181, 180f, 180t, 196
    hypokalemia, 175–177, 177b, 196, 237
    hypomagnesemia, 181–182, 182t
    hyponatremia, 173–174, 174t
    interventions for, 20
    in older adults, 173b
    physiologic consequences of, 20
    preoperative assessment of, 237
    prevention of, 20
    risk factors for, 19
    severe, 172
    total enteral nutrition as cause of, 1222–1223
    transfusion as cause of, 833
    types of, 20t, 164t
Electromyography
    description of, 854
    musculoskeletal system evaluations using, 1013
    myasthenia gravis evaluations using, 918
    renal system evaluations, 1340
Electromyoneurography, 918
Electronic health record
    description of, 8
    intraoperative review of, 263–264
    preoperative review of, 246–247
Electronic infusion devices, 211
Electronic infusion pumps, 211
Electronic medical record, 8
Electronic nicotine delivery systems, 514
Electronic patient record, 8
Electronystagmography, 991
Electroretinography, 967
Elevation, 1010f
Elimination
    assessment of, 19
    bowel, 18, 18f
    changes in, 18–19
    definition of, 18
    interventions for, 19
    scope of, 18, 18f
    urinary, 18
E-mail, 5

Embolectomy, 621, 738, 936
Embolic stroke, 928–929, 929t, 934
Embolism
  blood clot, 1034b
  definition of, 15–16, 737
  fat, 1034, 1034b
  pulmonary. See Pulmonary
    embolism
Emergency care
  for amputation, 1053
  for drowning, 147
  for fractures, 1037–1038, 1038b
Emergency departments
  adverse events in, 121
  care environment of, 118–120,
    119f
  case management after, 125
  death in, 126–127
  dementia care in, 126b
  demographic data, 118
  disposition from, 124–127,
    130–131
  environment safety in, 120–121
  fall prevention in, 121
  family education in, 125–126
  forensic nurse examiners in, 118
  health care role of, 117–118
  health education, 125
  homelessness and, 127
  hospital-based, 117
  injury management in, 127
  interprofessional team in, 118–120
  language barriers in, 123b
  medical errors in, 121
  older adults in, 118b
  patient education in, 125–126
  patient identification in, 121
  patient safety in, 120b, 121–122
  physicians in, 119
  procedures commonly performed
    in, 122–123
  psychiatric crisis nurse team in,
    118–119
  skin integrity protection in, 121
  specialized nursing teams in,
    118–119
  staff in
    ancillary, 119–120
    professional, 119–120
    safety of, 120–121, 120b
  The Joint Commission metrics
    for, 117–118
  triage in, 123–124, 124t
  triage reception area in, 120–121
  vulnerable populations in, 118
Emergency management plan, 149
Emergency medical technicians, 119
Emergency medicine physician, 119
Emergency nurse
  communication by, 123
  core competencies of, 122–123
  description of, 119–120
  health teaching by, 125
  priority setting by, 122
Emergency Nurses Association, 124

Emergency nursing
  certifications for, 120t, 123
  core competencies of, 122–123
  principles of, 123–127
  scope of, 122–123
  training for, 120t, 123
Emergency operations center, 154
Emergency preparedness and
    response
  goal of, 151
  mass casualty triage, 151–153
  nursing's role in, 157
Emergency preparedness plan
  activation of, 153
  notification of, 153
  personal, 155
  The Joint Commission mandate
    for, 150
Emergency Severity Index, 124
Emergent surgery, 232t
Emergent triage, 124
Emetogenic, 398
EMLA, 65
Emmetropia, 960, 960f
Emotional abuse, of older adults, 39
Emotional lability, 934
Empagliflozin, 1292b–1293b
Emphysema, 83
  incidence of, 573
  pathophysiology of, 572–573,
    572f
  prevalence of, 573
Empyema, 604
EMR. See Electronic medical record
EMTs. See Emergency medical
    technicians
Enbrel. See Etanercept
Encephalitis, 883–884, 884b
End of life. See also Death; Dying
  advance directives for, 104–115
  agitation at, 111
  delirium at, 111
  grieving at, 112–114
  nausea and vomiting at, 111
  overview of, 103–104
  pain management during,
    108–109
  planning for, 104–115
  in prisoners, 106b
  psychosocial needs at, 111–112
  religious beliefs, 112t
  respiratory distress at, 110
  seizure management at, 111
  spiritual assessment at, 112–113
  spirituality during, 108
  symptom management at, 109
End stoma, 1132
Endocervical curettage, 1470
Endocrine disorders
  diabetes insipidus, 1250–1251,
    1250b
  hyperpituitarism, 1247–1250,
    1247f, 1248b
  hypopituitarism, 1245–1247,
    1246b

Endocrine disorders (Continued)
  psychosocial assessment of, 1242
  syndrome of inappropriate
    antidiuretic hormone,
    1251–1253, 1252t
Endocrine system
  adrenal glands, 1237–1238
  age-related changes in, 1240,
    1241b
  assays of, 1243
  assessment of, 1240–1243
  description of, 1234–1235
  diagnostic assessment of,
    1242–1243
  elimination affected by, 1241
  functions of, 1235
  genetic testing of, 1243
  glands of, 1234–1235, 1235f
  history-taking, 1240–1241
  hormones of, 1235t
  hypothalamus. See Hypothalamus
  imaging assessment of, 1243
  inspection of, 1241–1242
  laboratory assessment of,
    1242–1243, 1243b
  needle biopsy of, 1243
  in older adults, 1240, 1241b
  pancreas. See Pancreas
  parathyroid glands. See
    Parathyroid glands
  physical assessment of, 1241–1242
  pituitary gland. See Pituitary
    gland
  provocative testing of, 1243
  psychosocial assessment of, 1242
  suppression testing of, 1243
  thyroid gland. See Thyroid gland
  urine tests, 1243, 1243b
Endogenous osteomyelitis, 1022
Endolymph, 986
Endometrial biopsy, 1437–1438,
    1466
Endometrial cancer, 1465–1467,
    1465t, 1466b
Endorphins, 48
Endoscopes, 254, 255f
Endoscopic retrograde
    cholangiopancreatography
  acute pancreatitis diagnosis using,
    1194, 1199, 1201
  chronic pancreatitis diagnosis
    using, 1203
  description of, 1071, 1175
  pancreatic cancer evaluations,
    1206
Endoscopic sclerotherapy, 1177
Endoscopic ultrasound, for gastric
    cancer, 1116
Endoscopic variceal ligation, 1177
Endoscopy
  carpal tunnel release, 1058–1059
  definition of, 1070
  follow-up care for, 526
  gastroesophageal reflux disease
    treated with, 1091

Endoscopy (Continued)
  gastrointestinal system
    assessments using, 1070
  hemorrhage treated with, 1177
  pancreatic necrosectomy, 1204
  patient preparation for, 525
  procedure for, 525
  reproductive system assessments,
    1436–1437
  respiratory system assessment
    using, 524–526
  small bowel capsule, 1071–1072
  upper, 1089
  upper gastrointestinal bleeding
    treated with, 1113
Endothelin, 694
Endothelin-receptor agonists, 585
Endotoxins, 414
Endotracheal intubation
  description of, 561
  nursing care for, 629–630
  preparation for, 629
Endotracheal tube, 273
  complications of, 630
  description of, 628–629
  dislodgement of, 538, 629–630
  extubation of, 635–636
  obstruction of, 537–538
  placement of, 537, 628, 629f
  stabilization of, 629
Endovascular stent grafts, 739
Endoventricular circular patch
    cardioplasty, 702
ENDS. See Electronic nicotine
    delivery systems
End-stage kidney disease
  acute kidney injury progression
    to, 1398
  chronic kidney disease progression
    to, 1398–1399
  description of, 1286, 1379
  features of, 1403b
  treatment of, 1390
End-tidal carbon monoxide
    monitoring, 625
Enema, preoperative, 242
Energy balance, 1211
Enophthalmos, 963
Entacapone, 870
Entamoeba histolytica, 1165
Entecavir, 1185t
Enterostomal feeding tubes,
    1220–1221
Enteroviruses, 883
Enucleation, 982
Environmental emergencies
  altitude-related illnesses, 145–146,
    145b–146b
  drowning, 147, 147b
  frostbite, 144–145, 144b, 144f
  heat exhaustion, 133–134
  heat stroke, 133–135, 134b–135b
  hypothermia, 142–144, 143b
  lightning injuries, 141–142,
    141b

Environmental emergencies
  (Continued)
  snakebites, 135–137, 136b,
    136f–137f, 136t, 138t–140t
  spider bites, 136–137, 137b, 137f,
    138t–140t
  stings, 137, 137b, 137f, 138t–140t,
    141b
EOC. See Emergency operations
    center
Eosinophils
  function of, 797t
  in inflammation, 294
Epidermal growth factor, 1081
Epidermal growth factor/receptor
    inhibitors, 404t, 405, 549–550,
    1130
Epidermis
  age-related changes, 434b
  anatomy of, 432, 432f
  blood supply to, 432
  functions of, 433t
Epidural analgesia
  delivery of, 61, 61f
  patient-controlled, 55, 61
Epidural anesthesia, 261t, 262f, 275,
    275b
Epidural catheters, 226
Epidural hematoma, 226, 942, 942f,
    954
Epidural space, 225, 840
Epiglottis, 510, 510f
Epiglottitis, 491b
Epilepsy
  antiepileptic drugs for, 880
  definition of, 876
  health teaching for, 880b
Epinephrine, 1238
Epinephrine injectors, 363f, 364b,
    365
EpiPen, 363f
EpiPen Jr., 363f
Epistaxis, 557–558, 557b, 558f
Epithalamus, 840, 840f
Epitympanum, 984
Epoetin alfa, 310, 397, 402t
Epoprostenol, 585
EPR. See Electronic patient record
Epstein-Barr virus
  cancers associated with, 379t
  leukoplakia caused by, 1078–1079
Eptifibatide, 736–737
Equianalgesia, 58, 60t
Equilibrium testing, 849–850
ERCP. See Endoscopic retrograde
    cholangiopancreatography
Erectile dysfunction, 27, 1286,
    1484–1485, 1489–1490
Ergocalciferol, 1277–1278
Erlotinib, 589t
Eructation, 1089, 1193
Erythema migrans, 332
Erythrocyte(s), 290
  description of, 796
  growth pathway of, 797f

Erythrocyte count, 657
Erythrocyte sedimentation rate,
    320–321, 425
Erythrocyte-stimulating agents, 797
Erythroplakia, 548, 1079
Erythropoiesis, 797
Erythropoiesis-stimulating agents,
    397, 826
Erythropoietin, 290, 300t, 310,
    1327
Erythropoietin-stimulating agents,
    1410b
Eschar, 453, 466, 496f
Escharotomies, 484, 494–496, 496f
Escherichia coli
  diarrhea caused by, 1148t
  O157:H7, 427–428
Esophageal cancer
  description of, 1095
  physical assessment of, 1096
  risk factors for, 1095–1096
Esophageal disorders
  gastroesophageal reflux disease.
    See Gastroesophageal reflux
    disease
  tumors. See Esophageal tumors
Esophageal manometry, 1089
Esophageal speech, 552
Esophageal stricture, 1088, 1096
Esophageal tumors
  assessment of, 1096
  care coordination for, 1100–1101
  chemoradiation for, 1097
  chemotherapy for, 1097
  diagnostic assessment of, 1096
  features of, 1096b
  health care resources for,
    1100–1101
  history-taking for, 1096
  home care management for, 1100
  interventions for, 1097–1100,
    1099f
  nonsurgical management of,
    1097–1098
  nutrition therapy for, 1097
  pathophysiology of, 1095
  photodynamic therapy for,
    1098
  physical assessment of, 1096
  psychosocial assessment of,
    1096
  radiation therapy for, 1097
  self-management education for,
    1100
  squamous cell carcinoma, 1095
  surgical management of,
    1098–1100, 1099f
  swallowing therapy for, 1097
  targeted therapy for, 1097–1098
  transition management for,
    1100–1101
  wound management of, 1099
Esophageal ultrasound, 1096
Esophageal varices, 1170
Esophagectomy, 1098

Esophagitis, 347f
  reflux, 1087
Esophagogastroduodenoscopy
  cirrhosis evaluations using, 1175
  description of, 1089
  esophageal diverticula evaluations
    using, 1101
  esophageal tumor evaluations
    using, 1096
  gastric cancer diagnosed using,
    1116
  gastritis diagnosed using, 1105
  gastrointestinal uses of,
    1070–1071, 1071b, 1071f
  peptic ulcer disease diagnosed
    using, 1111
  sliding hernia evaluations using,
    1093
  upper gastrointestinal bleeding
    treated with, 1113
Esophagogastrostomy, 1098, 1099f
Esophagus
  anatomy of, 1062–1063, 1062f
  chemical injury to, 1101
  dilation of, 1098
  diverticula of, 1101
  functions of, 1087
  perforation of, 1101t
  trauma to, 1101–1102, 1101t
ESR. See Erythrocyte sedimentation
    rate
Essential hypertension, 721, 721t
Estrogen
  for male-to-female transgender
    patients, 1493–1494, 1493t,
    1497–1498, 1497t
  osteoblast stimulation by, 1006
Estrogen agonists/antagonists, 1021,
    1021b
ESWL. See Extracorporeal shock
    wave lithotripsy
Etanercept, 323b, 466b
Ethics
  attributes of, 9
  Code of, 9, 9t
  context of, 9
  definition of, 8–9
  in genetic testing, 81–82
  organizational, 9
  professional, 9
Ethmoid sinus, 509f
Ethnic minorities
  diabetes mellitus in, 1292b–1293b
  special needs of, 10
Euploid, 74
Euploidy, 373, 376–377
Eustachian tube, 509, 509f, 985,
    985f
Euthanasia, 114
Everolimus
  autoimmune diseases treated with,
    368–369
  immunosuppression uses of,
    302b
Eversion, 1010f

Evidence-based practice
  attributes of, 7
  context of, 7
  definition of, 6
  levels of evidence, 6, 6f
  scope of, 6–7
Evidence-based practice
    improvement, 7
Evisceration, wound, 277, 278f, 283,
    283b
Evoked potentials, 854–855
Ewing's sarcoma, 1025
Excisional biopsy, 445, 477
Excitability, 665
Exenatide, 1292b–1293b
Exercise
  aerobic, 32
  asthma managed with, 571
  by older adults, 31–32, 32f
  chronic obstructive pulmonary
    disease managed with, 579
  diabetes mellitus managed with,
    1300–1301, 1301b
  obesity treated with, 1228
  in osteoporosis prevention, 1020
  peripheral arterial disease
    managed with, 740
  swimming, 32
Exercise electrocardiography,
    659–660, 660f
Exercise testing
  for myocardial infarction, 774
  for peripheral arterial disease, 733
  for respiratory system assessment,
    524
  for valvular heart disease, 707
Exertional dyspnea, 695
Exertional heat stroke, 134, 135b
Exfoliative psoriasis, 464
Existential distress, 113
Exogenous osteomyelitis, 1022
Exophthalmos, 963, 1265, 1266f
Exotoxins, 414
Expedited partner therapy
  for chlamydia infection, 1512
  for gonorrhea, 1513
Exploratory laparotomy, 1125, 1146
Expressive aphasia, 938
Extended-care environment, 271
Extension, 1010f
External beam radiation therapy,
    388. See also Radiation therapy
  endometrial cancer treated with,
    1466–1467
  prostate cancer treated with, 1485
  testicular cancer treated with,
    1489
External disasters, 149–151
External ear, 984, 985f, 988
External fixator, 1043
External genitalia, 1428–1429
External hemorrhoids, 1139, 1140f
External otitis, 993–994, 993b, 994f
External trigeminal nerve stimulator,
    875

External urethral sphincter, 1327, 1327f
Extracellular fluid, 19, 160, 162, 164, 173, 188
Extracorporeal membrane oxygenation, 628
Extracorporeal shock wave lithotripsy, 1195, 1364
Extraocular muscles, 959, 959f, 960t, 964, 964f
Extravasation, 200b, 204, 217t–219t, 392–393
Extremity assessment, 652
Extremity pain, 651
Extrinsic factors, 798
Extubation, of endotracheal tube, 635–636
Eye(s). See also Vision
   age-related changes in, 961, 961b
   anatomy of, 957–959, 958f–959f
   blood vessels of, 959
   donation of, for corneal transplantation, 979
   electroretinography of, 967
   external structures of, 958–959, 959f
   extraocular muscles of, 959, 959f, 960t, 964, 964f
   fluorescein angiography of, 966–967
   foreign bodies in, 981
   function of, 960
   gonioscopy of, 967
   innervation of, 959
   lacerations to, 981–982
   layers of, 957–958, 958f
   muscles of, 959, 959f, 960t
   ophthalmoscopy evaluations, 966, 966f, 966t
   penetrating injuries to, 982
   refractive structures and media of, 958
   slit-lamp examination of, 965, 965f
   structure of, 957–959, 958f
   trauma to, 981–982
Eye disorders
   cataracts. See Cataract
   cornea
     abrasion of, 977
     infection of, 977
     opacities, 977–979, 978f
     ulceration of, 977
   glaucoma. See Glaucoma
   keratoconus, 977–979, 978f
   refractive errors, 960, 960f, 980–981
   retinal detachment, 979–980
   retinal holes, 979–980
   retinal tears, 979–980
Eye infections, 961–962, 962b
Eyedrops, 961–962, 962b, 966b, 971f
Eyelids
   anatomy of, 958, 959f
   eversion of, 435f
   laceration of, 981
Ezetimibe, 730

F
Face tent, 534–535, 534t
Facemasks
   nonrebreather, 532t, 533, 533f
   partial rebreather, 532–533, 532t, 533f
   simple, 532, 532t, 533f
FACES pain scale—revised, 50–52
Facial expression
   in myasthenia gravis, 917–918, 918f
   in Parkinson disease, 869, 869f
Facial nerve, 844t
Facial paralysis, 924–925
Facial trauma, 558–559
Facilitated diffusion, 162–163
Factor V Leiden, 619b
Factor VIII replacement, 831
Failed back surgery syndrome, 909
Failure to rescue, 8
Fall(s)
   definition of, 40–41
   home modifications for prevention of, 33, 33b
   in older adults, 33, 33b, 40–42
   preoperative assessment of, 236
   prevention of
     in alkalosis patients, 197
     description of, 33, 33b
     in emergency departments, 121
   risk factors for, 41b
   toileting-related, 41
Fallophobia, 33
Fallopian tubes, 1429
Familial adenomatous polyposis, 1065, 1126, 1127b, 1128
Familial clustering, 80
Family caregivers, 866, 866b
Family-centered care, 2
Fanconi's anemia, 815
Fasciculations, 919
Fasciotomies, 484, 738, 1044–1045
Fasting blood glucose, 1281f
Fasting plasma glucose, 1289
Fat emboli, 617
Fat embolism syndrome, 1034, 1034b
Fat malabsorption, 1202–1203
Fatigue
   in anemia, 802
   assessment of, 90
   in chronic kidney disease, 1409–1410
   definition of, 650
   in heart failure, 702
   hepatitis as cause of, 1184
   in leukemia, 825–826
   in pancreatic cancer, 1206
   in systemic lupus erythematosus, 327
   in tuberculosis, 610
Fatigue fracture, 1032
Fatty liver, 1185–1186
Fc fragment, 297, 297f

Fear, preoperative, 237
Febrile transfusion reaction, 835
Febuxostat, 331–332
Fecal fats, 1068–1070, 1141
Fecal immunochemical test, 1068
Fecal impaction, 1125, 1126b
Fecal incontinence, 18
Fecal microbiota transplantation, 428
Fecal occult blood test, 1068, 1128–1129, 1128b
Federal Emergency Management Agency, 153
Feeding tubes, 552–553. See also Endotracheal tube
Felty's syndrome, 321
FEMA. See Federal Emergency Management Agency
Female reproductive system
   anatomy of, 1428–1430, 1429f–1430f
   breasts, 1429–1430
   external genitalia, 1428–1429
   internal genitalia, 1429, 1429f
   in older adults, 1431b
   pelvic examination, 1433
   physical assessment of, 1433
   structure of, 1428–1430
Female-to-male transgender patients
   definition of, 1493–1494, 1493t
   drug therapy for, 1498
   masculinizing surgeries for, 1500–1501
   phalloplasty for, 1501
Femoral aneurysms, 740
Femoral fractures, 1048
Femoral hernia, 1137, 1137f
Fenoldopam, 783b
Fentanyl (Fentora)
   equianalgesic dosing of, 60t
   transdermal delivery of, 60, 60b
Ferumoxytol, 815–816
Fetal hemoglobin, 808, 811
Fetor hepaticus, 1173
Fever
   antipyretic drugs for, 426
   cooling methods for, 426
   dehydration and, 168–169
   as infection sign, 424b, 425–426
   interventions for, 425–426
Fiberglass cast, 1039, 1039f
Fibrin clot, 798–799
Fibrinogen, 796, 798t
Fibrinolysis, 800f
Fibrinolytic system, 15
Fibrinolytics, 777–778, 778t
   acute arterial occlusions treated with, 738
   anticoagulant action of, 801
   injury prevention in patients using, 623b
   mechanism of action, 801
   pulmonary embolism treated with, 621b
   stroke treated with, 935

Fibrin-stabilizing factor, 798t
Fibroadenoma, 1455, 1455t
Fibrocystic breast condition, 1455–1456, 1455t
Fibroids, 1459–1460
Fibromyalgia syndrome, 333–334
Fibrosarcoma, 1025
Fibrosis, 1441
Fibular fracture, 1048–1049
Fidelity, 9
Field block, 261f, 261t
"Fight or flight" mechanism, 18, 46–47, 1238
Filgrastim, 402t
Filtration
   definition of, 161
   diagram of, 161f
   in fluid balance, 161–162, 161f–162f
FIM. See Functional Independence Measure
Financial abuse, of older adults, 39
Finasteride, 1498
Fingolimod, 891
Fire, 150b
Fire safety, 252
Fire triangle, 252, 254f
First aid
   for drowning, 147
   for frostbite, 144
   for heat stroke, 134
   for hypothermia, 143
   for lightning injury, 142
First heart sound, 654
First-degree frostbite, 144
Fissures, 438f
Fistulae
   anal, 1165
   in Crohn's disease, 1158, 1158f, 1160, 1160b
   skin barriers around, 1161f
   in ulcerative colitis, 1151t, 1158
   after Whipple procedure, 1208
Flaccid bladder, 97–98, 98t
Flaccid paralysis, 933, 938
Flail chest, 637, 637f
Flash burns, 488
Flat bones, 1005
Flatulence, 1089, 1193
Flexion, 1010f
Fludrocortisone, 1255b
Fluid(s)
   composition of, 161
   description of, 19, 160
   electrolyte composition of, 173f
   extracellular, 19, 160, 162, 164
   functions of, 160–161
   intake regulation, 164, 165t
   interstitial, 160
   intracellular, 19, 160, 162, 164
   loss of, 164–165, 165t
   pH, 185–186
Fluid balance
   age-related changes in, 165b
   aldosterone regulation of, 165

Fluid balance (Continued)
    anatomy of, 160–164
    antidiuretic hormone regulation of, 165–166
    assessment of, 20
    definition of, 19
    diffusion in, 162–163, 162f
    filtration in, 161–162, 161f–162f
    homeostatic mechanisms in, 160
    hormonal regulation of, 165–166
    laboratory testing for, 20
    natriuretic peptide regulation by, 166
    osmosis in, 163–164, 163f
    physiology of, 160–164
    postoperative, 276
    promotion of, 20
    renin-angiotensin II pathway in, 166–167, 166f
    scope of, 19
Fluid compartments
    dehydration effects on, 168f
    fluid overload effects on, 171f
Fluid deficit, 20
Fluid excess, 20
Fluid imbalances
    after coronary artery bypass grafting, 787
    dehydration. See Dehydration
    diarrhea caused by, 18
    fluid shift as cause of, 485
    interventions for, 20
    parenteral nutrition as cause of, 1224
    physiologic consequences of, 20
    prevention of, 20
    risk factors for, 19
    total enteral nutrition as cause of, 1222–1223
    types of, 20t
Fluid overload
    assessment of, 171
    cardiac complications during, 171f
    description of, 20
    drug therapy for, 172
    features of, 172b
    fluid compartment changes associated with, 171f
    hypervolemia, 171
    interventions for, 171–172
    nutrition therapy for, 172
    pathophysiology of, 167t, 171
    in pulmonary edema, 172b
    respiratory complications during, 171f
    safety considerations in, 172
    in syndrome of inappropriate antidiuretic hormone, 1252
    total enteral nutrition as cause of, 1222
Fluid remobilization, 485
Fluid replacement
    dehydration treated with, 169–170, 170t

Fluid replacement (Continued)
    hyperglycemic-hyperosmolar state treated with, 1315
    kidney trauma treated with, 1387
Fluid restriction
    by older adults, 31b
    in chronic kidney disease, 1405
    syndrome of inappropriate antidiuretic hormone treated with, 1252
Fluid resuscitation
    burn injury treated with, 494–495, 495b
    intravenous therapy for, 758–759
Fluid retention
    in Cushing's disease, 1258
    weight gain as sign of, 172
Fluid volume management
    in chronic kidney disease, 1405, 1405b
    in cirrhosis, 1175–1177
Fluorescein angiography, 966–967
Fluorescent antinuclear antibody test, 320
Fluorescent treponemal antibody absorption test, 1509
Fluoroscopy, 527
5-Fluorouracil
    pancreatic cancer treated with, 1206–1207
    skin cancer treated with, 477
Flushing of catheters, 214–215
Fluticasone, 569b–570b
Focal brain injury, 941
FOCUS-Plan-Do-Study-Act model, 7
Folic acid deficiency anemia, 814–816, 814t
Follicle-stimulating hormone
    deficiency of, 1246, 1246b
    description of, 1237t, 1435
    overproduction of, 1248b
Follicular carcinoma, 1275
Folliculitis, 466, 467b
Food allergy, 234–235, 1212b
Foot care
    in diabetes mellitus, 1304–1307, 1305f–1306f, 1306b–1307b
    in peripheral vascular disease, 737b
Foot disorders
    description of, 1028–1029, 1028f, 1029t
    diabetes mellitus-related, 1304–1307, 1305f–1306f, 1306b
Foot drop, 267b
Foot fracture, 1038
Footwear, for diabetic patients, 1306
Forebrain, 840
Foreign bodies
    in ear, 994–995, 994b, 994f
    in eye, 981
Forensic nurse examiners, 118
Fosphenytoin, 879

Fourth-degree frostbite, 144
Fovea centralis, 958
Fraction of inspired oxygen, 529, 532–533, 618, 632
Fractional flow reserve, 659
Fractures
    ankle, 1043, 1049
    assessment of, 1035–1037
    bone reduction for, 1038
    care coordination for, 1045–1046
    casts for, 1039–1040, 1039f, 1045b
    chest, 1049–1050
    classification of, 1032
    closed, 1032, 1032f
    closed reduction and immobilization of, 1038–1040
    Colles', 1046, 1046f, 1057
    complete, 1032
    complications of, 1032–1035
        acute compartment syndrome, 1033–1034, 1034b, 1044–1045, 1044b
        avascular necrosis, 1035
        chronic, 1035
        complex regional pain syndrome, 1035, 1041–1042
        delayed union, 1035
        fat embolism syndrome, 1034, 1034b
        hemorrhagic shock, 1034
        hypovolemic shock, 1034
        infection, 1035, 1045
        venous thromboembolism, 1034–1035
    compound, 1032
    compression, 1032
    definition of, 1032
    delayed union of, 1035
    distal radius, 1046–1047, 1046f
    drug therapy for, 1041
    emergency care for, 1037–1038, 1038b
    etiology of, 1035
    fatigue, 1032
    femoral, 1048
    fibular, 1048–1049
    fragility, 1032
    genetic risks of, 1035
    healing stages for, 1032, 1033f
    health care resources for, 1045–1046
    health promotion and maintenance for, 1035
    hip, 1035b, 1047–1049, 1047f–1048f, 1049b
    history-taking for, 1035–1036
    home care management of, 1045
    humeral shaft, 1046
    imaging assessment of, 1037
    incidence of, 1035
    incomplete, 1032
    laboratory assessment of, 1037

Fractures (Continued)
    lower-extremity, 1047–1049, 1047f–1048f
    mandibular, 558
    metacarpal, 1047
    mobility promotion in, 1043–1044
    nasal, 556–557, 556f
    neurovascular compromise caused by
        interventions for, 1044–1045
        status assessments for prevention of, 1036b–1037b, 1044
    nonsurgical management of, 1038–1042
    nonunion of, 1035, 1043
    open, 1032, 1032f
    open reduction and internal fixation of, 1042–1043, 1042f, 1048
    orthopedic boots/shoes for, 1038, 1038f
    osteoporosis as risk factor for, 1016, 1018
    pain management of, 1037–1043
    pathologic, 1032
    pathophysiology of, 1032–1035
    pelvic, 1036, 1049–1050
    phalangeal, 1047, 1049
    physical assessment of, 1036
    physical therapy for, 1041
    prevalence of, 1035
    proximal femur, 1035b
    proximal humerus, 1046
    psychosocial assessment of, 1036–1037
    rib, 636–637
    self-management education for, 1045
    signs and symptoms of, 1036
    simple, 1032
    splints for, 1038
    stress, 1032
    surgical management of, 1042–1043, 1042f
    swelling associated with, 1036b
    tibial, 1048–1049
    traction for, 1040–1041, 1040t, 1041b, 1041f
    transition management for, 1045–1046
    types of, 1032, 1032f
    upper-extremity, 1046–1047, 1046f
    vertebral compression, 1036, 1050
    weight-bearing, 1050
Fragility fracture, 1032
Fremitus, 518–519, 587
Frequency (hearing), 990
Fresh frozen plasma, 832t, 835
Frontal lobe, 841t, 860
Frontal sinus, 509f
Frostbite, 144–145, 144b, 144f
Fructosamine, 1289

FSH. *See* Follicle-stimulating hormone
Full-body lift, 93, 95*f*
Full-thickness wound
    definition of, 27
    physiologic consequences of, 28
Fulmer SPICES framework, 40
Fulminant hepatitis, 1182
Functional ability, 23
    assessment of, 92
    definition of, 92
    rehabilitation for improving, 96
Functional electrical stimulation, for spinal cord injury, 902
Functional incontinence, 1344
Functional Independence Measure, 92
Functional magnetic resonance imaging, 853
Fungal infections
    antifungal agents for, 470
    cystitis caused by, 1356
    in HIV-infected patients, 346–347
    of skin, 467*b*, 468
    skin cultures for, 444
    treatment of, 1078
Furanocoumarins, 731*b*
Furosemide, 699, 1276
Furuncles, 466, 466*f*, 467*b*

G
Gabapentin, 63–64, 925
Gabapentinoids, 63–64
Gadolinium contrast, 852*b*
GAGs. *See* Glycosaminoglycans
Gait
    assessment of, 1009
    for crutches, 1044
    in Parkinson disease, 871
    testing of, 849–850
Gait training, 95–96, 95*b*, 95*f*
Galactorrhea, 1247–1248
Gallbladder
    anatomy of, 1063–1064, 1063*f*
    cholecystitis of. *See* Cholecystitis
Gallium scan, 1011
Gallops, 654
Gallstones
    acute pancreatitis caused by, 1201
    description of, 1191. *See also* Cholecystitis
    extracorporeal shock wave lithotripsy for, 1195
    sites of, 1192*f*
Gamma globulins, 298
Gamma knife, for brain tumors, 952, 952*f*
Gamma rays, 387, 387*f*
Gamma-glutamyl transpeptidase, 1174
Ganglion, 1028
Gardasil, 1469, 1511
Gas bloat syndrome, 1094–1095

Gas exchange
    assessment of, 21, 364–365
    breathing for, 509
    chronic obstructive pulmonary disease effects on, 21, 21*f*
    decreased, 21, 22*f*
    definition of, 20–21
    failure of, 625
    hematologic system in, 796*f*
    in human immunodeficiency virus infection, 353
    in hypothyroidism, 1272–1273
    improvement of, 195
    interventions for, 21
    patient positioning for, 1080
    in pneumonia, 604
    postoperative, 280–281, 1082*b*
    scope of, 21
Gastrectomy
    dumping syndrome secondary to, 1117–1119, 1118*t*
    gastric cancer treated with, 1117, 1117*f*
    in Whipple procedure, 1207, 1207*f*
Gastric bypass, 1229, 1230*f*
Gastric cancer
    advanced, 1116, 1116*b*
    assessment of, 1116
    care coordination for, 1118–1119
    chemotherapy for, 1116
    early, 1116, 1116*b*
    esophagogastroduodenoscopy diagnosis of, 1116
    etiology of, 1115
    gastrectomy for, 1117, 1117*f*
    genetic risk of, 1115
    health care resources for, 1119
    health promotion and maintenance for, 1116
    home care management of, 1119
    incidence of, 1115–1116
    interventions for, 1116–1118
    nonsurgical management of, 1116
    pathophysiology of, 1115–1116
    prevalence of, 1115–1116
    radiation therapy for, 1116
    self-management education for, 1119
    surgical management of, 1116–1118, 1117*f*
    transition management for, 1118–1119
Gastric distention, 1088
Gastric emptying, 1089, 1107
Gastric outlet obstruction, 1109
Gastric ulcers, 1107–1110, 1108*f*
Gastritis
    acute, 1104–1105, 1105*b*
    assessment of, 1105
    atrophic, 1104, 1115
    chronic, 1104–1105, 1105*b*
    complementary and integrative health for, 1107*t*
    definition of, 1103
    dietary prevention of, 1104–1105

Gastritis *(Continued)*
    esophagogastroduodenoscopy of, 1105
    etiology of, 1104
    features of, 1105*b*
    genetic risk of, 1104
    health promotion and maintenance of, 1104–1105
    Helicobacter pylori as cause of, 1104
    H_2-receptor antagonists for, 1105
    interventions for, 1105–1107, 1106*b*–1107*b*
    nonsteroidal anti-inflammatory drugs as cause of, 1104–1105
    pathophysiology of, 1103–1104
    prevention of, 1104*b*
    types of, 1104
Gastroenteritis, 1148–1150, 1148*t*, 1149*b*–1150*b*
Gastroesophageal reflux, 1087
Gastroesophageal reflux disease
    antacids for, 1090–1091
    assessment of, 1088–1089
    asthma triggered by, 565
    care coordination for, 1091–1092
    definition of, 1087
    diagnostic assessment of, 1089
    drug therapy for, 1090–1091
    dysphagia caused by, 1089
    endoscopic therapy for, 1091
    features of, 1088*b*
    health promotion and maintenance, 1088
    hiatal hernia and, 1088
    histamine receptor antagonists for, 1091
    interventions for, 1090–1091
    laparoscopic Nissen fundoplication for, 1091
    lifestyle changes for, 1090, 1090*b*
    lower esophageal sphincter in, 1088, 1088*t*
    nonsurgical management of, 1090–1091
    nutrition therapy for, 1090
    obesity and, 1090
    in older adults, 1089*b*
    pathophysiology of, 1087–1088
    physical assessment of, 1088–1089
    proton pump inhibitors for, 1090*b*, 1091
    reflux esophagitis secondary to, 1087
    risk factors for, 1088
    signs and symptoms of, 1088–1089
    Stretta procedure for, 1091, 1091*b*
    surgical management of, 1091
    transition management for, 1091–1092
Gastrointestinal bleeding
    in Cushing's disease, 1259
    lower, 1156, 1156*b*
    upper. *See* Upper gastrointestinal bleeding

Gastrointestinal system
    age-related changes in, 1064, 1064*b*
    anatomy of, 1061–1064
    assessment of, 90–91, 90*t*, 1065–1073
    burn injury effects on, 486, 492
    colonoscopy of, 1072–1073
    computed tomography of, 1070
    current health problems assessments, 1066
    diagnostic assessment of, 1068–1073, 1069*b*
    endoscopic retrograde cholangiopancreatography of, 1071
    endoscopy of, 1070
    esophagogastroduodenoscopy of, 1070–1071, 1071*b*, 1071*f*
    esophagus. *See* Esophagus
    family history assessments, 1066
    functions of, 1062–1064
    gallbladder, 1063–1064, 1063*f*
    history-taking, 1065–1066, 1065*b*
    imaging assessment of, 1070
    inspection of, 1067
    laboratory assessment of, 1068–1070, 1069*b*
    large intestine, 1064
    liver, 1063–1064, 1063*f*
    liver-spleen scan, 1073
    magnetic resonance imaging of, 1070
    nutrition assessments, 1213*b*
    nutrition history, 1065–1066
    oral cavity. *See* Oral cavity
    palpation of, 1067–1068
    pancreas. *See* Pancreas
    percussion of, 1067
    physical assessment of, 1066–1068
    postoperative assessment of, 276–277
    psychosocial assessment of, 1068
    radiographic assessments of, 1070
    sigmoidoscopy of, 1073
    small bowel capsule endoscopy of, 1071–1072
    small intestine, 1064
    stomach. *See* Stomach
    stool tests, 1068–1070
    structure of, 1061–1062, 1062*f*
    ultrasonography of, 1073
    urine tests, 1068
Gastrointestinal tract
    anatomy of, 1061
    functions of, 1061–1062
    infection transmission, 415
    lumen of, 1061–1062
    tumors of, 385
Gastrojejunostomy, 1207
Gastroparesis, 1285
Gastrostomy, 1221
Gaviscon, 1091

GCS. *See* Glasgow Coma Scale
G-CSF. *See* Granulocyte colony-stimulating factor
Gel phenomenon, 319
Gender dysphoria, 1493, 1493*t*
Gender identity, 11*t*, 123*b*, 1492–1493, 1493*t*
Gender reassignment surgery
  definition of, 1493*t*, 1499
  for male-to-female patients, 1499–1500
Genderqueer, 1493*t*
Gene(s)
  alleles, 74–75, 75*f*, 79
  in chromosomes, 72
  composition of, 72
  definition of, 72
  function of, 74–76
  genotype of, 76
  penetrance of, 79
  phenotype of, 75–76
  protein synthesis, 76
  purpose of, 71–72
  structure of, 74–76
  susceptibility, 76
  variations in, 76–77
Gene expression, 76
Gene mutations, 76–77
Gene products, 76
Gene sequences, 76
Gene therapy
  cystic fibrosis treated with, 583
  heart failure treated with, 701
General anesthesia, 257–260, 258*t*–259*t*, 260*b*, 275
General appearance, 651
Generalized osteoporosis, 1016
Generalized peritonitis, 1145
Generalized seizures, 876
Genetic counseling
  communication during, 82–83
  confidentiality of, 81, 83
  description of, 81
  medical-surgical nurse's role in, 82–83
  patient advocacy and support during, 83
  privacy of, 83
  steps for, 82*b*
Genetic disorders, 72
Genetic testing
  benefits of, 80–81
  for cancer, 380–382
  ethical issues in, 81–82
  purpose of, 80, 81*t*
  risks of, 80–81
  steps for, 82*b*
Genetics
  competencies in, 72, 72*t*
  genes. *See* Gene(s)
  genomics versus, 71
  inheritance patterns
    autosomal dominant, 78–79, 78*t*
    autosomal recessive, 78*t*, 79, 79*f*

Genetics (*Continued*)
    complex, 78*t*, 80
    overview of, 77–80
    pedigree, 77–78, 78*f*–79*f*
    sex-linked recessive, 78*t*, 79–80, 80*f*
  purpose of, 71
Genital herpes, 1506–1508, 1507*b*
Genital warts. *See* Condylomata acuminata
Genitourinary system
  nutrition assessments, 1213*b*
  trauma to, 1387*b*
Genome, 72
Genomics, 71
Genotype, 76
Gentamicin sulfate, 501*b*
Genu valgum, 1010
Genu varum, 1010
GER. *See* Gastroesophageal reflux
GERD. *See* Gastroesophageal reflux disease
Geriatric Depression Scale, 850–851
Geriatric Depression Scale—Short form, 36–37, 37*f*
Geriatric failure to thrive, 31
Geriatric syndromes
  decreased mobility, 31–32
  decreased nutrition and hydration, 30–31
  definition of, 29–30
Germline mutations, 76
GFTT. *See* Geriatric failure to thrive
Ghrelin, 1225
Giant cell tumor, 1025
Giardia lamblia, 1165
Giardiasis, 1165–1166
Gigantism, 1006
Ginkgo biloba, 801–802
Glans penis, 1430
Glasgow Coma Scale
  decreases in, 851*b*
  description of, 130, 850
  illustration of, 850*f*
Glass bottles, for infusion therapy, 208
Glatiramer acetate, 891, 891*b*
Glaucoma
  assessment of, 972–974
  carbonic anhydrase inhibitors for, 974–975
  care coordination for, 975–976
  concept map for, 972*f*–973*f*
  definition of, 972
  drug therapy for, 26, 974–975
  etiology of, 972
  eye injury as risk factor for, 961
  eyedrops for, 966*b*, 975*f*
  genetic risks of, 972
  health care resources for, 976
  health promotion and maintenance for, 972
  home care management of, 975

Glaucoma (*Continued*)
  incidence of, 972
  laser trabeculoplasty for, 975
  nonsurgical management of, 974–975
  pathophysiology of, 958, 962*t*, 972
  physical assessment of, 972–974
  prevalence of, 972
  primary angle-closure, 972
  primary open-angle, 972
  self-management education for, 975–976
  signs and symptoms of, 972–974
  surgical management of, 975
  trabeculectomy for, 975
  transition management for, 975–976
  types of, 962*t*, 972
Glimepiride, 1292*b*–1293*b*
Glipizide, 1292*b*–1293*b*
Global aphasia, 938
Globulins, 796
Glomerular filtration, 1324
Glomerular filtration rate
  in acute kidney injury, 1391
  age-related declines in, 1328, 1328*b*
  creatinine clearance used to estimate, 1335–1336
  description of, 1324
  in nephrotic syndrome, 1379
Glomerulonephritis
  acute, 1376–1378, 1376*t*
  chronic, 1378
  rapidly progressive, 1377–1378
Glomerulus
  anatomy of, 1323, 1323*f*
  capillary wall, 1324*f*
Glossectomy, 1082
Glossitis, 814, 815*f*
Glossopharyngeal nerve, 844*t*
Glottis, 510, 510*f*
Gloves, 418*b*, 419*t*
Gloving, 256, 257*f*
Glucagon, 1240, 1281
Glucagon-like peptide-1, 1293
Glucocorticoids
  Crohn's disease treated with, 1160
  Cushing's disease treated with, 1258–1259
  endogenous, 1237–1238, 1238*t*
  functions of, 1238*t*
  production of, 1237–1238
  release of, 1238
  rheumatoid arthritis treated with, 322–323
  ulcerative colitis treated with, 1152–1153
Gluconeogenesis, 1282
Glucosamine, 308–309, 309*b*
Glucose
  blood. *See* Blood glucose
  counterregulatory hormone effects on, 1282
  fasting blood, 1281*f*, 1282
  fasting plasma, 1289

Glucose (*Continued*)
  function of, 1281
  incomplete breakdown of, 188
Glucose regulation
  definition of, 1280–1281
  insulin for, 1282
  poor, 1283
Glucose-6-phosphate dehydrogenase deficiency anemia, 814*t*, 815–816
Glutamate, 864
Gluten-free diet, 1164
Glyburide, 1292*b*–1293*b*
Glycocalyx, 421
Glycogenesis, 1282
Glycogenolysis, 1282
Glycoprotein IIb/IIIa inhibitors, 776
Glycosaminoglycans, 1271
Glycosylated hemoglobin, 1243, 1289, 1289*t*, 1291
GM-CSF. *See* Granulocyte-macrophage colony-stimulating factor
Goiter, 1265, 1266*f*, 1266*t*, 1271
Goldmann applanation tonometer, 965, 965*f*
Golimumab, 323*b*, 333
Gonadotropin-releasing hormone agonists, 1498
Gonadotropins
  deficiency of, 1246*b*
  description of, 1246
  overproduction of, 1248*b*
Gonads, 1237
Goniometer, 1010
Gonorrhea, 1512–1514, 1513*f*
Good death, 103, 113
Gout, 330–332, 331*f*
Gowning, 256, 257*f*
gp120, 338
Graduated compression stockings
  varicose veins treated with, 748
  venous insufficiency treated with, 747*b*
Graft occlusion, 736*b*
Graft-versus-host-disease
  after hematopoietic stem cell transplantation, 824–825, 825*f*
  transfusion-associated, 836
Granulocyte colony-stimulating factor, 293, 300*t*
Granulocyte-macrophage colony-stimulating factor, 293, 300*t*
Granulocytes, 292–293
Granulomatous thyroiditis, 1275
Graves' disease, 1265, 1267, 1270
Gray, 387–388
Gray matter, 840
Grief/grieving
  in colorectal cancer patients, 1132–1133
  definition of, 112
  at end of life, 112–114

Grommet, 992, 992f
Groshong valve, 205
Ground substance, 431–432
Group homes, 88
Growth factors
    definition of, 1081
    in oral cancer treatment, 1081
    types of, 300t
Growth hormone
    deficiency of, 1246, 1246b
    description of, 1006, 1237t
    overproduction of, 1247, 1247f, 1248b
Guaiac fecal occult blood test, 1068
Guanylate cyclase stimulators, for pulmonary arterial hypertension, 585
Guardian, 36
Guillain-Barré syndrome
    assessment of, 914
    care coordination for, 916–917
    clinical features of, 914b
    cranial nerve involvement in, 914
    definition of, 912
    description of, 849
    diagnostic assessment of, 914
    electrophysiologic studies of, 914
    etiology of, 913–914
    health care resources for, 917
    home care management of, 916–917
    incidence of, 914
    interventions for, 914–916
    intravenous immunoglobulin for, 915
    mobility manifestations of, 914, 914b, 916
    pathophysiology of, 912–914
    physical assessment of, 914
    plasmapheresis for, 914–915, 915b
    prevalence of, 914
    signs and symptoms of, 914
    stages of, 913, 916b
    transition management of, 916–917
Gum chewing, in postoperative period, 286
Gynecologic disorders
    cervical cancer, 1469–1470, 1470b
    endometrial cancer, 1465–1467, 1465t, 1466b
    ovarian cancer, 1467–1469, 1467t
    overview of, 1459
    pelvic organ prolapse, 1464–1465, 1464f
    toxic shock syndrome, 1471, 1471b
    uterine leiomyoma. See Uterine leiomyoma
    vulvovaginitis, 1470–1471, 1471b
Gynecomastia, 407, 1173, 1247, 1386, 1441

H
Habit training, for urinary incontinence, 1351, 1351b

HACE. See High-altitude cerebral edema
HAD. See High-altitude disease
Hageman factor, 798t
Hair
    age-related changes, 434b
    anatomy of, 432
    assessment of, 441
    growth of, 432
    preoperative removal of, 242, 243f
Half-life, 58–59
Halitosis, 1096
Hallux valgus, 1028, 1028f, 1304
Halo fixator device, 899, 899b
"Halo" sign, 946
Hammertoe, 1029, 1029f
Hand
    disorders of, 1028, 1028f
    Dupuytren's contracture of, 1028, 1028f
    ganglion of, 1028
    joints of, 1009, 1009f
Hand hygiene, 418, 418b
Hand strength, 848, 848f
Hand-off communication, 119–120, 317
Hand-off report, 271b
Handrails, 325, 325f
Hantavirus, 423
Hantavirus pulmonary syndrome, 423
HAPE. See High-altitude pulmonary edema
Hashimoto's disease, 1275
Hashimoto's thyroiditis, 1265
Haversian system, 1005, 1005f
Hazardous materials (HAZMAT) training, 150, 151f
HCOs. See Health care organizations
Head
    assessment of, 802
    cancer of. See Head and neck cancer
Head and neck cancer
    airway obstruction caused by, 549–553
    anxiety management in, 553
    aspiration prevention in, 553
    assessment of, 548–549
    biotherapy for, 549–550
    care coordination for, 554–555
    chemotherapy for, 549
    communication issues in, 550b, 555
    composite resections for, 552–553
    etiology of, 548
    health care resources for, 555
    history-taking for, 548
    home care management of, 554, 554b
    imaging assessment of, 548
    incidence of, 548
    interventions for, 549–553
    laboratory assessment of, 548

Head and neck cancer (Continued)
    metastasis of, 548
    neck dissection for, 550
    nonsurgical management of, 549–550
    nutrition alterations in, 552
    pain management in, 551–552
    pathophysiology of, 547–548
    prevalence of, 548
    psychosocial assessment of, 548
    psychosocial preparation for, 555
    radiation therapy for, 549
    salivary glands, 549
    self-esteem support in, 553–554
    self-management education of, 554–555
    signs and symptoms of, 548, 548t
    speech and language rehabilitation in, 552
    staging of, 548
    surgical management of, 550–553
    transition management for, 554–555
Headache
    medication overuse, 874
    migraine. See Migraine headaches
    rebound, 874
Health Canada, 1212
Health care disparities, 10–11, 11t
Health care organizations
    attributes of, 10
    context of, 10
    critical care access hospitals, 9
    definition of, 9
    scope of, 9–10
Health care workers, HIV transmission to, 343, 344f, 345b
Health care-associated infection
    biofilms and, 421
    definition of, 417
    in long-term care settings, 417
    risks for, 421
Health care-associated methicillin-resistant Staphylococcus aureus, 422, 422b
Health care-associated pneumonia, 599t–600t
Health Professions Education: A Bridge to Quality, 2
Health-enhancing behaviors, 30b
Health-protecting behaviors, 30b
Healthy People 2020
    description of, 694b, 695t
    health care disparities, 10, 11t
    heart disease, 722t
    lesbian, gay, bisexual, transgender, and queer population, 10, 1495
    medication assessments, 35
    nutrition, 1226t
    sexually transmitted infection objectives of, 1505, 1506t
    stroke, 722t
    syphilis objectives, 1505, 1506t

Hearing. See also Ear(s)
    age-related changes, 986, 987b
    assessment of, 986, 989–991, 1002
    audiometry assessments of, 990–991
    diagnostic assessment of, 990–991
    history-taking, 986–988
    psychosocial assessment of, 990
    voice test for, 989
Hearing aids
    assessment of, 987–988
    care of, 999b
    definition of, 999
    description of, 26, 27f
Hearing loss
    anxiety associated with, 1001
    assessment of, 997–998, 998b
    assistive devices for, 999
    care coordination for, 1001–1002
    causes of, 26
    clinical manifestations of, 998, 998b
    cochlear implantation for, 999
    communication in, 998b, 1001
    conductive, 989, 996–997, 997t
    family history of, 988
    genetic risk of, 988, 988b
    health care resources for, 1002
    health promotion and maintenance for, 997
    history-taking for, 997–998
    home care management of, 1001
    imaging assessment of, 998–1001
    incidence of, 997
    interventions for, 999–1001
    laboratory assessment of, 998
    in Ménière's disease, 996
    mixed conductive-sensorineural, 989, 996
    nonsurgical management of, 999–1001
    pathophysiology of, 996–997
    physical assessment of, 998
    prevalence of, 997
    psychosocial assessment of, 998
    self-management education for, 1002
    sensorineural, 989, 997, 997t
    stapedectomy for, 1000–1001, 1000f
    surgical management of, 999–1001
    totally implanted devices for, 1001
    transition management for, 1001–1002
    tuning fork tests for, 989–990, 998
    tympanoplasty for, 999–1000, 1000f
Heart. See also Cardiovascular system
    anatomy of, 642–644, 642f–643f
    blood flow in, 642
    conduction system of, 664–665, 665f
    coronary arterial system of, 643, 643f

Heart (Continued)
function of, 644–645
mechanical properties of, 645
structure of, 642–644, 642f–643f
valves of, 642, 643f
Heart attack. See Cardiac arrest
Heart failure
activity schedule for, 704–705
advance directives in, 705
aldosterone antagonists for, 700
assessment of, 695–697
beta-blockers for, 700
cardiac resynchronization therapy for, 701
care coordination for, 703–705
in chronic kidney disease, 1401
in chronic obstructive pulmonary disease, 573–574
classification of, 692, 781–782, 782t
compensatory mechanisms for, 692–694, 693f
congestive, 692
continuous positive airway pressure for, 701
definition of, 691
diagnostic assessment of, 697
diastolic, 692, 701
digoxin for, 700
diuretics for, 699
drug therapy for, 697–701, 698t, 704–705, 705b
dyspnea in, 695
edema in, 696b
electrical cardioversion for, 680–681
etiology of, 694, 694t
fatigue in, 702
gas exchange in, 697
gene therapy for, 701
health care resources for, 705
heart transplantation for, 705
home care management of, 703
hyperpolarization-activated cyclic nucleotide-gated channel blocker for, 701
imaging assessment of, 697
incidence of, 694
infective endocarditis as cause of, 711
inotropic drugs for, 700
interventions for, 680–681
intra-aortic balloon pump for, 782
laboratory assessment of, 696–697
left-sided, 651, 692, 695–696, 780–782
nitrates for, 699
nonsurgical management of, 697–701, 698t
nutrition therapy for, 698–699, 705
in older adults, 694b

Heart failure (Continued)
partial left ventriculectomy for, 702
pathophysiology of, 691–694
prevalence of, 694
psychosocial assessment of, 696
pulmonary edema in, 702–703, 702b
re-hospitalization for, 704
right-sided, 651, 692, 694–695, 782
self-management education for, 703–705, 704t
staging of, 692
surgical management of, 701–702
sympathetic nervous system stimulation from, 692
systolic, 692
transition management for, 703–705
types of, 692
ventricular assist devices for, 701–702, 701f
Heart rate, 645, 670
Heart sounds, 654–655, 696, 773
Heart transplantation
cardiomyopathy treated with, 716–717, 717f
discharge planning for, 717
heart failure treated with, 705
operative procedures for, 716, 717f
postoperative care for, 716–717
preoperative care for, 716
rejection of, 716b
survival rates after, 717
Heart valve replacement, 709–710, 709f
Heat exhaustion, 133–134
Heat stroke, 133–135, 134b–135b
Heat-related illnesses
environmental factors, 133
heat exhaustion, 133–134
heat stroke, 133–135, 134b–135b
prevention of, 134b
risk factors for, 133
Heberden's nodes, 306, 306f
Height measurements, 1213–1215
Heimlich maneuver. See Abdominal thrust maneuver
Helicobacter pylori
drug therapy for, 1111–1112
gastric cancer risks associated with, 1115
gastritis caused by, 1104
in older adults, 1111b
peptic ulcers caused by, 1107, 1109, 1111–1112
Helicopters, 119f
Helper/inducer T-cells, 299, 797t
Hematemesis, 1105, 1108, 1170
Hematochezia, 1128
Hematocrit, 803, 810–811, 813
Hematogenous tuberculosis, 605–606

Hematologic disorders
anemia. See Anemia
autoimmune thrombocytopenic purpura, 830–831
hemophilia, 831, 832t
heparin-induced thrombocytopenia, 832
hereditary hemochromatosis, 817
idiopathic thrombocytopenic purpura, 830–831
leukemia. See Leukemia
lymphomas, 828–829, 829t
multiple myeloma, 829–830
polycythemia vera, 816–817, 817b
sickle cell disease. See Sickle cell disease
thrombotic thrombocytopenic purpura, 831
Hematologic system
age-related changes in, 800, 800b
anatomy of, 795–800
assessment of, 800–806
bone marrow, 795–796, 796f
current health problems that affect, 802
diagnostic assessment of, 803–806, 804b
drugs that affect, 801t
functions of, 808
in gas exchange, 796f
imaging assessment of, 806
laboratory assessment of, 803–806, 804b
in older adults, 800b
physical assessment of, 802–803
psychosocial assessment of, 803
Hematoma
epidural, 226, 942, 942f
subdural, 942–943, 942f
Hematopoiesis, 1005
Hematopoietic stem cell transplantation
aplastic anemia treated with, 816
bone marrow harvesting for, 823
chronic lymphoblastic leukemia treated with, 821
complications of, 824–825
conditioning regimen for, 823–824, 823f
cord blood harvesting, 823
engraftment of, 824
graft-versus-host-disease secondary to, 824–825, 825f
leukemia treated with, 822–825, 822t
myelodysplastic syndromes treated with, 817
peripheral blood stem cell harvesting, 823
sickle cell disease treated with, 812
stem cells for, 822–823
steps of, 823f
transplantation procedure for, 824
transplants, 822t
veno-occlusive disease secondary to, 825

Hematuria, 16, 803, 1303, 1341, 1358, 1361, 1482
Hemianopsia, 934, 934f
Hemiarthroplasty, 316, 1047, 1048b
Hemilaryngectomy, 551t
Hemiparesis, 933–934
Hemiplegia, 933–934
Hemoconcentration, 485, 1283
Hemodialysis
anticoagulation during, 1413
arteriovenous fistulas, 1413, 1414f–1415f, 1414t–1415t, 1415b
arteriovenous grafts, 1413, 1414f, 1414t–1415t, 1415b
arteriovenous shunt for, 1414f
cardiac events during, 1417
care after, 1416, 1416b
catheters for, 208, 1414t
complications of, 1416–1417
description of, 1397, 1411
dialyzers, 1412–1413, 1412f, 1417
hemofiltration versus, 1413f
home care management of, 1424
infectious disease transmission during, 1417
nursing care during, 1416
patient selection, 1411–1412
peritoneal dialysis versus, 1411t
procedure, 1412–1413, 1412f–1413f
self-management education for, 1424–1425
settings, 1412
subclavian vein catheterization for, 1414f
temporary vascular access, 1416
vascular access, 1413–1416, 1414f, 1414t–1415t
Hemofiltration
description of, 1397–1398
hemodialysis versus, 1413f
Hemoglobin
definition of, 796
fetal, 808, 811
formation of, 797
glycosylated, 1243, 1289, 1289t
in malnutrition, 1217
oxygen delivery to tissue by, 512
Hemoglobin A, 808, 809f
Hemoglobin electrophoresis, 805
Hemoglobin S, 809–810, 809f
Hemolytic transfusion reaction, 835
Hemophilia, 831, 832t
Hemoptysis, 559–560, 618
Hemorrhage. See also Bleeding
in cirrhosis, 1177–1178
drug therapy for, 1177
external, 129–130
intracerebral, 943
postpartum, 1246
postsurgical, 551
spinal cord, 894

Hemorrhage (Continued)
  subarachnoid
    cerebral vasospasm after, 937
    description of, 929, 931
    traumatic brain injury as cause of, 944–950
Hemorrhagic shock, 1034
Hemorrhagic stroke, 16, 929, 929t
Hemorrhoidectomy, 1140
Hemorrhoids, 1139–1140, 1140f
Hemostasis, 798
Hemothorax, 637–638
Hemovac drain, 278, 279f, 282
Hendrich II Fall Risk Model, 41
Heparin
  with hemodialysis catheters, 208, 1413
  low-molecular-weight, 744–745
  pulmonary embolism treated with, 617–618, 620, 621b
  unfractionated, 744
Heparin-induced thrombocytopenia, 744, 832
Hepatic arterial infusion, for liver cancer, 1187
Hepatic artery embolization, 1187
Hepatic encephalopathy, 1170–1171, 1171t, 1178–1179
Hepatitis
  assessment of, 1183–1184
  care coordination for, 1185
  carriers of, 1181
  chronic, 1182
  classification of, 1180–1181
  complications of, 1182
  delta, 1181
  drug therapy for, 1185t
  drug-induced, 1180
  etiology of, 1180–1181
  fatigue caused by, 1184
  fulminant, 1182
  health promotion and maintenance for, 1182
  incidence of, 1182
  jaundice in, 1183
  liver biopsy for, 1184
  nutrition promotion in, 1184
  pathophysiology of, 1180–1182
  prevalence of, 1182
  self-management education for, 1185b
  toxic, 1180
  transition management for, 1185
  viral, 1180, 1182b, 1185b
Hepatitis A, 1180–1182, 1184
Hepatitis B
  cancers associated with, 379t
  carriers of, 1181
  in chronic kidney disease patients, 1417
  cirrhosis caused by, 1172
  drug therapy for, 1185t
  symptoms of, 1181
  transmission of, 1181
  vaccines for, 1182

Hepatitis C
  cancers associated with, 379t
  in chronic kidney disease patients, 1417
  cirrhosis caused by, 1172
  diagnosis of, 1184
  drug therapy for, 1185t
  transmission of, 1181
  in veterans, 1183b
Hepatitis D, 1181, 1184
Hepatitis E, 1181, 1184
Hepatobiliary scan, 1194
Hepatocellular carcinoma, 1186
Hepatomegaly, 1067, 1173, 1205
Hepatopulmonary syndrome, 1177
Hepatorenal syndrome, 1171
Herbs, 232–233
Hereditary angioedema, 362
Hereditary chronic pancreatitis, 1202
Hereditary hemochromatosis, 817
Hereditary nonpolyposis colorectal cancer, 1126, 1127b, 1466
Heritability, 72
Hernia
  abdominal, 1137–1138, 1137f
  assessment of, 1138
  direct inguinal, 1137, 1137f
  examination for, 1138
  femoral, 1137, 1137f
  hiatal. See Hiatal hernias
  incisional, 1137f, 1138
  indirect inguinal, 1137–1138, 1137f
  interventions for, 1138–1139
  irreducible, 1138
  minimally invasive repair of, 1138–1139, 1139b
  nonsurgical management of, 1138
  pathophysiology of, 1137–1138
  reducible, 1138
  strangulated, 1138
  surgical management of, 1138–1139
  types of, 1137–1138, 1137f
  umbilical, 1137, 1137f
Herniated nucleus pulposus, 903, 903f
Hernioplasty, 1138
Herniorrhaphy, 1138
Herpes simplex virus
  in AIDS-infected patients, 347, 355
  assessment of, 1506
  description of, 467b, 468, 881
  drug therapy for, 1507
  encephalitis caused by, 883
  genital, 1506–1508, 1507b
  HSV-1, 1506
  HSV-2, 1506
  pathophysiology of, 1506
  self-management of, 1507b
Herpes zoster, 467b, 468, 468f
Herpetic whitlow, 468
Heterografts, 499, 499f
Heterotopic ossification, 897, 900
Heterozygous, 75

Hiatal hernias
  assessment of, 1093
  care coordination for, 1095
  definition of, 1092
  features of, 1093b
  gastroesophageal reflux disease risks, 1088
  nonsurgical management of, 1093
  paraesophageal, 1092, 1093b
  pathophysiology of, 1092, 1092f
  rolling, 1092–1093, 1092f
  sliding, 1092, 1092f
  surgical management of, 1093–1095
  transition management for, 1095
Hiccups, 1123
HICS. See Hospital Incident Command System
Hierarchy of Pain Measures, 53, 53t
High-altitude cerebral edema, 145–146, 145b–146b
High-altitude disease, 145–146, 145b–146b
High-altitude pulmonary edema, 145–146, 145b–146b
High-density lipoprotein cholesterol, 730
High-density lipoproteins, 656
High-flow nasal cannula, 534–535
High-frequency chest wall oscillation, 583, 583f
High-frequency oscillatory ventilation, 627
Highly sensitive C-reactive protein
  description of, 656
  in rheumatoid arthritis, 321
Hinge joints, 1007
Hip(s)
  arthroplasty of. See Total hip arthroplasty
  dislocation of, after total hip arthroplasty, 311–312
  flexion contractures of, 1052
  fracture of, 1047–1049, 1047f–1048f, 1049b
  mobility evaluations, 1010
Hip resurfacing, 310
Hirsutism, 441, 1242, 1256
Hispanics
  Alzheimer's disease in, 866b
  older adults, 39b
Histamine, 293–294, 361, 361f, 364
Histamine receptor antagonists
  gastritis treated with, 1105
  gastroesophageal reflux disease treated with, 1091
  peptic ulcer disease treated with, 1112
Histoplasmosis, 347
HIT. See Heparin-induced thrombocytopenia
HIV infection. See Human immunodeficiency virus infection

HIV-associated nephropathy, 348
HIV-associated neurocognitive disorder, 348
HLAs. See Human leukocyte antigens
HMG-CoA reductase inhibitors, 730
H1N1, 597
H5N1, 597–598
H7N9, 597
H1N1 virus, 151
Hodgkin's lymphoma, 828
Homans' sign, 742–743
Home care management
  for acute pancreatitis, 1202
  for amputation, 1055, 1056b
  for benign prostatic hyperplasia, 1481
  for bone tumors, 1027
  for breast cancer, 1452–1453
  for breast cancer surgery, 1453b
  for burn injury, 505
  for cataract, 962b, 971, 971f
  for central venous catheter, 826b
  for chronic obstructive pulmonary disease, 581, 581b
  for cirrhosis, 1179, 1179b
  for colorectal cancer, 1133
  for Cushing's disease, 1260
  for diabetes mellitus, 1317–1318, 1318b
  for esophageal tumors, 1100
  for fractures, 1045
  for gastric cancer, 1119
  for glaucoma, 975
  for head and neck cancer, 554, 554b
  health care resources in, 101
  for hearing loss, 1001
  for heart failure, 703
  for hypertension, 727
  for hypoglycemia, 1310b
  for hypothyroidism, 1273–1274
  for infection, 426
  for intestinal obstructions, 1125
  for laryngectomy, 554b
  leave-of-absence visit, 100–101
  for leukemia, 826
  for malnutrition, 1224
  for myasthenia gravis, 921–922
  for myocardial infarction, 789–790, 790b
  for obesity, 1231
  for oral cancer, 1083, 1083b
  for osteoarthritis, 317
  for osteoporosis, 1022
  for otitis media, 993
  for oxygen therapy, 536
  for pain, 67
  for pancreatic cancer, 1209
  for pelvic inflammatory disease, 1516
  for peptic ulcer disease, 1114, 1115b
  for peritonitis, 1146

Home care management (Continued)
  for pneumonia, 605
  postoperative, 286
  for pressure injuries, 459–460
  for prostate cancer, 1485–1486
  for pulmonary embolism, 623, 624b
  for pyelonephritis, 1375
  in rehabilitation, 100
  for rheumatoid arthritis, 325
  for stomatitis, 1078
  for stroke, 939
  for tracheostomy, 544
  for tuberculosis, 610
  for ulcerative colitis, 1156
  for urinary incontinence, 1353
  for uterine leiomyomas, 1463
  for valvular heart disease, 710
Home infusion therapy, 67
Homelessness
  emergency department care and, 127
  impact of, 127
  in older adults, 30
Homeostasis, 1235
Homocysteine, 656
Homografts, 499
Homonymous hemianopsia, 934, 934f
Homozygous, 75
Honeybee stings, 137
Hookah smoking, 514
Hormonal manipulation, for cancer, 406–407, 406t
Hormones. See also specific hormone
  appetite regulation by, 1225
  definition of, 1234–1235
  endocrine, 1235t
  "lock and key" model of, 1235, 1235f
  male reproductive, 1430
  positive and negative feedback control of, 1236f
  receptor binding by, 1235, 1235f
  thyroid gland, 1235t, 1239t
Hospice care, 106, 106b, 107t, 113–114, 593
Hospital(s)
  critical access, 117
  emergency preparedness in
    infrastructure of, 152–153
    nurse's role in, 154–156
    personnel roles and responsibilities, 153–156, 154t
  older adults in, 39–42
  restraints used by, 41, 42b
Hospital care
  drowning, 147
  frostbite, 144–145
  heat stroke, 134–135
  hypothermia, 143
  lightning injury, 142
Hospital Elder Life Program, 38

Hospital Incident Command System, 153–154
Hospital incident commander, 154, 154t
Hospital-acquired infection, 122, 216
Hospitalist, 8
Hostile patients, 121b
Hot packs, 323–324
Huber noncoring needle, 208
Human B-type natriuretic peptides, 698
Human immunodeficiency virus infection. See also Acquired immunodeficiency syndrome
  acquired immunodeficiency syndrome and, 338, 340
  in African-American women, 345b
  anal intercourse as risk factor for, 342
  antibody-antigen tests, 349
  archiving in, 350
  care coordination for, 356–357
  classification of, 339–340
  cognition enhancements in, 355
  complementary and integrative health for, 353–354
  counseling about, 341–342
  course of, 344–345
  diarrhea management in, 354
  "docking" proteins of, 338f
  drug therapy for
    antiretroviral drugs, 350–353
    CCR5 antagonists, 351b–352b
    combination antiretroviral therapy, 342–343, 350–353
    integrase inhibitors, 351b–352b
    non-nucleoside reverse transcriptase inhibitors, 338, 351b–352b
    nucleoside reverse transcriptase inhibitors, 338, 351b–352b
    protease inhibitors, 338, 348, 351b–352b
  effects of, 338
  endocrine complications of, 348
  etiology of, 337–340
  gas exchange in, 353
  gender differences, 342
  genetic risk for, 337–340
  health care resources for, 357
  health care worker exposure to, 343, 344f, 345b
  health promotion and maintenance for, 340–343
  history-taking, 345–346
  home care management of, 356
  home testing kits for, 350
  incidence of, 340
  increased intracranial pressure in, 355
  infectious process of, 337–339
  in injection drug users, 343
  laboratory assessments in, 349
  long-term nonprogressors, 338b

Human immunodeficiency virus infection (Continued)
  lymphocyte count in, 349
  malignancies associated with, 347–348, 348f
  mouth care in, 354
  nutrition promotion in, 354
  occupational exposure to, 343
  opportunistic infections associated with
    description of, 339, 346–347, 347f
    prevention of, 350–353
  pain management in, 353–354
  parenteral transmission of, 341, 343
  particle features of, 337–338, 338f
  pathophysiology of, 337–340
  perinatal transmission of, 341, 343
  postexposure prophylaxis for, 342–343, 344f
  pre-exposure prophylaxis for, 342
  in pregnancy
    outcomes affected by, 340
    perinatal transmission, 341, 343
  prevalence of, 340
  progression of, 340
  psychosocial assessment, 348
  psychosocial distress caused by, 355–356
  as retrovirus, 338
  schematic diagram of, 338f
  screening for, 341, 341b
  self-management education for, 356, 357b
  sexual transmission of, 341–343
  signs and symptoms of, 339
  skin integrity in, 354–355
  stages of, 339–340
  testing for, 341–342, 341b, 349
  transition management for, 356–357
  transmission of
    needlestick injuries as cause of, 343
    parenteral, 341, 343
    perinatal, 341, 343
    sexual, 341–343
  in veterans, 341b
  viral load, 342, 349
  virus-host interactions, 338
  in women, 340b, 345b
Human immunodeficiency virus protease, 338
Human leukocyte antigens
  B5701 allele test, 350b
  description of, 290, 294
  rheumatoid arthritis and, 318b
Human lymphotrophic virus type I, 379t
Human lymphotrophic virus type II, 379t

Human papilloma virus, 348
  cancers associated with, 379t
  cervical cancer risks, 1469
  condylomata acuminata caused by, 1510–1511, 1510f
  oral cancer associated with, 1079
  test for, 1434–1435
  vaccinations for, 382, 1469, 1511
Human trafficking, 131
Human waste management, 157
Humeral shaft fracture, 1046
Humidified oxygen, 531, 531f
Humira. See Adalimumab
Humoral immunity, 295. See also Antibody-mediated immunity
Huntington disease, 72, 79–81
  clinical features of, 868t
  definition of, 868
  Parkinson disease versus, 868t
Hurricane Katrina, 151
Hyaluronic acid, 308
Hyaluronidase, 223
Hydration
  in chronic obstructive pulmonary disease, 579
  peristalsis and, 286
  postoperative assessment of, 276
Hydrocephalus
  brain tumors as cause of, 954
  description of, 882, 937, 943
Hydrocodone
  equianalgesic dosing of, 60t
  pain management uses of, 60, 60t
Hydrocortisone, 1255b
Hydrogen breath test, 1136
Hydrogen ions
  bicarbonate effects on, 187
  carbon dioxide and, 187–188
  description of, 186
  overproduction of, 191
  underelimination of, 192
Hydromorphone
  equianalgesic dosing of, 60t
  pain management uses of, 60, 60t
  postoperative pain management using, 284b
Hydronephrosis, 1361, 1382–1384, 1383f, 1474
Hydrophilic dressing, 457
Hydrophobic dressing, 457
Hydrostatic pressure, 161
Hydrotherapy, 498–499
Hydroureter, 1361, 1382–1384, 1474
Hydroxychloroquine, 322, 327–328
17-Hydroxycorticosteroids, 1254, 1257
Hydroxyurea, 811
Hygiene
  hand, 418, 418b
  oral. See Oral hygiene
  of surgical team, 255
Hyoscyamine, 110, 1359b
Hyperactive reflexes, 849
Hyperacusis, 988
Hyperacute rejection, 301

Hyperaldosteronism, 1260–1261
Hyperbaric oxygen therapy
  description of, 458
  osteomyelitis treated with, 1024
Hypercalcemia
  cancer-induced, 408
  characteristics of, 181, 181t
  in chronic kidney disease, 1409
Hypercalciuria, 1365
Hypercapnia, 177, 646
Hypercarbia, 530, 576, 944–945
Hypercoagulability, 15
Hypercortisolism. See Cushing's
  disease
Hyperemia, 144, 294
Hyperextension spinal cord injury,
  894, 895f
Hyperflexion spinal cord injury, 894,
  894f
Hyperglycemia
  description of, 1265
  in hospitalized patients, 1301
  hypoglycemia versus, 1309t
  injury from, 1291–1303
  insulin absence as cause of,
    1282–1283
  metabolic syndrome risks, 1287
  vision complications of, 1284
Hyperglycemic-hyperosmolar state,
  1300b, 1313t, 1314–1316, 1314b,
  1315f
Hyperinsulinemia, 1300
Hyperkalemia
  burn injury as cause of, 485
  in chronic kidney disease, 1400
  definition of, 1254
  description of, 178–179, 178t,
    179b, 192, 237
  management of, 1253b
  potassium-sparing diuretic as
    cause of, 1261
Hyperkinetic pulse, 653
Hyperleptinemia, 1225
Hyperlipidemia, 729
  in chronic kidney disease, 1401
  metabolic syndrome risks, 1287
Hypermagnesemia, 182, 182t
Hypernatremia, 174–175, 175t, 953
Hyperopia, 960, 960f, 980–981
Hyperosmotic fluid, 163
Hyperoxaluria, 1362t
Hyperparathyroidism, 1275–1277,
  1276b, 1276t
Hyperperfusion syndrome, 936
Hyperphosphatemia, 1378, 1400,
  1409
Hyperpituitarism, 1247–1250, 1247f,
  1248b
Hyperpolarization-activated cyclic
  nucleotide-gated channel
  blocker, 701
Hypersensitivity reactions, 23.
  See also Allergy
  definition of, 360
  histamine in, 361, 361f

Hypersensitivity reactions
  (Continued)
  type I
    allergic rhinosinusitis,
      365–366
    anaphylaxis as. See Anaphylaxis
    angioedema as, 361–366, 362b,
      362f
    description of, 360–361
    examples of, 361t
    mechanism of action, 361t
  type II
    description of, 366
    examples of, 361t
    mechanism of action, 361t
  type III
    description of, 366
    examples of, 361t
    immune complex in, 366,
      366f
    mechanism of action, 361t
  type IV
    description of, 367
    examples of, 361t
    mechanism of action, 361t
Hypertension. See also Blood
  pressure
  adrenal-mediated, 721
  in African Americans, 722b
  assessment of, 722–728
  care coordination for, 727–728
  in chronic kidney disease, 1401,
    1407
  classification of, 721
  complementary and integrative
    health for, 723
  concept map for, 724f
  after coronary artery bypass
    grafting, 787–788
  definition of, 652, 720
  diagnostic assessment of, 723
  drug therapy for, 723–727, 725b
    angiotensin II receptor blockers,
      725b, 726–727
    angiotensin-converting enzyme
      inhibitors, 725b, 726
    beta blockers, 725b, 727
    calcium channel blockers, 725b,
      726
    diuretics, 725b, 726
  end-stage kidney disease caused
    by, 1379
  essential, 721, 721t
  etiology of, 721, 721t
  gender differences in, 722b
  health care resources for, 728
  health promotion and
    maintenance for, 722, 722t
  home care management of, 727
  incidence of, 722
  interventions for, 723–727,
    725b–726b, 726t, 916
  ischemic heart disease with, 727
  lifestyle changes for, 723
  malignant, 721

Hypertension (Continued)
  management of
    angiotensin receptor blockers
      for, 167
    angiotensin-converting enzyme
      inhibitors for, 167
    renin-angiotensin II pathway in,
      167
  metabolic syndrome risks, 1287
  pathophysiology of, 720–722
  in pheochromocytoma,
    1261–1262
  in polycystic kidney disease, 1380
  portal, 1170
  prevalence of, 722, 722b
  psychosocial assessment of, 723
  pulmonary arterial, 584–585, 585t
  renovascular, 721
  secondary, 721, 721t
  self-management education for,
    727
  signs and symptoms of, 722–723
  transition management for,
    727–728
Hypertensive crisis, 727, 727b
Hypertensive urgency, 727
Hyperthermia, 425
  malignant, 258–259, 259b–260b
Hyperthyroidism
  assessment of, 1265–1267
  drug therapy for, 1267–1268,
    1268b
  etiology of, 1265
  exogenous, 1265
  exophthalmos in, 1265, 1266f
  eye problems associated with,
    1266
  features of, 1265, 1265b
  genetic risk of, 1265
  goiter associated with, 1265, 1266f,
    1266t
  history-taking for, 1265–1266
  incidence of, 1265
  interventions for, 1267–1270
  iodine preparations for,
    1267–1268
  laboratory assessment of, 1266,
    1267b
  nonsurgical management of,
    1267–1268
  pathophysiology of, 1264–1265
  physical assessment of, 1266
  prevalence of, 1265
  psychosocial assessment of, 1266
  radioactive iodine therapy for,
    1266–1269, 1269b
  signs and symptoms of, 1266
  surgical management of,
    1269–1270
Hypertonia, 933
Hypertonic fluid, 163
Hypertonic saline, 1252
Hypertonic solution, 200
Hypertrophic cardiomyopathy,
  714–716, 715t

Hypertrophic ungual labium, 1029t
Hyperuricemia, 331, 1362t
Hyperventilation, 189, 196, 854
Hypervolemia, 171, 174
Hypnotics, 258
Hypoactive delirium, 111
Hypoactive reflexes, 849
Hypocalcemia, 179–181, 180f, 180t,
  196, 657, 1269, 1400
Hypocapnia, 145
Hypocarbia, 944–945
Hypochromic, 803–804
Hypodermoclysis, 223
Hypoglossal nerve, 844t
Hypoglycemia
  drug therapy for, 1311
  glucagon effects on, 1281
  hyperglycemia versus, 1309t
  management of, 1253b
  nutrition therapy for, 1310–1311
  in older adults, 1309, 1312b
  patient and family education
    about, 1311
  prevention of, 1302, 1308–1311
  signs and symptoms of, 1309
Hypoglycemic unawareness, 1309
Hypokalemia
  burn injury as cause of, 485
  characteristics of, 175–177, 177b
  description of, 18, 196, 237
Hypokinetic pulse, 653
Hypomagnesemia, 181–182, 182t,
  1277
Hyponatremia
  burn injury as cause of, 485
  in chronic kidney disease, 1400
  definition of, 1254
  description of, 173–174, 174t
  dilutional, 1252
Hypo-osmotic fluid, 163
Hypoparathyroidism, 1277–1278
Hypophysectomy, 1249–1250, 1249b,
  1258
Hypopituitarism, 1245–1247, 1246b
Hypotension
  brain injury caused by, 941
  description of, 20
  drug therapy for, 621–622
  monitoring for, 1423b
  orthostatic, 121, 134b, 168,
    174–175, 652, 723, 726b, 901,
    1285
  postural, 652
  in pulmonary embolism, 621–622
Hypothalamic-hypophysial portal
  system, 1236
Hypothalamus
  anatomy of, 840, 840f, 1236–1237
  function of, 1236
  hormones produced by, 1235t
Hypothermia, 142–144, 143b
  after coronary artery bypass
    grafting, 787
  shivering caused by, 280
  in trauma patients, 130

Hypothyroid crisis, 1271
Hypothyroidism
  assessment of, 1272
  care coordination for, 1273–1274
  cognition support in, 1273
  etiology of, 1271, 1272t
  features of, 1271b
  gas exchange in, 1272–1273
  health care resources for, 1274
  home care management of,
      1273–1274
  hypotension prevention in, 1273
  incidence of, 1271
  interventions for, 1273
  laboratory assessment of, 1272
  levothyroxine sodium for, 1273
  myxedema coma in, 1271, 1273,
      1273b–1274b
  pathophysiology of, 1270–1271
  physical assessment of, 1272
  prevalence of, 1271
  psychosocial assessment of, 1272
  self-management education of,
      1274
  signs and symptoms of, 1271b, 1272
  transition management for,
      1273–1274
Hypotonia, 933
Hypotonic fluid, 163
Hypotonic solution, 200
Hypoventilation
  description of, 189–190, 625
  intraoperative, 267–268
  oxygen-induced, 530
Hypovolemia, 167–168, 174, 1113,
    1283
Hypovolemic shock
  adaptive responses and events
      during, 754t
  assessment of, 756–758
  in burn injury, 494–496
  care coordination for, 760
  concept map for, 756f–757f
  drug therapy for, 495, 759b
  etiology of, 752–753, 755
  in fractures, 1034
  health promotion and
      maintenance for, 756
  incidence of, 755
  laboratory assessment of, 758,
      758b
  nonsurgical management of,
      758–760, 759b
  pathophysiology of, 754–755
  peritonitis as cause of, 1145
  physical assessment of, 756–758
  prevalence of, 755
  risk factors for, 752t, 756b
  signs and symptoms of, 756–758
  surgical management of, 760
  transition management for, 760
Hypoxemia, 177
  in asthma, 566–567
  in chronic obstructive pulmonary
      disease, 573, 576

Hypoxemia (Continued)
  definition of, 529, 617
  home care management of, 581
  management of, 619–621
  oxygen therapy for, 626, 775
  in pulmonary embolism,
      619–621
  pulse oximetry for, 603
  severe, 536
  traumatic brain injury as cause of,
      947
Hypoxia, 1283
  brain injury caused by, 941
  definition of, 529, 797, 809
  in drowning, 147
  prevention of, 541
  in tracheostomy, 541
Hypoxic-ventilatory response, 145
Hysterectomy, 1461–1463, 1461t,
    1462b–1463b, 1466
Hysterosalpingography, 1435
Hysteroscopy, 1437

I
IADLs. See Instrumental activities of
    daily living
Iatrogenic hypoparathyroidism,
    1277
Ibandronate, 1021
IBS. See Irritable bowel syndrome
Ibuprofen, 284b
Ibutilide, 677b–678b
Icterus, 1192
Idarucizumab, 745, 801
Ideal body weight, 1215, 1225
Idiopathic chronic pancreatitis,
    1202
Idiopathic hypoparathyroidism,
    1277
Idiopathic pulmonary fibrosis,
    585–586
Idiopathic thrombocytopenic
    purpura, 830–831
Ileo pouch-anal anastomosis,
    restorative proctocolectomy
    with, 1154–1155, 1154f
Ileostomy
  dietary considerations in, 1156
  health care resources for, 1157
  self-management education for,
      1157b
  stoma for, 1153, 1154b
  total proctocolectomy with
      permanent ileostomy, 1154,
      1155f
  ulcerative colitis treated with,
      1153–1154
Ilizarov technique, 1043
Iloprost, 585
Imagery, 67
Imatinib mesylate, 821
Immobility, 1044
Immune complexes, 297f, 366, 366f
Immune reconstitution
    inflammatory syndrome, 353

Immune status
  environmental factors that affect,
      414–415
  infection risks and, 414
Immune system
  age-related changes in, 291b
  antibody-mediated, 417
  burn injury effects on, 486
  leukocytes, 290–291, 292t
  organization of, 290–291
Immunity
  acquired, 295, 298
  active, 21–22, 298, 414
  age-related changes in, 290, 300
  antibody-mediated, 22, 290–291
  assessment of, 22–23
  cancer effects on, 385
  cell-mediated, 22, 290–291
  changes in, 22–23
  chronic kidney disease effects on,
      1401
  definition of, 21–23, 289, 414,
      605
  development of, 367
  divisions of, 290–291, 292f
  functions of, 379
  in hospitalized patients, 351b
  human leukocyte antigens,
      290
  inflammation. See Inflammation
  innate-naive, 291–292
  natural, 291–292
  non-self proteins, 289–290,
      290f
  passive, 21–22, 298–299, 414
  promotion of, 23
  risk factors for, 22
  scope of, 22
  self cells, 289–290, 290f
  specific, 295–300
  sustained, 298
Immunocompetent, 289–291
Immunoglobulin A, 298t
Immunoglobulin D, 298t
Immunoglobulin E, 298t
Immunoglobulin G, 298, 298t
Immunoglobulin M, 298, 298t
Immunoglobulins, 298, 298t
Immunohemolytic anemia,
    815–816
Immunologic assays, 1243
Immunomodulators, 1153
Immunosuppressants/
    immunosuppressive therapy
  autoimmune diseases treated with,
      368–369, 370b
  idiopathic pulmonary fibrosis
      treated with, 586
  in kidney transplantation patients,
      1424
  myasthenia gravis treated with,
      920
  systemic lupus erythematosus
      treated with, 328, 328b
  after transplantation, 302b

Immunotherapy
  allergic rhinosinusitis treated with,
      365–366
  cancer treated with, 401–403,
      402t
Impact of Event Scale—Revised, 158,
    158b
Impaired cellular regulation, 14–15
Impedance, 645
Impedance plethysmography, 743
Impermeable membrane, 162
Implantable cardioverter/
    defibrillator, 687–688, 688b
Implanted ports, 207–208, 207f–208f
IMRT. See Intensity-modulated
    radiation therapy
Incentive spirometry, 243–244, 244f,
    604, 1094
Incisional hernia, 1137f, 1138
Incomplete fracture, 1032
Incontinence
  age-related, 18
  definition of, 18, 1330, 1343–1344
  fecal, 18
  in older adults, 31
  pressure injuries and, 451
  urinary. See Urinary incontinence
Incontinence-associated dermatitis,
    1352
Increased intracranial pressure
  brain tumors as cause of, 954
  edema as cause of, 942
  in human immunodeficiency
      virus infection, 355
  management of, 937
  stroke as cause of, 936–937, 936b
  traumatic brain injury as cause of,
      941–942, 946
Incretin, 1282
Incretin mimetics, 1292b–1293b,
    1293
Incus, 984, 985f–986f
Indacaterol, 569b–570b
Indirect contact transmission, 416
Indirect Coombs' test, 805
Indirect inguinal hernia, 1137–1138,
    1137f
Indirect thrombin inhibitors, 801
Induration, 607
Infarction
  definition of, 928
  myocardial. See Myocardial
      infarction
Infection(s)
  airborne transmission of, 416
  antimicrobial therapy inadequacy
      for, 423–427
  antimicrobial-resistant, 421,
      421b
  assessment of, 423–425
  bloodstream, 416, 423
  care coordination for, 426
  CDC information about, 414
  communicable, 414
  contact transmission of, 416

Infection(s) (Continued)
corneal, 977
in Cushing's disease, 1259–1260
directly observed therapy for, 423
droplet transmission of, 416
ear, 1000b
emerging types of, 427–428, 427t
environmental exposure to, 423
fever associated with, 424b,
    425–426
food contamination as source of,
    427–428
fractures as risk factor for, 1035,
    1045
fungal. See Fungal infections
gastrointestinal tract transmission
    of, 415
health care resources for, 426
health promotion and
    maintenance for, 417–421
history-taking for, 423–424
home care management for, 426
hospital-acquired, 122
host factors in development of,
    414t
imaging assessment of, 425
immune status and, 414
inflammation and, 292
intraoperative, 267, 268f
laboratory assessment of, 424–425
in leukemia, 821–822, 821b
lymphadenopathy associated with,
    424
mechanical ventilation-related,
    635
multidrug-resistant organism
    carbapenem-resistant
        Enterobacteriaceae,
        422–423
    contact precautions for, 419
    methicillin-resistant
        Staphylococcus aureus, 422
    types of, 421–422
    vancomycin-resistant
        Enterococcus, 422
occupational exposure to, 423
opportunistic
    description of, 339, 346–347,
        347f
    prevention of, 350–353
oxygen therapy as cause of, 531
pandemic, 427
physical assessment of, 424
physiologic defenses for, 416–417
portal of exit for, 416
prevention of. See Infection
    prevention
psychosocial assessment of, 424
reservoirs of, 414
respiratory tract transmission of,
    415
risks of, 414, 415b, 417b
self-management education for,
    426
sepsis caused by, 760–761

Infection(s) (Continued)
sexually transmitted. See Sexually
    transmitted infections
signs and symptoms of, 424
skin. See Skin infections
skin barrier against, 415
surgical site. See Surgical site
    infections
tracheostomy as cause of, 539
transition management for, 426
transmission of
    description of, 414–416
    precautions based on, 419, 420t
    routes of, 415–416
urinary tract. See Urinary tract
    infections
Infection control
disinfection for, 418
hand hygiene for, 418, 418b
in health care settings, 417
methods of, 417–421
patient placement for, 421
for patient transfer, 421
staff considerations, 421
Standard Precautions for,
    418–419, 419t
sterilization for, 418
transmission-based precautions
    for, 419, 420t
Infection prevention
after amputation, 1054
description of, 397b
disinfection for, 418
methods of, 417–421, 827b
patient placement for, 421
in pressure injuries, 459
staff considerations, 421
Standard Precautions for,
    418–419, 419t
transmission-based precautions
    for, 419, 420t
Infectious cystitis, 1355
Infective endocarditis, 711–712,
    711b
Inferior oblique muscle, 960t
Inferior rectus muscle, 960t
Inferior vena cava filter, 618, 621,
    745
Inferior wall myocardial infarction,
    771
Infertility, 1517
Infiltrating ductal carcinoma, 1441
Infiltration, 200, 217t–219t, 221t
Infiltration Scale, 221t
Inflammation
asthma caused by, 565
basophils in, 293–294
cells involved in, 292–294, 292t
complement system in, 294
as defense mechanism, 417
eosinophils in, 294
five cardinal symptoms of, 294
infection and, 292
leukocytes in, 292, 292t
leukocytes involved in, 797t

Inflammation (Continued)
macrophages in, 293–295
neutrophils in, 292–293, 292t
phagocytosis in, 294
pneumonia caused by, 599
sequence of, 294–295
stages of, 294–295
tissue mast cells in, 294
Inflammatory bowel disease. See
    Crohn's disease; Ulcerative
    colitis
Inflammatory breast cancer, 1441
Inflammatory cytokines, 1225
Infliximab, 323b, 466b, 1160b
Influenza
pandemic, 597–598
pandemic outbreaks of, 151
seasonal, 596–597
Informatics
attributes of, 8
context of, 8
definition of, 7
scope of, 8
Informed consent
for cardiac catheterization, 658
preoperative, 239–241, 240f
Infratentorial lesion, 840
Infratentorial tumors, 950
Infusate, 200
Infusion nurses, 199–200
Infusion Nurses Society, 200
Infusion pressure, 214
Infusion therapy. See also
    Intravenous therapy
administration sets for
    add-on devices, 209–210
    definition of, 209
    filters used with, 210
    intermittent, 209
    needleless connection devices,
        210–211, 210f, 214
    secondary, 209, 209f
    slip lock, 210
ambulatory pumps, 211
blood and blood components, 200
containers used in, 208–209
definition of, 199
dose-track technology for, 211
drugs, 201
electronic infusion devices for, 211
electronic infusion pumps, 211
fluids used in, 200
indications for, 199
intra-arterial, 224–225
intraosseous, 223–224, 224f
intraperitoneal, 225
intraspinal, 225–226
intrathecal, 225–226
intravenous. See Intravenous
    therapy
intravenous solutions, 200
mechanically regulated devices for,
    211, 212f
overview of, 199–202
prescribing of, 201

Infusion therapy (Continued)
rate-controlling devices, 211
smart pumps for, 211
subcutaneous, 223
syringe pumps, 211
vascular access devices for,
    201–202
Ingrown nail, 1029t
Inguinal hernia, 1137, 1137f
Inhalant irritants, 515
Inhalation anthrax, 611–612, 612b
Inheritance patterns
autosomal dominant, 78–79, 78t
autosomal recessive, 78t, 79, 79f
complex, 78t, 80
overview of, 77–80
pedigree, 77–78, 78f–79f
sex-linked recessive, 78t, 79–80,
    80f
Inherited mutation, 76
Injection drug users, 343
Injection sclerotherapy, 1177
In-line filter, for intraspinal
    infusions, 226
Inner ear, 985–986
Inner maxillary fixation, 558–559
Inpatient rehabilitation facility, 87
Inpatient rehabilitation facility
    patient assessment instrument,
    92
Inpatient surgery, 229–230
INR. See International normalized
    ratio
Insensible water loss, 165
Inspection
of abdomen, 1067
of endocrine system, 1241–1242
of myocardium, 653, 654f
of skeletal system, 1009–1010,
    1009f
of skin, 436–439
Institute for Safe Medication
    Practices, 1297–1298
Institute of Medicine Health
    Professions Education: A Bridge
    to Quality, 2
Instrumental activities of daily
    living, 1217
    definition of, 92
    self-management education for
        performing, 100
Insufflation, 254
Insulin
absence of, 1282–1283, 1283t
absorption of, 1295–1296
complications of, 1296, 1296f
continuous subcutaneous infusion
    of, 1294, 1296, 1296f, 1313
functions of, 1236, 1240
gene for, 72
injection areas and sites for, 1295f
injection devices for, 1297
Lispro, 1294
long-acting, 1295t
metabolic effects of, 1282

Insulin (Continued)
mixing of, 1296
pen-type injectors for, 1297–1298
preoperative administration of, 242
rapid-acting, 1295t, 1296
regimens, 1294–1295
secretion of, 1281
sensitizers of, 1291, 1292b–1293b
short-acting, 1295t
stimulators of, 1291–1294, 1292b–1293b
storage of, 1297
structure of, 76, 1281, 1282f
subcutaneous administration of, 1297b
syringes for, 1297
Insulin pump, 1296f
Insulin resistance, 1286–1287
Insulin-dependent diabetes mellitus. See Diabetes mellitus, type 1
Integrase, 337–340
Integrase inhibitors, 351b–352b
Integrative care, 3
Integrative therapies, 3t
Integumentary system
assessment of, before rehabilitation, 90t, 91
components of, 431
hair, 432–433
nails, 432–433, 432f
nutrition assessments, 1213b
skin. See Skin
Intensity, of sound, 990
Intensity-modulated radiation therapy, 388, 549, 556
Intensivist, 8
Intention tremors, 848, 889
Interbody cage fusion surgery, 906
Intercostal space, 518
Interferons
cancer treated with, 402, 402t
multiple sclerosis treated with, 891b
Interleukins
-1, 300t
-2, 300t
-6, 300t
cancer treated with, 402, 402t
Intermittent catheterization, 98
Intermittent claudication, 651, 732, 735
Intermittent hemodialysis. See Hemodialysis
Intermittent self-catheterization, 1352
Internal carotid artery, 841
Internal cerebral artery, 933b
Internal derangement, 1056
Internal hemorrhoids, 1139, 1140f
Internal mammary artery, 784–786
Internal urethral sphincter, 1327, 1327f
International Critical Incident Stress Foundation, 156

International normalized ratio, 16, 622b, 657, 805, 1174
International Prostate Symptom Score, 1474, 1475f–1476f
International Society of Blood Transfusion, 200, 201f
Interprofessional collaboration
attributes of, 5
definition of, 5
scope of, 5
Interprofessional communication, 5–6
competencies for, 5t
e-mail for, 5
goals of, 5
SBAR process for, 5–6
Interprofessional Education Collaborative Expert Panel, 5
Interprofessional team
in emergency departments, 118–120
members of, 5
in rehabilitation settings, 88–89, 88t, 89f
Interrupted sutures, 268f
Interstitial brachytherapy, 1451
Interstitial cystitis, 1354, 1356
Interstitial edema, 942
Interstitial fluid, 160
Intestinal disorders
appendicitis, 1147–1148, 1147b, 1148f
bacterial overgrowth, 1142
celiac disease, 1164, 1164b
colorectal cancer. See Colorectal cancer
Crohn's disease. See Crohn's disease
diverticular disease, 1162–1164, 1162f, 1163b
gastroenteritis, 1148–1150, 1148t, 1149b–1150b
hemorrhoids, 1139–1140, 1140f
hernia, 1137–1139, 1137f
inflammatory, 1144–1168
irritable bowel syndrome, 1135–1137
malabsorption syndrome, 1141–1142
noninflammatory, 1121–1143
obstruction. See Intestinal obstructions
peritonitis. See Peritonitis
polyps, 1126
ulcerative colitis. See Ulcerative colitis
Intestinal ischemia, 1122
Intestinal obstructions
assessment of, 1123
care coordination for, 1125–1126
closed-loop, 1122
complications of, 1122
diagnostic assessment of, 1123
exploratory laparotomy for, 1125
features of, 1123b

Intestinal obstructions (Continued)
fecal impaction as cause of, 1125, 1126b
fluid replacement and maintenance for, 1124
health care resources for, 1126
history-taking for, 1123
home care management for, 1125
imaging assessment of, 1123
interventions for, 1123–1125
intussusception, 1122, 1122f
laboratory assessment of, 1123
large-bowel, 1123b
mechanical, 1122–1123, 1122f
minimally invasive surgery for, 1125
nasogastric tubes for, 1124, 1134b
nonmechanical, 1122–1123
nonsurgical management of, 1124–1125
nursing care for, 1124b
pain associated with, 1123
pathophysiology of, 1121–1122
physical assessment of, 1123
postoperative ileus, 1122, 1124
self-management education for, 1126
signs and symptoms of, 1123
small-bowel, 1123b
strangulated, 1122, 1125
surgical management of, 1125
transition management for, 1125–1126
types of, 1122
volvulus, 1122, 1122f
Intestinal tract, 1144
Intestinal villi, 1064
Intestine. See also Large intestine; Small intestine
contents of, 1122
obstruction of. See Intestinal obstruction
preoperative preparation of, 242
Intimate partner violence, 118
Intra-aortic balloon pump, 782
Intra-arterial infusion therapy, 224–225
Intra-arterial thrombolytic therapy, 736
Intracellular fluid, 19, 160, 162, 164
Intracerebral hemorrhage, 929, 943
Intracranial pressure
in encephalitis, 884b
after hypophysectomy, 1249
increased. See Increased intracranial pressure
normal level of, 941
Intraductal papilloma, 1455t
Intrahepatic obstructive jaundice, 1170
Intraocular pressure
activities that increase, 961t
definition of, 958

Intraocular pressure (Continued)
in glaucoma, 972
normal, 972
tonometry of, 965, 965f–966f
Intraoperative period
advance directives, 263
anesthesia
allergies to, 263
definition of, 256
general, 257–260, 258t–259t, 260b
local, 260–261
moderate sedation, 261–262, 262t
providers of, 256–257
regional, 260–261, 261f–262f, 261t
selection criteria for, 256–257
description of, 228
diagnostic tests, 263–264
electronic health record review in, 263–264
history-taking in, 262–263
hypoventilation prevention, 267–268
infection prevention, 267, 268f
laboratory testing, 263–264
moderate sedation, 261–262, 262t
nursing interventions, 264b
onset of, 251–252
overview of, 251–268
patient positioning, 264–267, 265f, 267b
retained surgical items, 267
surgical attire, 256, 256f
surgical scrub, 256, 257f
surgical team, 252, 253t. See also Surgical team
Intraosseous infusion therapy, 223–224, 224f
Intraperitoneal infusion therapy, 225
Intraspinal analgesia, 61–62
Intraspinal infusion therapy, 225–226
Intrathecal analgesia, 61–62, 62b
Intrathecal baclofen, 891, 900
Intrathecal contrast-enhanced computed tomography scan, 853
Intrathecal infusion, 225–226
Intravascular ultrasonography, 659
Intravenous immunoglobulin, 915
Intravenous pumps, 211
Intravenous solutions, 170, 170t, 200
Intravenous therapy
administration sets for
add-on devices, 209–210
changing of, 214
definition of, 209
filters used with, 210
intermittent, 209
needleless connection devices, 210–211, 210f, 214
secondary, 209, 209f
slip lock, 210

Intravenous therapy (Continued)
    catheters used in
        blood samples obtained from,
            215
        dressings with, 212–214
        flushing of, 214–215
        hemodialysis, 208
        peripherally inserted central,
            205–206, 205f, 206b,
            212–213
        securing of, 212–214, 213f, 222b
        short peripheral, 202–204,
            202f–203f, 202t, 203b,
            214–215
    central
        hemodialysis catheters, 208
        implanted ports, 207–208,
            207f–208f
        peripherally inserted central
            catheters, 205–206, 205f,
            206b, 212–213
        tunneled central venous
            catheters, 207, 207f, 213,
            226
        vascular access devices for, 205
    complications of
        catheter embolism, 219t–220t
        catheter-related bloodstream
            infection, 204–206,
            211–212, 216, 216t,
            220t–221t
        circulatory overload, 219t–220t
        ecchymosis, 217t–219t
        extravasation, 217t–219t
        hematoma, 217t–219t
        infiltration, 217t–219t, 221t
        local, 216, 217t–219t
        nerve damage, 217t–219t
        phlebitis, 217t–219t
        site infection, 217t–219t
        speed shock, 219t–220t
        systemic, 216, 219t–220t
        thrombophlebitis, 217t–219t
        thrombosis, 217t–219t
        venous spasm, 217t–219t
    documentation of, 216
    drug delivery using, 201
    nursing assessment for, 212
    nursing care for, 211–216
    in older adults
        cardiac changes, 222–223
        catheter selection for, 222
        renal changes, 222–223
        skin care, 216–222
        vein selection for, 222
        venous distention, 222
    patient education about, 211–212
    peripheral
        midline catheters for, 204–205,
            204f, 213
        short peripheral catheters for,
            202–204, 202f–203f, 202t,
            203b, 214–215
        site selection for, 203–204, 203f,
            204b
        skin preparation for, 203–204

Intravenous therapy (Continued)
        ultrasound applications in,
            202–203
        vein selection for, 203–204,
            203f, 204b
    skin care in, 216–222
    in trauma patients, 130
Intrinsic factor, 798, 814, 1063
Intrinsic renal failure, 1392
Intubation
    complications of, 260
    endotracheal. See Endotracheal
        intubation
Intussusception, 1122, 1122f
Inversion, 1010f
Iodine, 1239
Iodoform gauze, 1000
Iontophoresis, 1041
IPEC Expert Panel. See
        Interprofessional Education
        Collaborative Expert Panel
Ipratropium, 569b–570b, 571
IPV. See Intimate partner violence
IRF. See Inpatient rehabilitation
        facility
IRF-PAI. See Inpatient rehabilitation
        facility patient assessment
        instrument
Iris
    age-related changes in, 961b
    anatomy of, 957, 958f
Iron, 796
Iron deficiency anemia, 814–816,
        814t, 815b
Irreducible hernia, 1138
Irregular bones, 1005
Irrigation
    external ear canal, 994b, 994f
Irritability, 174–175
Irritable bowel syndrome, 1068,
        1135–1137
I-SBAR, 5
I-SBAR-R, 5
ISBT. See International Society of
        Blood Transfusion
Ischemia-edema cycle, 1033
Ischemic heart disease, 727
Ischemic stroke, 927–929, 929t, 935
Ishihara chart, 964
Islam, 112t
Islet cell transplantation, 1303
Islets of Langerhans, 1063, 1239,
        1240f, 1281
Isoelectric line, 666
Isosmotic fluids, 163
Isosthenuria, 1399–1400
Isotonic dehydration, 167–168
Isotonic fluids, 163
Isotonic solution, 200
Ivabradine, 701

J

Jacknife position, 265f
Jackson-Pratt drain, 278, 279f, 282,
        1500
Jaeger card, 964

Janus kinases, 367, 369
Jarisch-Herxheimer reaction, 1510
Jaundice
    cholecystitis as cause of, 1192
    cirrhosis as cause of, 1170, 1171f
    in dark-skin patients, 444
    definition of, 1170
    in hepatitis, 1183
    intrahepatic obstructive, 1170
    obstructive, 1192
    in sickle cell disease, 810
Jaw osteonecrosis,
        bisphosphonate-related, 1021
Jehovah's Witnesses, 123b
Jejunostomy, 1221
Jejunum, 1064
Jitter, 918
Job analysis, 92
Joint(s)
    anatomy of, 1006–1007
    ball-and-socket, 1007
    definition of, 1006
    dislocation of, 1057t
    hand, 1009, 1009f
    hinge, 1007
    pivot, 1007
    synovial, 1006–1007
    types of, 1006
Joint effusions
    mobility affected by, 1010
    in osteoarthritis, 306–307
    in rheumatoid arthritis, 319
J-pouch, 1154, 1154f
Judaism, 112t
Jugular venous distention, 653
Juxtaglomerular complex, 1323,
        1323f
Juxtamedullary nephrons, 1323
JVD. See Jugular venous distention

K

Kallidin, 1197
Kaposi's sarcoma, 347, 348f, 354–355
Karyotype, 74, 75f, 1079
Keratin, 432
Keratinocytes, 432
Keratoconus, 977–979, 978f
Keratoplasty, 978
Keraunographic markings, 142
Keraunoparalysis, 142
Ketoacids, 191
Ketogenesis, 1282
Ketone bodies, 1283, 1301, 1335
Ketorolac tromethamine, 284b, 1195
Kidney(s). See also Renal system
    in acid-base balance, 189t, 190
    acute injury of. See Acute kidney
        injury
    age-related changes in, 234b, 1328
    anatomy of, 1322–1323,
        1322f–1323f
    assessment of, 803, 1330–1331,
        1331f
    bicarbonate movement by, 190
    biopsy of, 1340–1341, 1394
    in blood pressure regulation, 646

Kidney(s) (Continued)
    blood supply to, 1322, 1328
    burn injury-related assessment of,
        491–492
    capsule of, 1322, 1322f
    dehydration effects on, 169
    functions of, 1321, 1323–1327,
        1372, 1390
    gross anatomy of, 1322–1323,
        1322f–1323f
    hormonal functions of,
        1326–1327, 1326t
    microscopic anatomy of, 1323,
        1323f–1324f
    nephrons, 1323, 1323f, 1325t
    nephrotoxic substances for, 1393t
    in older adults, 222–223, 1328b
    palpation of, 1330–1331, 1331f
    postoperative assessment of, 276
    preoperative assessment of, 236
    regulatory functions of,
        1323–1326
    scarring of, 1373–1374
    sickle cell disease effects on, 810
    structure of, 1322–1323,
        1322f–1323f
    trauma to, 1387–1388, 1387b
    tubular reabsorption, 1325
    tubular secretion, 1326
    tumors of, 1385, 1385t
Kidney, ureter, and bladder x-rays,
        1337, 1337t
Kidney disease
    chronic. See Chronic kidney
        disease
    diabetes mellitus as cause of, 1308
    polycystic. See Polycystic kidney
        disease
    terms used for, 1330
Kidney disorders
    acute glomerulonephritis,
        1376–1378, 1376t
    chronic glomerulonephritis, 1378
    diabetic nephropathy, 1286,
        1384–1385
    hydronephrosis, 1361, 1382–1384,
        1383f
    hydroureter, 1361, 1382–1384
    nephrosclerosis, 1379
    nephrotic syndrome, 1378–1379,
        1379b
    polycystic kidney disease. See
        Polycystic kidney disease
    pyelonephritis. See Pyelonephritis
    renal cell carcinoma, 1385–1386
    renovascular disease, 1384
Kidney replacement therapies
    acute kidney injury treated with,
        1397–1398, 1397f
    chronic kidney disease treated
        with, 1411–1424, 1411t,
        1412f–1415f
Kidney stones, 1362t
Kidney transplantation
    acute rejection, 1423–1424, 1423t
    assessments after, 1425b

Kidney transplantation (Continued)
  candidate selection criteria, 1421
  chronic rejection, 1423–1424, 1423t
  complications of, 1423–1424, 1423t
  donors, 1421–1422, 1422f
  hyperacute rejection, 1423–1424, 1423t
  immunosuppressive drug therapy in, 1424
  incidence of, 1421
  living related donors, 1421, 1423
  operative procedures, 1422–1423, 1422f
  postoperative care, 1423
  preoperative care, 1422
  rejection, 1423–1424, 1423t
  self-management education after, 1425
Killip Classification, 651, 781, 782t
Kineret. See Anakinra
Kinins, 293–294
Klebsiella pneumoniae, 422
Knee
  arthroplasty of. See Total knee arthroplasty
  effusion of, 1010
  internal derangement of, 1056
  sports-related injuries of, 1056, 1056b, 1057f, 1057t
Knee height caliper, 1213
Knee immobilizer, 1057f
Knowledge, skills, attitudes, and abilities, 2
Kock's pouch, 1369
Koilonychia, 443t
Kupffer cells, 1063–1064
Kussmaul respiration, 193, 1283, 1312–1313, 1400, 1404
Kwashiorkor, 1215
Kyphoplasty, 1050
Kyphosis, 1009f

L
Labia majora, 1429
Labia minora, 1429
Laboratory technicians, 119–120
Labyrinthectomy, 996
Lacerations
  corneal, 982
  ocular, 981–982
Lacrimal gland, 959, 959f
Lactase deficiency, 1141
Lactate dehydrogenase, 1174
Lactic acidosis, 191–192
Lacto-ovo-vegetarian, 1212
Lactose intolerance, 1212b
Lactose tolerance test, 1141
Lacto-vegetarian, 1212
Lactulose, 1178
Laennec's cirrhosis, 1170
Lamellar keratoplasty, 978
Laminectomy, 906
Lamivudine, 1185t
Language assessment, 847

Lanreotide, 1248–1249
Laparoscopes, 254, 255f
Laparoscopic adjustable gastric band, 1229, 1230f
Laparoscopic Nissen fundoplication, 1091, 1093, 1093f, 1094b
Laparoscopic sleeve gastrectomy, 1229
Laparoscopy
  appendectomy through, 1148
  cholecystectomy, 1195–1196
  radical prostatectomy, 1484
  reproductive system assessments using, 1436–1437, 1437f
  Whipple procedure via, 1207
Laparotomy, 1148
Large intestine
  anatomy of, 1064
  cecum, 1064
  functions of, 1064
  obstruction of, 1123b
Large-volume parenteral infusions, 224
Laryngeal cancer
  description of, 549
  surgical management of, 550, 551t
Laryngeal edema, 363
Laryngeal stridor, 1269–1270
Laryngectomee, 552
Laryngectomy, 550, 554b
Laryngofissure, 551t
Laryngopharynx, 510
Laryngoscopy, 524–525
Larynx
  age-related changes in, 513b
  anatomy of, 509f, 510
  trauma to, 559–560
Laser in-situ keratomileusis, 981
Laser trabeculoplasty, 975
Laser-assisted laparoscopic lumbar diskectomy, 906
LASIK. See Laser in-situ keratomileusis
Late adulthood, 30
Latency period, 375
Latent syphilis, 1508
Latent tuberculosis, 606
Lateral position, 265f
Lateral rectus muscle, 960t
Latex allergy, 234–235, 419
Laxatives, 1136
Lead axis, 666, 666f
Leave-of-absence visit, 100–101
LEEP. See Loop electrosurgical excision procedure
Leflunomide, 322
Left atrial appendage, 681
Left hemisphere stroke, 932–933, 933b
Left main coronary artery, 643, 643f
Left shift, 280, 293
Left ventricular failure
  description of, 695b
  after myocardial infarction, 780–782

Left-sided cardiac catheterization, 658, 658f
Left-sided heart failure, 651, 692, 695–696, 780–782
Legal competence, 36
Leiomyomas, uterine
  assessment of, 1460
  bleeding in, 1461–1463
  care coordination for, 1463
  classification of, 1460f
  etiology of, 1460
  genetic risk of, 1460
  health care resources for, 1463
  home care management of, 1463
  hysterectomy for, 1461–1463, 1461t, 1462b–1463b
  incidence of, 1460
  interventions for, 1461–1463
  pathophysiology of, 1459–1460
  physical assessment of, 1460
  prevalence of, 1460
  psychosocial assessment of, 1460
  self-management education for, 1463
  signs and symptoms of, 1460
  submucosal, 1459–1460, 1460f
  subserosal, 1459–1460, 1460f
  surgical management of, 1461–1463
  transcervical endometrial resection for, 1461
  transition management for, 1463
  transvaginal ultrasound of, 1460
  uterine artery embolization for, 1461, 1461b
Lens
  age-related changes in, 961b
  anatomy of, 958, 958f
Leptin, 1225, 1226b
Leptin resistance, 1225
LES. See Lower esophageal sphincter
Lesbian, gay, bisexual, transgender, and queer population, 1492–1493. See also Transgender patients/health
  description of, 10–11, 11t, 1495
  environment for, 1495b
  sexually transmitted infections in, 1509b
  smoking in, 514b
  The Joint Commission recommendations for, 1495, 1495b
Lethargic, 846
Leukemia, 380b
  acute
    consolidation therapy for, 820–821
    description of, 817, 819b
    drug therapy for, 820–821
    induction therapy for, 820
  acute lymphocytic, 814t
  acute myelogenous, 814t, 820
  acute promyelocytic, 814t
  assessment of, 818–820
  biphenotypic, 818

Leukemia (Continued)
  bleeding precautions in, 825, 825b
  bone marrow aspiration and biopsy for, 820, 820f
  care coordination for, 826–827, 827b
  chronic lymphocytic, 814t, 821
  chronic myelogenous, 814t
  classification of, 818
  drug therapy for, 820–821
  energy conservation in, 826, 826b
  etiology of, 818
  fatigue in, 825–826
  genetic risks of, 818
  genetic syndromes associated with, 818
  health care resources for, 827
  hematopoietic stem cell transplantation for
    bone marrow harvesting for, 823
    complications of, 824–825
    conditioning regimen for, 823–824, 823f
    cord blood harvesting, 823
    engraftment of, 824
    graft-versus-host-disease secondary to, 824–825, 825f
    leukemia treated with, 822–825, 822t
    peripheral blood stem cell harvesting, 823
    stem cells for, 822–823
    steps of, 823f
    transplantation procedure for, 824
    transplants, 822t
    veno-occlusive disease secondary to, 825
  history-taking for, 818–819
  home care management of, 826
  imaging assessment of, 820
  incidence of, 818
  infection protection in, 821–822, 821b
  injury minimization in, 825
  interventions for, 820–825
  laboratory assessment of, 819
  lymphoblastic, 818, 818t
  lymphocytic, 818, 818t
  myelocytic, 818, 818t
  myelogenous, 818, 818t
  nutrition therapy in, 825–826
  pathophysiology of, 817–818
  physical assessment of, 819
  platelet function in, 819
  prevalence of, 818
  psychosocial assessment of, 819
  psychosocial preparation for, 827
  risk factors for, 818
  self-management education for, 826–827, 826b–827b
  transition management for, 826–827, 827b

Leukocyte alkaline phosphatase, 805
Leukocytes
    definition of, 290–291
    functions of, 797t
    in inflammation, 292, 292t
Leukoesterase, 1335
Leukopenia, 815
Leukoplakia, 548, 1078–1079
Leukotriene modifiers, 569b–570b,
    571
Level I trauma center, 127, 128t
Level II trauma center, 127–128, 128t
Level III trauma center, 128, 128t
Level IV trauma center, 128, 128t
Level of consciousness
    assessment of, 130, 896
    definition of, 846
    during dying, 107
    postoperative assessment of,
        274–275
    in stroke patients, 931–932
    in traumatic brain injury patients,
        946
Levels of evidence, 6, 6f
Levodopa/carbidopa, 870
Levosimendan, 700
Levothyroxine sodium, 1273
LGBTQ population. See Lesbian, gay,
    bisexual, transgender, and queer
    population
LH. See Luteinizing hormone
Libido, 1265
Lichenifications, 438f
Lichtenberg figures, 142
Lidocaine patch, 65
Life planning, 100
Life review, 112
Life Safety Code, 150
Ligament tear, 1057t
Light therapy, 465
Lightning injuries, 141–142, 141b
Linagliptin, 1292b–1293b
Linear scleroderma, 329
Lipase, 1068, 1197, 1200
Lipids, 728–729
Lipoatrophy, 348
Lipodystrophy, 348
Lipophilicity, 60
Lipoprotein-a, 656
Liposomal bupivacaine, 65
Lip-reading, 1001
Liquid formula diet, 1227
Liquid oxygen, 536–537, 537f
Liraglutide, 1228, 1292b–1293b
Lispro insulin, 1294
Lithotomy position, 265f
Liver
    anatomy of, 1063–1064, 1063f
    cancer of, 1186–1187
    functions of, 1063
    palpation of, 803
    transplantation of, 1187–1189,
        1188t, 1189b
    trauma to, 1186, 1186b
    in vitamin K formation, 798

Liver disorders
    cancer, 1186–1187
    cirrhosis. See Cirrhosis
    fatty liver, 1185–1186
    hepatitis. See Hepatitis
Liver-spleen scan, 1073
Living will, 104–106
Lixisenatide, 1292b–1293b
LMX-4, 65
Lobar pneumonia, 599
Lobectomy, 589
Lobular carcinoma in situ, 1441
Local anesthesia, 260–261
Local anesthetics, 64–65
Localized pain, 50
Localized peritonitis, 1145
"Lock and key" model, 1235,
    1235f
Locus, 72
Loneliness, 31
Long bones, 1005, 1005f
Long-acting beta₂ agonists,
    569b–571b, 570–571
Long-term care settings
    description of, 30
    health care-associated infections
        in, 417
    older adults in
        care coordination and
            transition management
            for, 42
        health issues for, 39–42
        restorative aids in, 89
Long-term nonprogressors, 338b
Loop diuretics, 699b, 701
Loop electrosurgical excision
    procedure, 1470
Loop of Henle, 1323
Lorazepam, 110, 879
Lorcaserin, 1228
Lordosis, 1009, 1009f
Lovaza, 731
Low back pain. See also Back pain
    assessment of, 904–905
    care coordination for, 908–909
    contributing factors for, 904b
    exercises for, 906b
    health care resources for, 909
    health promotion and
        maintenance for, 904
    herniated nucleus pulposus as
        cause of, 903, 903f
    imaging assessment of, 905
    nonsurgical management of,
        905–906, 906b
    pathophysiology of, 903–904
    physical assessment of, 904–905
    prevention of, 904b, 908b
    signs and symptoms of, 904–905
    surgical management of, 906–908,
        907b
    transition management for,
        908–909
    weight reduction for, 905–906
Low-density lipoprotein, 656

Low-density lipoprotein cholesterol,
    730
Low-energy diets, 1228
Lower esophageal sphincter,
    1062–1063, 1087–1088, 1092
Lower extremity
    amputation of, 1051, 1051b, 1051f
    arterial disease of, 731
    fractures of, 1047–1049,
        1047f–1048f
    traction for, 1040t
Lower gastrointestinal bleeding,
    1156, 1156b
Lower motor neuron, 842
Lower motor neuron disease, 99
Lower respiratory tract, 510–511,
    511f
Lower urinary tract symptoms, 1474,
    1477
Low-intensity pulsed ultrasound,
    1043
Low-molecular-weight heparin,
    744–745
Low-profile gastrostomy device,
    1220f, 1221
Lubiprostone, 1136
Luer-Lok connection, 210
Lukens tube, 601f–602f
Lumacaftor/ivacaftor, 583
Lumbar puncture, 855
Lung(s)
    age-related changes in, 513b
    anatomy of, 510–511, 511f
    assessment of, 518–521
    auscultation of, 519, 520f
    inspection of, 518, 518f
    percussion of, 519, 519f–520f,
        519t
Lung biopsy
    follow-up care for, 527
    patient preparation for, 526–527
    percutaneous, 527
    procedure for, 527
    respiratory system assessments
        using, 526–527
Lung cancer
    assessment of, 380b, 587–588
    chemotherapy for, 588
    deaths caused by, 586
    diagnostic assessment of, 588
    dyspnea management in, 593
    etiology of, 587
    genetic risk of, 587
    history-taking for, 587
    hospice care for, 593
    incidence of, 587
    interventions for, 588–593
    metastasis of, 586
    metastatic sites of, 376t
    nonsurgical management of,
        588–593
    pain management in, 593
    palliative interventions for, 593
    paraneoplastic syndromes
        associated with, 586, 586t

Lung cancer (Continued)
    pathophysiology of, 586–587
    photodynamic therapy for, 589
    physical assessment of, 587–588
    prevalence of, 587
    primary prevention of, 587
    psychosocial assessment of, 588
    radiation therapy for, 588–589,
        593
    signs and symptoms of, 587–588,
        587t
    staging of, 586–587
    surgical management of,
        589–593
    targeted therapy for, 588, 589t
Lung transplantation
    cystic fibrosis treated with,
        583–584
    pulmonary arterial hypertension
        treated with, 585
Lunula, 432–433, 432f
Lupus erythematosus
    discoid, 326–328, 328b
    pathophysiology of, 326
    systemic. See Systemic lupus
        erythematosus
Lupus nephritis, 326
Lurch, 1009
Lutein, 979
Luteinizing hormone
    deficiency of, 1246, 1246b
    description of, 1237t
    overproduction of, 1248b
Luteinizing hormone-releasing
    hormone agonists, 1485
Lyme disease, 332, 333b
Lymph nodes, cervical, 1080, 1080f
Lymphadenopathy, 424
Lymphangiography, 1487
Lymphedema, 652, 1454, 1454b
Lymphokines, 299
Lymphomas
    in AIDS-infected patients,
        347–348
    assessment of, 828–829
    classification of, 827, 829t
    Hodgkin's, 828
    indolent, 828
    interventions for, 829
    mucosa-associated lymphoid
        tissue, 1115
    non-Hodgkin's, 828–829
    pathophysiology of, 828
    staging of, 828, 829t
    treatment of, 829
Lynch syndrome, 1127b, 1128
Lyrica. See Pregabalin
Lysis, 297

M
Macitentan, 585
Macrocytic, 803–804
Macrophages
    function of, 797t
    in inflammation, 293–295

Macula densa, 1323, 1323f
Macula lutea, 958
Macular degeneration, 979
Macular rash, 440
Macules, 438f
Maculopapular rash, 881
Mafenide acetate, 501b
MAG3, 1394
Magnesium
    description of, 181–182
    hypermagnesemia, 182, 182t
    hypomagnesemia, 181–182,
        182t
    in older adults, 165b
    serum levels of, 164t
Magnesium hydroxide, 1091,
    1106b–1107b
Magnesium sulfate, 182, 686, 1277
Magnetic resonance angiography
    description of, 853
    renovascular disease evaluations,
        1384
    stroke assessments using, 935
Magnetic resonance arthrography,
    1013
Magnetic resonance
    cholangiopancreatography,
    1070, 1194
Magnetic resonance enterography
    Crohn's disease assessments using,
        1159
    ulcerative colitis assessments
        using, 1152
Magnetic resonance imaging
    cardiovascular system evaluations
        using, 661
    cognition assessments with, 17
    contraindications for, 853
    ear assessments using, 990
    functional, 853
    gastrointestinal system
        assessments, 1070
    hyperpituitarism evaluations,
        1248
    multiple sclerosis evaluations, 890,
        890f
    musculoskeletal system
        evaluations using, 1012–1013,
        1013b
    neurologic system evaluations
        using, 853
    osteoporosis evaluations, 1019
    patient preparation for, 1013b
    renal system assessments using,
        1337t, 1338
    reproductive system assessments,
        1436
    traumatic brain injury
        evaluations, 946
    vision assessments, 965
Magnetic resonance spectroscopy
    description of, 853
    osteoporosis evaluations, 1019
Magnetoencephalography, 854
Malabsorption syndrome, 1141–1142

Male reproductive disorders
    benign prostatic hyperplasia. See
        Benign prostatic hyperplasia
    erectile dysfunction, 27, 1286,
        1484–1485, 1489–1490
    overview of, 1473
    testicular cancer. See Testicular
        cancer
Male reproductive system
    function of, 1430–1431
    genitalia, 1430f
    hormones of, 1430
    in older adults, 1431b
    physical assessment of, 1433
    structure of, 1430–1431
Male-to-female transgender patients
    definition of, 1493–1494, 1493t
    drug therapy for, 1497–1499, 1497t
    gender reassignment surgery for,
        1499–1500
    vaginoplasty for, 1499–1500
Malignant hypertension, 721
Malignant hyperthermia, 258–259,
    259b–260b
Malignant otitis, 993
Malleus, 984, 985f–986f
Malnutrition
    assessment of, 25, 1217
    care coordination for, 1224–1225
    complications of, 1215–1216
    description of, 24
    drug therapy for, 1219
    dysphagia as cause of, 1217b
    eating disorders as cause of, 1216
    health care resources for,
        1224–1225
    health promotion and
        maintenance for, 1216
    history-taking for, 1217
    home care management of, 1224
    inadequate nutrient intake as
        cause of, 1216
    incidence of, 1216
    infection risks associated with,
        414–415
    interventions for, 1217–1224
    laboratory assessment of, 1217
    manifestations of, 1218t
    meal management for, 1218
    nutrition supplements for,
        1218–1219
    in older adults, 40, 1216b
    partial parenteral nutrition for,
        1223–1224
    pathophysiology of, 1215–1216
    physical assessment of, 1217
    prevalence of, 1216
    protein-calorie, 1215
    protein-energy, 1215
    psychosocial assessment of, 1217
    risk assessment for, 1216b
    self-management education for,
        1224
    signs and symptoms of,
        1215–1217

Malnutrition (Continued)
    total enteral nutrition for
        abdominal distention caused by,
            1222
        administration of, 1220–1221,
            1220f
        complications of, 1221–1223
        description of, 1219–1223
        diarrhea secondary to, 1223
        electrolyte imbalances caused
            by, 1222–1223
        enterostomal feeding tubes used
            in, 1220–1221
        fluid imbalances caused by,
            1222–1223
        gastrostomy for, 1221
        jejunostomy for, 1221
        nasoduodenal tube delivery of,
            1220
        nasoenteric tube delivery of,
            1220, 1220f
        nasogastric tube delivery of,
            1220
        nausea and vomiting caused by,
            1222
        refeeding syndrome caused by,
            1221–1222
        tube misplacement and
            dislodgement, 1222
    total parenteral nutrition for,
        1224
    transition management for,
        1224–1225
Malunion, of fracture, 1035
Mammalian target of rapamycin, 405
Mammography, 382, 1435–1436,
    1443, 1446
MammoSite, 1451
Mandibular fractures, 558
Mandibulectomy, 1082
Mannitol, for traumatic brain injury,
    948, 948b
Marasmic-kwashiorkor, 1215
Marasmus, 1215
Marfan syndrome, 334t, 740
Mass casualty event
    acute stress disorder after, 156,
        156b, 158
    definition of, 149–150
    nurse's role in, 155
    post-traumatic stress disorder
        after, 156b
    resolution of, 156–157
    survivors to, psychosocial response
        of, 157–158
    triage for, 151–153, 152t
Massage, 109
Massive hemothorax, 637
Mast cells, 294, 361, 361f, 565
Mastectomy
    breast reconstruction after,
        1449–1450, 1450t, 1451b
    exercises after, 1451b
    lymphedema after, 1454
    modified radical, 1448, 1448f

Mastectomy (Continued)
    postoperative teaching for,
        1453–1454
    prophylactic, 1443–1444
    total, 1448f
Mastication, 1062
Mastoid process, 984, 988
Mastoiditis, 995
Mattress overlays, 97
Maxillary sinus, 509f
Maze procedure, 681
McBurney's point, 1147–1148, 1148f
McGill-Melzack Pain Questionnaire,
    50–52, 51f
MCH. See Mean corpuscular
    hemoglobin
MCV. See Mean corpuscular volume
Meal planning, for diabetes mellitus,
    1300
Mean arterial pressure, 643–644, 752,
    753f, 754, 756
Mean corpuscular hemoglobin,
    803–804
Mean corpuscular volume, 803–804
Mechanical débridement, 457, 457t
Mechanical obstruction, 1122–1123,
    1122f
Mechanical ventilation
    care for patient receiving, 630b
    complications of, 634–635
    dependence on, 635
    indications for, 628
    infections caused by, 635
    modes of, 631
    nursing management of, 632–635
    pain assessments in patients
        receiving, 54
    patient's response to, monitoring
        of, 632–633
    purposes of, 630
    respiratory acidosis and, 192, 195
    upper airway obstruction treated
        with, 561
    ventilators
        controls and settings for, 631–633
        types of, 631, 633
        ventilator-associated events,
            634, 634t
    weaning from, 635, 636t
Mechanically regulated devices, for
    infusion therapy, 211, 212f
Mechanism of injury, 128–129
Medial rectus muscle, 960t
Median nerve, 1057
Mediastinitis, 788–789, 1099
Mediastinoscopy, 524–525
Medical command physician, 154, 154t
Medical emergency team, 8
Medical history, 233–234
Medical nutrition supplements,
    1218–1219
Medical nutrition therapy, for
    diabetes mellitus, 1299–1300
Medical Reserve Corps, 153
Medical-surgical nursing, 1–2

Medicare, 32
Medicare Hospice Benefit, 106
Medication administration records, 201
Medication errors
    in emergency departments, 121
    in older adults, 35
Medication overuse headache, 874
Medication reconciliation
    definition of, 3
    information used for, 3
    nurse-led protocol for, 4b
Medicine wheel, 113f
Medullary carcinoma, 1275
Megaloblastic anemia, 814
Meglitinide analogs, 1291, 1292b–1293b
Melanin, 432
Melanocytes, 432
Melanocyte-stimulating hormone, 1237t, 1254
Melanoma, 376t, 475t, 476, 476f
Melatonin, 923
Melena, 1105, 1108, 1170
Memantine, 864
Memory, 16
    Alzheimer's disease-related impairments in, 860
    assessment of, 847
Memory cells, 297–298, 797t
Ménière's disease, 986–987, 995–996
Meniett device, 996
Meninges, 840
Meningiomas, 951
Meningitis
    aseptic, 881
    care for, 882b
    Cryptococcus neoformans, 881
    definition of, 954
    interventions for, 882–883
    meningococcal, 881
    pathophysiology of, 880–881
    viral, 881
Meningococcal meningitis, 881
Meniscus tear, 1057t
Menopause, 27
Mental status
    age-related changes in, 845
    assessment of, 846–847
    in heat stroke victims, 134
Meperidine, 59b, 61, 1047
Mepilex Ag, 501b
MERS. *See* Middle East respiratory syndrome
Mesalamine, 1152b
Mesenteric artery thrombosis, 16b
MET. *See* Medical emergency team
Metabolic acidosis, 13, 191, 191t, 193–195, 193b, 1122
Metabolic alkalosis, 13, 193b, 196, 196t, 1122
Metabolic syndrome
    clinical features of, 1287
    description of, 771, 772t
    type 2 diabetes mellitus risks, 1287

Metabolic/respiratory acidosis, 192
Metabolism
    burn injury effects on, 486
    chronic kidney disease effects on, 1400–1401, 1400f
    insulin effects on, 1282
    liver's function in, 1064
Metacarpal fractures, 1047
Metacarpophalangeal joint, 1009, 1009f
Metaproterenol, 365
Metastasis. *See also* Cancer
    bloodborne, 375
    brain tumors caused by, 951
    breast cancer, 1440–1441, 1446–1452
    cervical lymph node, 1082
    colorectal cancer, 1127, 1129–1132
    definition of, 375, 384–385
    esophageal cancer, 1095
    head and neck cancer, 548
    lung cancer, 586
    lymphatic spread for, 375
    prostate cancer, 1483–1485
    sites of, 376t, 1440–1441
    steps of, 376f
Metastatic calcifications, 1401
Metered dose inhaler, 568–570, 570b, 570f
Metformin, 1291, 1291b, 1338
Methacholine, 567
Methadone, 61
Methemoglobinemia, 525
Methicillin-resistant *Staphylococcus aureus*
    community-associated, 422
    contact precautions for, 419
    description of, 422
    health care-associated, 422, 422b
    in osteomyelitis, 1023
    prevention of, 468–469, 469b
    skin infections caused by, 466
    stool culture and sensitivity for, 19
Methimazole, 1268b
Methotrexate
    pregnancy contraindications with, 322
    for rheumatoid arthritis, 322
Metronidazole, 1166, 1179
Metyrapone, 1258
Microalbuminuria, 656, 697, 1308, 1335, 1399
Microbiome, 77, 414b
Microcytic, 803–804, 814
Microdiskectomy, for back pain, 906
Microhemagglutination assay, 1509
Microorganisms
    antimicrobial sensitivity testing of, 424
    culture of, 424
Microprocessor ventilators, 631, 631f
Microvascular bone transfers, 1024
Microvascular decompression, 924
Microwave ablation, 1026, 1386
Micturition, 1327

Midarm circumference, 1215
Midarm muscle mass, 1215
MIDCAB. *See* Minimally invasive coronary artery bypass grafting
Mid-clavicular catheter, 205
Middle cerebral artery
    anatomy of, 841
    stroke involving, 933b
Middle ear, 984–985, 985f
Middle East respiratory syndrome, 598
Midline catheters, 204–205, 204f, 213
Midrin, 875
Mifepristone, 1258, 1258b
Miglitol, 1292b–1293b
Migraine headaches
    abortive therapy for, 874–875
    assessment of, 873–874
    atypical, 873–874, 874b
    with aura, 873–874, 874b
    categories of, 873–874
    complementary and integrative health for, 875–876
    definition of, 873
    diagnosis of, 874
    drug therapy for, 874–875
    ergotamine preparations for, 875
    external trigeminal nerve stimulator for, 875
    neuroimaging of, 874
    nortriptyline for, 875
    pathophysiology of, 873
    preventive therapy for, 875
    triggers for, 873, 875, 876b
    triptans for, 874–875, 875b
    without aura, 873–874, 874b
Migratory arthritis, 318–319
Miliary tuberculosis, 605–606
Milrinone, 700, 783b
Mindfulness, 67
Mineralocorticoids, 1237
Mini Nutritional Assessment, 1213, 1214f
Minimally invasive coronary artery bypass grafting, 789
Minimally invasive esophagectomy, 1098
Minimally invasive inguinal hernia repair, 1138–1139, 1139b
Minimally invasive surgery
    back pain treated with, 906, 910
    bariatric surgery using, 1229
    benefits of, 252–254
    brain tumors treated with, 953
    colorectal cancer treated with, 1130, 1132
    description of, 232t, 235, 252–254
    endoscopes used in, 254, 255f
    gastroesophageal reflux disease treated with, 1091
    home care management of, 908
    injuries during, 255
    insufflation in, 254
    intestinal obstruction managed with, 1125

Minimally invasive surgery (Continued)
    nasogastric tubes in, 1125
    pancreatic cancer treated with, 1207
    peptic ulcer disease treated with, 1114
    prostate cancer treated with, 1484
    testicular cancer treated with, 1488
    thymomas treated with, 921
    total hip arthroplasty, 310
    total knee arthroplasty, 314
    urolithiasis treated with, 1364
    Whipple procedure, 1207
Mini-Mental State Examination, 860–861
Miosis, 960, 960f
Mirabegron, 1349
Mistriage, 124
Mitosis, 73–74
Mitoxantrone, 891
Mitraclip, 709
Mitral regurgitation, 706, 706b
Mitral stenosis, 705–706, 706b, 710b
Mitral valve
    anatomy of, 642–643, 643f
    annuloplasty of, 709
    prolapse of, 706
Mitral valvuloplasty, 708
Mixed agonists/antagonists, 57
Mixed aphasia, 938
Mixed conductive-sensorineural hearing loss, 989
Mixed incontinence, 1345t
Mixed urinary incontinence, 1345t, 1352
MMSE. *See* Mini-Mental State Examination
MNA. *See* Mini Nutritional Assessment
Mobility
    assessment of, 23, 94f, 1009–1010
    cane for, 1044
    crutches for, 1043–1044, 1044f
    decreased
        description of, 23–24, 23t
        in older adults, 31–32
        rehabilitation for, 93–96
    definition of, 23
    Guillain-Barré syndrome effects on, 914, 914b, 916
    in multiple sclerosis, 891–892
    musculoskeletal trauma effects on, 1032
    postoperative, 245
    promotion of
        after amputation, 1053–1054
        in burn injury patients, 502–504
        description of, 23–24
        in fracture patients, 1043–1044
        in myasthenia gravis patients, 919

Mobility *(Continued)*
  in osteoarthritis patients, 316
  in rheumatoid arthritis patients, 324
  scope of, 23
  spinal cord injury effects on, 23, 896, 900–901
  stroke-related changes in, 933–934, 938
  walker for, 1044
Moderate sedation, 261–262, 262*t*
Modified radical mastectomy, 1448, 1448*f*
Modified-release opioids, 58–59, 59*b*
MODS. *See* Multiple organ dysfunction score
Mohs' surgery, 477
Moist heat, 486
Moniliasis, 1076
Monoamine oxidase type B inhibitors, 870
Monoclonal antibodies
  cancer treated with, 402–403
  immunosuppression uses of, 302*b*
  mechanism of action, 402–403
  skin cancer treated with, 477
  ulcerative colitis treated with, 1153
Monoclonal gammopathy of undetermined significance, 830
Monocytes, 797*t*
Monogenic traits, 74
Monokines, 299
Monounsaturated fatty acids, 1299
Montelukast, 569*b*–570*b*
Montgomery straps, 278, 278*f*, 282
Morbid obesity, 1225
Morbidity, 235
Morphine sulfate
  acute coronary syndrome applications of, 775
  description of, 59–60
  dyspnea treated with, 110
  equianalgesic dosing of, 60*t*
  heart failure applications of, 699
  postoperative pain management using, 284*b*
Mortality, 235
Motor aphasia, 938
Motor end plate, 1007
Motor function assessments, 848
Motor neurons, 839–840
Motor vehicle accidents
  by older adults, 34, 34*b*
  spinal cord injury caused by, 895
  traumatic brain injury caused by, 943. *See also* Traumatic brain injury
Mourning, 112
MRSA. *See* Methicillin-resistant *Staphylococcus aureus*
MSH2 gene, 382

mTOR. *See* Mammalian target of rapamycin
Mu agonists, 56–57
Mucosa-associated lymphoid tissue lymphoma, 1115
Mucosal barrier fortifiers, 1105, 1106*b*–1107*b*, 1112
Mucositis, chemotherapy-related, 399–400, 400*b*, 588
Mucous fistula, 1132
Mucous membranes, 520, 530–531
Multi-casualty event, 149–152
Multidrug-resistant organism infections
  carbapenem-resistant *Enterobacteriaceae*, 422–423
  contact precautions for, 419
  methicillin-resistant *Staphylococcus aureus*, 422
  in osteomyelitis, 1023
  types of, 421–422
  vancomycin-resistant *Enterococcus*, 422
Multidrug-resistant tuberculosis, 609
Multigated blood pool scanning, 661, 697
Multi-infarct dementia, 37
Multikinase inhibitors, 404*t*, 405
Multimodal analgesia
  continuous, 54
  pain managed with, 54–55
Multimodal therapy, for oral cancer, 1080
Multiple endocrine neoplasia, 1246*b*
Multiple myeloma, 829–830
Multiple organ dysfunction score, 104
Multiple organ dysfunction syndrome, 754–755, 755*b*, 762
Multiple sclerosis
  amyotrophic lateral sclerosis versus, 889*t*
  assessment of, 888–890
  care coordination for, 892–894
  clinical features of, 889*b*
  cognitive impairment in, 892*b*
  complementary and integrative health for, 892
  concept map for, 892*f*–893*f*
  definition of, 888
  diagnostic assessment of, 890, 890*f*
  etiology of, 888
  familial patterns of, 888*b*
  health care resources for, 894
  history-taking for, 888
  home care management of, 892
  incidence of, 888
  infection prevention in, 890–891
  intention tremor associated with, 889
  interventions for, 890–891
  laboratory assessment of, 890
  magnetic resonance imaging of, 890, 890*f*
  mobility interventions in, 891–892

Multiple sclerosis *(Continued)*
  muscle spasticity in, 891
  pathophysiology of, 888
  plaques associated with, 890, 890*f*
  prevalence of, 888
  primary progressive, 888
  progressive-relapsing, 888
  psychosocial assessment of, 889–890
  relapsing-remitting, 888, 890–891
  secondary progressive, 888
  self-management education for, 892
  sexuality affected by, 890, 892
  transition management for, 892–894
  visual system manifestations of, 889, 892
Murmurs, 654–655
Muromonab-CD3, 302*b*
Muscarinic-receptor antagonists, 1137
Muscle biopsy, 1013
Muscle enzymes, 1011
Muscle fibers, 1007
Muscle spasticity, 891
Muscle strength, 1011, 1011*t*
Muscle-specific kinase, 918
Muscular system
  anatomy of, 1007
  assessment of, 1011
Musculoskeletal disorders
  bone tumors. *See* Bone tumors
  foot disorders, 1028–1029, 1028*f*, 1029*t*
  hand disorders, 1028, 1028*f*
  osteomyelitis, 1022–1024, 1023*b*, 1023*f*, 1035
  osteoporosis. *See* Osteoporosis
  overview of, 1015
Musculoskeletal system
  age-related changes in, 234*b*, 1007–1008, 1007*b*
  arthroscopy applications for, 1013–1014, 1013*f*
  assessment of, 90*t*, 91, 803, 1008–1014
  biopsies of, 1013, 1013*b*
  bone. *See* Bone
  computed tomography of, 1011
  current health problems that affect, 1008–1009
  diagnostic assessment of, 1011–1014
  electromyography of, 1013
  ethnic differences in, 1005*t*
  functional assessments of, 1009–1010
  gait assessments, 1009
  health promotion and maintenance of, 1007–1008
  history-taking, 1008–1009
  hypernatremia effects on, 175
  hypocalcemia effects on, 180
  hypokalemia effects on, 176

Musculoskeletal system *(Continued)*
  imaging assessment of, 1011–1013
  inspection of, 1009–1010, 1009*f*
  joints, 1006–1007
  laboratory assessment of, 1011, 1012*b*
  magnetic resonance imaging of, 1012–1013, 1013*b*
  mobility assessments, 1009–1010
  muscular system
    anatomy of, 1007
    assessment of, 1011
    strength grading, 1011, 1011*t*
  neurovascular assessment of, 1010, 1010*b*
  nuclear scans of, 1011–1012
  nutrition history, 1008
  overview of, 1004–1005
  posture assessments, 1009, 1009*f*
  preoperative assessment of, 236
  psychosocial assessment of, 1011
  radiography of, 1011
  range of motion assessments of, 1010, 1010*f*
  sickle cell disease effects on, 810
  skeletal system
    anatomy of, 1005–1007, 1005*f*
    assessment of, 1009–1010
    bone. *See* Bone
  ultrasonography of, 1013
Musculoskeletal trauma
  amputation. *See* Amputation
  carpal tunnel syndrome, 1057–1059, 1058*b*
  description of, 1032
  fractures. *See* Fractures
  knee injuries, 1056, 1056*b*, 1057*f*, 1057*t*
  mobility affected by, 1032
  rotator cuff injuries, 1059
Music therapy, 109, 111
Mutations
  gene, 76–77
  somatic, 76
Myasthenia gravis
  acetylcholine receptors in, 917
  assessment of, 917–919
  care coordination for, 921–922
  cholinesterase inhibitors for, 919–920
  clinical features of, 917*b*
  definition of, 917
  diagnostic assessment of, 918–919
  drug therapy for, 919–921
  Eaton-Lambert syndrome, 918
  electromyography for, 918
  facial expression in, 917–918, 918*f*
  factors that worsen or precipitate, 922*t*
  health care resources for, 922
  home care management of, 921–922
  immunosuppressants for, 920
  interventions for, 919–921

Myasthenia gravis (Continued)
  mobility promotion in, 919
  nonsurgical management of, 919–921
  nutrition in, 921b
  pathophysiology of, 917
  plasmapheresis for, 920–921
  repetitive nerve stimulation for, 918
  respiratory support in, 919
  self-management education of, 922, 922b
  single-fiber electromyography for, 918
  surgical management of, 921
  thymoma associated with, 918
  transition management for, 921–922
Myasthenic crisis, 918–920, 920t
Mycobacterium avium complex, 347
Mycobacterium tuberculosis, 605–606
Mycophenolate
  autoimmune diseases treated with, 368
  immunosuppression uses of, 302b
Mydriasis, 960, 960f
Myelin sheath, 840
Myeloablation, 824
Myelodysplastic syndromes
  hematopoietic stem cell transplantation for, 817
  leukemia. See Leukemia
  in older adults, 817
  pathophysiology of, 817
  risk factors for, 817
Myelosuppression, chemotherapy-induced, 396–398
Myocardial contractility, 645
Myocardial hypertrophy, 694
Myocardial infarction
  anterior wall, 771
  aspirin for, 776–777
  beta blockers for, 777
  cardiac rehabilitation for, 790
  care coordination for, 789–792
  chest discomfort associated with, 650t
  complementary and integrative health after, 791
  coronary artery bypass graft for. See Coronary artery bypass graft
  drug therapy for, 774–778, 776b, 791
  electrocardiographic changes and patterns associated with, 770f
  emergency care for, 774–775
  features of, 773b
  gender and, 772b
  glycoprotein IIb/IIIa inhibitors for, 776
  heart failure after
    classification of, 781–782, 782t
    drug therapy for, 782

Myocardial infarction (Continued)
  hemodynamic monitoring of, 780
    left ventricular, 780–782
    right-ventricular, 782
  home care management of, 789–790, 790b
  imaging assessment of, 773–774
  incidence of, 772
  inferior wall, 771
  interventions for, 774–778
  laboratory assessment of, 773
  lateral wall, 771
  medical assistance indications in, 791–792
  nitroglycerin for, 774
  non–ST-segment elevation, 770
  pathophysiology of, 770
  percutaneous coronary intervention for, 783–784, 784f
  posterior wall, 771
  prevalence of, 772
  psychosocial assessment of, 773
  reperfusion therapy for, 777–778
  risk factor modification for, 790–791
  serum markers of, 655
  sexual activity after, 791
  ST-elevation, 770
  surgical complications caused by, 233
  thrombolytic therapy for, 777–778, 778t
  transition management for, 789–792
Myocardial nuclear perfusion imaging, 661
Myocardium
  coronary artery blood flow to, 643–644
  functions of, 641
Myoclonic seizures, 876
Myoglobin, 492
Myoglobinuria, 258–259
Myomas, 1459–1460
Myopathy, 1008–1009
Myopia, 960, 960f, 980–981
Myosplint, 702
Myotomes, 896
MyPlate, 1211–1212, 1212f
Myringoplasty, 999
Myringotomy, 992–993, 992f
Myxedema, 1265, 1271, 1271f
Myxedema coma, 1271, 1273, 1273b–1274b

N
NAFLD. See Nonalcoholic fatty liver disease
Nails
  age-related changes, 435f
  anatomy of, 432–433, 432f
  assessment of, 441–442, 442f, 442t
  clubbing of, 443t, 652

Nails (Continued)
  consistency of, 441
  dystrophic, 441
  ingrown, 1029t
  lesions of, 441–442
  pigmentation of, 441, 442f
  shape of, 441, 443t
Naloxone, 64b, 284
Naltrexone SR/bupropion SR, 1228
Narcan. See Naloxone
Nasal cannula, 531–532, 532f, 532t, 604
Nasal polyps, 517
Nasoduodenal tube, 1220
Nasoenteric tube, 1220, 1220f
Nasogastric tube
  aspiration risks associated with, 553
  in bariatric surgery patients, 1230b
  complications of, 277
  in esophageal surgery patients, 1100, 1100b
  intestinal obstruction managed with, 1124, 1134b
  postoperative monitoring of, 277
  total enteral nutrition delivery using, 1220
  upper gastrointestinal bleeding managed with, 1113
Nasopharyngeal secretions, 560
Nasopharynx, 509, 509f
Nasoseptoplasty, 557
Natal sex, 1493, 1493t
Natalizumab, 891
Nateglinide, 1292b–1293b
National Comprehensive Cancer Network Distress Thermometer, 395, 395f
National Fire Protection Association, 150
National Institute for Occupational Safety and Health safe patient handling guidelines, 93
National Institute on Aging, 38
National Institutes of Health Stroke Scale, 931, 931t–932t
National Patient Safety Goals
  blood components, 200, 833
  blood donation, 235
  description of, 4–5, 8
  drug safety, 201
  for falls, 40–41, 1018, 1020
  hand-off communication, 120, 317
  hand-off report, 271
  handwashing, 882, 1100
  infection control, 417
  influenza vaccine, 596–597
  informed consent, 658
  nutrition screening, 1212
  patient identification, 247, 262–263, 262b
  preoperative requirements, 238–239

National Patient Safety Goals (Continued)
  pressure injuries, 448–449
  for pressure injuries, 42
  surgical communication, 229
  tracheostomy communication, 544
  transfusion therapy, 833
  warfarin monitoring, 745
Natriuresis, 698
Natriuretic peptides
  B-type, 694, 697
  definition of, 694
  fluid balance regulation by, 166
Natural immunity, 291–292
Natural killer cells, 299, 797t
Natural orifice transluminal endoscopic surgery, 1148, 1153, 1196, 1204
Nausea and vomiting
  chemotherapy-induced, 398–399, 399b
  at end of life, 111
  opioid analgesics as cause of, 63t
  postoperative, 276
  total enteral nutrition as cause of, 1222
Near point of vision, 961
Near vision, 964
Near-drowning, 147
Near-syncope, 650–651
Necitumumab, 589t
Neck
  assessment of, 802
  cancer of. See Head and neck cancer
Neck dissection, 550
Neck veins, 168
Necrotic tissue
  debridement of, in frostbite patients, 145
  description of, 28
Necrotizing hemorrhagic pancreatitis, 1197–1198
Necrotizing otitis, 993
Nedocromil, 569b–570b
Needle biopsy, 1243
Needle thoracostomy, 638
Needleless connection devices, 210–211, 210f, 214
Needlestick injuries, 343
Needlestick Safety and Prevention Act, 210
Negative feedback, 1235–1236, 1236f
Negative nitrogen balance, 1265
Negative-pressure wound therapy, 278, 458, 1160
Neisseria gonorrhoeae, 1512
Neisseria meningitidis, 414
Neobladder, 1368, 1369b
Neodermis, 499
Neovascularization, 1284
Nephrectomy, 1375, 1386

Nephrogenic diabetes insipidus, 1250, 1250b
Nephrolithiasis, 1361
Nephrolithotomy, 1364
Nephrons, 1323, 1323f, 1325t
Nephrosclerosis, 1379
Nephrostomy, 1383
Nephrotic syndrome, 1378–1379, 1379b
Nerve block, 261f, 261t
Nervous system. See also Brain; Neurologic system; Spinal cord
  assessment of, 846–855
  autonomic, 842–844
  cells of, 839–840
  central. See Central nervous system
  complete assessment of, 846–850
  computed tomography–magnetic resonance imaging of, 853–854
  divisions of, 839
  history-taking for, 846
  imaging assessment of, 851–855
  laboratory assessment of, 851
  magnetic resonance imaging of, 853
  peripheral, 842
  physical assessment of, 846–850
  psychosocial assessment of, 850–851
  rapid/focused assessment of, 850
Nesiritide, 698, 698b
Neuritic plaques, 858, 859f
Neurofibrillary tangles, 858, 859f
Neurogenic bladder, 98t
Neurogenic bowel, 99t
Neurogenic diabetes insipidus, 1250
Neurogenic pulmonary edema, 954
Neurogenic shock, 898
Neuroglia cells, 840
Neurohypophysis, 1236, 1237f
Neurokinin receptor antagonists, for chemotherapy-induced nausea and vomiting, 399b
Neurologic disorders
  Alzheimer's disease. See Alzheimer's disease
  encephalitis, 883–884, 884b
  meningitis. See Meningitis
  migraine headaches. See Migraine headaches
  Parkinson disease. See Parkinson disease
  seizures. See Seizures
Neurologic system. See also Nervous system
  age-related changes in, 234b, 844–845, 845b
  assessment of, 90t, 91, 846–855
  auditory evoked potentials of, 855
  cerebral angiography evaluations of, 852–853, 852b
  complete assessment of, 846–850
  computed tomography of, 853

Neurologic system (Continued)
  computed tomography–magnetic resonance imaging of, 853–854
  dehydration effects on, 168–169
  electroencephalography of, 854
  electromyography of, 854
  evoked potentials of, 854–855
  health promotion and maintenance of, 845–846
  imaging assessment of, 851–855
  laboratory assessment of, 851
  lumbar puncture of, 855
  magnetic resonance imaging of, 853
  magnetoencephalography of, 854
  postoperative assessment of, 274–275, 274t
  psychosocial assessment of, 850–851
  rapid/focused assessment of, 850
  single-photon emission computed tomography of, 854
  somatosensory evoked potentials of, 855
  transcranial Doppler ultrasonography of, 855
  visual evoked potentials of, 855
  x-rays of, 851
Neuroma
  acoustic, 951, 996
  definition of, 1050
Neuromodulation therapy, 1349
Neuromuscular blocking agents, 258
Neuromuscular system
  acidosis effects on, 193, 193b
  alkalosis effects on, 196, 196b
  hypercalcemia effects on, 181
  hyperkalemia effects on, 178
  hypocalcemia effects on, 180
  hypomagnesemia effects on, 182
  hyponatremia-related changes, 174
Neuron
  afferent, 840
  efferent, 840
  functions of, 839–840
  motor, 839–840
  sensory, 839–840
  structure of, 839–840, 840f
  synapse in, 840
Neurontin. See Gabapentin
Neuropathic pain, 48, 48t, 1307
Neuropathy, 1008–1009
Neurotransmitters
  definition of, 840
  in Parkinson disease, 868
Neutropenia
  chemotherapy-induced, 395, 396b
  definition of, 817
Neutrophilia, 295
Neutrophils
  functions of, 293, 797t
  in inflammation, 292–293, 292t

New York Heart Association Functional Classification, 651, 651t
New-onset angina, 770
Nicotine replacement therapies, 514–515
Nifedipine, 146
NIOSH. See National Institute for Occupational Safety and Health
Nitrates
  acute coronary syndromes treated with, 776b, 783b
  heart failure treated with, 699
Nitrites, 1335
Nitrofurazone, 501b
Nitroglycerin
  for angina pectoris, 774–775
  drug interactions for, 775b
  for myocardial infarction, 783b
  sublingual, 791b
Nitroprusside sodium, 783b
Nivolumab, 477, 589t
NMDA receptor antagonists, 864
NNRTIs. See Non-nucleoside reverse transcriptase inhibitors
Nociception
  processes of, 47–48, 49f
  schematic diagram of, 49f
Nociceptive pain, 47–48, 48t
Nociceptors, 47, 873
Nocturia, 41, 91, 236, 1328b, 1330, 1381, 1474, 1482
Nocturnal polyuria, 1328
Nodes of Ranvier, 840
Nodules, 438f
Nonabsorbable sutures, 267
Nonalcoholic fatty liver disease, 1172, 1185–1186
Nonalcoholic steatohepatitis, 1185
Noncommunicating hydrocephalus, 943
Noncompliance, 423
Non-Hodgkin's lymphoma, 828–829
Noninfectious cystitis, 1356
Noninsulin-dependent diabetes mellitus. See Diabetes mellitus, type 2
Noninvasive positive-pressure ventilation
  description of, 535, 535b, 536f
  obstructive sleep apnea treated with, 535, 559
Nonmaleficence, 9
Nonmechanical obstruction, 1122–1123
Non-nucleoside reverse transcriptase inhibitors
  mechanism of action, 338
  types of, 351b–352b
Nonrebreather masks, 532t, 533, 533f
Non-self cells, 380
Non-self proteins, 289–290, 290f
Nonseminomas, 1487

Nonsteroidal anti-inflammatory drugs
  adverse effects of, 56, 56b
  cardiovascular risks, 791b
  carpal tunnel syndrome managed with, 1058
  fibromyalgia managed with, 334
  gastritis caused by, 1104–1105
  in older adults, 56b
  pain management uses of, 55–56, 56b, 284b, 307–308, 1364
  peptic ulcer disease caused by, 1109
  postoperative pain management using, 284b
  rheumatoid arthritis managed with, 321
  topical, 308
Non–ST-segment elevation myocardial infarction, 770
Nonsustained ventricular tachycardia, 683
Nontunneled percutaneous central venous catheters, 206–207, 206f, 215
Nonunion, of fracture, 1035, 1043
Nonurgent triage, 124
Norco. See Hydrocodone
Norepinephrine, 1238
Normal sinus rhythm, 671, 671f
Normotonic fluids, 163
Norovirus, 1148t, 1149
Nortriptyline, for migraine headaches, 875
Nose
  anatomy of, 509, 509f
  assessment of, 517
  cancer of, 556
  epistaxis of, 557–558, 557b, 558f
  fractures of, 556–557, 556f
Novel oral anticoagulants
  clinical uses of, 680, 708, 710
  deep vein thrombosis treated with, 745
Novelty diets, 1228
NPO status, 241
NPPV. See Noninvasive positive-pressure ventilation
NPSGs. See National Patient Safety Goals
NPWT. See Negative-pressure wound therapy
NRS. See Numeric rating scale
NRTIs. see Nucleoside reverse transcriptase inhibitors
Nuclear, biologic, and chemical threats, 150
Nuclear scans
  gastrointestinal bleeding evaluations using, 1111
  musculoskeletal system evaluations using, 1011–1012
Nuclear-to-cytoplasmic ratio, 373–374

Nucleic acid amplification test, 347, 1513
Nucleoside reverse transcriptase inhibitors
    mechanism of action, 338
    types of, 351b–352b
Nucynta. See Tapentadol
Numeric rating scale, 50
Nurse
    emergency. See Emergency
    health care facility emergency preparedness role of, 154–156
    perioperative, 229
    postanesthesia care unit, 271
    registered, 123–124, 253t
    rehabilitation, 88, 88t
Nursing assistants, 88
Nursing technicians, 88
Nutrition. See also Diet
    in acute pancreatitis, 1201
    for acute respiratory distress syndrome, 628
    age-related changes in, 31
    in cholecystitis, 1194
    in chronic kidney disease, 1407–1408, 1407t
    clotting affected by, 802
    decreased
        description of, 23t, 24–25
        in older adults, 30–31
    definition of, 24
    ethnic preferences, 1212b
    gastrectomy effects on, 1118
    gout treated with, 332
    head and neck cancer effects on, 552
    for health promotion and maintenance, 1211–1212
    Healthy People 2020 objectives for, 1226t
    in hepatitis, 1184
    in human immunodeficiency virus infection, 354
    laboratory testing for, 25
    malabsorption managed with, 1142
    in myasthenia gravis, 921b
    in older adults, 1219b
    preoperative assessment of, 236–237
    promotion of, 25, 1219b
    scope of, 24
    socioeconomic influences on, 1065–1066
    in tracheostomy, 543
    in tuberculosis, 610
    in wound healing, 97, 287
Nutrition assessment
    anthropometric measurements, 1213–1215
    before rehabilitation, 90–91, 90t
    body mass index, 1215, 1215b
    description of, 25
    nutrition screening, 1212–1213
    nutrition status, 1212, 1213b

Nutrition history
    cardiovascular system, 648–649
    description of, 1227, 1240
    gastrointestinal system, 1065–1066
    musculoskeletal system, 1008
    renal system, 1329
    reproductive system, 1432
    vision, 962–963
Nutrition screening
    description of, 1212–1213, 1213b
    for older adults, 31b
Nutrition status
    definition of, 1212
    evaluation of, 1212
    pressure injuries and, 449–451
Nutrition supplements, 1218–1219
Nutrition therapy. See also Total enteral nutrition; Total parenteral nutrition
    acute kidney injury treated with, 1396–1397
    atherosclerosis treated with, 730
    cirrhosis managed with, 1175, 1178
    Crohn's disease treated with, 1159–1160
    Cushing's disease treated with, 1258
    esophageal tumors treated with, 1097
    fluid overload treated with, 172
    gastroesophageal reflux disease treated with, 1090
    heart failure treated with, 698–699, 705
    hyperkalemia treated with, 179b
    hypernatremia treated with, 175
    hypocalcemia treated with, 181
    hypoglycemia treated with, 1310–1311
    hypokalemia treated with, 177
    hyponatremia treated with, 174
    leukemia treated with, 825–826
    obesity treated with, 1228
    osteoporosis treated with, 1020
    peptic ulcer disease managed with, 1112
    pressure injury wound healing through, 458
    ulcerative colitis managed with, 1153
    urinary incontinence treated with, 1348
Nutritionally balanced diet, 1228
Nystagmus
    description of, 934, 964, 996
    electronystagmography of, 991

O
Obesity
    assessment of, 1227
    bariatric surgery for, 1229–1231
    behavioral management of, 1229
    body fat distribution in, 1225
    care coordination for, 1231

Obesity (Continued)
    complementary and integrative health for, 1229
    complications of, 1225, 1225t
    definition of, 648, 1225
    diet programs for, 1227–1228
    dietary causes of, 1225–1226
    drug therapy for, 1228–1229
    drugs that cause, 1226
    etiology of, 1225–1226
    exercise for, 1228
    familial factors, 1226b
    gastric bypass for, 1229, 1230f
    gastroesophageal reflux disease risks, 1090
    genetic risk of, 1225–1226, 1226b
    health care resources for, 1231
    history-taking, 1227
    home care management of, 1231
    insulin resistance caused by, 1286–1287
    interventions for, 25
    laparoscopic adjustable gastric band for, 1229, 1230f
    malnutrition associated with, 236–237
    morbid, 1225
    nonsurgical management of, 1227–1229
    nutrition history for, 1227
    nutrition therapy for, 1228
    obstructive sleep apnea risks, 236
    overweight versus, 1225
    pathophysiology of, 1225–1226
    physical assessment of, 1227
    physical inactivity as cause of, 1226
    prevalence of, 1225
    Roux-en-Y gastric bypass for, 1229, 1230f
    self-management education for, 1231
    signs and symptoms of, 1227
    surgical management of, 1229–1231, 1230f, 1231b
    sympathomimetic drugs for, 1228–1229
    transition management for, 1231
    wound healing affected by, 236–237
Obligatory solute excretion, 1336
Obligatory urine output, 165
Obstipation, 18, 1123
Obstructive jaundice, 1192
Obstructive sleep apnea
    assessment of, 559
    interventions for, 559
    noninvasive positive-pressure ventilation for, 535, 559
    in obese patients, 236
    pathophysiology of, 559
Occipital lobe, 841t
Occupational Safety and Health Administration, 423
Occupational therapists, 89, 93

Occupational therapy assistants, 89
Octreotide, 1118, 1177, 1248–1249, 1311
Ocular trauma, 981–982
Oculomotor nerve, 844t, 847–848
Odynophagia, 1089, 1096
Off-pump coronary artery bypass, 789
OGTT. See Oral glucose tolerance testing
Older adults. See also Aging
    abuse of, 39, 39t
    acute kidney injury in, 1394b
    acute pancreatitis in, 1199
    adjuvant analgesics in, 64b
    adverse drug events in, 35t
    anemia in, 803
    brain in, 858
    burn injury in, 490b
    cancer in, 380b
    candidiasis in, 1076b
    cardiac changes in, 222–223
    cardiovascular system in, 647b
    cerumen impaction in, 995b
    chronic respiratory disorder in, 564b
    in community-based settings, 30–39
    constipation in, 31
    coping by, 32–33
    coronary artery bypass grafting in, 790b
    dehydration in, 167b, 1194b
    diabetic retinopathy in, 1284b
    diverticulitis in, 1164b
    driving safety for, 34, 34b
    drugs in
        adverse drug events, 35t
        age-related changes, 34
        assessment of, 35, 36b
        self-administration of, 35, 35f
        use and misuse of, 34–35, 35f, 35t
    dysrhythmias in, 682b
    electrolyte imbalances in, 173b
    electrolyte levels in, 165b
    emergency department care for, 118b
    endocrine system in, 1240, 1241b
    exercise for, 31–32, 32f
    fecal impaction in, 1126b
    fluid restriction by, 31b
    fractures in, 1047–1048, 1047b
    gastroesophageal reflux disease in, 1089b
    gastrointestinal system in, 1064b
    glomerular filtration rate in, 1328b
    health care for, 32
    health care-associated methicillin-resistant Staphylococcus aureus in, 422b
    health issues for
        abuse, 39, 39t
        accidents, 33–34
        alcoholism, 38

Older adults (Continued)
  cognition-related, 35–38
  in community-based settings,
      30–39
  confusion, 40–42
  delirium, 38
  dementia, 37
  depression, 36–37, 37f
  drug use and misuse, 34–35,
      35f, 35t
  falls, 33, 33b, 40–42
  in hospitals, 39–42
  hydration-related, 30–31
  in long-term care settings,
      39–42
  loss, 32–33
  malnutrition, 40
  mobility-related, 31–32
  neglect, 39, 39t
  nutrition-related, 30–31
  pressure injuries, 42
  sleep disorders, 40
  stress, 32–33
  substance use, 38–39
heart failure in, 694b
Helicobacter pylori in, 1111b
hematologic system in, 800b
hip fractures in, 1047–1048, 1047b
Hispanic, 39b
history-taking in, 122b
homelessness in, 30
in hospitals, 39–42
hydration in, 30–31
hyperglycemic-hyperosmolar state
    in, 1300b, 1314b
hypoglycemia in, 1309, 1312b
incontinence in, 31
iron deficiency anemia in, 815b
kidneys in, 1328b
living arrangements for, 30
loneliness in, 31
in long-term care settings
  care coordination and transition
      management for, 42
  health issues for, 39–42
malnutrition in, 1216b
meal management in, 1219b
motor vehicle accidents by, 34, 34b
musculoskeletal system in, 1007b
myelodysplastic syndromes in, 817
neglect of, 39, 39t
nutrition in, 30–31, 1219b
nutritional screening for, 31b
opioid analgesics in, 64b, 279b
oral cancer in, 1082b
oral candidiasis in, 1076b
orthostatic hypotension in, 134b
overview of, 30
pain in, 52b, 56b, 59b
patient-controlled analgesia in, 284b
peritonitis in, 1163b
physical activity by, 31–32, 32f
pneumonia in, 603b
population growth of, 29
preoperative care of, 236b

Older adults (Continued)
  protein-energy malnutrition in,
      1216b
  in rehabilitation settings, 90b
  relocation stress syndrome in,
      30–31, 33b
  renal changes in, 222–223
  renal system in, 1328b
  reproductive system in, 1431b
  sensory changes in, 844
  sexually transmitted infections in,
      1505b
  special needs of, 10
  subgroups of, 30
  surgery in, 232
  thyroid disorders in, 1274b
  transfusion in, 834b
  transgender, 1497b
  traumatic brain injury in, 944b
  tricyclic antidepressants in, 37b
  urinary incontinence in, 1344b
  urinary tract infections in, 91
  vision impairments in, 963b
  water intake by, 1212b
  wellness promotion in, 30b
  wound infection in, 954
Olfactory nerve, 844t
Oligomenorrhea, 1256
Oligospermia, 1487–1488
Oliguria, 18, 236, 1362, 1392, 1423
Onabotulinumtoxin A, 875, 1349
Oncofetal antigens, 1068
Oncogenes, 378–379, 380b
Oncogenesis, 375
Oncologic emergencies
  description of, 385, 407–410
  disseminated intravascular
      coagulation, 407
  hypercalcemia, 408
  sepsis, 407
  spinal cord compression, 408
  superior vena cava syndrome,
      408–409, 409f
  syndrome of inappropriate
      antidiuretic hormone,
      407–408
  tumor lysis syndrome, 409–410,
      409f
Oncoviruses, 379
On-Q PainBuster, 211, 212f
Onycholysis, 441–442
Oophorectomy, 1444–1445
Open fracture, 1032, 1032f
Open reduction and internal
    fixation, 1042–1043, 1042f,
    1047–1048
Open reduction with internal
    fixation, 558
Open thoracotomy, 638
Operating rooms
  fire safety in, 252
  layout of, 252
  occupational hazards in, 252
  safety in, 252
  surgical attire in, 256, 256f

Ophthalmic artery, 959
Ophthalmic ointment, 961b, 970
Ophthalmoscopy, 966, 966f
Opioid analgesics
  addiction to, 58
  administration of, 57–58
  adverse effects of, 62–63, 63t
  age considerations in dosing of,
      58b
  in chronic kidney disease patients,
      1409
  chronic pain managed with, 225
  classification of, 56–57
  complications of, 284
  constipation caused by, 1147
  controlled release, 58–59
  description of, 55–56
  dosing of, 57, 59
  drug formulation terminology for,
      58–59
  dual mechanism, 61
  dyspnea treated with, 110
  in end-of-life patients, 108–109
  epidural delivery of, 61, 61f, 225
  equianalgesia for, 58, 60t
  fast acting, 58
  fentanyl, 60, 60t
  general anesthesia use of, 258
  in human immunodeficiency
      virus infection, 354
  hydrocodone, 60, 60t
  hydromorphone, 60, 60t
  immediate release, 58
  intraspinal delivery of, 61–62
  intrathecal delivery of, 61–62, 62b
  lipophilicity of, 60
  mechanism of action, 56–57
  methadone, 61
  mixed agonists/antagonists, 57
  modified release, 58–59, 59b
  morphine, 59–60, 60t
  mu agonists, 56–57
  in older adults, 279b
  overdose of, 285b
  oxycodone, 60, 60t
  partial agonists, 57
  phantom limb pain managed
      with, 1053
  physical dependence on, 58
  postoperative ileus caused by, 286
  postoperative pain management
      using, 283–284, 284b
  respiratory depression caused by,
      62–63, 63t, 64b, 524b
  sedation caused by, 62–63, 63t–64t
  short acting, 58
  side effects of, 63t, 64b
  sustained release, 58–59
  tapentadol, 61
  titration of, 57
  tolerance to, 58
  tramadol, 61
  types to avoid, 61
Opioid antagonists, 57, 64b, 284
Opioid naïve, 58

Opioid tolerant, 58
Opportunistic infections
  description of, 339, 346–347, 347f
  prevention of, 350–353
Oprelvekin, 398, 402t
Opsonins, 294
Optic disc, 958
Optic fundus, 958
Optic nerve
  description of, 844t
  ultrasonic imaging of, 967
Oral cancer
  assessment of, 1079–1080
  basal cell carcinoma, 1079
  brachytherapy for, 1081
  care coordination for, 1083–1084
  chemotherapy for, 1080–1081
  cryotherapy for, 1081
  features of, 1080b
  genetic mutations in, 1079b
  health care resources for, 1084
  home care management of, 1083,
      1083b
  interventions for, 1080–1083
  multimodal therapy for, 1080
  nonsurgical management of,
      1080–1081
  in older adults, 1082b
  pathophysiology of, 1079
  prevention of, 1079
  radiation therapy for, 1081
  self-management education for,
      1083, 1083b
  squamous cell carcinomas, 1079
  surgical management of,
      1081–1083
  targeted therapy for, 1081
  taste changes after, 1083
  transition management for,
      1083–1084
Oral candidiasis, 1076–1077, 1076b
Oral cavity
  anatomy of, 1062, 1075–1076
  examination of, 1080
  health of, 1076b
  masticatory function of, 1062
  teeth, 1062
Oral cavity disorders
  erythroplakia, 1079
  high-risk patients for, 1075–1076
  leukoplakia, 1078–1079
  oral cancer. See Oral cancer
  oral tumors, 1078–1084
  stomatitis, 1076–1078
Oral glucose tolerance testing, 1289
Oral hairy leukoplakia, 1078
Oral hygiene
  mucositis managed with, 400
  in oral cancer patients, 1080–1081
  routine for, 1080–1081
  in tracheostomy, 543
Oral rehydration solutions
  dehydration treated with, 170
  gastroenteritis treated with, 1149
Oral tumors, 1078–1084

OralCDx, 1080

Orbit, 957

Orchiectomy
in male-to-female gender reassignment surgery, 1499
testicular cancer treated with, 1488–1489

Orchitis, 1431

Orencia. *See* Abatacept

Orexins, 1225

Organ of Corti, 986

Organizational ethics, 9

Orientation, assessment of, 846–847

ORIF. *See* Open reduction and internal fixation

Orlistat, 1228

Oropharynx, 509, 509f

Ortho checks, 168

Orthopedic boots/shoes, 1038, 1038f

Orthopnea, 517, 574, 576f, 625, 649–650, 695

Orthostatic hypotension, 121, 134b, 168, 174–175, 652, 723, 726b, 901, 1285

Oseltamivir, 597–598

OSHA. *See* Occupational Safety and Health Administration

Osmolality, 163

Osmolarity
blood, 1332
description of, 163, 1222–1223
urine, 1336

Osmoreceptors, 164

Osmosis, 163–164, 163f, 1412

Ossiculoplasty, 999

Osteoarthritis
care coordination for, 316–317
clinical features of, 306t
definition of, 305
etiology of, 305
exercises for, 317b
gender differences in, 305b
genetic risk of, 305
health care resources for, 317
health promotion and maintenance for, 305–306
history-taking, 306
home care management of, 317
incidence of, 305
joint changes in, 305f
joint effusions associated with, 306–307
laboratory assessment of, 307
mobility improvements in, 316
pain management in
complementary and integrative health for, 308–309
drugs for, 307–308
hyaluronic acid for, 308
nonpharmacologic interventions, 308
nonsteroidal anti-inflammatory drugs, 307–308
surgical options for, 309–316

Osteoarthritis (*Continued*)
pathophysiology of, 305–306, 1007
physical assessment of, 306–307, 306f
physical therapy for, 316
prevalence of, 305
primary, 305
psychosocial assessment of, 307
rheumatoid arthritis versus, 306t
secondary, 305
self-management education for, 317, 317b
signs and symptoms of, 306–307, 306f
spinal involvement by, 307
total hip arthroplasty for
anesthesia used in, 310
complications of, 311t, 312–313
components of, 310–311, 310f
hip dislocation after, 311–312
hip resurfacing versus, 310
low-molecular-weight heparin uses, 312
minimally invasive, 310
mobility after, 313–314, 313f
operative procedures, 310–311
pain management after, 312b, 313
patient positioning after, 311, 313f
postoperative care, 311–314, 311b
preoperative care, 309–310
primary, 309
quadriceps-setting exercises after, 312–313
rehabilitation, 314
revision, 309
self-management education, 312b, 314
venous thromboembolism risks after, 310, 312–313
weight-bearing restrictions, 313–314
total joint arthroplasty for, 309
total knee arthroplasty for
complications of, 316
continuous passive motion machine, 315, 315f, 316b
cryotherapy after, 315
description of, 314–316
discharge instructions, 316
minimally invasive, 314
operative procedures, 315
pain management after, 315–316
postoperative care, 315–316, 315f
preoperative care, 314–315
rehabilitation after, 316
total shoulder arthroplasty for, 316
transition management for, 316–317

Osteoblasts, 1005

Osteochondroma, 1024

Osteoclasts, 1005

Osteocytes, 1005

Osteomalacia
definition of, 1016
osteoporosis versus, 1016t

Osteomyelitis, 1022–1024, 1023b, 1023f, 1035

Osteonecrosis
bone healing affected by, 1032
of jaw, bisphosphonate-related, 1021
in systemic lupus erythematosus, 327

Osteopenia, 1007, 1016

Osteoporosis
assessment of, 1018–1020
bisphosphonates for, 1021, 1021b
bone turnover markers in, 1019, 1019t
calcium intake for, 1020–1021, 1021b
care coordination for, 1022
computed tomography-based absorptiometry of, 1019
in Crohn's disease patients, 1151t
definition of, 1007, 1015–1016
denosumab for, 1021
description of, 24–25
dietary supplements for, 1020–1021, 1021b
dowager's hump associated with, 1018, 1018f
drug therapy for, 1020–1022
dual x-ray absorptiometry of, 1019
estrogen agonists/antagonists for, 1021, 1021b
etiology of, 1016–1017
fallophobia risks, 33
falls secondary to, 1020
fractures caused by, 1016, 1018, 1047
generalized, 1016
genetic risk of, 1016–1017, 1017b
growth hormone deficiency as cause of, 1246
health care resources for, 1022
health promotion and maintenance for, 1017–1018
hip fracture risks associated with, 1047
home care management of, 1022
imaging assessment of, 1019–1020
immune factors in, 1017b
incidence of, 1017
interventions for, 1020–1022
laboratory assessment of, 1019, 1019t
lifestyle changes for, 1020
magnetic resonance imaging of, 1019
magnetic resonance spectroscopy of, 1019

Osteoporosis (*Continued*)
nutrition therapy for, 1020
osteomalacia versus, 1016t
pathophysiology of, 1016–1017
physical assessment of, 1018–1019, 1018f
prevalence of, 1017
prevention of, 1018
primary, 1017b
psychosocial assessment of, 1019
regional, 1016
risk factors for, 1017b
salmon calcitonin for, 1022
secondary, 1016
self-management education for, 1022
teriparatide for, 1022
transition management for, 1022
vertebral imaging of, 1019
vitamin D$_3$ for, 1020–1021

Osteosarcoma, 1012, 1025

Osteotomy, 1028–1029

Ostomate, 1153

Ostomy, 1154

Otezla. *See* Apremilast

Otitis media, 991–993, 992f, 1023b

Otorrhea, 880–881

Otosclerosis, 986–987, 996–997

Otoscope, 988, 989f

Otoscopic examination
description of, 988–989, 989f, 998
otitis media on, 992f
tympanic membrane perforation on, 992f

Outpatient surgery, 229–230

Ova and parasites testing, 1068–1070

Ovarian cancer, 1467–1469, 1467t

Ovaries
anatomy of, 1429, 1429f
hormones produced by, 1235t

Overactive bladder, 97–98, 1344, 1349

Overflow incontinence, 1344, 1345t, 1351–1352

Overhydration. *See* Fluid overload

Overweight, 648, 1225

Ovoid pupil, 946

Oxybutynin, 98

Oxycodone
equianalgesic dosing of, 60t
pain management uses of, 60, 60t
postoperative pain management using, 284b

Oxygen
humidified, 531, 531f
liquid, 536–537, 537f
tissue delivery of, 512

Oxygen concentrator, 537

Oxygen tanks, 536, 536f

Oxygen therapy
absorptive atelectasis caused by, 530, 531b
acute respiratory failure treated with, 626

Oxygen therapy (Continued)
  asthma treated with, 571
  burn injury treated with, 494
  care coordination for, 536–537
  chronic obstructive pulmonary
      disease treated with, 578
  combustion caused by, 530
  complications of, 530–531
  delivery systems for
      description of, 531–536
      face tent, 534–535, 534t
      facemasks, 532–533, 532t, 533f,
          604
      high-flow, 533–535, 534t
      low-flow, 531–533, 532f, 532t
      nasal cannula, 531–532, 532f,
          532t, 604
      T-piece, 534–535, 534t, 535f
      Venturi masks, 533–534, 534f,
          534t
  dyspnea treated with, 110
  hazards of, 530–531
  home care management of, 536
  home care preparation for,
      536–537, 536f
  humidified oxygen, 531, 531f
  hypoventilation caused by, 530
  hypoxemia treated with, 626, 775
  indications for, 529
  infection risks, 531
  mucous membrane drying caused
      by, 530–531
  noninvasive positive-pressure
      ventilation, 535, 535b, 536f
  overview of, 529
  patient safety in, 530b
  in pneumonia, 604
  postoperative, 280–281
  purpose of, 529
  respiratory acidosis treated with,
      195
  safety in, 530b
  self-management education for,
      536
  septic shock managed with,
      765
  toxicity caused by, 530
  transition management for,
      536–537
  transtracheal, 536
Oxygen toxicity, 530
Oxygenation, in burn injury
    patients, 493–497
Oxygen-hemoglobin dissociation
    curve, 512, 512f
Oxymorphone, 60t
Oxytocin, 1237t

P
P wave, 667
Pacemaker, permanent, 675, 675f,
    676b
Pacing
  asynchronous, 675
  biventricular, 681

Pacing (Continued)
  sinus bradycardia treated with,
      674–675
  synchronous, 675
  temporary, 674–675
  transcutaneous, 674, 674f
Packed red blood cells, 200
Pack-years, 514
PACU. See Postanesthesia care unit
Pain
  abdominal. See Abdominal pain
  acute, 46–47, 46t, 52
  amputation-related, 1051, 1053
  back. See Back pain
  breakthrough, 54–55
  cancer
      chronic, 47
      intrathecal pump for, 62b
      self-management education for,
          68
  categorization of, 46–48
  chronic
      description of, 46–47
      epidural infusion for, 225
      in older adults, 56b
      psychosocial factors that affect,
          52
      self-management education for,
          68
  definition of, 46
  drug therapy for. See Pain
      management
  duodenal ulcers as cause of, 1110
  duration-based categorization of,
      46–47
  extremity, 651
  gastric ulcers as cause of, 1110
  inadequate management of, 46
  intestinal obstruction-related,
      1123
  irritable bowel syndrome as cause
      of, 1136
  localized, 50
  low back. See Back pain
  mechanism-based categorization
      of, 46–48
  modulation of, 48, 49f
  neuropathic, 48, 48t, 1307
  nociceptive, 47–48, 48t
  in older adults, 52b, 59b
  overview of, 45–68
  perception of, 48, 49f
  persistent, 46–47
  phantom limb, 1051, 1053
  professional organizations for, 46
  projected, 50
  psychosocial factors, 52–53
  radiating, 50
  rectal, 1164
  referred, 50
  scope of problem, 45–46
  self-reports of, 48
  somatic, 48
  surgery-related, 47
  transduction of, 47, 49f

Pain (Continued)
  transmission of, 47–48, 49f
  treatment of. See Pain
      management
  unrelieved, impact of, 46, 46t
  visceral, 48
Pain assessment
  challenges for, 53–54
  components of, 50–52
  in delirium, 53–54, 53t
  in dementia, 53–54, 53t
  description of, 1008
  Hierarchy of Pain Measures, 53,
      53t
  locations of pain, 50–52, 51f
  McGill-Melzack Pain
      Questionnaire for, 50–52, 51f
  in mechanically ventilated
      patients, 54
  in older adults, 59b
  overview of, 49–50
  postoperative, 278
  psychosocial assessments as part
      of, 52–53
Pain Assessment in Advanced
    Dementia scale, 54
Pain management
  in acute pancreatitis, 1199–1201
  analgesics for
      acetaminophen, 55
      adjuvant, 55, 63–65
      anticonvulsants as, 63–64
      antidepressants as, 63–64
      around-the-clock dosing of,
          54–55, 59b
      local anesthetics as, 64–65
      nonopioid, 55–56
      nonsteroidal anti-inflammatory
          drugs, 55–56, 56b, 284b,
          1364
      opioid. See Opioid analgesics
      routes of administration, 54
  in bone tumors, 1027–1028
  in burn injury, 491
  care coordination and transition
      management, 67–68
  in cholecystitis, 1194–1197
  after coronary artery bypass
      grafting, 788
  during dying, 108–109
  in fractures, 1037–1043
  in head and neck cancer, 551–552
  health care resources for, 68
  home care management in, 67
  in human immunodeficiency
      virus infection, 353–354
  in lung cancer, 593
  multimodal analgesia, 54–55
  nonpharmacologic
      cognitive-behavioral therapy,
          66–67
      complementary and alternative
          therapies, 109, 285, 496
      cryotherapy, 66
      description of, 65

Pain management (Continued)
  interventions for, 65
      physical modalities, 65–66
      spinal cord stimulation, 66
      tactile stimulation, 496
      transcutaneous electrical nerve
          stimulation, 66, 66f
  in older adults, 59b
  after oral cancer surgery, 1083
  patient-controlled analgesia, 55, 497
  in peritonitis, 1146
  placebos for, 65, 65b
  in polycystic kidney disease, 1382
  postoperative, 283–285,
      284b–285b
  preemptive analgesia, 54
  in pyelonephritis, 1375
  referrals in, 68
  regional anesthesia for, 65
  in rheumatoid arthritis, 321–324
  self-management education as
      part of, 68
  in sickle cell disease, 811–812
  total hip arthroplasty-related,
      312b, 313
  total knee arthroplasty-related,
      315–316
  in ulcerative colitis, 1155–1156,
      1156b
  in urolithiasis, 1363–1365
Pain perception assessments, 849
Pain rating scales, 50–52, 50t, 52f
Pain resource nurse programs, 45
PAINAD scale. See Pain Assessment
    in Advanced Dementia scale
Palatine tonsils, 509
Palliation, 106
Palliative care
  description of, 106, 107t, 113
  in lung cancer, 593
  for Parkinson disease, 873
Palliative surgery, 386
Pallor, 443, 651, 802b
Palmoplantar pustulosis, 464
Palpation
  of chest, 518–519
  of gastrointestinal system,
      1067–1068
  of kidneys, 1330–1331, 1331f
  of skin, 440–441, 440t
  of testes, 1242
  of thyroid gland, 1242, 1242b
Palpitations, 650, 671
Pamidronate, 1021, 1026
Pancreas
  abscess of, 1205
  alpha cells of, 1281
  anatomy of, 1063, 1063f
  beta cells of, 1281
  cancer of. See Pancreatic cancer
  endocrine, 1197, 1202, 1239, 1281
  exocrine, 1197, 1239, 1281
  functions of, 1197
  hormones produced by, 1235t
  insulin production by, 1281

Pancreas (Continued)
  islets of Langerhans, 1063, 1239, 1240f
  necrosis of, 1197
  pseudocyst of, 1205
  tumors of, 1205
Pancreatectomy, 1207
Pancreatic cancer
  abdominal pain associated with, 1206
  assessment of, 1206
  care coordination for, 1208–1209
  chemotherapy for, 1206–1207
  endoscopic retrograde cholangiopancreatography of, 1206
  features of, 1206b
  genetic risk for, 1205b
  health care resources for, 1209
  home care management of, 1209
  laboratory assessment of, 1206
  nonsurgical management of, 1206–1207
  pathophysiology of, 1205–1206
  radiation therapy for, 1207
  risk factors for, 1206
  self-management education for, 1209
  signs and symptoms of, 1205–1206
  surgical management of, 1207–1208, 1207f
  transition management for, 1208–1209
  venous thromboembolism secondary to, 1205
  Whipple procedure for, 1207, 1207f, 1208t
Pancreatic insufficiency, 1202
Pancreatic transplantation
  complications of, 1303
  description of, 1204
  diabetes mellitus treated with, 1302–1303
  rejection of, 1302–1303
Pancreatic-enzyme replacement therapy, 1203
Pancreaticojejunostomy, 1207
Pancreatitis
  acute
    abdominal pain associated with, 1199–1201
    alcohol consumption as cause of, 1200
    assessment of, 1199–1200
    autodigestion in, 1198f
    care coordination for, 1202
    complications of, 1197–1198, 1198t, 1201
    death caused by, 1199
    definition of, 1197
    drug therapy for, 1200–1201
    endoscopic retrograde cholangiopancreatography-related trauma as cause of, 1199

Pancreatitis (Continued)
    etiology of, 1199
    gallstones as cause of, 1201
    genetic risk of, 1199
    history-taking for, 1199
    home care management of, 1202
    imaging assessment of, 1200
    incidence of, 1199
    interventions for, 1200–1201
    laboratory assessment of, 1200, 1200t
    multi-system organ failure caused by, 1198
    nonsurgical management of, 1200–1201
    nutrition promotion in, 1201
    in older adults, 1199
    paralytic ileus secondary to, 1201b
    pathophysiology of, 1197–1199
    physical assessment of, 1199
    prevalence of, 1199
    psychosocial assessment of, 1200
    respiratory status monitoring in, 1201b
    shock caused by, 1198, 1199b
    signs and symptoms of, 1199
    surgical management of, 1201
    transition management for, 1202
    ultrasonography of, 1200
  chronic, 1202–1204, 1203b–1204b
  necrotizing hemorrhagic, 1197–1198
Pancytopenia, 327, 815
Pandemic, 151, 427, 597
Pandemic influenza, 597–598
Panendoscopy, 549
Panhysterectomy, 1461t
Panitumumab, 1130
Panniculitis, 1227
Panniculus, 1227
Pao₂. See Partial pressure of arterial oxygen
Papanicolaou test, 1433–1434, 1469
Papillae, 1062
Papillary carcinoma, 1275
Papilledema, 946, 951
Papillotomy, 1071
Papular rash, 440
Papules, 438f
Paracentesis, 1175–1177, 1177b
Paradoxical blood pressure, 652–653
Paradoxical chest wall movement, 637, 637f
Paradoxical pulse, 713
Paradoxical splitting, 654
Paraesophageal hiatal hernias, 1092, 1093b
Paraffin dips, 323
Paralysis, 91
Paralytic ileus, 176, 277, 1122, 1201b
Paranasal sinuses
  anatomy of, 509, 509f
  cancer of, 556
Paraneoplastic syndromes, 1385
Paraprotein, 830

Parasitic disorders/infections
  bedbugs, 471
  description of, 1165–1166
  pediculosis, 470–471
  scabies, 470–471, 471f
Parasympathetic nervous system, 842
Parathyroid disorders
  hyperparathyroidism, 1275–1277, 1276b, 1276t
  hypoparathyroidism, 1277–1278
Parathyroid glands
  anatomy of, 1239
  hormones produced by, 1235t
Parathyroid hormone
  calcium levels affected by, 179, 1239
  description of, 1006
  functions of, 1239, 1239f
  phosphorus levels regulated by, 1400, 1400f
Parathyroid hormone modulator, 1410b
Parathyroidectomy, 1277
Parent cells, 372
Parenteral nutrition, 204–205. See also Total parenteral nutrition
Paresis, 91
Paresthesia, 178, 904–905, 914, 934, 1261
Paresthesias, 319
Parietal cells, 1063
Parietal lobe, 841t
Parkinson disease
  anticholinergics for, 871
  assessment of, 869–870
  care coordination for, 872–873
  care for, 870b
  catechol O-methyltransferase inhibitors for, 870
  clinical features of, 868t
  deep brain stimulation for, 872
  dietary considerations for, 871
  dopamine agonists for, 870–871, 870b
  drug therapy for, 870–871
  dyskinesias associated with, 870, 872
  etiology of, 869
  facial expression changes associated with, 869, 869f
  fetal tissue transplantation for, 872
  gait in, 871
  genetic risk of, 869
  health care resources for, 872–873
  home care preparation for, 872
  Huntington disease versus, 868t
  imaging assessment of, 869–870
  incidence of, 869
  laboratory assessment of, 869–870
  monoamine oxidase type B inhibitors for, 870
  neurotransmitters in, 868
  nonsurgical management of, 870–872
  palliative care for, 873

Parkinson disease (Continued)
  pathophysiology of, 868–869
  physical assessment of, 869
  postural instability associated with, 871
  prevalence of, 869
  rigidity associated with, 869
  self-esteem promotion in, 872
  self-management education for, 872
  signs and symptoms of, 868–869, 869f, 871
  speech difficulties associated with, 871–872
  stages of, 868–869, 869t
  stereotactic pallidotomy for, 872
  substantia nigra degeneration in, 868
  surgical management of, 872
  transition management for, 872–873
Parkland formula, 494–495
Paromomycin, 1166
Paronychia, 442
Parotidectomy, 1085
Paroxysmal nocturnal dyspnea, 517, 650, 695
Paroxysmal supraventricular tachycardia, 676
Partial agonists, 57
Partial breast irradiation, 1451
Partial corpus callosotomy, 880
Partial left ventriculectomy, 702
Partial pancreatectomy, 1207
Partial parenteral nutrition, 1223–1224
Partial pressure of arterial oxygen, 194, 624, 646
Partial pressure of carbon dioxide, 14, 624
Partial pressure of end-tidal carbon dioxide, 523
Partial rebreather mask, 532–533, 532t, 533f
Partial seizures, 876–877, 878b
Partial thromboplastin time, 619–620, 622b, 657, 805
Partial-thickness wound, 473
  definition of, 27
  physiologic consequences of, 28
PAS. See Physician-assisted suicide
Pasero Opioid-Induced Sedation Scale, 64t
Pasireotide, 1258
Passive immunity, 21–22, 298–299, 414
Passive range of motion, 1010
Passive smoking, 514
Patches, 438f
Patellofemoral pain syndrome, 1057t
Pathogen
  definition of, 414
  transmission methods for, 416

Pathogenicity, 414

Pathologic fracture, 1032

Patient harm and error, 3–4

Patient identification
  in emergency departments, 121
  intraoperative, 262–263
  preoperative, 241, 247

Patient safety, 4

Patient Self-Determination Act, 104, 241

Patient transfer, 421

Patient-centered care
  attributes of, 2
  context of, 3
  definition of, 2
  for older veterans, 36b
  scope of, 2

Patient-controlled analgesia, 55, 283–284, 497, 592

Patient-controlled epidural analgesia, 55, 61

Patient-controlled regional anesthesia, 65

Patterns of inheritance. See Inheritance patterns

PAWP. See Pulmonary artery wedge pressure

PCA. See Patient-controlled analgesia

PCEA. See Patient-controlled epidural analgesia

PCRA. See Patient-controlled regional anesthesia

PCSK9 inhibitors, 730–731

Peaceful death, 103

Peak airway (inspiratory) pressure, 632

Peak expiratory flow, 567–568

Peak expiratory flow rate, 567

Peak flow meter, 568b, 568f, 577

Peau d'orange, 1441, 1441f, 1445

Pediatric advanced life support, 120t, 123

Pediculosis, 470–471

Pediculosis capitis, 470

Pediculosis corporis, 470

Pediculosis pubis, 470, 1470

Pedigree, 77–78, 78f–79f

PEEP. See Positive end-expiratory pressure

Pegfilgrastim, 402t

PEG-INF/RBV, 1185t

Pegloticase, 332

Pegvisomant, 1248–1249

Pelvic examination, 1433

Pelvic fractures, 1036, 1049–1050

Pelvic inflammatory disease
  abdominal ultrasonography of, 1515
  antibiotics for, 1516, 1516b
  assessment of, 1514–1515
  care coordination for, 1516–1517
  diagnostic criteria for, 1515t
  health care resources for, 1517
  home care management of, 1516
  infertility caused by, 1514, 1517

Pelvic inflammatory disease (Continued)
  interventions for, 1515–1516, 1516b
  laboratory assessment of, 1515
  pathogens that cause, 1514
  pathophysiology of, 1514, 1514f
  physical assessment of, 1515
  psychosocial assessment of, 1515
  risk factors for, 1515
  self-management education for, 1516–1517
  signs and symptoms of, 1515
  transition management for, 1516–1517

Pelvic muscle exercises, 1347, 1347b, 1351, 1464

Pelvic organ prolapse, 1464–1465, 1464f

Pelvic pouch, 1154, 1154f

PEM. See Protein-energy malnutrition

Pembrolizumab, 477

Penetrance, 79

Penetrating keratoplasty, 978, 978f

Penetrating trauma
  description of, 129
  ocular, 982
  osteomyelitis secondary to, 1023
  spinal cord injury caused by, 894

Penile implants, 1490

Penis, 1430, 1430f

Penrose drain, 278, 279f, 282

Pentamidine isethionate, 353

Pentoxifylline, 734

Peptic ulcer(s)
  complications of, 1108–1109
  definition of, 1107
  duodenal ulcers, 1107–1108, 1108f, 1110
  gastric ulcers, 1107–1110, 1108f
  Helicobacter pylori as cause of, 1107, 1109
  perforation of, 1108–1109
  stress ulcers, 1108
  types of, 1107–1108

Peptic ulcer disease
  antacids for, 1112
  assessment of, 1109–1111
  care coordination for, 1114–1115
  complementary and integrative health for, 1107t, 1112–1113
  complications of, 1108–1109
  definition of, 1107
  dietary considerations in, 1112, 1112b
  drug therapy for, 1106b–1107b, 1111–1112
  dyspepsia associated with, 1110
  esophagogastroduodenoscopy for, 1111
  etiology of, 1109
  genetic risk of, 1109
  health care resources for, 1115

Peptic ulcer disease (Continued)
  Helicobacter pylori as cause of, 1107, 1109
  histamine receptor antagonists for, 1112
  home care management of, 1114, 1115b
  imaging assessment of, 1111
  incidence of, 1109
  interventions for, 1111–1113
  laboratory assessment of, 1111
  minimally invasive surgery for, 1114
  nonsteroidal anti-inflammatory drugs as cause of, 1109
  nutrition therapy for, 1112
  pain caused by, 1111–1113
  pathophysiology of, 1107–1109, 1108f
  physical assessment of, 1110
  prevalence of, 1109
  psychosocial assessment of, 1111
  self-management education for, 1114–1115
  signs and symptoms of, 1110
  surgical management of, 1114
  transition management for, 1114–1115
  upper gastrointestinal bleeding caused by
    acid suppression for rebleeding prevention, 1114
    description of, 1108, 1109b
    endoscopic therapy for, 1113
    fluid replacement for, 1113
    hypovolemia concerns secondary to, 1113
    interventional radiologic procedures for, 1113–1114
    interventions for, 1113–1114
    nasogastric tube for, 1113
    nonsurgical management of, 1113–1114
  in uremia, 1401

Percussion
  of chest, 519, 519f–520f, 519t
  of gastrointestinal system, 1067

Percutaneous alcohol septal ablation, 716

Percutaneous cervical diskectomy, 910

Percutaneous coronary intervention
  acute coronary syndromes treated with, 778
  myocardial infarction treated with, 783–784, 784f

Percutaneous endoscopic gastrostomy, 1221

Percutaneous lung biopsy, 527

Percutaneous stereotactic rhizotomy, for trigeminal neuralgia, 924

Percutaneous transhepatic biliary catheter, 1195

Percutaneous transhepatic biliary drain, 1206

Percutaneous ureterolithotomy, 1364

Percutaneous vascular intervention, for peripheral arterial disease, 735, 735b

Perfusion
  central, 25
  decreased, 25–26
  definition of, 25, 795
  inadequate, 104
  peripheral, 25
  sickle cell disease effects on, 809

Perfusionist, 253t

Pericardial friction rub, 655, 713

Pericardiectomy, 713

Pericardiocentesis, 713–714

Pericarditis, 650t, 712–714, 712b, 1401

Pericardium, 642

Perilymph, 986

Perimetry, 964

Perineal wound, 1133b

Perineometer, 1347

Periodontal disease, 1079

Perioperative nurse, 229

Perioperative nursing data set, 229

Perioperative period
  definition of, 228
  patient safety in, 228–229
  patient-focused model, 229, 229f

Peripheral arterial disease
  aortofemoral bypass surgery for, 735, 736f
  assessment of, 731–733
  axillofemoral bypass surgery for, 735–736, 736f
  chronic, 732b
  drug therapy for, 734–735
  exercise for, 740
  exercise tolerance testing for, 733
  features of, 732b, 733f
  home care management of, 737b
  inflow disease, 732
  intermittent claudication associated with, 732
  interventions for, 733–737
  magnetic resonance angiography for, 733
  nonsurgical management of, 733–737
  obstructions associated with, 731, 732f
  outflow disease, 732
  pathophysiology of, 731
  patient positioning for, 740
  percutaneous vascular intervention for, 735, 735b
  surgical management of, 735–737
  ulcers associated with, 732–733, 734b
  vasodilation promotion in, 740–741

Peripheral artery aneurysms, 740

Peripheral blood smear, 803

Peripheral blood stem cell harvesting, 823

Peripheral chemoreceptors, 646
Peripheral cyanosis, 652
Peripheral intravenous therapy
    midline catheters for, 204–205,
        204f, 213
    short peripheral catheters for,
        202–204, 202f–203f, 202t,
        203b, 214–215
    site selection for, 203–204, 203f,
        204b
    skin preparation for, 203–204
    ultrasound applications in,
        202–203
    vein selection for, 203–204, 203f,
        204b
Peripheral nerves
    cancer effects on, 385
    distribution of, 913f
Peripheral nervous system
    description of, 842
    facial paralysis, 924–925
    Guillain-Barré syndrome. See
        Guillain-Barré syndrome
    myasthenia gravis. See Myasthenia
        gravis
    restless legs syndrome, 922–923
    trigeminal neuralgia, 923–924,
        923f
Peripheral neuropathy
    chemotherapy-induced, 385
    definition of, 912
    diabetic, 1284–1285, 1285t,
        1304–1307, 1305f
Peripheral perfusion, 25
Peripheral vascular disease
    description of, 731
    foot care in, 737b
Peripheral venous disease
    description of, 741–748
    venous thromboembolism. See
        Venous thromboembolism
Peripherally inserted central
        catheters, 205–206, 205f, 206b,
        212–213
Peristalsis
    peritonitis effects on, 1145
    in postoperative period, 285–286
Peristaltic contractions, 1064
Peritoneal dialysis
    automated, 1419–1420,
        1419f–1420f
    catheters, 1418f, 1420b
    chronic kidney disease treated
        with, 1408
    complications of, 1420–1421
    continuous ambulatory, 1418,
        1419f
    continuous-cycle, 1419
    description of, 1408, 1417
    dialysate additives, 1418
    dialysate leakage during, 1420
    hemodialysis versus, 1411t
    home care management of, 1424
    intermittent, 1420
    nursing care during, 1421

Peritoneal dialysis (Continued)
    nutrition needs for, 1408
    patient selection, 1417
    peritonitis caused by, 1420,
        1420b
    procedure, 1417–1418, 1418f
    self-management education for,
        1425
    types of, 1418–1420, 1418f–
        1419f
Peritonitis
    abdominal x-rays of, 1146
    assessment of, 1145–1146
    care coordination for, 1146–1147
    cholecystitis as cause of, 1192
    definition of, 1144
    etiology of, 1145, 1420
    features of, 1145b
    fluid volume restoration in, 1146
    generalized, 1145
    home care management of, 1146
    imaging assessment of, 1146
    incidence of, 1145
    interventions for, 1146
    laboratory assessment of, 1146
    localized, 1145
    nonsurgical management of, 1146
    in older adults, 1163b
    pain management in, 1146
    pathophysiology of, 1144–1145
    peptic ulcers as cause of,
        1108–1109
    peristalsis affected by, 1145
    peritoneal dialysis as cause of,
        1420, 1420b
    physical assessment of, 1145,
        1145b
    prevalence of, 1145
    psychosocial assessment of, 1145
    signs and symptoms of, 1145,
        1145b
    spontaneous bacterial, 1171, 1175
    surgical management of, 1146
    transition management for,
        1146–1147
Peritonsillar abscess, 611
Periungual lesions, 319
Permeable membrane, 161
Pernicious anemia, 814, 1104–1105
PERRLA, 847–848, 963
Persistent pain, 46–47
Personal emergency preparedness
        plan, 155
Personal protective equipment
    definition of, 418
    illustration of, 420f
    recommendation for, 419t
Personal readiness supplies, 155b,
        156t
Personality
    Alzheimer's disease-related
        changes in, 861
    description of, 16
Pertussis, 613
Pessary, 1348, 1352

Petechiae
    definition of, 802
    description of, 439, 440f, 1173
    infective endocarditis as cause of,
        711
PFPS. See Patellofemoral pain
        syndrome
pH
    acidic, 186f
    alkaline, 187f
    blood, 13–14, 188
    body fluids, 185–186
    gastric contents, 1222
    urine, 1333
pH monitoring examination, 1089
Phacoemulsification, 970, 970f
Phagocytosis, 293–294, 294f, 417
Phalangeal fractures, 1047, 1049
Phalen's maneuver, 1058
Phalloplasty, 1501
Phantom limb pain, 1051, 1053
Pharmacists, 89
Pharmacokinetics, 57b
Pharmacologic stress
        echocardiogram, 660
Pharynx
    age-related changes in, 513b
    anatomy of, 509–510
Phenazopyridine, 1359, 1359b
Phenotype, 75–76
Phenoxybenzamine, 1262
Phentermine-topiramate, 1228
Phenytoin, 952
Pheochromocytomas, 721, 1261–1262
"Philadelphia" chromosome,
        376–377, 820
Phlebitis, 200, 217t–219t, 742
Phlebitis Scale, 221t
Phlebostatic axis, 780b
Phlebothrombosis, 742
Phonophobia, 874, 881
Phosphodiesterase inhibitors, 700
    high-altitude pulmonary edema
        treated with, 146
    nitroglycerin and, interactions
        between, 775b
Phosphodiesterase-5 inhibitors, 1489
Phosphorus
    in bone, 1006
    chronic kidney disease effects on,
        1400, 1400f
Photodynamic therapy
    description of, 405–406
    esophageal tumors treated with,
        1098
    lung cancer treated with, 589
Photophobia, 874, 881, 1266, 1270
Photopsia, 979
Photoreceptors, 957–958
Physiatrists, 88
Physical abuse, of older adults, 39
Physical activity, 31–32, 32f. See also
        Exercise
Physical dependence, 58
Physical inactivity, 1226

Physical therapists, 88–89, 89f, 93
Physical therapy
    fractures treated with, 1041
    osteoarthritis uses of, 316
    wound care applications of, 458
Physical therapy assistants, 88–89
Physician assistants, 88
Physician-assisted suicide, 114
Physicians
    emergency medicine, 119
    medical command, 154, 154t
    in rehabilitation settings, 88
Physiotherapists, 88–89
Pia mater, 840
PICC. See Peripherally inserted
        central catheters
Pick's disease, 857–858
Piggyback set, 209, 209f
Pill boxes, 34
Pinna, 984, 985f, 988
Pioglitazone, 1291, 1292b–1293b
Pit vipers, 136, 136f, 136t, 138t–140t
Pitting edema, 171f, 652f
Pituitary adenoma, 1247
Pituitary gland
    anatomy of, 1236–1237
    anterior. See Anterior pituitary
        gland
    hormones produced by, 1235t
    magnetic resonance imaging of,
        1243
    posterior. See Posterior pituitary
        gland
Pituitary gland disorders
    hyperpituitarism, 1247–1250,
        1247f, 1248b
    hypopituitarism, 1245–1247, 1246b
Pituitary tumors, 951
Pivot joints, 1007
Placebos, 65, 65b
Plague, 428
Plan-Do-Study-Act model, 7
Plantar fasciitis, 1029
Plaques, 438f, 928
Plasma
    electrolyte levels in, 165b
    transfusion of, 835
Plasma cells, 297, 797t, 829
Plasma thromboplastin, 798t
Plasmapheresis, 366
    complications of, 915b
    Guillain-Barré syndrome treated
        with, 914–915, 915b
    myasthenia gravis treated with,
        920–921
Plasmin, 801
Plasminogen, 801
Plastic containers, for infusion
        therapy, 208–209
Platelet(s)
    activation of, 798
    aggregation of, 798, 805
    in clotting, 15
    definition of, 797
    leukemia effects on, 819

Platelet count, 805, 825
Platelet plugs, 798
Platelet transfusions
    idiopathic thrombocytopenic
        purpura treated with, 831
    indications for, 832t, 835
    reaction to, 835
Platelet-derived growth factor, 458
Plethysmography, 733
Pleura, 510
Pleural effusion, 1405
    description of, 518–519
    in lung cancer patients, 593
    thoracentesis for, 593
Pleural friction rub, 521t
Pleur-evac system, 590, 591f
Plexuses, 842
PMI. See Point of maximal impulse
PNDS. See Perioperative nursing
    data set
Pneumatic compression devices, 245,
    245f
Pneumocystis jiroveci pneumonia,
    346, 353
Pneumonectomy
    complications of, 593
    definition of, 589
    incisions for, 589f
    pain management after, 592
    postoperative care for, 590–593
    preoperative care for, 589
    respiratory management after,
        592–593
Pneumonia
    airway obstruction in, 604
    assessment of, 601–603
    care coordination for, 604–605
    chest x-rays for, 603
    community-acquired, 599t–600t
    empyema management in, 604
    etiology of, 599
    gas exchange in, 604
    health care resources for, 605
    health care-associated, 599t–600t
    health promotion and
        maintenance for, 599–601
    history-taking for, 601
    home care management of, 605
    hospital-acquired, 599t–600t
    imaging assessment of, 603
    incentive spirometry in, 604
    incidence of, 599
    inflammation as cause of, 599
    laboratory assessment of, 603,
        603f
    lobar, 599
    in older adults, 603b
    oxygen therapy in, 604
    pathophysiology of, 598–599,
        603t
    physical assessment of, 601–603
    prevalence of, 599
    prevention of, 600b
    psychosocial assessment of, 603
    risk factors for, 599, 599t

Pneumonia (Continued)
    self-management education for,
        605
    sepsis prevention in, 604
    signs and symptoms of, 601–603,
        603t
    transition management for,
        604–605
    vaccines/vaccination for, 599, 601
    ventilator-associated, 600t, 601,
        633
Pneumonia Severity Index, 603
Pneumothorax, 539, 637–638
Pneumovax, 599
PNS. See Parasympathetic nervous
    system
Podagra, 331
Podofilox, 1511
Point of maximal impulse, 654
Point-of-care testing, 656
Polyclonal antibodies, 302b
Polycystic kidney disease
    assessment of, 1381–1382
    autosomal-dominant, 1380, 1380b,
        1380f
    blood pressure management in,
        1381–1382
    care coordination for, 1382
    chronic kidney disease progression
        of, 1382
    constipation in, 1382
    definition of, 1379
    etiology of, 1380
    features of, 1379–1380, 1380f,
        1381b
    genetic risk of, 1380, 1380f
    health care resources for, 1382
    history-taking for, 1381
    incidence of, 1381
    interventions for, 1381–1382
    pain management in, 1382
    pathophysiology of, 1379–1381
    physical assessment of, 1381
    prevalence of, 1381
    self-management education for,
        1382b
    signs and symptoms of, 1381
    transition management for, 1382
Polycythemia vera, 15, 576–577,
    816–817, 817b
Polydipsia, 1261, 1283
PolyMem, 501b
Polymorphisms, 76–77
Polymorphonuclear cells, 292–293
Polymorphonuclear leukocytes, 417
Polymyalgia rheumatica, 334t
Polymyositis, 334t
Polymyxin B-bacitracin, 501b
Polypectomy, 1072, 1126
Polyphagia, 1283
Polyps
    hyperplastic, 1126
    intestinal, 1126
    nasal, 517
    screening for, 1070

Polyuria, 1261, 1283
PONV. See Postoperative nausea and
    vomiting
Pores, 162
Porfimer sodium, 1098
Portal hypertension, 1170
Portal hypertensive gastropathy,
    1170
Portal-systemic encephalopathy,
    1170–1171
Positive end-expiratory pressure,
    627, 632
Positive end-expiratory volume, 497
Positive inotropic agents, 622,
    699–700, 782
Positive-pressure valve, 210
Positive-pressure ventilation, 535,
    535b, 536f
Positron emission tomography
    cardiovascular system evaluations
        using, 661
    metastatic disease evaluations,
        1096
Post-acute care, 87, 92
Postanesthesia care unit
    description of, 270
    discharge from, 272, 272b
    pain assessment in, 278
Postanesthesia care unit nurse, 271
Postanesthesia care unit record, 273f
Postcholecystectomy syndrome,
    1196, 1196t
Postembolectomy syndrome, 1461b
Posterior cerebral artery
    anatomy of, 841
    stroke involving, 933b
Posterior colporrhaphy, 1465
Posterior nasal bleeding, 557
Posterior pituitary gland
    diabetes insipidus, 1250–1251,
        1250b
    hormones produced by, 1235t,
        1236–1237, 1237t
    syndrome of inappropriate
        antidiuretic hormone,
        1251–1253, 1252t
Posterior vitreous detachment, 979
Postherpetic neuralgia, 468
Post-irradiation sialadenitis, 1085
Postmenopausal women, 180b
Postmortem care, 114, 114b
Postnecrotic cirrhosis, 1170
Postoperative ileus, 285–286, 1122,
    1124
Postoperative nausea and vomiting,
    276
Postoperative period
    acid-base balance in, 276
    airway maintenance in, 280
    arterial blood gas tests in, 280
    breathing exercises in, 281
    cardiac monitoring in, 274
    cardiovascular system in
        assessment of, 274
        complications involving, 244–246

Postoperative period (Continued)
    care coordination in, 286–287
    comfort alterations in, 278
    complications in, 272t
    constipation in, 277
    definition of, 270
    description of, 228
    drains used in, 277–278, 279f,
        282
    dressings used in, 277–278,
        281–282
    drug reconciliation in, 287
    electrolyte balance in, 276
    fluid balance in, 276
    gas exchange in, 280–281
    gastrointestinal system, 276–277
    gum chewing in, 286
    hand-off report, 271b
    health care resources, 287
    history-taking, 271
    home care management, 286
    hydration status assessments, 276
    incentive spirometry in, 243–244,
        244f
    intake and output measurements,
        276
    kidneys in, 276
    laboratory assessment in, 280
    leg exercises in, 245, 245b
    mobility in, 245
    movement in, 281
    nasogastric tube monitoring, 277
    neurologic system, 274–275, 274t
    oxygen saturation monitoring in,
        280
    oxygen therapy in, 280–281
    pain in
        assessment of, 278
        management of, 283–285,
            284b–285b
    peripheral vascular assessment in,
        274
    peristalsis in, 285–286
    phases of, 270–271
    physical assessments, 272–278
    pressure injuries in, 283
    psychosocial assessment in,
        278–280
    renal system in, 276
    respiratory system in
        assessment of, 273–274
        complications involving,
            242–244
    self-management education in,
        286–287
    skin assessments, 277–278, 278f
    skin care, 281b
    total knee arthroplasty, 315–316,
        315f
    transition management in,
        286–287
    urinary system, 276
    venous thromboembolism
        prevention, 274, 281
    vital signs, 274

Postoperative period (Continued)
  wound
    dehiscence of, 277, 278f, 282–283
    drains, 277–278, 279f, 282
    dressings for, 277–278, 281–282
    evisceration of, 277, 278f, 283, 283b
    healing of, 277, 278f
    nonsurgical management of, 281–282
    staple closure of, 282
    suture closure of, 282
    wound infection prevention in, 281–283
Postpartum hemorrhage, 1246
Postpericardiotomy syndrome, 789
Postrenal failure, 1392
Posttraumatic stress disorder
  after mass casualty event, 156b
  in transgender patients, 1494
Postural hypotension, 121, 168, 652
Posture
  assessments of, 1009, 1009f
  instability, in Parkinson disease, 871
Post-void residual, 98
Potassium
  in acidosis, 194
  bicarbonate ion and, 194f
  dietary sources of, 175
  extracellular fluid, 175
  laboratory testing for, 1069b
  in older adults, 165b
  replacement of, for hypokalemia, 176
  restriction of, in chronic kidney disease, 1408
  serum levels of, 164t, 175
Potassium imbalances
  hyperkalemia, 178–179, 178t, 179b, 192, 237
  hypokalemia, 175–177, 177b, 196, 237
Potassium-sparing diuretics, 177, 699, 701
Povidone-iodine allergy, 234–235
Powered air-purifying respirator, 120, 416
PPE. See Personal protective equipment
PQRST, 1066
PR interval, 669–670, 669f
PR segment, 667–669, 669f
Pramlintide, 1292b–1293b
Prasugrel, 783–784
Prealbumin, 25, 1217
Precipitation, 297
Precordium, 653–654, 654f
Prediabetes, 1287
Prednisolone, 302b
Prednisone, 1255b
  asthma treated with, 569b–570b
  immunosuppression uses of, 302b
  rheumatoid arthritis treated with, 322–323

Prednisone (Continued)
  ulcerative colitis treated with, 1152–1153
Preemptive analgesia, 54
Pregabalin, 63–64
Pregnancy
  human immunodeficiency virus infection effects on, 340
  methotrexate contraindications for, 322
  in sickle cell disease patients, 813b
Prehospital care providers, 119, 119f
Pre-infarction angina, 770
Preload
  definition of, 645
  drugs that affect, 699–701
  interventions that reduce, 698
Premature atrial complexes, 676
Premature complexes, 671
Premature ventricular complexes, 683–684, 683f, 779
Premature ventricular contractions, 683
Preoperative period
  administering regularly scheduled drugs, 241–242
  antibiotic prophylaxis in, 247
  anxiety in, 237, 246
  bowel preparation, 242
  checklist for, 247–249, 248f
  definition of, 229
  description of, 228
  dietary restrictions in, 241
  discharge planning in, 235
  drains, 242
  drugs in, 241–242, 247, 257
  electrocardiogram in, 238
  electronic health record review in, 246–247
  expected outcomes in, 238
  family members, 246
  fear in, 237
  focused assessment in, 238b
  hair removal, 242, 243f
  history-taking in, 230–235
  imaging assessments in, 237
  informed consent, 239–241, 240f
  interventions in, 238–246
  intestinal preparation, 242
  laboratory assessments in, 237
  medical history, 233–234
  National Patient Safety Goal requirements, 238–239
  older adults, 236b
  patient preparation in, 247
  patient self-determination, 241
  patient transfer to surgical suite, 247–249
  physical assessments in, 235–237
  postoperative procedures and exercises
    antiembolism stockings, 244
    for cardiovascular complications, 244–246
    coughing and splinting, 244

Preoperative period (Continued)
  incentive spirometry, 243–244, 244f
  leg exercises, 245, 245b
  overview of, 244
  pneumatic compression devices, 245, 245f
  for respiratory complications, 242–244
  psychosocial assessments, 237
  rest in, 246
  skin preparation, 242, 243f
  studies of, 239b
  teaching in, 239t, 246
  total hip arthroplasty, 309–310
  total knee arthroplasty, 314–315
  tubes, 242
  urinalysis, 237
  vascular access preparations, 242
Prerenal failure, 1392
Presbycusis, 26, 997
Presbyopia, 26, 33, 980–981
Presence, 112
Pressure dressings, 267
Pressure injuries
  assessment of, 91
  Braden scale for, 457t
  care coordination for, 459–461
  Concept Map for, 455f–456f
  definition of, 447
  description of, 27
  features of, 452b
  friction in, 448
  health care resources for, 461
  health promotion and maintenance for, 448–452
  high-risk patients for, 448–451, 461b
  home care management of, 459–460
  incidence of, 448
  incontinence and, 451
  infection prevention in, 459
  laboratory assessment of, 455
  mechanical forces that cause, 448
  nutrition status and, 449–451
  in older adults, 42
  pathophysiology of, 447–448
  patient positioning for, 452
  physical assessment of, 453
  postoperative, 283
  pressure-redistribution techniques for, 451–452
  prevalence of, 448
  prevention of, 96–97, 449, 449b, 900
  psychosocial assessment of, 455
  self-care management of, 460–461
  shearing forces as cause of, 448, 448f
  signs and symptoms of, 453
  skin integrity care bundle for, 449b
  in spinal cord injury patients, 901–903
  stages of, 452b, 454f

Pressure injuries (Continued)
  support surfaces and devices for, 451
  transition management for, 459–461
  wound caused by
    assessment of, 453–455
    best practices for, 460b
    dressings for, 457–458
    drug therapy for, 458
    electrical stimulation for, 458–459
    hyperbaric oxygen therapy for, 458
    management of, 455–459, 457b
    negative-pressure wound therapy for, 458
    nonsurgical management of, 457–459
    nutrition therapy for, 458
    physical therapy for, 458
    skin substitutes for, 458
    surgical management of, 459
    ultrasound-assisted wound therapy for, 458–459
Pressure support ventilation, 636t
Pressure-activated safety valve, 205
Pressure-cycled ventilators, 631
Pressure-reducing devices, 97
Pressure-relieving devices, 97
Pretibial myxedema, 1265, 1271f
Priapism, 810
Primary aldosteronism, 721
Primary angle-closure glaucoma, 972
Primary biliary cirrhosis, 1170
Primary gout, 330–331
Primary lesions, 436, 438f
Primary open-angle glaucoma, 972
Primary prevention
  of cancer, 381–382
  of impaired cellular regulation, 15
  of sensory perception changes, 26
Primary progressive multiple sclerosis, 888
Primary survey and resuscitation interventions, 129–130, 131t
Primary syphilis, 1508
Primary tumor, 375
Prinzmetal's angina, 770
Priority setting, 122
Privacy, of genetic counseling, 83
Proaccelerin, 798t
Probenecid, 332
Probiotics, for irritable bowel syndrome, 1137
Procainamide hydrochloride, 685
Proctocolectomy
  with ileo pouch-anal anastomosis, 1154–1155, 1154f
  total proctocolectomy with permanent ileostomy, 1154, 1155f
Professional ethics, 9

Progressive multifocal leukoencephalopathy, 891
Progressive-relapsing multiple sclerosis, 888
Proinsulin, 1281, 1282f
Projected pain, 50
Prokinetic agents, for chemotherapy-induced nausea and vomiting, 399b
Prolactin, 1237t, 1248b
Prolactin-secreting tumors, 1247
Proliferative diabetic retinopathy, 1284
Pronation, 1010f
Pronator drift, 848
Prone position, 265f
Prophylactic mastectomy, 1443–1444
Prophylactic surgery, for cancer, 386
Proportionate palliative sedation, 111
Proprioception, 850, 932–933
Propylthiouracil, 1267, 1268b
Prostacyclin agents, 585
Prostaglandin agonists, for glaucoma, 966b
Prostaglandin analogs, 1106b–1107b
Prostaglandin-5 inhibitors, 892
Prostaglandins, 873, 1103, 1326–1327
Prostate artery embolization, 1479
Prostate cancer
    active surveillance of, 1483–1484
    anti-androgen drugs for, 1485
    assessment of, 380b, 1482–1483
    benign prostatic hyperplasia and, 1482f
    care coordination for, 1485–1486
    chemotherapy for, 1485
    etiology of, 1482
    health care resources for, 1486
    health promotion and maintenance for, 1482
    history-taking for, 1482
    home care management of, 1485–1486
    incidence of, 1482
    interventions for, 1483–1485
    laboratory assessment of, 1483
    laparoscopic radical prostatectomy for, 1484
    metastasis of, 376t, 1483–1485
    nonsurgical management of, 1485
    pathophysiology of, 1481–1482, 1482f
    physical assessment of, 1482–1483
    prevalence of, 1482
    psychosocial assessment of, 1483
    radiation therapy for, 1485
    risk factors for, 1482
    self-management education for, 1486, 1486b
    signs and symptoms of, 1482–1483

Prostate cancer (Continued)
    surgical management of, 1484–1485, 1484b
    transition management for, 1485–1486
    transrectal ultrasound for, 1483, 1483b
Prostate gland
    anatomy of, 1431
    benign hyperplasia of. See Benign prostatic hyperplasia
    biopsy of, 1438
    digital rectal examination of, 382, 1346–1347, 1474
Prostate-specific antigen, 1435, 1477, 1483
Prostatic intraepithelial neoplasia, 1481–1482
Prostatic stents, 1479
Prostatitis, 1474–1476
Prosthetic heart valves, 709–710
Protamine sulfate, 744
Protease inhibitors, 338, 348, 351b–352b
Proteases, 572
Proteasome inhibitors, 404t, 405
Protein
    restriction of, in chronic kidney disease, 1407–1408
    in urine, 1333
Protein buffers, 188–189
Protein C, 764
Protein malabsorption, 1202–1203
Protein synthesis, 76
Protein-calorie malnutrition, 414–415, 1215
Protein-energy malnutrition, 1215
Proteinuria, 1333–1335, 1377, 1381
Proteolysis, 1197
Prothrombin, 798t
Prothrombin time, 622b, 657, 805, 1068, 1174
Proton pump inhibitors
    gastritis treated with, 1105
    gastroesophageal reflux disease treated with, 1090b, 1091
    peptic ulcer disease treated with, 1106b–1107b, 1111–1112
Proto-oncogenes, 375
Proximal convoluted tubule, 1323–1324
Proximal femur fractures, 1035b
Proximal humerus fractures, 1046
Proximal interphalangeal joint, 1009, 1009f
Pruritus, 436, 461–462, 1192
PSDA. See Patient Self-determination Act
Pseudoaddiction, 58
Pseudocyst, pancreatic, 1205
Pseudomonas aeruginosa, 1023, 1135–1136
Psoralen and ultraviolet A therapy, 465

Psoriasis
    assessment of, 464
    collaborative care for, 463–465
    corticosteroids for, 464
    definition of, 463
    drug therapy for, 466b
    emotional support for, 465
    exfoliative, 464
    history-taking for, 464
    light therapy for, 465
    pathophysiology of, 463
    systemic therapy for, 465
    tar preparations for, 464
    topical therapy for, 464–465
Psoriasis vulgaris, 464, 464f
Psoriatic arthritis, 332–333, 463
PSVT. See Paroxysmal supraventricular tachycardia
Psychiatric crisis nurse team, 118–119
Ptosis, 917, 934, 963
Ptyalin, 1062
Pubovaginal sling procedure, 1349t
Pulmonary arterial hypertension, 584–585, 585t
Pulmonary artery, 511, 511f
Pulmonary artery occlusive pressure, 780
Pulmonary artery pressure, 697
Pulmonary artery wedge pressure, 697, 780–782
Pulmonary autographs, 709
Pulmonary circulation, 511
Pulmonary contusion, 636
Pulmonary edema
    in chronic kidney disease, 1405–1407
    fluid overload in, 172b
    in heart failure, 702–703, 702b
    high-altitude, 145–146, 145b–146b
    neurogenic, 954
    prevention of, 1405–1407
Pulmonary embolism
    anxiety management in, 622–623
    assessment of, 618–619
    in atrial fibrillation, 680b
    bleeding management in, 622
    care coordination for, 623–624
    collaborative care for, 618–624
    definition of, 616–617
    drug therapy for, 619–620, 620b
    fractures as risk factor for, 1034–1035
    health care resources for, 623–624
    health promotion and maintenance for, 617–618
    heparin for, 617–618, 620, 621b
    home care management of, 623, 624b
    hypotension, 621–622
    hypoxemia in, 619–621
    imaging assessment of, 619
    laboratory assessment of, 618–619
    lifestyle changes for prevention of, 617

Pulmonary embolism (Continued)
    nonsurgical management of, 619–621, 619b
    pathophysiology of, 616–617
    physical assessment of, 618
    prevention of, 617b
    psychosocial assessment of, 618
    risk factors for, 617
    self-management education for, 623, 623b
    severity of, 620t
    signs and symptoms of, 618, 618b
    surgical management of, 620–621
    transition management for, 623–624
    venous thromboembolism as cause of, 617, 716
Pulmonary fibrosis, idiopathic, 585–586
Pulmonary fluid overload, 491
Pulmonary function tests
    for asthma, 567
    description of, 523–524, 525t
Pulmonary rehabilitation, 579
Pulmonary tuberculosis. See Tuberculosis
Pulmonary vein isolation, 681
Pulmonic valve, 643
Pulse
    description of, 653
    palpation of, 729
Pulse antibiotic therapy, for urinary tract infections, 98
Pulse deficit, 672
Pulse oximetry
    description of, 247, 273
    respiratory system assessment using, 523, 523f
Pulse pressure, 652–653
Pulse therapy, 322
Pulsus alternans, 696
Pulsus paradoxus, 713
Punch biopsy, 445
Punctal occlusion, 975, 975f
Pupil(s)
    age-related changes in, 961b
    assessment of, 963
    constriction of, 847–848, 960
    definition of, 957
    dilation of, 960
Pupil testing
    description of, 847–848
    in traumatic brain injury patients, 946
Pure-tone air-conduction testing, 990
Pure-tone audiometry, 990–991
Pure-tone bone-conduction testing, 991
Purified protein derivative test, 322, 347, 367
Purkinje cells, 665
Purpura, 439
Pursed-lip breathing, 578, 578b
Pustules, 438f

PVCs. *See* Premature ventricular complexes
Pyelogram, 1339
Pyelolithotomy, 1375
Pyelonephritis, 1359*b*
  acute, 1372–1373, 1374*b*
  assessment of, 1374
  care coordination for, 1375–1376
  chronic, 1372–1373, 1374*b*
  definition of, 1372
  diagnostic assessment of, 1374
  health care resources for, 1376
  history-taking for, 1374
  home care management for, 1375
  imaging assessment of, 1374
  interventions for, 1375
  laboratory assessment of, 1374
  nonsurgical management of, 1375
  pain management in, 1375
  pathophysiology of, 1372–1374, 1373*f*
  physical assessment of, 1374
  psychosocial assessment of, 1374
  self-management education for, 1376
  signs and symptoms of, 1374
  surgical management of, 1375
  transition management for, 1375–1376
Pyloric obstruction, 1109, 1114
Pyloromyotomy, 1098
Pyuria, 1358

Q
QRS complex, 669–670
QRS duration, 669–670
QSEN initiative, 2
QSEN Institute, 2
QT interval, 669*f*, 670–671
Quadriceps-setting exercises, 312–313
Quadrigeminy, 671
Quadriparesis, 933–934
Quality and safety education, 2
Quality improvement
  attributes of, 7
  continuous, 7
  definition of, 7
  scope of, 7
QuantiFERON-TB Gold In-Tube test, 607

R
Radial nerve compression, 267*b*
Radiating pain, 50
Radiation dermatitis, 389
Radiation dose, 387–388
Radiation exposure, 379
Radiation injuries, 488
Radiation proctitis, 1485
Radiation therapy. *See also* Brachytherapy; External beam radiation therapy
  bone tumors treated with, 1026
  brachytherapy, 388

Radiation therapy (*Continued*)
  breast cancer treated with, 1451
  cervical cancer treated with, 1470
  colorectal cancer treated with, 1129–1130
  delivery methods and devices for, 388–389
  endometrial cancer treated with, 1466–1467
  esophageal tumors treated with, 1097
  external beam, 388
  gastric cancer treated with, 1116
  head and neck cancer treated with, 549
  high-dose rate implants, 388–389, 389*b*
  hoarseness secondary to, 549
  hyperpituitarism treated with, 1249
  intensity of, 388
  intensity-modulated, 388
  low-dose rate implants, 388–389, 389*b*
  lung cancer treated with, 588–589, 593
  oral cancer treated with, 1081
  overview of, 387–388
  prostate cancer treated with, 1485
  side effects of, 389–390, 389*t*, 1116, 1119
  skin cancer treated with, 477
  skin protection during, 390*b*
  stereotactic body, 388
  tissue effects of, 387
  xerostomia caused by, 1084–1085
Radical cystectomy, 1366
Radical hysterectomy, 1461*t*, 1466
Radical prostatectomy
  laparoscopic, 1484
  open, 1484*b*
Radical surgery, 232*t*
Radiculopathies, 905
Radioactive iodine therapy
  hyperthyroidism treated with, 1266–1269, 1269*b*
  thyroid cancer treated with, 1275
Radiofrequency ablation
  description of, 681
  liver cancer treated with, 1187
  supraventricular tachycardia treated with, 676–678
Radiofrequency identification, 8
Radiographs
  chest. *See* Chest x-rays
  gastrointestinal system assessments, 1070
  skeletal system assessments using, 1011
Radioisotope scanning, 965
Radiosurgery, for trigeminal neuralgia, 924
Rales, 521*t*
Raloxifene, 1021

Ramsay Sedation Scale, 261, 262*t*
Ramucirumab, 589*t*
Range of motion
  active, 1010
  assessments of, 1010, 1010*f*
  mobility rehabilitation exercises, 96, 503
  passive, 1010
Ranibizumab, 1284
Rapid influenza diagnostic test, 597
Rapid plasma reagin, 1509
Rapid response teams, 8
Rapid urease testing, 1105
Rapidly progressive glomerulonephritis, 1377–1378
Rattlesnake bites, 136, 138*t*–140*t*
Raynaud's disease, 741*t*
Raynaud's phenomenon, 329–330, 741*t*
Reasoning, 16
Rebound headache, 874
Rebound phenomenon, 146
Receptive aphasia, 938
Recombinant human bone morphogenetic protein-2, 1045
Reconstructive surgery, 386
Recreational therapists, 89
Rectal pain, 1164
Rectal tumors, 1130*t*
Rectocele, 1464, 1464*f*
Recurrent aphthous ulcers, 1076–1078
Red blood cells
  description of, 796
  gender differences, 800*b*
  production of, 797
  transfusion of
    compatibility determinations for, 834, 834*t*
    indications for, 832*t*, 834–835
    sickle cell disease treated with, 812
Red reflex, 966
Reducible hernia, 1138
Reduction mammoplasty, 1456
Reed-Sternberg cells, 828
Re-epithelialization, 473–474, 474*f*
Refeeding syndrome, 1221–1222
Referred pain, 50
Reflex arc, 842, 843*f*
Reflex incontinence, 1344, 1345*t*
Reflex sympathetic dystrophy, 1035
Reflexes
  assessment of, 848–849
  asymmetry of, 849, 849*f*
  components of, 842
  cutaneous, 848
  deep tendon, 848
  hyperactive, 849
  hypoactive, 849
Reflux, 1373
Reflux esophagitis, 1087
Refraction
  definition of, 960, 980
  errors of, 960, 960*f*, 980–981

Regional anesthesia, 65, 260–261, 261*f*–262*f*, 261*t*
Regional osteoporosis, 1016
Registered dietitians, 89
Registered nurse, 123–124, 253*t*
Regurgitation, 1089
Rehabilitation
  ambulatory care, 88
  for bowel continence, 99
  after cancer surgery, 387
  cognitive assessments before, 91
  continuum of care, 87
  definition of, 86
  desired outcome of, 88
  for functional abilities, 96
  functional ability assessments before, 92
  history-taking, 89–90
  home care preparation after, 100
  inpatient, 87
  interprofessional team for, 88–89, 88*t*, 89*f*
  for mobility issues, 93–96
  for pressure injury prevention, 96–97
  safe patient handling and mobility practices during, 93–95, 93*b*
  for spinal cord injury, 901–902
  telerehabilitation, 101
  for urinary continence, 97–98
Rehabilitation assistants, 89
Rehabilitation case manager, 88
Rehabilitation nurses, 88, 88*t*
Rehabilitation settings
  care coordination and transition management in, 99–101
  description of, 87–88
  gait training in, 95–96, 95*b*, 95*f*
  interprofessional team in, 88–89, 88*t*, 89*f*
  leave-of-absence visit, 100
  older adults in, 90*b*
  physical assessments in
    bowel elimination, 90*t*, 91
    cardiovascular system, 90, 90*t*
    gastrointestinal system, 90–91, 90*t*
    integumentary system, 90*t*, 91
    musculoskeletal system, 90*t*, 91
    neurologic system, 90*t*, 91
    nutrition, 90–91, 90*t*
    overview of, 90*t*
    renal system, 90*t*, 91
    respiratory system, 90, 90*t*
    skin, 90*t*, 91
    tissue integrity, 90*t*, 91
    urinary system, 90*t*, 91
  predischarge assessments, 100
  psychosocial assessments in, 92
  safe patient handling and mobility practices in, 93–95, 93*b*
  staff members in, work-related musculoskeletal disorders to, 93
  vocational assessments in, 92

Rehabilitation therapists, 89

Rehabilitative surgery, 386

Rehydration, 170

Reiter's syndrome, 334t

Relapsing-remitting multiple sclerosis, 888, 890–891

Relative alkalosis, 195

Relative dehydration, 167

Relative potency, 58

Relaxation techniques, 67, 285

Religion
  death rituals based on, 112t
  emergency department care affected by, 123b

Relocation stress syndrome, 30–31, 33b

Remicade. See Infliximab

Reminiscence/reminiscence therapy, 112, 862

Renal arteriography, 1339

Renal artery bypass surgery, 1384

Renal artery stenosis, 721, 1384, 1423–1424

Renal cell carcinoma, 1385–1386

Renal colic, 1330, 1362

Renal columns, 1322

Renal cortex, 1322

Renal medulla, 1322

Renal osteodystrophy, 1400–1401, 1404

Renal replacement therapies
  acute kidney injury treated with, 1397–1398, 1397f
  chronic kidney disease treated with, 1411–1424, 1411t, 1412f–1415f

Renal scan, 1339

Renal system. See also Kidney(s)
  age-related changes in, 234b, 1328–1329, 1328b
  assessment of
    blood tests, 1331–1332
    computed tomography, 1337–1338, 1337t, 1338b
    current health problems, 1330
    cystography, 1337t, 1339
    cystometrography, 1340
    cystoscopy, 1337t, 1339
    cystourethrography, 1337t, 1339
    cystourethroscopy, 1339
    description of, 90t, 91
    diagnostic, 1331–1341
    electromyography, 1340
    family history, 1330
    genetic risks, 1330
    history-taking, 1329–1330
    imaging, 1337–1341
    kidney, ureter, and bladder x-rays, 1337, 1337t
    kidney biopsy, 1340–1341
    laboratory, 1331–1341
    magnetic resonance imaging, 1337t, 1338
    medication history, 1329–1330
    nutrition history, 1329

Renal system (Continued)
    physical, 1330–1331
    positron emission tomography, 1337t
    psychosocial, 1331
    renal arteriography, 1339
    renal scan, 1339
    retrograde procedures, 1339–1340
    ultrasonography, 1337t, 1338
    urine tests. See Urine tests
    urodynamic studies, 1340
  dehydration effects on, 169
  description of, 1321
  kidneys. See Kidney(s)
  physical assessment of, 1330–1331
  postoperative assessment of, 276
  preoperative assessment of, 236
  ureters, 1327, 1327f
  urethra, 1327–1328
  urinary bladder, 1327, 1327f

Renal threshold, 1325

Renal transplantation. See Kidney transplantation

Renin, 166–167, 721, 1237, 1323, 1326

Renin-angiotensin II pathway
  in fluid balance, 166–167, 166f
  in hypertension management, 167

Renin-angiotensin system
  activation of, 694
  angiotensin receptor blockers effect on, 698
  angiotensin-converting enzyme inhibitors effect on, 698
  description of, 166

Renin-angiotension-aldosterone system
  activation of, 692
  blood pressure regulation by, 721
  chronic kidney disease effects on, 1401

Renovascular disease, 1384

Renovascular hypertension, 721

Repaglinide, 1292b–1293b

Reperfusion therapy, for myocardial infarction, 777–778

Repetitive nerve stimulation, for myasthenia gravis, 918

Repetitive stress injury, 1057

Replication, of DNA, 73–74, 74f

Reproductive system
  age-related changes in, 1431, 1431b
  assessment of, 1431–1438
  biopsy studies of, 1437–1438, 1437b
  colposcopy of, 1436
  current health problems in, 1432–1433
  diagnostic assessment of, 1433–1438
  endoscopic studies of, 1436–1437
  family history of, 1432

Reproductive system (Continued)
  female. See Female reproductive system
  genetic risk of, 1432
  health promotion and maintenance for, 1431
  history-taking for, 1431–1433
  hysteroscopy of, 1437
  imaging assessment of, 1435–1436
  laboratory assessment of, 1433–1435, 1434b
  laparoscopy of, 1436–1437, 1437f
  magnetic resonance imaging of, 1436
  male. See Male reproductive system
  nutrition history for, 1432
  in older adults, 1431b
  physical assessment of, 1433
  psychosocial assessment of, 1433
  ultrasonography of, 1436

Residents, of skilled nursing facilities, 87, 87f

Resistin, 1225

Respect, 2, 9

Respiration
  accessory muscles of, 511
  assessment of, 63b
  neural regulation of, 189f

Respiratory acidosis, 13, 191t, 192, 194–195

Respiratory alkalosis, 13, 196, 196t

Respiratory bronchioles, 511f

Respiratory depression
  opioid analgesics as cause of, 62–63, 63t, 64b, 524b
  respiratory acidosis as cause of, 192

Respiratory hygiene/cough etiquette, 419, 419t

Respiratory infections, 573, 581

Respiratory system. See also Lung(s)
  in acid-base balance, 189–190, 189f, 189t
  acidosis effects on, 193, 193b
  age-related changes in, 234b, 512, 513b
  alkalosis effects on, 196, 196b
  anatomy of
    airways, 510, 511f
    alveolar ducts, 510
    bronchi, 510, 511f
    bronchioles, 510, 511f
    description of, 508–512
    larynx, 509f, 510, 517–518
    lungs, 510–511, 511f, 518–521
    nose, 509, 509f, 517, 556
    paranasal sinuses, 509, 509f, 517, 556
    pharynx, 509–510, 517–518
    sinuses, 509, 509f, 517, 556
    thorax, 518–521
    trachea, 510, 511f, 517–518
  assessment of
    capnography, 523, 523f, 524b
    capnometry, 523

Respiratory system (Continued)
    chest pain, 517
    chest x-rays, 521
    computed tomography, 521–522
    current health problems, 516–517
    description of, 90, 90t, 802
    diagnostic, 521–527
    dyspnea, 517, 517t
    endoscopy, 524–526
    exercise testing, 524
    family history, 516
    genetic risks, 516
    history-taking, 515–517
    imaging, 521–524
    laboratory, 521, 522b
    lung biopsy, 526–527
    orthopnea, 517
    physical, 517–521
    psychosocial, 521
    pulmonary function tests, 523–524, 525t
    pulse oximetry, 523, 523f
    in spinal cord injury, 896
    thoracentesis, 526, 526f
  dehydration effects on, 168
  description of, 508
  drug use effects on, 516
  fluid overload effects on, 171f
  health promotion and maintenance of, 512–515
  hypokalemia effects on, 176
  inhalant irritants that affect, 515
  leukemia effects on, 819
  nutrition assessments, 1213b
  oxygen delivery by, 512
  oxygen-hemoglobin dissociation curve, 512, 512f
  postoperative assessments of, 273–274
  postoperative procedures and exercises
    coughing and splinting, 244
    incentive spirometry, 243–244, 244f
  preoperative assessment of, 236
  respiratory adequacy indicators, 520–521
  sickle cell disease effects on, 810
  smoking effects on, 514

Respiratory system disorders
  acute respiratory distress syndrome. See Acute respiratory distress syndrome
  acute respiratory failure, 624–626, 625t
  asthma. See Asthma
  chronic obstructive pulmonary disease. See Chronic obstructive pulmonary disease
  coccidioidomycosis, 613
  cystic fibrosis. See Cystic fibrosis

Respiratory system disorders
  (Continued)
  idiopathic pulmonary fibrosis,
    585–586
  influenza. See Influenza
  inhalation anthrax, 611–612,
    612b
  Middle East respiratory syndrome,
    598
  peritonsillar abscess, 611
  pertussis, 613
  pulmonary arterial hypertension,
    584–585, 585t
  pulmonary embolism. See
    Pulmonary embolism
  rhinosinusitis, 610–611
  tuberculosis. See Tuberculosis
Respiratory tract
  infection transmission, 415
  lower, 510–511, 511f
  upper, 509–510, 509f
Respite care, 866, 949
Resting metabolic rate, 1228
Restless legs syndrome, 922–923
Restorative aides, 89
Restorative nursing programs, 96
Restorative proctocolectomy with
  ileo pouch-anal anastomosis,
  1154–1155, 1154f
Restraints
  alternatives to, 42b
  chemical, 41
  definition of, 41
  hospital use of, 41
Restrictive cardiomyopathy, 714–715,
  715t
Retained surgical items, 267
Rete pegs, 432, 432f
Retention sutures, 267
Reticular activating system, 841
Reticulocyte count, 804–805
Retina
  anatomy of, 957–958
  detachment of, 979–980
  holes of, 979–980
  macular degeneration of, 979
  tears of, 979–980
  ultrasonic imaging of, 967
Retinitis pigmentosa, 980
Retrograde pyelography, 1358
Retroperitoneal lymph node
  dissection, 1489
Retropubic suspension, 1349t
Retrovirus, 338
Reverse transcriptase, 337–340
Rewarming
  frostbite treated with, 144–145
  hypothermia treated with, 143
RFID. See Radiofrequency
  identification
Rh antigen system, 835
Rheumatic carditis, 714
Rheumatic disease, 304
Rheumatic endocarditis, 714
Rheumatic fever, 714

Rheumatoid arthritis
  arthrocentesis for, 321
  care coordination for, 325
  cervical, 319b
  clinical features of, 306t
  complementary and integrative
    health interventions for, 324
  coping strategies for patients with,
    325
  definition of, 318
  diagnostic assessments for, 321, 321b
  drug therapy for
    biological response modifiers,
      321–322, 323b
    disease-modifying
      antirheumatic drugs, 322
    nonsteroidal anti-inflammatory
      drugs, 321
  early stage of, 318–319
  etiology of, 318
  exercises for, 317b
  extra-articular manifestations of,
    319
  features of, 318b
  genetic risk of, 318
  health care resources for, 325
  home care management of, 325
  human leukocyte antigens and,
    318b
  incidence of, 318
  joint deformities associated with,
    319, 319f
  laboratory assessment of, 320–321,
    320b
  mobility interventions in, 324
  nonpharmacologic interventions
    for, 323–324
  osteoarthritis versus, 306t
  pain management in, 321–324
  pathophysiology of, 318
  prevalence of, 318
  psychosocial assessment of,
    319–320
  referrals for, 319
  self-esteem promotion in, 324–325
  self-management education for,
    325
  signs and symptoms of, 318–319,
    319f
  subcutaneous nodules associated
    with, 319
  transition management of, 325
  vasculitis associated with, 319
Rheumatoid factor, 320
Rheumatology, 304
Rhinoplasty, 556–557, 556f
Rhinorrhea, 880–881
Rhinosinusitis, 610–611
Rhonchi, 521t
Rib fracture, 636–637
Rifater, 608
Rifaximin, 1137
Right atrial pressure, 780
Right atrium, 642
Right coronary artery, 643–644, 643f

Right hemisphere stroke, 932–933,
  933b
Right ventricle, 642
Right ventricular failure, 696, 696b,
  782
Right-sided heart failure, 651, 692,
  694–695
Rigidity, 869
Rinne tuning fork test, 989–990
Risedronate, 1021
Rituximab (Rituxan), 323b
Rivastigmine, 871
Robotic surgery, 254–255, 789
Rods, 957–958
Rollator, 95
Rolling hiatal hernias, 1092–1093,
  1092f
Romberg sign, 850
Rosenbaum Pocket Vision Screener,
  964
Rosiglitazone, 1291, 1292b–1293b
Rotation, 1010f
Rotator cuff injuries, 1059
Rotigotine, 870
Roux-en-Y gastric bypass, 1229,
  1230f
RRTs. See Rapid response teams
Rubor, 652
Rule of nines, 492, 492f

S
Sacubitril/valsartan, 698, 704–705
Safe patient handling and mobility,
  93–95, 93b
Safer sex practices, 1505–1506
SAFEs. See Sexual assault forensic
  examiners
Safety
  attributes of, 4
  context of, 4–5
  culture of, 4–5
  definition of, 3
  in dehydration patients, 170
  emergency department staff,
    120–121, 120b
  in fluid overload, 172
  oxygen therapy, 530b
  scope of, 3–4
  surgical checklist for, 228–229,
    230f
Safety promotion, 2
Salem sump tube, 1124
Saline lock, 203
Salivary glands
  acute sialadenitis of, 1084–1085
  disorders involving, 1084–1085
  radiation therapy effects on,
    549
  tumors of, 1085
Salmeterol, 569b–570b, 570–571
Salmon calcitonin, 1022
Salpingitis, 1431, 1512
Salt tablets, 134
Salt water drowning, 147
Same-day admission, 229–230

SANE. See Sexual assault nurse
  examiners
Sarcoma
  Ewing's, 1025
  fibrosarcoma, 1025
  Kaposi's, 347, 348f, 354–355
  osteosarcoma, 1012, 1025
Sargramostim, 402t
SARS. See Severe acute respiratory
  syndrome
Saxagliptin, 1292b–1293b
SBAR, 5–6, 895
SBRT. See Stereotactic body
  radiotherapy
Scabies, 470–471, 471f, 1470
Scald injuries, 486
Scales, 438f
Schilling test, 1141
Schwartz-Bartter syndrome, 1251
SCIP. See Surgical Care Improvement
  Project
Sclera
  anatomy of, 957
  assessment of, 963
Scleral buckling, 980
Scleroderma, 329
Scoliosis, 1009, 1009f
Scorpion stings, 136–137, 137b, 137f,
  138t–140t
Scrotum, 1430
Seasonal influenza, 596–597
Sebaceous glands, 433
Sebum, 433
Second heart sound, 654
Secondary administration set, 209,
  209f
Secondary gout, 331
Secondary hypertension, 721, 721t
Secondary lesions, 436, 438f
Secondary prevention
  of cancer, 382
  of impaired cellular regulation, 15
  of sensory perception changes, 26
Secondary progressive multiple
  sclerosis, 888
Secondary survey and resuscitation
  interventions, 130
Secondary syphilis, 1508
Secondary tuberculosis, 606
Secondary tumors, 375
Second-degree frostbite, 144
Secondhand smoke, 514
Secukinumab, 369, 370b, 466b
Sedation
  moderate, 261–262, 262t
  opioid analgesics as cause of,
    62–63, 63t–64t
Segmented neutrophils, 292–293,
  293f
Seizures
  in acquired immunodeficiency
    syndrome, 355
  antiepileptic drugs for, 877–878,
    878b
  assessment of, 877

Seizures (Continued)
  care coordination for, 880
  definition of, 876
  drug therapy for, 877–878
  emergency care for, 879
  at end of life, 111
  etiology of, 877
  generalized, 876
  genetic risk for, 877
  management of, 878
  myoclonic, 876
  nonsurgical management of,
      877–879
  partial, 876–877, 878b
  partial corpus callosotomy for,
      880
  pathophysiology of, 876
  precautions for, 878
  prevention of, 877t
  surgical management of, 879–880
  tonic-clonic, 876, 878b–879b
  transition management for, 880
  types of, 876–877
  unclassified, 877
  vagal nerve stimulation for, 879
Selective estrogen receptor
    modulators, 1452, 1456. See also
    Estrogen agonists/antagonists
Selective internal radiation therapy,
    1187
Selective serotonin reuptake
    inhibitors
  depression treated with, 37
  tramadol interactions with, 61
Self cells, 289–290, 290f
Self-determination, 9
Self-esteem
  in amputation patients,
      1054–1055
  in burn injury patients, 504
  in head and neck cancer patients,
      553–554
  in Parkinson disease patients, 872
  in rheumatoid arthritis patients,
      324–325
Self-management, 9
Self-management education
  for activities of daily living, 100
  for Alzheimer's disease, 866–867
  for amputation, 1055–1056
  for asthma, 567–568, 568b, 568f
  for back pain, 908–909
  for benign prostatic hyperplasia,
      1481
  for bone tumors, 1027–1028
  for burn injury, 505
  for cataracts, 971
  for chronic kidney disease,
      1424–1425
  for chronic obstructive pulmonary
      disease, 581
  for cirrhosis, 1179–1180, 1179b
  for colorectal cancer, 1133–1135
  for deep vein thrombosis, 746,
      746b

Self-management education
    (Continued)
  for dysrhythmias, 682
  for esophageal tumors, 1100
  for fractures, 1045
  for gastric cancer, 1119
  for glaucoma, 975–976
  for gonorrhea, 1514
  for head and neck cancer, 554–555
  for hearing loss, 1002
  for heart failure, 703–705, 704t
  for hepatitis, 1185b
  for human immunodeficiency
      virus infection, 356, 357b
  for hypothyroidism, 1274
  for ileostomy, 1157b
  for infection, 426
  for instrumental activities of daily
      living, 100
  for intestinal obstructions, 1126
  for leukemia, 826–827, 826b–827b
  for low back pain, 908–909
  for malnutrition, 1224
  for multiple sclerosis, 892
  for myasthenia gravis, 922, 922b
  for obesity, 1231
  for oral cancer, 1083, 1083b
  for osteoarthritis, 317, 317b
  for osteoporosis, 1022
  for otitis media, 993
  for oxygen therapy, 536
  for pain, 68
  for pancreatic cancer, 1209
  for Parkinson disease, 872
  for pelvic inflammatory disease,
      1516–1517
  for peptic ulcer disease,
      1114–1115
  for pneumonia, 605
  in postoperative period, 286–287
  for prostate cancer, 1486, 1486b
  for pulmonary embolism, 623,
      623b
  for pyelonephritis, 1376
  for rheumatoid arthritis, 325
  for sepsis, 766
  for spinal cord injury, 902
  for stomatitis, 1078
  for stroke, 939–940, 940f
  for systemic lupus erythematosus,
      328
  for total hip arthroplasty, 312b
  for tracheostomy, 544
  for traumatic brain injury, 949,
      949b
  for tuberculosis, 610
  for ulcerative colitis, 1156–1157
  for urinary incontinence, 1353,
      1353b
  for urolithiasis, 1366b
  for uterine leiomyomas, 1463
  for valvular heart disease, 710,
      710b
Self-monitoring of blood glucose,
    1298, 1317

Self-tolerance, 289–290
Sella turcica, 1243
Semicircular canals, 985–986
Semi-Fowlers position, 21
Semilunar valves, 643, 643f
Seminoma, 1487, 1487t
Semipermeable membrane, 163
Semmes-Weinstein monofilaments,
    1305–1306, 1306f
Senile angiomas, 439f
Sensorineural hearing loss, 989, 997,
    997t
Sensory function assessments, 849
Sensory neurons, 839–840
Sensory perception
  auditory. See Ear(s); Hearing
  cancer effects on, 385
  definition of, 957
  description of, 26–27, 27f
  fall risks caused by changes in, 33
  in spinal cord injury, 896, 896b
  stroke-related changes in, 934, 939
  after traumatic brain injury,
      948–949
  visual. See Eye(s); Vision
Sensory receptors, 842
Sentinel events, 4–5
Sepsis
  assessment of, 763–764
  burn wound, 497–498, 498t
  care coordination for, 765–766
  definition of, 407, 753, 760–761
  description of, 28
  diagnostic criteria for, 762t
  etiology of, 762
  health promotion and
      maintenance for, 763
  home care management of, 766,
      766b
  inadequate antimicrobial therapy
      as cause of, 423
  incidence of, 762
  indicators of, 498t
  infection as cause of, 760–761
  interventions for, 765, 765t
  laboratory assessment of, 764
  as oncologic emergency, 407
  pathophysiology of, 760–762
  in pneumonia, 604
  predisposing factors for, 762t
  prevalence of, 762
  prevention of, 604, 812, 1101
  psychosocial assessment of, 764
  self-management education for,
      766
  in sickle cell disease, 812
  signs and symptoms of, 763–764
  Surviving Sepsis Campaign for, 765
  transition management for,
      765–766
September 11, 2001, 150
Septic shock
  assessment of, 763–764
  definition of, 753, 762
  description of, 423

Septic shock (Continued)
  health promotion and
      maintenance for, 763
  interventions for, 765
  predisposing factors for, 762t
  progression of, 760, 760f
  signs and symptoms of, 763–764
Septicemia, 407
Sequestrectomy, 1024
Sequestrum, 1022
Serologic testing, 425
Serosanguineous drainage, 277
Serotonin antagonists, for
    chemotherapy-induced nausea
    and vomiting, 399b
Serous drainage, 277
Serum creatinine, 1331, 1332b
Serum ferritin test, 805
Serum protein electrophoresis, 918
Serum sickness, 366
Severe acute respiratory syndrome,
    598
Sex, 1493, 1493t
Sex chromosomes, 74, 75f
Sex hormones, 1238
Sex-linked recessive pattern of
    inheritance, 78t, 79–80, 80f
Sexual assault forensic examiners, 118
Sexual assault nurse examiners, 118
Sexual disinhibition, 861
Sexual dysfunction, 1286
Sexual orientation, 11t
Sexual transmission, of HIV
    infection, 341–343
Sexuality
  assessment of, 90
  breast cancer and, 1445
  description of, 27–28
  hysterectomy effects on, 1462b
  multiple sclerosis effects on, 890,
      892
  spinal cord injury effects on,
      901–902
Sexually transmitted infections
  assessment of, 1507b
  chlamydia infection, 1511–1512
  complications caused by, 1505t
  condylomata acuminata,
      1510–1511, 1510f
  genital herpes, 1506–1508, 1507b
  gonorrhea, 1512–1514, 1513f
  health promotion and
      maintenance for, 1505–1506,
      1506t
  Healthy People 2020 objectives for,
      1505, 1506t
  interventions for, 27
  in lesbian, gay, bisexual,
      transgender, and queer
      population, 1509b
  in older adults, 1505b
  overview of, 1504–1505
  pelvic inflammatory disease
      secondary to. See Pelvic
      inflammatory disease

Sexually transmitted infections (Continued)
  prevalence of, 1504–1505, 1505b
  safer sex practices for prevention of, 1505–1506
  screening for, 27
  syphilis, 1508–1510, 1508f
Shave biopsy, 445
Shearing forces, 448, 448f
Sheehan's syndrome, 1246
Shigellosis, 1148t, 1149
Shingles. See Herpes zoster
Shivering, 135, 280
Shock
  acute pancreatitis as cause of, 1198, 1199b
  cardiogenic
    acute coronary syndrome as cause of, 782
    etiology of, 753
    risk factors for, 752t, 756b
  classification of, 751
  clinical features of, 752b
  definition of, 751
  distributive
    chemical-induced, 753
    etiology of, 753
    risk factors for, 752t, 756b
  hypovolemic
    adaptive responses and events during, 754t
    assessment of, 756–758
    care coordination for, 760
    concept map for, 756f–757f
    drug therapy for, 759b
    etiology of, 752–753, 755
    in fractures, 1034
    health promotion and maintenance for, 756
    incidence of, 755
    laboratory assessment of, 758, 758b
    nonsurgical management of, 758–760, 759b
    pathophysiology of, 754–755
    physical assessment of, 756–758
    prevalence of, 755
    risk factors for, 752t, 756b
    signs and symptoms of, 756–758
    surgical management of, 760
    transition management for, 760
  multiple organ dysfunction syndrome secondary to, 754–755, 755b
  obstructive
    etiology of, 753
    risk factors for, 752t
  overview of, 751–754
  risk factors for, 756b
  septic. See Septic shock
  signs and symptoms of, 752, 752b
  stages of, 754–755
  types of, 752–754
Short bones, 1005

Short Michigan Alcoholism Screening Test—Geriatric Version, 38
Short peripheral catheters, 202–204, 202f–203f, 202t, 203b, 214–215
Short-acting beta₂ agonists, 568–570, 569b–570b
SIADH. See Syndrome of inappropriate antidiuretic hormone
Sialadenitis
  acute, 1084–1085
  post-irradiation, 1085
Sickle cell anemia. See Sickle cell disease
Sickle cell disease
  acute chest syndrome in, 810, 812
  assessment of, 809–811
  care coordination for, 812–813
  crises in, 809, 811, 812b
  definition of, 808
  etiology of, 809
  genetic risk of, 809
  hematopoietic stem cell transplantation for, 812
  history-taking for, 809–810
  hydroxyurea in, 811
  imaging assessment of, 811
  incidence of, 809
  jaundice associated with, 810
  laboratory assessment of, 810–811
  pain management in, 811–812
  pathophysiology of, 808–809
  perfusion affected by, 809
  physical assessment of, 810
  pregnancy in, 813b
  prevalence of, 809
  priapism in, 810
  psychosocial assessment of, 810
  red blood cell transfusion for, 812
  self-management education for, 812–813, 813b
  sepsis prevention in, 812
  signs and symptoms of, 810
  transition management for, 812–813
  ulcers associated with, 810
  vaso-occlusive events, 809
Sickle cell trait, 79, 809
Sigmoid colon, 1064
Sigmoid colostomy, 1131f, 1134
Sigmoidoscopy
  colorectal cancer diagnosis using, 1128b, 1129
  description of, 1073
Sigmoidostomy, 1368f
Sign language, 1001
Sildenafil, 146, 1489
Silver sulfadiazine, 501b
Simple facemask, 532, 532t, 533f
Simple fracture, 1032
Simple hemothorax, 637
Simple surgery, 232t
Simponi. See Golimumab

SIMV. See Synchronized intermittent mandatory ventilation
Sinemet, 870, 923
Single gene traits, 74
Single nucleotide polymorphisms, 76–77
Single-fiber electromyography, for myasthenia gravis, 918
Single-incision laparoscopic cholecystectomy, 1195
Single-photon emission computed tomography, 854
Singultus, 1123
Sinoatrial node, 664, 672–673
Sinus(es)
  anatomy of, 509, 509f
  assessment of, 517
  cancer of, 556
Sinus arrhythmia, 671
Sinus dysrhythmias, 672–675
Sinus tachycardia, 673, 673f
Sipuleucel-T, 402t
Sirolimus
  autoimmune diseases treated with, 368
  immunosuppression uses of, 302b
SIRS. See Systemic inflammatory response syndrome
Sitagliptin, 1292b–1293b
Situational awareness, 157
Situational depression, 36
Sjögren's syndrome, 319–320
Skeletal system. See also Musculoskeletal system
  anatomy of, 1005–1007, 1005f
  assessment of, 1009–1010
  bone. See Bone
  imaging assessment of, 1011–1013
  radiography of, 1011
Skeletal traction, 1040
Skene's glands, 1429
Skilled nursing facilities
  rehabilitation in, 87
  residents of, 87, 87f
Skin
  age-related changes in, 234b, 433, 652, 800b
  anatomy of, 431–432, 432f
  assessment of, 90t, 91, 433–445, 651–652, 802
  barrier functions of, 415
  burn injury-related changes to, 481–485, 484f, 491
  cleanliness of, 439
  in dark-skin patients, 443–444, 444b
  dehydration effects on, 168
  diagnostic assessment of, 444–445
  edema effects on, 437
  functions of, 433, 433t, 482
  history-taking for, 433–436, 435b
  hydration effects on, 436
  inflammation of, 443
  inspection of, 436–439
  laboratory testing of, 444–445

Skin (Continued)
  leukemia effects on, 819
  nutrition assessments, 1213b
  palpation of, 440–441, 440t
  postoperative assessments of, 277–278, 278f
  preoperative assessment of, 237
  psychosocial assessment of, 444
  radiation therapy effects on, 1084
  sebaceous glands of, 433
  self-examination of, 476
  sepsis manifestations of, 764
  sickle cell disease effects on, 810
  structure of, 431–432, 432f
  sweat glands of, 433
  systemic lupus erythematosus manifestations of, 326–328, 327f
  temperature of, 652
  trauma to
    collaborative management of, 474
    pathophysiology of, 471–474
  turgor of, 441
  Wood's light examination of, 445
Skin biopsy, 445
Skin cancer, 380b
  assessment of, 436–437, 477
  basal cell carcinoma, 475t, 476, 476f
  collaborative care for, 476–477
  drug therapy for, 477
  etiology of, 475–476
  genetic risk of, 475–476
  health promotion and maintenance for, 476
  incidence of, 476
  melanoma, 475t, 476, 476f
  nonsurgical management of, 477
  pathophysiology of, 474–476
  prevalence of, 476
  prevention of, 476b
  radiation therapy for, 477
  squamous cell carcinoma, 475–476, 475f, 475t
  surgical management of, 477
  types of, 475f, 475t
Skin care
  in diarrhea patients, 1142b
  infection spread prevention through, 469
  in older adults, 216–222
  postoperative, 281b
  for pressure injury prevention, 97
  in systemic lupus erythematosus patients, 328
  for ulcerative colitis, 1156b
Skin color, 436, 437t
Skin disorders
  inflammatory, 458–459, 462–463, 463b
  pressure injuries. See Pressure injuries

Skin disorders (Continued)
pruritus, 461–462
psoriasis. See Psoriasis
Stevens-Johnson syndrome, 478, 478f
toxic epidermal necrolysis, 478
urticaria, 462
Skin grafts, for burn wound management, 500–501
Skin infections
assessment of, 469
bacterial, 466–468, 466f, 467b
cutaneous anthrax, 466, 467f
drug therapy for, 470
folliculitis, 466, 467b
fungal, 467b, 468
furuncles, 466, 466f, 467b
health promotion and maintenance for, 468–469
history-taking for, 469
methicillin-resistant Staphylococcus aureus as cause of, 466
pathophysiology of, 466–470
transmission-based precautions for, 469–470
viral, 467b, 468
Skin lesions
configuration of, 439t
primary, 436, 438f
secondary, 436, 438f
Skin substitutes, 458
Skin traction, 1040, 1041f
Skin turgor, 168, 169f
Skinfold measurements, 1215
Sleep deprivation, 845–846
Sleep disorders, 40
Sliding board, 901
Sliding hiatal hernias, 1092, 1092f
Slip lock, 210
Slit-lamp examination, 965, 965f
Slow continuous ultrafiltration, 1398
SLPs. See Speech-language pathologists
Small bowel capsule endoscopy, 1071–1072
Small intestine
anatomy of, 1064
functions of, 1064
obstruction of, 1123b
Small molecule inhibitor targeted therapy, 403–405, 403f–404f, 404t
Smart pumps, for infusion therapy, 211
SMAST-G. See Short Michigan Alcoholism Screening Test—Geriatric Version
Smoke detectors, 488–489
Smoke poisoning, 491
Smoking
assessment of, 514
carboxyhemoglobin levels, 233–234

Smoking (Continued)
cardiovascular disease risks, 512–514, 647
cessation of, 514–515, 515b, 555, 1308
chronic obstructive pulmonary disease caused by, 14, 21, 573
hookah, 514
pack-years for, 514
passive, 514
pneumonia risks secondary to, 605
prevalence of, 514b
secondhand smoke, 514
social, 514
surgical risks associated with, 232–233
in transgender community, 1494
Smooth muscle, 1007
Snakebites, 135–137, 136b, 136f–137f, 136t, 138t–140t
Snellen eye chart, 963–964
SNFs. See Skilled nursing facilities
SNP. See Single nucleotide polymorphism
SNS. See Sympathetic nervous system
Social justice, 9
Social smokers, 514
Social workers
in emergency departments, 119–120
in rehabilitation settings, 89
Sodium
description of, 173–175
in older adults, 165b
restriction of
in chronic kidney disease, 1408
cirrhosis managed with, 1175
serum levels of, 164t
Sodium channel blockers, 677b–678b
Sodium imbalances
hypernatremia, 174–175, 175t
hyponatremia, 173–174, 174t
Sodium lauryl sulfate, 1077
Sodium polystyrene sulfonate, for hyperkalemia, 20
Sodium-glucose cotransport inhibitors, 1292b–1293b, 1294
Solar keratosis, 475, 475t
Solifenacin, 98
Solutes, 161
Solvent, 161
Somatic mutations, 76
Somatic pain, 48
Somatomedins, 1246
Somatosensory evoked potentials, 855
Somatostatin, 1239–1240
Somogyi phenomenon, 1296
Soriatane. See Acitretin
Sotalol, 677b–678b, 685
Sound
decibel scale for, 990
intensity of, 990

Sound judgment, 8
Spastic paralysis, 933, 938
Specific gravity, 1332–1333
Specific morphology, 373
SPECT. See Single-photon emission computed tomography
Speech
assessment of, 847
in Parkinson disease patients, 871–872
Speech and language rehabilitation, 552
Speech audiometry, 991
Speech discrimination testing, 991
Speech reception threshold, 991
Speech-language pathologist, 89
Speech-language pathologist assistants, 89
Sphenoid sinus, 509f
Sphincter of Oddi, 1064, 1192
Sphincterotomy, 1201
Spider angiomas, 1173
Spider bites, 136–137, 137b, 137f, 138t–140t
Spinal anesthesia, 261t, 262f, 275, 275b
Spinal column, 225
Spinal cord
functions of, 842, 887
hemorrhage of, 894
multiple sclerosis. See Multiple sclerosis
Spinal cord compression, 408
Spinal cord injury
aging and, 902b
airway management in, 897–898
assessment of, 895–897
autonomic dysreflexia in, 896, 896b, 898, 898b
axial loading as cause of, 894, 895f
cardiovascular assessment in, 896
care coordination for, 901–903, 901f
cervical, 896–897
cervical collar for, 899, 899f
complete, 894
complications of, 897
contractures secondary to, 900–901
"cough assist" technique in, 897–898, 898f
drug therapy for, 900
etiology of, 895
functional electrical stimulation for, 902
gastrointestinal assessment in, 896–897
genitourinary assessment in, 896–897
halo fixator device for, 899, 899b
health care resources for, 903
history-taking for, 895
home care management of, 901–902
hydration for, 898

Spinal cord injury (Continued)
hyperextension as cause of, 894, 895f
hyperflexion as cause of, 894, 894f
imaging assessment of, 897
incidence of, 895
incomplete, 894
laboratory assessment of, 897
mechanism of injury, 894–895, 894f–895f
mobility affected by, 23, 896, 900–901
neurogenic shock after, 898
pathophysiology of, 894–895
penetrating trauma as cause of, 894
physical assessment of, 896–897
pressure injury risks secondary to, 901–903
prevalence of, 895
psychosocial adaptation for, 901
psychosocial assessment of, 897
rehabilitation for, 901–902
respiratory assessment in, 896
respiratory secretion management in, 897
secondary, 894, 899–900, 899b, 899f
self-management education for, 902
sensory perception assessments in, 896, 896b
sexuality affected by, 901–902
signs and symptoms of, 896–897
spinal immobilization and stabilization after, 899–900, 899b, 899f–900f
surgical management of, 900
traction for, 899
transition management for, 901–903, 901f
venous thromboembolism risks secondary to, 897
vertical compression as cause of, 894, 895f
in veterans, 903b
Spinal cord stimulation, 66, 909, 909b
Spinal fusion, 906, 908
Spinal nerves, 842
Spinal osteoarthritis, 307
Spinal shock, 896
Spine board, 945
Spine stabilization, 147
SPINK1 gene, 1202
Spiritual counselors, 89
Spiritual distress, 113
Spirituality, 108
Spironolactone, 1261, 1498
Spleen
in blood formation, 797
liver-spleen scan, 1073
red pulp of, 797
white pulp of, 797
Splenectomy, 797, 831, 1207

Splenic infarction, 711
Splenomegaly, 1067, 1170
Splint(s), 1038
Splinter hemorrhages, 711
Spondee, 991
Spontaneous bacterial peritonitis, 1171, 1175
Spores, 612
Sports-related injuries, 1056, 1056b, 1057f, 1057t
S-pouch, 1154, 1154f
Sprain, 1057t
Sputum, 516
Squamous cell carcinoma
    description of, 475–476, 475f, 475t
    esophageal, 1095
    oral, 1079
Squamous metaplasia, 548
St. John's wort, 701, 801–802
ST segment, 669, 669f
Staff nurses, 155
Staff safety, 4
Staffing, infection control through, 421
Standard Precautions, 418–419, 419t, 1358
Stapedectomy, 1000–1001, 1000f
Stapes, 984, 985f
Staphylococcal endotoxin, 1105
Staples, 268f
Starling's law, 645, 692–694
Starvation, 1221–1222
Statins
    for atherosclerosis, 731b
    myocardial infarction treated with, 777
Status asthmaticus, 572
Status epilepticus, 879
Stay sutures, 268f
Steal syndrome, 1415
Steatorrhea, 1068–1070, 1141, 1159, 1194, 1203
Steatosis, 1185–1186
Stelara. See Ustekinumab
ST-elevation myocardial infarction, 770
Stem cell transplantation, for breast cancer, 1452
Stem cells. See also Hematopoietic stem cell transplantation
    bone marrow production of, 290, 291f
    differentiation and maturation of, 290, 291f, 293
Stents, 783
Stereotactic body radiotherapy, 388
Stereotactic pallidotomy, for Parkinson disease, 872
Stereotactic radiosurgery, 952, 952f
Sterilization, 418
Sternal split procedure, 921
Sternal wound infection, 785, 788–789
Stevens-Johnson syndrome, 478, 478f, 1359b

Stings, 137, 137b, 137f, 138t–140t, 141b
Stoma
    colostomy, 1131–1132, 1132f
    home care management of, 1134b
    ileostomy, 1153, 1154b
    measurement of, 1134
    after total laryngectomy, 551, 554–555
Stomach
    anatomy of, 1063
    description of, 1103
    ulcers of, 1107–1109, 1108f
Stomach disorders
    cancer. See Gastric cancer
    gastritis. See Gastritis
    peptic ulcer disease. See Peptic ulcer(s); Peptic ulcer disease
Stomatitis, 399–400, 820, 1076–1078, 1401
Stool tests, 1068–1070, 1111
STOP-Bang Sleep Apnea Questionnaire, 559
Storytelling, during dying, 112
Strain, 1057t
Strangulated hernia, 1138
Strangulated obstruction, 1122, 1125
Stratum corneum, 432, 432f
Stratum germinativum, 432, 432f
Stratum granulosum, 432, 432f
Stratum lucidum, 432
Stress
    coping with, 32–33
    family caregiver, 866b
    management of, 1137
    in older adults, 32–33
    in transgender patients, 1494
Stress debriefing, 157
Stress fracture, 1032
Stress incontinence, 1344, 1348, 1349t, 1464
Stress testing, 659–660, 660f
Stress ulcers, 1108
Stretta procedure, 1091, 1091b
Striae, 1242, 1257
Striated muscle, 1007
Strictures
    bowel, 1161
    esophageal, 1088, 1096
    urinary tract, 1383
Stricturoplasty, 1161
Stridor, 274, 364, 636
Stroke. See also Transient ischemic attack
    anterior cerebral artery, 933b
    antithrombotics for, 937
    aphasia after, 938, 938t
    assessment of, 930–935
    in atrial fibrillation, 16
    cardiovascular assessment in, 934
    care coordination for, 939–940
    carotid artery angioplasty with stenting for, 936
    cerebral perfusion in, 935–938

Stroke (Continued)
    cognitive changes associated with, 932–933
    communication promotion after, 938
    complications of, 937
    cranial nerve function assessments after, 934
    definition of, 928
    depression after, 939
    diabetes mellitus as risk factor for, 1284
    drug therapy for, 937–938
    embolectomy for, 936
    embolic, 928–929, 929t, 934
    emotional lability assessments in, 934
    endovascular interventions for, 936
    etiology of, 929
    fibrinolytic therapy for, 935
    genetic risk of, 929
    health care resources for, 940
    health promotion and maintenance for, 930
    hemorrhagic, 929, 929t
    history-taking for, 930–931
    home care management of, 939
    imaging assessment of, 935
    incidence of, 929–930
    increased intracranial pressure monitoring after, 936–937, 936b
    internal cerebral artery, 933b
    interventions for, 935–938
    intracranial bleeding-induced, 831
    ischemic, 927–929, 929t, 935
    laboratory assessment of, 934–935
    left hemisphere, 932–933, 933b
    level of consciousness assessments in, 931–932
    magnetic resonance angiography of, 935
    middle cerebral artery, 933b
    mobility after, 933–934, 938
    National Institutes of Health Stroke Scale, 931, 931t–932t
    nonsurgical management of, 935–938
    pathophysiology of, 928–930
    physical assessment of, 931–935
    posterior cerebral artery, 933b
    prevalence of, 929–930
    psychosocial assessment of, 934
    racial predilection for, 930b
    recurrence of, 940
    right hemisphere, 932–933, 933b
    risk factors for, 930b
    self-management education for, 939–940, 940f
    sensory changes caused by, 934
    sensory perception changes after, 934, 939
    signs and symptoms of, 931–935
    thrombotic, 928, 929t

Stroke (Continued)
    transition management for, 939–940
    types of, 928–929, 928f, 929t
    vertebrobasilar artery, 933b
    visual loss secondary to, 934, 934f
    in women, 935b
Stroke center, 930, 939
Stroke syndromes, 933b
Stroke volume, 645, 692–694
Stromelysin, 305
Strong acid, 186
Strong bases, 186
Struvite stones, 1364
Stuart-Prower factor, 798t
Stuporous, 846
Subacute thyroiditis, 1275
Subarachnoid hemorrhage
    cerebral vasospasm after, 937
    description of, 929, 931
Subarachnoid space, 225, 840
Subclavian dialysis catheters, 1397f
Subclavian steal, 741t
Subcutaneous emphysema, 518
    definition of, 1036
    in fracture patients, 1036
    laryngeal trauma as cause of, 559–560
    tracheostomy as cause of, 539
Subcutaneous fat, 431, 432f
Subcutaneous infusion therapy, 223
Subcutaneous nodules, in rheumatoid arthritis, 319
Subdural hematoma, 942–943, 942f, 954
Subdural space, 840
Sublimaze. See Fentanyl
Submucous resection, 557
Substance P, 56–57
Substance use, 38–39
Substantia nigra, 868
Subsys. See Fentanyl
Subtotal thyroidectomy, 1269
Sucralfate, 1112
Suctioning
    of artificial airway, 541–542, 541b
    in chronic obstructive pulmonary disease, 579
Sulfamethoxazole/trimethoprim, 1359b–1360b
Sulfasalazine, 1152, 1152b
Sulfonylureas, 1291, 1292b–1293b
Sundowning, 861
Superior oblique muscle, 960t
Superior rectus muscle, 960t
Superior vena cava, 408–409
Superior vena cava syndrome, 408–409, 409f
Superstorm Sandy, 151
Supervision
    definition of, 6
    of unlicensed assistive personnel, 6
Supination, 1010f
Supine position, 265, 265f
Support systems, 92b

Suppressor genes, 378
Suppressor T-cells, 299
Suppurative cholangitis, 1192
Supraglottic partial laryngectomy, 551t
Supratentorial lesion, 840
Supratentorial tumors, 950
Supraventricular tachycardia, 676–678
Surfactant, 147, 510
Surgeon, 253t
Surgery
  administering regularly scheduled drugs before, 241–242
  American Society of Anesthesiologists Physical Status Classification system, 230–232, 233t, 257
  antibiotic prophylaxis before, 247
  appendicitis treated with, 1148
  back pain treated with, 906–908, 907b
  benign prostatic hyperplasia treated with, 1479–1480, 1480b, 1480f
  blood donation for, 235
  brain tumors treated with, 952–954
  breast cancer treated with, 1447–1452, 1448f, 1453b
  breast-conserving, 1447, 1448f
  cancer treated with, 386–387
  cataracts treated with, 969–971, 970f
  categories of, 232t
  cholecystitis treated with, 1195–1197
  chronic obstructive pulmonary disease managed with, 579–580
  complications of, 272t
    pulmonary, 233–234
    risk factors for, 233t
  consent for, 239–241, 240f
  cost reduction in, 228
  Crohn's disease treated with, 1161
  Cushing's disease treated with, 1258–1259
  cystic fibrosis treated with, 583–584
  discharge planning before, 235
  elective, 232t
  emergent, 232t
  esophageal tumors treated with, 1098–1100, 1099f
  fractures managed with, 1042–1043, 1042f
  gastric cancer treated with, 1116–1118, 1117f
  gastroesophageal reflux disease treated with, 1091
  glaucoma treated with, 975
  head and neck cancer treated with, 550–553

Surgery (Continued)
  hearing loss treated with, 999–1001
  hernia treated with, 1138–1139
  hiatal hernias treated with, 1093–1095
  history-taking before, 230–235
  hyperpituitarism treated with, 1249–1250
  informed consent for, 239–241, 240f
  low back pain treated with, 906–908, 907b
  lung cancer treated with, 589–593
  medical history before, 233–234
  minimally invasive. See Minimally invasive surgery
  myasthenia gravis treated with, 921
  NPO status before, 241
  obesity treated with, 1229–1231, 1230f, 1231b
  in older adults, 232
  oral cancer treated with, 1081–1083
  overview of, 229–249
  pain caused by, 47
  pancreatic cancer treated with, 1207–1208, 1207f
  patient identification before, 241
  patient positioning for, 264–267, 265f, 267b
  pelvic organ prolapse treated with, 1464–1465
  peritonitis treated with, 1146
  postoperative period. See Postoperative period
  preoperative period. See Preoperative period
  previous procedures, 234
  radical, 232t
  readiness for, 229
  reasons for, 232t
  robotic, 254–255
  safety checklist for, 228–229, 230f
  same-day admission, 229–230
  simple, 232t
  skin cancer treated with, 477
  skin preparation before, 242, 243f
  Surgical Care Improvement Project measures, 229, 231t, 244, 282
  trigeminal neuralgia treated with, 924
  types of, 232t
  ulcerative colitis treated with, 1153–1155, 1155f
  urgency of, 232t
  urgent, 232t
  urinary incontinence treated with, 1348–1349, 1349t
  urolithiasis treated with, 1364–1365
Surgical assistant, 253t

Surgical attire, 256, 256f
Surgical Care Improvement Project, 229, 231t, 244, 282
Surgical scrub, 256, 257f
Surgical settings
  inpatient, 229–230
  outpatient, 229–230
Surgical site infections
  after coronary artery bypass grafting, 786b
  definition of, 267
  after oral cancer surgery, 1083
  predisposing factors for, 242
  Surgical Care Improvement Project measures for, 229
Surgical suite
  fire safety in, 252
  layout of, 252
  occupational hazards in, 252
  patient transfer to, 247–249
  safety in, 252–256
  surgical attire in, 256, 256f
Surgical team
  gloving of, 256, 257f
  gowning of, 256, 257f
  health and hygiene of, 255
  members of, 252, 253t
  safety of, 252–256
  surgical attire worn by, 256, 256f
  surgical scrub by, 256, 257f
Surviving Sepsis Campaign, 765
Susceptibility genes, 76
Sustained immunity, 298
Sutures
  absorbable, 267
  nonabsorbable, 267
SVT. See Supraventricular tachycardia
Swallowing, 1062
  aspiration prevention during, 543b, 553
  evaluation of, 553
  supraglottic method of, 553, 553b
Swallowing therapy, 1097
Swimmer's ear. See External otitis
Swimming, 32
Syme amputation, 1051, 1051f
Sympathectomy, 1042
Sympathetic nervous system, 842
  burn injury compensation, 486, 487f
  heart failure stimulation of, 692
Sympathetic tone, 752
Sympathomimetics
  acute coronary syndromes treated with, 783b
  description of, 1228–1229
Synapse, 840
Synaptic cleft, 840
Synaptic knob, 840
Synarthrodial joints, 1006
Synchronized intermittent mandatory ventilation, 631, 636t
Syncope
  definition of, 650–651, 1285
  description of, 618, 706

Syndrome of inappropriate antidiuretic hormone
  characteristics of, 1251–1253, 1252t
  as oncologic emergency, 407–408
  signs and symptoms of, 954
Syndrome X, 771
Syngeneic stem cells, 822
Synovial joint, 1006–1007
Synovitis, 1006–1007, 1057
Syphilis, 1508–1510, 1508f
Syringe pumps, 211
Systemic inflammatory response syndrome, 761–762, 761f, 762t, 763b, 881
Systemic lupus erythematosus
  care coordination of, 328
  definition of, 326
  drug therapy for, 327–328
  features of, 326b
  laboratory assessment of, 327
  pathophysiology of, 326
  psychosocial assessment of, 327
  self-management education for, 328
  signs and symptoms of, 326–327, 327f
  skin manifestations of, 326–327, 327f
  skin protection in, 328, 328b
  transition management of, 328
Systemic necrotizing vasculitis, 334t
Systemic sclerosis, 326b, 329–330, 330b
Systole, 644, 706
Systolic blood pressure, 646
Systolic heart failure, 692
Systolic murmurs, 655

T
T$_3$. See Triiodothyronine
T$_4$. See Thyroxine
T cells
  differentiation of, 295f
  subsets of, 299
T wave, 669, 669f, 671
Tachycardia
  heart rate in, 670
  paroxysmal supraventricular, 676
  sinus, 673, 673f
  supraventricular, 676–678
  ventricular, 684, 684f
Tachydysrhythmias, 668b, 672
Tacrolimus, 302b, 1303
Tactile fremitus, 518–519
Tactile stimulation, for pain management, 496
Tadalafil, 146
Tamponade effect, 1341
Tapentadol, 61
Tar preparations, 464
Target tissues, 1234–1235
Targeted therapy
  breast cancer treated with, 1452
  esophageal tumors treated with, 1097–1098

Targeted therapy (Continued)
  oral cancer treated with, 1081
  pancreatic cancer treated with, 1207
  renal cell carcinoma treated with, 1386
Taste sense
  age-related changes in, 31
  oral cancer effects on, 1083
Tattoos, 439
Tbo-filgrastim, 402t
TBPI. See Toe brachial pressure index
TBSA. See Total body surface area
TeamSTEPPS, 6
Teamwork
  attributes of, 5
  definition of, 5
  scope of, 5
Technetium scan, 661
Technology
  attributes of, 8
  context of, 8
  definition of, 7
  scope of, 8
Telangiectasias, 748
Telaprevir, 1185t
Telehealth, 101
Telemetry, 667
Teleneurology, 935
Telerehabilitation, 101
Teletherapy, 388
Temporal arteritis, 334t
Temporal lobe, 841t
Temporary pacing, 674–675
Tendons
  definition of, 1007
  rupture of, 1057t
Tenesmus, 1150, 1166
Tenofovir, 1185t
TENS. See Transcutaneous electrical nerve stimulation
Tension pneumothorax, 637–638
Tentorium, 840
Teriparatide, 1022
Terminal dehydration, 115
Terminal delirium, 111
Terminal knob, 840
Terminally ill patients, withholding food in, 1219
Tertiary syphilis, 1508–1509
Testes
  anatomy of, 1430, 1430f
  hormones produced by, 1235t
  palpation of, 1242
  self-examination of, 1486b
Testicular cancer
  assessment of, 1487
  chemotherapy for, 1488–1489
  classification of, 1486–1487, 1487t
  laboratory assessment of, 1487
  pathophysiology of, 1486–1487
  psychosocial assessment of, 1487
  surgical management of, 1488
Testicular self-examination, 1486b

Testicular tumors, 1486–1487, 1487t
Testosterone, 1430, 1481–1482, 1498
Tetanus, 145
Tetany, 1269
Thalamus, 840, 840f
Thalidomide, 369
Thallium imaging, 661
Thallium scan, 1011–1012
The Joint Commission
  care coordination recommendations, 3
  emergency department metrics, 117–118
  emergency preparedness plan, 150
  family-centered care, 2
  interprofessional communication strategies, 5
  lesbian, gay, bisexual, transgender, and queer population, 1495, 1495b
  medication reconciliation requirements, 4b
  National Patient Safety Goals
    blood components, 200, 833
    blood donation, 235
    description of, 4–5, 8
    drug safety, 201
    for falls, 40–41, 1018, 1020
    hand-off communication, 120, 317
    hand-off report, 271
    handwashing, 882, 1100
    infection control, 417
    influenza vaccine, 596–597
    informed consent, 658
    nutrition screening, 1212
    patient identification, 247, 262–263, 262b
    preoperative requirements, 238–239
    pressure injuries, 448–449
    surgical communication, 229
    tracheostomy communication, 544
    transfusion therapy, 833
    warfarin monitoring, 745
  restraints used by hospitals, 41
  sentinel event reporting requirements, 4–5
  tobacco use screening, 514–515
Therapeutic hypothermia, 947
Therapeutic Touch, 109
Thermal burns, 488, 491
Thermoregulation, 135b
Thiazide diuretics, 699, 725b
Thiazolidinediones, 1291, 1292b–1293b
Third space fluid, 19
Third spacing, 485, 1145, 1170
Third-degree frostbite, 144
Thirst, 164
Thoracentesis, 526, 526f, 593

Thoracic aortic aneurysms, 738–739
Thoracic outlet syndrome, 741t
Thoracotomy, 638
Thorax assessments, 518–521
Threshold (hearing), 990
Thrombectomy, 736, 738, 745
Thrombocytopenia
  chemotherapy as cause of, 395, 397–398, 588
  definition of, 815, 817
  description of, 15
  heparin-induced, 832
  injury prevention in patients with, 398b
  management of, 825b
  platelet count in, 805
Thrombocytosis, 321
Thrombolytic therapy
  contraindications for, 778t
  deep vein thrombosis treated with, 745
  myocardial infarction treated with, 777–778, 778t
Thrombophlebitis
  definition of, 742
  intravenous therapy as cause of, 217t–219t
  management of, 743
Thrombopoietin, 300t, 797
Thrombosis
  arterial, 16b
  deep vein. See Deep vein thrombosis
  definition of, 15–16
  intravenous therapy as cause of, 217t–219t
  mesenteric artery, 16b
  vascular stasis as cause of, 816
  venous, 15–16
Thrombotic stroke, 928, 929t
Thrombotic thrombocytopenic purpura, 831
Thromboxane A$_2$, 798
Thrombus. See also Thrombosis
  definition of, 742
  etiology of, 742
  stroke caused by, 928
Thrush, 347f, 468
Thymoma, 918
Thyrocalcitonin, 179, 1239
Thyroid cancer, 1275
Thyroid cartilage, 510
Thyroid crisis, 1270
Thyroid disorders
  hyperthyroidism. See Hyperthyroidism
  hypothyroidism. See Hypothyroidism
  in older adults, 1274b
  thyroiditis, 1275
Thyroid gland
  anatomy of, 1238–1239, 1239f
  hormones produced by, 1235t, 1239t, 1264–1265
  palpation of, 1242, 1242b

Thyroid storm, 1267, 1270, 1270b
Thyroidectomy, 1269, 1275
Thyroiditis, 1275
Thyroid-stimulating hormone
  deficiency of, 1246, 1246b
  description of, 1237t, 1239, 1271
  overproduction of, 1248b
Thyroid-stimulating hormone receptors, 1265
Thyroid-stimulating immunoglobulins, 1265
Thyrotoxic periodic paralysis, 1268b
Thyrotoxicosis, 918, 1264–1265, 1268b
Thyrotropin-releasing hormone, 1239
Thyroxine, 697b, 1006, 1238, 1247, 1266, 1272
TIBC. See Total iron-binding capacity
Tibial fracture, 1048–1049
Tibial nerve, 267b
Tic douloureux. See Trigeminal neuralgia
Tidal volume, 631
Time-cycled ventilators, 631
Time-out, 265, 266f
Tinea capitis, 468
Tinea corporis, 468
Tinea cruris, 468
Tinea manus, 468
Tinea pedis, 468
Tinel's sign, 1058
Tinnitus, 987, 995
TIPS. See Transjugular intrahepatic portal-systemic shunt
Tirofiban, 736–737
Tissue integrity
  assessment of, before rehabilitation, 90t, 91
  description of, 27–28
Tissue mast cells, 294
Tissue perfusion
  after amputation, 1053
  hematologic system in, 796f
Tissue plasminogen activator, 736–738
Tissue thromboplastin, 798t
TJC. See The Joint Commission
TLS. See Tumor lysis syndrome
Tobacco, 379. See also Smoking
Tocilizumab, 323b, 369, 370b
Toe brachial pressure index, 653
Toe fracture, 1038
Tofacitinib, 369
Toileting-related falls, 41
Tolerance, 58
Toll-like receptors, 290, 300
Tolterodine, 98
Tolvaptan, 954, 1252, 1252b
Tongue, 1062
Tonic-clonic seizures, 876, 878b–879b
Tonometry, 965
Tono-Pen, 965, 966f

Tooth loss, 31
Topiramate, 875
Topoisomerase inhibitors, 391, 391t
Torsade de pointes, 657
Total abdominal hysterectomy, 1462, 1462b–1463b
Total body irradiation, 387
Total body surface area, 489, 492
Total body water, 160, 161f
Total enteral nutrition
    abdominal distention caused by, 1222
    administration of, 1220–1221, 1220f
    complications of, 1221–1223
    description of, 1219–1223
    diarrhea secondary to, 1223
    electrolyte imbalances caused by, 1222–1223
    enterostomal feeding tubes used in, 1220–1221
    fluid imbalances caused by, 1222–1223
    gastrostomy for, 1221
    jejunostomy for, 1221
    nasoduodenal tube delivery of, 1220
    nasoenteric tube delivery of, 1220, 1220f
    nasogastric tube delivery of, 1220
    nausea and vomiting caused by, 1222
    refeeding syndrome caused by, 1221–1222
    tube misplacement and dislodgement, 1222
Total hip arthroplasty
    anesthesia used in, 310
    complications of, 311t, 312–313
    components of, 310–311, 310f
    hip dislocation after, 311–312
    hip resurfacing versus, 310
    low-molecular-weight heparin uses, 312
    minimally invasive, 310
    mobility after, 313–314, 313f
    operative procedures, 310–311
    pain management after, 312b, 313
    patient positioning after, 311, 313f
    postoperative care, 311–314, 311b
    preoperative care, 309–310
    primary, 309
    quadriceps-setting exercises after, 312–313
    rehabilitation, 314
    revision, 309
    self-management education, 312b, 314
    venous thromboembolism risks after, 310, 312–313
    weight-bearing restrictions, 313–314
Total iron-binding capacity, 805

Total joint arthroplasty
    hip. See Total hip arthroplasty
    hospital length of stay after, 314b
    osteoarthritis treated with, 309
Total knee arthroplasty
    complications of, 316
    continuous passive motion machine, 315, 315f, 316b
    cryotherapy after, 315
    description of, 314–316
    discharge instructions, 316
    minimally invasive, 314
    operative procedures, 315
    pain management after, 315–316
    postoperative care, 315–316, 315f
    preoperative care, 314–315
    rehabilitation after, 316
Total laryngectomy, 551, 551t, 555
Total lymphocyte count, 1217
Total parenteral nutrition
    complications of, 1224
    fluid imbalance risks, 1224
    malnutrition treated with, 1224
    solutions for, 200
Total proctocolectomy with permanent ileostomy for, 1154, 1155f
Total shoulder arthroplasty, 316
Total thyroidectomy, 1269
Total vaginal hysterectomy, 1462, 1463b
Touch discrimination assessments, 849
Touch sense, 33
Tourniquets, 129–130, 222
Toxic diffuse goiter, 1265
Toxic epidermal necrolysis, 478
Toxic hepatitis, 1180
Toxic megacolon, 1151t, 1153
Toxic multinodular goiter, 1265
Toxic shock syndrome, 1471, 1471b
Toxicity
    digoxin, 700b
    oxygen, 530
Toxins, 414
Toxoplasma gondii, 346
Toxoplasmosis encephalitis, 346
T-piece, 534–535, 534t, 535f, 636t
Trabeculation, 1358
Trabeculectomy, 975
Trachea, 510, 511f
Trachea–innominate artery fistula, 538t
Tracheal stenosis, 538t
Tracheobronchial tree, 510
Tracheoesophageal fistula, 538t
Tracheoesophageal puncture, 552
Tracheomalacia, 538t
Tracheostomy
    air warming in, 540–541
    aspiration prevention during swallowing, 543b
    assessments in, 542b
    bronchial hygiene in, 543
    care coordination for, 544

Tracheostomy (Continued)
    care issues for patients with, 539–544
    care of, 542–543, 542b
    caregiver anxiety in, 555b
    communication issues during, 543–544
    complications of, 537–539, 538t
    definition of, 537
    dressings for, 543, 543f
    health care resources for, 544
    home care management of, 544
    humidification in, 540–541
    in laryngeal cancer, 550
    minimal leak technique in, 540
    nutrition in, 543
    operative procedures for, 537, 538f
    oral hygiene in, 543
    overview of, 537
    psychosocial needs in, 544
    self-concept needs in, 544
    self-management education for, 544
    suctioning of, 541–542, 541b
    tissue damage in, 539–540, 541f
    transition management for, 544
    tubes used in, 539, 540f, 543
    weaning from, 544
Tracheostomy button, 544
Tracheotomy, 494, 553, 561
Traction
    fractures treated with, 1040–1041, 1040t, 1041b, 1041f
    lower-extremity, 1040t
    skeletal, 1040
    skin, 1040, 1041f
    spinal cord injury treated with, 899
    upper-extremity, 1040t
Trafficking, human See Human trafficking
Training
    bladder, 1350–1351, 1351b
    for emergency nursing, 120t, 123
    gait, 95–96, 95b, 95f
    habit, 1351, 1351b
TRALI. See Transfusion-related acute lung injury
TRAM flap, 1449–1450
Transarterial chemoembolization, for liver cancer, 1187
Transbronchial biopsy, 526
Transbronchial needle aspiration, 526
Transcatheter aortic valve replacement, 708–709, 708f
Transcervical endometrial resection, 1461
Transcranial Doppler ultrasonography, 855
Transcutaneous electrical nerve stimulation, 66, 66f
Transcutaneous oxygen pressure, 1052
Transcutaneous pacing, 674, 674f

Transesophageal echocardiography
    description of, 660
    valvular heart disease evaluations, 707
Transfer belts, 95
Transferrin, 805, 1217
Transfusion
    acute reactions to, 835–836
    allergies to, 263, 836
    autologous blood, 836
    bacterial reactions to, 836
    cell savers, 235, 310
    febrile reactions to, 835
    hemolytic reactions to, 835
    indications for, 832t
    infusion therapy for, 200
    in older adults, 834b
    plasma, 835
    platelet
        idiopathic thrombocytopenic purpura treated with, 831
        indications for, 832t, 835
        reaction to, 835
    reactions to, 835–836
    red blood cells, 834–835
        compatibility determinations for, 834, 834t
        indications for, 832t, 834–835
        sickle cell disease treated with, 812
    reinfusion system, 310
    responsibilities in, 832–834
    safety in, 833b
    setup for, 832, 834f
    types of, 834–835
    white blood cells, 832t, 835
Transfusion-associated circulatory overload, 836
Transfusion-associated graft-versus-host-disease, 836
Transfusion-related acute lung injury, 626, 836
Transgender patients/health
    assessment of, 1495–1497
    care coordination for, 1501
    communication therapy for, 1499
    definition of, 1493
    drug therapy for, 1497–1498
    environment for, 1495b
    estrogen for, 1497–1498
    female-to-male
        definition of, 1493–1494, 1493t
        drug therapy for, 1498
        masculinizing surgeries for, 1500–1501
        phalloplasty for, 1501
    gonadotropin-releasing hormone agonists, 1498
    health care for, 1494–1501, 1496t
    history-taking of, 1496–1497
    issues in, 1494
    male-to-female
        definition of, 1493–1494, 1493t
        drug therapy for, 1497–1499, 1497t

Transgender patients/health (Continued)
 gender reassignment surgery for, 1499–1500
 vaginoplasty for, 1499–1500
 nonsurgical management of, 1497–1499
 older adults as, 1497b
 physical assessment of, 1497
 pronoun usage for, 1495–1496
 psychosocial assessment of, 1497
 reproductive health options in, 1499
 stress experienced by, 1494
 surgical management of, 1499–1501
 terminology associated with, 1493–1494, 1493t
 transition management for, 1501
 violence and verbal harassment of, 1494
 voice therapy for, 1499
Transient ischemic attack, 927–928, 928b. See also Stroke
Transition management, 3. See also specific disorder, transition management for
Transition (transgender), 1493t
Transjugular intrahepatic portal-systemic shunt, 1177–1178
Transmission-based precautions
 for infection control, 419, 420t
 for skin infections, 469–470
Transmyocardial laser revascularization, 789
Transparent film dressings, 499, 500f
Transplantation
 bone marrow, 822
 heart
  cardiomyopathy treated with, 716–717, 717f
  discharge planning for, 717
  heart failure treated with, 705
  operative procedures for, 716, 717f
  postoperative care for, 716–717
  preoperative care for, 716
  rejection of, 716b
  survival rates after, 717
 hematopoietic stem cell. See Hematopoietic stem cell transplantation
 immunosuppression after, 302b
 islet cell, 1303
 kidney. See Kidney transplantation
 liver, 1187–1189, 1188t, 1189b
 lung
  cystic fibrosis treated with, 583–584
  pulmonary arterial hypertension treated with, 585
 pancreatic
  complications of, 1303

Transplantation (Continued)
 description of, 1204
 diabetes mellitus treated with, 1302–1303
 rejection of, 1302–1303
 rejection of
  acute, 301
  causes of, 300–301
  chronic, 301
  drugs for, 302b
  hyperacute, 301
  management of, 301, 302b
  renal. See Kidney transplantation
Transport maximum, 1325
Transrectal ultrasonography, 1436, 1483, 1483b
Transsexual, 1493–1494, 1493t
Transtracheal oxygen therapy, 536
Transurethral resection of the bladder tumor, 1368
Transurethral resection of the prostate, 1479–1480, 1480b, 1480f, 1483
Transvaginal ultrasonography
 description of, 1436
 uterine leiomyoma evaluations, 1460
Transverse colostomy, 1131f
Trastuzumab, 405, 1097–1098
Trauma. See also Accidents; Motor vehicle accidents
 amputations caused by, 1050, 1053
 bladder, 1369
 blunt, 129
 chest
  flail chest, 637, 637f
  fractures caused by, 1049–1050
  pulmonary contusion, 636
  rib fracture, 636–637
 definition of, 127
 ear, 995, 1000b
 esophageal, 1101–1102, 1101t
 eye, 981–982
 facial, 558–559
 kidney, 1387–1388, 1387b
 laryngeal, 559–560
 liver, 1186, 1186b
 mechanism of injury, 128–129
 ocular, 981–982
 penetrating
  description of, 129
  ocular, 982
  osteomyelitis secondary to, 1023
  spinal cord injury caused by, 894
Trauma centers, 127–128, 128f, 128t, 130–131
Trauma nursing
 mechanism of injury, 128–129
 primary survey and resuscitation interventions, 129–130, 131t
 principles of, 127–131
 secondary survey and resuscitation interventions, 130

Trauma systems, 128
Traumatic brain injury
 acceleration-deceleration mechanism of, 941, 941f
 airway assessments in, 948–949
 Alzheimer's disease risks, 858–859
 assessment of, 944–946
 brain death after, 947
 breathing pattern assessments in, 948–949
 care coordination for, 949–950, 949b
 cognitive rehabilitation for, 948
 death after, 947
 definition of, 940
 drug therapy for, 948, 948b
 epidural hematoma secondary to, 942, 942f
 etiology of, 943
 features of, 945b
 health care resources for, 950
 health promotion and maintenance for, 943–944
 hemorrhage caused by, 944–950
 home care management of, 949
 hydrocephalus caused by, 943
 hypotension secondary to, 941
 hypoxemia after, 947
 hypoxia secondary to, 941
 imaging assessment of, 946
 incidence of, 943
 increased intracranial pressure after, 941–942, 946
 interventions for, 947–950
 laboratory assessment of, 946
 level of consciousness assessments in, 946
 magnetic resonance imaging of, 946
 mannitol for, 948, 948b
 mild, 944t, 945b
 moderate, 944t, 949
 neurogenic pulmonary edema caused by, 954
 neurologic assessment of, 945–946
 nonsurgical management of, 947–948
 in older adults, 944b
 pathophysiology of, 940–943
 patient positioning in, 947b
 physical assessment of, 944–946
 prevalence of, 943
 primary, 941
 psychosocial assessment of, 946
 secondary brain injuries caused by, 941–943, 947
 self-management education for, 949, 949b
 sensory perception after, 948–949
 severe, 941, 944t, 947, 949
 severity of, 941, 944t, 947
 signs and symptoms of, 944–946
 spine precautions with, 945
 subdural hematoma secondary to, 942–943, 942f

Traumatic brain injury (Continued)
 therapeutic hypothermia for, 947
 transition management for, 949–950, 949b
 in veterans, 845–846, 950b
 vital signs assessment in, 945
Traumatic relocation syndrome, 861
Trendelenburg position, 265f
Treponema pallidum, 415–416, 1508
Treprostinil, 585
TRH. See Thyrotropin-releasing hormone
Triage
 automated tracking systems for, 152–153
 "civilian", 151–153
 in culturally competent care, 152b
 disaster triage tag system, 152, 152b
 in emergency departments, 123–124, 124t
 green-tagged patients, 152
 mass casualty event, 151–153, 152t
 radiofrequency technology for, 152–153
 red-tagged patients, 152
 yellow-tagged patients, 152
Triage officer, 154, 154t
Trichloroacetic acid, 1511
Trichomonas, 1356
Tricuspid valve, 642–643, 643f
Tricyclic antidepressants
 in Alzheimer's disease, 864
 fibromyalgia treated with, 334
 in older adults, 37b
 pain management uses of, 64
 side effects of, 64
Trigeminal nerve
 description of, 844t
 external stimulator for, 875
Trigeminal neuralgia, 923–924, 923f
Trigeminy, 671
Trigger points, 333
Triglycerides, 656
Triiodothyronine, 1238, 1247, 1266, 1272
Trimethoprim/sulfamethoxazole, 1359b–1360b
Triptans, for migraine headaches, 874–875, 875b
Trochlear nerve, 844t
Troponin, 656
Trousseau's sign, 180, 180f, 182, 1201, 1277
Truss, 1138
Truvada, 342
Trypanosoma cruzi, 1166
Trypsin, 1197
TSH. See Thyroid-stimulating hormone
T-SPOT TB test, 607
TTP. See Thrombotic thrombocytopenic purpura
T-tube drain, 278, 279f

Tube feedings
    administration of, 1221
    bolus feeding, 1221
    care and maintenance in, 1221b–1222b
    continuous, 1221
    cyclic, 1221
    enterostomal, 1220–1221
    tube misplacement and dislodgement, 1222
Tuberculin skin test, 607, 607f
Tuberculosis
    in AIDS-infected patients, 347
    airborne precautions for, 609
    airway clearance in, 607–608
    anxiety management in, 609
    assessment of, 606–607
    care coordination for, 610
    diagnostic assessment of, 607
    drug therapy for, 608–609
    etiology of, 606
    fatigue management in, 610
    health care resources for, 610
    health promotion and maintenance for, 606
    hematogenous, 605–606
    history-taking for, 606–607
    home care management of, 610
    imaging assessment of, 607
    latent, 606
    miliary, 605–606
    multidrug-resistant, 609
    nutrition in, 610
    pathophysiology of, 605–606
    physical assessment of, 607
    psychosocial assessment of, 607
    screening for, 607
    secondary, 606
    self-management education for, 610
    signs and symptoms of, 607
    sputum culture for, 607
    transition management for, 610
    tuberculin skin test for, 607, 607f
Tumor(s). See also Cancer
    bone. See Bone tumors
    brain. See Brain tumors
    doubling time of, 377
    esophageal. See Esophageal tumors
    grading of, 377t
    growth assessments, 377
    kidney, 1385, 1385t
    oral, 1078–1084
    pancreatic, 1205
    primary, 375
    rectal, 1130t
    salivary glands, 1085
    secondary, 375
    testicular, 1486–1487, 1487t
Tumor, node, metastasis system, 377, 378t
Tumor cells, 373–374
Tumor lysis syndrome, 409–410, 409f
Tumor necrosis factor, 300t

Tuning fork tests, 989–990, 998
Tunneled central venous catheters, 207, 207f, 213, 226
Turbinates, 509, 509f
Turgor, 441
24-hour urine collection, 1334t, 1336b
Two-point discrimination, 849
Tympanic membrane
    anatomy of, 984, 985f–986f
    perforation of, 992f
Tympanometry, 991
Tympanoplasty, 999–1000, 1000f
Tympany, 519t
Type 1 diabetes mellitus. See Diabetes mellitus, type 1
Type 2 diabetes mellitus. See Diabetes mellitus, type 2
Type A chronic gastritis, 1104
Type B chronic gastritis, 1104
Type II pneumocytes, 510, 626
Tyrosine, 1239
Tyrosine kinase inhibitors, 330, 404t, 405, 1207
Tyrosine kinases, 403
Tzanck smear, 445

U
U wave, 669–670, 669f
UAP. See Unlicensed assistive personnel
UC. See Ulcerative colitis
UES. See Upper esophageal sphincter
Ulcer(s)
    description of, 438f, 448
    duodenal, 1107–1108, 1108f
    foot, 1305
    gastric, 1107, 1108f, 1110
    peptic. See Peptic ulcer(s)
    stress, 1108
Ulcerative colitis
    activity restrictions for, 1153
    American College of Gastroenterologists classification of, 1150t
    assessment of, 1151–1152
    blood loss monitoring in, 1156b
    care coordination for, 1156–1157
    colonoscopy of, 1152
    complementary and integrative health for, 1153
    complications of, 1151t
    Crohn's disease versus, 1150t
    cultural considerations for, 1151b
    definition of, 1150
    diagnostic assessment of, 1151–1152
    diarrhea management in, 1152–1155
    drug therapy for, 1152–1153
    etiology of, 1150–1151
    genetic risk of, 1150–1151
    health care resources for, 1157
    history-taking for, 1151
    home care management of, 1156

Ulcerative colitis (Continued)
    ileostomy for, 1153–1154
    immunomodulators for, 1153
    incidence of, 1151
    interventions for, 1152–1155
    laboratory assessment of, 1151–1152
    lower gastrointestinal bleeding in, 1156, 1156b
    magnetic resonance enterography for, 1152
    nonsurgical management of, 1152–1153
    nutrition therapy for, 1153
    pain management in, 1155–1156, 1156b
    pathophysiology of, 1150–1151
    physical assessment of, 1151
    prevalence of, 1151
    psychosocial assessment of, 1151
    restorative proctocolectomy with ileo pouch-anal anastomosis, 1154, 1154f
    self-management education for, 1156–1157
    severity of, 1150, 1150t
    signs and symptoms of, 1151
    skin care for, 1156b
    surgical management of, 1153–1155, 1155f
    total proctocolectomy with permanent ileostomy for, 1154, 1155f
    transition management for, 1156–1157
Ultrafiltration, 1397–1398
Ultram. See Tramadol
Ultrasonography
    abdominal, 1123
    acute pancreatitis evaluations, 1200
    breast evaluations, 1446
    cholecystitis evaluations, 1194
    gastrointestinal system assessments using, 1073
    malabsorption evaluations, 1141
    musculoskeletal system evaluations using, 1013
    peripheral intravenous therapy applications of, 202–203
    renal system assessments, 1337t, 1338
    reproductive system assessments, 1436
    transrectal, 1436
    transvaginal, 1436
    vision assessments, 965
Ultrasound-assisted wound therapy, 458–459
Ultraviolet light therapy, 465
Ultraviolet radiation, 379
Umbilical hernia, 1137, 1137f
Umbo, 985f
Uncal herniation, 943, 943f
Undernutrition. See Malnutrition
Unfractionated heparin, 744

Unilateral inattention syndrome, 934, 939
Unintentional injury, 127
Unlicensed assistive personnel
    delegation of tasks to, 6
    fluid replacement therapy by, 169
    pressure injury prevention by, 42b
    skin care by, 97
    supervision of, 6
Unna boot, 747–748
Unstable angina pectoris, 769–770
Upper airway
    edema of, 490, 491b
    obstruction of, 560–561, 561f
    structures of, 547
Upper endoscopy, 1089
Upper esophageal sphincter, 1062–1063, 1087–1088
Upper extremity
    amputations of, 1050
    fractures of, 1046–1047, 1046f
    traction for, 1040t
Upper gastrointestinal bleeding
    acid suppression for rebleeding prevention, 1114
    description of, 1108, 1109b
    endoscopic therapy for, 1113
    fluid replacement for, 1113
    hypovolemia concerns secondary to, 1113
    interventional radiologic procedures for, 1113–1114
    interventions for, 1113–1114
    nasogastric tube for, 1113
    nonsurgical management of, 1113–1114
Upper gastrointestinal radiographic series, 1070
Upper respiratory tract, 509–510, 509f
Urea breath test, 1111
Urease, 1401
Uremia, 1330, 1398b
Uremic cardiomyopathy, 1401
Uremic encephalopathy, 1403
Uremic frost, 1404
Uremic syndrome, 1398
Ureter(s)
    anatomy of, 1327, 1327f
    assessment of, 1330–1331
Ureterolithiasis, 1361
Ureterolithotomy, 1364
Ureteropelvic junction, 1338
Ureteroplasty, 1375
Ureteroscopy, 1364
Ureterostomy, 1368f
Urethra
    anatomy of, 1327–1328, 1430
    assessment of, 1331
Urethral occlusion devices, 1348
Urethral pressure profile, 1340
Urethral sphincter, 1327, 1327f
Urethritis, 1359–1361
Urethrogram, 1339

Urge incontinence, 1344, 1345*t*, 1349–1351, 1350*b*, 1484–1485
Urgency, 1328, 1330
Urgent surgery, 232*t*
Urgent triage, 124
Urinalysis, 1332–1335, 1333*b*
  preoperative, 237
  urolithiasis evaluations, 1362–1363
Urinary bladder. *See* Bladder
Urinary diversion, 1368, 1368*f*
Urinary elimination, 18
Urinary incontinence
  areflexic bladder as cause of, 97–98, 98*t*
  assessment of, 1346–1347, 1346*b*
  behavioral interventions for, 1352
  bladder training for, 1350–1351, 1351*b*
  care coordination for, 1353–1354, 1353*b*
  contributing factors, 1346*b*
  description of, 19
  drug therapy for, 98, 1348, 1350*b*, 1352
  electrical stimulation for, 1348
  etiology of, 1344
  flaccid bladder as cause of, 97–98, 98*t*
  functional, 1352
  habit training for, 1351, 1351*b*
  health care resources for, 1353–1354
  history-taking for, 1346
  home care management of, 1353
  incidence of, 1344–1346
  intermittent catheterization for, 98, 1352
  interventions for, 1347–1349, 1347*b*
  magnetic resonance therapy for, 1348
  mixed, 1345*t*, 1352
  nonpharmacologic management of, 97–98
  nonsurgical management of, 1347–1348
  nutrition therapy for, 1348, 1350
  in older adults, 1344*b*
  overactive spastic bladder as cause of, 97
  overflow, 1344, 1345*t*, 1351–1352
  pathophysiology of, 1343
  pelvic muscle exercises for, 1347, 1347*b*, 1351
  pessary for, 1348, 1352
  physical assessment of, 1346–1347
  prevalence of, 1344–1346
  psychosocial preparation for, 1353
  rehabilitation for, 97–98
  risk factors for, 1344–1346
  self-management education for, 1353, 1353*b*
  signs and symptoms of, 1346–1347
  stress, 1344, 1348, 1349*t*, 1464

Urinary incontinence *(Continued)*
  surgical management of, 1348–1349, 1349*t*
  transition management for, 1353–1354, 1353*b*
  types of, 1345*t*
  urge, 1344, 1345*t*, 1349–1351, 1350*b*, 1484–1485
  vaginal cone weight therapy for, 1348, 1348*f*
Urinary retention, 18
Urinary stones. *See* Urolithiasis
Urinary system
  age-related changes in, 234*b*, 1328–1329
  assessment of, 90*t*, 91, 803
  burn injury-related assessment of, 491–492
  postoperative assessment of, 276
  sickle cell disease effects on, 810
  ureters, 1327
Urinary system disorders
  urethritis, 1359–1361
  urinary tract infection. *See* Urinary tract infections
  urolithiasis. *See* Urolithiasis
Urinary tract
  anatomy of, 1321, 1322*f*, 1343
  obstruction of, 1365
Urinary tract infections. *See also* Cystitis
  assessment of, 1357–1359
  asymptomatic bacterial, 1354
  care coordination for, 1359
  catheter-associated, 415, 415*b*, 1355–1356, 1356*b*, 1423, 1500
  comfort measures for, 1359
  complicated, 1354
  contributing factors for, 1355*t*
  definition of, 1354
  diagnostic assessment of, 1358–1359
  drug therapy for, 98, 1359, 1360*b*
  etiology of, 1354–1357
  features of, 1358*b*
  fluid intake for, 1359
  genetic risk of, 1354–1357
  nonsurgical management of, 1359
  in older adults, 91
  risk factors for, 1354
  signs and symptoms of, 98, 1358
  surgical management of, 1359
  transition management for, 1359
  uncomplicated, 1354
Urine
  casts in, 1335
  color of, 1332
  composition of, 18
  culture and sensitivity of, 1335
  early, 1324
  electrolytes in, 1336
  glucose in, 1335
  nitrites in, 1335
  osmolarity of, 1336

Urine *(Continued)*
  pH, 1333
  post-void residual, 98
  protein in, 1333
  sediment in, 1335
  specific gravity of, 1332–1333
Urine collections, 1335
Urine output, obligatory, 165
Urine specimens, 1334*t*
Urine stream testing, 1340
Urine tests
  description of, 1068, 1243, 1243*b*
  urinalysis, 1332–1335, 1333*b*
Urobilinogen, 1068, 1192
Urodynamic studies, 1340
Urolithiasis
  assessment of, 1362–1363
  computed tomography of, 1363*f*
  definition of, 1361
  dietary treatment of, 1365, 1366*t*
  etiology of, 1361–1362
  extracorporeal shock wave lithotripsy for, 1364
  genetic risk of, 1361–1362, 1362*b*
  incidence of, 1362
  infection prevention in, 1365
  interventions for, 1363–1365, 1363*f*
  minimally invasive surgery for, 1364
  nonsurgical management of, 1363–1364
  pain management in, 1363–1365
  pathophysiology of, 1361–1362
  prevalence of, 1362
  self-management education for, 1366*b*
  surgical management of, 1364–1365
  urinary obstruction caused by, 1365
Urosepsis, 1356–1357
Urothelial cancer
  assessment of, 1367–1369
  health promotion and maintenance of, 1366–1367
  interventions for, 1367–1369, 1368*f*
  pathophysiology of, 1366
Urothelium, 1327
Urticaria, 462, 1261
Ustekinumab, 333, 369, 370*b*, 466*b*
USWT. *See* Ultrasound-assisted wound therapy
Uterine artery embolization, 1461, 1461*b*
Uterine leiomyomas
  assessment of, 1460
  bleeding in, 1461–1463
  care coordination for, 1463
  classification of, 1460*f*
  etiology of, 1460
  genetic risk of, 1460
  health care resources for, 1463
  home care management of, 1463

Uterine leiomyomas *(Continued)*
  hysterectomy for, 1461–1463, 1461*t*, 1462*b*–1463*b*
  incidence of, 1460
  interventions for, 1461–1463
  pathophysiology of, 1459–1460
  physical assessment of, 1460
  prevalence of, 1460
  psychosocial assessment of, 1460
  self-management education for, 1463
  signs and symptoms of, 1460
  submucosal, 1459–1460, 1460*f*
  subserosal, 1459–1460, 1460*f*
  surgical management of, 1461–1463
  transcervical endometrial resection for, 1461
  transition management for, 1463
  transvaginal ultrasound of, 1460
  uterine artery embolization for, 1461, 1461*b*
Uterus
  anatomy of, 1429
  prolapse of, 1464
Uvea, 957
Uvulopalatopharyngoplasty, 559

V
Vaccines, influenza, 596–597
Vacutainer needle holder, 215, 215*f*
Vacuum constriction device, 1490
VAD. *See* Vascular access devices
Vagal maneuvers, 678
Vagal nerve stimulation, 542, 879
Vagina
  anatomy of, 1429
  bleeding from, 1469
Vaginal cone weight therapy, 1348, 1348*f*
Vaginoplasty, 1499–1500, 1501*t*
Vagus nerve, 844*t*
Validation therapy, 863
Valsalva maneuver, 98, 634, 1301, 1352
Valvular heart disease
  antibiotic prophylaxis for, 707*b*
  aortic regurgitation, 706*b*, 707
  aortic stenosis, 706–707, 706*b*
  assessment of, 707
  atrial fibrillation and, 708
  balloon valvuloplasty for, 708
  cardiac output in, 708
  care coordination for, 710–711
  direct commissurotomy for, 709
  drug therapy for, 707–708
  echocardiography of, 707
  health care resources for, 711–712
  heart valve replacement procedures for, 709–710, 709*f*
  home care management of, 710
  interventions for, 707–710
  mitral regurgitation, 706, 706*b*
  mitral stenosis, 705–706, 706*b*, 710*b*
  mitral valve annuloplasty for, 709

Valvular heart disease *(Continued)*
  mitral valve prolapse, 706
  noninvasive reparative procedures
    for, 708–709, 708*f*
  nonsurgical management of,
    707–709
  pathophysiology of, 705–707
  self-management education for,
    710, 710*b*
  surgical management of, 709–710
  transcatheter aortic valve
    replacement for, 708–709,
    708*f*
  transition management for,
    710–711
Vancomycin, 200*b*
Vancomycin-intermediate
    Staphylococcus aureus, 421–422
Vancomycin-resistant *Enterococcus*
  contact precautions for, 419
  description of, 422
Vancomycin-resistant *Staphylococcus
    aureus*, 421–422
Vaping, 514
Vardenafil, 1489
Varenicline, for smoking cessation,
    515, 515*b*
Variant angina, 770, 774
Varicella-zoster virus infection, 347
Varicose veins, 748
Vas deferens, 1430–1431
Vascular access
  hemodialysis, 1413–1416, 1414*f*,
    1414*t*–1415*t*
  preoperative preparation for, 242
Vascular access devices
  central intravenous therapy, 205,
    212
  definition of, 201–202
  removing of, 215
  securing of, 213*b*
  tunneled central venous catheters,
    207, 207*f*, 213
Vascular dementia
  Alzheimer's disease versus, 858*t*
  pathophysiology of, 857–858
Vascular endothelial growth factor,
    375, 784
Vascular endothelial growth factor/
    receptor inhibitors
  colorectal cancer treated with,
    1130
  description of, 404*t*, 405
  macular degeneration treated
    with, 979
Vascular leak syndrome, 293–294
Vascular system
  arterial system, 645–646
  purposes of, 645–646
Vasculitis
  in rheumatoid arthritis, 318–319
  systemic necrotizing, 334*t*
Vasoconstriction, 752
Vasodilators, for acute coronary
    syndromes, 783*b*

Vasogenic edema, 942
Vaso-occlusive events, 809
Vasopressin, 1237*t*, 1245, 1246*b*,
    1332. *See also* Antidiuretic
    hormone
VATS. *See* Video-assisted
    thoracoscopic surgery
Vaughn-Williams classification, 685
Vedolizumab, 1153
Vegetarians, 1212
Veins, 646
Venereal Disease Research
    Laboratory serum test, 1509
Veno-occlusive disease, 825
Venous beading, 1284
Venous distention, 222
Venous duplex ultrasonography, 743
Venous insufficiency
  assessment of, 747
  chronic, 746–747
  description of, 716
  graduated compression stockings
    for, 747*b*
  interventions for, 747–748, 747*b*
  pathophysiology of, 746–747
Venous pulse, 653
Venous system, 646
Venous thromboembolism. *See also*
    Deep vein thrombosis;
    Pulmonary embolism
  assessment of, 742–743
  Core Measure Set for, 742, 742*t*,
    746, 938
  diagnostic assessment of, 743
  etiology of, 742
  fractures as risk factor for,
    1034–1035
  heparin prophylaxis for, 617–618
  history-taking for, 742
  inadequate clotting secondary to, 15
  incidence of, 742
  pancreatic cancer as cause of, 1205
  pathophysiology of, 742
  physical assessment of, 742–743
  postoperative, 244, 274, 281
  preoperative prophylactic
    interventions for, 274
  prevalence of, 742
  prevention of, 23, 281, 312–313
  pulmonary embolism caused by,
    617, 716
  risk factors for, 244, 617
  signs and symptoms of, 742–743
  in spinal cord injury patients, 897
  thrombus in, 742
  after total hip arthroplasty, 310,
    312–313
Venous thrombosis, 15–16
Venous ulcers, 732–733, 734*b*, 747
Venous vasodilators, 699
Ventilation
  mechanical. *See* Mechanical
    ventilation
  noninvasive positive-pressure, 535,
    535*b*, 536*f*

Ventilation/perfusion mismatch, 625
Ventilator(s), 631–633
Ventilator-associated events, 634,
    634*t*
Ventilator-associated lung injury, 635
Ventilator-associated pneumonia
  description of, 600*t*, 601
  noninvasive positive-pressure
    ventilation for prevention of,
    535
  prevention of, 897
Ventilator-induced lung injury, 635
Ventilatory failure, 624–625, 625*t*
Ventricular assist devices, for heart
    failure, 701–702, 701*f*
Ventricular asystole, 686–688
Ventricular dysrhythmias
  description of, 683–688
  premature ventricular complexes,
    683–684, 683*f*
  ventricular asystole, 686–688
  ventricular fibrillation, 684–686,
    685*f*
  ventricular tachycardia, 684, 684*f*
Ventricular fibrillation, 684–686, 685*f*
Ventricular gallop, 654–655
Ventricular remodeling, 694, 771
Ventricular tachycardia, 684, 684*f*
Ventriculomyomectomy, 716
Venturi masks, 533–534, 534*f*, 534*t*
Veracity, 9
Vermiform appendix, 1064
Vertebral compression fractures,
    1036, 1050
Vertebrobasilar artery stroke, 933*b*
Vertebroplasty, 1050, 1050*b*
Vertical compression, of spine, 894,
    895*f*
Vertigo, 987, 995–996, 1001
Very-low-calorie diets, 1227
Vesicants, 204, 392
Vesicles, 438*f*
Vesicoureteral reflux, 1355*t*
Vesicular sounds, 520*t*
Vestibulocochlear nerve, 844*t*
Veterans
  Alzheimer's disease in, 859*b*, 867*b*
  chronic pain in, 36*b*, 47*b*
  cognitive-behavioral therapy for,
    67*b*
  dementia in, 126*b*
  depression in, 36*b*
  diabetes mellitus in, 1291*b*
  hepatitis C in, 1183*b*
  lower-extremity amputation in,
    1051*b*
  smoking in, 515*b*
  spinal cord injury in, 903*b*
  traumatic brain injury in,
    845–846, 950*b*
  type 2 diabetes mellitus in, 1291*b*
Veterans Administration
  description of, 9–10
  safe patient handling and mobility
    practices, 93, 95*f*

Vibratory positive expiratory
    pressure device, for chronic
    obstructive pulmonary disease,
    579, 579*f*
Vicodin. *See* Hydrocodone
Video-assisted thoracoscopic surgery,
    589
Viral carcinogenesis, 378*t*, 379
Viral gastroenteritis, 1148*t*, 1149
Viral hepatitis, 1180, 1185*b*
Viral infections
  of skin, 467*b*, 468
  skin cultures for, 444–445
Viral meningitis, 881
Virchow's triad, 742
Virtual colonoscopy, 1073
Virulence, 414
Visceral pain, 48
Visceral proteins, 1217
Vision. *See also* Eye(s)
  acuity of, 26
  assessment of, 962–967
  diagnostic assessment of, 965–967
  health promotion and
    maintenance of, 961–962
  imaging assessment of, 965
  impairment of, in older adults, 963*b*
  laboratory assessment of, 965
  loss of, 26, 934*f*
  near, 964
  near point of, 961
  psychosocial assessment of,
    964–965
  testing of, 963–964, 964*f*
Vision loss
  diabetes mellitus as cause of,
    1307–1308
  environmental management of,
    1307–1308
Visual acuity tests, 963–964
Visual analog dyspnea scale, 576, 576*f*
Visual evoked potentials, 855
Visual field testing, 964
Vital signs
  postoperative assessment of, 274
  in traumatic brain injury, 945
Vitamin B$_{12}$
  absorption of, 1141
  deficiency of
    anemia caused by, 814, 814*t*,
      815*f*, 816
    central nervous system affected
      by, 803
    in vegetarians, 1212
  pernicious anemia and, 1105
Vitamin D
  activation of, 1327
  deficiency of, 1277–1278
  description of, 432, 482, 1006
Vitamin D$_3$, 1020–1021
Vitamin K, 745*b*, 798
Vitamin K antagonists
  mechanism of action, 801
  pulmonary embolism treated
    with, 621*b*

Vitiligo, 1242
Vitreous body, 958, 958f
Vocal fremitus, 518–519
Vocational assessments, 92
Vocational counselors, 89
Voice sounds, 519
Voided urine, 1334t
Voiding
    facilitating techniques for, 98
    post-void residual urine after, 98
    toileting routines to re-establish,
        98
Volkmann's contractures, 1034
Volume fraction, 803
Volume-cycled ventilators, 631
Voluntary stopping of eating and
        drinking, 115
Volutrauma, 635
Volvulus, 1092, 1122, 1122f
Vomiting. See Nausea and vomiting
VSED. See Voluntary stopping of
        eating and drinking
VTE. See Venous thromboembolism
Vulnerable populations, 118
Vulva, 1428–1429
Vulvovaginitis, 1470–1471, 1471b

W
Waist circumference, 1225
Waist-to-hip ratio, 1225
Walker, 1044
Wandering, 864, 864b
Warfarin
    antidote for, 745b
    deep vein thrombosis treated with,
        745
    drug interactions with, 746b
    food interactions with, 746b
    genetic testing before using, 620b
    in mechanical valve patients, 710
Warm antibody anemia, 815
Wasp stings, 137, 137b, 138t–140t
Water brash, 1089
Water pressure, 161
Water-seal chest drainage system,
        590–591, 590b
Weak acid, 186, 186f
Weak bases, 186
Weakness
    assessment of, 1008–1009
    during dying, 109
    in systemic lupus erythematosus,
        327

Weaning
    from mechanical ventilation, 635,
        636t
    from tracheostomy, 544
Weapons of mass destruction, 153
Wearable cardioverter/defibrillator,
        688
Weber tuning fork test, 989–990
Wedge resection, 589
Weight
    assessment of, 1213b
    ideal body, 1215, 1225
    measurement of, 1213–1215
Weight gain
    fluid retention as cause of, 172
    mobility affected by, 93–95
Weight loss
    in burn injury patients, 502
    in chronic obstructive pulmonary
        disease, 580
    dehydration and, 168
    unintentional, 1215
Weight-bearing fractures, 1050
Wellness promotion, 30b
Wernicke's aphasia, 938
West Nile virus, 883, 884b
Wet age-related macular
        degeneration, 979
Wheelchair, 95
Wheelchair pushups, 97
Wheezes, 521t, 601
Whipple procedure, 1207, 1207f,
        1208t
White blood cell(s)
    description of, 290–291
    formation of, 797
    transfusion of, 832t, 835
White blood cell count, 657
White blood cell count with
        differential, 424–425
White blood cell differential, 293,
        293t
"White clot syndrome", 744
White matter, 840
Wild-type gene sequence, 76
Williams position, 905
Winged needles, 203–204
Withdrawing or withholding
        life-sustaining therapy, 114–115
Women
    carpal tunnel syndrome in, 1057b
    coronary artery disease in, 772b
    dehydration in, 164b

Women (Continued)
    human immunodeficiency virus
        infection in, 340b, 345b
    stroke in, 935b
Wong-Baker FACES pain rating
        scale, 50, 52f
Wood's light examination, 445
Work-arounds, 4
Work-related musculoskeletal
        disorders, 93
Wound
    breakdown of, 551
    chemical débridement of, 457,
        457t
    closure of, 267, 268f
    colostomy, 1132
    contraction of, 474f
    débridement of, 457, 457t
    dehiscence of, 277, 278f, 282–283,
        1099
    drains, 277–278, 279f, 282
    dressings for. See Dressings
    enzymatic débridement of, 499
    evisceration of, 277, 278f, 283,
        283b
    full-thickness, 473–474
    mechanical débridement of, 457,
        457t, 498–499
    partial-thickness, 473
    perineal, 1133b
    pressure injury
        assessment of, 453–455
        best practices for, 460b
        dressings for, 457–458
        drug therapy for, 458
        electrical stimulation for,
            458–459
        hyperbaric oxygen therapy for,
            458
        management of, 455–459,
            457b
        negative-pressure wound
            therapy for, 458
        nonsurgical management of,
            457–459
        nutrition therapy for, 458
        physical therapy for, 458
        skin substitutes for, 458
        surgical management of, 459
        ultrasound-assisted wound
            therapy for, 458–459
    staple closure of, 282
    suture closure of, 282

Wound exudate, 453t
Wound healing
    delayed primary intention, 278
    impaired, 277, 278f, 474t
    mechanisms of, 473–474
    normal, 471t
    nutrition for, 97, 287
    obesity effects on, 236–237
    phases of, 466f, 471–473, 471t
    postoperative, 277, 278f
    promotion of, 28
Wound infection
    drug therapy for, 282
    in older adults, 954
    postoperative prevention of,
        281–283
Wrist
    carpal tunnel syndrome of,
        1057–1059, 1058b
    Colles' fracture of, 1046, 1046f,
        1057
Wrist drop, 267b

X
X chromosome, 74
Xanthine oxidase inhibitors, 331–332
Xanthines, 571
Xeljanz. See Tofacitinib
Xenografts, 499, 499f, 709
Xerosis, 449b, 461
Xerostomia, 319, 549, 1084–1085
Xylose absorption, 1069b

Y
Y chromosome, 72, 74
Y-tubing, 832

Z
Zanamivir, 597–598
Zeaxanthin, 979
Zegerid, 1091
Zenker's diverticula, 1101
Ziconotide, 905, 905b
Zika virus, 416
Zohydro. See Hydrocodone
Zoledronic acid, 1026
Zostavax, 469